NO_2	nitrous oxide
NPO	nothing by mouth
NP	nasopharyngeal
NPV	negative pressure ventilation
O_2	oxygen
O_2Hb	oxygenated hemoglobin
OH^-	hydroxide ions
OHDC	oxyhemoglobin dissociation curve
P	pressure
ΔP	change in pressure
P_{50}	PO_2 at which 50% saturation of hemoglobin occurs
P_{100}	Pressure on inspiration measured at 100 milliseconds
P_A	alveolar pressure
Pa	arterial pressure
PA	pulmonary artery
$P(A\text{-}a)O_2$	alveolar-to-arterial partial pressure of oxygen
P_ACO2	partial pressure of carbon dioxide in the alveoli
P_aCO_2	partial pressure of carbon dioxide in the arteries
Palv	alveolar pressure
P_AO_2	partial pressure of oxygen in the alveoli
PaO_2	partial pressure of oxygen in the arteries
PaO_2/F_IO_2	ratio of arterial PO_2 to F_IO_2
PaO_2/P_AO_2	ratio of arterial PO_2 to alveolar PO_2
PAP	pulmonary artery pressure
$\overline{PAP}$	mean pulmonary artery pressure
$P(a\text{-}et)CO_2$	Arterial-to-end-tidal partial pressure of carbon dioxide also, a-et PCO_2
PAGE	perfluorocarbon associated gas exchange
PAug	pressure augmentation
PAV	proportional assist ventilation
P_{aw}	airway pressure
$\bar{P}aw$	mean airway pressure
P_{awo}	airway opening pressure
PB	barometric pressure
P_{bs}	pressure at the body's surface
PCEF	peak cough expiratory flow
PCIRV	pressure control inverse ratio ventilation
PCO_2	partial pressure of carbon dioxide
PCV	pressure control ventilation
PCWP	pulmonary capillary wedge pressure
$PCWP_{tm}$	transmural pulmonary capillary wedge pressure
PDA	patent ductus arteriosus
PEA	pulseless electrical activity
$P_{\bar{E}}CO_2$	partial pressure of mixed expired carbon dioxide
PEEP	positive end expiratory pressure
$PEEP_E$	extrinsic PEEP (set-PEEP)
$PEEP_I$	intrinsic PEEP (auto-PEEP)
$PEEP_{total}$	total PEEP (the sum of intrinsic and extrinsic PEEP)
PEFR	peak expiratory flow rate
P_{es}	esophageal pressure
$P_{ET}CO_2$	partial pressure of end-tidal carbon dioxide; also $PetCO_2$
P_{FLEX}	pressure at the inflection point of a pressure/volume curve
P_{GA}	gastric pressure
P_{high}	high pressure during APRV
PHY	permissive hypercapnia
PIE	pulmonary interstitial edema
PIF	pulmonary interstitial fibrosis
P_{Imax}	maximum inspiratory pressure; also MIP, MIF, NIF
P_{inside}	inside pressure
$P_{intrapleural}$	intrapleural pressure; also P_{pl}
P_IO_2	partial pressure of inspired oxygen
PIP	peak inspiratory pressure; also P_{peak}
P_L	transpulmonary pressure
P_{low}	low pressure during APRV
PLV	partial liquid ventilation
P_M	mouth pressure
P*mus*	muscle pressure
PO_2	partial pressure of oxygen
$P_{outside}$	pressure outside
P_{Peak}	peak inspiratory pressure; also PIP
PPHS	persistent pulmonary hypertension in the newborn
P_{pl}	intrapleural pressure
$P_{plateau}$	plateau pressure
ppm	parts per million
PPST	premature pressure-support termination
PPV	positive pressure ventilation
PRA	plasma renin activity
PRVC	pressure regulated volume control
PS	pressure support
Pset	set pressure
PSmax	maximum pressure support
PSV	pressure support ventilation
psi	pounds per square inch
psig	pounds per square inch gauge
P_{TA}	transairway pressure
$PtcCO_2$	transcutaneous PCO_2
$PtcO_2$	transcutaneous PO_2
P_{TM}	transmural pressure
P_{TR}	transrespiratory pressure
P_{TT}	transthoracic pressure; also P_W
PV	pressure ventilation
PVCs	premature ventricular contractions
$P_{\bar{v}}O_2$	partial pressure of oxygen in mixed venous blood
PVR	pulmonary vascular resistance
PVS	partial ventilatory support
P_W	transthoracic pressure; also P_{TT}
Q2H	every two hours
$\dot{Q}_T$	cardiac output
$\dot{Q}_s/\dot{Q}_T$	shunt
R	respiratory exchange ratio
RAM	random access memory
RAP	right atrial pressure
Raw	airway resistance
RCP	respiratory care practitioner
RDS	respiratory distress syndrome
Re	Reynold's number
R_E	expiratory resistance
REE	resting energy expenditure
R_I	inspiratory resistance
ROM	read only memory
RQ	respiratory quotient
RT	respiratory therapist
RV	right ventricle
RVP	right ventricular pressure
RVEDP	right ventricular end-diastolic pressure
RVEDV	right ventricular end-diastolic volume
SA	sinoatrial
SaO_2	arterial oxygen saturation
S.I.	system internationale (international system)
SIMV	synchronized intermittent mandatory ventilation
Sine	sinusoidal
sp.	species
sPEEP	spontaneous PEEP
SpO_2	oxygen saturation measured by pulse oximeter
STPD	standard temperature, pressure saturated; zero degrees Celsius, 760 mm Hg, dry
SV	stroke volume
SVC	slow vital capacity
$S\bar{v}O_2$	mixed venous oxygen saturation
SVN	small volume nebulizer
SVR	systemic vascular resistance
T	temperature
TCT	total cycle time
T_E	expiratory time
TGI	tracheal gas insufflation
T_I	inspiratory time
TID	three times a day
T_I/TCT	duty cycle
T_{high}	time for high pressure delivery in APRV
T_{low}	time for low pressure delivery in APRV
TLV	total liquid ventilation
torr	measurement of pressure equivalent to mm Hg
TPTV	time-triggered, pressure-limited, time-cycled ventilaion
U	unit
UN	urinary nitrogen
V	volume
$\dot{V}$	flow
$\dot{V}_A$	alveolar ventilation per minute
VA	venoarterial
VAI	ventilator-assisted individuals
VAPS	volume assured pressure support
VC	vital capacity
V_C	volume lost to tubing compressibility
VCIRV	volume controlled inverse ratio ventilation
$\dot{V}CO_2$	carbon dioxide production per minute
V_D	volume of dead space
$\dot{V}_D$	dead space ventilation per minute
V_{Dalv}	alveolar dead space
V_{Danat}	anatomical dead space
V_{Dmech}	mechanical dead space
$\dot{V}_E$	minute ventilation
VEDV	ventricular end-diastolic volume
$\dot{V}O_2$	oxygen consumption per minute
VS	volume support
V_T	tidal volume
V_D/V_T	dead space-to-tidal volume ratio
vol%	volume per 100 mL of blood
$\dot{V}/\dot{Q}$	ventilation/perfusion ratio
VV	volume ventilation; also venovenous
W	work
WOB	work of breathing
WOBi	imposed work of breathing
yr	year

Mosby's
Respiratory Care Equipment

Mosby's Respiratory Care Equipment

J.M. Cairo, PhD, RRT
Professor of Cardiopulmonary Science and Physiology
Department Head, Cardiopulmonary Science,
School of Allied Health Professions,
Louisiana State University Medical Center,
New Orleans, Louisiana

Susan P. Pilbeam, MS, RRT
Program Director, Respiratory Care,
Edison Community College,
Fort Myers, Florida
Educational Consultant,
Estero, Florida

Sixth Edition

with 703 illustrations

Mosby

St. Louis Baltimore Boston Carlsbad Chicago Naples New York Philadelphia Portland
London Madrid Mexico City Singapore Sydney Tokyo Toronto Wiesbaden

Mosby
Dedicated to Publishing Excellence

Editor-in-Chief: Andrew M. Allen
Editor: Janet Russell
Developmental Editor: Dina Shourd
Project Manager: Mark Spann
Production Editor: Jodi Everding
Designer: Judi Lang
Manufacturing Manager: Dave Graybill
Cover Designer: Scott Tjaden

SIXTH EDITION

Composition by Carlisle Communications, Inc.
Printing/binding by Von Hoffman Press

Mosby, Inc.
11830 Westline Industrial Drive
St. Louis, Missouri 64146

Library of Congress Cataloging in Publication Data

Cairo, Jimmy M.
Mosby's respiratory care equipment.—6th ed. / J. M. Cairo, Susan P. Pilbeam.
p. cm.
Rev. ed. of: Respiratory care equipment / Steven P. McPherson. 5th ed. c1995.
Includes bibliographical references and index.
ISBN 0-8151-2148-2 (alk. paper)
1. Respiratory therapy—Equipment and supplies. 2. Respiratory intensive care—Equipment and supplies. I. Cairo, J. M. II. Pilbeam, Susan P. Respiratory care equipment. III. Title. IV. Title: Respiratory care equipment.
[DNLM: 1. Respiratory Therapy—instrumentation. WF 26 C136m 1999]
RC735.I5M43 1999
615.8'36'028—dc21
DNLM/DLC
for Library of Congress 98-55692
CIP

99 00 01 / 9 8 7 6 5 4 3 2 1

To Rhonda, Allyson, and Brooke for their unselfish love and support throughout this project;

And to my first teachers, Johnny, Mary, John, and Charlie Cairo.

JMC

To Bob Wazgar for always being there for me;

And to the memory of my brother, Phillip D. Pritchard, for being my spiritual guidepost.

SPP

CONTRIBUTORS

Charles G. Durbin, Jr., MD, FCCM
Professor of Anesthesiology,
Medical Director, Respiratory Care Department,
University of Virginia,
Charlottesville, Virginia

Michelle Lilley, AAS, RRT
Respiratory Therapist,
Department of Respiratory Care,
Children's Hospital,
Boston, Massachusetts

Kevin Lord, BS, RRT
Instructor,
Department of Cardiopulmonary Science,
School of Allied Health Professions,
Louisiana State University
New Orleans, Louisiana

Kenneth F. Watson, RRT
Respiratory Therapist,
Children's Hospital,
Boston, Massachusetts

Dennis R. Wissing, PhD, RRT
Associate Professor and Program Coordinator
Department of Cardiopulmonary Science,
School of Allied Health Professions,
Louisiana State University Medical Center
Shreveport, Louisiana

REVIEWERS

Robert Beckerman, MD, FAAP, FCCP
Professor of Pediatrics and Physiology,
Skip Kaufman Chair in Pediatric Pulmonology,
Section Chief Pediatric Pulmonology,
Tulane University Medical Center/Tulane Hospital for Children,
Tulane University
New Orleans, Louisiana

Ken Drechny, RRT, RCP
Clinical Technical Supervisor,
University of Chicago-Mitchell Hospital,
Chicago, Illinois

Jim Fink, MS, RRT
Administrative Director, Respiratory Sciences,
Edward Hines Jr. VA Hospital,
Hines, Illinois

Theresa Gramlich, RRT, MS
Assistant Professor,
Department of Respiratory Care,
University of Arkansas for Medical Sciences,
Education Coordinator,
Veteran's Administration Medical Center,
Little Rock, Arkansas

Robert Hirnle, MS, RRT
Program Director,
Highline Community College,
Des Moines, Washington

Chris Kallus, MEd, RRT
Program Director,
Respiratory Care Program,
The Victoria College,
Victoria, Texas

Sindee Karpel, MPA
Assistant Professor,
Allied Health Sciences,
Borough of Manhattan Community College,
New York, New York

Joe Koss, MS, RRT
Director of Clinical Education,
Respiratory Therapy Program,
Indiana University,
Indianapolis, Indiana

S. Gregory Marshall, PhD
Associate Professor,
Department of Respiratory Care,
Southwest Texas State University,
San Marco, Texas

Timothy Op't Holt, EdD, RRT
Associate Professor,
Cardiorespiratory Care Program,
University of South Alabama,
Mobile, Alabama

Fran Piedalue, RRT
Clinical Coordinator of Respiratory Care,
University Hospital,
University of Colorado,
Denver, Colorado

Joe Ross, MS, RRT
Program Director,
Respiratory Care Program,
Baltimore City Community College,
Baltimore, Maryland

James R. Sills, MEd, CPFT, RRT
Director, Respiratory Care Programs,
Rock Valley College,
Rockford, Illinois

FOREWORD

I am very pleased to write the foreword to a work that will make a major contribution to respiratory care. Jim Cairo and Sue Pilbeam, with contributions from other experts in the field, have written the sixth edition of Mosby's Respiratory Care Equipment, which was formerly authored by Steven McPherson. While maintaining the scope of the previous editions, the new authors have significantly altered content and made many additions and improvements. They have achieved the seemingly impossible, making an ordinarily dry-as-dust subject both readable and interesting. It is readable because the authors have substituted a personal style for the usually arid didactic style, and it is interesting because it encompasses an absolutely critical area.

Of the many changes, I would like to mention only a few. This edition spans the entire spectrum of respiratory care equipment, from the most basic to the most sophisticated and most recent. Indeed, equipment and techniques are described that are entirely new to the American market and some even that are still considered to be experimental at the time of printing. A new and very interesting chapter is devoted to sleep and the various diagnostic steps used in identifying sleep problems. Each chapter is profusely illustrated and has a number of special boxes. Some boxes highlight the most important or most complex aspect of the equipment under discussion. Another set of boxes contains Decision Making & Problem Solving questions that should test and improve the student's understanding in a clinical, decision-making format. Each chapter is followed by a number of review questions that test the student's understanding and recall. A new feature of every chapter is the inclusion of a number of Internet references, bringing both the textbook and the student to the cutting edge of the science. These references should make it possible for future students to use this text profitably.

This book contains an enormous amount of material. In order to digest it, the student will have to pay careful attention to the lectures and laboratory exercises concerned with equipment. With this background, all readers will find that this textbook opens a clear and panoramic view of the large and increasingly complex field of respiratory care equipment. This is particularly important, because regardless of how much theoretical knowledge the students or practitioners may have, a thorough understanding of the equipment used at the bed-side is essential because they must be prepared to treat patients entrusted to their care. It is the thorough and honest understanding of the equipment that will allow respiratory care students and practitioners to put their theoretical knowledge to the test in service of their patients.

A textbook like this will bridge the information gap between knowledge and practice and enable the respiratory care practitioner to become a responsible and effective health care deliverer.

The field of respiratory care is fortunate indeed in having authors of this caliber. I am proud to have been asked to make this minuscule contribution to a great textbook.

Thomas J. DeKornfeld, MD
Professor Emeritus of Anesthesiology
Brentwood, Tennessee

PREFACE

This latest edition of Mosby's Respiratory Care Equipment represents a continuing effort to provide a comprehensive review of the devices and techniques used by respiratory therapists to treat patients with cardiopulmonary dysfunction. In previous editions of this text, Stephen McPherson skillfully presented a detailed analysis of various types of equipment that respiratory care practitioners encounter daily. His efforts in these earlier editions helped to establish a framework for discussing respiratory care equipment in the classroom and in the clinic.

In this edition of Mosby's Respiratory Care Equipment, we have tried to maintain the comprehensive nature of this text, but have adjusted the focus to make the information more clinically applicable. Additionally, we have attempted to present this material in a concise and readable fashion. The style that we have used is a reflection of our experiences as teachers of respiratory care students. We have used a number of pedagogical aids to help readers see applications for the various devices and concepts described. Each chapter begins with a chapter outline and learning objectives along with a list of key terms used in the chapter. Decision making and problem solving exercises, summaries of AARC Clinical Practice Guidelines, expanded reference lists that include computer and Internet resources, and national board-style review questions are also included in every chapter. Figures and tables are used extensively throughout the text. Every effort has been made to provide the reader with high-quality photographs and illustrations that are descriptive and easy to follow.

The text begins with a review of the physical principles that readers will encounter in later chapters. Our intent is to provide an overview of physics that is sufficient to understand the clinical applications of respiratory care equipment. Chapters 2 and 3 provide a detailed discussion of the devices and concepts that are used in medical gas therapy. We have included the most current modes of medical gas therapy, including nitric oxide, Heliox, and hyperbaric oxygen therapy.

Chapter 4 describes basic concepts and equipment related to the administration of aerosols and humidity therapy. Particular emphasis has been placed on providing strategies for selecting, applying, and troubleshooting these devices. Chapter 5 presents an up-to-date and clinically useful approach to airway management and includes an extensive review of various artificial airways and related ancillary equipment. The indications, applications, and contraindications (including complications) associated with the use of each device are also included. Manual resuscitators, incentive spirometers, IPPB apparatuses, and chest physiotherapy devices are reviewed in a concise manner in Chapter 6 (Lung Expansion Therapy). Regarding IPPB, earlier editions focussed to a large extent on the specific internal mechanical function of the various types of machines that are used to administer this type of therapy. We have chosen to use a different approach in our presentation of these devices because current practice requires respiratory therapists to understand the clinical applications of IPPB rather than how to repair these machines. We have condensed this material to an appropriate and teachable level that addresses the basic theories of operation for each device without going into the extensive detail required in a maintenance and repair environment.

Chapters 7 and 8 provide detailed descriptions of the devices that are routinely used by respiratory care practitioners to monitor various aspects of physiologic function, including volume-, flow-, and pressure-measuring devices, indirect calorimeters and metabolic monitoring units, capnographs, transcutaneous monitors, pulse oximeters, and

CO-oximeters. We have included a discussion of the theory of operation and the clinical application of each device. This discussion includes not only how these devices record, but also how information derived from these measurements is used in the care of patients.

The chapters on mechanical ventilators have been completely reorganized. Chapter 9 reviews basic technical operation and physical function of ventilator components and includes coverage of subjects such as fluidics, ventilator graphics, and the basic function of high-frequency ventilators. Chapter 9 does not attempt to cover management of the patient-ventilator system, which is handled in other texts. Chapter 10 reviews multipurpose ventilators that are used in pediatric and adult respiratory care and, in some cases, neonatal care. It is subdivided so that each section targets a specific ventilator and contains objectives, content, and review questions relevant to that device. In this way readers can elect to study a particular machine used in their part of the country and have all the study components included within the section.

Choosing what ventilators to include in Chapter 10 was not easy; we did not attempt to cover all of them. You will notice that older ventilators have not been included. For example, we decided not to include the MA-1. Although it is very simple to operate and is still used in some facilities, it is reasonable to assume that most hospitals and extended care facilities rely on more modern mechanical ventilators for patient care. You will also notice that we have included several more recently developed ventilators, such as the Servo 300, Drager E-4, and the Hamilton GALILEO to mention just a few. We encourage our readers to let us know additional ventilators that we might include. Units that are used specifically for infants and pediatric patients are discussed in Chapter 11, and those ventilators that are more commonly used for transport and in the home-care setting are discussed in Chapter 12.

We're sure that our readers are aware that software changes are now common to microprocessor-controlled ventilators; however, trying to keep up with these rapid changes is approaching the limitations of the printed word. No sooner is a unit installed in a hospital than the manufacturer has added new features, often times before even the operating manual can be updated. It is essential for clinicians using these devices to stay informed. We have relied upon information provided by the product specialist for the manufactured piece of equipment.

The final two chapters are new additions to Mosby's Respiratory Care Equipment. Chapter 13 provides information about infection control procedures that apply to respiratory care equipment. This information includes the most current recommendations from the Centers for Disease Control on methods to reduce the risk of infection to both patients and respiratory care practitioners. Chapter 14 contains a review of the equipment and procedures used in sleep diagnostics. It was not our intent to present an exhaustive review of this subject, but rather to provide a basic overview of both normal and abnormal sleep patterns and the types of monitors and evaluation equipment used in the diagnosis of sleep disorders. Graphic plots of EEG, respiratory flow, chest-wall motion, and oxygen saturation are included to illustrate these concepts.

Our intent in writing this book was to provide students, teachers, practicing respiratory therapists, and other members of the health care team with a text that is comprehensive, up-to-date, and easy to read. Every attempt was made to provide clinically applicable information that could help practitioners provide better patient care.

ACKNOWLEDGMENTS

There were a number of individuals who generously contributed to this project. We are particularly grateful to Charles Durbin, MD; Dennis Wissing, PhD, RRT; Ken Watson, MS, RRT; Michelle Lilley, AAS, RRT; Kevin Lord, BS, RRT; and Theresa Gramlich, MS, RRT for their insightful contributions and dedication to purpose in their specialty areas.

We also want to recognize those individuals who graciously provided technical assistance during this project. They include Tom Baxter, MA, RRT; Catherine E. DeJong, RRT, RPsgT; Yvon Dupuis, MS, RRT; Demitirus Frazier; Barbara Gair; Kay Givens, MEd, RRT; Vincent Guttuso, BS, RRT; William Hunt, Jr., MD; Lisa Kinoshita, RRT; Tom Lotz, MEd, RRT; Valerie Mohrman, BS, RRT; Andy Pellett, PhD; Vicki Wissing, MSN, RN; and John Zamjahn, MHS, RRT.

The reviews of Fran Piedalue, RRT; Chris Kallus, MEd, RRT; Robert Beckerman, MD, FAAP, FCCP; Ken Drechny, RRT, RCP; Jim Fink, MS, RRT; Theresa Gramlich, RRT, MS; Robert Hirnle, MS, RRT; Sindee Karpel, MPA; Joe Koss, MS, RRT; S. Gregory Marshall, PhD; Timothy Op't Holt, EdD, RRT; Joe Ross, MS, RRT; and James R. Sills, MEd, CPFT, RRT were extremely valuable to us in terms of technical detail and keeping the text focused in the right direction, that is, toward our students and their needs.

We would like to offer a special thanks to all of the manufacturers and distributors represented in this text and for their tremendous cooperation. They include Glen and Helen Philmon, Asepsis Product Consultants, Inc.; Aequitron Corporation; Greg Oliver, Former Product Manager, and Robert Swan, Bear Medical Products; Dan Fleming and L'Oris Hunter, Bird Products Corporation; Bunnell, Inc.; Geoffrey F. Lear, RRT and Bradford M. Saunders, Dräger, Inc.; Bruce Bray, RRT, Beth Keifer, RRT, Tim Rossman, RRT, and David Thompson, RRT, Hamilton Medical; Keith Glaeser and Duke Johns, Medical Specialties, Inc.; Kathy Lovett, MHA, RRT, Jeff Henk, Diane Huttmann, Bud Reeves, RRT, Barbara Sullivan, RRT, Vance Wilson, and Lisa Farrar, Nellcor Puritan Bennett (Mallinckrodt); Cyndy Miller and Jim Yap, Newport Medical; O. "Skip" Drumheller, PhD, RRT, Respironics; Mike MacGregor, RRT, Bruce Damman, Siemens Medical Systems, Inc.; and Univent, Corporation.

We believe you will be pleased with significant changes made to the illustrations in this edition thanks to the exceptional artistic talents of Donald O'Connor who has managed to accurately convey important technical detail in a manner that is at the same time creative and attractive to the eye. A special note of thanks goes to Brandy L. Durbin for providing drawings that inspired the new line art in Chapter 5. We also want to thank two talented and creative photographers, Don Price and Joe Walsh from the University of Michigan, who photographed equipment provided by Ron Dechert, MS, RRT; Mike Becker, RRT; Kent Miller, RRT; and the University of Michigan. Many of the fine photographs in this text are due to their efforts.

Throughout the course of this project, we were blessed with outstanding editorial support from Mosby. Jennifer Roche brought us together to write this text and convinced us that this would be an intellectually rewarding process. She was right! Mindy Copeland organized the reviews, and Jodi Everding copyedited our manuscript with finesse. Janet Russell and Dina Shourd gently guided us through the publishing process making sure that we stayed on track and on time. To Janet and Dina, we want you to know that we have thoroughly enjoyed working with you and offer you our heartfelt thanks for all of your work.

The foreword for this text was written by someone we both very much admire and respect. He is an individual who has and continues to dedicate his life to helping the medical profession and the profession of respiratory care. Dr. Thomas DeKornfeld took on the Herculean task of reading the entire manuscript before he wrote the foreword. This speaks volumes about the caring and tireless effort of this wonderful scholar who helped us throughout the arduous task of editing. His contribution helped to refine the quality of the finished copy that you see.

Finally, we would like our readers to know that this project was a wonderful experience for both of us. We have grown both personally and professionally from working together. Becoming part of each other's family during the course of writing this book may be the greatest reward of all for us.

Jim Cairo
New Orleans, Louisiana

Sue Pilbeam
Fort Myers, Florida

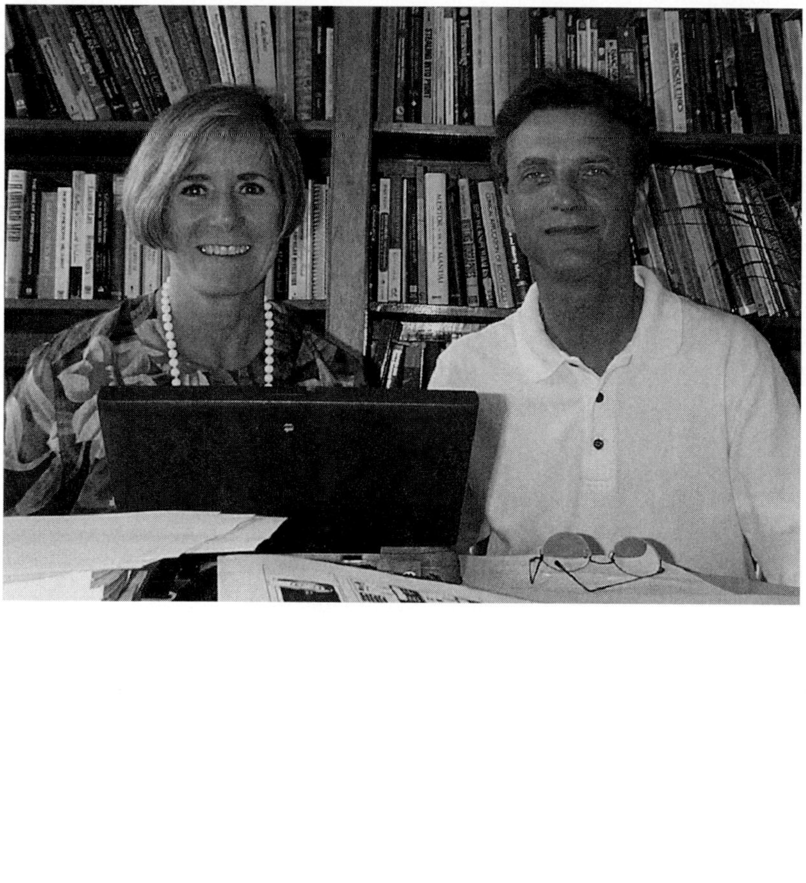

CONTENTS IN BRIEF

DETAILED CONTENTS

CHAPTER 11

CHAPTER 12

American Association for Respiratory Care Clinical Practice Guideline Excerpts Included in the 6th Edition of Mosby's Respiratory Care Equipment

Mosby's
Respiratory Care Equipment

CHAPTER 1

CHAPTER OUTLINE

Energy and Matter
- Energy and Work
- Kinetic and Potential Energy

States of Matter
- Change of State

Physical Properties of Liquids and Gases
- Temperature
- Pressure
- Buoyancy
- Viscosity
- Surface Tension
- Density

The Gas Laws
- Boyle's Law
- Charles's and Gay-Lussac's Laws
- Combined Gas Law
- Avogadro's Law
- Laws of Diffusion

Fluid Mechanics
- Patterns of Flow
- Poiseuille's Law
- Reynolds's Number
- Bernoulli Principle
- Venturi Principle
- Coanda Effect

Principles of Electricity
- Principles of Electronics
- Ohm's Law
- Electrical Circuits
- Electrical Safety
- Preventing Electrical Hazards

KEY TERMS

Absolute Humidity
Acoustics
Adhesive Forces
Ammeter
Amorphous Solids
Ampere
Archimedes's Principle
Atomic Theory
Atoms
Avogadro's Number
Boiling Point
Boltzman's Universal Gas Constant
Chemical Potential Energy
Cohesive Forces
Compounds
Condensation
Critical Pressure
Critical Temperature
Diffusion
Dipole-Dipole Interactions
Elastic Potential Energy
Electricity and Magnetism
Electromotive Force
Elements
Evaporation
Fahrenheit
Fluids
Freezing Point
Gravitational Potential Energy
Horsepower
Hydrogen Bonding
Hydrometer
Insulators
Joules
Kelvin
Kilowatt
Kinetic Energy
Latent Heat
Macroshock
Mechanics
Melting Point
Microshock
Molecules
Mixtures
Newtons
Ohm
Optics
Potential Energy
Power
Relative Humidity
Resistors
Sublimation
Supercooled Liquids
Systèm International
Thermistor
Thermodynamics
Thermometers (Electrical and Nonelectrical)
Van der Waals Forces
Vaporization
Vapor Pressure
Vapors
Volt
Voltmeter
Watt
Wheatstone Bridge

Basic Physics for the Respiratory Therapist

J. M. Cairo

CHAPTER LEARNING OBJECTIVES

Upon completion of this chapter, the reader should be able to:

1. Differentiate between kinetic and potential energy.
2. Compare the physical and chemical properties of the three primary states of matter.
3. Explain why large amounts of energy are required to accomplish the changes associated with solid-liquid and liquid-gas phase transitions.
4. Convert temperature measurements from the Kelvin, Celsius, and Fahrenheit temperature scales.
5. Define pressure and describe two devices that are commonly used to measure it.
6. List various pressure equivalents for 1 atmosphere (atm).
7. Calculate the density and specific gravity of liquids and gases.
8. Explain how changes in pressure, volume, temperature, and mass affect the behavior of an ideal gas.
9. Calculate the partial pressure of oxygen in a room air sample of gas obtained at 1 atm.
10. List the physical variables that influence the flow of a gas through a tube.
11. Explain how the pressure, velocity, and flow of a gas change as it moves from part of a tube with a large radius to another part with a small radius.
12. Describe the Venturi and Coanda effects and how both can be used in the design of respiratory care equipment.
13. State Ohm's law and relate how changes in voltage and resistance affect current flow in a direct-current series circuit.
14. Describe three strategies that can be used to protect patients from electrical hazards.

"Physics is the most fundamental and all-inclusive of all the sciences, and has had a profound effect on all scientific development. In fact, physics is the present-day equivalent of what used to be called natural philosophy, from which most of our modern sciences arose. Students of many fields find themselves studying physics because of the basic role it plays in all phenomena."[1]

RICHARD P. FEYNMAN
Six Easy Pieces

Physics is the branch of science that deals with the interactions of matter and energy. Classical physics comprises the fields of **mechanics, optics, acoustics, electricity** and **magnetism,** and **thermodynamics.** The laws of classical physics describe the behavior of matter and energy under ordinary, everyday conditions. Modern physics, which began at the end of the nineteenth century, seeks to explain the interactions of matter and energy under extraordinary conditions, such as in extreme temperatures or when moving near the speed of light. Modern physics is also concerned with the interactions of matter and energy on a very small scale (i.e., nuclear and elementary particle physics). It is noteworthy that at the subatomic level, the laws of classical physics governing space, time, matter, and energy are no longer valid.

Knowing the principles of classical physics is fundamental to having a clear understanding of how various types of respiratory care equipment operate. Indeed, this chapter began with a quote from Nobel laureate Richard Feynman to underscore the idea that physics is not only part of the foundation of respiratory care but also serves the same function in all of the clinical sciences.

This chapter presents a review of classical physics applicable to respiratory care equipment. It is not intended to present a compendium of physics, but rather focuses its discussion on how these physical principles are commonly encountered in respiratory care equipment. A list of several physics textbooks is included in the reference list at the end of the chapter to facilitate a more detailed study of physics.[2,3,4]

ENERGY AND MATTER

Energy and Work

The concepts of energy and work are closely related. In fact, energy is usually defined as the ability to do work, where work (W) equals the product of a force (F) acting on an object to move it a distance (d), or

$$W = F \times d.$$

Note that this definition is more specific than our everyday description of work. In everyday life, we say that work is anything that requires the exertion of effort. In physics, work is performed *only* when the effort produces a change in the position of the matter (i.e., the matter moves in the direction of the force). In the **Systèm International** (SI) of measurements, energy and work are expressed in **joules** (J), where 1 J equals the force of 1 **newton** (N) acting on a 1-kilogram (kg) object to move it 1 meter (m). **Power** (P), which is a measure of the rate at which work is being performed (P = W/t), is expressed in **watts** (W), with 1 W equivalent to 1 J/second. Because the watt is a relatively small number, we rely more on the **kilowatt** (kW), which equals 1000 watts [e.g., a 2-kilowatt motor can perform work at a rate of 2000 joules per second]. Another common term used for power is **horsepower** (hp). Approximately, 1 unit of horsepower equals 746 W of power, or 0.746 kW.

The energy required to perform work can exist in various forms, including mechanical energy, thermal energy, chemical energy, sound energy, nuclear energy, and electrical energy. According to the law of conservation of energy, energy cannot be created or destroyed but can only be transferred. For example, a fossil fuel such as coal, which is a form of chemical energy, can be converted to electrical energy, which, in turn, can provide the power to operate a fan or compressor. Therefore we can think of work as the transfer of energy by mechanical means. As such, mechanical energy is usually divided into two categories: **kinetic energy** and **potential energy.**

Kinetic and Potential Energy

Kinetic energy is the energy that an object possesses when it is in motion; potential energy is stored energy, or the energy that an object possesses because of its position. The kinetic energy (KE) of an object can be quantified with the formula:

$$KE = 1/2(mv^2),$$

where m is the mass of the object and v is the velocity at which it is traveling. Intuitively, one might guess that the greater the mass, the greater the kinetic energy. It is not necessarily obvious that the kinetic energy of the substance increases to a greater extent with similar increases in the velocity at which the object is traveling. In fact, when looking at the formula, one can see that the kinetic energy increases exponentially when velocity increases. That is, kinetic energy is proportional to the square of the velocity at which the object is moving (e.g., a twofold increase in mass increases the kinetic energy twofold, and a twofold increase in velocity results in a fourfold increase in the kinetic energy).

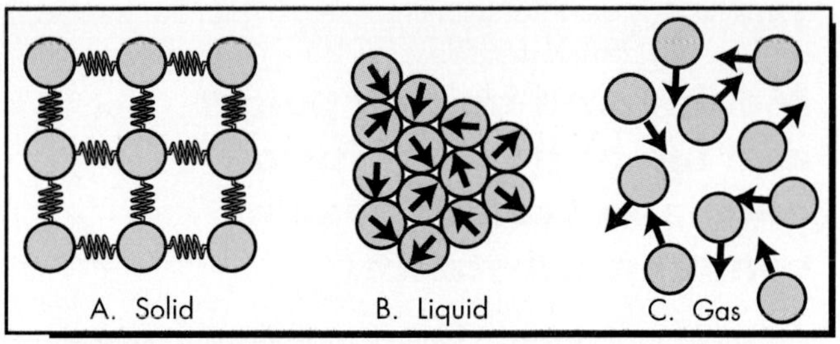

Figure 1-1 Simplified models illustrating the three states of matter: *A*, solid; *B*, liquid; *C*, gas.

One can think of potential energy as the energy that an object has by virtue of its position. For example, a weight raised above your head has the potential to exert a force when it falls. The energy that the weight gains as it falls is the result of gravity. (In this example, however, potential energy is more correctly referred to as **gravitational potential energy.**) The amount of potential energy (PE) that an object possesses can be calculated as:

$$PE = mgh,$$

where m is the mass of the object, g is the force of gravity (32 feet/sec^2), and h is the height that the object is raised. Potential energy can also be stored in a compressed spring or a chemical bond. With a spring, energy is required for compression. This **elastic potential energy** is then converted into kinetic energy when the spring is allowed to uncoil. Petroleum reserves of coal, oil, and gas, which represent **chemical potential energy** stores, can be converted to kinetic energy to provide the power required to operate lights, automobiles, and other devices we use in our daily lives.

STATES OF MATTER

Matter is generally defined as anything that has mass and occupies space. The **atomic theory** states that all matter is composed of tiny particles called **atoms.** Although it can appear in various forms, all matter is made up of only about 100 different types of atoms called **elements.**[5,6] These elements can combine in fixed proportions to form **molecules,** which in turn can form **compounds** and **mixtures.**

All matter can exist in three distinct states: **solid, liquid,** and **gas.** The physical properties of each of these states can be explained by the **kinetic theory,** which states that the atoms and molecules that make up matter are in constant motion. Figure 1-1 is a schematic illustrating the three states of matter. Solids are usually characterized as either crystalline or amorphous. Notice that crystalline solids are highly organized structures whose atoms and molecules are arranged in a lattice. Amorphous solids, such as glass or margarine, have constituent particles that are less rigidly arranged. Amorphous solids are sometimes called **supercooled** liquids because of this random arrangement.

Of the three states of matter, solids possess the least amount of kinetic energy. Most of their internal energy is potential energy that is contained in the intermolecular forces holding the individual particles of solids together. In solids, these forces are strong enough to limit the motion of the atoms and molecules to what appear to be vibrations or oscillations about a fixed point. Because of these features, solids are characterized as incompressible substances that can maintain their volume and shape.

Liquids possess attractive forces like solids, but the cohesive forces in liquids are not as strong. Liquid molecules have greater freedom of movement and possess more kinetic energy than those of solids. It is difficult to illustrate exactly how liquid particles move, but one can envision that these particles can slide past each other, thus giving liquids fluidity, or the ability to flow. Although the intermolecular forces holding liquids together are relatively weak when compared with solids, these forces lend enough cohesiveness to liquid molecules to allow them to maintain their volumes. Liquids are essentially incompressible. That is, a liquid can be made to occupy a smaller volume only if an incredible amount of force is exerted upon it.

Gases have very weak—if any—cohesive forces between their constituent particles. Therefore gases possess the greatest amount of kinetic energy of the three states of matter, though their potential energy is minimal compared with the other two states of matter. The motion of the atoms and molecules that make up gases is random. Gases do not maintain their shapes and volumes but expand to fill the available space. Gases are similar to liquids in that the particles composing them can move freely, thus giving gases the ability to flow. For this reason, gases and liquids are described as **fluids.**

Box 1-1 lists some of the more common substances that normally exist as gases at room temperature. Most of the gases encountered in everyday life (i.e., nitrogen, oxygen, carbon dioxide, and carbon monoxide) are colorless

BOX 1-1

Substances Existing as Gases at Room Temperature and 1 atm

Oxygen
Nitrogen
Helium
Hydrogen
Chlorine
Nitrogen dioxide

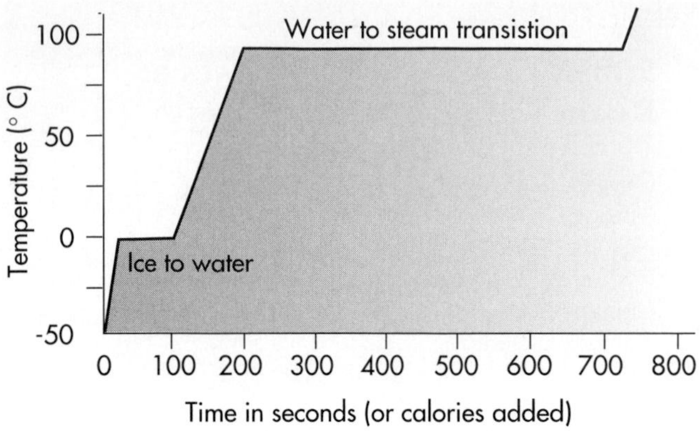

Figure 1-2 Energy-temperature relationship for the conversion of solid ice to liquid water to steam. Energy is added at a rate of 1 cal/sec. (Redrawn from Nave CR and Nave BC: Physics for the health sciences, ed 3, Philadelphia, 1985, Saunders.)

and odorless; however, a notable exception is nitrogen dioxide (NO_2), which is an atmospheric pollutant that is dark brown and has a pungent odor. The properties of individual medical gases are discussed in Chapter 2.

Change of State

It should be apparent from the discussion so far that thc physical state of any substance is determined from the relation of its kinetic energy content and the potential energy stored in its intermolecular bonds. Changes of state involve the interconversions of solids, liquids, and gases, which can be accomplished by altering the relationship between the kinetic and potential energy of a substance, such as by changing its temperature (i.e., by adding or removing heat). Consider the example of converting the solid form of water, ice, to liquid and then to steam. Adding heat to ice increases the kinetic activity (i.e., vibration of the water molecules) in ice, thus melting or weakening the intermolecular attractive forces and producing liquid water. (Freezing, which is the opposite of melting, can be accomplished by transferring the kinetic energy of a substance to its surroundings, such as when a substance is exposed to cold temperatures.) Adding more heat causes the liquid water molecules to move more vigorously and escape into the gaseous state, or vaporize (**evaporation**). The temperature at which a solid converts to a liquid is a substance's **melting point.** (Note that the **freezing point** is the same temperature as the melting point, that is, the temperature at which a liquid is changed to a solid state.) The temperature at which a liquid converts to a gaseous state is its **boiling point.**

Figure 1-2 shows the phase changes associated with the conversion of 1 gram (g) of ice to steam.[7] As heat is added, ice begins to change to liquid at a temperature of 0° C. Note that although the addition of heat effects a change in state, the temperature of the water does not change immediately (i.e., there is a plateau in temperature). The temperature will change *only* after all of the ice is converted to liquid. The amount of heat that must be added to a substance to cause a complete change of state is called the **latent heat** of fusion and is expressed in calories per gram. Therefore the amount of heat that must be added to effect the change from solid to liquid is called the latent heat of melting. In the case of water, approximately 80 calories (cal)/g of ice must be added to completely liquefy ice when the temperature reaches 0° C. Once the ice has been completely liquefied, the temperature will increase 1° C per second if heat continues to be added at a rate of 1 cal/sec. This same type of phenomenon occurs at the substance's boiling point when water is converted to steam. The amount of heat that must be supplied to completely change liquid to steam (i.e., vaporize water) is the latent heat of vaporization. As one can see, a considerably greater amount of heat (540 cal/g) must be added to convert water to steam when compared with the amount of heat that must be added to melt ice into water. More energy is required in the process of vaporization because intermolecular forces must be essentially removed to allow the molecules to break loose and enter into the gaseous state.[8] Table 1-1 lists the melting and boiling points along with the latent heats of fusion and vaporization for some commonly used substances.

TABLE 1-1

Melting and boiling points and latent heats of fusion and vaporization of some common substances

Substance	Melting point (° C)	Heat of fusion (cal/g)	Boiling point (° C)*	Heat of vaporization (cal/g)
Water	0	80	100	540
Ammonia	−75	108	−33	327
Ethyl alcohol	−114	26	78	204
Nitrogen	−210	6.2	−196	48
Oxygen	−219	3.3	−183	51
Lead	327	5.9	1620	208
Mercury	−39	2.7	357	68

*At standard atmospheric pressure of 760 mm Hg.

From Scanlan CL, Spearman CB, and Sheldon RL: Egan's fundamentals of respiratory care, ed 6, St Louis, 1995, Mosby.

Sublimation

Under certain conditions, solid molecules can completely bypass the liquid state and change to gas. This process, called **sublimation,** occurs when the heat content of a substance

BOX 1-2

Evaporation and Condensation

A fairly common example that can be used to illustrate concepts of evaporation and condensation relates to the water-vapor content, or humidity, of the air surrounding us. This concept is obvious to anyone who has ever spent a hot August day somewhere in the southern part of the United States, such as New Orleans. As stated in the section on evaporation, one of the main factors influencing evaporation is temperature. Temperature increases water evaporation (in New Orleans, the water is from the lakes and bayous all around the city) by increasing the molecular activity of the water and increasing the capacity of the air to hold water vapor. If the actual amount of water vapor in the air is to be measured, the water-vapor content must be determined. The amount or weight of water that can be contained (to capacity) in the air is called the **absolute humidity** and is expressed in grams of water vapor per cubic meter (gm/m^3) or milligrams per liter (mg/L). (The absolute humidity can be measured or it can be computed with tables supplied by the United States Weather Bureau.[8]) Note that at a temperature of 37° C (98.6° F), which is a typical temperature in New Orleans during August, air that is 100% saturated will contain 43.80 mg of water per liter of air. In most cases, the air is not fully saturated but is *only* 90% saturated with water vapor; that is it only contains 0.90 × 43.80 mg/L, or 39.42 mg of water in every liter of air. For this reason, the National Weather Service chooses to report **relative humidity,** or the ratio of actual water content to its saturated capacity, at a given temperature (in this case, the relative humidity would be 90%).

One might ask how condensation can be included in this example, but consider that nearly every afternoon between 4 and 5 PM it rains in New Orleans. The rain occurs because the air cools (the sun begins to set), and the capacity of the air to hold water decreases. This decreased capacity to hold water vapor causes condensation, and rain results.

increases to a point where the molecules in the solid state gain enough energy to break loose and enter the gaseous state while remaining below its melting point. The conversion of solid carbon dioxide (i.e., dry ice) to gaseous carbon dioxide is the most common example of this process.

Evaporation

The conversion of a liquid to the gaseous state has been discussed in terms of boiling (e.g., the transition from water to steam occurs at a temperature of 100° C). Although it may not be obvious, this phase transition (evaporation) begins at temperatures between 0° C and 100° C. Evaporation occurs when some of the liquid molecules gain enough kinetic energy to break through the surface of the liquid and convert to free gaseous molecules. The rate of evaporation increases with an increase in temperature, an increase in surface area, and/or a decrease in pressure.

Two forces must be overcome for evaporation to occur: the mass attraction of the molecules for each other (i.e., **dipole-dipole interactions, hydrogen bonding**, and **van der Waals forces**) and the pressure of the gas above the liquid. We can enhance the process of evaporation by either increasing the kinetic energy of the liquid molecules or reducing the pressure above the liquid. Raising the temperature of a liquid increases the velocity and the force of the molecules hitting each other and moves them farther apart. This increased kinetic activity increases the force that these molecules possess as they hit the surface of the liquid, thus allowing the liquid molecules to escape more easily and frequently. **Vapor pressure** is a measure of the force that molecules exert as they hit the surface of the liquid and escape into the gaseous phase.

The concept of vapor pressure can be used to define the boiling point of a liquid in more precise terms. That is, the boiling point is the temperature at which the vapor pressure of a liquid equals the atmospheric pressure. Reducing the pressure above the liquid lowers its boiling point because the forces opposing the escape of molecules from the liquid are decreased. This concept explains why water boils at a lower temperature at high altitudes. It also explains the process of freeze-drying as a means of food preservation. In the latter procedure, a substance is placed in a vacuum, thus reducing the opposition that liquid molecules must overcome to evaporate, so any liquid present boils off.

The opposite of evaporation is condensation, which is simply defined as the conversion of a substance from a gas to a liquid. In evaporation, heat energy is removed from the air surrounding a liquid and transferred to the liquid, thus cooling the air. In contrast, during condensation, heat is removed from the liquid and transferred to the surrounding air, warming it. Box 1-2 contains an example of how evaporation and condensation can affect a person's daily life.

Evaporation and condensation are essential components in respiration. Specifically, effective ventilation requires that there is a balance between the evaporation and condensation of the moisture of respired gases so that airway mucosa is not dried and irritated. Therapeutic procedures, such as administration of dry medical gases or insertion of an endotracheal tube into the patient's airway to provide mechanical ventilatory support, can severely interfere with the patient's ability to maintain this balance. The potential problems

TABLE 1-2

Critical temperatures and pressures required for maintaining the liquid state of gases at room temperature

	Critical temperature		Critical pressure		Approximate pressure in commercial cylinder at room temperature	
Gas	°C	°F	atm	psi	atm	psi
Cyclopropane	125	257	54.2	797	5.4	79
Nitrous oxide	36.5	97.7	71.8	1054	50.6	745
Carbon dioxide	31.1	87.9	73.0	1071	57.0	838

From Scanlan CL, Spearman CB, and Sheldon RL: Egan's fundamentals of respiratory care, ed 6, St Louis, 1995, Mosby.

associated with bypassing the body's mechanisms for humidifying inspired gases can be minimized by ensuring that all gases delivered to the patient are adequately humidified. Devices, such as cascade humidifiers and hygroscopic condenser filters, or artificial noses, are two examples of devices that can be used to ensure adequate humidification of inspired gases. We will revisit these concepts in our discussion of humidity and aerosol therapy (see Chapter 4).

Critical Temperature and Critical Pressure

When a liquid is placed in a closed container, the force of the molecules trying to escape from the liquid eventually equilibrate with the force or pressure of the liquid molecules that have entered into the gaseous state, and no more liquid molecules will escape. If the temperature of the liquid is raised, however, the velocity its molecules are traveling will increase, while the mass attraction between its constituent molecules is reduced. Raising the temperature also increases the capacity of the air above the liquid to hold liquid vapor. Thus the vapor pressure also increases with increases in temperature, necessitating a higher opposing force to equilibrate the molecule's escape from the liquid state. At its boiling point, the force of the molecules in the liquid equals the surrounding pressure, and the molecules may fail to escape. So, in essence, the boiling point is the temperature at which the force exerted by the molecule of the liquid trying to escape equals the forces opposing its escape (i.e., atmospheric pressure and mass attraction). As gas molecules are heated above the boiling point, the force (pressure) required for converting them back to a liquid also increases. Ultimately, a temperature is reached above which gaseous molecules of a substance cannot be converted back to a liquid, no matter what pressure is exerted on them. This temperature is called the **critical temperature.**[7] Therefore the critical temperature can be thought of as the highest temperature at which a substance can exist in a liquid state. **Critical pressure** is the pressure that must be applied to the substance at its critical temperature to maintain equilibrium between the liquid and gas phases.[8] The term ***critical point*** is used to describe the critical temperature and the critical pressure of a substance. Substances that exist as liquids at ambient conditions have critical temperatures that are greater than room temperature (i.e., 20° C to 25° C). Substances that normally exist as gases at ambient conditions have critical temperatures that are usually well below room temperature. (Table 1-2 lists critical temperatures and pressures of some commonly encountered substances.)

Two commonly encountered substances can be used to demonstrate the principles of critical temperature and critical pressure. For example, water boils at 100° C and has a critical temperature of 374° C. At temperatures below 100° C, water exists as a liquid. As its temperature is raised above 100° C, water converts to a gas, steam. Between 100° C and 374° C, steam can be converted back into liquid by applying progressively greater amounts of pressure to it. In fact, to maintain equilibrium between the liquid and gaseous states of water at 374° C, 218 atm of pressure must be applied. Furthermore, above 374° C, water can only exist as a gas—no matter how much pressure is applied. Oxygen has a boiling point of −183° C and a critical temperature of about −119° C. At temperatures below −183° C, oxygen can exist as a liquid. Once its temperature is raised above −183° C, liquid oxygen becomes a gas. At temperatures between −183° C and −119° C, the gaseous oxygen can be converted back to a liquid by compression. As with water, greater amounts of pressure must be applied to cause this conversion until the critical temperature of −119° C is reached. At oxygen's critical temperature, a pressure of 49.7 atm must be applied to maintain equilibrium between the gaseous and liquid phases of oxygen. Once the temperature is raised above the critical temperature, oxygen cannot be converted to a liquid no matter how much pressure is applied to it.

Application of the concepts of critical temperature and critical pressure can be seen in medical gas therapy. As discussed in Chapters 2 and 3, medical gases can be supplied in cylinders and bulk storage systems. Substances such as nitrous oxide and carbon dioxide have critical temperatures above room temperature and thus can exist as vapors (i.e., as a mixture of liquid and gas when placed in a compressed-gas cylinder [gases and vapors will be discussed in the next section of this chapter]). Air, oxygen, and helium, on the other hand, have critical temperatures well below room temperature and exist as gases when placed under pressure in a compressed-gas cylinder. Liquid air and oxygen, which must be kept at very low temperatures (i.e., below their boiling points), are stored in specially insulated containers. When needed, the liquid oxygen or air is allowed to exceed its critical temperature and convert to gas.[8]

Gases vs. Vapors

A gas is a state of matter that is above its critical temperature. Free molecules of the same substance below its critical temperature are a vapor. Simply stated, a vapor is the gaseous form of any substance that can exist as a liquid or a solid at ordinary pressures and temperatures. For example, under normal conditions, oxygen exists in the gaseous state above its critical temperature (− 183° C) and is therefore classified as a true gas. Water, on the other hand, is below its critical temperature (374° C) and is considered a vapor. Water vapor can be converted back to liquid or ice if sufficient pressure is applied.

Two commonly used vapors are carbon dioxide and nitrous oxide. Both of these substances can be converted to liquid at room temperature if enough pressure is applied. In fact, both gases are supplied to hospitals in pressurized cylinders in which most of the vapor is converted to liquid. As will be discussed in Chapter 2 (Manufacture, Storage, and Transport of Medical Gases), the amount of carbon dioxide or nitrous oxide remaining in cylinders containing substances below their critical temperature (liquids) must be determined by weighing the cylinders instead of reading the pressure level within the cylinder. Gases such as oxygen, nitrogen, and helium are examples of substances that are usually supplied in compressed-gas cylinders above their critical temperatures. In these cases, the pressure gauge gives an accurate estimate of amount of gas remaining in the cylinder.

PHYSICAL PROPERTIES OF LIQUIDS AND GASES

Temperature

As already stated, temperature is a measure of the average kinetic energy of the molecules of an object,[9] but it is also a measure of the relative warmth or coolness of a substance. Recall that adding heat to a substance changes its physical properties. This phenomenon of changing physical properties can be used in temperature measurements and in designing temperature scales.[10]

Thermometers are devices used to measure temperature. They are made with materials that undergo physical changes as their temperature changes. Thermometers are generally classified as **nonelectrical** and **electrical thermometers.**[10] The most commonly used nonelectrical devices are mercury and alcohol thermometers. Resistance thermometers, thermistors, and thermocouples are examples of electrical thermometers.

The mercury thermometer is probably the best known example of a nonelectric thermometer. This device is the product of Gabriel Daniel Fahrenheit's work on temperature measurement during the early part of the 18th century. Fahrenheit (1686-1736) used mercury because he found that it expands and contracts as its temperature changes. He constructed the first thermometer and ultimately the first mercury temperature scale (i.e., the Fahrenheit temperature scale).

Electrical thermometers operate on the principle that the electrical resistance of metal increases linearly with increases in temperature.[10] A typical resistance thermometer consists of a platinum wire resistor, a battery, and an ammeter for measuring current flow. Because the amount of current flowing through the platinum wire is directly related to the resistance of the wire, the ammeter can detect temperature changes by measuring the changes in current flow that occur when the resistor's temperature is changed.*

Another common example of an electrical thermometer is the **thermistor.** It is typically a metal oxide bead, whose resistance changes as its temperature rises and falls. An ammeter connected to an electrical circuit measures temperature in a manner similar to that described for the resistance thermometer. Thermistors are incorporated into a number of medical devices, including mechanical ventilators, spirometers, capnographs, and metabolic monitors. Thermistors are also an integral part of the balloon-flotation catheters that are used with thermodilution cardiac output monitors. All of these devices will be discussed in more detail in Chapter 7 when monitoring physiological function is considered.

Temperature Scales

A temperature scale is constructed by choosing two reference temperatures and dividing the difference between these points into a certain number of degrees. The size of the degree depends on the particular temperature scale being used. The most common reference temperatures are the melting point of ice and the boiling point of water because recognizable changes take place and thus can be given a value against which other temperatures can be measured.

Three temperature scales are routinely used in science and medicine: the absolute (**Kelvin**) scale, the **Celsius** scale, and the **Fahrenheit** scale. A fourth temperature scale, the **Rankine** scale is used in the engineering

*Actually, the electrical circuit consists of multiple resistors arranged in a configuration called a **Wheatstone bridge**. We will limit our discussion of electrical circuits at this point because we will discuss the principles of electricity later in this chapter.

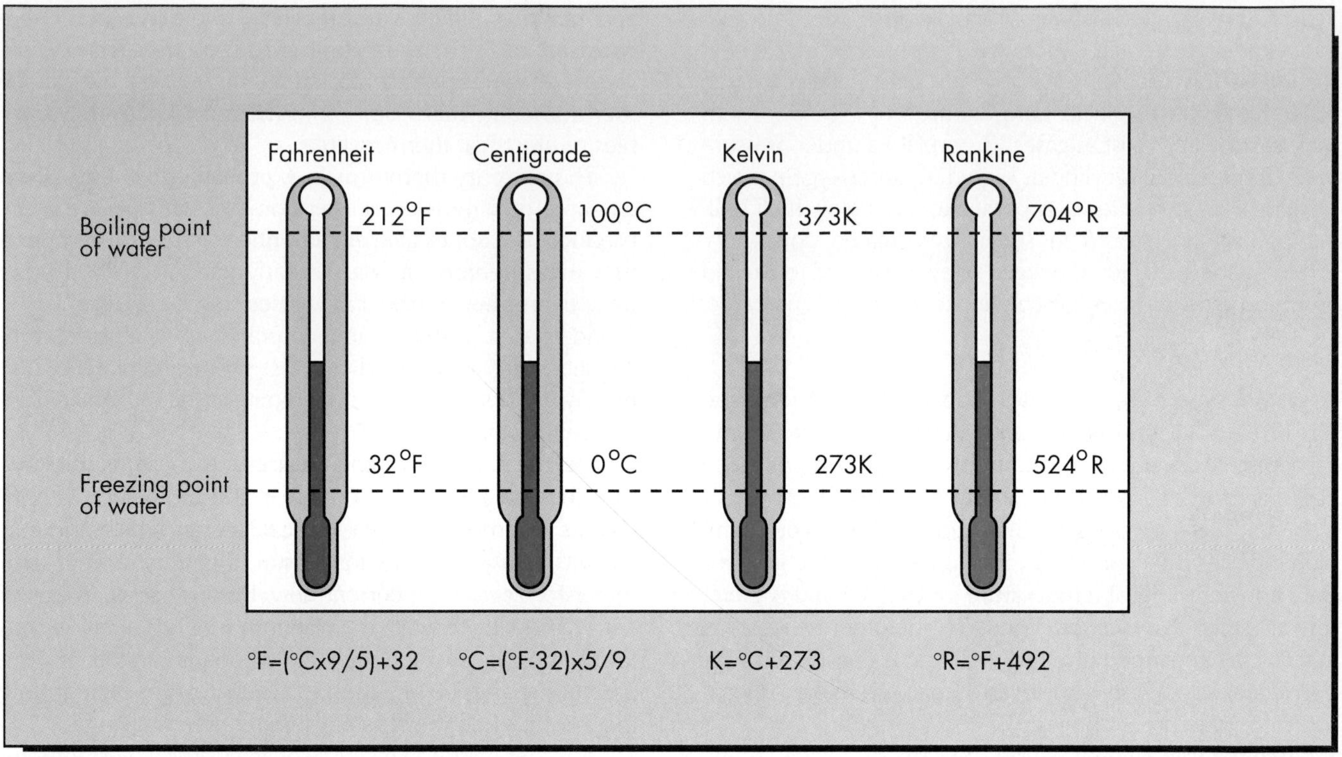

Figure 1-3 Temperature scales.

sciences.[7] Figure 1-3 shows the scalar relationships between the Kelvin, Celsius, and Fahrenheit scales.

The **Systèm International** (SI) units for temperature are based on the Kelvin scale, with the zero point equal to 0 K or absolute zero, and the boiling point equal to 100 K. Theoretically, absolute zero is the temperature at which all molecular motion stops. Notice that the Kelvin scale is described as a centigrade scale because there are 100 divisions between the freezing and boiling points of water.

The metric or centimeter-gram-second (cgs) system is based on the Celsius scale, which can also be characterized as a centigrade scale. In the Celsius scale, the freezing point for water is designated as 0° C, while the boiling point of water equals 100° C. It is important to recognize that although the Celsius and Kelvin scales are both considered centigrade scales, the same temperature will have different values on each. Notice in Figure 1-3 that a temperature of 0 K (i.e., absolute zero or the temperature at which all of the kinetic activity of a substance stops) corresponds to a temperature of −273° C, and that the zero point on the Celsius scale (0° C; i.e., the freezing point of water) therefore corresponds to a temperature of 273 K on the Kelvin scale. Similarly, the boiling point of water on the Celsius scale (100°C) corresponds to a temperature of 373 K.

The Fahrenheit scale, which is used in British or the foot-pound-second (fps) system sets the freezing point of water at 32° F and the boiling point of water equals 212° F. The Fahrenheit scale has 180 divisions between the freezing and the boiling points of water, and therefore cannot be considered a centigrade scale.

Box 1-3 contains formulae for converting temperatures between the various scales. As will be seen later in this chapter, the Kelvin scale is used when the gas and other physical laws are described; and although there is increased emphasis on using the Celsius scale in the scientific literature and clinical medicine, clinicians in the United States continue to use the Fahrenheit scale for recording patient temperatures.

Pressure

When gas molecules collide with solid or liquid surfaces, they exert a pressure. Pressure (P) is usually defined as the force that a gas exerts over a given area (P = Force/Area). Pressure measurements are reported in a variety of units, including pounds per square inch (psi, or lb/in^2), millimeters of mercury (mm Hg), torr, centimeters of water (cm H_2O), and kilopascals (kPa).[11] Box 1-4 contains formulae for converting pressure units.

Atmospheric pressure is the pressure that atmospheric gases exert on objects within the earth's atmosphere. It exists because the gases that make up the atmosphere are attracted to the earth's surface by gravity, thus forming a column of air around the earth. Notice that atmospheric pressure is highest near the earth's surface; at sea level at-

BOX 1-3

Temperature Scales

Conversions between the Kelvin and Celsius Scales

$$K = °C + 273$$
$$°C = K - 273$$

Example 1

37° C equals how many Kelvin?

$$K = 37° C + 273$$
$$= 310\ K$$

(Note that Kelvin is not preceded by the symbol for degrees)

Example 2

373 K equals how many degrees Celsius?

$$°C = 373\ K - 273$$
$$= 100° C$$

Conversions between the Celsius and Fahrenheit Scales

$$°C = 5/9\ (°F - 32)$$
$$°F = (9/5 \times °C) + 32$$

Example 1

98.6° F equals how many degrees Celsius?

$$°C = 5/9(98.6° F - 32)$$
$$= 5/9(66.6)$$
$$= 37° C$$

Example 2

25° C equals how many degrees Fahrenheit?

$$°F = (9/5 \times 25) + 32$$
$$= 45 + 32$$
$$= 77° F$$

mospheric pressure equals 760 mm Hg. As you move away from the surface of the earth, the atmospheric pressure decreases because of a reduction in the force of gravity pulling air molecules towards the earth. For example, the atmospheric pressure in Chicago, which is located at sea level, averages around 760 mm Hg. The atmospheric pressure in Denver, which is located 1 mile above sea level averages about 630 mm Hg.

Atmospheric pressure can be measured with a barometer similar to the one shown in Figure 1-4. The mercury barometer, which was invented by Evangelista Torricelli (c. 1608-1647), is the most commonly used device for measuring atmospheric pressure. (Torricelli was the first person to recognize the existence of atmospheric pressure; the pressure measurement *torr* is named in his honor.) The mercury barometer uses the weight of a column of mercury to equilibrate with the force of the gas molecules hitting the surface of a mercury reservoir. A column is completely filled with mercury and erected with its open end below the surface of a mercury reservoir. The mercury in the column tries to return to the reservoir as a result of gravity. The force, which gas molecules exert as they hit the surface of the reservoir, counteracts the force of gravity and pushes the mercury upward in the tube. The atmospheric pressure equals the height of the mercury column.

The aneroid barometer (Figure 1-5) measures atmospheric pressure by equilibrating the atmospheric gas pressure with a mechanical force, or the expansion force of an evacuated metal container. As atmospheric pressure increases, the pressure on the surface of the metal container tends to compress it. The change in the container's dimensions is recorded by a gearing mechanism, which changes the location of an indicator on the recording dial. Likewise, a decrease in atmospheric pressure surrounding the container allows the metal container to expand toward its normal shape.

Buoyancy

When an object is immersed in a fluid, it appears to weigh less than it does in air. This effect, ***buoyancy,*** can be explained by **Archimedes's principle.**[7,8,9] Archimedes's principle states that when an object is submerged in a fluid, it will be buoyed up by a force equal to the weight of the fluid that is displaced by the object. The weight of the displaced liquid can be calculated as the product of the volume (V) of displaced liquid and the weight density (d_w) of the liquid:

$$F_{buoyancy} = Vd_w.$$

Consider what happens when an object is submerged in water. Water has a weight density of 1 gm/cm^3. If the weight density of the object being submerged is less than the weight density of water, the object will float. If the weight density of the submerged object is greater than that of water, the object will sink. Figure 1-6 illustrates a practical example of this concept that is commonly encountered by patients who use metered dose inhalers (MDIs) for delivery of medication. In this case, the weight density of the cannister varies with the amount of medication contained in it. That is, the more medication that is in the cannister, the greater the weight density of the cannister. It should be apparent from this example that an empty cannister has a weight density less than water and floats, whereas a full cannister has a weight density greater than water, and sinks.

The measurement of the specific gravity of a liquid or a gas represents another practical application of Archimedes's principle. Specific gravity is a comparison of a substance's weight density relative to a standard. For liquids, water is used as the standard, and gases are compared to oxygen or

BOX 1-4

Pressure Conversions

Pressure can be measured in a variety of units, including:

- Centimeters of water (cm H_2O)
- Millimeters of mercury (mm Hg), or torr
- Pounds per square inch (lb/in^2, or psi)
- Atmospheres (atm)
- Kilopascals (kPa)

The following formulae enable conversions between these units:

- cm $H_2O \times 0.7355$ = mm Hg (torr)
- mm Hg (torr)/0.7355 = cm H_2O
- cm $H_2O \times 0.098$ = kPa
- kPa/0.098 = cm H_2O
- mm Hg $\times$ 0.1333 = kPa
- kPa/0.1333 = mm Hg
- mm Hg $\div$ 760 = atm
- atm $\times$ 14.7 = lb/in^2 (psi)

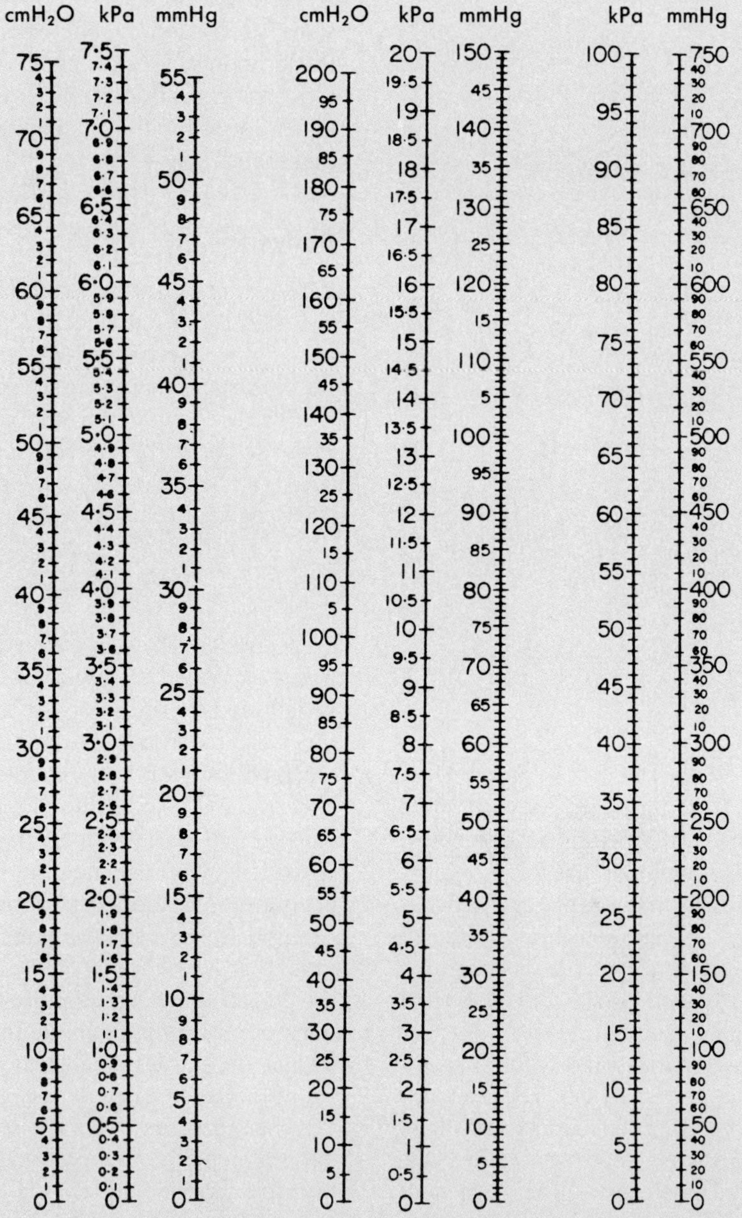

Figure from Sykes MK, McNichols MW, and Camp EJM: Respiratory failure, ed 2, London, 1976, Blackwell Scientific Publications.

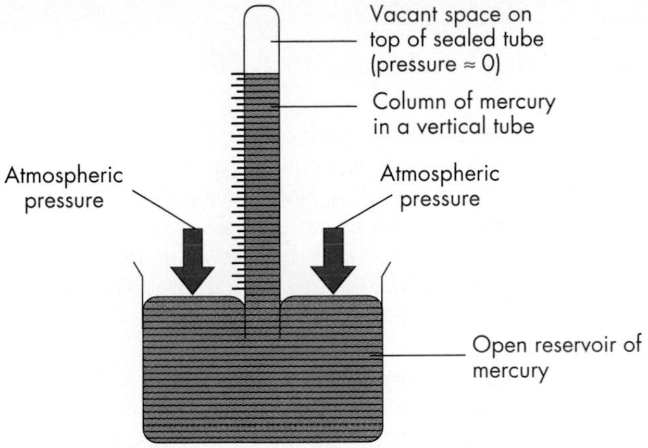

Figure 1-4 A mercury barometer. (From Eubanks DH and Bone RC: Comprehensive respiratory care, ed 2, St Louis, 1990, Mosby.)

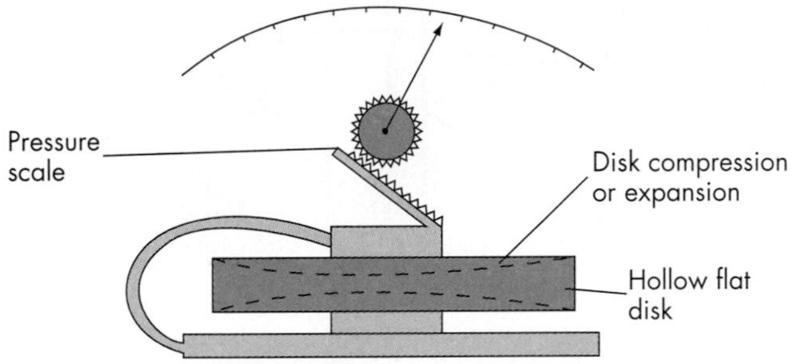

Figure 1-5 An aneroid barometer. (From Eubanks DH and Bone RC: Comprehensive respiratory care, ed 2, St Louis, 1990, Mosby.)

hydrogen.[6] The device shown in Figure 1-7, a **hydrometer,** is used clinically to measure the weight density or specific gravity of liquids, such as urine. The density of a liquid is measured by the level at which the hydrometer floats in the liquid. Thus if the liquid is very dense, the hydrometer floats near the surface because only a small volume of liquid needs to be displaced to equal the weight of the hydrometer. Notice in Figure 1-7 that the specific gravity can be read from the tube. Thus a reading of 1.030 indicates that the urine weighs 1.030 times more than water.[8]

Viscosity

Viscosity can be defined as the force opposing deformation of a fluid. The viscosity of a fluid is dependent on its density, as well as on the cohesive forces between its constituent molecules (i.e., as the cohesive forces of a fluid increase, so does its viscosity).

Viscosity is manifest differently in liquids and gases.[9] The viscosity of a liquid is primarily determined by the cohesive forces between its molecules, whereas the viscosity of a gas is determined by the number of collisions of the gas molecules. For example, raising the temperature of a liquid such as cooking oil weakens the cohesive forces between its molecules and decreases its viscosity. As the oil is heated and its temperature increases, it flows more freely than at a lower temperature (e.g., room temperature). Conversely, increasing the temperature of a gas increases its kinetic energy (i.e., the frequency of collisions

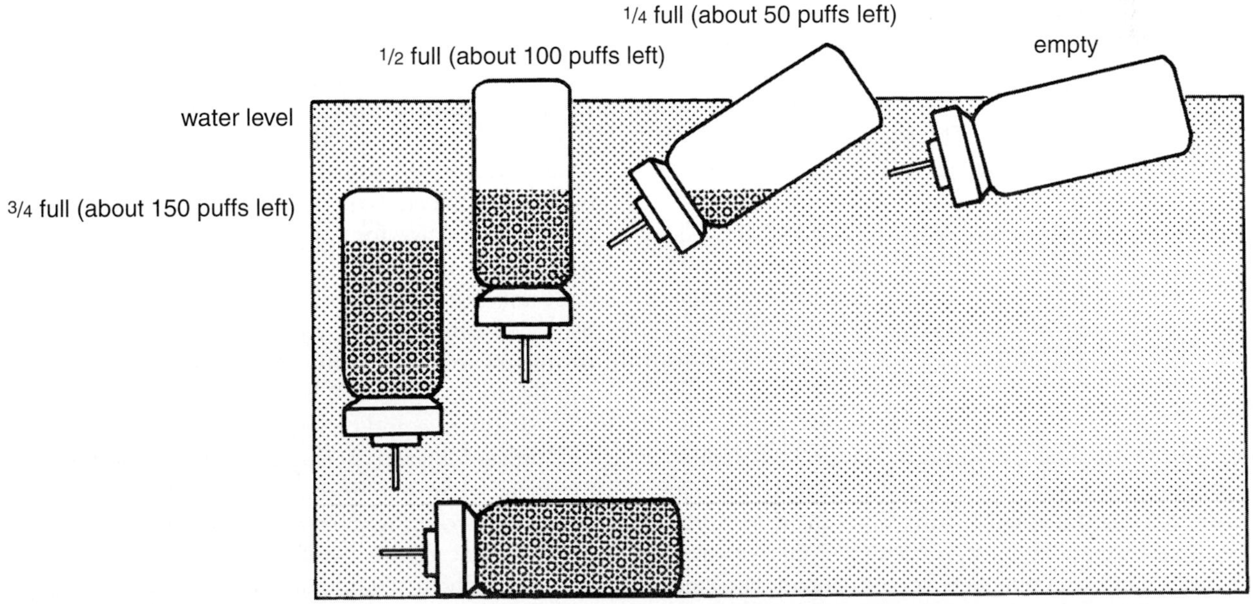

Figure 1-6 Determining how much medication is left in a MDI cannister is a common problem for patients who use MDIs. A float test can be used to determine how much medication is present. This test is performed by placing the cannister in a basin of room temperature water and observing its position in the basin, as illustrated above. (Modified from *Nursing 93*, Springhouse Corp., Springhouse, Pa.)

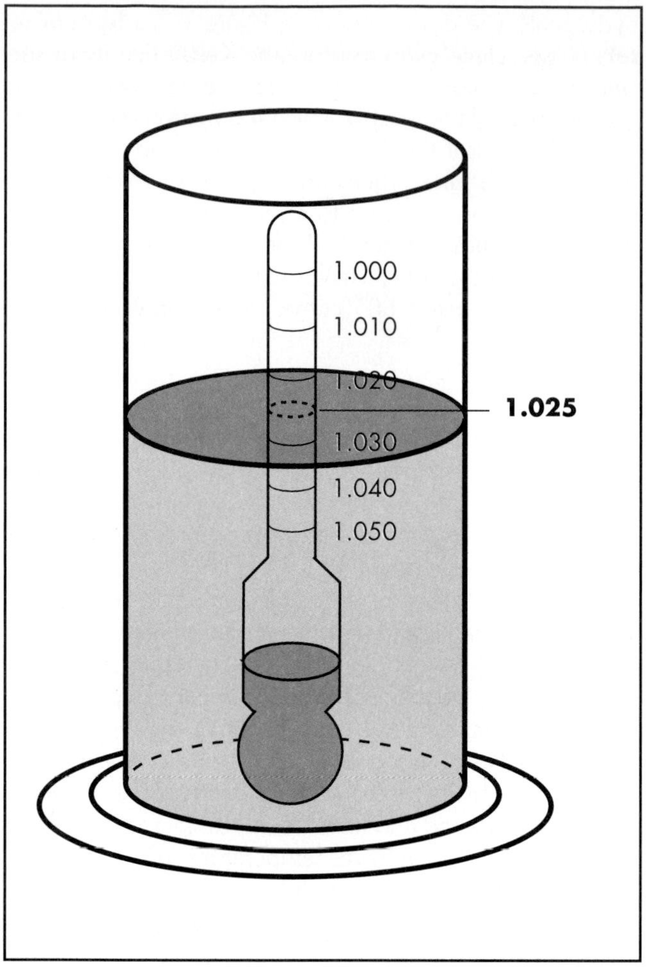

Figure 1-7 A hydrometer for measuring the specific gravity of liquids. The specific gravity can be read directly from the calibrated tube. (Modified from Nave CR and Nave BC: Physics for the health sciences, ed 3, Philadelphia, 1985,

BOX 1-5

Adhesive and Cohesive Forces

The properties of adhesion and cohesion can be demonstrated by placing liquid in a small-diameter glass tube like those shown below. Notice that at the top of the column of liquid, the liquid forms a curved surface, or meniscus. In Tube A, which contains water, the meniscus is concave; but in Tube B, which contains mercury, the meniscus is convex. In Tube A, the meniscus is turned up because the attractive, adhesive forces between the water and the glass cause the water to adhere to the wall of the tube. In Tube B, the meniscus is turned down because the cohesive forces within the mercury are stronger than the adhesive forces between the mercury and the glass.

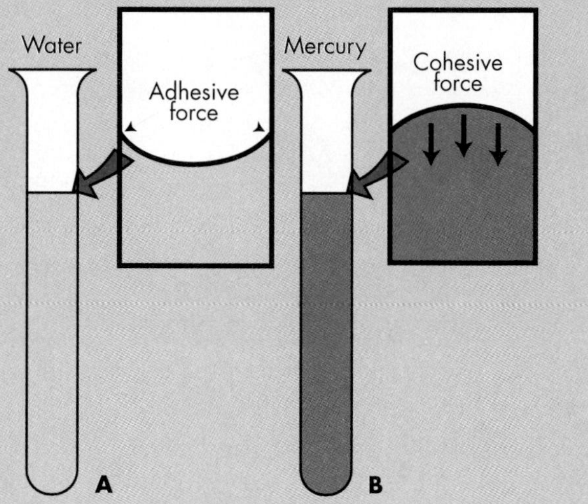

of its constituent molecules). The greater number of collisions results in a higher internal friction, and thus an increase in viscosity.

Viscosity is an important factor to consider when describing laminar or streamlined flow. How viscosity influences fluid mechanics, specifically as it relates to Poiseuille's law, will be discussed later in this chapter.

Surface Tension

Before the phenomenon of surface tension is described, the difference between **adhesive** and **cohesive** forces should be discussed. Adhesive forces are attractive forces between two different kinds of molecules. Cohesive forces, on the other hand, are attractive forces between like kinds of molecules. The difference between these two forces can be envisioned by taking two dishes and filling one with water and the other with mercury. If a paper towel is gently submerged into each liquid, the results will be different. When the towel is placed in the water dish, it absorbs the water. This is because the attractive, *adhesive* forces between the molecules of the towel and the water are greater than the attractive forces of the water molecules for each other. When the towel is submerged in the mercury dish, it does not absorb the mercury because the attractive, *cohesive* forces between the mercury molecules are greater than the attractive forces between the molecules of the towel and the mercury. (See Box 1-5 for another application involving adhesive and cohesive forces.)

Surface tension is generated by the cohesive forces between liquid molecules at a gas-liquid interface or at the interface of two immiscible (i.e., unable to mix) liquids like oil and water. Figure 1-8 illustrates the molecular basis of surface tension at a gas-liquid interface. At some depth, the molecules within a liquid are attracted equally from all sides, whereas the molecules near the surface experience unequal attractions.[10] Notice that near the surface of the liquid, some of the forces in the liquid act in a direction that

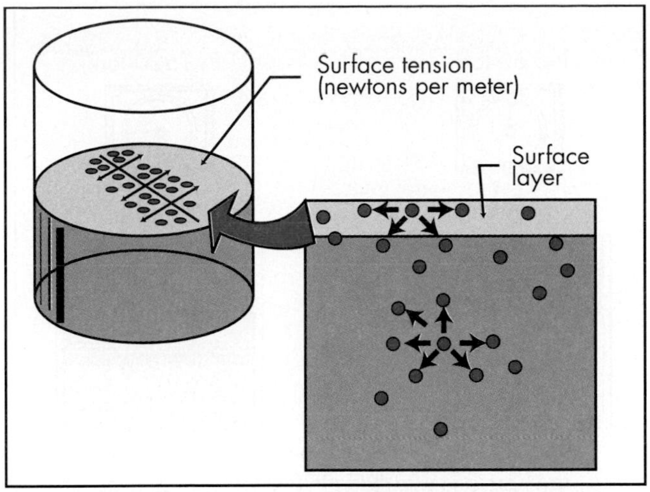

Figure 1-8 The molecular basis for surface tension. See text for explanation.

TABLE 1-3

Examples of surface tension

Substance	°C	Surface tension (dynes/cm)
Water	20	73
Water	37	70
Tissue fluid	37	50
Whole blood	37	58
Plasma	37	73
Ethyl alcohol	20	22
Mercury	17	547

From Scanlan CL, Wilkins RL, and Stoller JK: Egan's fundamentals of respiratory care, ed 7, St Louis, 1999, Mosby.

is parallel to the surface, while others are drawn toward the center of the liquid mass by this net force. Those forces acting parallel to the surface of the liquid cause the liquid to behave as though a film is present at the gas-liquid interface. The forces drawn toward the center of the liquid tend to reduce its exposed surface to the smallest possible area, which is usually a sphere.

We can measure the surface tension of a liquid by determining the force that must be applied to produce a "tear" in this film.[7] As such, in the SI system of measurements, surface tension is usually expressed in dynes per centimeter (dyn/cm). Table 1-3 lists surface tensions for several liquids that are commonly encountered in respiratory care. Note that the surface tension of a given liquid varies inversely with its temperature. Thus surface tension decreases as the temperature of a liquid increases.

Laplace's Law

As just stated, surface tension forces cause a liquid to have a tendency to occupy the smallest possible area, which is usually a sphere. The pressure within a liquid sphere should be influenced both by the surface tension forces offered by the liquid and by the size of the sphere. Indeed, Pierre-Simon Laplace (1749-1827), a French astronomer and mathematician, found that pressure within a sphere is directly related to the surface tension of the liquid and inversely related to the radius of the sphere, or:

$$P = 2(ST/r),$$

where *P* is the pressure within the sphere, *ST* is the surface tension of the liquid, and *r* is the radius of the sphere.

The examples shown in Figure 1-9 should help to illustrate this principle. In Figure 1-9, *A*, two droplets of water are shown. One droplet has a radius of 2 cm and the other droplet has a radius of 4 cm. If we assume that the surface

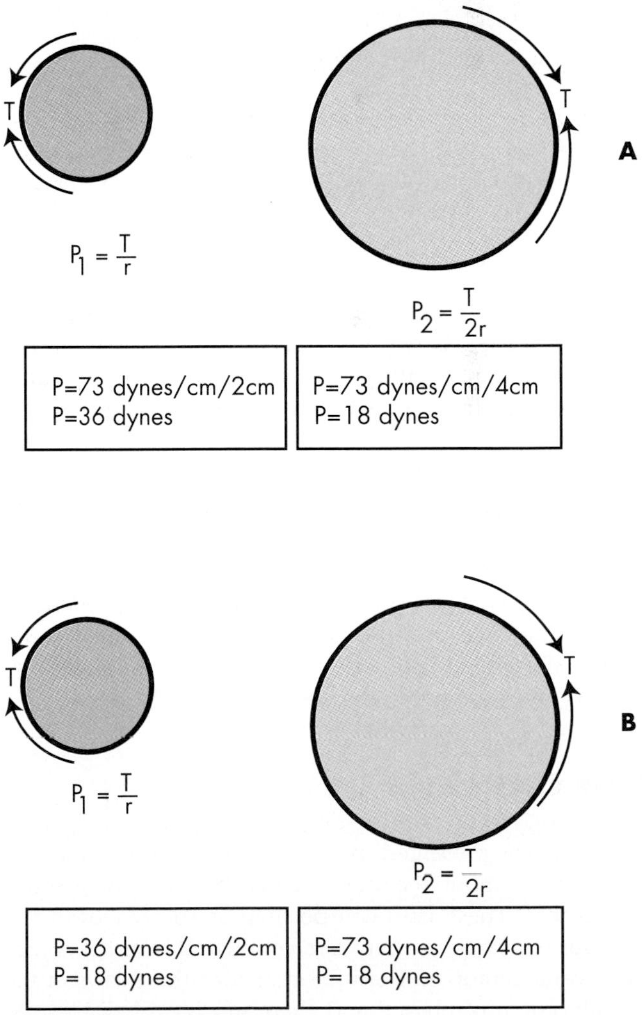

Figure 1-9 LaPlace's law. (*A*, water bubble; *B*, soap bubble). See text for discussion.

tension is equal in both droplets (i.e., the surface tension of water is 73 dyn/cm), then the pressure in the smaller droplet is twice that of the larger droplet.

Now consider what happens when the surface tension of the smaller droplet is reduced by, for example, adding a surface-active agent (i.e., soap) to the water. As shown in Figure 1-9, *B,* the surface tension of the larger water droplet remains at 73 dyn/cm, but the surface tension of the smaller soap bubble is reduced by half as much. (36 dyn/cm). By a simple calculation, one can see that the pressures within both of the spheres are now equal.

Applications of Laplace's law can be found in the discussion of aerosol therapy in Chapter 4. As will be seen, surface tension explains why liquid particles retain their spherical shape when suspended in an aerosol suspension.

Density

Density (d) is the measure of a substance's mass per unit volume under specific conditions of pressure and temperature, or:

$$d = \text{mass/volume.}$$

For measurements taken near the surface of the earth, mass may be replaced by a substance's weight, so that **weight density** (d_w) equals weight divided by its volume, or:

$$d_w = \text{weight/volume.}$$

As one travels away from the surface of the earth, the force of gravity diminishes, and thus the relationship between mass and weight changes (i.e., as the force of gravity decreases, so does weight, even though mass stays the same).

For solids and liquids, density can be expressed in grams per liter (g/L) or in grams per cubic centimeter (g/cm^3). The density of gases is also expressed in grams per liter. Because of the influence of pressure and temperature on the density of gases, density is calculated under standard temperature and pressure conditions. The density of gases will be discussed in more detail with the discussion of Avogadro's law later in this chapter.

The Gas Laws

The gas laws presented in this section are important generalizations about the macroscopic behavior of gaseous substances. These laws can be seen as summaries of numerous experiments that were conducted over the course of several centuries. The importance of these laws in the development of physics and chemistry is undeniable, and their relevance to the practice of respiratory care cannot be overstated.

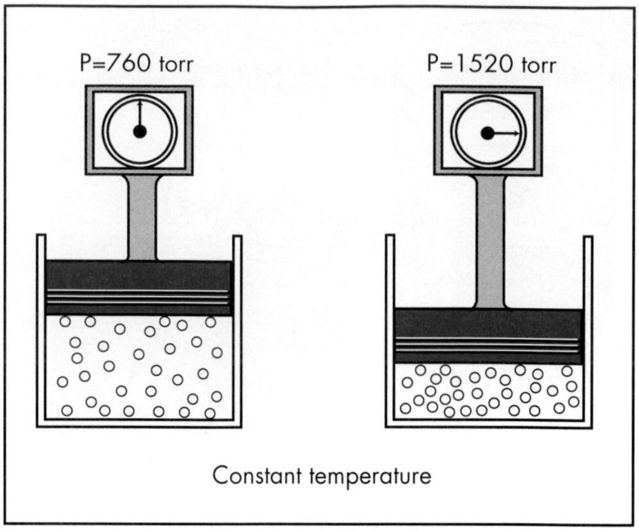

Figure 1-10 Boyle's law. (Redrawn from Levinsky MG, Cairo JM, and Hall SM: Introduction to respiratory care, Philadelphia, 1990, W.B. Saunders.)

Boyle's Law

Robert Boyle (1627-1691), a British chemist, was the first scientist to systematically investigate the pressure-volume relationships of a gas sample. Using an apparatus like the one shown in Figure 1-10, Boyle found that the volume that a gas occupies when it is maintained at a constant temperature is inversely proportional to the absolute pressure exerted on it, or:

$$V = 1/P, \text{ or } V = k(1/P).$$

Note that the absolute pressure of a gas equals the atmospheric pressure plus the pressure measured with a gauge. For example, the pressure of a gas compressed into a 10 L tank is measured to be 29.4 psi. The absolute pressure of the gas equals the atmospheric pressure (14.7 psi) plus the gauge pressure of 29.4 psi. Thus the absolute pressure of the gas is 44.1 psi.

Boyle's law can be expressed in a more useful form:

$$V_1P_1 = V_2P_2, \text{ or } V_1/V_2 = P_2/P_1,$$

which allows an unknown volume or pressure to be calculated when the other variables are known. For example, one can solve for an unknown volume by rearranging the equation to read:

$$V_2 = V_1P_1/P_2.$$

Applications of Boyle's law can be found in a number of topics included in this text, such as the mechanics of ventilation, medical gas therapy, blood-gas measurements, and pulmonary function testing, which includes spirometry and body plethysmography (see Chapter 7). Box 1-6 contains a problem-solving exercise involving Boyle's law.

BOX 1-6

Decision Making & Problem Solving

A snorkel diver is preparing to descend a freshwater pond to a depth of 66 ft. At sea level, his lungs contain about 3000 mL of air. As he descends below the surface of the water, what will happen to the gas volume in his lungs as he descends to 33 ft and then to 66 ft below the surface of the pond?

See Appendix A for the answer.

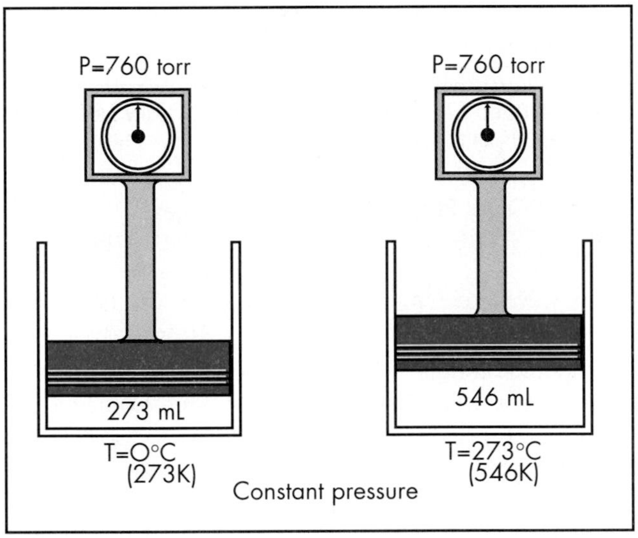

Figure 1-11 Charles's law. (Redrawn from Levinsky MG, Cairo JM, and Hall SM: Introduction to respiratory care, Philadelphia, 1990, W.B. Saunders.)

Charles's and Gay-Lussac's Laws

Jacques Charles (1746-1823), a French chemist, is recognized as the first scientist to demonstrate experimentally how the volume of a gas varies with changes in temperature. He showed that the volume of a given amount of gas held at a constant pressure increases proportionately with increases in the temperature of the gas[12] (Figure 1-11). The relationship between volume and temperature can be explained by the fact that as the temperature of the gas increases, the kinetic energy of the gas molecules increases. This increased kinetic energy content causes the gas molecules to move more vigorously, so the gas expands. Conversely, as the temperature of the gas decreases, its molecular activity diminishes, so the gas volume contracts.

William Thomson (Lord Kelvin, 1824-1907) realized the significance of these findings and suggested that there should theoretically be a temperature at which all molecular activity ceases and the associated gas volume is zero. This temperature is called *absolute zero* and has been calculated to be −273.15° C. Although the absolute zero of any substance has not been achieved in a laboratory setting, this temperature serves as a starting point for the Kelvin temperature scale. As mentioned earlier, 1° C corresponds to 1 K. Also, notice that temperature is expressed without degrees in the Kelvin scale (e.g., 0 K equals −273.15° C). Using the work of Kelvin, Charles's Law is now stated as: when the pressure of a gas is held constant, the volume of a gas varies directly with its absolute temperature expressed in Kelvins, or:

$$V/T = k, \text{ or } V_1/T_1 = V_2/T_2.$$

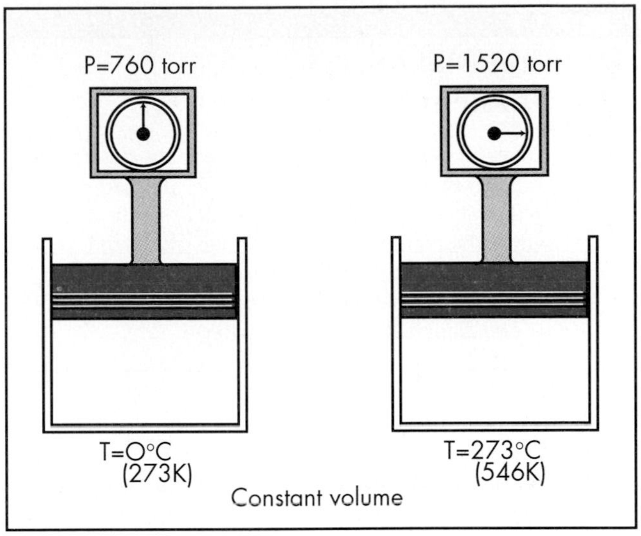

Figure 1-12 Gay-Lussac's law. (Redrawn from Levinsky MG, Cairo JM, and Hall SM: Introduction to respiratory care, Philadelphia, 1990, W.B. Saunders.)

Therefore, doubling the absolute temperature of a gas increases the volume of the gas two-fold. Conversely, reducing the temperature of a gas by half decreases the volume of the gas by half.

Joseph Gay-Lussac (1778-1850) extended Charles's work by showing that if the volume of a gas is held constant, the gas pressure rises as the absolute temperature of the gas increases, or:

$$P/T = k, \text{ or } P_1/T_1 = P_2/T_2.$$

Figure 1-12 illustrates Gay-Lussac's law. Box 1-7 contains an example of Gay-Lussac's law that might be encountered in clinical practice.

Combined Gas Law

In the discussions of the gas laws so far, it was assumed that one or more of the variables in each law were constant. For example, Boyle's law describes the relationship between pressure and volume when temperature is constant. Charles's law specifies the relationship between temperature and volume when pressure is constant; and Gay-Lussac's law describes the relationship between temperature and pressure while volume is constant.

BOX 1-7

Decision Making & Problem Solving

An alarm signals that there is a fire in the basement of the hospital. Although the fire is confined to an area that is approximately 300 ft from the room where the compressed-gas cylinders are stored, you are asked to move the cylinders to a safer location. Why is it necessary to move the cylinders?

See Appendix A for the answer.

The combined gas law describes the macroscopic behavior of gases when any or all of the variables change simultaneously. As such, the combined gas law states that the absolute pressure of a gas is inversely related to the volume it occupies and directly related to its absolute temperature, or:

$$PV/T = nR,$$

where *n* is the number of moles of gas (a mole is the atomic mass of the gas expressed in grams), and *R* is **Boltzmann's universal gas constant.**[7,8]

A more practical expression of the combined gas law equation that is used throughout this text is:

$$P_1V_1/T_1 = P_2V_2/T_2.$$

In this form of the combined gas law, the gas constant (R) and the mass (m) are not included because it is assumed that they will not be affected by changes in pressure, volume, and temperature. See Box 1-8 for an example of a calculation using this form of the combined gas law.

Applications of the combined gas law are found throughout this text. Pressure, volume, and temperature corrections are used extensively in arterial blood-gas measurements (see Chapter 8) and during pulmonary function testing (see Chapter 7).

Dalton's Law of Partial Pressures

Dalton's law states that the sum of the partial pressures of a gas mixture equals the total pressure of the system. Furthermore, the partial pressure of any gas within a gas mixture is proportional to its percentage of the mixture.[7,8] The partial pressure of a gas in a mixture can be calculated by multiplying the total pressure of the mixture by the percentage of the mixture that the gas in question occupies. For example, the partial pressure of oxygen in room air when the barometric pressure equals 1 atm (760 mm Hg) can be calculated by multiplying the total barometric pressure by the percentage of oxygen in the room air. (Note that oxygen makes up approximately 21% of the atmosphere, or 0.21.) Thus:

BOX 1-8

Decision Making & Problem Solving

What is the new volume of a 6 L gas sample existing at 273 K and 760 mm Hg when it is heated to 37° C (310 K) and subjected to 3 atm (2280 mm Hg) of pressure?

See Appendix A for the answer.

$$PO_2 = (760)\,(0.21)$$
$$PO_2 = 159.6 \text{ mm Hg}$$

Continuing with this example, the total atmospheric pressure equals the sum of the partial pressures for oxygen (21%), nitrogen (78%), carbon dioxide (0.03%), and other trace gases (~0.7%), or:

$$P_B = PO_2 + PN_2 + PCO_2 + P(\text{trace gases})$$
$$P_B = (760)\,(0.21) + (760)\,(0.78) + (760)\,(0.0003) + (760)\,(0.07)$$
$$P_B = 760 \text{ mm Hg}$$

It should be noted that water vapor pressure does not follow Dalton's law because such pressure primarily depends on temperature. Because water vapor displaces the partial pressure of other gases, the water vapor pressure (P_{H2O}) must be subtracted from the total pressure of the gas mixture when the partial pressure of a gas saturated with water vapor is calculated. For example, to calculate the partial pressure of oxygen in a sample of gas that is saturated with water vapor at 37° C, the following formula* is applied:

$$PO_2 = (P_B - P_{H20})\,(FIO_2)$$
$$PO_2 = (760 \text{ mm Hg} - 47 \text{ mm Hg})\,(0.21)$$
$$PO_2 = 149.73 \text{ mm Hg}$$

Avogadro's Law

This law states that equal volumes of gas at the same pressure and temperature contain the same number of molecules. It is based on the work of Amedeo Avogadro (1776-1856), who determined that 1 gram molecular weight (gmw), or mole, of any gas occupies 22.4 L at a temperature of 0° C (273 K) and a pressure of 1 atm. Subsequently, it was determined that 1 mole of gas at this volume contains 6.02×10^{23} molecules (**Avogadro's number**). For example, one mole of oxygen (mw = 32 g) occupies a volume of 22.4 L and contains 6.02×10^{23} molecules when measured at 0° C (273 K) and 1 atm.

*Note that the vapor pressure of water at 37°C is 47 mm Hg; Table 1-4 lists the vapor pressures for water at selected temperatures.

TABLE 1-4

Water-vapor pressure and content at selected temperatures and 760 mm Hg

°C	Vapor pressure (mm Hg)
0	4.58
10	9.21
11	9.84
12	10.52
13	11.23
14	11.99
15	12.79
16	13.63
17	14.53
18	15.48
19	16.48
20	17.54
21	18.65
22	19.83
23	21.07
24	22.38
25	23.76
26	25.21
27	26.74
28	28.35
29	30.04
30	31.82
31	33.70
32	35.66
33	37.73
34	39.90
35	42.18
36	44.56
37	47.07
38	49.70
39	52.44
40	55.32

A practical application of Avogadro's law is seen in the calculation of gas densities and specific gravity. The density of a gas per unit volume can be calculated with the following formula:

$$\text{Density (gm/L)} = \text{mw of gas}/22.4\text{ L}.$$

The specific gravity of a gas is defined as the ratio of the density of a gas relative to the density of a standard gas, such as air, oxygen, or hydrogen. Figure 1-13 shows the specific gravity of several gases used in respiratory care and anesthetics.

Laws of Diffusion

Up to this point, the discussion of gases has focused on the ability of a gas to expand and to be compressed. Another property that must be discussed in any analysis of gas behavior is **diffusion,** which can be defined as the net movement of gas molecules, by virtue of their kinetic properties, from an area of high concentration to an area of low concentration. Graham's law, Henry's law, and Fick's law will be used to describe diffusion and its applications in respiratory care.

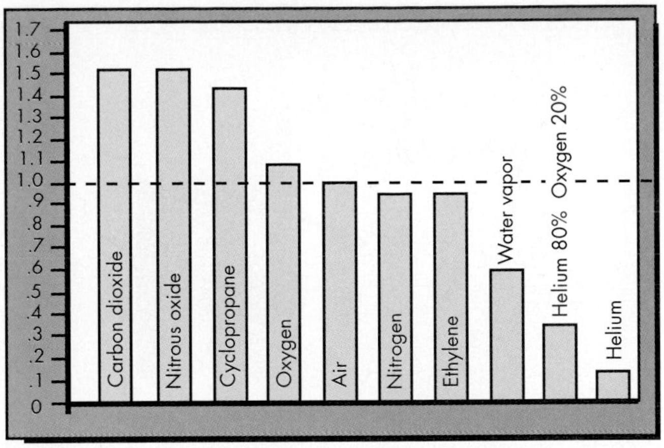

Figure 1-13 Specific gravity for several gases that are used in respiratory care and anesthetics. Comparisons have been made with air at 25° C and 1 atm. (Redrawn from Adriani J: The chemistry and physics of anesthesia, ed 3, Springfield, Ill., 1979, Charles C. Thomas.)

Graham's Law

In 1832, Thomas Graham (1805-1869) stated that when two gases are placed under the same temperature and pressure conditions, the rates of diffusion of the two gases are inversely proportional to the square root of their masses, or:

$$r_1/r_2 = \sqrt{M_1/M_2},$$

where r_1 and r_2 represent the diffusion rates of the respective gases, and M_1 and M_2 are the molar masses.

If the mass of a gas is considered directly proportional to its density at a constant temperature and pressure, then:

$$r_1/r_2 = \sqrt{d_1/d_2},$$

where d_1 and d_2 are the densities of the gases in question.

Henry's Law

When a gas is confined in a space adjacent to a liquid, a certain number of gas molecules dissolve in the liquid phase. Joseph Henry found that for a given temperature, the mass of a gas that dissolves (and does not combine chemically) in a specified volume of liquid is directly proportional to the product of the partial pressure of the gas and its solubility coefficient, or:

$$c \propto P \times S,$$

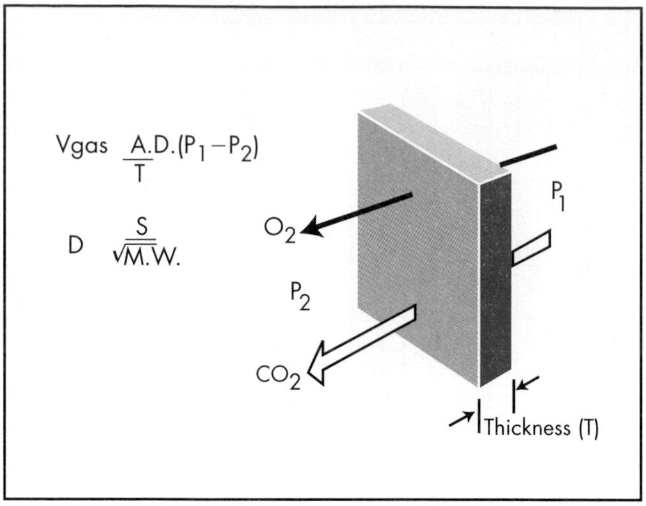

Figure 1-14 Fick's law of diffusion. (Modified from West JB: Respiratory physiology: the essentials, ed 3, Baltimore, 1985, Williams & Wilkins.)

where *c* is the molar concentration (in mol/L) of the dissolved gas, *P* is the pressure (in atm) of gas over the liquid, and *S* is the solubility coefficient (also known as Bunsen's coefficient) for the gas in that particular liquid (in L/atm or L/mm Hg). The solubility of a gas in a liquid is equal to the volume of gas (in liters) that will saturate 1 L of liquid at standard temperature and pressure (0° C and 1 atm). In respiratory care, Henry's law is encountered in discussions of the solubility of gases, such as oxygen, in blood. In the latter case, we express the solubility of a gas in milliliters of gas dissolved in milliliters of blood. For example, it is known that 0.023 mL of oxygen dissolve in every milliliter of blood at a temperature of 38° C and 1 atm of pressure.

Fick's Law of Diffusion

Thus far, the diffusion rate of a gas into another gas and the diffusion rate of a gas into a liquid have been discussed. In respiratory care, the diffusion of gases across semipermeable membranes (e.g., the diffusion of oxygen and carbon dioxide across the alveolar-capillary membrane) is also a concern.[12,13] A semipermeable membrane is not freely permeable to all components of a mixture. Thus the membrane may be impermeable to a substance because of its size or chemical composition (e.g., electrical charge).

Adolph Fick stated that the flow of a gas across a semipermeable membrane per unit time ($\dot{V}gas$) into a membrane fluid phase is directly proportional to the surface area (A) available for diffusion, the partial pressure gradient between the two compartments (ΔP), and the solubility of the gas (S). This flow is inversely proportional to the square root of the molecular weight of the gas ($\sqrt{MW}$) and the thickness of the membrane (T) (Figure 1-14). Fick's law can be shown as,

> **BOX 1-9**
> **Decision Making & Problem Solving**
>
> Using Fick's law of diffusion, describe several conditions during which the diffusion of oxygen across the alveolar-capillary membrane is reduced.
>
> See Appendix A for the answer.

$$\dot{V}gas = A \times S \times \Delta P/\sqrt{MW} \times T.$$

Considering that the diffusivity of a gas equals its solubility divided by the square root of its molecular weight, or

$$D = S \div \sqrt{MW},$$

where *D* is the diffusivity, *S* is the solubility, and *MW* is the molecular weight, then Fick's law can be restated as:

$$\dot{V}gas = A \times D \times \Delta P/T.$$

Test your understanding of the laws of diffusion by answering the question in Box 1-9.

Fluid Mechanics

Fluid mechanics is the branch of physics dealing with the properties and behavior of fluids in motion. This field mostly involves fluid dynamics, which is subdivided into hydrodynamics (the study of liquids in motion) and aerodynamics (the study of gases in motion). With diffusion, gas movement was described as being the result of the spontaneous intermingling of the individual gas molecules as a result of random thermal motion. In the section that follows, bulk gas flow, which deals with the transport of whole groups of molecules (i.e., a volume of gas) from one location to another rather than the movement of individual gas molecules, will be discussed.

Patterns of Flow

This text is primarily concerned with the flow of fluids through various types of tubes. Whether this flow involves the movement of liquids or gases, all fluid flow may be characterized as being laminar, turbulent, or transitional in nature. Figure 1-15 shows the three types of flow.

In laminar flow, the fluid flows in discrete cylindrical layers or streamlines.[8] Laminar flow is normally associated with the movement of fluids through tubes with smooth surfaces and fixed radii. With laminar flow, the pressure required to produce a given flow is directly related to the viscosity of the fluid and the length of the tube and inversely

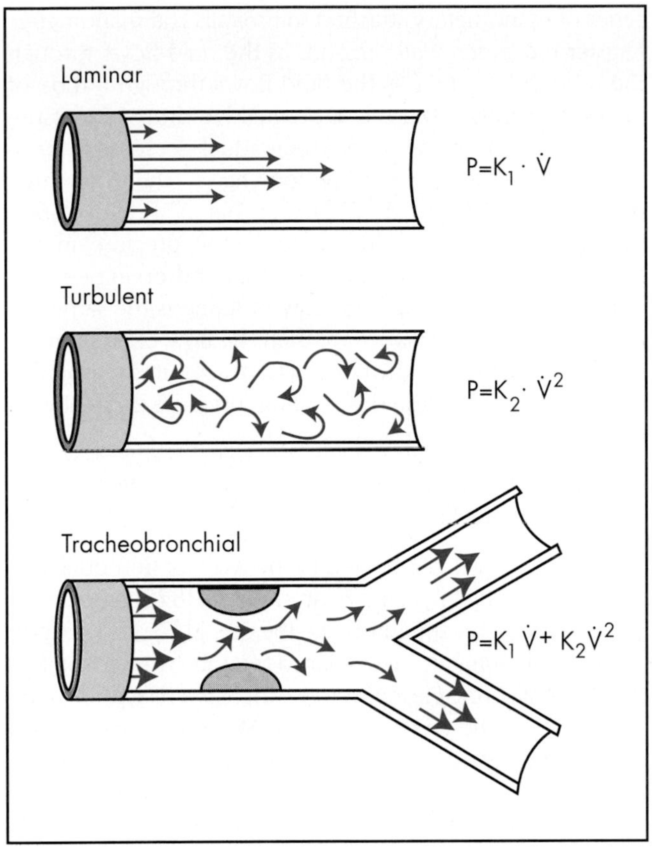

Figure 1-15 Three patterns of flow: laminar, turbulent, and transitional.

related to the radius of the tube. These relationships will be discussed in detail in the section on Poiseuille's law.

With turbulent flow, the movement of fluid molecules becomes chaotic and the orderly pattern of concentric layers seen with laminar flow is lost. As will be seen, Poiseuille's law cannot be used to predict the amount of pressure required for a given flow when turbulence is present. When turbulence is present, the pressure required to produce a given flow is influenced less by the viscosity of the fluid and more by its density. Additionally, the driving pressure required to achieve a given flow is proportional to the *square* of the flow. Turbulent flow occurs when there is a sharp increase in the velocity at which the fluid is moving, when the tube's radius varies, and when tubes have rough, uneven surfaces. The likelihood of developing turbulent flow can be predicted by Reynolds's number, which will be discussed shortly.

Transitional flow is simply a mixture of laminar and turbulent flows. In cases when laminar flow predominates, the driving pressure varies linearly with the flow. When turbulent flow dominates, the driving pressure varies with the *square* of the flow. As one might expect, the driving pressure is affected more by changes in the density of the fluid rather than its viscosity when turbulent flow exists. Transitional flow typically occurs at points where tubes divide into one or more branches. Figure 1-15 illustrates the types of flow that can be observed as gas flows into the lungs. Gas flow in the larger airways is turbulent, but laminar flow predominates in the smaller airways. Transitional flow (or tracheobronchial flow, as it appears in Figure 1-15) occurs at points where the airways divide (e.g., where the mainstem bronchi divide into the lobar bronchi).

Poiseuille's Law

When considering the flow of a liquid or gas through a tube, there are two factors that must be considered: the driving pressure forcing the fluid through the tube (i.e., the pressure gradient) and the resistance that the fluid must overcome as it flows through the tube. Jean L.M. Poiseuille (1797-1869), a French physiologist, described the interrelationships between pressure, flow, and resistance for a liquid flowing through an unbranched rigid tube with the formula:

$$\Delta P = \dot{Q} \times R,$$

where ΔP is the pressure gradient from the beginning to the end of the tube ($P_1 - P_2$), $\dot{Q}$ is the flow of the liquid through the tube, and *R* is the resistance opposing the flow of the liquid. (Note that in discussions of the mechanics of breathing, $\dot{Q}$ is replaced with $\dot{V}$, which is used to symbolize the flow of a gas.) The pressure gradient can be described as the difference in pressure at the entrance of the tube and the exit point, or $P_1 - P_2$. Poiseuille found that the factors determining resistance to flow include the viscosity of the fluid, as well as the length and radius of the tube, or

$$R = (8\eta l)/(\pi r^4),$$

where η is the viscosity of the liquid, *l* is the length of the tube, and *r* is the radius of the tube. Incorporating these findings, Poiseuille's law can be rewritten as,

$$\Delta P = \dot{Q} \times [(8\eta l)/(\pi r^4)].$$

Based on these equations, the following can be stated:

1. The more viscous a fluid, the greater the pressure gradient required to cause it to move through a given tube.
2. The resistance offered by a tube is directly proportional to its length; the pressure required to achieve a given flow through a tube must increase in direct proportion to the length of the tube.
3. Because the resistance to flow is inversely proportional to the fourth power of the radius, small changes in the radius of a tube will cause profound decreases in the flow of the fluid through the tube.

For example, decreasing the radius by one half increases the resistance sixteenfold.

Applications of Poiseuille's law are found in the discussion related to medical gas therapy, physiological pressure monitoring, and mechanical ventilation.

Reynold's Number

As discussed earlier, fluid flow becomes turbulent when there is a sharp increase in the velocity at which the liquid or gas molecules are traveling. Several other factors can also produce turbulent flow, including changes in the density and viscosity of the gas or in the diameter of the tube. These factors can be combined mathematically to determine Reynolds's number:

$$N_R = v \times d \times (2r/\eta),$$

where v is the velocity of flow, r is the radius of the tube, and d and η are the density and viscosity of the gas, respectively. Note that the Reynolds's number does not have units. Turbulent flow predominates when the Reynolds's number exceeds 2000, although turbulent flow may occur at lower Reynolds's numbers when the surface of the tube is rough or irregular.[8,14]

Turbulent flow is produced by an increase in the linear velocity of the gas, the density of the gas, or the radius of the tube; it can also be produced by reductions in the viscosity of the gas. Applications of Reynolds's number will be seen in the discussions of the mechanics of breathing and mechanical ventilation later in this text.

Bernoulli Principle

This principle is the result of work by Daniel Bernoulli (1700-1782), a Swiss mathematician who stated that as the forward velocity of a gas increases, its lateral pressure decreases and its forward pressure increases.[7,15] This can be demonstrated with an apparatus like that in Figure 1-16, which consists of a fluid flowing through a tube that has a series of manometers attached to its wall. The manometers register the lateral wall pressure as the fluid flows through the tube. Notice that as the fluid flows through a tube of uniform diameter, there is a progressive drop in pressure over the length of the tube. The gradual decrease in pressure can be determined by looking at the first three manometers in Figure 1-16. Notice that as the fluid flows through a constriction in the tube, the pressure in the fourth manometer shows an even greater drop in pressure. If it is assumed that the total flow of liquid is the same before and after the constriction, then the flow of liquid must accelerate as it enters the constriction. Thus it is reasonable to assume then that the drop in fluid pressure is directly related to the increase in fluid speed.

Venturi Principle

This principle, which is related to the work of Bernoulli, was first described by Giovanni Venturi (1746-1822) and can be illustrated with an apparatus like the one in Figure 1-17. Notice that this apparatus is similar to the tube used to explain the Bernoulli principle, except that there is a dilatation in the tube distal to the constriction. The Venturi principle states that the pressure drop that occurs distal to a constriction in a tube can be restored to the preconstriction pressure if there is a dilatation in the tube distal to the constriction with an angle of divergence not exceeding 15 degrees.[8]

Venturi tubes are used in many devices in respiratory care. Air entrainment masks, aerosol generators, and humidifiers are the most common examples. With these devices, a lateral port located just distal to the constriction is used to entrain the second gas into the main gas flow. The increased gas flow is accommodated by a dilatation located downstream of the constriction. Other applications of the Venturi principle are described throughout this text.

Coanda Effect

The Coanda effect, which is also based on the Bernoulli principle, is illustrated in Figure 1-18. As was already ex-

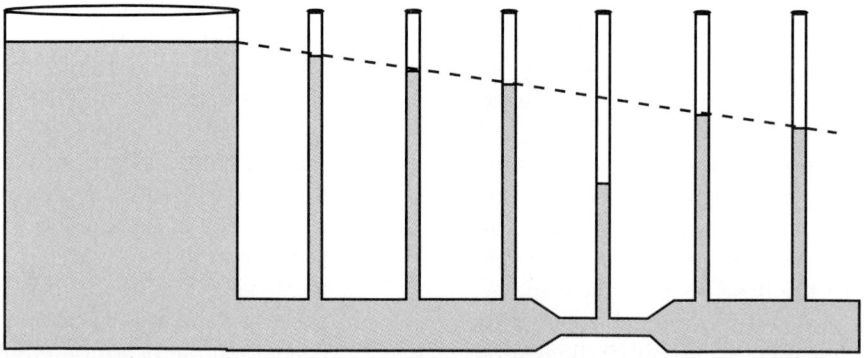

Figure 1-16 The Bernoulli Principle. (Redrawn from Nave CR and Nave BC: Physics for the health sciences, ed 3, Philadelphia, 1985, Saunders.

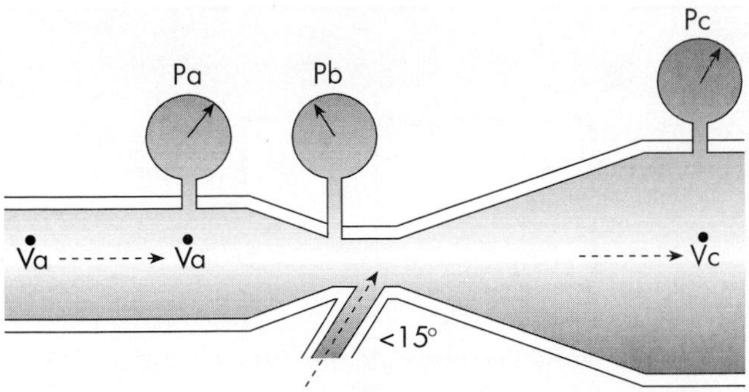

Figure 1-17 The Venturi Principle. See text for discussion. (From Scanlan CL, Wilkins BL, and Stoller JK: Egan's fundamentals of respiratory care, ed 7, St Louis, 1998, Mosby.)

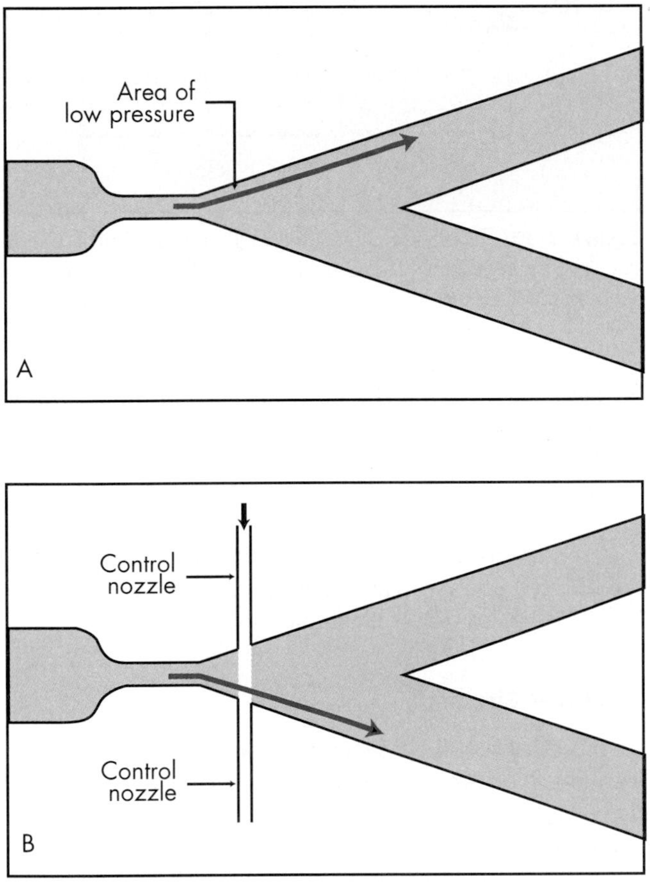

Figure 1-18 The Coanda effect.

plained, the lateral wall pressure of the tube decreases when the fluid flows through a narrowing of the tube. The reduction in lateral wall pressure results from an increase in the forward velocity of the fluid flow. If the wall does not have a side port for entraining another fluid, the low pressure adjacent to the wall draws the stream of fluid against the wall. When a specially contoured tube, such as the one in Figure 1-18, is attached distal to the narrow part of the tube, the flow exiting the narrow part of the tube tends to adhere to the wall of the contoured tube because of two factors: a negative pressure is generated past the constriction, thus drawing the fluid toward the curved extension; and the ambient pressure opposite the extension pushes the fluid stream against the wall, where it remains locked until interrupted by a counter-force, such as a pulse of air.[8] Using these findings, Coanda was able to demonstrate that with careful placement of the postconstriction extensions, he could deflect a stream of air through a full 180-degree turn by extending the wall contour.[10]

The Coanda effect is the basis for **fluidic** devices that are used in several mechanical ventilators (see Chapter 10). Such devices use gates that are regulated by gas flow from side jets, which operate on the principle that pulses of air are used to redirect the original gas stream. The main advantage of using these fluid logic devices is that they have fewer valves and moving parts that can break (i.e., gas flow is regulated by gas jets, not typical mechanical metal or plastic valves). The primary disadvantage is that these devices consume more gas than more conventional devices because gas flow is used to power the various fluid logic gates. Chapter 9 includes an extensive discussion of fluidic elements used in mechanical ventilators.

Principles of Electricity

Many respiratory care devices are powered by electricity and, in many cases, are also controlled by computers that use solid-state electronic circuitry. Mechanical ventilators, blood-gas analyzers, physiologic transducers and monitors, cathode ray tube displays, strip chart and X-Y recorders are some examples.[8] Because of the importance of these devices in respiratory care, it is essential to have a basic understanding of electronics and electrical safety.

Principles of Electronics

Electricity is produced by the flow of electrons through a conductive path or circuit. This flow, electric current, is influenced by: (1) the force pushing the electrons through a conductive path (i.e., electromotive force or voltage), and (2) the resistance that the electrons must overcome as they flow through the conductive path.

Electric current, which is symbolized as *I,* can be measured with an **ammeter.** The standard unit of measurement of electric current is the **ampere** (A), where 1 A is equivalent to 6.25×10^{18} electrons passing a point in 1 second. (Note that in electronics, the term *coulomb* is used as a shorthand notation for 6.25×10^{18} electrons. Thus 1 A equals 1 coulomb per second). Amperes can be subdivided into smaller quantities, such as milliamperes (μA, or milliamp) and microamperes (μA or microamp), using scientific notation. For example, 1 mA is 1/1000 of an ampere, and 1 μA is 1/1,000,000 of an ampere. Ammeters typically have scales calibrated in amperes, milliamperes, and microamperes.

As already stated, voltage is the electrical force (more correctly termed **electromotive force,** or emf) that drives electrons through the conductive path. In most physics textbooks, voltage is also described as the potential difference between two points. Voltage sources include batteries, hydroelectric generators, solar cells, and piezoelectric crystals.

Voltage is measured using a **voltmeter;** and the standard unit of measurement for voltage is the **volt** (V), which can be defined as the electrical potential required for 1 A of electricity to move through 1 ohm (Ω) of resistance. Like amperes, volts can be subdivided into smaller units, such as millivolts (mV) and microvolts (μV).

Resistance in electric circuits, like resistance in fluid circuits, is the opposition to flow. Resistance, which is measured in **ohms,** is a property of conductors that is influenced by its chemical composition or specific resistance (ρ), as well as by its length and cross-sectional area. Most metals and salt solutions are good conductors (i.e., they offer low resistance to current flow). Rubber, plastic, and glass are poor conductors because they offer high resistance to current flow. Because these materials are such poor conductors, they can be used as protective coverings on conductive wires. As such, these latter materials are often called **insulators.** With regard to physical dimensions, the resistance of a conductor increases as its length increases or its cross-sectional area decreases.

Resistance is not limited to conductors alone. Electronic components called **resistors** are manufactured to have specific amounts of resistance. Resistors serve to limit current and to develop voltages that are less than the source voltage.

Ohm's Law

The relationships between current, voltage, and resistance can be explained with **Ohm's law:**

$$V = I \times R.$$

According to Ohm's law, voltage and current are directly related, which simply means that if the resistance is constant, increases in voltage cause increases in current flow. Conversely, decreases in source voltage cause a reduction in current flow (assuming resistance is constant). Now consider how changes in resistance affect current flow. If voltage is held constant, increases in resistance will cause a decrease in current flow, whereas decreases in resistance will cause an increase in current flow. Thus current and resistance are inversely related.

It should be apparent from this discussion that any one variable can be solved for if the other two are known. Thus, by rearranging the above equation, the current can be solved for:

$$I = V/R.$$

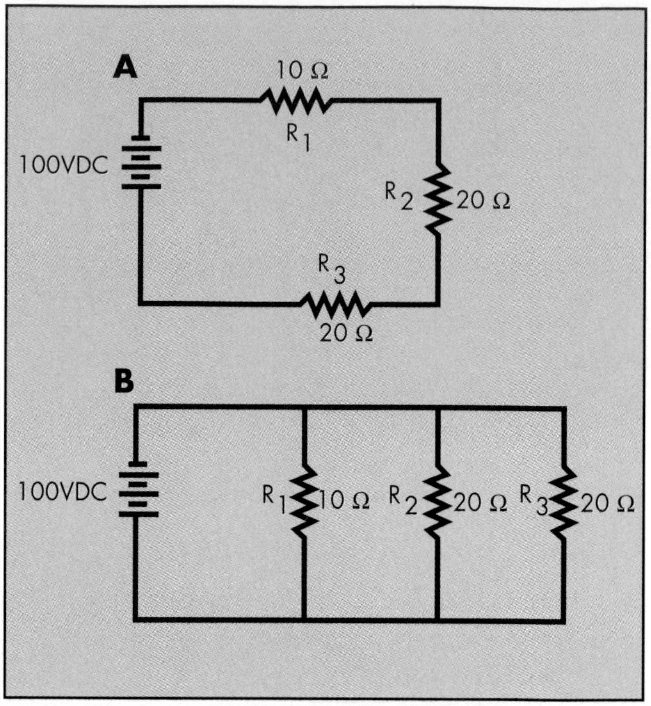

Figure 1-19 Schematic illustrating two types of electric circuits: *A,* direct current (DC) series circuit; *B,* direct current (DC) parallel circuit.

Similarly, resistance can be solved for with the following rearrangement:

$$R = V/I.$$

It is important to grasp these concepts in order to understand circuit analysis. These principles will now be applied in an analysis of simple electric circuits.

Electrical Circuits

An electrical circuit consists of a voltage source, a load, and a conductive path. An applied voltage causes a current to flow through a conductive path containing one or more loads before returning to the voltage source.

Figure 1-19 shows two types of electric circuits: series circuits and parallel circuits. Notice that in a series circuit, the current flows through one path. The current flows from the voltage source through the conductor and through a series of resistive loads, which are arranged end-to-end (i.e., through R1 then R2), and then back to the voltage source. This is contrasted by the parallel circuit, which may be depicted as two or more series circuits connected to a common voltage source.

There are several principles to remember when analyzing series and parallel circuits. These principles, which are referred to as Kirchhoff's laws, provide the framework for performing circuit analysis.

BOX 1-10

Electrical Circuit Analysis

Series Circuits

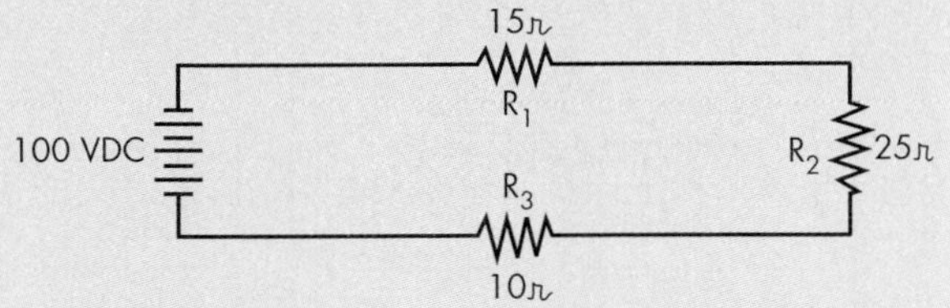

What is the total electrical resistance of this circuit?

$R_T = R_1 + R_2 + R_3$

$R_T = 1/(1/10\Omega) + 1/(1/20\Omega)$

$R_T = 50\Omega$

What is the total current through the circuit?

$I_T = V_T/R_T$

$I_T = 100\ V/50\Omega$

$I_T = 2\ A$

Parallel Circuits

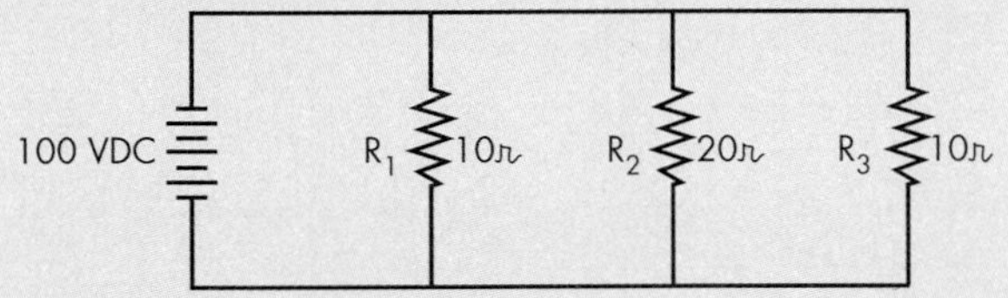

What is the total electrical resistance of this circuit?

$R_T = 1/1/R_1 + 1/R_2 + 1/R_3$

$R_T = 1\ /(1/10\Omega) + 1/(1/20\Omega) + 1/(1/10\Omega)$

$R_T = 4\Omega$

What is the current flow through each branch of the circuit?

$I_1 = 100\ V/10\Omega$

$I_1 = 10\ A$

$I_2 = 100\ V/20\Omega$

$I_2 = 5\ A$

$I_3 = 100\ V/10\Omega$

$I_3 = 10\ A$

What is the total current flow through the circuit?

$I_T = I_1 + I_2 + I_3$

$I_T = 25\ A$

The total current flow can also be calculated in the following manner:

$I_T = V_T/R_T$

$I_T = 100\ V/4\Omega$

$I_T = 25\ A$

Kirchhoff's laws governing series circuits may be summarized as follows:

1. A series circuit can have one or more voltage sources. The total source voltage equals the sum of the individual sources if their direction of polarity is the same.
2. In a series circuit, current is the same through all components.
3. The total resistance in a series circuit can be computed by finding the sum of all resistance in the circuit. That is, $R_T = R_1 + R_2 + R_3$...
4. The sum of voltage drops across resistance in the circuit equals the applied voltage, or $V_T = IR_1 + IR_2 + IR_3$...

Parallel circuits must adhere to the following guidelines:

1. All branches of parallel circuit have the same applied voltage.
2. Each branch of a parallel circuit may have a different current flow, depending on the resistance of the branch.
3. The total current flowing through a parallel circuit can be computed by finding the sum of the currents flowing through the various branches of the circuit. Thus, $I_T = I_1 + I_2 + I_3$...
4. The total resistance in a parallel circuit can be computed by finding the sum of the reciprocals for each resistance. That is, $R_T = 1/(1/R_1 + 1/R_2 + 1/R_3...)$.

Box 1-10 provides several examples of simple circuit analysis.

Electrical Safety

Electrical accidents occur when current from an electrical device interacts with body tissue, impairing physiologic function. It is important to recognize that electrical hazards only exist when the current path through the body is complete. That is, two connections to the body are required for an electrical shock to occur.[8,16] One connection (the "hot" wire) brings the current to the body while the second connection (the neutral wire) completes the circuit by sending the charge to a point of lower potential or ground (Figure 1-20).

The extent of impairment depends on the amount of current flowing through the body, the duration that the current is applied, and the path that the current takes through the body.[8] Figure 1-21 shows the approximate current ranges and the physiological effects of a 1-second exposure to various levels of 110 V, 60 Hz alternating currents applied externally to the body.[16]

Two types of electric shock hazards are usually described: **macroshock** and **microshock.** A macroshock occurs when a relatively high current is applied to the body surface. Generally, a current of 1 mA is required to elicit a macroshock. A microshock occurs when a low current

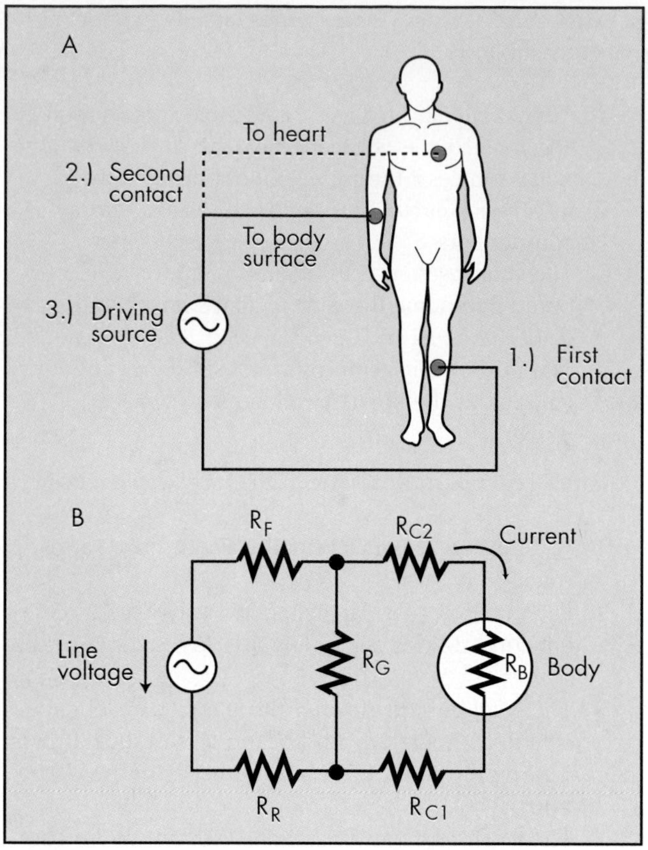

Figure 1-20 Schematic illustrating the necessary conditions for an electrical accident. (Redrawn from Cromwell L, Weibell FJ, and Pfeiffer EA: Biomedical instrumentation and measurements, ed 2, Englewood Cliffs, NJ, 1980, Prentice-Hall.)

(usually less than 1 mA) is allowed to bypass the body surface and flow directly into the body.

Electric current can damage body tissues by causing thermal burns and inadvertently stimulating excitable tissue, such as cardiac muscle. Burns are caused when electric energy dissipates in body tissues, causing the temperature of the tissues to rise. If the temperature gets high enough, it can cause burns. Inadvertent stimulation of excitable tissue can occur when an extraneous electric current of sufficient magnitude causes local voltages that can trigger action potentials. Action potentials triggered in sensory nerves cause a tingling sensation that is associated with electric shock. Action potentials generated in motor nerves and muscles result in muscle contractions, which—if the intensity of the stimulation is high enough—can cause tetanus or sustained contraction of the muscle.

It should be noted that the heart is the organ most susceptible to electrical hazards. Its susceptibility to electrical hazards arises from the fact that when current exceeds a certain value, extra systolic contractions can occur in cardiac muscle. Further increases in current can cause the heart to fibrillate and can ultimately cause sustained myocardial contraction.

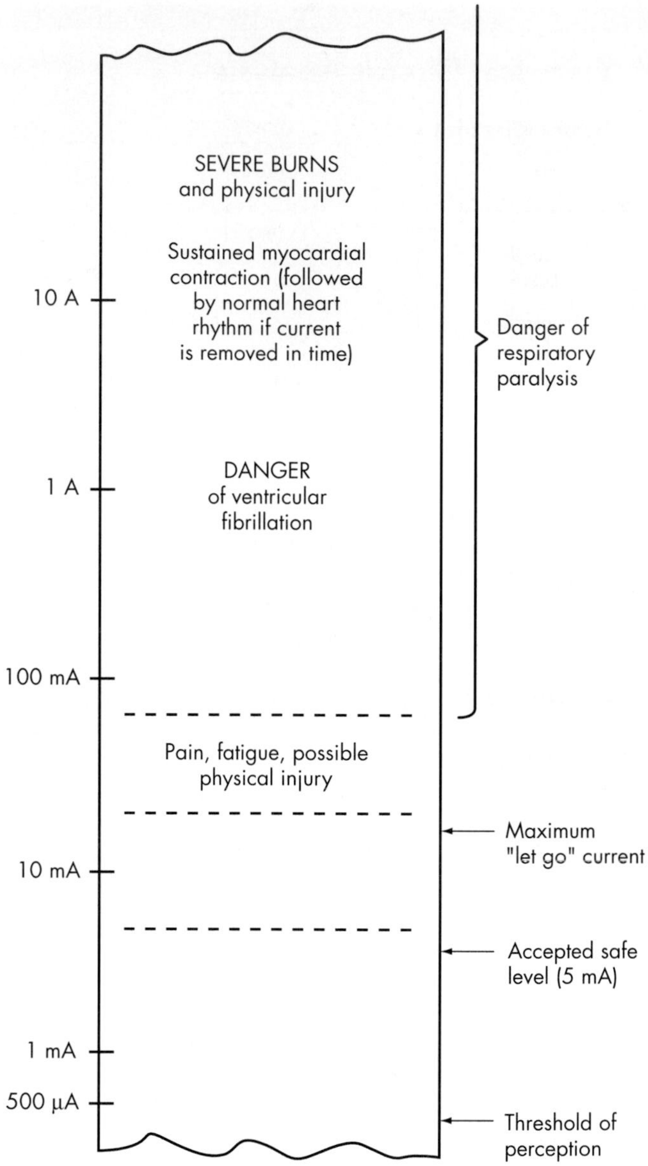

Figure 1-21 Physiological effects of electrical current associated with a 1-second external contact with a 110 VAC current at 60 Hz. (Redrawn from Cromwell L, Weibell FJ, and Pfeiffer EA: Biomedical instrumentation and measurements, ed 2, Englewood Cliffs, NJ, 1980, Prentice-Hall.)

Preventing Electrical Hazards

Various strategies should be employed to reduce the likelihood of electrical accidents. These include ensuring the proper grounding of medical equipment, installing ground-fault circuit interrupters, and avoiding contact with transcutaneous conductors.[16]

Grounding

The principle of this protection method for medical equipment is to provide a low-resistance conductive path that allows the majority of fault current to bypass the patient and re-

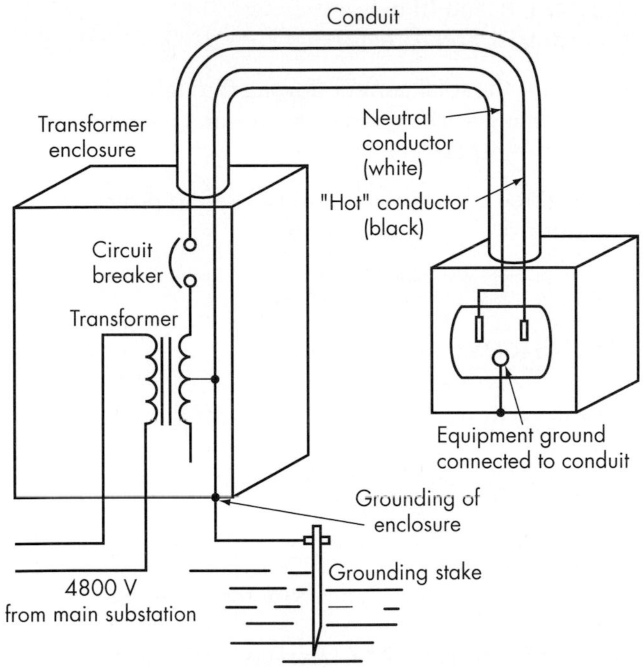

Figure 1-22 Electrical grounding of hospital outlets. (From Comwell, Wabel, and Pfeiffer: Biomedical instrumentation and measurements, ed 2, Englewood Cliffs, NJ, 1980, Prentice-Hall.)

turn to ground. In cord-connected electrical equipment, this ground connection is established by a third round or U-shaped contact in the plug, like the one shown in Figure 1-22.

It is important to recognize that grounding is only effective if a good ground connection exists. Worn or broken wires, inadvertent disconnection of ground wires from receptacles, as well as deliberate removal of ground contacts from plugs interfere with the protection associated with grounding. Because conventional receptacles, line cords, and plugs do not hold up to hospital use, most manufacturers provide hospital-grade receptacles and plugs that must meet Underwriters' laboratory specifications. Hospital-grade receptacles and plugs can usually be identified by a green dot.[16]

Ground-fault Circuit Interrupters

Normally, all of the power entering a device through the hot wire returns through the neutral wire. Circuit interrupters monitor the difference between the hot and neutral wires of the power line with a differential transformer and an electrical amplifier. When this difference exceeds a predetermined level (e.g., 5 mA), as occurs when the current bypasses the neutral wire and flows through the patient, the power is interrupted by a circuit breaker. Notice that this interruption occurs rapidly so that the patient does not encounter any harmful effects.

Avoiding Contact with Transcutaneous Conductors

The resistance offered by the skin represents the greatest part of the body's electrical resistance.[16] This resistance can be significantly reduced by permeating the skin with conductive fluid, by cuts and abrasions to the epithelium, or by the introduction of needles through the skin surface. Electrically conductive catheters inserted through a vein or artery can also bypass the natural electrical resistance offered by the skin.

It should be apparent from the discussion so far that these conditions can place patients in compromised states and make them susceptible to microshock hazards. These hazardous effects can be lessened if all electrical devices being used with a microshock-sensitive patient are well-insulated and connected to outlets with a common low-resistance ground.[8] Additionally, devices should be inspected regularly for frayed or bare wires.

Summary

Physics provides a basic framework for any discussion of respiratory care equipment. Under ordinary conditions, all matter behaves according to a group of physical laws, such as the gas laws and the laws of fluid dynamics. Medical application of these laws can be found in a variety of devices, including compressed-gas cylinders, oxygen therapy apparatuses, aerosol generators and humidifiers, mechanical ventilators, as well as spirometers and medical gas analyzers.

In the following chapters, the operational theories for various devices used in respiratory care will be described. A working knowledge of topics such as matter and energy, temperature and pressure measurements, the gas laws, fluid mechanics, and electricity is necessary to fully appreciate how various respiratory care devices operate.

Review Questions

See Appendix A for answers.

1. Convert the following temperature:
   - a. 37° C = _____ ° F
   - b. _____ ° C = 54° F
   - c. _____K = 98.6° F
   - d. 25° C = _____K
2. Perform the following pressure conversions:
   - a. _____kPa = 30 cm H_2O
   - b. 760 mm Hg = _____cm H_2O
   - c. _____cm H_2O = 25 mm Hg
   - d. 303.9 kPa = _____atm

3. Calculate the partial pressures of each of the following gases in room air when the barometric pressure is 750 mm Hg. (Assume that room air contains 21% oxygen, 78% nitrogen, and 0.03% carbon dioxide.):
   a. PO_2 = _____mm Hg
   b. PN_2 = _____mm Hg
   c. PCO_2 = _____mm Hg
4. What is the total pressure of a gas mixture if PO_2 = 90 mm Hg, PCO_2 = 40 mm Hg, PN_2 = 573 mm Hg, and P_{H2O} = 47 mm Hg?
   a. 573 mm Hg
   b. 713 mm Hg
   c. 750 mm Hg
   d. 760 mm Hg
5. A compressed-gas cylinder at 760 mm Hg and 25° C is moved into a room where the temperature is 38° C. What is the new pressure of the cylinder, assuming that the volume of gas within the cylinder remains constant?
6. A patient's lung capacity is measured to be 5 L at an initial temperature of 25° C and an ambient pressure of 760 mm Hg. What will be the new volume if the temperature increases to 37° C and the pressure to 1520 mm Hg?
7. Calculate the densities of oxygen and carbon dioxide. The molecular weight of oxygen is 32 gmw, and the molecular weight of carbon dioxide is 44 gmw.
8. According to Poiseuille's law, the gas flow through a tube is inversely proportional to the:
   I. Length of the tube
   II. Driving pressure of the gas through the tube
   III. Viscosity of the gas
   IV. Radius of the tube
      a. IV only
      b. I and III only
      c. I, II, and III only
      d. II, IV, and V only
9. Which of the following will increase the likelihood of generating turbulent airflow?
   a. increasing the linear velocity of gas flow
   b. decreasing the density of the gas
   c. decreasing the radius of the tube
   d. increasing the viscosity of the gas
10. Which of the following variables will lead to an increase in turbulent airflow?
    I. Increased density of the gas
    II. Decreased linear velocity of the gas flow
    III. Increased diameter of the conducting tube
    IV. Decreased viscosity of the gas
       a. I only
       b. II and II only
       c. I, II, and III only
       d. I, III, and IV only
11. What is the total current flowing through a DC circuit containing a 100 V power source and a total resistance of 50 Ω?
12. List three strategies that can be used to protect patients from electrical hazards.

References

1. Feynman R: Six easy pieces, Reading, Mass., 1995, Addison-Wesley.
2. Krauskoff KB and Beiser A: The physical universe, ed 7, New York, 1993, McGraw-Hill.
3. Asimov I: Understanding physics, New York, 1993, Barnes and Noble.
4. Kuhn KF: Basic physics, ed 2, New York, 1996, John Wiley & Sons.
5. Chang R: Chemistry, ed 3, New York, 1987, Random House.
6. Weast RC, editor: Handbook of chemistry and physics, ed 69, Cleveland, 1988, Chemical Rubber Co.
7. Nave CR and Nave BC: Physics for the health sciences, ed 3, Philadelphia, 1985, Saunders.
8. Scanlan CL: Physical principles in respiratory care. In Scanlan CL, Spearman CB, and Sheldon RL, editors: Egan's fundamentals of respiratory care, ed 6, St Louis, 1995, Mosby.
9. Wojciechowski WV: Respiratory care sciences, an integrated approach, ed 2, Albany, 1995, Delmar.
10. Davis PD, Parbrook GD, and Kenny, GNC: Basic physics and measurement in anaesthesia, ed 4, Oxford, 1995, Butterworth-Heinemann.
11. Adriani J: The chemistry and physics of anesthesia, ed 3, Springfield, Ill., 1979, Charles C. Thomas.
12. West JB: Respiratory physiology: the essentials, ed 3, Baltimore, 1985, Williams & Wilkins.
13. Guyton AC: Textbook of medical physiology, ed 9, Philadelphia, 1996, Saunders.
14. Cromwell L, Weibell FJ, and Pfeiffer EA: Biomedical instrumentation and measurements, ed 2, Englewood Cliffs, NJ, 1980, Prentice-Hall.
15. Levitzky MG, Cairo JM, Hall SM: Introduction to respiratory care, Philadelphia, 1990, Saunders.
16. Kacmarek RM, Mack CM, and Dimas S: The essentials of respiratory care, ed 3, St Louis, 1995, Mosby.

Internet Resources

1. The World Lecture Hall—Physics: http://www.utexas.edu/world/lecture/phy/
2. How Things Work—Louis A. Bloomfield: http://howthingswork.virginia.edu
3. Interactive Textbook of PHP 96: http://www.physics.upenn.edu/courses/gladney/mathphys/Contents.html

4. Physics Reference Guide:
   http://www.physlink.com
5. Physical Constants:
   http://physics.hallym.ac.kr:80/reference/reference.html
6. WWW Virtual Library: Biosciences—Medicine:
   http://www.ohsu.edu/cliniweb/wwwvl/all.html
7. College Physics for Students of Biology and Chemistry:
   http://www.rwc.uc.edu/koehler/biophys/text.html
8. University of Winnipeg Introductory Physics Notes:
   http://theory.uwinnipeg.ca/physics/
9. The Internet Public Library:
   http://www.ipl.org

CHAPTER 2

CHAPTER OUTLINE

Properties of Medical Gases
- Air
- Oxygen
- Carbon Dioxide
- Helium
- Nitric Oxide
- Nitrous Oxide

Storage and Transport of Medical Gases
- Cylinders
- Liquid Oxygen Systems
- Medical Air Supply
- Central Supply Systems
- Piping Systems
- Station Outlets
- Oxygen Concentrators

KEY TERMS

Alternating-Supply Systems
American Standards Association (ASA) indexing
Check Valves
Continuous-Supply Systems
Cryogenic
Cylinder Volume-Pressure Constants
Diameter Index Safety System (DISS)
Diaphragm Compressors
Diaphragm Valves
Direct-Acting Valves
Frangible (Rupture) Disks
Fusible Plugs
Fractional Distillation
Isolation Valve
Joule-Kelvin (Joule-Thompson) Effect
Liquefaction
Molecular Sieves
Oxygen Concentrators
Physical Separation
Pin Index Safety System (PISS)
Piston Compressors
Quick-Connect Adapters
Rotary Compressors
Semipermeable Membranes
Spring-Loaded Devices
Thorpe-Tube Flowmeter
Volume-Pressure Constant
Wood's Metal

Manufacture, Storage, and Transport of Medical Gases

J.M. Cairo

CHAPTER LEARNING OBJECTIVES

Upon completion of this chapter, the reader should be able to:

1. Describe the chemical and physical properties of the medical gases most often encountered in respiratory care.
2. Identify various types of medical gas cylinders (e.g., Types 3, 3A, 3AA, and 3AL).
3. Identify the following cylinder markings: Department of Transportation (DOT) specifications, service pressure, hydrostatic testing dates, manufacturer's identification, ownership mark, serial number, and cylinder size.
4. List the color codes used to identify medical gas cylinders.
5. Discuss United States Pharmacopia (USP) purity standards for medical gases.
6. Compare the operation of direct-acting cylinder valves with diaphragm type of cylinder valves.
7. Explain the American Standards Association (ASA) indexing, the Pin Index Safety System (PISS), and the Diameter Index Safety System (DISS).
8. Identify and correct a problem with cylinder valve assembly.
9. Calculate the gas volume remaining in a compressed-gas cylinder and estimate the duration of gas flow based on the cylinder's gauge pressure.
10. Describe the components of a bulk liquid oxygen system and discuss National Fire Protection Agency (NFPA) recommendations for the storage and use of liquid oxygen in bulk systems.
11. Discuss the operation of a portable liquid oxygen system and describe NFPA recommendations for these systems.
12. Calculate the duration of a portable liquid oxygen supply.
13. Identify three types of medical air compressors and describe the operational theory of each.
14. Summarize NFPA recommendations for medical air supply safety.
15. Compare continuous- and alternating-central–supply systems.
16. Identify a DISS station outlet and a quick-connect station outlet.
17. Compare the operational theory of a membrane oxygenator with that of a molecular sieve oxygenator.

Compressed gases are routinely used in the diagnosis and treatment of patients with cardiopulmonary dysfunction. The appropriate quality, purity, and potency of these medical gases are subject to government regulations. These regulations, along with recommendations proposed by the Compressed Gas Association (CGA) and other private agencies, provide guidelines for the manufacture, storage, and transport of compressed gases. As such, the primary purpose of these guidelines is to protect public safety. Respiratory therapists should be familiar with these regulations, as well as the indications, contraindications, and adverse effects associated with breathing medical gases.

TABLE 2-1

Composition of room air

Component	% by volume	% by weight
Nitrogen	78.084	75.5
Oxygen	20.946	23.2
Argon	0.934	1.33
Carbon Dioxide	0.0335	0.045
Neon	0.001818	—
Helium	0.000524	—
Methane	0.0002	—
Krypton	0.000114	—
Nitrous Oxide	0.00005	—
Xenon	0.0000087	—

From Compressed Gas Association, Inc: Handbook of compressed gases, ed. 3, New York, 1990, Van Nostrand Reinhold.

Properties of Medical Gases

Air

At normal atmospheric conditions, air is a colorless, odorless gas mixture that contains varying amounts of water vapor. For practical purposes, we can assume that atmospheric air contains about 78% nitrogen and 21% oxygen by volume. Trace gases, including argon, carbon dioxide, neon, helium, methane, krypton, nitrous oxide, and xenon, make up the remaining 1% of atmospheric air. Table 2-1 shows a typical analysis of dry air at sea level.

Air is a nonflammable gas but it supports combustion. It has a density of 1.2 kg/m^3 at 21.1° C (70° F) and 760 mm Hg.[1] Because air is used as a standard for measuring the specific gravity of other gases, it is assigned a value of 1 at 21.1° C and 1 atmosphere (atm).[1] At its freezing point, −195.6° C (−320° F), air is a transparent liquid with a pale bluish cast.

Compressed air is prepared synthetically from nitrogen and oxygen and shipped as a gas in cylinders at high pressure. Liquid air can be obtained through a process called **liquefaction** and shipped in bulk in specially designed **cryogenic** containers. For many medical applications, air is filtered and compressed at the point of use. The theory of operation of portable air compressors is described later in this chapter.

Oxygen (O_2)

Oxygen is an elemental gas that is colorless, odorless, and tasteless at normal temperatures and pressures. It makes up 20.9% of the earth's atmosphere by volume and 23.2% by weight. It constitutes about 50% of the earth's crust by weight. Oxygen is slightly heavier than air, having a density of 1.326 kg/m^3 at 21.1° C and 760 mm Hg (specific gravity = 1.105).[1] At temperatures less than −184° C (−300° F), oxygen exists as a pale bluish liquid that is slightly heavier than water.

Oxygen is classified as a nonflammable gas, but it readily supports combustion (i.e., the burning of flammable materials is accelerated in the presence of oxygen). Some combustibles, such as oil and grease, burn with nearly explosive violence if ignited in the presence of oxygen.[1] All elements except the inert gases combine with oxygen to form oxides; oxygen is therefore characterized as an oxidizer.

The two methods most commonly used to prepare oxygen are the **fractional distillation** of liquid air and the **physical separation** of atmospheric air. The fractional distillation of liquid air, which relies on the **Joule-Kelvin** or the **Joule-Thompson effect,** was introduced by Karl von Linde in 1907.[2] Box 2-1 describes the fractional distillation process; Figure 2-1 illustrates the components of a typical fractional distillation system. The fractional distillation process is used commercially to produce bulk oxygen, which can be stored as a liquid in cryogenic storage tanks or converted into a gas and shipped in metal cylinders.

The physical separation of atmospheric air is accomplished with devices that use **molecular sieves** and **semipermeable membranes** to filter room air. These devices, which are called **oxygen concentrators,** are primarily used to provide enriched oxygen mixtures for oxygen therapy in home-care settings. How oxygen concentrators operate will be discussed in more detail later in this chapter.

Carbon Dioxide (CO_2)

Carbon dioxide is a colorless, odorless gas at normal atmospheric temperatures and pressures. It has a density of 1.833 kg/m^3 at 21.1° C and 1 atm; it is therefore about 1.5 times heavier than air (specific gravity = 1.522).[1] Carbon dioxide is nonflammable and does not support combustion or life.

Carbon dioxide can exist as a solid, liquid, and gas at a temperature of −56.6° C (−69.9° F) and a pressure of 60.4 psig (the triple point of CO_2).[1] At temperatures and

BOX 2-1

Fractional Distillation of Liquid Air

1. Room air is drawn through scrubbers to remove dust and other impurities.
2. Air is cooled to near the freezing point of water (0°C) to remove water vapor.
3. Air is compressed to 200 atm, causing the temperature of the gas mixture to increase.
4. Compressed air is cooled to room temperature by passing nitrogen through coils surrounding the gas mixture.
5. As the temperature drops, the gas mixture expands. The temperature achieved is less than the critical temperature of nearly all gases in air, thus producing a liquid gas mixture.
6. The liquid air is transferred to a distilling column where it is warmed to room temperature. As the air warms, various gases boil off as their individual boiling points are reached.
7. Liquid oxygen is obtained by maintaining the temperature of the gas mixture just below the boiling point of oxygen (−183° C, or −297.3° F at 1 atm).
8. The process is repeated until the liquid oxygen mixture is 99% pure with no toxic impurities.
9. The liquid oxygen is then transferred to cold converters for storage and later transported either in bulk as a liquid or in compressed gas cylinders as a gas.

pressures below its triple point,* carbon dioxide exists as a solid ("dry ice") or a gas, depending on the temperature. At temperatures and pressures above its triple point but below its critical temperature (31.1° C or 87.9° F), carbon dioxide can exist as a liquid or as a gas. Thus when carbon dioxide is stored at these temperatures in a pressurized container, such as a metal cylinder, the liquid and gaseous forms of carbon dioxide exist in equilibrium. Above 31.1° C, carbon dioxide cannot exist as a liquid, regardless of the pressure.[1]

Unrefined carbon dioxide can be obtained from the combustion of coal, natural gas, or other carbonaceous fuels.[1] Carbon dioxide can also be obtained as a byproduct in the production of ammonia, lime, and kilns, among other products. Purified carbon dioxide is prepared through the liquefaction and fractional distillation processes.

Solid carbon dioxide is used to refrigerate perishable materials while in transport (e.g., food and laboratory specimens). Liquid carbon dioxide can be used as an expendable refrigerant[1] and is used extensively as a fire-extinguishing agent in portable and stationary fire-extinguishing systems. Gaseous carbon dioxide is used in food processing (e.g., carbonation of beverages), water treatment, and as a growth stimulant for plants.[1]

Carbon dioxide is primarily used for the treatment of singultus (hiccups) and as a stimulant/depressant of the central nervous system (CNS). It is also used as a standard calibration gas for blood-gas analyzers, transcutaneous partial pressure of carbon dioxide (PCO_2) electrodes, and capnographs. Because carbon dioxide cannot support life, it must be combined with oxygen before being administered to patients. Carbon dioxide/oxygen mixtures (carbogen mixtures) are prepared by combining 5% to 10% carbon dioxide with 90% to 95% oxygen. The United States Food and Drug Administration (USFDA) purity standard requires that carbon dioxide used for medical purposes is 99.0% pure.[3]

Helium (He)

Helium is the second lightest element, having a density of 0.165 kg/m^3 at 21.1° C and 1 atm (specific gravity = 0.138).[1] It is an inert gas that has no color, odor, or taste. Helium is only slightly soluble in water and is a good conductor of heat, sound, and electricity.[4]

Helium occurs naturally in the atmosphere in very small quantities (see Table 2-1). It can be prepared commercially from natural gas, which contains as much as 2% helium.[1] Helium can also be obtained by heating uranium ore. Purity standards for the preparation of helium require that commercially available helium be 95% pure. Helium is chemically and physiologically inert and is classified as a nonflammable gas that will not support combustion or life. Breathing 100% helium will lead to severe hypoxemia. Because of its low density, helium is combined with oxygen (i.e., heliox is a mixture of 80% helium and 20% oxygen) to deliver oxygen therapy to patients with severe airway obstruction (i.e., it decreases the work of breathing by decreasing turbulent airflow). It is also used in pulmonary function testing for measuring residual volume and diffusing capacity.

Nitric Oxide (NO)

Nitric oxide is a diatomic molecule that exists as colorless gas at room temperature. It is nonflammable and will support combustion. It has a density of 1.245 kg/m^3 and a specific gravity of 1.04 (21.1° C, 760 mm Hg).[1] Nitric oxide is highly unstable in the atmosphere and can exist in three biologically active forms in tissues: nitrosonium (NO^+), nitroxyl anions (NO^-), and as a free radical ($NO^\cdot$).

In the presence of air, nitric oxide combines with oxygen to form brown fumes of nitrogen dioxide (NO_2), which is a strong oxidizing agent. It is not corrosive, and most structural materials are unaffected; in the presence of moisture, however, it can form nitrous and nitric acids, both of which

*Remember that the triple point is a specific combination of temperature and pressure in which a substance can exist in all three states of matter in a dynamic equilibrium.

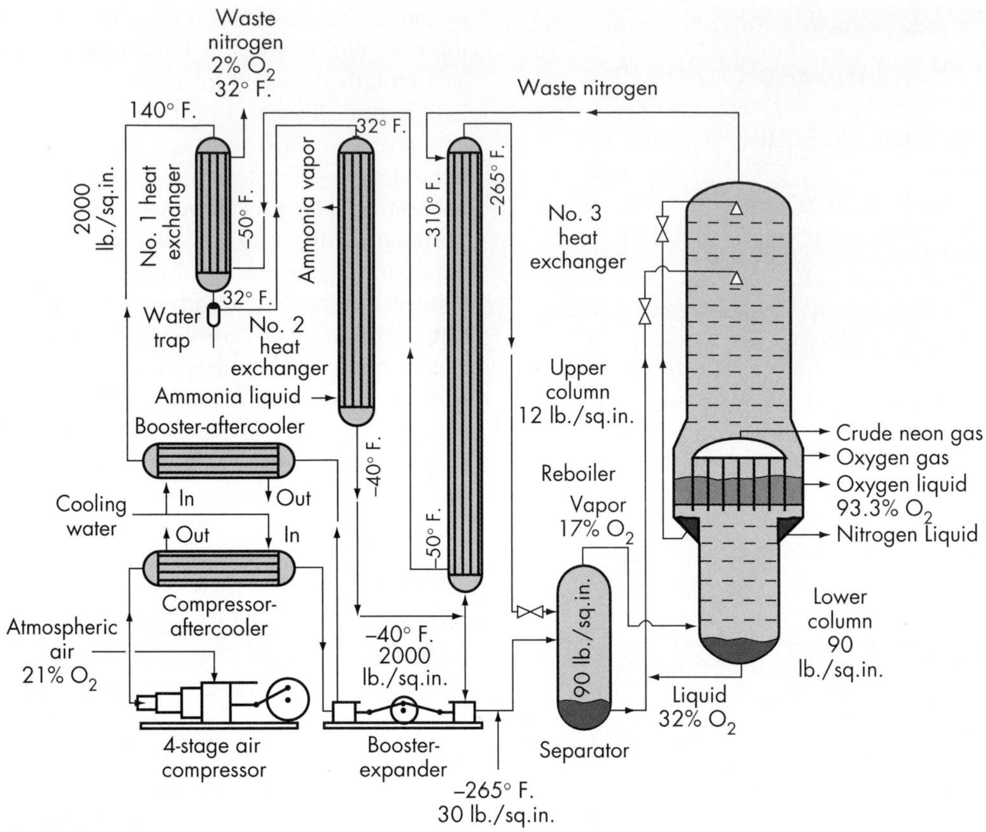

Figure 2-1 Fractional distillation apparatus for producing liquid oxygen. (Courtesy Nellcor Puritan Bennett, Pleasanton, Calif.)

can cause corrosion. Nitric oxide and nitrogen dioxide combined form a potent irritant that can cause chemical pneumonitis and pulmonary edema.[4]

Nitric oxide can be prepared by oxidizing ammonia at high temperatures (500° C) in the presence of a platinum catalyst or by reducing acid solutions of nitrates.[1] Chemiluminescent analysis is used to determine the final concentration of nitric oxide and nitrogen dioxide with a stated accuracy of ±2% (see Chapter 7 for a discussion of chemiluminescent analysis of nitrogen oxides). Nitric oxide is supplied with nitrogen in compressed-gas aluminum alloy cylinders.[5] Before 1997, nitric oxide was supplied in cylinders with a volume capacity of 152 ft^3 with 660 CGA valve outlets. It is now supplied in smaller cylinders (82 ft^3) with 626 CGA valve outlets.

Although nitric oxide is toxic in high concentrations, experimental results suggest that low doses of it are a powerful pulmonary vasodilator.[5] Very low concentrations (2 to 80 parts per million [ppm]) combined with oxygen have been used successfully to treat persistent pulmonary hypertension of the newborn (PPHN)[6] and adult respiratory distress syndrome (ARDS).[7] Although many investigators have suggested that inhalation of low-dose nitric oxide is relatively safe, special precautions apply. Specifically, the levels of nitrogen dioxide and nitrogen trioxide, as well as the patient's methemoglobin levels, should be monitored throughout the procedure.[5]

Nitrous Oxide (N_2O)

Nitrous oxide is a colorless gas at normal temperatures and atmospheric pressures. It is odorless, tasteless, and nonflammable but will support combustion, and is slightly soluble in water, alcohol, and oils. Nitrous oxide is noncorrosive and may therefore be stored in commercially available cylinders. Because it is an oxidizing agent, it will react with oils, grease, and other combustible materials.

Nitrous oxide is prepared commercially by the thermal decomposition of ammonium nitrate and as a by-product from adipic acid manufacturing processes.[1] At elevated temperatures (>649° C), it decomposes into nitrogen and oxygen.

The major use of nitrous oxide is as a CNS depressant (i.e., an anesthetic). As such, it is a potent anesthetic when administered in high concentrations; in low concentrations, other depressant drugs must be used concomitantly to achieve effective anesthesia. (Nitrous oxide is often called "laughing gas," a term that was coined in 1840.[8]) Note that inhalation of nitrous oxide without provision of a sufficient oxygen supply may cause brain damage or be fatal.

Long-term exposure of health-care workers to nitrous oxide has been associated with adverse side effects, including neuropathy and feto-toxic effects (spontaneous abortions).[1] The National Institute of Occupational Safety and Health (NIOSH) has recommended limits for expo-

TABLE 2-2

Properties of commonly used medical gases

Medical gas	Chemical symbol	Molecular weight	Physical characteristics: Color	Odor	Taste	Boiling point °C (1 atm)	Critical temperature °C (1 atm)	Physical state	Combustion characteristics
Air	Air	28.97	colorless	odorless	tasteless	−194.3	−140.6	gas/liquid	NF*/SC**
Oxygen	O_2	31.99	colorless	odorless	tasteless	−182.9	−118.4	gas/liquid	NF/SC
Carbon dioxide	CO_2	44.01	colorless	odorless	slightly acid	−78.5	+31	liquid	NF
Carbon monoxide	CO	28.01	colorless	odorless	tasteless	−191.5	−140.2	gas	F***
Nitrous oxide	N_2O	44.01	colorless	odorless	tasteless	−88.5	+36.4	liquid	NF
Nitric oxide	NO	30.01	colorless	odorless	tasteless	−151.8	−92.9	gas	NF
Helium	He	4.00	colorless	odorless	tasteless	−268.9	−267	gas	NF

*NF = Nonflammable
**SC = Supports combustion
***F = Flammable

BOX 2-2

Decision Making & Problem Solving

Based on the discussion of compressed gases, name the appropriate gas for each of the following situations:

1. As a refrigerant.
2. For reducing the work of breathing in a patient with airway obstruction.
3. To treat hypoxemia in a patient with COPD.
4. For reducing pulmonary vasoconstriction, such as occurs in PPHN.

See Appendix A for answers.

sure to nitrous oxide of health-care providers working in surgical suites and dental offices. Systems to trap exhaled nitrous oxide are used to capture any unused gas, preventing inadvertent exposure of health-care workers.

Table 2-2 provides a summary of the properties of commonly used medical gases. Box 2-2 contains a list of problems involving the uses of medical gases.

STORAGE AND TRANSPORT OF MEDICAL GASES

Medical gases can be classified as nonliquefied and liquefied. Nonliquefied gases are stored and transported under high pressure in metal cylinders. Liquefied gases are stored and transported in specially designed bulk liquid storage units. The design of compressed gas cylinders, bulk storage containers, and their valve outlets, as well as their transportation, testing, and periodic examination, are subject to national standards and regulations.[9] Box 2-3 contains a list of agencies that provide recommendations and regulations for the manufacture, storage, transport, and use of medical gases.

Cylinders

Metal cylinders have been used for storing compressed gases since 1888.[10] Federal regulations issued by the Department of Transportation (DOT) require that all cylinders used to store and transport compressed gases conform to well-defined specifications.* These specifications, along with recommendations from the NFPA and the CGA, provide industry standards for cylinder design and maintenance and the safe use of compressed gases. Appendix 2-1 contains a summary of NFPA and CGA recommendations for compressed-gas cylinders.

Construction and Maintenance of Compressed-Gas Cylinders

Compressed-gas cylinders are constructed of seamless, high-quality steel, chrome-molybdenum, or aluminum that is either stamped into shape using a punch-press die or spun into shape by wrapping heated steel bands around specially designed molds. The bottom of the cylinder is welded closed and the top of the cylinder is threaded and fitted with a valve stem (Figure 2-2).

Type 3AA cylinders are produced from heat-treated, high-strength steel; type 3A cylinders are made of carbon-steel (non-heat–treated). Type 3AL cylinders are constructed of specially prescribed seamless aluminum alloys. Type 3 cylinders, which are made of low-carbon steel, are

*Prior to 1970, the Interstate Commerce Commission served as the regulatory agency for the construction, transport, and maintenance of compressed gases, but in 1970 the DOT took over this responsibility.

BOX 2-3

Agencies Regulating Manufacture, Storage, and Transport of Medical Gases

Regulating Agencies

Bureau of Medical Devices (BMD)

An agency of the FDA that provides standards for medical devices.

Department of Health and Human Services (HHS)

Department of the federal government that oversees health-care delivery in the United States. Formerly known as the Department of Health, Education, and Welfare (HEW).

Department of Transportation (DOT)

Provides regulations for the manufacture, storage, and transport of compressed gases. Before 1970, this responsibility was vested with the Interstate Commerce Commission (ICC).

Food and Drug Administration (FDA)

An agency of the Department of Health and Human Services (HHS) that sets purity standards for medical gases.

Occupational Safety and Health Administration (OSHA)

An agency of the Department of Labor that oversees safety issues related to the work environment.

Recommending Agencies

American National Standards Institute (ANSI)

Private, nonprofit organization that coordinates the voluntary developments of national standards in the United States. Represents U.S. interests in international standards.

Compressed Gas Association (CGA)

Comprises companies involved in the manufacture, storage, and transport of compressed gases. Provides standards and safety systems for compressed-gas systems.

International Standards Organization (ISO)

International agency that provides standards for technology.

National Fire Protection Association (NFPA)

Independent agency that provides information on fire protection and safety.

Z-79 Committee

ANSI committee for establishing standards for anesthetic and ventilatory devices, including anesthetic machines, reservoir bags, tracheal tubes, humidifiers, nebulizers, and other oxygen-related equipment.

From Scanlan CL, Spearman CB, and Sheldon RL: Egan's fundamentals of respiratory care, ed 6, St Louis, 1995, Mosby.

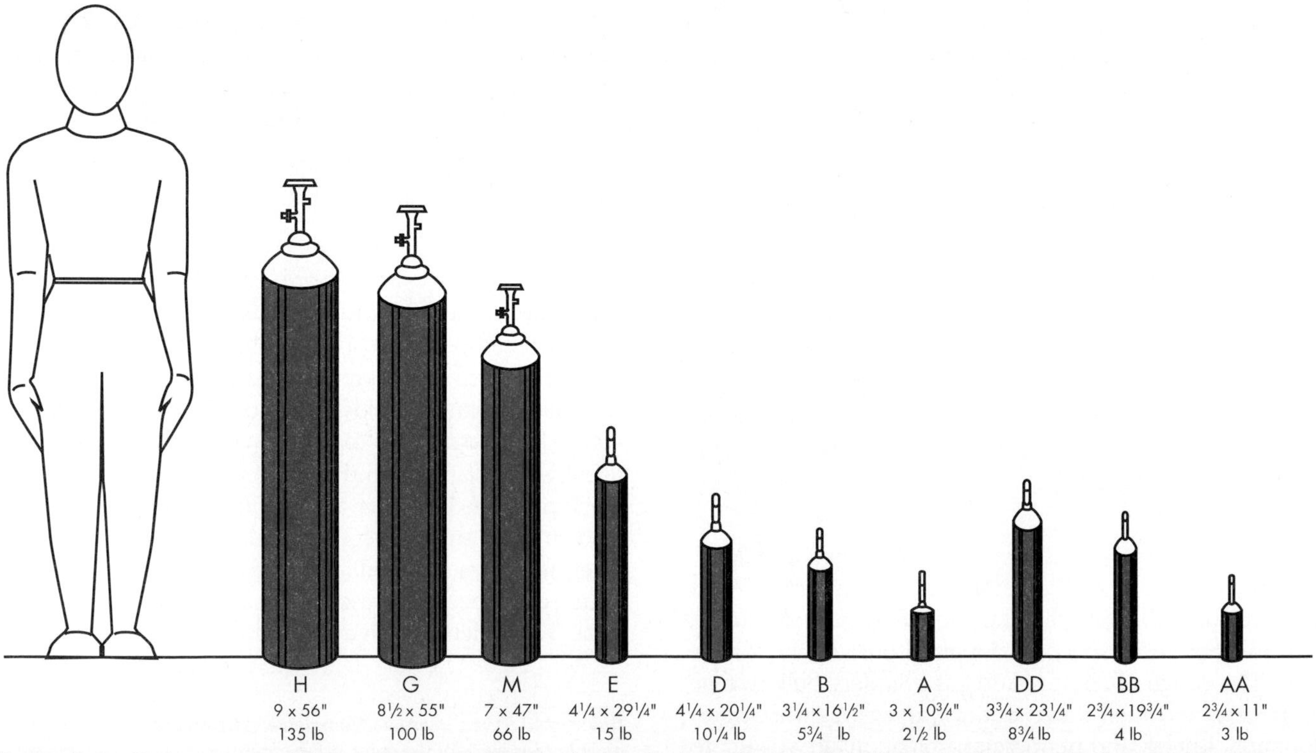

Figure 2-2 Various types of high-pressure cylinders used in medical gas therapy. (Modified from Barnes TA: Core textbook of respiratory care practice, ed 2, St Louis, 1994, Mosby.)

no longer produced. Note that the steel used in the construction of cylinders must meet the chemical and physical standards set by the DOT. (In Canada, the specifications for the construction of cylinders are set by the Board of Transport Commissioners.[10])

Compressed-gas cylinders should be capable of holding up to 10% more than the maximum filling pressure as marked.[11,12] This added capacity is required because of variations in cylinder pressure that occur with changes in ambient temperature. The Bureau of Explosives requires that all cylinders contain a pressure-relief mechanism to prevent explosion.[13]

Type 3AA and 3A cylinders must be hydrostatically reexamined every 5 years (unless otherwise specified) to determine their expansion characteristics. (Some cylinders must be retested every 10 years; an asterisk following the reexamination date on the cylinder markings [see Figure 2-4] indicates that the cylinder must be retested every 10 years.[11]) Hydrostatic examination involves measuring a cylinder's expansion characteristics when it is filled to a pressure of five-thirds its working pressure. This examination consists of placing a cylinder filled with water in a vessel that is also filled with water. When pressure is applied to the interior of the cylinder, the cylinder expands, displacing water from the jacket surrounding the cylinder. The volume of water displaced when pressure is applied equals the total expansion of the cylinder. The permanent expansion of the cylinder equals the volume of water displaced when the pressure is released. This information is then used to calculate the elastic expansion of the cylinder, which is directly related to the thickness of the cylinder. Increases in the elastic expansion of a cylinder indicate a reduction in the wall thickness. Reductions in wall thickness can occur when the cylinder is physically damaged or is attacked by corrosion.[1] Figure 2-3 is a schematic illustrating an example of an apparatus for testing cylinders.

Cylinder Sizes and Capacities

Table 2-3 summarizes the weights and volume capacities for various cylinders and gases that are used in respiratory care. The most commonly used are the "E," "G," and "H" types of cylinders.

"E" cylinders are frequently used as a source of oxygen in emergency situations (e.g., CPR carts, etc.) and for

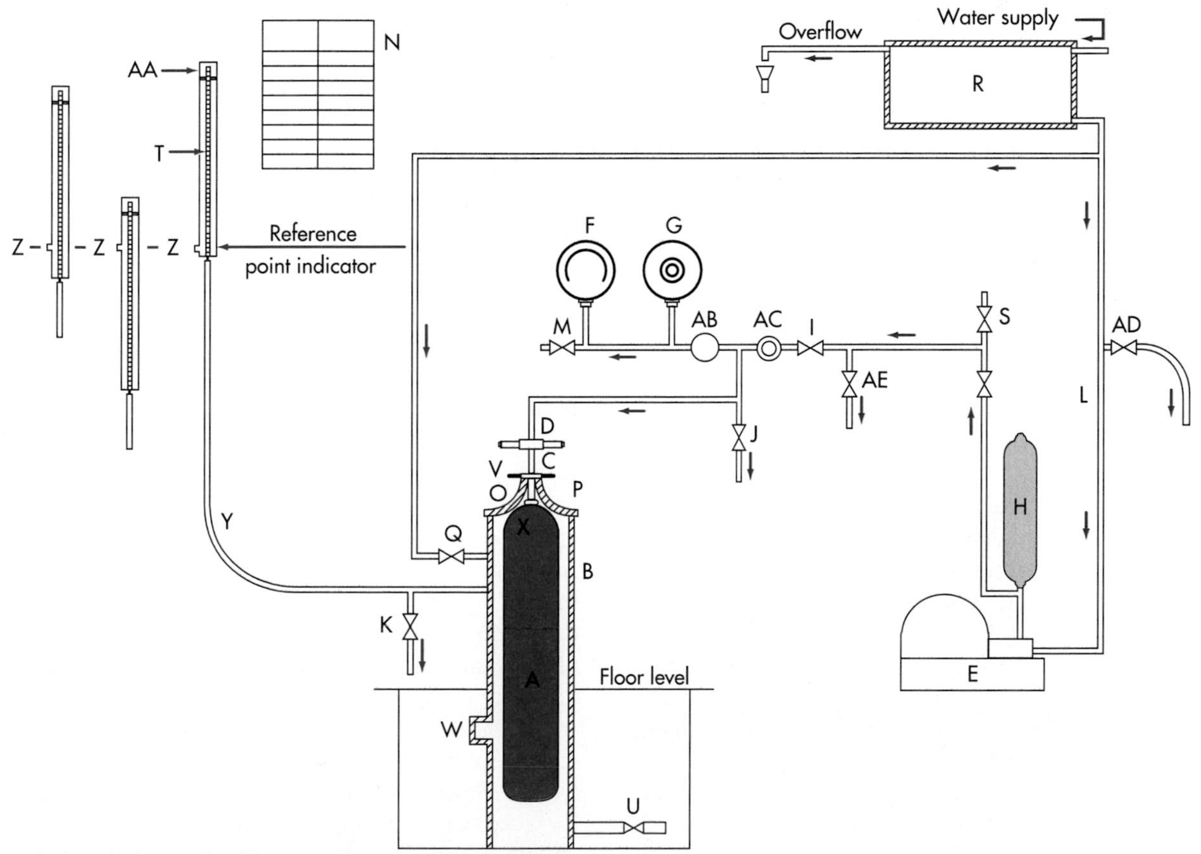

Figure 2-3 System for hydrostatic testing of compressed gas cylinders: *A,* cylinder; *B,* water jacket; *C,* cylinder connection; *D,* pressure connection; *E,* hydraulic pressure source; *F* and *G,* pressure gauges; *H,* pressure surge chamber; *N,* log sheet; *O,* water jacket; *R,* water reservoir; *S,* safety-relief valve; *T,* burrette (calibrated in cubic centimeters). (Modified from Klein BR: Health care facilities handbook, ed 4, Quincy, Mass., 1993, National Fire Protection Association.)

TABLE 2-3

Common cylinder sizes and gases used in respiratory care

	Gas (cylinder pressure at 21.11° C [70° F] [psig*])							
Cylinder sizes	Carbon dioxide (840)	Cyclopropane (80)	Ethylene (1250)	Helium (1650 to 2000)	Nitrous oxide (745)	Oxygen (1800 to 2400)	Helium-oxygen mixtures (1650 to 2000)	Carbon dioxide mixtures (1500 to 2200)
D: Contents weight (lb)	4.0	3.3	2.0	0.1	4.0	1.0	—	—
Gas volume at 21.11° C (70° F) and 14.7 psia†								
Cubic feet	33.0	30.0	26.6	10.6	34.5	12.6	11.0	12.6
Liters	934.0	848.0	752.0	300.0	975.0	356.0	310.0	356.0
E: Contents weight (lb)	6.6	—	3.3	0.2	6.6	2.0	—	—
Gas volume at 21.11° C (70° F) and 14.7 psia								
Cubic feet	56.0	—	44.0	17.0	57.0	22.0	18.0	22.0
Liters	1585.0	—	1245.0	480.0	1610.0	622.0	510.0	622.0
G: Contents weight (lb)	50.0	—		1.5	56.0	16.0	—	—
Gas volume at 21.11° C (70° F) and 14.7 psia								
Cubic feet	425.0	—	372.0	146.0	485.0	186.0	150.0	186.0
Liters	12,000.0	—	10,500.0	4130.0	13,750.0	5260.0	4250.0	5260.0
H-K: Contents weight (lb)	—	—	—	—	64.0	20.0	—	—
Gas volume at 21.11° C (70° F) and 14.7 psia								
Cubic feet	—	—	—	—	557.0	244.0	—	—
Liters	—	—	—	—	15,800.0	6900.0	—	—

*Pounds per square inch gauge.
†Pounds per square inch absolute.

From the Standard for Nonflammable Medical Gas Systems (NFPA 56 F), 1973, copyright National Fire Protection Association, Quincy, Mass.

transporting patients requiring oxygen therapy. These smaller cylinders also store gases used in anesthetics, as well as calibration gases for portable diagnostic equipment (e.g., capnographs and pulse oximeters).

"G" and "H" types of cylinders are used as the primary source of oxygen and other medical gases in smaller hospitals without bulk liquid systems (see the following section). Hospitals and other facilities with bulk liquid oxygen systems use these larger cylinders as a secondary or reserve source of medical gases. Large cylinders are frequently used for home-care patients requiring long-term oxygen therapy. These larger cylinders are also routinely used to store calibration gases that are required in the blood-gas and pulmonary function laboratories.

Cylinder Identification

Cylinders are engraved with information that is primarily designed to identify where the cylinder was manufactured, the type of material used in its construction (i.e., 3AA, 3A, or 3AL), the service pressure of the cylinder, the date of its original hydrostatic test, as well as its reexamination dates.[1] Additionally, the manufacturer's name, the owner's identification number, and the size of cylinder are usually engraved on the cylinder. Figure 2-4 illustrates the standard markings that appear on compressed-gas cylinders. Note that a "+" following the stamped hydrostatic examination date indicates that the cylinder complied with requirement of the examination. A "+" does not follow the reexamination date on aluminum cylinders.

Medical gas cylinders are color-coded for easy identification. Table 2-4 shows the color codes prescribed by the United States National Formulary (USNF).[3] Generally, these colors conform to the international cylinder color-coding system. Two major exceptions in the international system are oxygen cylinders, which are painted white, and compressed-air cylinders, which are painted yellow or black and white. Cylinders containing gas mixtures, such as helium-oxygen and carbon dioxide-oxygen are divided into

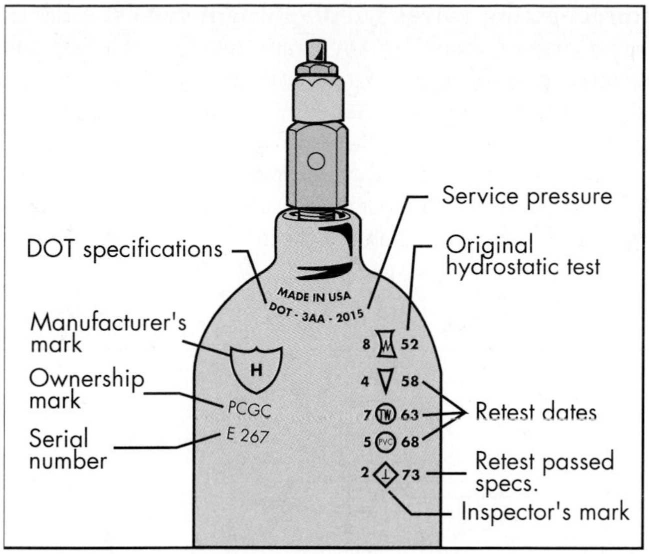

Figure 2-4 Standard markings for compressed gas cylinders. (Modified from Nellcor Puritan Bennett, Pleasanton, Calif.)

TABLE 2-4

Color codes for medical gases

Gas	Chemical symbol	Purity*	Color code
Air	—	99.0	yellow or black and white[†]
Carbon dioxide	CO_2	99.0	gray
Carbon dioxide/oxygen	CO_2/O_2	99.0	gray and green[‡]
Cyclopropane	C_3H_6	99.0	orange
Ethylene	C_2H_4	99.0	red
Helium	He	99.0	brown
Helium/oxygen	He/O_2	99.0	brown and green[‡]
Nitrogen	N_2	99.0	black
Nitrous oxide	N_2O	97.0	light blue
Oxygen	O_2	99.0	green or white[†]

*National Formulary Standards
[†]International color code system.
[‡]Always check labels to determine the percentages of each gas.

two categories of color-coding, each based on the percentage of gases contained. For example, cylinders of carbon dioxide-oxygen mixtures that contain more than 7% carbon dioxide are predominantly gray with the shoulder of the tank painted green. Cylinders containing carbon dioxide-oxygen mixtures with less than 7% carbon dioxide are predominantly green with a gray shoulder. Helium-oxygen cylinders containing more than 80% helium are painted brown with a green shoulder. Cylinders of helium-oxygen mixtures containing less than 80% helium (balanced with oxygen) are predominantly green with a brown shoulder.

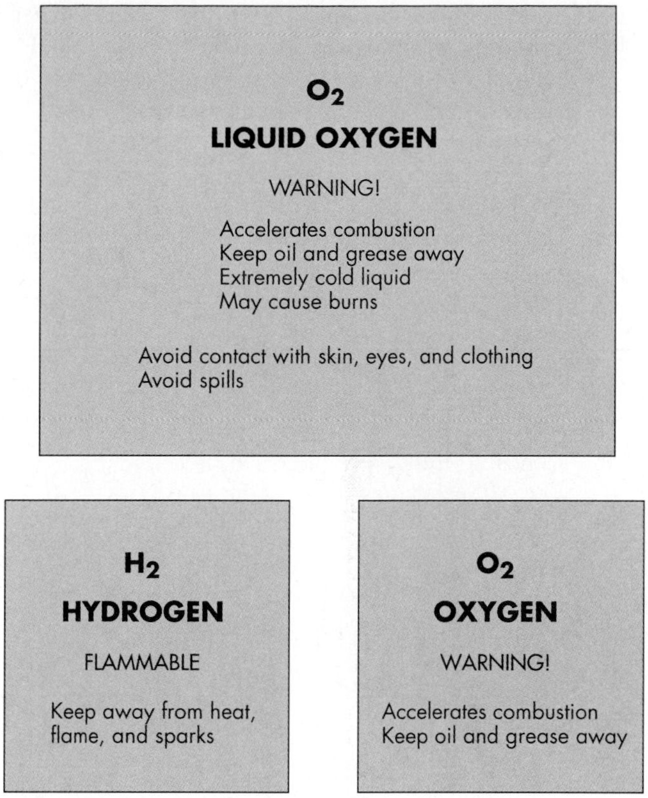

Figure 2-5 Example of gas labels. (Modified from McPherson S: Respiratory care equipment, ed 5, St Louis, 1995, Mosby.)

Color codes are only a guide; printed labels are still the primary way to identify the contents of a gas cylinder. Figure 2-5 is a standard label for an oxygen cylinder. The CGA and the ASA specify that all labels should include the name and chemical symbol of the gas in the cylinder. The label should also show the volume of the cylinder (in liters) at a temperature of 21.1° C (70° F).[1] Generally, labels will also include any specific hazards related to use of the gas, as well as precautionary measures and instructions in case of accidental exposure or contact with the contents.

The USFDA requires that compressed gases used for medical purposes meet certain minimum requirements for purity, and the purity of the gas must be indicated on the label identifying the contents of the cylinder. These standards are listed in the NF/USP. (See Table 2-4 for a list of these purity requirements.) The USFDA also requires that the names of the manufacturer, packer, and distributor be included on the label.

Cylinder Valves

Cylinder valves are control devices that seal the contents of a compressed cylinder until it is ready for use. A cylinder valve is composed of the following elements:

1. A chrome-plated, brass body
2. A threaded inlet connector for attachment to the cylinder

3. A stem that opens and closes the cylinder when turned by a handwheel or handle
4. An outlet connection that allows for attachment of regulators and pressure-reducing valves
5. A pressure-relief valve

Figure 2-6 shows the two different types of cylinder valves that are affixed to compressed medical gas cylinders: **direct-acting valves** and **diaphragm valves.** A direct-acting valve (Figure 2-6 **A**) contains two fiber washers and a Teflon packing to prevent gas leakage around the threads. The term *direct-acting* is derived from the arrangement of movements in the valve wheel. These movements are directly reflected in the valve seat because it is one piece moved by threads. Direct-acting valves can withstand high pressures (i.e., more than 1500 psi).

A

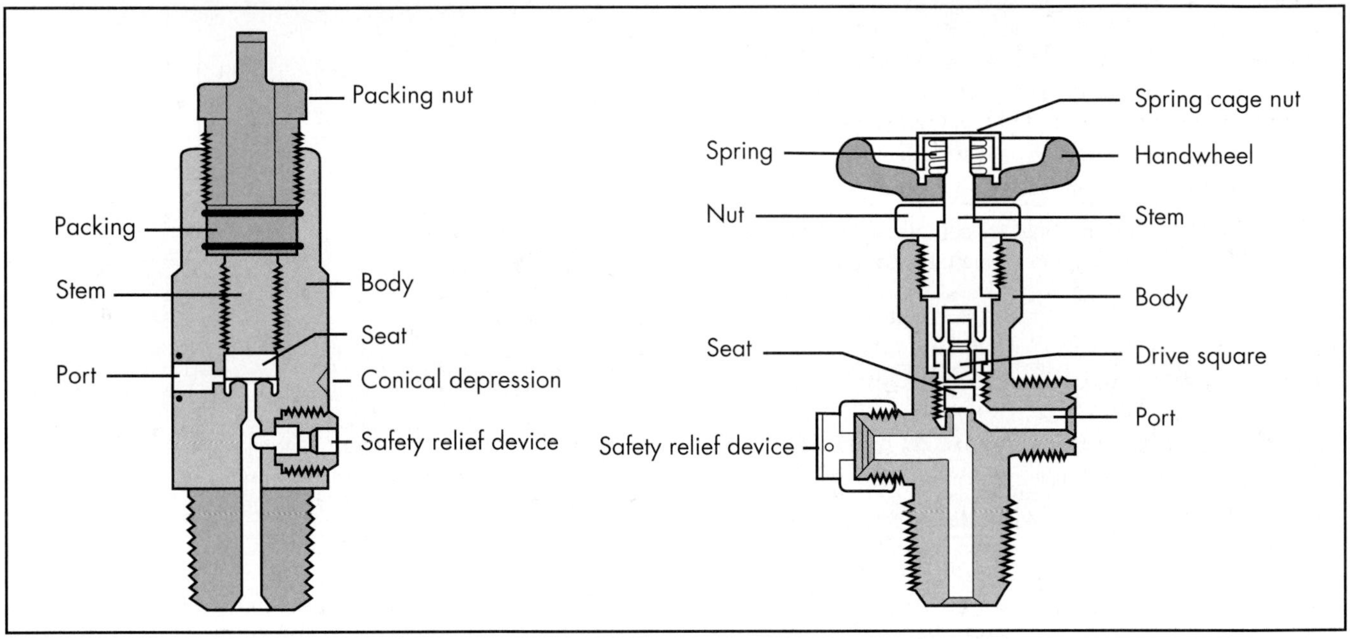

B

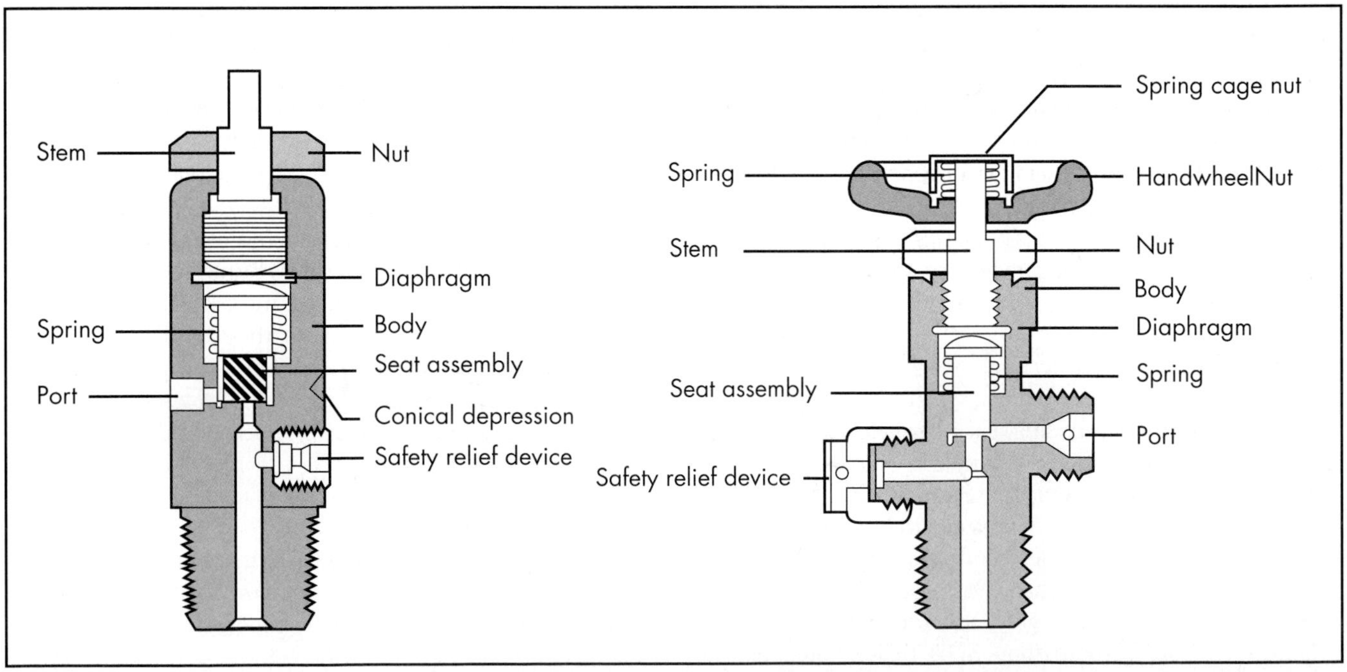

Figure 2-6 Cylinder valves: **A,** direct-acting valve; **B,** diaphragm valve. (Courtesy Nellcor Puritan Bennett, Pleasanton, Calif.)

Diaphragm type of valves (Figure 2-6 **B**) use a threaded stem in place of the packing found on the direct-acting valves. The stem is separated from the valve seat and spring by two diaphragms, one made of steel and one made of copper. When the stem is turned counterclockwise and raised because of the threading, the diaphragm is pushed upward with the stem by the valve seat and spring, causing the valve to open. Turning the stem clockwise resets the diaphragm and closes the valve.

Diaphragm type of valves have several advantages, including: (1) the valve seat does not turn and is therefore resistance to scoring, which could cause leakage; (2) no stem leakage can occur because of the diaphragm; and (3) the stem can be opened with a partial rotation rather than with two turns of the wheel as in direct-acting type of valves. Diaphragm valves are generally preferable when pressures are relatively low (i.e., less than 1500 psi). They are also ideal for situations where no gas leaks can be allowed, such as with flammable anesthetics.

Pressure Relief Valves. Figure 2-7 illustrates three types of pressure-relief mechanisms: **rupture disks, fusible plugs,** and **spring-loaded devices.**[1] A rupture disk (also called a frangible disk) is a thin, metal disk that ruptures or buckles when the pressure inside the cylinder exceeds a certain predetermined limit. A fusible plug is made of a metal alloy that melts when the temperature of the gas in the tank exceeds a predetermined temperature. Fusible plugs operate on the principle that as the pressure in a tank increases, the temperature of the gas increases, causing the plug to melt. Once the plug melts, excess pressure is released.* Spring-loaded devices are designed to release excessive cylinder pressure and reseal, preventing further release of gas from the cylinder after the cause of the excessive pressure is removed.[1] With these devices, a metal seal is held in place by an adjustable spring. The amount of pressure required to force the seal open depends on the tension of the spring holding the metal seal in place. Spring-loaded devices are usually more susceptible to leakage around the metal seal than rupture disks and fusible plugs.[1] Note that spring-loaded devices may also be affected by changes in environmental conditions (i.e., freezing, sticking).

Safety Systems. Outlet connections of cylinder valves are indexed according to standards that were designed by the CGA and adopted by the ASA and the Canadian Standards Association. American Standard connections are *noninterchangeable* to prevent the interchange of regulating equipment between gases that are not compatible.

*A commonly used metal alloy is called **Wood's metal;** fusible plugs made of this alloy generally have melting temperatures of 208° to 220° F.

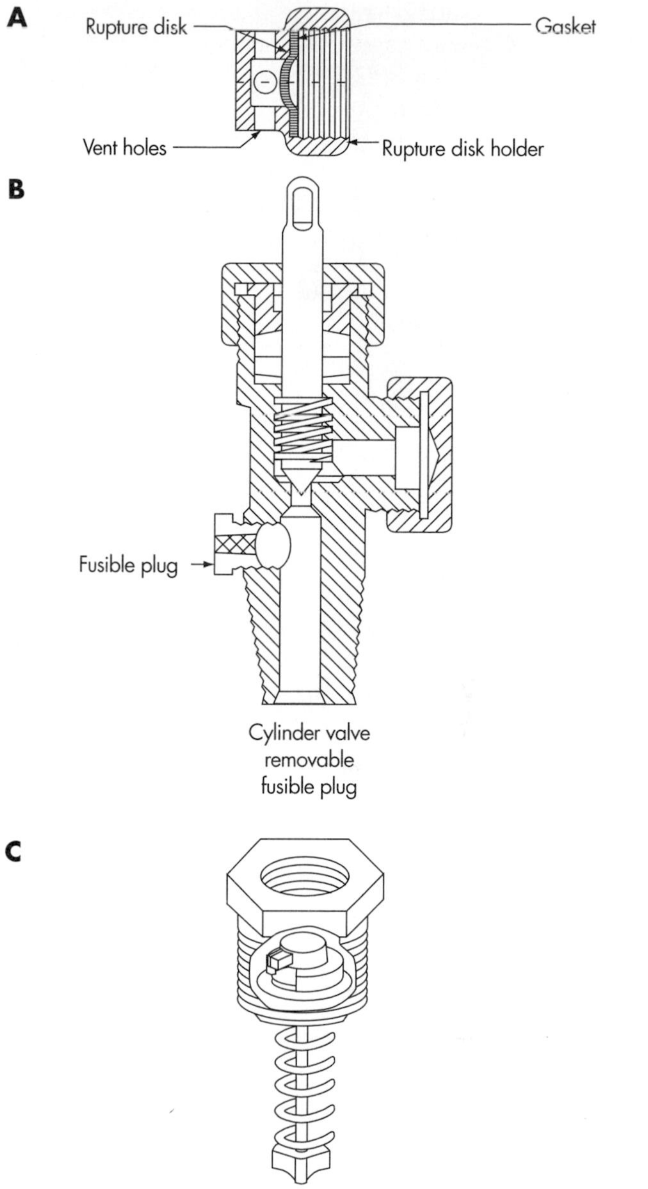

Figure 2-7 Pressure-relief valves: **A,** rupture (frangible) disks; **B,** fusible plug; **C,** spring-loaded device. (Redrawn from Compressed Gas Association: Handbook of compressed gases, ed 3, New York, 1990, Van Nostrand Reinhold.)

American Standard indexing includes separate systems for large and small cylinders. Large cylinder-valve outlets and connections (e.g., for sizes G, H, and K) are indexed by thread type, thread size, right- or left-handed threading, external or internal threading, and nipple-seat design.[12] Figure 2-8 illustrates the American Standard connections for medical gases that are commonly used in respiratory care. Look at the oxygen connection shown in this figure. The diameter of the cylinder's outlet is listed in thousandths of inches (e.g., oxygen connection is 0.903 in). The letters following these numbers indicate the type of threading used

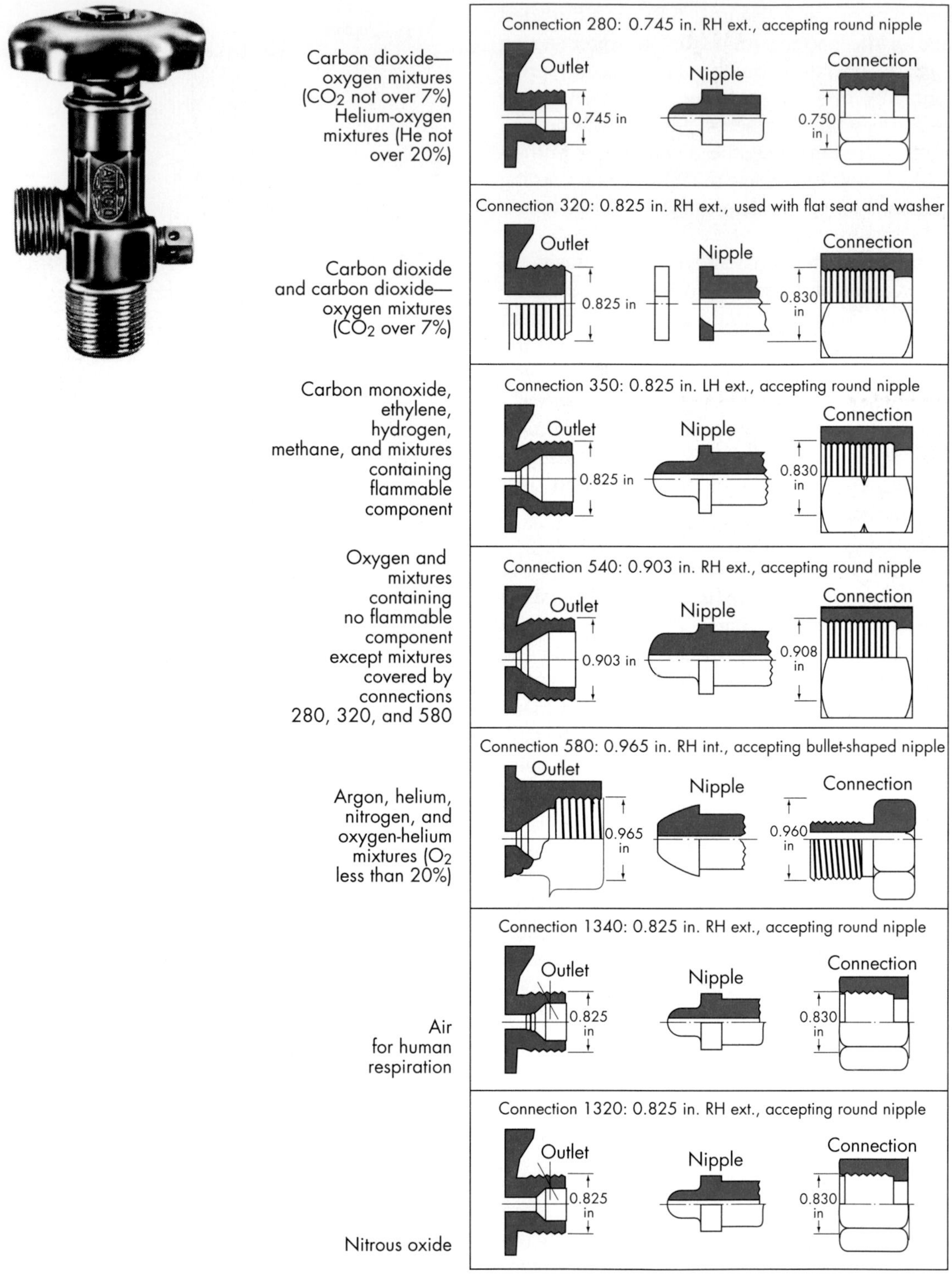

Figure 2-8 American Standard system for large cylinders. (Courtesy Datex-Ohmeda, Madison, Wisconsin.)

(i.e., right-handed [RH] vs. left-handed [LH]). The abbreviations *Ext* and *Int* specify whether the threads are external or internal. Note that the connections for oxygen and other life-support gases are right-handed and external. The remaining information indicates if the outlet requires a nipple attachment. Oxygen valves require a rounded nipple.

Small cylinders (e.g., sizes A to E) with post type of valves use a different American Standard indexing called the **Pin Index Safety System (PISS).** In this system, indexing is accomplished by the exact placement of two pins into holes in the post valve. Note that the hole positions are numbered from 1 to 6; each medical gas uses a specified

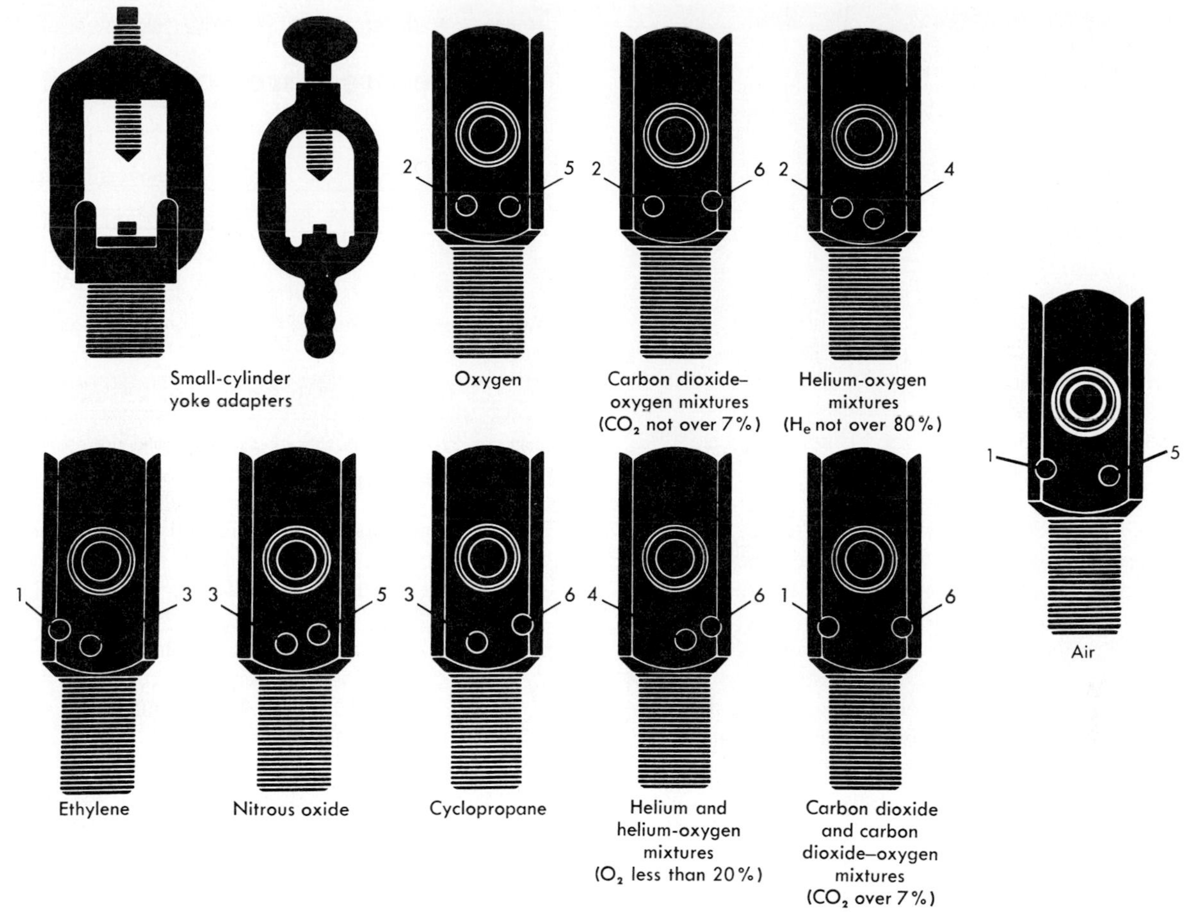

Figure 2-9 PISS system for small cylinders. (Courtesy Datex-Ohmeda, Madison, Wisconsin.)

pin sequence. Figure 2-9 shows the different combinations that are used to differentiate the most commonly used medical gases. For example, the pins for an oxygen regulator must be placed in the 2 and 5 positions for it to attach to the oxygen cylinder's post valve. Cylinder regulators will be discussed in Chapter 3.

Setting Up and Troubleshooting of Compressed-Gas Cylinders

Box 2-4 contains the steps that should be followed when setting up a compressed-gas cylinder.[14] The following is a list of simple suggestions that should be kept in mind when handling compressed gas cylinders:

1. Cylinder contents should be clearly labeled. If the contents of a cylinder are questionable, do not use it.
2. Full and empty cylinders should be appropriately labeled and kept separate.
3. Cylinder valves should be fully opened when in use and always closed when the gas contained in the cylinder is not being used. Cylinder valves should be closed if the cylinder is empty.
4. Large cylinders have a protective cap that fits over the valve stem. This cap should be kept on cylinders when moving or storing them. Small cylinders with PISS valve stems do not have protective caps but have an outlet seal that must be removed before the appropriate regulator is attached.
5. Regulators and other appliances intended for use with a specific gas should not be used with other gases.
6. Cylinders should be properly secured at all times either in a stand, chained to a wall, or in a cart to prevent them from tipping over.

Most problems encountered with cylinders and regulators involve: (1) gas leakage at the valve stem or in the regulator, and (2) failure to achieve adequate gas flow at the cylinder regulator outlet. Leaks typically occur from large cylinders because of loose connections between the regulator and the cylinder valve. Gas leaks from small cylinders are most often associated with damage to the plastic washer that fits between the valve stem and the regulator. Gas leaks at the regulator outlet can be caused by a loose connection between the regulator and attached equipment. Box 2-5 is a problem-solving exercise involving regulators. Failure to achieve a desired gas flow from a cylinder regulator can result from inadequate pressure (e.g., low gauge pressure) or from an obstruction at the regulator outlet.

BOX 2-4

Procedure for Setting up a Compressed-Gas Cylinder

1. Make sure that the cylinder is properly secured.
2. Remove the protective cap or wrap and inspect the cylinder valve to ensure that it is free of dirt, debris, or oil.
3. Alert others nearby that you are about to "crack" the cylinder valve, making a loud noise. Turn the cylinder valve away from anyone present. Then quickly open and close the valve to remove dirt or small debris from the valve outlet.
4. Inspect the inlet of the device to be attached to ensure that it is free of dirt and debris.
5. Securely tighten—but do not force—the device onto the cylinder outlet. Use appropriate wrenches that are free of oil and grease; never use pipe wrenches. Remember to only use cylinder valve connections that conform to ANSI and PISS B57. Low- pressure, threaded connections must comply with DISS or must be noninterchangeable, low-pressure, quick-connecting devices. Never connect fixed or adjustable orifices or metering devices directly to a cylinder without a pressure-reducing valve.
6. Be certain that the regulator or reducing valve is in the closed position, and then slowly open the cylinder valve to pressurize the reducing valve or regulator that is attached. Once pressurization has occurred, open the cylinder valve completely and turn it back a quarter- to a half-turn to prevent "valve freeze" (i.e., when the valve cannot be turned).

BOX 2-5

Decision Making & Problem Solving

A respiratory therapist "cracks" an H cylinder of oxygen and then attaches an oxygen regulator to the cylinder outlet. She slowly opens the valve stem and hears a sudden, loud hissing sound coming from the connection between the cylinder outlet and the regulator. What should she do?

See Appendix A for answer.

Determining the Volume of Gas Remaining in a Cylinder and the Duration of Cylinder Gas Flow. Calculating the gas volume remaining in a cylinder requires knowledge of either the pressure or the weight of the cylinder. (See Table 2-3 for a list of values for commonly used medical gas cylinders.) For nonliquefied gas cylinders (e.g., compressed air, oxygen, helium), the gas volume contained in a cylinder is directly related to the regulator's gauge pressure. Table 2-5 shows these constants, or "tank factors," for the more commonly used medical gas cylinders. The volume of gas remaining in a cylinder can then be calculated by multiplying the cylinder's **volume-pressure constant** by the gauge pressure. Box 2-6 is an example of this calculation. The resultant volume can then be divided by the flow rate of gas being used to determine the duration of gas flow remaining in minutes.

Determining the gas volume remaining in a liquefied gas cylinder (e.g., carbon dioxide and nitrous oxide) is more of a challenge. The gas volume remaining in a liquefied gas cylinder cannot be determined by the method just described because the liquid remains in equilibrium with the gas above it until the liquid is depleted. The volume of liquefied gas remaining is best determined by weighing the

TABLE 2-5

Volume-pressure conversion factors

Cylinder size	Conversion factor		
E	622.0 L/2200 psi	=	0.28
G	5269.0 L/2200 psi	=	2.41
H to K	6600.0 L/2200 psi	=	3.14

BOX 2-6

Estimating the Duration of a Medical Gas Cylinder Supply

The amount of time that it will take a cylinder filled with compressed gas to provide a set flow rate of gas can be calculated with the following formula:

$$\frac{\text{cylinder pressure (psi)} \times \text{cylinder factor*}}{\text{flow rate of gas (L/min)}}$$
$$= \text{duration of flow in min}$$

Example:

You are asked to transport a patient who is receiving oxygen from a nasal cannula at 4 L/min. The pressure gauge on the cylinder reads 1800 psi. How long will the cylinder provide the appropriate oxygen flow?

$$1800 \text{ psi} \times (0.28 \div 4 \text{ L/min})$$
$$= 126 \text{ min, or about 2 hours}$$

*The cylinder factor represents the relationship between cylinder volume and gauge pressure. Thus an E cylinder can hold 622 L of gas at a filling pressure of 2200 psi. The volume-pressure cylinder factor for E cylinders equals 622 L/2200 psi, or 0.28 L/psi. Table 2-5 shows the cylinder factors for the several commonly used cylinders.

cylinder before and after it is filled. Thus the volume of liquid gas remaining in the cylinder is directly related to the weight of the cylinder. Once the volume is determined, the duration of gas flow can be calculated by dividing that volume by the flow rate of gas being used.

Liquid Oxygen Systems

Hospitals and larger health-care facilities typically rely on bulk liquid supply systems for medical air and oxygen needs. The increased use of bulk liquid supply systems is the result of a couple of factors: (1) gases shipped in bulk are less expensive than gases shipped in cylinders, and (2) liquefied oxygen occupies a fraction of the space required to store gaseous oxygen. Note that gaseous oxygen occupies a volume 860 times that of liquid oxygen.

Construction of bulk gas systems is regulated by the NFPA and the American Society of Mechanical Engineers (ASME). The Bureau of Explosives of the United States Department of the Treasury provides regulations for the design and operation of pressure-release valves.[1,13]

Bulk Liquid Oxygen Systems

The NFPA defines a bulk oxygen system as more than 20,000 ft^3 of oxygen (at atmospheric temperature and pressure), including unconnected reserves, that are on hand at the site.[13] Figure 2-10 illustrates the major components of a bulk oxygen system. It consists of an insulated reservoir, a vaporizer with associated tubing attached to the reservoir, a pressure-reducing valve, and an appropriate pressure-release valve. The reservoir stores a mixture of liquid and gaseous oxygen. The vaporizer acts a heat exchanger where heat is absorbed from the environment and used to warm the liquid oxygen to room temperature, thus forming gaseous oxygen. The pressure-reducing valve serves to reduce the working pressure of the gas to a desired level (usually 50 psi for hospitals and other health-care facilities) before it enters the hospital's compressed gas piping system (see Figure 2-20 for a description of piping systems). The pressure-release valve allows some of the gas on top of the liquid to escape if the contents are warmed too much. This release of gas allows the gas within the container to expand, thus lowering the temperature (see Gay-Lussac's law in Chapter 1). This maintains the gas under pressure between its boiling point and its critical temperature so that the majority of the reservoir's contents will be maintained in the liquid state.

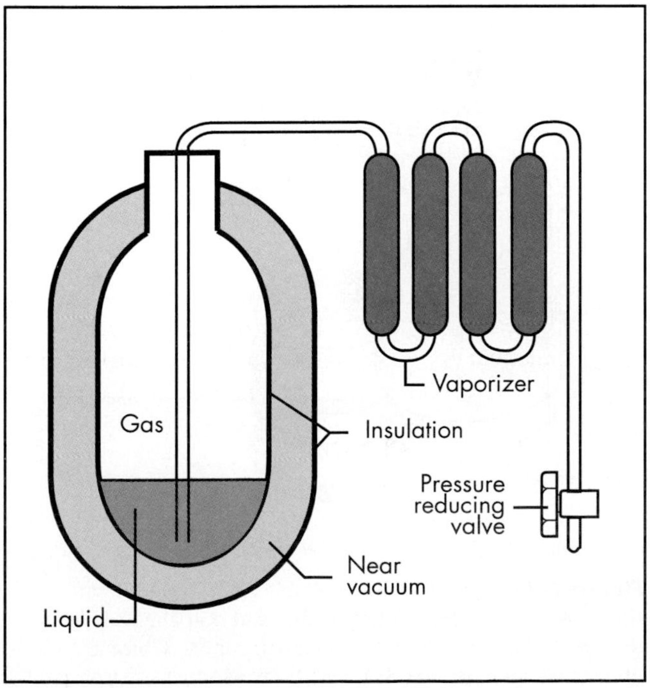

Figure 2-10 Components of a bulk oxygen supply.

As previously stated, bulk reservoir systems must meet specifications provided by the NFPA.[13] Appendix 2-1 contains a summary of the NFPA recommendations and regulations for bulk oxygen systems. Proper installment of these systems is critical to maintain public safety. Figure 2-11 illustrates the minimum distances between bulk oxygen storage facilities and other structures.

Portable Liquid Oxygen Systems. Smaller versions of the bulk oxygen system are available for home-care settings. Figure 2-12 illustrates the Linde PC 500/Walker unit (Union Carbide). Figure 2-13 shows the Linde/Walker portable unit. The main unit contains a liquid reservoir, a vaporizer coil, and a pressure-relief valve. The smaller, portable device, which has a similar design, is filled from the main unit. Most portable systems are designed to provide a working pressure of 20 psi. The Linde unit, however, can provide a working pressure of 90 psi.

Bulk systems used in home care can provide an economical source of oxygen for patients requiring long-term oxygen therapy. These systems generally can provide a reliable source of oxygen for 4 to 6 weeks, depending on the demand. Portable units can provide an 8 to 12 hour supply of oxygen for patients during times of greater mobility. As will be discussed in Chapter 3, oxygen-conserving devices can increase the amount of time that these smaller systems can provide oxygen. Box 2-7 shows how to calculate the duration of a liquid oxygen supply. Remember that the amount of time that a supply will last depends on the weight of the liquid remaining in the reservoir—not the pressure, as for cylinders. Because 1 L of liquid oxygen weighs 2.5 lb, the number of liters of liquid oxygen present can be calculated by dividing the weight of the liquid oxygen by 2.5. Considering that oxygen expands to 860 times its liquid volume at 25° C and 1 atm, the total volume of gaseous oxygen available can be calculated by multiplying the number of liters of liquid oxygen by 860. Then the amount of time in minutes that the supply will last can be determined by dividing this volume by the flow rate of the gas being delivered.

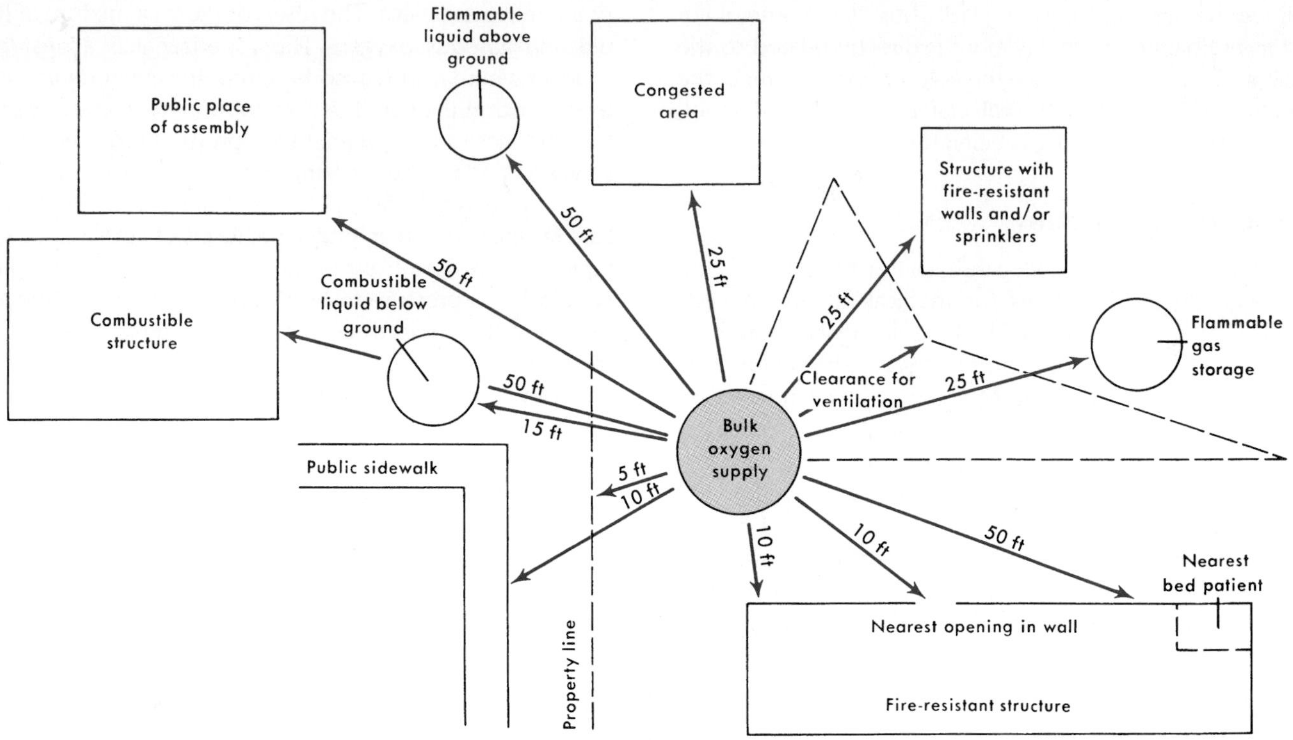

Figure 2-11 Minimum distances for locating structures around a bulk oxygen supply.

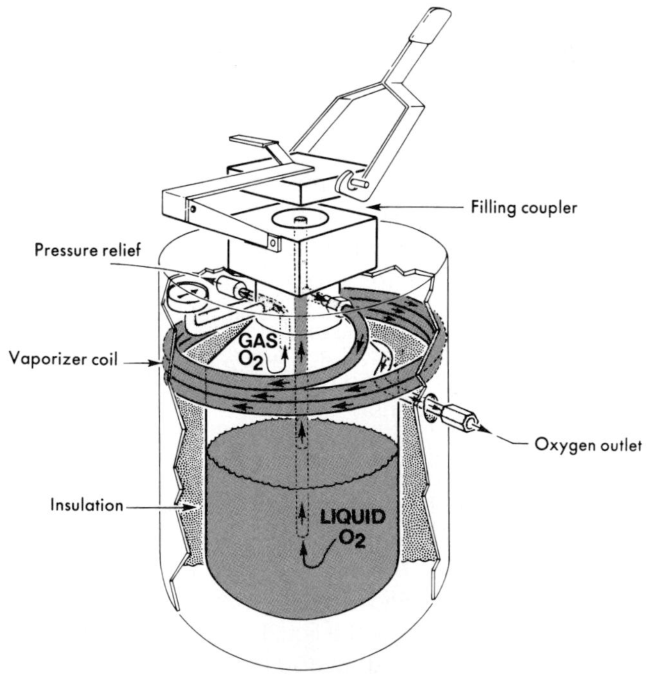

Figure 2-12 Linde PC500/Walker liquid oxygen system. (Modified from Lampton LM: Home and outpatient oxygen therapy. In Brasher RE and Rhodes MI, editors: Chronic obstructive lung disease, St Louis, 1978, Mosby.)

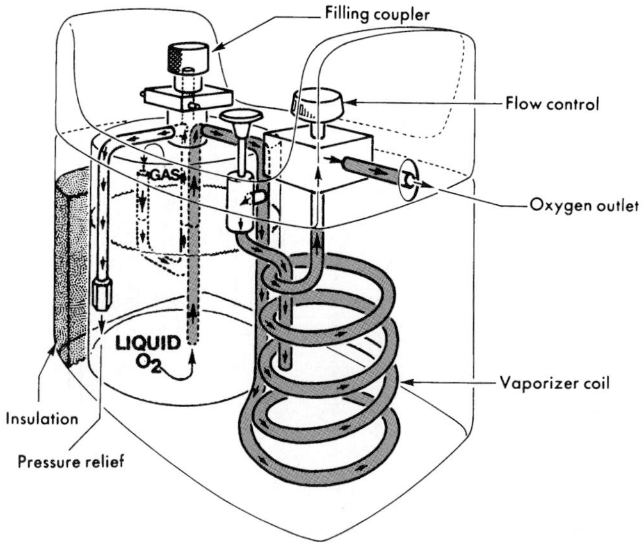

Figure 2-13 Linde/Walker portable liquid oxygen unit. (Modified from Lampton LM: Home and outpatient oxygen therapy. In Brasher RE and Rhodes MI, editors: Chronic obstructive lung disease, St Louis, 1978, Mosby.)

BOX 2-7

Calculating the Duration of a Liquid Oxygen Supply

1. A liter of liquid oxygen weighs 2.5 lbs, so:
   liquid weight/2.5 = # of liters of liquid oxygen.
2. Gaseous oxygen occupies a volume that is 860 times the volume of liquid oxygen, so:
   liters of liquid × 860 = liters of gas.
3. Duration of supply (minutes) = gas supply remaining (in liters) ÷ flow (liters/minute).
   Example:
   How long would a liquid oxygen supply weighing 10 lbs last if a patient were receiving oxygen through a nasal cannula at 2 L/min?

Amount of gas (liters) = (10 lb ÷ 2.5 lb/L) × 860
Amount of gas = 3440 L
Duration of supply (minutes)
= amount of gas ÷ flow (in liters)
Duration of supply = 3440 L ÷ (2 L/min)
Duration of supply = 1720 min,
or about 28 hours and 40 min

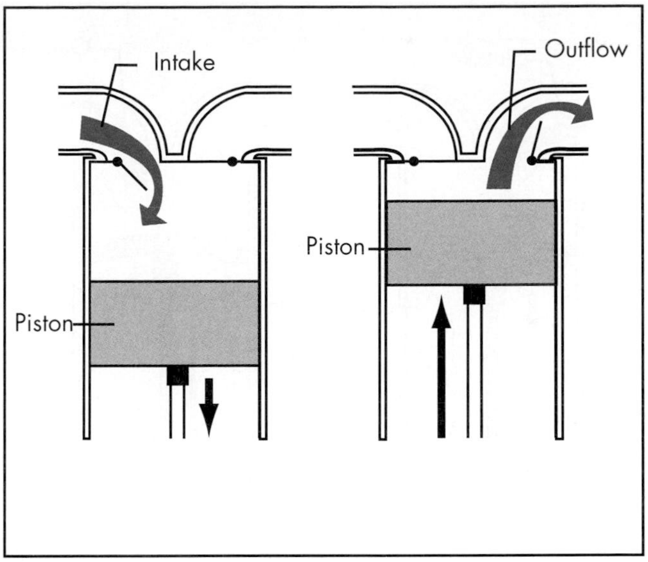

Figure 2-14 Piston air compressor.

It is important to know the operating pressure of the device before attaching flowmeters or restrictors to control gas flow out of the system. Failure to recognize the actual delivery pressure of these devices can result in injury to the patient and/or damage to the attached equipment. The actual flow delivered can be determined with a calibrated **Thorpe-tube flowmeter** (see Chapter 3 for a discussion of flowmeters). Appendix 2-3 lists the NFPA safety recommendations for portable oxygen systems.

Medical Air Supply

Portable Air Compressors

Compressed air is used to power many respiratory care devices. In many cases, air can be compressed at the point of administration by portable air compressors. Larger portable systems can produce compressed air with a standard working pressure of 50 psi; these units can therefore be used to power devices such as pneumatically powered ventilators. Smaller portable compressors, which are unable to achieve these high working pressures, are used for bedside applications (e.g., powering small-volume nebulizers).

Three types of compressors are currently available: piston, diaphragm, and rotary units. **Piston compressors** use the action of a motor-driven piston to compress atmospheric air. The piston is seated within a cylinder casing and is sealed to it with a carbon or Teflon ring. Figure 2-14 illustrates the operational principle of a typical piston air compressor used to power a mechanical ventilator. As the piston retracts, atmospheric air is drawn in through a one-way intake valve. When the piston protracts, the intake valve closes, and gas leaves through a one-way outflow valve. A small gas reservoir is placed in a coiled tube to allow the hot, compressed gas to cool to room temperature before it is delivered to the output valve. The reservoir also removes some of the humidity from the intake gas. There is usually a water drain near the compressor's output, and it is recommended that a water trap be placed between the output and the device to be attached to the compressor to avoid problems with moisture accumulation. Examples of portable piston compressors include the Bennett MC-1 and MC-2 compressors, the Ohio High Performance Compressor, and the Timemeter PCS-1 units.

Diaphragm compressors (Figure 2-15) use a flexible diaphragm attached to a piston to compress gas. As the piston moves down, the diaphragm is bent outward, and gas is drawn through a one-way valve into the cylinder. Upward movement of the piston forces the gas out of the cylinder through a separate one-way outflow valve. Examples of diaphragm compressors are the Air Shields Diapump and the DeVilbiss small nebulizer compressor.

Rotary compressors use a rotating vane to compress air from an intake valve. As the rotating vane turns, gas is drawn into the cylinder through a one-way valve (Figure 2-16). While the rotor turns, the gas is compressed as the oval-shaped cylinder becomes smaller. The compressed gas is then forced out of the compressor through another one-way outflow valve. Low-pressure, rotary compressors are used in ventilators like the Bennett MA-1.

Bulk Air Supply Systems

Bulk systems of compressed air for hospitals and other healthcare facilities can be supplied by a system like the one shown in Figure 2-17. Most bulk air systems use two compressors that

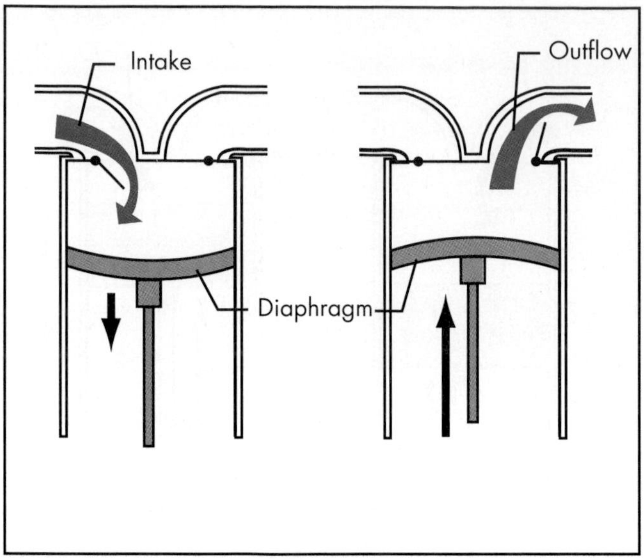

Figure 2-15 Diaphragm compressor.

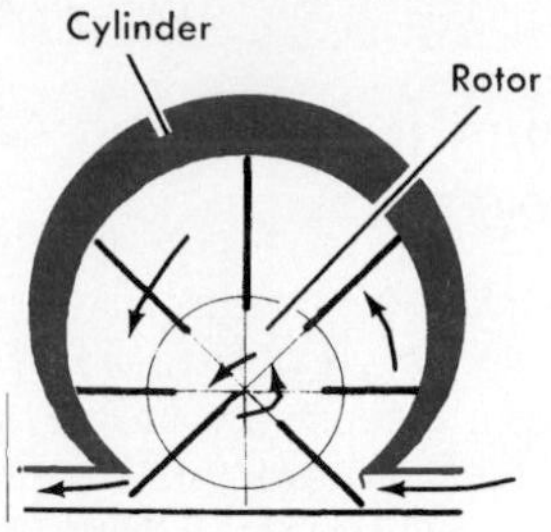

Figure 2-16 Rotary compressor.

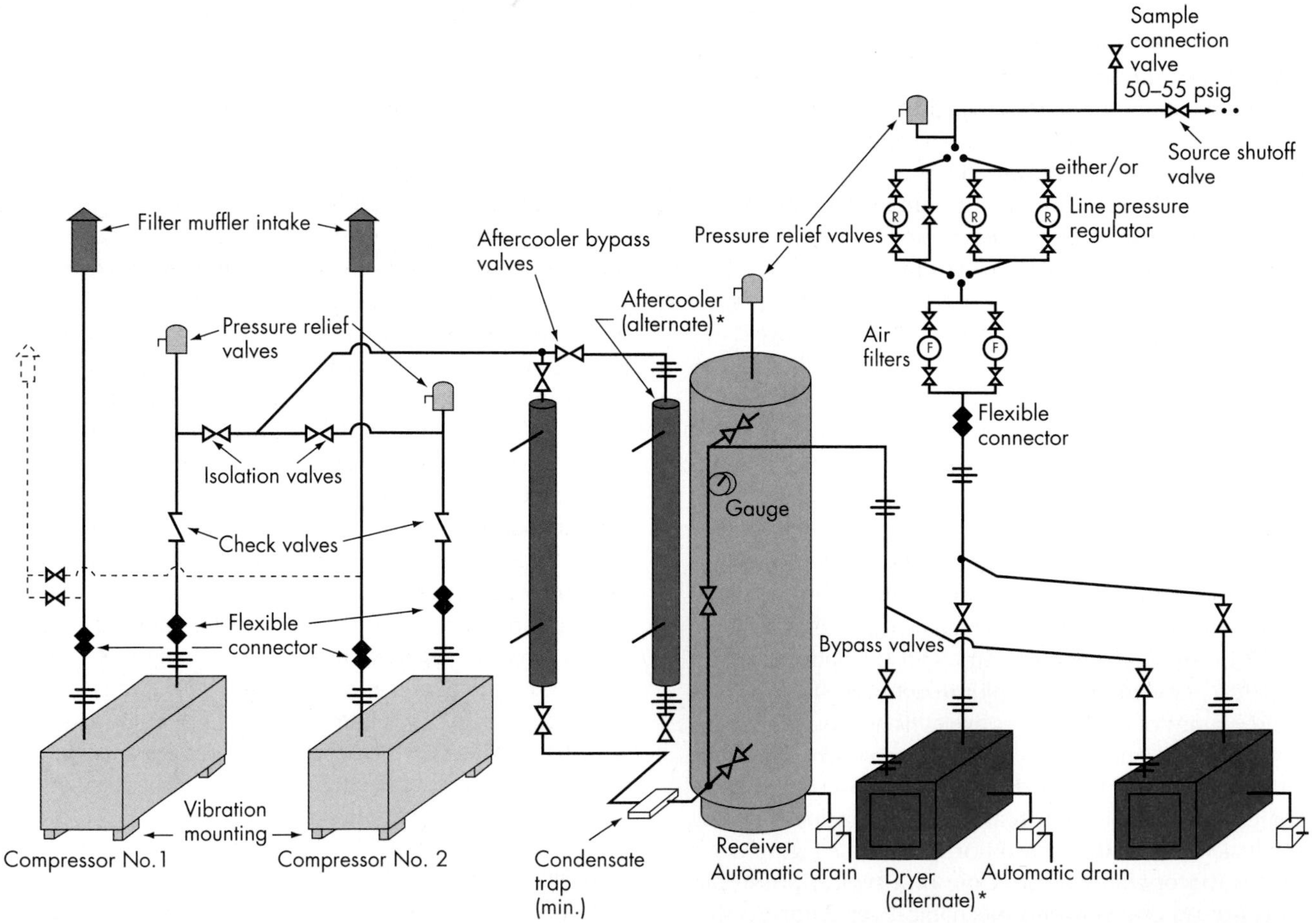

Figure 2-17 Bulk medical air supply. (Modified from Standard for health care facilities, [NFPA99], 1996, copyright National Fire Protection Association, Quincy, Mass.)

BOX 2-8

NFPA Recommendations for Medical Air Supply

1. The source of medical air must be from the outside atmosphere and should not contain contaminants such as particulate matter, odor, or other gases.
2. The air-intake port must be located outdoors, above roof level, at a minimum distance above the ground, and 10 ft from any door, window, or other intake opening in the building. Intake ports must be turned downward and screened.
3. Air taken into the system must contain no contamination from engine exhaust, fuel storage vents, vacuum system discharges, or other particulate matter because odor of any type can be drawn into the system.
4. A minimum of two oil-free compressors must be duplexed together, with provisions for operating alternately or simultaneously, depending on the demand. Each compressor or duplex must be capable of maintaining the air supply to the system at peak demand.
5. Backflow through compressors that are cycled off must be prevented automatically.
6. Each duplex system should be provided with disconnection switches, motor-starting devices with overload protection, and a means of automatically alternating the compressor(s). Use of the compressors should be divided evenly and automatic means of activating additional compressor(s) should be provided in case the supply source unit becomes incapable of maintaining adequate pressure.
7. Air storage tanks or receivers must have a safety valve, an automatic drain, a pressure gauge, and the capacity to ensure practical on-off operation.
8. The type of medical air compressor and the local atmospheric conditions govern the need for intake filters/mufflers, after-coolers for air dryers, and additional downstream regulators.
9. Antivibration mountings are to be installed (in accordance with manufacturer's recommendations) under the components and flexible couplings that connect the air compressors, receivers, and intake and supply lines.
10. A maintenance program must be established following the manufacturer's recommendations.

From Compressed Gas Association: Handbook of compressed gases, ed 3, New York, 1990, Van Nostrand Reinhold.

can operate together or independently, depending on the demand for compressed air. Each compressor should also be able to deliver 100% of the average peak demand if the other compressor is turned off for maintenance or fails to operate. Box 2-8 summarizes the NFPA recommendations for safely operating medical air-supply systems.

Air compressors used in bulk supply systems are usually piston or rotary compressors. Large piston compressors can typically provide a high-flow output and working pressures of at least 50 psi. A reservoir is incorporated into the design of the compressor unit to accommodate varying peak flow needs. The reservoir receives the compressed air and stores it at a higher pressure than in the piping system. A dryer attached to the outflow of the reservoir removes humidity (from refrigeration) from the air entering the piping system. A reducing valve on the reservoir outflow line reduces the pressure to 50 psi or the desired working pressure. In most cases, a pneumatic sensing unit turns the compressor off when the reservoir pressure reaches a preset high level. This sensing unit also turns the compressor back on when the reservoir pressure falls below 50 psi.

High-pressure rotary units require a liquid sealant to efficiency produce high pressures. These systems typically include a reservoir for storing gas under high pressure, a dryer to remove humidity, and a pressure-relief valve to control the output pressure of the compressed gas. A pneumatic sensing unit like those used in piston type of compressors is also used to maintain a constant working pressure of 50 psi and avoid unnecessary high pressures.

Central-Supply Systems

Hospitals and other health-care facilities, such as free-standing clinics, rehabilitation centers, and diagnostic laboratories, typically rely on central-supply systems to provide medical gases to multiple sites within the institution. Two types of central-supply systems are described by the NFPA: **continuous-** and **alternating-supply systems.**[13]

Large hospitals usually rely on continuous supply systems like the one shown in Figure 2-18. A continuous-supply system contains two sources of oxygen supply, one of which serves as a reserve source for use only in an emergency.[13] The primary source is usually a large liquid oxygen or air reservoir, whereas the reserve supply is a smaller liquid reservoir or a bank of compressed-gas cylinders. The primary source must be refilled at regular intervals. NFPA regulations require that the reserve supply contain an average day's supply of oxygen. The NFPA also requires that these systems include a pressure regulator, **check valves,** and a pressure-relief valve between each gas supply and main piping system.

Alternating-supply systems usually consist of two banks of cylinders, one designated as the primary source and the other as the secondary source. Figure 2-19, *A*, illustrates an alternating system without a reserve supply. Each bank of cylinders must contain a minimum of two cylinders or at least an average day's supply of oxygen or air. Once the primary source is depleted or unable to meet system demands, the secondary system automatically becomes the primary source of oxygen or air. The empty

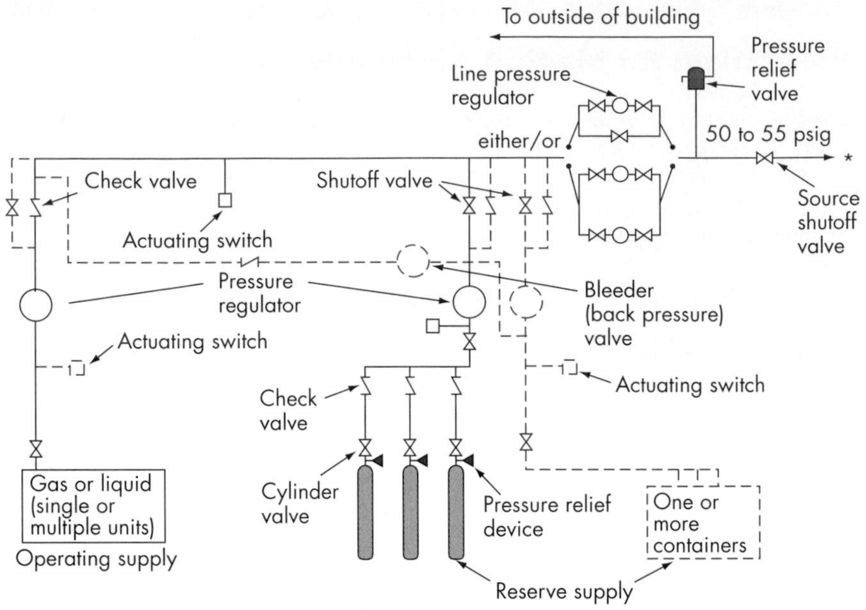

Figure 2-18 Continuous supply system for medical air or oxygen. (Modified from Standard for health care facilities, [NFPA99], 1996, copyright National Fire Protection Association, Quincy, Mass.)

bank is simply refilled or replaced. As a safety feature, an actuating switch must be connected to the master control panel to indicate when the change to the secondary bank is about to occur.[13] Check valves are installed between each cylinder and the manifold to prevent the loss of gas from the manifold cylinders in the event the pressure-relief devices on an individual cylinder functions or a cylinder lead fails.

Figure 2-19 **B** illustrates an alternating system that contains liquid oxygen cylinders as the primary and secondary oxygen sources, along with a reserve oxygen supply of compressed-gas cylinders. The reserve supply, which must include a minimum of three cylinders or an average day's supply of oxygen, is used only when the primary and secondary sources are unable to supply system demands.[13] Note that the system must contain check valves and pressure-relief devices between the gas source and the main supply line. As with the previously described alternating system, an actuating switch signals when the changeover from the primary to the secondary source occurs.

Piping Systems

Gases stored in central-supply units are distributed to various sites or zones within a hospital or health-care facility via a piping system like the one shown in Figure 2-20. NFPA regulations govern the construction, installation, and testing of these systems.[13] Pipes used to transport gases must be seamless type K or L (ASTMB-8) copper tubing or standard weight brass pipe. The size of the pipes must be sufficient to maintain proper delivery volumes and to conform to good engineering practices. The gas contents of the pipeline must be labeled at least every 20 ft and at least once in each room and/or story through which the pipeline travels.

Pressure-regulating devices located between the bulk and the main supply lines must be capable of maintaining a minimum delivery pressure of 50 psi to all station outlets at the maximum delivery-line flow. Pressure-relief valves should be installed downstream from the mainline pressure regulator. A pressure-relief valve should also be installed upstream of any zone valve to prevent excessive pressure in a zone where the shutoff valve is closed. All pressure-relief valves are set 50% higher than the system working pressure (e.g., 75 psi for a 50-psi system pressure).

As already stated, piping systems in hospitals are organized into zones, which allow for quick isolation of all independent areas if maintenance is required. In case of fire, affected zones can be isolated, thus preventing the problem from spreading to other areas of the hospital (Box 2-9). Shutoff valves are located at the point where the mainline enters the hospital, at each riser, and between each zone and the main supply line. Zone shutoff valves for oxygen must be located outside of each critical care unit. Shutoff valves for every oxygen or nitrous oxide line must also be located outside of each surgical suite.

Shutoff valves are generally located in a large box with removable windows large enough to permit manual operation

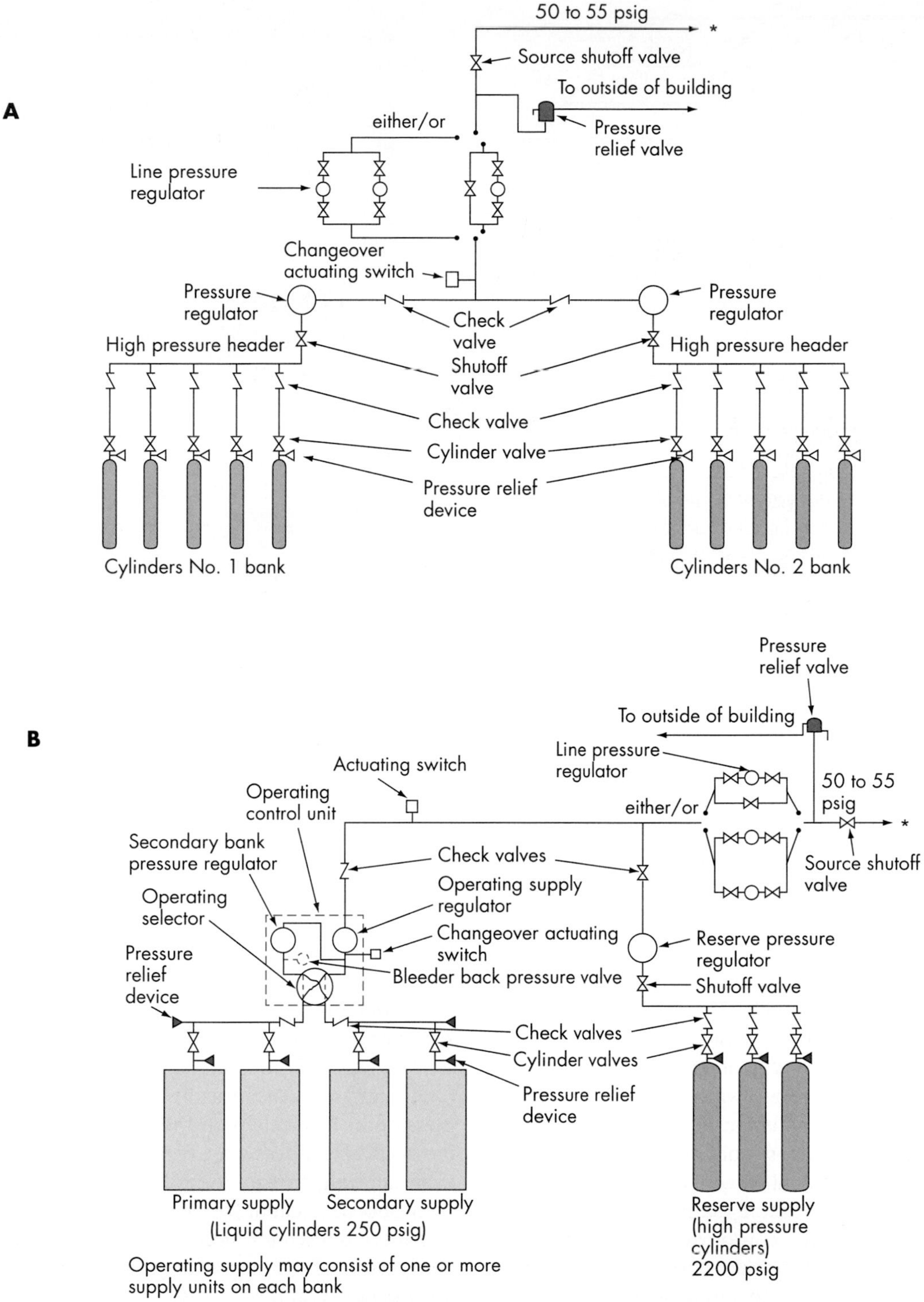

Figure 2-19 Alternating supply systems for medical air or oxygen: **A,** alternating supply without reserve supply; **B,** alternating supply with primary and secondary cylinders. (Modified from Standard for health care facilities, [NFPA99], 1996, copyright National Fire Protection Association, Quincy, Mass.)

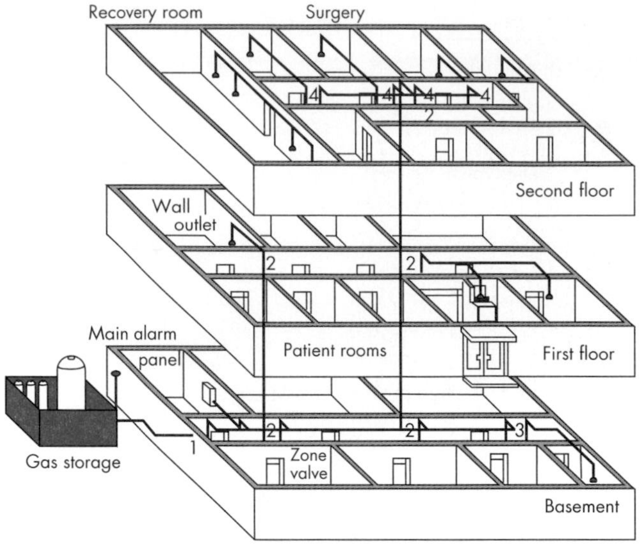

Figure 2-20 Hospital piping system. Zone valves must be placed (1) at the entrance to the hospital, (2) at each riser, (3) at each branch supplying an area, and (4) at each operating room. (Courtesy Nellcor Puritan Bennett, Pleasanton, Calif.)

BOX 2-9

Decision Making & Problem Solving

A fire occurs on the north wing of the fifth floor of the hospital where you work. How should you respond to this emergency?

See Appendix A for answer.

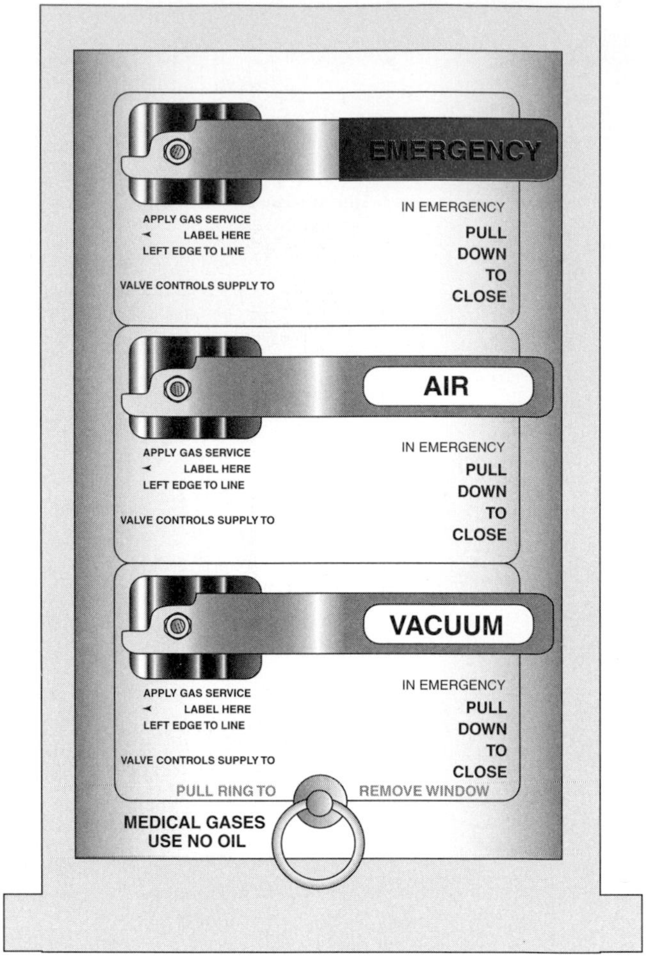

Figure 2-21 Zone shutoff valves for a bulk oxygen supply.

of the valve. They should be installed at a height where they can be operated from the standing position in an emergency. All valves must be labeled as shown in Figure 2-21.

Piping systems must be tested for leaks and to ensure that gas-supply lines have not become crossed. Visual inspection of the system can identify obvious problems, such as worn or loose connections, damaged pipes, pipes soiled with oil, grease, or other oxidizable materials, and crossing of gas supplies (e.g., crossing of compressed air and oxygen supply lines). Crossing of supply lines can be checked by reducing the system pressure to atmospheric and then purging each supply line separately with oil-free dry air or nitrogen. It can also be determined if the gas lines are crossed by analyzing gas samples from the appropriate station outlets. Gases used to purge the supply lines should be passed through a white filter at a flow of 100 L/min to determine if the purge gas is clean and odor-free. The content of gas lines should be tested for purity with the appropriate gas analysis.

All medical gas supply lines should contain alarm systems that alert hospital personnel of system malfunctions (e.g., loss of system pressure, change from the primary system supply source to the secondary and reserve supplies, and reduction in reserve supply below an average day's amount). Alarm panels should include visual and audible alerting signals and should be placed in locations that allow for continuous surveillance (e.g., in the engineering department of the hospital). Alarm systems should also be located in critical-care areas where life-support systems such as mechanical ventilators are used. The Joint Commission on Accreditation of Healthcare Organizations (JCAHO) requires that there is a written policy for responding to alarms and that personnel working in areas where alarms are located are instructed on how to respond.[15] Failure to respond appropriately can end in disaster. Response plans should include ensuring that all patient equipment is working properly and that appropriate personnel (i.e., respiratory care services and engineering) are immediately notified.

Station Outlets

Station outlets provide connections for gas-delivery devices, such as flowmeters and mechanical ventilators. These outlets consist of a body mounted to the supply line, an

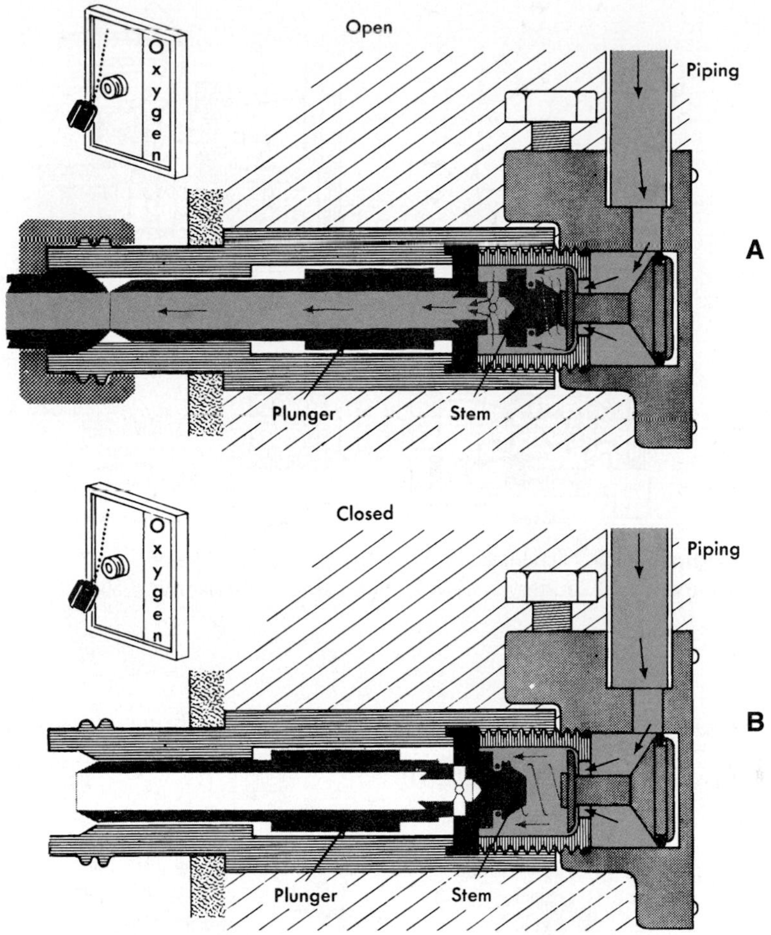

Figure 2-22 Station outlets for a DISS system. (Courtesy Nellcor Puritan Bennett, Pleasanton, Calif.)

outlet faceplate, and primary and secondary check valves, which are safety valves that open when the delivery device's adapter is inserted into the station outlet and which close automatically when the adapter is disengaged from the outlet. Station outlets must not be supplied directly from a riser unless they are supplied through the manual shutoff valve located in the same story as the outlet. Outlet faceplates must be labeled with the name and/or symbol of the delivered gas. They may also be color-coded for easy identification.

Station outlets are designed with safety systems that prevent connection of incompatible devices. Two safety systems are currently available: the **Diameter Index Safety System (DISS)** and **quick-connect adapters.** Figure 2-22 shows an outlet that uses DISS. This system, which was designed by the CGA, uses noninterchangeable, threaded fittings to connect gas-powered devices to station outlets. Each outlet must be fitted with a cap on a chain or installed in a recessed box that is equipped with a door to protect the outlet when not in use. Outlets are typically located about 5 ft above the floor or are recessed to prevent physical damage to the valve or control equipment. Delivery lines that serve anesthetic devices must have a backflow of gas into the system, and the check valves must be able to hold a minimum of 2400 psi.[1,13,15]

Figure 2-23 shows a schematic of a quick-connect type of connection, and Figure 2-24 shows examples of quick-connect adapters. These connections use a plunger that is held forward by a spring to prevent gas from leaving the outlet. Inserting the appropriate adapter pushes the plunger backward, allowing gas to flow into the striker and into the equipment that is attached to the adapter. When the adapter is removed, the spring resets the plunger and closes the outlet.

Oxygen Concentrators

Oxygen concentrators are devices that produce enriched oxygen from atmospheric air. They provide an alternative to compressed-gas cylinders, particularly in the delivery of respiratory therapy to home-care patients. Two types of concentrators are currently available: those using semipermeable plastic membranes and those using molecular sieves.

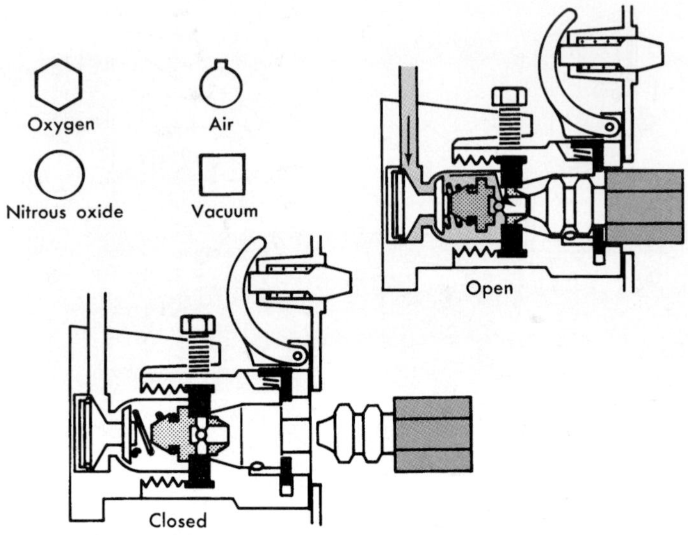

Figure 2-23 Schematic of typical quick-connect type of connection. (Courtesy Nellcor Puritan Bennett, Pleasanton, Calif.)

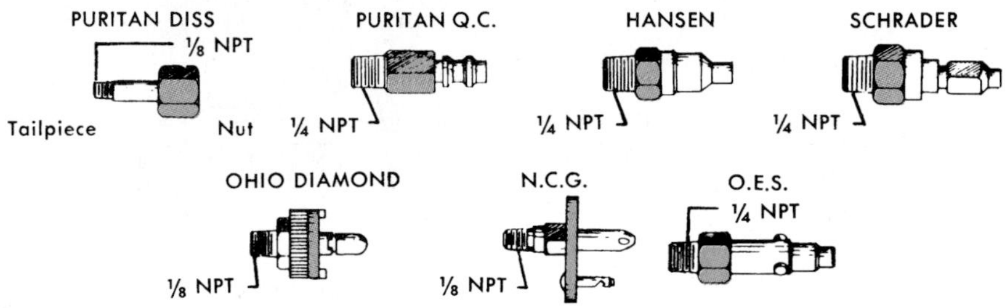

Figure 2-24 Common types of quick-connect adapters. (Courtesy Nellcor Puritan Bennett, Pleasanton, Calif.)

Concentrators using semipermeable membranes to separate oxygen from room air are composed of plastic membranes containing pores that are 1 μm in diameter (1 μm = 1/25,000 in). Atmospheric gases diffuse through the membrane at different rates. The rate at which a gas diffuses depends on its diffusion constant and solubility for the plastic membrane and the pressure gradient for the gas across the membrane. A diaphragm compressor is used to provide a constant vacuum across the membrane.

Oxygen and water vapor diffuse through these membranes faster than nitrogen. Generally, a constant flow of humidified 40% oxygen can be provided for 1 to 10 L/min.[16] The Oxygen Enrichment Company produces two models of concentrators that use this principle of oxygen concentration. Figure 2-25 is a functional diagram of an oxygen concentrator that uses a semipermeable membrane.

Figure 2-26 shows an oxygen concentrator that relies on molecular sieves to produce an enriched oxygen mixture. Such systems use a compressor to pump room air to one of two sets of sieves. Nitrogen is removed by passing room air through sodium-aluminum silicate pellets. Because oxygen passes readily through the pellets, the output contains an enriched oxygen gas. The concentration of oxygen leaving the system depends on the flow rate set. For example, at a flow of 2 L/min, the gas is about 90% oxygen, whereas a flow of 10 L/min contains about 50% oxygen. The DeVO_2/44 (DeVilbiss Company) and the Marx O_2 (Respiratory Support Systems) are examples of molecular sieve concentrators.

Figure 2-27 is a picture of a large concentrating system for producing enriched oxygen mixtures in bulk. This system contains a compressor that supplies air to a refrigerated drying system. Gas exits the refrigeration unit and passes through a 0.015 μm filter. Part of the air flows through a molecular sieve bed at 120 psi. The resulting gas that leaves the molecular sieve contains 92% to 95% oxygen. Air and oxygen are reduced to 50 psi and stored in reservoir tanks. These systems are available for smaller hospitals as well as for recharging oxygen cylinders on site.

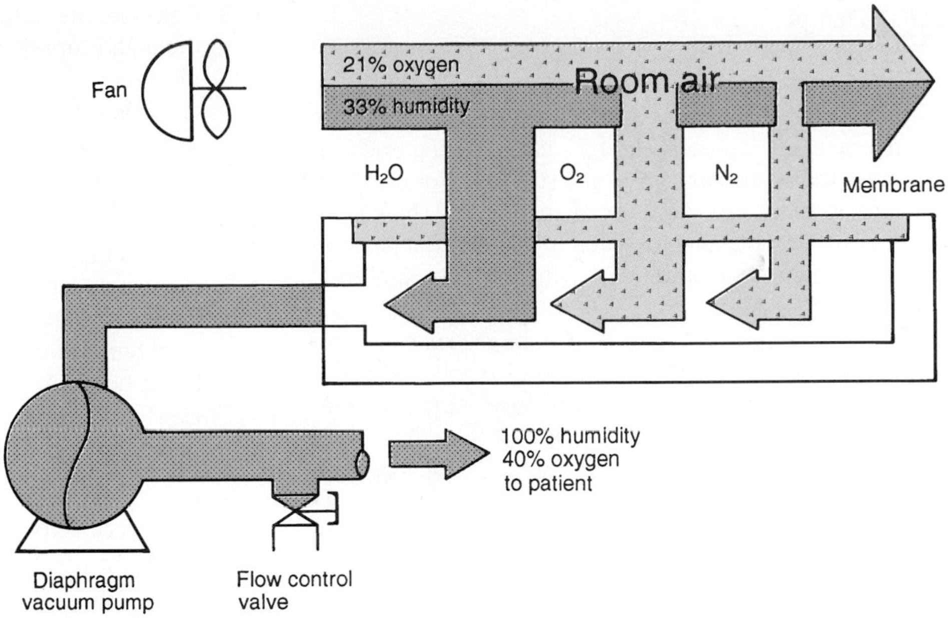

Figure 2-25 Oxygen concentrator that uses semipermeable membrane. (Courtesy Oxygen Enrichment Co, Schenectady, New York.)

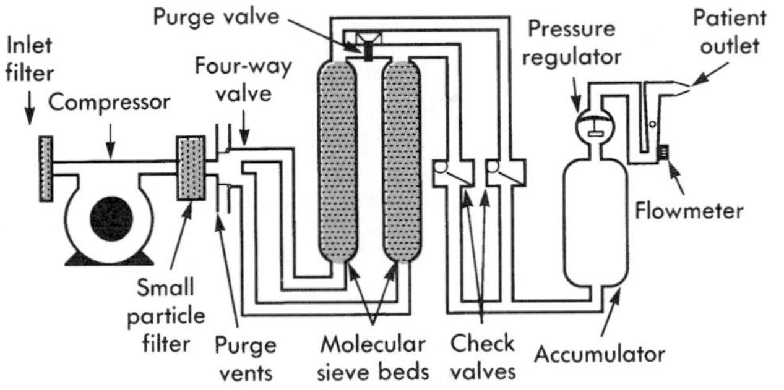

Figure 2-26 Oxygen concentrator that relies on a molecular sieve.

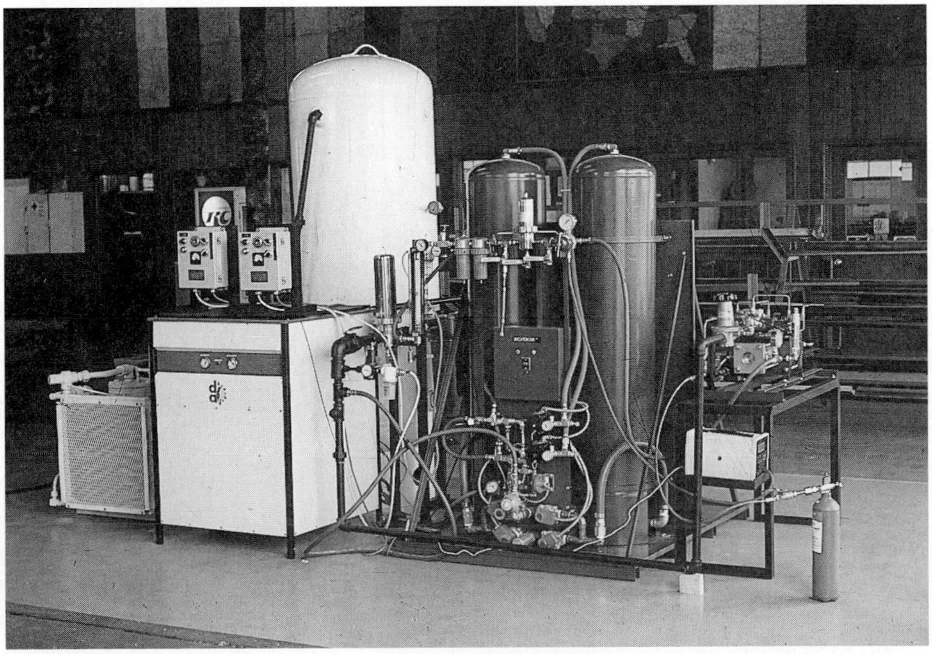

Figure 2-27 Large oxygen concentrator for producing bulk oxygen for a hospital. (Courtesy Dri-Aire, Columbus, California.)

Summary

The information contained in this chapter represents some of the basic principles of respiratory care. Respiratory care practitioners are responsible for administering medical gases and therefore must know the standards for the manufacture, storage, and transport of such gases. These standards provide guidelines for safely using medical gases in the diagnosis and treatment of patients with cardiopulmonary dysfunctions.

Compressed-gas cylinders and bulk gas supplies provide the source gas for the operation of many respiratory care devices. Oxygen concentrators have added another dimension to the home treatment of patients with chronic cardiovascular and pulmonary diseases. Respiratory care practitioners should understand the theory of operation of medical gas supply systems and be able to identify malfunctions that can interfere with the proper delivery of medical gases.

Review Questions

See Appendix A for answers.

1. Which of the following is classified as a nonflammable gas that does not support combustion?
   a. oxygen
   b. carbon dioxide
   c. helium
   d. nitric oxide

2. Medical gas cylinders are color-coded for easy identification. E cylinders of carbon dioxide are painted:
   a. yellow
   b. green
   c. black
   d. gray

3. A respiratory therapist is having trouble attaching a regulator to an E cylinder. One possible cause might be that the:
   a. outlet threads of the cylinder do not match the threads of the regulator
   b. regulator diaphragm is jammed
   c. pin positions of the regulator are not the same as the cylinder
   d. cylinder has not been cracked

4. Bulk liquid oxygen supplies should not be closer than ______ to public sidewalks.
   a. 2 ft
   b. 4 ft
   c. 7 ft
   d. 10 ft

5. Calculate the duration of the liquid oxygen supply if the liquid supply weighs 30 lb and the oxygen demand is 4 L/min.
   a. 10 hours
   b. 23 hours
   c. 35 hours
   d. 43 hours

6. What is the duration of oxygen flow from an H cylinder containing 1200 psi of oxygen when the flow to a nasal cannula is 4 L/min?
   a. 9 hours and 42 minutes
   b. 12 hours and 15 minutes
   c. 15 hours and 42 minutes
   d. 16 hours and 10 minutes

7. Large-piston air compressors employed in bulk supply systems can typically provide working pressures of:
   a. 50 psi
   b. 75 psi
   c. 100 psi
   d. 120 psi

8. Alternating supply systems for medical gases that are used in hospitals should include a reserve supply for oxygen in case the primary system fails. How much reserve oxygen should be available?
   a. an average 8-hour supply
   b. an average day's supply
   c. an average 3-day supply
   d. an average week's supply

9. Oxygen concentrators that use semipermeable membranes can usually provide what percentage of oxygen at flows of 1 to 10 L/min?
   a. 24%
   b. 40%
   c. 60%
   d. 100%

10. The percentage of oxygen delivery provided by molecular sieve O_2 concentrators depends on which of the following factors?
    I. The size of the concentrator
    II. The rate of gas flow
    III. The temperature of the refrigeration unit
    IV. The age of the sieve beds
    a. II only
    b. I and IV only
    c. I, II, and III only
    d. I, II, and IV only

11. The pressure inside a cylinder increases dramatically when the cylinder is exposed to extremely high temperatures. What prevents cylinders with frangible discs from exploding when exposed to extremely high temperatures?

a. the frangible disc will rupture from the increased pressure, allowing gas to escape from the cylinder
b. the cylinder stem will blow off when the temperature reaches 200° F
c. the stem diaphragm will rupture, allowing gas to escape
d. the frangible disc will melt when the temperature reaches 100° F

12. A respiratory therapist is checking cylinder markings to determine if any of the cylinders need to be tested. The labeling reads as follows:

9	83+
6	94+

This information indicates:
a. the cylinder is due for retesting
b. the time between the test dates shown exceeds recommendations
c. the cylinder is made of aluminum
d. the owner of the cylinder

13. Before using an H cylinder of oxygen, a respiratory therapist opens it, and gas at high pressure comes out of the cylinder outlet. Which of the following statements is true?
a. this was an accident and should not be repeated
b. allowing gas to escape from the cylinder lets the therapist smell the gas to ensure it is oxygen
c. this action clears debris from the connector
d. this action should be performed after a regulator is attached to the cylinder outlet

14. A respiratory therapist is helping design a new hospital wing. Which of the following agencies should be contacted so that the piping system of oxygen and air is correctly installed?
a. NFPA
b. FDA
c. HHS
d. DOT

15. A hospital uses a large air compressor system to supply air through its piped gas lines. This gas will be free from pollutants found in the local environment—true or false? Why?

References

1. Compressed Gas Association, Inc: Handbook of compressed gases, ed. 3, New York, 1990, Van Nostrand Reinhold.
2. McPherson S: Respiratory care equipment, ed 4, St Louis, 1990, Mosby.
3. Dorsch JA and Dorsch SE: Understanding anesthesia equipment: construction, care, and complications, Baltimore, 1975, Williams & Wilkins.
4. Scanlan CL, Spearman CB, and Sheldon RL: Egan's fundamentals of respiratory care, ed 6, St Louis, 1995, Mosby.
5. Howder CL: Cardiopulmonary pharmacology, ed 2, Baltimore, 1996, Williams & Wilkins.
6. Kinsella JP, et al: Clinical response to prolonged treatment of persistent pulmonary hypertension of the newborn with low doses of inhaled nitric oxide, J Pediatr 123(1): 103, 1993.
7. Gerlach H, et al: Long term inhalation with evaluated low doses of nitric oxide for improvement of oxygenation in patients with adult respiratory distress syndrome, Intensive Care Med 19(8): 443, 1993.
8. Hunsinger DL, et al: Respiratory technology: a procedure manual, ed 2, Reston, Virginia, 1976, Prentice Hall.
9. Schreiber P: Anesthetic equipment, New York, 1972, Springer-Verlag.
10. McPherson S: Respiratory care equipment, ed 5, St Louis, 1995, Mosby.
11. Code of Federal Regulations: Title 49, Parts 1-199, Washington, DC, 1974, US Government Printing Office.
12. Compressed Gas Association: Handbook of compressed gases, New York, 1965, Holt-Reinhold.
13. National Fire Protection Association: Standard for health care facilities, New York, 1993, ANSI/NFPA 99.
14. Blaze C: Quick reference to respiratory care equipment assembly and troubleshooting, St Louis, 1995, Mosby.
15. Klein BR, editor: Health care facilities handbook, ed 4, Quincy, Mass., 1993 National Fire Protection Association.
16. Lampton LM: Home and outpatient oxygen therapy. In Harchear RE and Rhodes MI, editors: Chronic obstructive lung disease: clinical treatment and management. St Louis, 1978, Mosby.

Internet Resources

1. American Association for Respiratory Care:
http://www.aarc.org
2. Joint Commission on Health Care Organizations:
http://www.jcaho.org
3. The RT Corner, A Website for the Respiratory Therapy Student:
http://www.rtcorner.com
4. GasNet—Global Anesthesiology Server Network:
http://gasnet.med.yale.edu
5. Susquehanna Micro Inc.:
http://www.susquemicro.com/frames/smi_a.html
6. Nellcor Puritan Bennett:
http://www.nellcorpb.com
7. Ohmeda Medical:
http://www.ohmedamedical.com

APPENDIX 2-1

NFPA and CGA Recommendations for Cylinders

Storage

1. Storage rooms must be dry, cool, and well-ventilated. Cylinders should not be stored in an area where the temperature exceeds 51.67° C (125° F).
2. No flames should have the potential of coming in contact with the cylinders.
3. The storage facility should be fire-resistant where practical.
4. Cylinders must not be stored near flammable or combustible substances.
5. Those gases supporting combustion must be stored in a separate location from those that are combustible.
6. The storage area must be permanently posted.
7. Cylinders must be grouped by content.
8. Full and empty cylinders must be segregated in the storage areas.
9. Below-ground storage should be avoided.
10. Cylinders should never be stored in the operating room.
11. Large cylinders must be stored upright.
12. Cylinders must be protected from being cut or abraded.
13. Cylinders must be protected from extreme weather to prevent rusting, excessive temperatures, and accumulations of snow and ice.
14. Cylinders should not be exposed to continuous dampness or corrosive substances that could promote rusting of the cylinder and its valve.
15. Cylinders should be protected from tampering.
16. Valves on empty cylinders should be kept closed at all times.
17. Cylinders must be stored with protective caps in place.
18. Cylinders must not be stored in a confined space, such as a closet or the trunk of a car.

Transportation

1. If protective valve caps are supplied, they should be used whenever cylinders are in transport and until they are ready for use.
2. Cylinders must not be dropped, dragged, slid, or allowed to strike each other violently.
3. Cylinders must be transported on an appropriate cart secured by a chain or strap.

Use

1. Before connecting equipment to a cylinder, be certain that connections are free of foreign materials.
2. Turn valve outlet away from personnel, and crack cylinder valve to remove any dust or debris from outlet.
3. Cylinder valve outlet connections must be American Standard or CGA pin indexed, and low-pressure connections must be CGA diameter indexed.
4. Cylinders must be secured at the administration site and not to any movable objects or heat radiators.
5. Outlets and connections must only be tightened with appropriate wrenches and must never be forced on.
6. Equipment designed to use one gas should not be used with another.
7. Never use medical cylinder gases when contamination by backflow of other gases may occur.
8. Regulators should be off when the cylinder is turned on, and the cylinder valve should be opened slowly.
9. Before equipment is disconnected from a cylinder, the cylinder valve should be closed and the pressure released from the device.
10. Cylinder valves should be closed at all times, except when in use.
11. Do not transfill cylinders because this is hazardous.
12. Cylinders may be refilled only if permission is secured from the owner.
13. Cylinders must not be lifted by the cap.
14. Equipment connected to cylinders containing gaseous oxygen should be labeled: OXYGEN–USE NO OIL.
15. Enclosures intended to contain patients must have the minimum text regarding NO SMOKING (as indicated in Figure 2-5, and the labels must be located (1) in a

position to be read by the patients and (2) on two or more opposing sides visible from the exterior. It should be noted that oxygen hoods fall under the classification of oxygen enclosures and require these labels as well. In addition, another label is required that instructs visitors to get approval from hospital personnel before placing toys into an oxygen enclosure.

16. High-pressure oxygen equipment must not be sterilized with flammable agents (for example, alcohol and ethylene oxide), and the agents used must be oil-free and nondamaging.
17. Polyethylene bags must not be used to wrap sterilized high-pressure oxygen equipment because when flexed, polyethylene releases pure hydrocarbons that are highly flammable.
18. Oxygen equipment exposed to pressures of less than 60 psi may be sterilized with either a nonflammable mixture of ethylene oxide and carbon dioxide or with fluorocarbons.
19. Cylinders must not be handled with oily or greasy hands, gloves, or clothing.
20. *Never lubricate* valve outlets or connecting equipment. (Oxygen and oil under pressure cause an explosive oxidation reaction.)
21. Do not flame test for leaks. (Usually a soap solution is used.)
22. When in use, open valve fully and then turn it back a quarter- to a half-turn.
23. Replace cap on empty cylinder.
24. Position the cylinder so that the label is clearly visible. The label must not be defaced, altered, or removed.
25. Check label *before* use; it should always match the color code.
26. No sources of open flames should be permitted in the area of administration. A NO SMOKING sign must be posted at the administration site. It must be legible from a distance of 5 ft and displayed in a conspicuous location.
27. Inform all area occupants of the hazards of smoking and of the regulations.
28. Equipment designated for use with a specific gas must be clearly and permanently labeled accordingly. The name of the manufacturer should be clearly marked on the device. If calibration or accuracy is dependent on gas density, the device must be labeled with the proper supply pressure.
29. Cylinder carts must be of a self-supporting design with appropriate casters and wheels, and those intended for use in surgery where flammable anesthetics are used must be grounded.
30. Cold cylinders must be handled with care to avoid hand injury resulting from tissue freezing caused by rapid gas expansion.
31. Safety-relief mechanisms, uninterchangeable connections, and other safety features must not be removed or altered.
32. Control valves on equipment must be closed both before connection and when not in use.

REPAIR AND MAINTENANCE

1. Use only the service manuals, operator manuals, instructions, procedures, and repair parts that are provided or recommended by the manufacturer.
2. Allow only qualified personnel to maintain the equipment.
3. Designate and set aside an area clean and free of oil and grease for the maintenance of oxygen equipment. Do not use this area for the repair and maintenance of other types of equipment.
4. Follow a scheduled preventive maintenance program.

APPENDIX 2-2

NFPA Recommendations and Regulations for Bulk Oxygen Systems

1. Containers that are permanently installed should be mounted on noncombustible supports and foundations.
2. Liquid oxygen containers should be constructed from materials that meet the impact test requirements of paragraph UG-48 of the ASME Boiler and Pressure Vessel Codes, Section VII, and must be in accordance with DOT specifications and regulations for 4 L liquid oxygen containers. Containers operating above 15 psi must be designed and tested in accordance with the ASME Boiler and Pressure Vessel Code, Section VII, and the insulation of the liquid oxygen container must be of noncombustible material.
3. All high-pressure gaseous oxygen containers must comply with the construction and test requirements of ASME Boiler and Pressure Vessel Code, Section VIII.
4. Bulk oxygen storage containers must be equipped with safety-release devices as required by ASME Code IV and the provisions of ASME S-1.3 or DOT specifications for both the container and safety releases.
5. Isolation casings on liquid oxygen containers shall be equipped with suitable safety-release devices. These devices must be designed or located so that moisture cannot either freeze the unit or interfere in any manner with its proper operation.
6. The vaporizing columns and connecting pipes shall be anchored and/or sufficiently flexible to provide for expansion and contraction as a result of temperature changes. The column must also have a safety-release device to properly protect it.
7. Any heat supplied to oxygen vaporizers must be done in an indirect fashion, such as with steam, air, water, or water solutions that do not react with oxygen. If liquid heaters are used to provide the primary source of heat, the vaporizers must be electrically grounded.
8. All equipment composing the bulk system must be cleaned to remove oxidizable material before the system is placed into service.
9. All joints and connections in the tubing should be made by welding or using flanged, threaded slip, or compressed fittings; and any gaskets or thread seals must be of suitable substance for oxygen service. Any valves, gauges, or regulators placed into the system must be designed for oxygen service. The piping must conform to ANSI B 31.3; piping that operates below −20° F must be composed of materials meeting ASME Code, Section VIII.
10. Storage containers, piping valves, and regulating equipment must be protected from physical damage and tampering.
11. Any enclosure containing oxygen control or operating equipment must be adequately ventilated.
12. The location shall be permanently posted to indicate "OXYGEN–NO SMOKING–NO OPEN FLAMES" or an equivalent warning.
13. All bulk systems must be regularly inspected by qualified representatives of the oxygen supplier.
14. Weeds and tall grass must be kept a minimum of 15 ft from any bulk oxygen container. The bulk oxygen system must be located so that its distance provides maximum safety for other areas surrounding it. The minimum distances for location of a bulk oxygen system near the following structures (Figure 2-11) are as follows:
    a. 50 ft from any combustible structure.
    b. 25 ft from any structure that consists of fire-resistant exterior walls or buildings of other construction that have sprinklers.
    c. 10 ft from any opening in the adjacent walls of fire-resistant structures.
    d. 50 ft from flammable liquid storage above ground that is less than 1000 gallons in capacity, or 90 ft from these storage areas if the quantity is in excess of 1000 gallons.
    e. 15 ft from an underground flammable liquid storage that is less than 1000 gallons, or 30 ft from one in excess of 1000 gallons capacity. The distance from the oxygen storage containers to connections used for filling and venting of flammable liquid must be at least 50 ft.
    f. 25 ft from combustible gas storage above ground that is less than 1000 gallons capacity, or 50 ft from the storage of over 1000 gallons capacity.

g. 15 ft from combustible liquid storage underground and 40 ft from the vent or filling connections.
h. 50 ft from flammable gas storage less than 5000 ft^3; 90 ft from flammable gas in excess of 5000 ft^3 NTP.
i. 25 ft from solid materials that burn slowly (e.g., coal and heavy timber).
j. 75 ft away in one direction and 35 ft away at an approximately 90-degree angle from confining walls unless they are made from a fire-resistant material and are less than 20 ft high. (This is to provide adequate ventilation in the area in case venting occurs.)
k. 50 ft from places of public assembly.
l. 50 ft from nonambulatory patients.
m. 10 ft from public sidewalks.
n. 5 ft from any adjoining property line.
o. Must be accessible by a mobile transport unit that fills the supply system.

15. The permanent installation of a liquid oxygen system must be supervised by personnel familiar with the proper installation and construction as outlined in the NFPA 50.
16. The oxygen supply must have an inlet for the connection of a temporary supply in emergency and maintenance situations. The inlet must be physically protected to prevent tampering or unauthorized use and must be labeled: "EMERGENCY LOW-PRESSURE GASEOUS OXYGEN INLET." The inlet is to be installed downstream from the main supply line shutoff valve and must have the necessary valves to provide the emergency supply of oxygen as well as isolate the pipeline to the normal source of supply. There must be a check valve in the main line between the inlet connection and the main shutoff valve and another check valve between the inlet connection and the emergency supply shutoff valve. The inlet connection must have a pressure-relief valve of adequate size to protect the downstream piping from pressures in excess of 50% above normal pipeline operating pressure.
17. The bulk oxygen system must be mounted on noncombustible supports and foundations.
18. A surface of noncombustible material must extend at least 3 ft beyond the reach of liquid oxygen leaks during system operation or filling. Asphalt or bitumastic paving is prohibited. The slope of the area must be considered in the sizing of the surface.
19. The same type of surface must extend at least the full width of the vehicle that fills the bulk unit and at least 8 ft in the transverse direction.
20. No part of the bulk system should be underneath electrical power lines or within reach of a downed power line.
21. No part of the system can be exposed to flammable gases or to piping containing any class of flammable or combustible liquids.
22. The system must be located so as to be readily accessible to mobile supply equipment at ground level as well as to authorized personnel.
23. Warning and alarm systems are required to monitor the operation and condition of the supply system. Alarms and gauges are to be located for the best possible surveillance, and each alarm and gauge must be appropriately labeled.
24. The master alarm system must monitor the source of supply, the reserve (if any), and the mainline pressure of the gas system. The power source for warning systems must meet the essentials of NFPA 76A.
25. All alarm conditions must be evaluated, and necessary measures taken to establish or ensure the proper function of the supply system.
26. Two master alarm panels, with alarms that cannot be canceled, are to be located in separate locations to ensure continuous observation. One signal must alert the user to a changeover from one operating supply to another, and an additional signal must provide notification that the reserve is supplying the system.
27. If check valves are not installed in the cylinder leads and headers, another alarm signal should be initiated when the reserve reaches a 1-day supply.
28. All piping systems must have both audible and visible signals that cannot be canceled to indicate when the mainline pressure increases or decreases 20% from the normal supply pressure. A pressure gauge must be installed and appropriately labeled adjacent to the switch that generates the pressure alarm conditions.
29. All warning systems must be tested before being placed in service or being added to existing service. Periodic retesting and appropriate recordkeeping are required.

APPENDIX 2-3

NFPA Safety Recommendations and Regulations for Portable Liquid Oxygen Systems

1. Liquid oxygen units will vent gas when not in use, creating an oxygen-enriched environment. This can be particularly hazardous in the following situations:
   a. When the unit is stored in a closed space.
   b. When the unit is tipped over.
   c. When the oxygen is transferred to another container.
2. Liquid oxygen units should not be located adjacent to heat sources, which can accelerate the venting of oxygen.
3. The unit surface should not be contaminated with oil or grease.
4. Verify the contents of liquid containers when setting up the equipment, changing the containers, or refilling the containers at the home.
5. Connections for containers are to be made with the manufacturer's operating instructions.
6. The patient and family must be familiar with the proper operation of the liquid devices along with all precautions, safeguards, and troubleshooting methods.
7. Transfill one unit from another in compliance with CGA pamphlet P-26, "Transfilling of Low Pressure Liquid Oxygen to be Used for Respiration," and in accordance with the manufacturer's operating instructions.
8. All connections for filling must conform to CGA V-1, and the hose assembly must have a pressure release set no higher than the container's rated pressure.
9. Liquid containers must have a pressure release to limit the container pressure to the rated level, and a device must also be incorporated to limit the amount of oxygen introduced into a container to the manufacturer's specified capacity.
10. Delivery vehicles should be well-vented to prevent the buildup of high oxygen levels, and transfilling should take place with the delivery vehicle doors wide open.
11. "No smoking" signs must be posted, and there can be no sources of ignition within 5 ft.
12. The transfiller must affix the labels required by DOT and FDA regulations, and records must be kept stating the content and purity. Instructions must be on the container, and the color-coding and labeling must meet CGA and NFPA standards.
13. All devices used with liquid oxygen containers must be moisture-free, and pressure releases must be positioned correctly to prevent freezing and the buildup of high pressures.
14. When liquid oxygen is spilled, both the liquid and gas that escape are very cold and will cause frostbite or eye injury. When filling liquid oxygen containers, wear safety goggles with side shields, along with loose-fitting, properly insulated gloves. High-top boots with cuffless pants worn outside of the boots are recommended.
15. Items exposed to liquid oxygen should not be touched because they cannot only cause frostbite, but can stick to the skin. Materials that are pliable at room temperature become brittle at the extreme temperatures of liquid oxygen.
16. If a liquid oxygen spill occurs, the cold liquid and resulting gas condense the moisture in the air, creating a fog. Normally, the fog will extend over an area that is larger than the area of contact danger, except in extremely dry climates.
17. In the event of a spill, measures should be taken to prevent anyone from walking on the surface or wheeling equipment across the area for at least 15 minutes. All sources of ignition must be kept away from the area.
18. Liquid oxygen spilled onto asphalt or oil-soaked concrete constitutes an extreme hazard because an explosive reaction can occur.
19. If liquid oxygen or gas comes in contact with the skin, remove any clothing that may constrict blood flow to the frozen area. Warm the affected area with water at about body temperature until medical personnel arrive. Seek immediate medical attention for eye contact or blistering of the skin.
20. Immediately remove contaminated clothing and air it away from sources of ignition for at least an hour.

CHAPTER 3

CHAPTER OUTLINE

KEY TERMS

Adjustable, Multiple-Orifice Flow Restrictors
Adjustable Regulators
Back Pressure-Compensated
Boothby-Lovelace-Bulbulian (BLB) Mask
Bourdon Flowmeters
Carbogen
Fixed-Performance Oxygen Delivery System
Fixed-Orifice Flow Restrictors
Fixed-Performance Devices
Flow-Restrictor Multistage Regulators
Flow Restrictors
French
Heliox
Monoplace Hyperbaric Chamber
Multiplace Hyperbaric Chamber
Multistage Regulators
Mustache Cannula
Non-Pressure–Compensated
Oxygen Adder
Oxygen Blender
Pendant Cannula
Pulse-Demand Oxygen Delivery System
Preset Regulators
Pressure-Compensated
Single-Stage Regulators
Thorpe-Tube Flowmeters
Variable-Performance Oxygen Delivery System

Administering Medical Gases: Regulators, Flowmeters, and Controlling Devices

J. M. Cairo

CHAPTER LEARNING OBJECTIVES

Upon completion of this chapter, the reader should be able to:

1. Compare the design and operation of single-stage and multistage regulators.
2. Identify the components of preset and adjustable regulators.
3. Explain the operational theory of a Thorpe-tube flowmeter, a Bourdon flowmeter, and a flow restrictor.
4. Demonstrate a method for determining if a flowmeter is pressure-compensated.
5. Compare low-flow and high-flow oxygen delivery systems.
6. Name several commonly used low-flow oxygen delivery systems.
7. Discuss the advantages and disadvantages of oxygen-conserving devices.
8. Explain the operational theory of air-entrainment devices.
9. Compare the operation of oxygen blenders with that of oxygen mixers and adders.
10. Describe the physiological effects of hyperbaric oxygen therapy.
11. List the indications and contraindications of nitric oxide therapy.
12. Describe the appropriate use of mixed-gas (e.g., heliox, carbogen) therapy.

Administering medical gases is one of the primary responsibilities of respiratory therapists. This responsibility stems from work that began in several 18th century physiology laboratories and came to fruition in the clinical settings of the middle of the 20th century. Barcroft, Davies and Gilchrist, Barach, and others made significant contributions to the theory and practice of oxygen therapy by designing apparatuses to deliver oxygen to dyspneic patients.[1] Cogent studies performed by these and other scientists demonstrated the value of oxygen therapy and laid the foundation for respiratory care professions.

As the responsibilities of respiratory therapists continue to grow, all practitioners must understand the principles of oxygen therapy, as well as other forms of medical gas therapy, including nitric oxide and hyperbaric oxygen therapy. Therefore, this chapter will review the operational principles of devices commonly used to administer medical gases.

Regulators and Flowmeters

Regulators (or reducing valves) are devices that reduce high-pressure gases from cylinders or bulk storage units to lower working pressures, usually to 50 psi. Flowmeters are devices that control and indicate the gas flow delivered to patients.

Regulators

Regulators are generally classified as **single-stage** or **multistage**. They can be further divided into **preset** and **adjustable regulators**. Preset regulators deliver a specific outlet pressure; adjustable regulators can deliver a range of outlet pressures.

Single-Stage Regulators

Figure 3-1 shows the components of a typical preset single-stage regulator, which consists of a body that is divided in half by a flexible metal diaphragm. The area above the diaphragm is a high-pressure chamber. The lower chamber has a spring attached to the lower surface of the diaphragm and is exposed to ambient pressure. A valve stem attached to the upper half of the diaphragm sits on the high-pressure inlet to the upper chamber. Note that excess pressures in the upper chamber can be released through a pressure-relief valve that opens if the regulator malfunctions and the pressure inside the high-pressure chamber rises to 200 psig.

The gas flow into the high-pressure side of the regulator is dependent upon the effects of two opposing forces: gas pressure above the diaphragm and spring tension below the diaphragm. When the force offered by the high-pressure gas above the diaphragm equals the force offered by spring tension, the diaphragm is straight and the inlet valve is closed. If the force offered by the spring exceeds

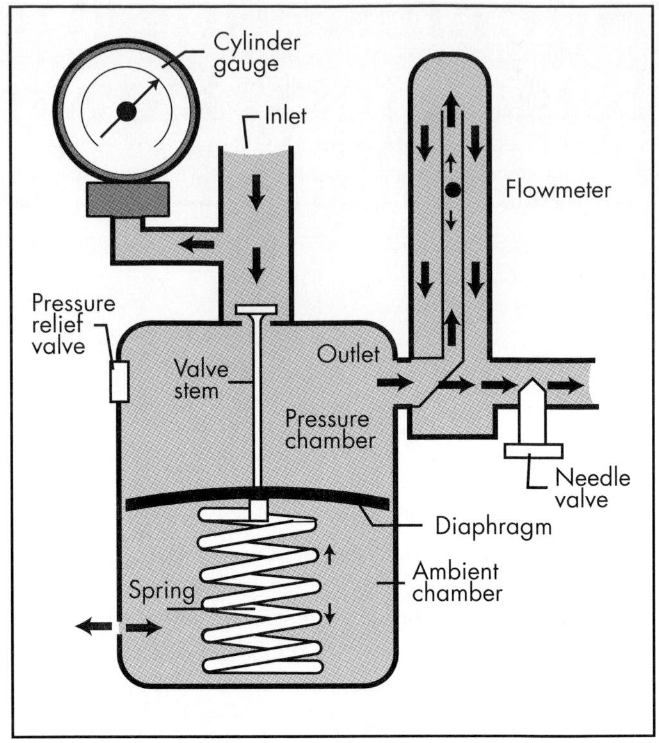

Figure 3-1 Components of a single-stage regulator. (Redrawn from Persing G: Entry level respiratory care review, Philadelphia, 1992, Saunders.)

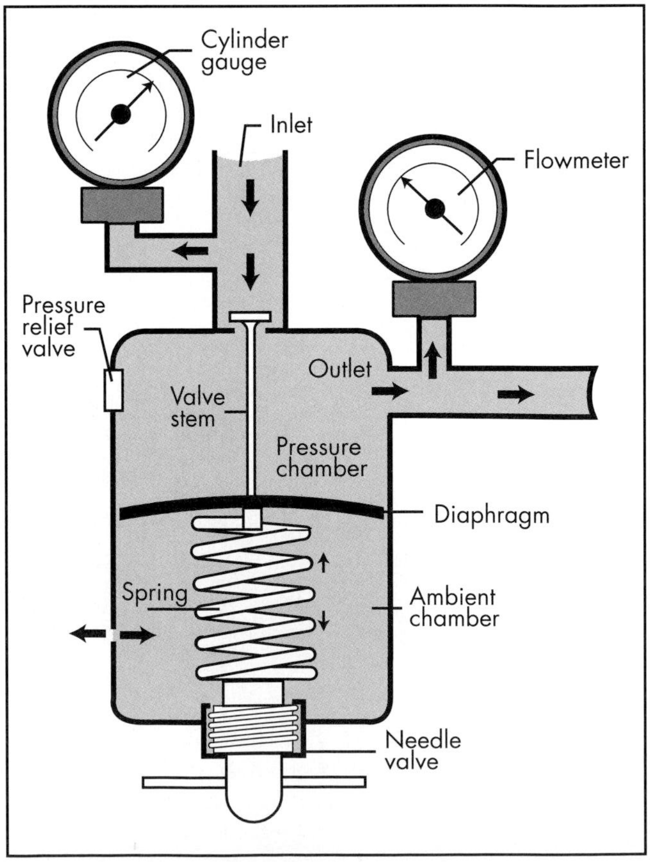

Figure 3-2 Components of an adjustable, single-stage regulator. (Redrawn from Persing G: Entry level respiratory care review, Philadelphia, 1992, Saunders.)

the force offered by the gas pressure, the spring expands the diaphragm and opens the inlet valve.

For a preset single-stage regulator, the spring tension is calibrated to deliver gas at a preset pressure (usually 50 psig). Adjustable regulators like the one in Figure 3-2 allow the operator to adjust the spring tension (and thus control the outlet pressure) by using a threaded hand control attached to the spring-diaphragm apparatus. Most adjustable regulators can be set to deliver pressures between 0 and 100 psig.

Multistage Regulators

Multistage regulators are simply two or more single-stage regulators in a series. Figure 3-3 is a schematic of a two-stage

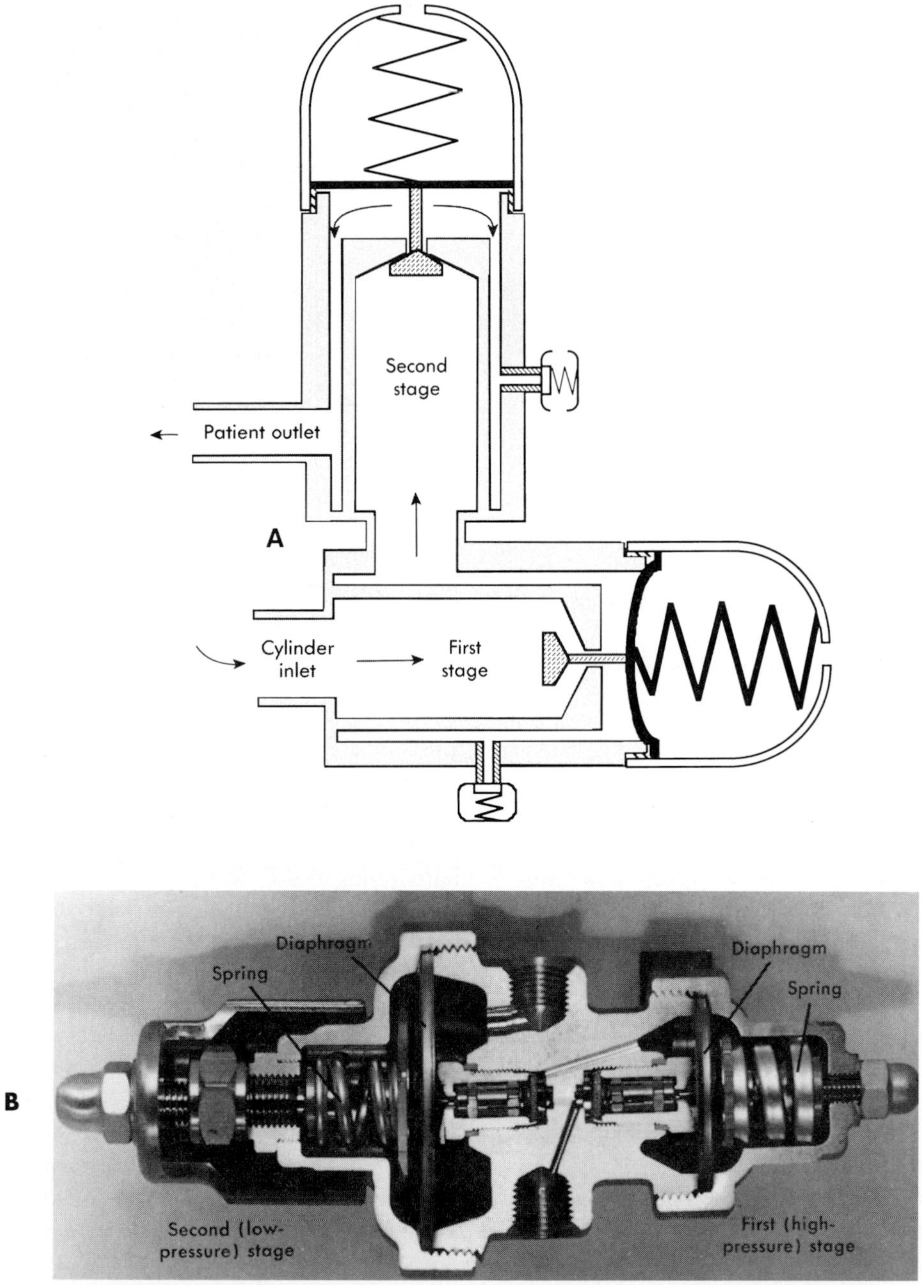

Figure 3-3 **A**, Multistage reducing valve. Double-stage valve is functionally two single-stage reducing valves in tandem. Gas enters the first stage (first reducing valve) and its pressure is lowered. Gas then enters the second stage (second reducing valve), and pressure is lowered to the desired working pressure (usually 50 psig). A three-stage reducing valve would have one more reducing valve in the series. **B**, National double-stage reducing valve. (Courtesy National Welding Equipment Co., Richmond, Calif.)

regulator. Notice that the tension of the spring in the first stage of the regulator is usually preset by the manufacturer, but the spring tension in the second stage is typically adjustable. Each stage of the regulator contains a pressure-relief valve to release excess pressure if there is a malfunction in either stage. (The number of stages of a regulator can be determined by counting the number of pressure-relief valves on the regulator.)

Multistage regulators operate on the principle that gas pressure is gradually reduced as gas flows from a high-pressure source through a series of stages to the outlet. For example, gas from a compressed cylinder (e.g., 2200 psig) enters the first stage of a two-stage regulator, and the gas pressure is reduced to an intermediate pressure (e.g., 700 psig). This lower pressure gas then enters into the second stage of the regulator, where the gas pressure is further reduced to the desired working pressure (e.g., 50 psig) before the gas reaches the outlet.

Multistage regulators can control gas pressures with more precision than single-stage regulators because the pressure is gradually reduced. Additionally, multistage regulators produce gas flow that is much smoother than that from single-stage regulators. Multistage regulators are more expensive and larger than single-stage regulators, so they are usually reserved for tasks requiring precise gas flow (e.g., for research purposes).

Flowmeters

As mentioned earlier, flowmeters are devices that control and indicate flow. Three types are usually described: **Thorpe-tube flowmeters, Bourdon flowmeters,** and **flow restrictors**.

Thorpe-Tube Flowmeters

Thorpe tubes are the most common flowmeters used in respiratory care. As Figure 3-4 shows, these devices consist of a tapered, hollow tube engraved with a calibrated scale (usually in L/min), a float, and a needle valve for controlling the flow rate of gas. (Flowmeters used in neonatal and pediatric care may be calibrated in mL/min.) The flow rate of gas delivered is read by locating the float on the calibrated scale. It is important to use the center of the float as the reference point when reading flow rates on the calibrated scale. This is particularly evident when trying to adjust flows of 1 to 3 L/min.

The operational principle for these devices can be explained in the following manner. As gas flows through the unit, it pushes the ball float higher. As the ball float moves higher in the tube, more gas is allowed to travel around it as a result of the gradually increasing diameter of the indicator tube. The height that the ball float is raised depends on the force of gravity pulling down on it and the force of the molecules trying to push it up. The ball float will rise until enough molecules can go around it to restore the equilibrium between gravity and the number of molecules hitting the bottom of the ball float.

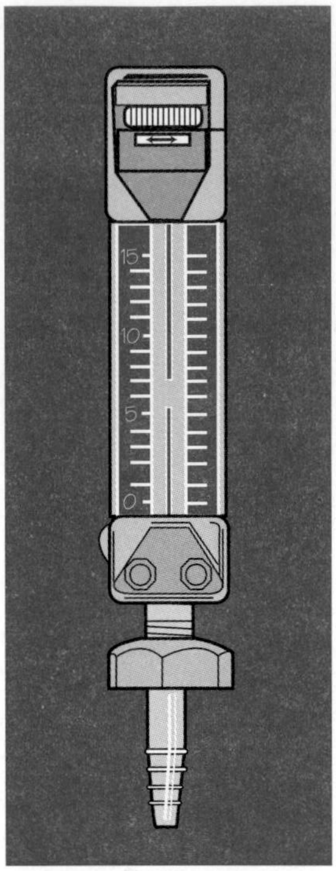

Figure 3-4 A Thorpe-tube flowmeter.

Back Pressure Compensation. Thorpe-tube flowmeters are usually described as being **pressure-compensated** and **non-pressure–compensated**. On pressure-compensated flowmeters (Figure 3-5), the needle valve controlling gas flow out of the flowmeter is located distal to the Thorpe tube. This arrangement allows the pressure in the indicator tube to be maintained at the source gas pressure (i.e., 50 psig). Pressure-compensated flowmeters provide accurate estimates of flow, regardless of the downstream pressure. (Note that pressure-compensated flowmeters indicate actual flow unless the source gas pressure varies, the flowmeter is set to deliver a higher flow than is actually available from its source gas supply, or the float in the tube is not set in a vertical position.[1]) The following example may help to illustrate how these devices operate. When a restriction or high-resistance device is attached to a pressure-compensated flowmeter, the pressure gradient between the source gas pressure and the outlet pressure is decreased. The float within the Thorpe tube registers the true gas flow out of the flowmeter because back pressure created by a downstream resistance only increases the pressure distal to the needle valve. It should be apparent, however, that if the back pressure exceeds the source gas pressure (e.g., 50 psig), gas flow stops.

In the case of non-pressure–compensated flowmeters (Figure 3-6), the needle valve is located before the indicator tube. Restriction or high-resistance devices attached to the outlet of a non-pressure–compensated Thorpe-tube flowmeter create back pressure, which is transmitted back to the needle valve. Because the needle valve is located proximal

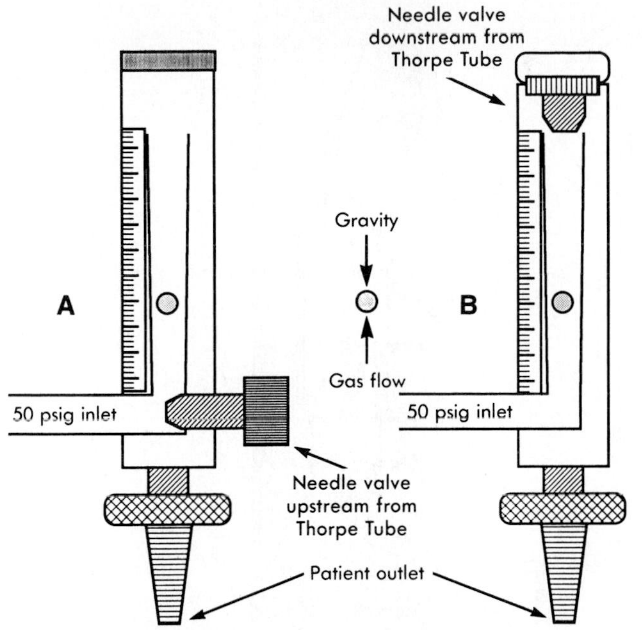

Figure 3-5 **A,** Thorpe-tube flowmeter. **B,** The two opposing forces are (*1*) gravity pulling the float downward and (*2*) the driving pressure of the gas flow pushing the float upward. When these two forces reach a balance (equilibrium), the float remains stationary, "floating" in the gas column. Because the gas column consists of a tapered tube, as the gas flow increases and the float is displaced upward, greater volumes of gas pass by the float and enter the patient outlet. Needle valve placement determines if the device is back-pressure–compensated.

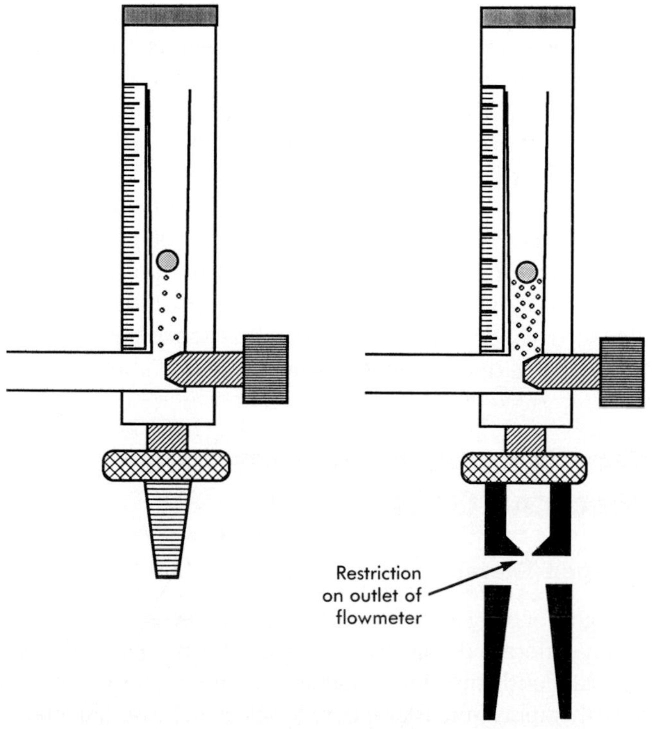

Figure 3-6 Non-pressure–compensated Thorpe-tube flowmeter.

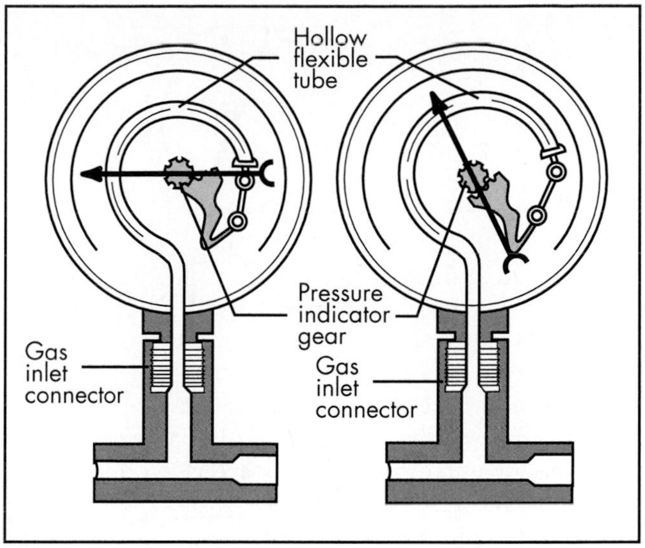

Figure 3-7 Schematic of a Bourdon flowmeter. (Redrawn from Persing G: Entry level respiratory care review, 1992, Philadelphia, Saunders.)

to the Thorpe tube, the back pressure causes the float to fall to a level that indicates a flow lower than the actual flow.

Pressure-compensated flowmeters are usually labeled as such on the back of the flowmeter. A flowmeter can also be determined to be pressure-compensated if the following test is performed. With the needle valve closed, the flowmeter is plugged into a high-pressure gas source (i.e., bulk storage wall outlet). If the float in the indicator tube jumps and then falls to zero, the flowmeter is pressure-compensated. This float movement occurs because the source gas must pass through the indicator tube before it reaches the needle valve.[1]

The most common problem associated with Thorpe-tube flowmeters is gas leakage because of faulty valve seats. This problem is usually detected when the flowmeter is turned off completely, but gas can be heard continuing to flow from the flowmeter outlet; the flowmeter should be replaced.

Bourdon Flowmeters

As Figure 3-7 shows, the Bourdon flowmeter is actually a reducing valve that controls the pressure gradient across an outlet with a fixed orifice. The operational principle of this device is simple: as the driving pressure is increased, the flow from the flowmeter outlet increases.

The flow rate of gas can be measured because the Bourdon flowmeter gauge is calibrated in liters per minute. As long as the pressure distal to or downstream from the orifice remains atmospheric, the indicated flow is accurate. As resistance to flow increases, the indicated flow reading becomes inaccurate (i.e., these devices are not back-pressure–compensated). Figure 3-8 demonstrates how increasing resistance at the gas outlet affects the flow reading. Note that although the outlet becomes totally occluded, the flow reading remains constant. Figure 3-9 is a picture of a commonly used Bourdon flowmeter.

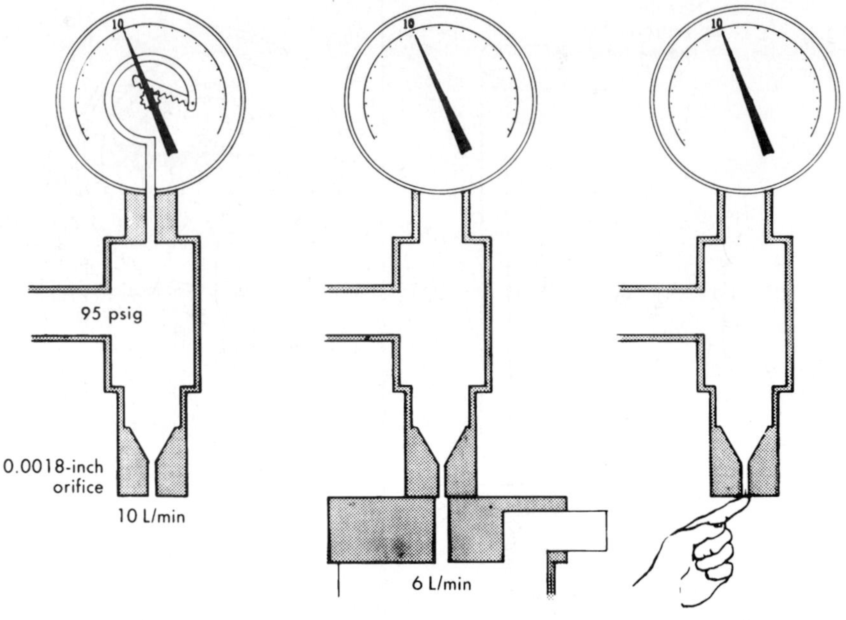

Figure 3-8 Bourdon gauge (*A*) with resistance (*B*) downstream. If resistance is placed on the outlet of the Bourdon regulator, the postrestriction pressure is no longer constant because it will be somewhat higher than atmospheric. Pressure gradient is then decreased; because only prerestriction pressure—not actual pressure gradient—is monitored, the reading will be erroneously high (*C*). (Courtesy Nellcor Puritan Bennett, Pleasanton, Calif.)

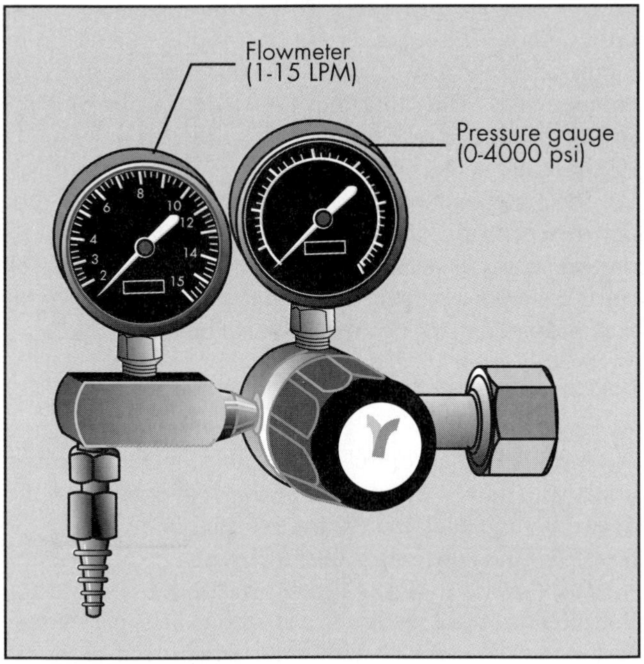

Figure 3-9 A Bourdon gauge flowmeter.

Flow Restrictors

These devices operate on the same principle as Bourdon flowmeters (i.e., the gas flow through these devices can be increased by raising the driving pressure across a fixed resistance). Like Bourdon flowmeters, flow-rate readings are inaccurate when resistance increases downstream from the gas outlet. There are two types of flow restrictors: **fixed-orifice** and **adjustable, multiple-orifice** types. Figure 3-10 shows several fixed-orifice flow restrictors, each calibrated for a specific flow. It is essential to use the appropriate operating pressure for these devices to function properly. Some are designed for use with hospital gas sources (i.e., 50-psi gas sources), whereas others are designed to work on portable liquid oxygen used in home-care settings (i.e., 20-psi gas source).

The adjustable, multiple-orifice type of flow restrictor employs a series of calibrated openings in a disc that can be adjusted to deliver different flows. As with the fixed-orifice type of flow restrictor, the operating pressure is crucial to the accuracy of the device. Figure 3-11 shows an example of a variable-orifice flow restrictor.

Devices for Administering Medical Gases

Oxygen Therapy

The goal of oxygen therapy is to treat or prevent hypoxemia. Many different devices can be used to achieve this goal in spontaneously breathing patients. It is important that respiratory therapists understand how to select and assemble these devices, as well as ensure that they are working properly. The American Association for Respiratory Care (AARC) has

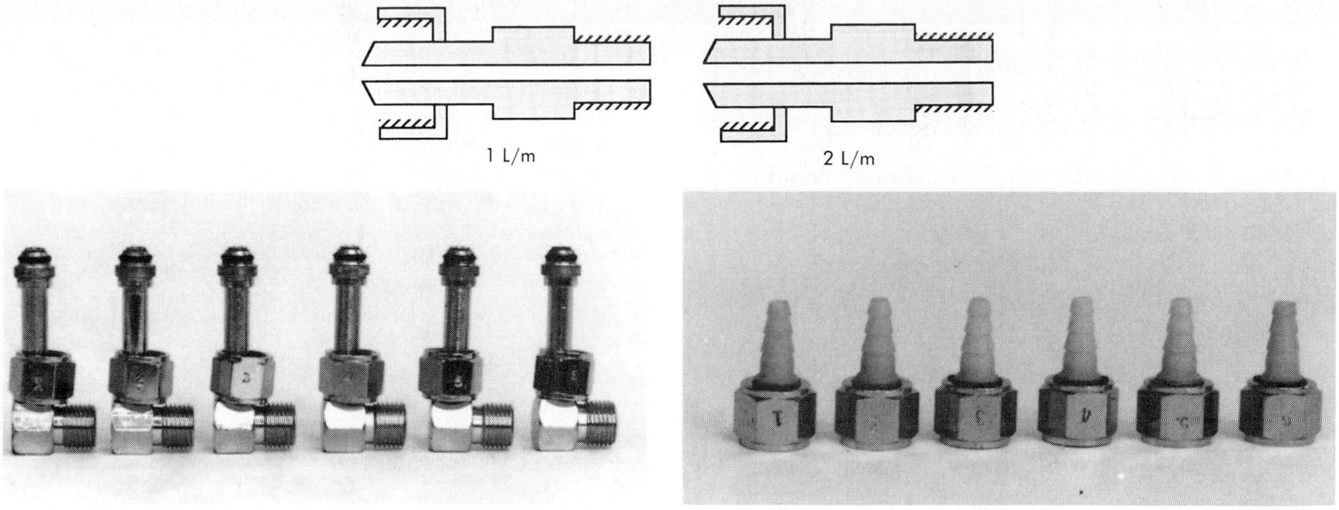

Figure 3-10 Examples of fixed-orifice flow restrictors. These devices are calibrated to deliver a set flow at a designated delivery pressure. Per NFPA requirements, the delivery pressure is included on the device label. (Courtesy of Erie Medical, Milwaukee.)

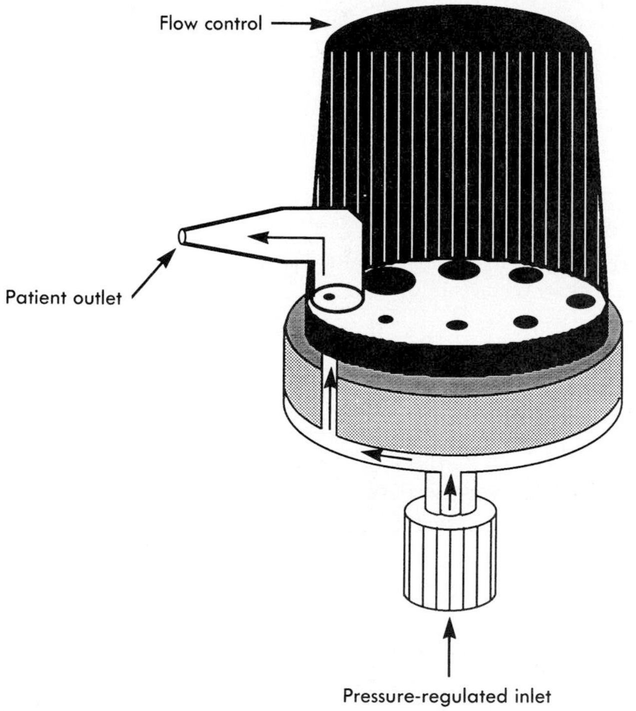

Figure 3-11 Schematic of a variable-orifice flow restrictor. These devices employ a series of calibrated ports to deliver a set flow at a designated pressure. Per NFPA requirements, the delivery pressure is included on the restrictor label.

developed clinical practice guidelines for oxygen administration in hospitals and in home- and extended-care facilities.[2,3] These guidelines inform practitioners of indications, contraindications, precautions, and possible complications of oxygen therapy. Each guideline lists the devices that can be used to administer oxygen to spontaneously breathing patients, along with a brief description of criteria that should be used to assess the need for and the outcome of oxygen therapy. These guidelines should be reviewed and used as a resource when treating patients who require oxygen therapy. Boxes 3-1 and 3-2 summarize the major points of each clinical practice guideline.

Low- vs. High-Flow Devices

Oxygen therapy systems are generally classified as **low-flow** and **high-flow devices**.[4] Low-flow devices supply oxygen at flow rates that are lower than a patient's inspiratory demands; thus varying amounts of room air must be added to provide part of the inspired volume.[5] These devices are often referred to as **variable-performance devices**. Low-flow devices deliver FiO_2s that can vary from 0.22 to approximately 0.60, depending on the patient's inspiratory flow, tidal volume, and the oxygen flow used. Nasal cannulas and catheters (Box 3-3), transtracheal catheters, simple oxygen masks, partial-rebreathing reservoir masks, and nonrebreathing reservoir masks are examples of low-flow oxygen therapy devices.

High-flow devices provide oxygen at flow rates high enough to completely satisfy a patient's inspiratory demands. Such devices supply the inspiratory demands of the patient either by entraining fixed quantities of ambient air or by using high-flow rates and reservoirs. Thus these devices are commonly called **fixed-performance devices**. The most important characteristic of high-flow devices is that they can deliver fixed FiO_2s (i.e., FiO_2s from 0.24 to 1.00), regardless of the patient's breathing pattern. Air-entrainment masks, incubators, oxygen tents, and oxygen hoods are high-flow systems. High-volume aerosol devices and humidifiers that are used to provide continuous humidification through face masks and tracheostomy collars incorporate air-entrainment devices and thus can also be considered high-flow oxygen therapy devices.

BOX 3-1

Clinical Practice Guidelines

Oxygen Therapy in the Acute-Care Hospital*

Definition/Description

Oxygen therapy is the administration of oxygen at concentrations greater than ambient air with the intent of treating or preventing the symptoms and manifestations of hypoxia.

Indications: Documented Hypoxemia

- In adults, children, and infants older than 28 days: partial pressure of arterial oxygen (P_aO_2) < 60 torr, or arterial oxygen saturation (SaO_2) < 90% in subjects breathing room air or with a P_aO_2 or SaO_2 below desirable range for specific clinical situation
- An acute situation in which hypoxemia is suspected
- Severe trauma
- Acute myocardial infarction
- Short-term therapy (postanesthesia)

Precautions and/or Complications

- With a $P_aO_2 \geq 60$ torr, ventilatory depression may occur in spontaneously breathing patients with chronically elevated partial pressure of arterial carbon dioxide ($PaCO_2$).
- With $FiO_2 \geq 0.50$, absorption atelectasis, oxygen toxicity, and/or depression of ciliary and/or leukocyte function may occur.
- In infants (particularly those born prematurely) avoid P_aO_2s > 80 torr to decrease the possibility of retinopathy of prematurity; increased P_aO_2 can contribute to closure or constriction of the arterial duct, a possible concern in infants with heart lesions dependent on this duct.
- Oxygen administration should be administered with caution to patients suffering from paraquat poisoning.
- During laser bronchoscopy, minimal levels of supplemental oxygen should be used to avoid intratracheal ignition.

Limitations

- Oxygen therapy has only limited benefit for the treatment of hypoxia due to anemia and may be of limited benefit with circulatory disturbances.
- Oxygen therapy should not be used in lieu of, but in addition to mechanical ventilation when ventilatory support is indicated.

Monitoring

- Patient monitoring should include clinical assessment along with oxygen tension or saturation measurements. This should be done at the following times: when therapy is initiated; within 12 hours of initiation of therapy for FiO_2s < 0.40; within 8 hours for FiO_2s > 0.40; within 72 hours of an acute myocardial infarction; within 2 hours for patients diagnosed with COPD; and within 1 hour for infants.
- All oxygen delivery systems should be checked at least once per day. More frequent checks with calibrated analyzers are indicated for systems susceptible to variations in FiO_2.

*For a copy of the complete AARC Clinical Practice Guideline, see Respiratory Care 36:1410, 1991.

It is a common misconception that low-flow systems can only deliver low FiO_2s and that high-flow systems can only deliver high FiO_2s. As will be seen, both low- and high-flow systems can deliver a wide range of FiO_2s. **Do not confuse the terms *low flow* and *high flow* with the terms *low FiO_2* and *high FiO_2*.**

Low-Flow Devices

Nasal Cannulas. Nasal cannulas (Figure 3-12) are used extensively to treat spontaneously breathing, hypoxemic patients in emergency rooms, in general- and critical-care units, during exercise in cardiopulmonary rehabilitation, and for long-term oxygen therapy in home-care settings.[6] The standard nasal cannula is a blind-ended, soft plastic tube that contains two prongs that fit into the patient's external nares. The prongs, which are approximately a half inch long, can be straight or curved. The cannula is held in place either with an elastic band that fits over the ears and around the head or with two small-diameter pieces of tubing that fit over the ears and can be tightened with a bolo tie type of device that fits under the chin. Cannulas are available in infant, child, and adult sizes.

The most common problems with these devices are related to (1) nasopharyngeal-mucosal irritation, (2) twisting of the connective tubing between the patient and the oxygen flowmeter, and (3) skin irritation at pressure points where the tubing holding the cannula in place touches the patient's face and ears. Irritation of the nasal mucosa and the paranasal sinuses occurs most often when high flow rates of oxygen are used. The problem appears to be increased with nasal cannulas that use straight instead of curved prongs. With straight prongs, oxygen flow is directed toward the superior aspects of the nasal cavity, thus promoting turbulent flow; with curved prongs, oxygen entering the nose is directed across the nasal turbinate, thus enhancing laminar flow as the gas flows through the nasal cavity. Twisting of connective tubing is an insidious problem that is difficult to prevent. Avoiding excessive lengths

BOX 3-2

Clinical Practice Guidelines

Oxygen Therapy in the Home or Extended-Care Facility*

Setting

This guideline is confined to oxygen administration in the home or extended care facility.

Indications: Documented Hypoxemia

- In adults, children, and infants older than 28 days: P_aO_2 < 55 torr, or $SaO_2 < 88\%$ in subjects breathing room air.
- P_aO_2 of 56 to 59 torr, or SaO_2 or $SpO_2 < 89\%$ in association with specific clinical conditions (e.g., cor pulmonale, congestive heart failure, or erythrocythemia with hematocrit $>56\%$).
- Some patients may not qualify for oxygen therapy at rest but will qualify for oxygen during ambulation, sleep, or exercise; oxygen therapy is indicated during these specific activities when the S_aO_2 falls to less than 88%.

Precautions and/or Complications

These are the same as those cited for oxygen therapy in the acute care hospital.

Limitations

These are the same as those cited for oxygen therapy in the acute-care hospital.

Monitoring

- Clinical assessment should be performed by the patient and/or the caregiver to determine changes in clinical status (e.g., dyspnea scales or diary cards).
- Baseline oxygen tension and saturation must be measured before oxygen therapy is begun; these measurements should be repeated when clinically indicated or following the course of the disease.
- SpO_2 may be made to determine appropriate oxygen flow for ambulation, exercise, or sleep.
- All oxygen delivery equipment should be checked at least once daily by the patient or caregiver. Checks should include proper equipment function, prescribed flow rates, fractional concentration of delivered oxygen (FDO_2), remaining liquid or compressed gas content, and backup supply. During monthly visits, a respiratory care practitioner should reinforce appropriate practices and performance by the patient and/or caregiver and assure that the oxygen equipment is maintained in accordance with manufacturer's recommendations.

Frequency

Oxygen should be administered continuously, unless it has been shown only to be necessary in specific situations (e.g., exercise, sleep).

Infection Control

Normally, low-flow oxygen systems without humidifiers do not present a clinically important risk of infection and need not be routinely replaced. High-flow systems that employ heated humidifiers or aerosol generators, especially when applied to patients with artificial airways, should be cleaned and disinfected on a regular basis.

*For a complete copy of this guideline see Respiratory Care 37:918-922, 1992.

of connective tubing, as well as periodically checking for patency appear to be the most reliable means of dealing with this problem. The problems of skin irritation and pressure-point soreness associated with using these devices can be minimized by placing cotton gauze padding between the tubing and the patient's face and ears.

For adult patients, nasal cannulas can theoretically produce FiO_2s of 0.24 to 0.44 with oxygen flow rates of 1 to 6 L/min. Oxygen flows higher than 6 L/min do not produce significantly higher FiO_2s and are poorly tolerated by patients because they cause nasal bleeding and drying of the nasal mucosa. For neonates, oxygen flows of 0.25 to 1.0 L/min can produce FiO_2s of 0.35 to 0.70.[6,7] Keep in mind that the actual FiO_2 delivered is influenced by the patient's tidal volume and respiratory rate and whether breathing is predominantly occurring through the nose or the mouth.

Table 3-1 lists the approximate FiO_2s delivered by flow rates of 1 to 6 L/min. Generally, the FiO_2 increases by about 4% for each liter of flow increase. Box 3-4 contains a problem-solving exercise for calculating the approximate FiO_2 when using a variable-performance device such as a nasal cannula. It should be emphasized that this is simply an estimate and that the actual delivered FiO_2 for any given oxygen flow rate may be significantly different.[2] In a clinical setting, adjusting the flow rate of oxygen delivered to the patient is generally an empirical process (i.e., it is adjusted according to the patient's oxygen needs). This empirical approach should be based on observations of the patient's breathing pattern and level of comfort, as well as pulse oximetry or arterial blood gas data, if available.

Oxygen-Conserving Devices Transtracheal oxygen (TTO) catheters, reservoir cannulas, and pulse-demand oxygen

BOX 3-3

Historical Note

Nasal Catheters

Nasal catheters were introduced by Lane in 1907.[1,6] It is important to recognize that although they are still available, they are used infrequently. Nasal catheters consist of a hollow, soft plastic tube that contains a blind distal tip with a series of side holes. They are available in 8 to 10 French (F) for children and 12 to 14 F for adults. Note that the term ***French*** is a method of sizing catheters according to the outside diameters (OD). Each unit in the French scale is approximately 0.33 mm. Thus an 8 F tube has an outside diameter of approximately 2.6 mm; a 10 F catheter has an outside diameter of 3.3 mm, etc.

The catheter can be placed with relative ease and minimal patient discomfort if done properly. First, it should be coated with a water-soluble lubricant, and its patency should be checked (by observing if oxygen flows through it unobstructed). Once the patency has been confirmed, the catheter is inserted into an external naris and advanced along the floor of the nasal cavity until it can be seen at the back of the patient's oropharynx. It should then be positioned just behind the uvula. For blind insertion, the distance that the catheter must be inserted can be estimated by measuring the distance from the tip of the patient's nose to the earlobe, which can then be marked on the catheter with a small piece of surgical tape. The catheter can be held in place by taping it to the nose.

Nasal catheters can deliver FiO_2s of approximately 0.22 to 0.24 when the oxygen flow is set at 2 to 5 L/min. Higher FiO_2s can be obtained by increasing the oxygen flow to the patient. Notice that the actual FiO_2 varies considerably depending on the patient's tidal volume and respiratory rate and whether respiration is occurring primarily through the nose or the mouth.

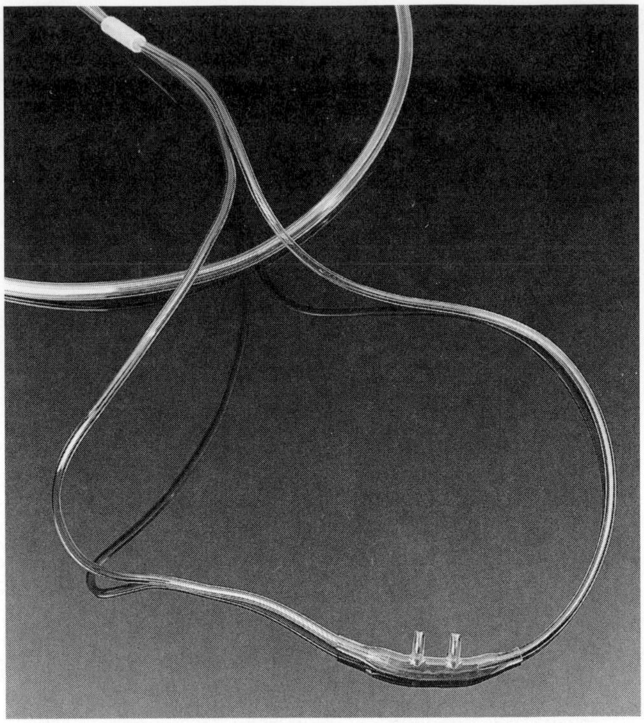

Figure 3-12 Nasal cannula.

TABLE 3-1

Guidelines for estimating FiO_2 with low-flow oxygen delivery systems

100% Oxygen Flow Rate (L)	FiO_2
Nasal cannula or catheter	
1	0.24
2	0.28
3	0.32
4	0.36
5	0.40
6	0.44
Oxygen mask	
5-6	0.40
6-7	0.50
7-8	0.60
Mask with reservoir bag	
6	0.60
7	0.70
8	0.80
9	0.80+
10	0.80+

From Shapiro, BA, et al: Clinical application of respiratory care, ed 4, St Louis, 1991, Mosby.

delivery systems are recent developments that have significantly improved the delivery of oxygen therapy, especially with regard to conserving oxygen supplies during long-term oxygen therapy.

Transtracheal Catheters. The concept of TTO therapy was first described by Heimlich in 1982.[8] The guiding principle of such oxygen therapy is that oxygen delivered directly into the trachea should provide the patient with adequate oxygen, while reducing the amount of oxygen used. That is, the direct delivery of oxygen into the trachea reduces dilution with room air on inspiration because the upper airways (the anatomical reservoir) are filled with oxygen. Consequently, lower oxygen flows from the source gas (e.g., 0.25 to 2 L/min) are required to achieve a desired

BOX 3-4

Decision Making & Problem Solving

A Simple Method for Estimating Theoretical FiO_2

A 150-lb, spontaneously breathing patient is receiving oxygen at 6 L/min through a nasal cannula. The patient's tidal volume is 500 mL and respiratory rate is 20 breaths per minute (inspiratory time = 1 second; expiratory time = 2 seconds). Estimate the theoretical FiO_2.

See Appendix A for the answer.

level of oxygenation. Indeed, TTO catheters can produce overall oxygen savings of 54% to 59%.[1]

Catheter placement requires minor surgery. A small, plastic stent is inserted into the patient's trachea between the second and third tracheal rings.[1,9] The stent remains in place for about a week to ensure that a permanent tract is formed between the trachea and the outer skin. Removal of the stent is accomplished over a guide wire. After the stent is removed, a 9 F, Teflon catheter is inserted into the tract over the guide wire. The catheter is held in place with a neck chain to prevent inadvertent dislodgment or removal (Figure 3-13). It is recommended that catheters are replaced at 90 days or earlier before they become cracked, kinked, or occluded by pus or mucus.[1,9,10] Patients must be educated on proper care of these devices to avoid complications. Routine care should include cleaning, lavage, and use of a cleaning rod to remove mucus that can occlude the lumen of the catheter.[9,10]

As previously stated, transtracheal catheters reduce oxygen costs by requiring lower oxygen flows to prevent hypoxemia. Therefore patients can purchase smaller, lighter cylinders or reservoirs for greater convenience. Using special, low-flow regulators or flow restrictors may also lead to greater cost savings.[1,10] Other important advantages of transtracheal catheters include improved patient compliance with oxygen therapy because of cosmetic appearance (these devices are relatively inconspicuous), increased patient mobility, and the avoidance of nasal irritation associated with the use of nasal cannulas. Finally, it should be mentioned that TTO devices use standard oxygen therapy equipment, which is important because if there is a problem with the catheter, emergency equipment (e.g., a conventional nasal cannula) can be easily set up and used by the patient.

The primary disadvantage of using transtracheal catheters is related to complications associated with minor

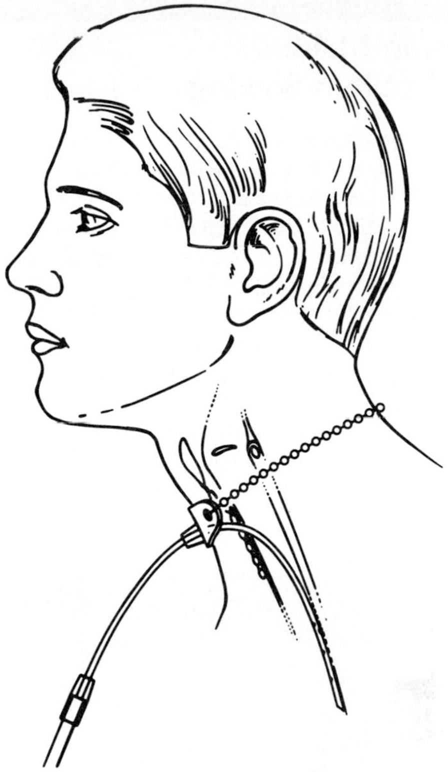

Figure 3-13 Transtracheal catheter. (From Scanlan CL, Spearman CB, and Sheldon RL: Egan's fundamentals of respiratory care, ed 6, St Louis, 1995, Mosby.)

surgery (i.e., hemoptysis, infection, and subcutaneous emphysema).[9,10] Mucous obstruction and occlusion of the distal end of the tube can also present complications, which can be minimized with proper care, including saline instillation and periodic clearing of the catheter lumen with a guide wire or cleaning rod. Box 3-5 illustrates a common example of how TTO can increase patient compliance with oxygen therapy.

Reservoir Cannulas. Figures 3-14 and 3-15 show two commercially available reservoir cannulas: the **mustache cannula** and the **pendant cannula**. The mustache cannula can hold about 20 mL of gas and works in the following manner. During the early part of exhalation, gas derived from the patient's dead space inflates the reservoir. As exhalation continues, oxygen from the source gas (e.g., 100% oxygen from a 50-psi source) flows into the lateral aspects of the cannula, forcing the dead space gas medial and out of the nasal prongs and filling the reservoir with 100% oxygen. On inspiration, the initial part of the inhaled gas entering the patient's airway is drawn from this reservoir. As the reservoir collapses, the device then functions like a conventional nasal cannula. Thus the reservoir adds 20 mL of 100% oxygen as a bolus in addition to the continuous oxygen flow from the supply source. The added bolus of gas therefore reduces the amount of oxygen that

BOX 3-5

Decision Making & Problem Solving

A home-care patient requiring continuous oxygen therapy is instructed to use a nasal cannula at a flow of 2 L/min. After a short period of time, the patient is admitted to the hospital with signs of hypoxemia. When asked if he had been using the prescribed oxygen, the patient explains that he used it only intermittently because it was uncomfortable, and furthermore he felt subconscious about wearing it in public. What would you suggest to help this patient overcome the problems he described?

See Appendix A for the answer.

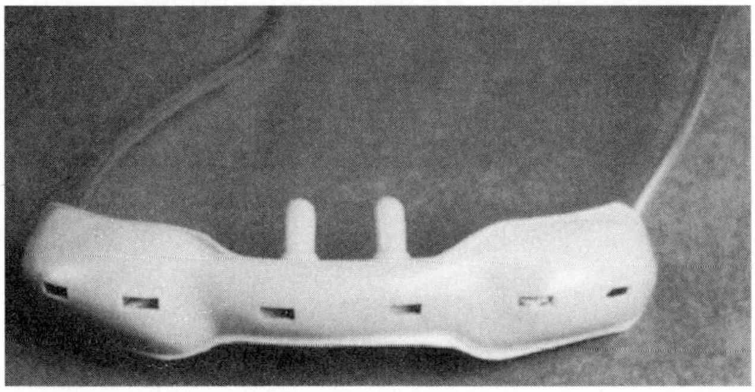

Figure 3-14 A mustache reservoir cannula. (Courtesy of Chad Therapeutics, Chatsworth, Calif.)

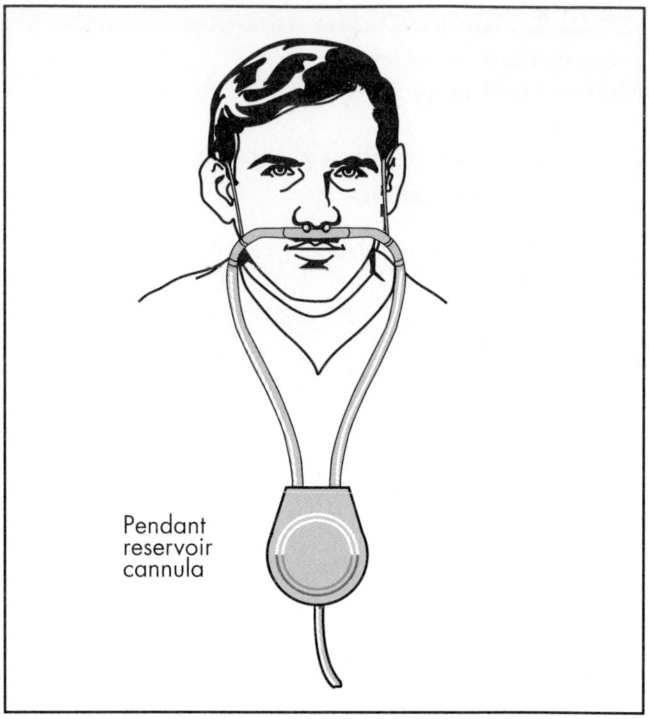

Figure 3-15 A pendant reservoir cannula.

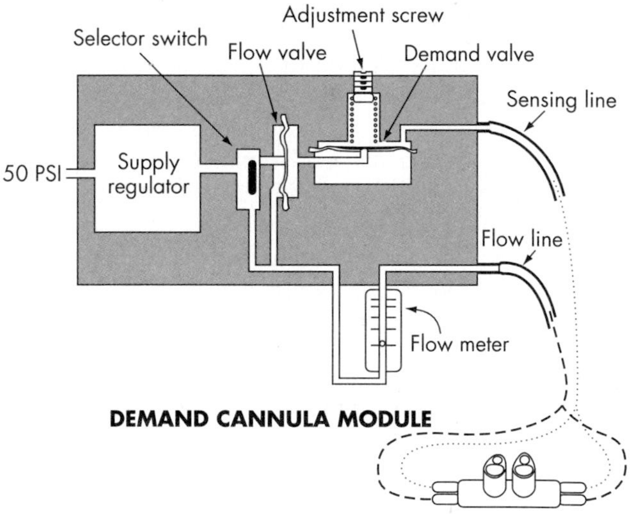

Figure 3-16 Pulse-demand oxygen-delivery system for nasal cannula. (Redrawn from Barnes TA: Core textbook of respiratory care practice, ed 2, St Louis, 1994, Mosby.)

must be derived from the continuous-flow source to achieve a desired FiO_2.

Pendant cannulas operate in a similar manner, except that the reservoir is attached with connective tubing that serves as a conduit to a pendant that hangs below the chin. The added tubing between the reservoir and the pendant increases the amount of gas that can be stored so that these types of devices can hold nearly 40 mL of 100% oxygen. As with mustache cannulas, the main advantage of these devices is their ability to conserve gas flow.

Mustache and pendant cannulas can significantly reduce oxygen supply use compared with continuous-flow nasal cannulas. Studies indicate that mustache and pendant systems may reduce oxygen supply use by 50%,[11] though the cost of reservoir cannulas is higher than that of standard nasal cannulas. Also, many patients feel that mustache type of cannulas are heavier, larger, and more obvious than conventional nasal cannulas. Pendant cannulas, however, can be concealed by the patient's clothing.

Pulse-Demand Oxygen Delivery Systems. As the name implies, these systems deliver oxygen to the patient on demand. That is, they provide oxygen only during inspiration. Electronic, fluidic, and combined electronic-fluidic sensors are used to control gas delivery to the patient. Demand systems can operate with nasal catheters, nasal cannulas, and transtracheal catheters.[11,12] Figure 3-16 is a schematic of a demand system for a nasal cannula.[1] With this type of system, oxygen is delivered to the patient only after a sufficient inspiratory effort is made (i.e., <-1 cm H_2O). Once activated, the demand valve opens, delivering oxygen at a preset flow rate, and closes during exhalation to conserve oxygen. The demand valve connects directly to the oxygen source (50 psig), therefore replacing the flowmeter that is used with continuous-flow cannulas. Note that demand systems can function as pulsed or continuous-flow sources of oxygen. Settings allow the operator to select the equivalent of 1 to 5 L/min of oxygen flow from a conventional flowmeter. Shigeoka and Bonnekat[12] calculated that a patient receives about 17 mL of oxygen at the 1 L/min setting, 35 mL at the 2 L/min setting, 51 mL at the 3 L/min setting, etc. It should be pointed out that oxygen delivered from these devices is not humidified because the system is delivering small pulses of oxygen. Thus humidification is not necessary because drying of the mucous membranes, as might occur with continuous-flow delivery systems, does not occur with these devices.

A common problem encountered with demand devices involves improper placement of the sensor. This type of problem can interfere with detection of an inspiratory effort, malfunction of the demand (solenoid) valve, and inadequate inspiratory flows. Improper placement of the sensor and malfunction of the demand valve can usually be detected by carefully observing the patient during initial set-up. Determining the adequacy of inspiratory flow requires feedback from the patient, either through verbal comments or oximetric analysis.

Simple Oxygen Mask. Although modern oxygen masks are made of different materials than earlier masks, their overall design has hardly changed since their introduction in the late 18th century.[4,6] Modern oxygen masks, like the one shown in Figure 3-17, are cone-shaped devices that fit over the patient's nose and mouth and are held in place with an elastic band that fits around the patient's head. During inspiration, the patient draws gases both from oxygen flowing into the mask through small-bore tubing connected to the base of the mask, as well as from room air via ports on the sides of the mask. These ports also serve as exhalation ports. A typical adult oxygen mask has a volume of approximately 100 to 200 mL and may be thought of as an extension of the anatomical reservoir because the patient will inhale its contents during the early part of inspiration. As such, simple oxygen masks can deliver higher FiO_2s than nasal cannulas because of a "reservoir effect." Note that the oxygen flow into the mask must be sufficient to wash out exhaled carbon dioxide, which can accumulate in this potential reservoir.

Generally, simple oxygen masks can deliver FiO_2s of 35% to 50% at oxygen flows of 5 to 10 L/min. The FiO_2 that is actually delivered to the patient depends on the flow of oxygen to the mask, the size of the mask, and the patient's breathing pattern. See Table 3-1 for a list of approximate FiO_2s for flows of 6 to 8 L/min. Simple oxygen masks are reliable and easy to set up. Disposable plastic masks are available in infant, child, and adult sizes. They are ideal for

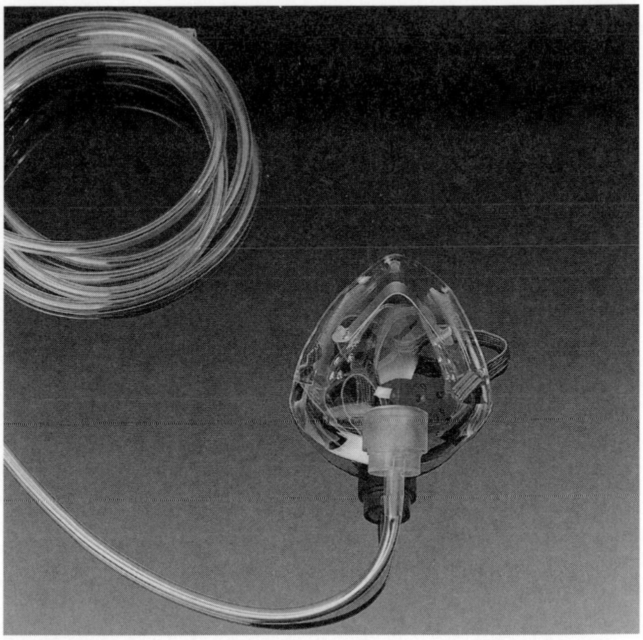

Figure 3-17 Simple oxygen mask.

delivering oxygen during minor surgical procedures and emergency situations.

There are, however, several disadvantages to using oxygen masks. For example, the delivered FiO_2 can vary significantly, thus limiting the use of these devices for patients who require well-defined inspired oxygen concentrations. Carbon dioxide rebreathing can occur if the oxygen flow to the mask is not sufficient to wash out the patient's exhaled gases. For this reason, it is generally recommended that the minimum flow set on an oxygen mask is 5 L/min. Oxygen masks are confining and may not be well-tolerated by some patients. Furthermore, they must be removed during eating, drinking, and facial and airway care. Patients often complain that these oxygen masks cause skin irritation, especially when they are tightly fitted. Finally, aspiration of vomitus may be more likely when the mask is in place.

Partial-Rebreathing Masks. The partial-rebreathing mask is derived from the **Boothby-Lovelace-Bulbulian (BLB) mask,** which was introduced by Boothby and associates in 1940.[13] As Figure 3-18 shows, the partial-rebreathing mask consists of a facepiece, which is similar to the simple oxygen mask described above, and a reservoir bag that is attached to the base of the mask. In a typical, adult partial-rebreathing mask, the reservoir bag has a volume capacity of about 300 to 500 mL. Gas flow from the oxygen source is directed into mask and the reservoir via small-bore tubing that connects at the junction of the mask and bag.

The operational theory of these devices is fairly straightforward. When the patient inhales, gas is drawn from the bag, the source gas flowing into the mask, and potentially from the room air through the exhalation ports. As the

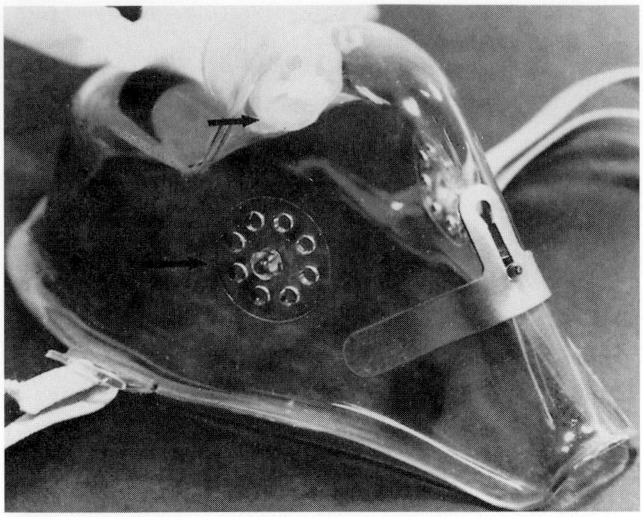

Figure 3-18 Partial-rebreathing mask. (From Gilmore TJ and Shoup CA: Laboratory exercises in respiratory care, ed 3, St Louis, 1988, Mosby.)

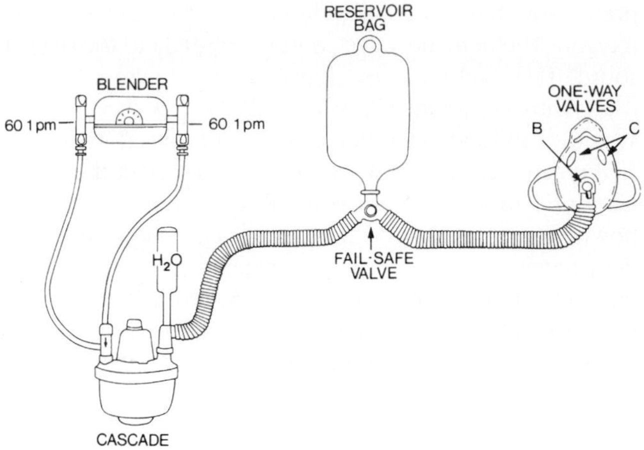

Figure 3-19 Nonrebreathing mask. (From Foust GN, et al: Chest 99:1346, 1991.)

patient exhales, the first third of the exhaled gas fills the reservoir bag, and the last two thirds of the exhaled gas are vented through the exhalation ports. Notice that the volume that fills the reservoir bag is roughly equivalent to the volume of the patient's anatomical dead space volume. Because the volume that fills the reservoir bag represents gas that has not participated in gas exchange, it will have a high partial pressure of oxygen (PO_2) and a low partial pressure of carbon dioxide (PCO_2). Thus the patient inhales this gas mixture during the next breath.

Partial-rebreathing masks can deliver FiO_2s of 0.60 to 0.80 for oxygen flows of 6 to 10 L/min (see Table 3-1). The actual percentage of oxygen delivered is also influenced by the patient's ventilatory pattern. Note that the minimum flow rate of oxygen should be sufficient to ensure that the bag does not completely deflate when the patient is inhaling.[14] Partial-rebreathing masks are available in child and adult sizes.

Nonrebreathing Masks. These masks look very similar to the partial-rebreathing masks except that they contain two valves (Figure 3-19). The first set of valves is a one-way valve (*B*) located between the reservoir bag and the base of the mask. This valve allows gas flow to enter the mask from the reservoir bag when the patient inhales and prevents gas flow from the mask back into the reservoir bag during the patient's exhalation, as occurs with the partial-rebreathing mask. The second set of valves is at the exhalation ports (*C*). The one-way valves placed there prevent room air from entering the mask during inhalation. They also allow the patient's exhaled gases to exit the mask on exhalation.

Nonrebreathing masks can theoretically deliver 100% oxygen, assuming that the mask fits snugly on the patient's face and the only source of gas being inhaled by the patient is derived from the oxygen flowing into the mask-reservoir system. In actual practice, disposable nonrebreathing masks can deliver FiO_2s of 0.6 to 0.8.[14] The discrepancy between disposable nonrebreathing masks and the original BLB masks is primarily related to the fact that manufacturers usually supply disposable masks with one of the exhalation valves removed. The valve is removed as a precaution in case the oxygen flow to the mask is interrupted or inadequate for the patient's needs (i.e., safety regulations require that the patient can still entrain room air if there is an interruption in source gas flow). Original BLB masks contain a spring-disk safety valve that opens if oxygen flow to the mask is interrupted.

Nonrebreathing masks are effective for administering high FiO_2s to spontaneously breathing patients for short periods. Prolonged use of these masks can be associated with valve malfunctions (i.e., sticking due to moisture accumulation, or deformity from wear).

High-Flow Oxygen System

Air-Entrainment Masks. Air-entrainment masks are the result of the pioneering work of Barach and associates[15,16,17] from the 1930s to the 1960s. Figure 3-20 is a schematic of a typical air-entrainment mask. It consists of a plastic mask connected to a jet nozzle, which is encased within a plastic housing that contains air-entrainment ports. Oxygen flowing through the nozzle "drags" in room air through the entrainment ports as a result of viscous, shearing forces between the gas exiting the jet nozzle outlet and the surrounding ambient air.[18] The amount of room air entrained, and therefore the concentration of oxygen delivered to the patient, depends on the flow rate of oxygen exiting the jet nozzle, the size of the jet nozzle outlet, and the size of the entrainment port.

For most commercially available masks, the concentration is varied by changing the size of the nozzle outlet or the

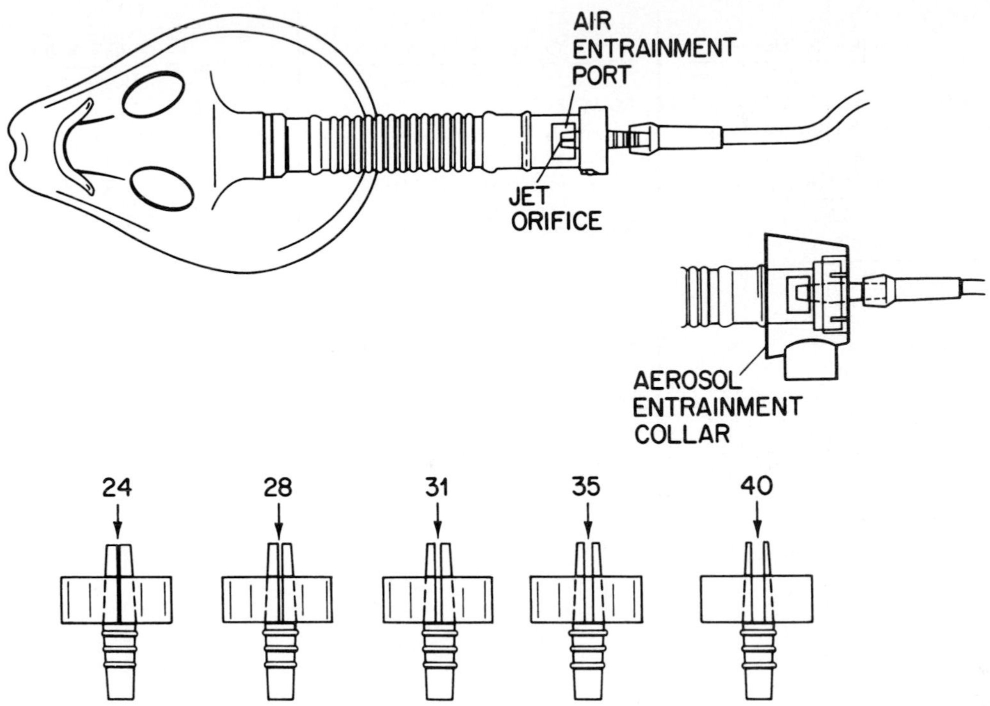

Figure 3-20 Schematic illustrating the components of an air-entrainment mask. Aerosol collar allows high humidity or aerosol entrainment from an air source. (From Kacmarek RM: In-hospital O_2 therapy. In Kacmarek RM and Stoller J, editors: Current respiratory care, Toronto, 1988, B.C. Decker.)

entrainment ports. The flow rate of oxygen to the nozzle is constant and set to a minimum value, usually between 2 and 10 L/min. Note that partial obstruction of oxygen flow downstream of the jet orifice or partial obstruction of the entrainment ports will decrease the amount of room air entrained, thus raising the FiO_2 of the delivered gas.[19,20,21]

Figure 3-21 presents a simple method for calculating the air:oxygen entrainment ratio and the total gas flow delivered for a given FiO_2.[20] Table 3-2 contains a list of the air:oxygen entrainment ratios required to achieve a given FiO_2, evidencing that the total flow of gas delivered is greater for low FiO_2s than it is for high FiO_2s. Air-entrainment masks are able to function much better as fixed-performance devices at low FiO_2s (<0.4) than at higher FiO_2s (>0.4).[19,21,22] The discrepancy between the set FiO_2 and the actual delivered FiO_2 is exaggerated by abrupt increases in inspiratory flow. Campbell and associates[23] suggest that many commercially available masks produce variable FiO_2s when patients generate high inspiratory flows due to insufficient mask volume.

Air-entrainment masks are excellent for providing oxygen therapy to hypoxemic chronic obstructive pulmonary disease (COPD) patients, who typically require fixed FiO_2s between 0.24 and 0.35.[17] The total flow rate of gas delivered (oxygen plus air) by such masks for lower FiO_2s is usually sufficient to meet ventilatory demands for these patients. Supplemental humidification of the delivered gas is usually not required when the oxygen flow is low (e.g., <4 L/min) because the oxygen flow is a small percentage of the total flow. Increased moisture can be delivered by attaching a compressed, air-driven aerosol to the air-entrainment port via an open, plastic collar. (Such collars work best with masks that have large air-entrainment ports.[20]) Alternatively, high humidity can be delivered with fixed FiO_2s with large-volume aerosol nebulizers and humidifier units that use air-entrainment devices, which can provide increased levels of moisture at several fixed oxygen percentage settings (e.g., 0.4, 0.6, and 1.0). A number of appliances, including aerosol masks, face tents, T-tubes, and tracheostomy collars, can be used to deliver these moisture-rich gases. Care should be taken not to allow moisture to accumulate in the tubing downstream from the air-entrainment device. Accumulated moisture acts as an obstruction, which can decrease the amount of room air entrained and raise the FiO_2 delivered to the patient. Notice that the total flow of gas provided by this type of apparatus may not be sufficient to meet patients' high ventilatory demands. Thus the FiO_2 may vary considerably in these situations because the patient will be forced to entrain room air to meet increased ventilatory needs.[24,25] Large-volume nebulizers and humidifiers will be discussed in more detail in Chapter 4.

A

$$O_2 \text{ flow} = \frac{\text{Total flow} \times (FIO_2 - 0.2)}{0.8}$$

EXAMPLE:

Known: Total flow = 10 L/min
$FIO_2 = 0.4$

$$O_2 \text{ flow} = \frac{10 \times (0.4 - 0.2)}{0.8}$$

$$O_2 \text{ flow} = \frac{10 \times 0.2}{0.8}$$

$$O_2 \text{ flow} = \frac{2}{0.8}$$

O_2 flow = 2.5 L/min

(Air flow = Total flow − O_2 flow)

B

$$FIO_2 = \frac{O_2 \text{ flow} + (0.2 \times \text{Air flow})}{\text{Total flow}}$$

EXAMPLE:

Known: O_2 flow = 2.5 L/min
Air flow = 7.5 L/min
Total flow = 10 L/min

$$FIO_2 = \frac{2.5 + (0.2 \times 7.5)}{10}$$

$$FIO_2 = \frac{2.5 + 1.5}{10}$$

$$FIO_2 = \frac{4}{10}$$

$FIO_2 = 0.4$

C

$$\text{Total flow} = \frac{O_2 \text{ flow} \times 0.8}{FIO_2 - 0.2}$$

EXAMPLE:

Known: O_2 flow = 2.5 L/min
$FIO_2 = 0.4$

$$\text{Total flow} = \frac{2.5 \times 0.8}{0.4 - 0.2}$$

$$\text{Total flow} = \frac{2}{0.2}$$

Total flow = 10 L/min

D

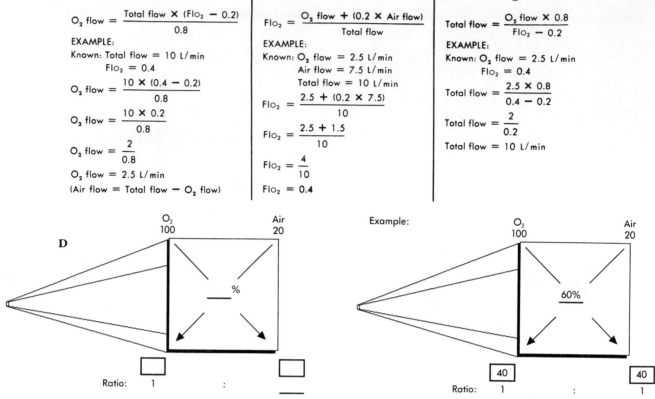

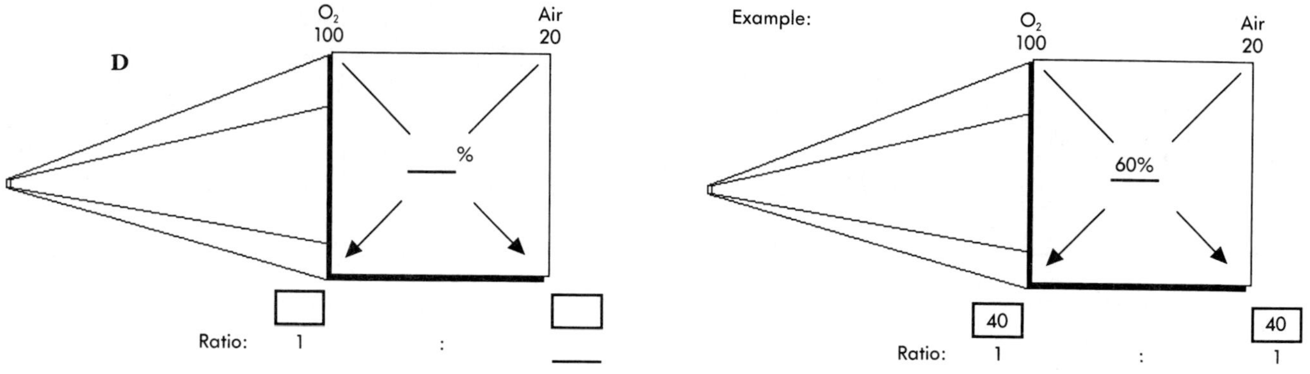

Figure 3-21 Method for calculating air-oxygen entrainment ratios.

Oxygen Hoods. Oxygen hoods were introduced in the 1970s as a means of maintaining a relatively constant FIO_2 to infants requiring supplemental oxygen. Figure 3-22 shows a typical hood used to deliver oxygen therapy to pediatric patients. It is a clear plastic enclosure that is placed around the patient's head. Fixed oxygen concentrations (from an air-entrainment device or an oxygen/air blender [see the section on oxygen blenders later in this chapter]) can be connected to the hood via an inlet port that is located at the rear of the hood. The flow rate of gas entering the hood is set to ensure that the exhaled carbon dioxide is flushed out (i.e., the flow rate should be approximately 5 to 10 L/min).

The FIO_2 must be measured intermittently or monitored continuously with an oxygen analyzer. Several studies have shown that in hoods, the O_2 seems to be layered, with the highest concentration near the bottom of the hood. The partial pressure of arterial oxygen (PaO_2) should also be measured by arterial blood gas analysis at regular intervals. The noise levels inside these devices can present problems, and every effort should be made to minimize this effect.[26]

TABLE 3-2

Approximate entrainment ratios for commonly used oxygen concentrations (assuming FIO_2 is 20.9%)

Oxygen percentage	Air:oxygen ratio	Total parts*
100	0:1	1
70	0.6:1	1.6
60	1:1	2
50	1.7:1	2.7
40	3:1	4
35	5:1	6
30	8:1	9
28	10:1	11
24	25:1	26

*Total parts × Oxygen flow = Total flow estimate

Incubators. Incubators, along with oxygen tents, can be classified as environmental delivery systems because they provide large volumes of oxygen-enriched gas to the atmosphere immediately surrounding the patient. The first

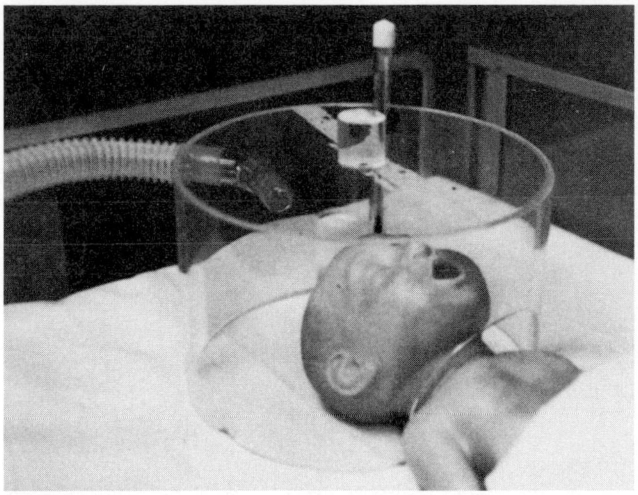

Figure 3-22 Oxygen hood. (From Scanlan CL, Wilkins RL, and Stoller JK: Egan's fundamentals of respiratory care, ed 7, St Louis, 1999, Mosby.)

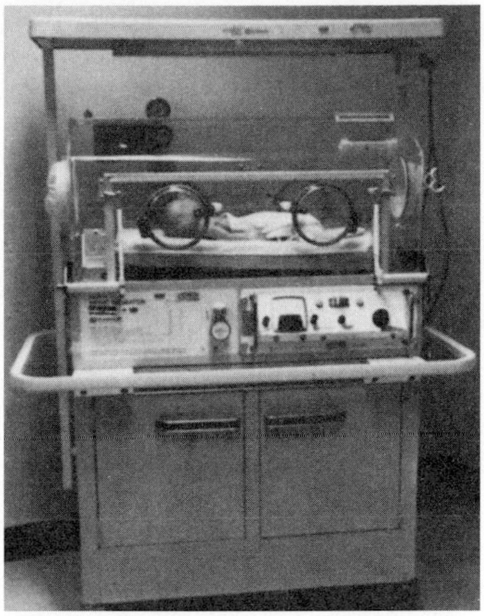

Figure 3-23 Infant incubator. (From Scanlan CL, Wilkins RL, and Stoller JK: Egan's fundamentals of respiratory care, ed 7, St Louis, 1999, Mosby.)

incubator was designed by Denuce in 1857.[20] Several years later (c. 1880), Tarnier designed an enclosed incubator to provide a warm environment for premature infants.[20] Current incubators (Figure 3-23) allow for variable control of the environmental temperature, humidity, and FiO_2. The temperature and humidity of the gas within the incubator are controlled by a servo-controlled mechanism connected to a fan that circulates environmental gas over heating coils and a blow-by humidifier. Supplemental oxygen can be provided by connecting a heated humidifier directly to the incubator.

The FiO_2 is controlled with an air-entrainment apparatus that allows the selection of high and low FiO_2s. Generally, when the air-entrainment port remains open, an FiO_2 of 0.4 or less is delivered. The port must be occluded to deliver higher FiO_2s. (Opening and closing of the port is accomplished by moving an occluder that is attached to a red metal flag. This feature is incorporated into the design of the system to alert the medical staff that high concentrations of oxygen are being delivered.)

It is important to remember that the actual concentration of oxygen delivered to the patient can vary considerably when the enclosure is opened for nursing-care procedures. Because of the variability in oxygen concentrations that can occur when oxygen is provided through the incubator's oxygen inlet, it may be necessary to deliver oxygen directly to the infant via an oxyhood placed directly over the infant's head inside the incubator.[9] Regardless of the method used to deliver oxygen to the infant, the actual FiO_2 in the incubator should be intermittently measured or continuously monitored. Additionally, blood gases should be sampled at regular intervals to ensure that the infant is receiving the appropriate oxygen therapy. (The partial pressure of arterial oxygen should be monitored in infants receiving oxygen therapy. High PaO_2 values in these patients are associated with a high incidence of retinopathy and loss of sight.)

Recent studies have demonstrated that noise levels within incubators can be quite high.[26] Although noise may be a difficult problem to control, every effort must be made to minimize noise levels within these devices.

Oxygen Tents. Sir Leonard Hill is credited as being the first clinician to use the oxygen tent,[3] but Alvin Barach improved the operation of these devices by conditioning the air within the tent.[4] (Barach accomplished this early form of air conditioning by adding a fan to circulate the air over a cooling tower containing ice.) During the early 1900s, oxygen tents were often used to provide oxygen to hypoxemic adults and children. Modern oxygen tents are primarily used for pediatric patients requiring enriched oxygen and high humidity levels. Today's oxygen tents can provide environmental control of (1) oxygen concentration, (2) humidity, and (3) temperature (Figure 3-24). The FiO_2 and the humidity content delivered to the patient are controlled by a high-flow aerosol unit, which is incorporated into the tent. Ultrasonic nebulizers (see Chapter 4) can also be used to increase the humidity inside of the tent. Temperature is controlled with refrigeration coils containing Freon. These systems can typically reduce the temperature inside of the tent from 10° to 12° F below room temperature.

Oxygen Proportioners

Oxygen Adders. The simplest example of an oxygen proportioner is an **oxygen adder**, such as the one shown in Figure 3-25. This system consists of two flowmeters: one

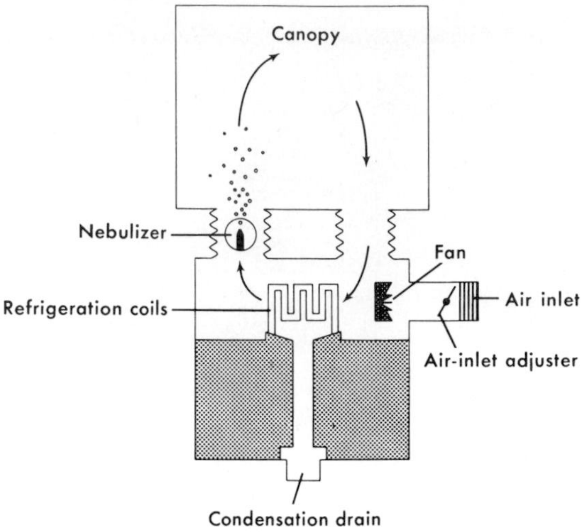

Figure 3-24 Oxygen tent.

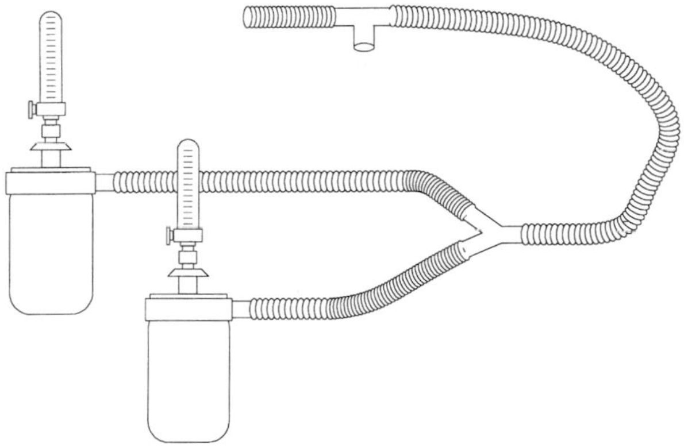

Figure 3-25 Schematic of an oxygen adder. (From Scanlan CL, Wilkins RL, and Stoller JK: Egan's fundamentals of respiratory care, ed 7, St Louis, 1998, Mosby.)

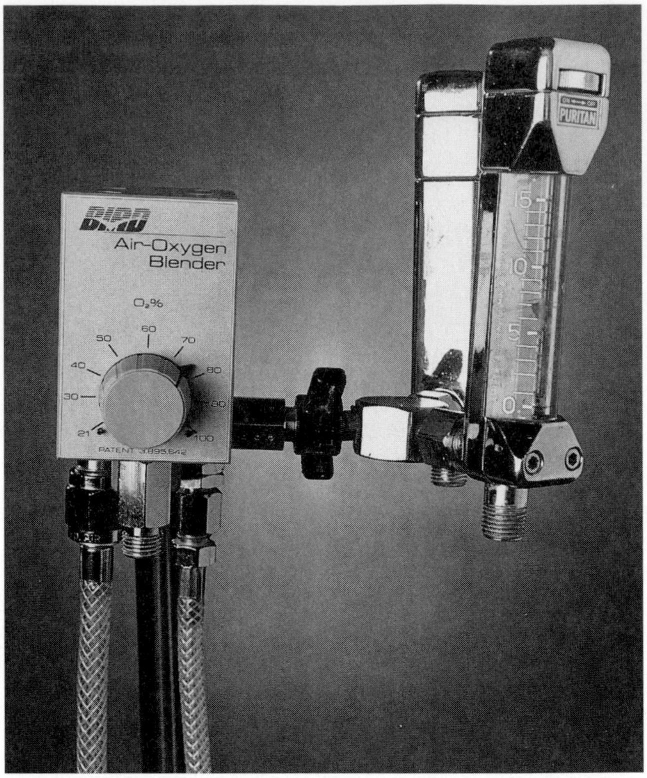

Figure 3-26 Oxygen blender.

attached to an oxygen supply and the another attached to an air supply. The outputs of the two flowmeters are directed to humidifiers and then to the patient via any of the delivery systems previously described. The FiO_2 of the gas delivered to the patient depends on the ratio of air:oxygen flow. The concentration can be calculated using the same principle as for calculating air:oxygen entrainment ratios for air-entrainment masks. For example, if the air and oxygen flowmeters are each set to deliver 15 L/min, then the ratio is 1:1, which corresponds to an FiO_2 of 0.60. However, if the air flowmeter was set to 15 L/min and the oxygen flowmeter was set to 5 L/min, then the air:oxygen entrainment ratio would be 3:1, corresponding to an FiO_2 of 0.40.

Oxygen Blenders and Mixers. A more sophisticated device for accomplishing air-oxygen mixing is the **oxygen blender** (or oxygen mixer). Figure 3-26 illustrates a typical oxygen blender and its components. Compressed air and oxygen from a high-pressure source enter into a chamber where the pressures of the two gases are equalized. (An alarm system is incorporated into the design of these devices to alert the practitioner if the pressures of the source gases are not comparable [i.e., >10 psi difference between the air and oxygen pressures].) Unequal source gas pressures can cause the blender to malfunction and deliver unreliable FiO_2s. This is accomplished by reducing the higher pressure gas to match the lower pressure gas, which is usually 50 psig. The gases are then routed to a precise metering device that controls the amount of each gas reaching the outlet. This metering device can be adjusted with a rotary mixing-control knob on the faceplate. Turning the knob counterclockwise decreases the amount of oxygen reaching the outlet, therefore reducing the delivered FiO_2. Conversely, turning the knob clockwise reduces the amount of air reaching the outlet, thus increasing the FiO_2.

Oxygen blenders are a reliable means of providing a variety of FiO_2s. Flowmeters can be connected to the blender's outlet, as can ventilators or any other devices that use 50 psig source gas. Because moisture and particulate matter introduced into the blender by the source gases can cause the blender to malfunction, it is important to filter the gas before it enters the blender housing.

Hyperbaric Oxygen Therapy

Hyperbaric oxygen therapy exposes patients to a pressure greater than atmospheric while they breathe 100% oxygen either continuously or intermittently. Historically, hyperbaric therapy has been used most often to treat subjects with decompression sickness and air embolism associated with deep sea diving. More recently, it has been successfully used to treat patients with a variety of disorders, including carbon monoxide poisoning and smoke inhalation, anaerobic infections that are refractory to conventional therapy, thermal injuries, skin grafts, and refractory osteomyelitis. Although hyperbaric oxygen therapy has increased significantly during the past decade, its use is somewhat limited because it is expensive to purchase and maintain hyperbaric units. A brief discussion of the physiological basis of hyperbaric oxygen therapy and a description of the equipment required follow. For a more detailed analysis of hyperbaric oxygen therapy, consult the references at the end of this chapter.[27,28,29]

Physiological Principles

Effects on Respiratory Function. Exposure to elevated barometric pressures during hyperbaric oxygen therapy can directly affect a number of physiologic parameters related to respiration, including lung volume, arterial and alveolar partial pressures for oxygen, the temperature of the gases being breathed, and the work of breathing.

Lung Volumes. The effects on lung volume can be explained by Boyle's law, which states that if the temperature of a gas remains constant, the volume of a gas is inversely related to its pressure. That is, as pressure exerted on the container increases, the gas volume decreases. Thus when a person is exposed to elevated pressures, the gas volume contained in any body cavity tends to be compressed. For example, as the ambient pressure is doubled (1520 mm Hg, or 2 atm), the air volume in the lung is reduced to half of what it would occupy at normal ambient pressures (760 mm Hg, or 1 atm). Figure 3-27 illustrates pressure/volume relationships that are typically encountered during hyperbaric oxygen therapy.

Depth in feet	Pressure in ATA	Relative volume	Relative diameter
0	1	100%	100%
33	2	50%	79.3%
66	3	33.3%	69.3%
99	4	25%	63%
132	5	20%	58.5%
165	6	16.6%	55%

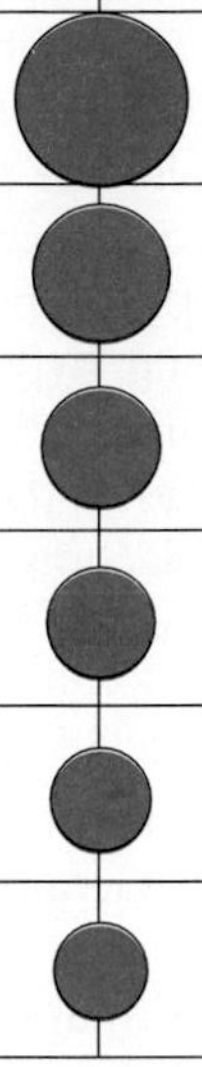

Figure 3-27 Pressure-volume relationships during hyperbaric oxygen therapy. (Redrawn from Davis JC, Hunt TK: Hyperbaric oxygen therapy, 1977, Kensington, Md., Undersea Medical Society.)

Alveolar and Arterial Partial Pressures of Oxygen. The effect of increased ambient pressure on the partial pressure of alveolar oxygen (P_AO_2) can be explained by Dalton's law, which states that the total pressure of a gas mixture, such as air, equals the sum of the partial pressures of each of the constituent gases in the mixture. Considering that air is 21% oxygen and 79% nitrogen, then ambient air (assuming that the barometric pressure is 760 torr) will have a partial oxygen pressure (PO_2) of about 160 torr (0.21 × 760 torr) and a partial nitrogen pressure (PN_2) of about 600 torr (0.79 × 760 torr). This same logic can be applied to the alveolar air equation for calculating the P_AO_2 that follows:

$$P_AO_2 = (P_{bar} - P_{H_2O})\ FiO_2 - P_aCO_2/0.8$$

Therefore, if the barometric pressure (P_{bar}) equals 760 torr and the FiO_2 equals 0.21, then the P_AO_2 would be about 100 torr. Consider if the barometric pressure is doubled to 1520 torr, or 2 atm. If all other variables in the equation remain constant, then the P_AO_2 would equal 333 torr.

Henry's law is used to explain the changes in the P_aO_2 that occur with exposure to elevated ambient pressures. It states that the degree to which a gas enters into physical solution in body fluids is directly proportional to the partial pressure of gas to which the fluid is exposed. Remember that Henry's law states that the relative quantities of gas entering a fluid are related to the pressure of gas exerted on the fluid and the solubility of the gas in the fluid in question. Thus oxygen's solubility in plasma is about 0.003 vol % (mL of oxygen/100 mL of whole blood) for every torr of P_aO_2. If it is assumed that the ventilation-perfusion relationship for a patient's lungs is normal, then the P_aO_2 would be slightly less than 100 torr when the patient is breathing room air at 1 atm. Furthermore, the P_aO_2 would be approximately 333 torr for breathing room air when the ambient pressure is increased to 2 atm. Then it can be calculated that as the P_aO_2 increases from about 100 torr (at 1 atm) to approximately 333 torr (at 2 atm), the amount of dissolved oxygen increases from 0.3 vol % (100 torr × 0.003 vol %/torr) to 1.0 vol % (333 torr × 0.003 vol %/mm Hg). So, the oxygen-carrying capacity of plasma increases considerably under hyperbaric conditions. It is therefore reasonable to assume that this form of therapy is beneficial to the treatment of patients who have abnormally functioning hemoglobin and thus a reduced ability to carry oxygen attached to hemoglobin, such as occurs with carbon monoxide poisoning.

Gas Temperatures. According to Gay-Lussac's law, if the volume of a gas remains constant, there is a direct relationship between the absolute pressure of a gas and its temperature. It is reasonable to suggest that if the volume of a hyperbaric chamber remains constant, increasing the pressure would raise the temperature inside of the chamber. (Indeed, this problem should limit the usefulness of this form of therapy.) In practice, gas temperature changes encountered during hyperbaric therapy are easily controlled by regulating the rates at which pressures are increased and decreased, the temperature of the air used for compression and decompression, and the flow rate of ventilation used to dissipate heat.[27]

Work of Breathing. As the barometric pressure increases, there is an increase in the density of the gas being breathed. The increase in gas density results in an increased work of breathing, which is not noticeable and can easily be accommodated in normal subjects. In patients with reduced lung reserves, however, this increased work may present problems and require ventilatory support. It is also important to recognize that many ventilators will malfunction when placed in a hyperbaric chamber.[30]

Vascular Function. A number of studies have demonstrated that hyperbaric oxygen therapy increases the synthetic ability of tissues by increasing collagen deposition, thus enhancing the growth of new blood vessels in damaged tissues as well as the revascularization of these tissues.[27] This effect has been used to successfully treat patients with skin grafts.

Immunologic Function. It is well-established that leukocyte function is enhanced during hyperbaric oxygen therapy. This improved function is thought to be related to an increase in the oxygen available for microbicidal metabolism (i.e., H_2O_2, OH^-). Coupled with this enhanced microbicidal activity of leukocytes, oxygen appears to directly inhibit the growth of certain bacteria, particularly those involved in anaerobic infections, such as *Clostridia* sp., which are responsible for gas gangrene.

Equipment

Hyperbaric chambers are generally classified as either monoplace or multiplace units (Figure 3-28). **Monoplace hyperbaric chambers** are specified by the NFPA as Class B chambers and are rated for single occupancy.[27] There are a number of monoplace units available commercially. Although they differ considerably in appearance, they all use the same principle of operation, generally relying on a single gas source for compression and respiration. (Some newer systems provide connections for a separate source gas for respiration.)

A typical chamber is generally about 8 to 10 ft long and 3 ft in diameter. The outer shell of the unit is constructed of steel and clear, double-thick acrylic. Some newer units contain a separate chamber compartment to accommodate attendants working with the patient. Most units are mounted on wheels for portability but are usually treated as stationary systems; therefore they are placed in a room that is designated for the purposes of hyperbaric therapy.

Multiplace hyperbaric chambers are walk-in units that provide enough space to treat two or more patients simultaneously. They vary in size (2 to 13 occupants) but usually contain a main chamber for treating patients and a smaller chamber allowing attendants to enter and leave without altering the pressure within the main chamber. Multiplace chambers provide two gas sources: one for compression and one for respiration. Hyperbaric oxygenation is achieved by having the patient breathe oxygen by mask or through a specially designed hood while being exposed to elevated barometric pressures in the compressed air chamber. Treatment schedules (i.e., the amount of time that the patient breathes 100% oxygen vs. air) are tailored to the specific needs of the patient. Generally, patients are placed on schedules in which intermittent air breathing periods of 5 minutes or more are programmed approximately every 20 minutes. This intermittent air breathing is used to prevent oxygen toxicity.

Monitoring Devices. All hyperbaric facilities should have the capability to monitor the oxygenation status of patients undergoing hyperbaric oxygen therapy. Transcutaneous monitoring has proven to be valuable in assessing the overall oxygenation status of a patient undergoing hyperbaric therapy. Selective placement of the probe can also provide information on the localized effects of hyperbaric oxygen therapy on ischemic tissue.

Arterial blood gas monitoring can provide information on the oxygenation status of patients receiving hyperbaric therapy and is also an indication of their ventilatory status. Arterial blood samples can be drawn from patients and removed from the chamber for analysis. Care must be taken to ensure that the sample remains tightly sealed until it is analyzed. Transcutaneous monitoring and arterial blood gas analysis is discussed further in Chapters 7 and 8.

Indications and Contraindications for Hyperbaric Oxygen Therapy

As stated earlier, hyperbaric oxygen therapy is most often associated with the treatment of individuals who have experienced decompression sickness and other maladies associated with deep-sea diving. Box 3-6 lists several other conditions that have been successfully treated with this type of oxygen therapy.[31,32,33] Although the effectiveness of hyperbaric oxygen therapy may vary among patients, patients with any of these conditions should respond to it.

Box 3-7 lists some of the known contraindications for hyperbaric oxygen therapy. The only absolute contraindication is pneumothorax. If pneumothorax occurs during hyperbaric treatment, chest tubes should be immediately inserted; failure to treat pneumothorax can have dire

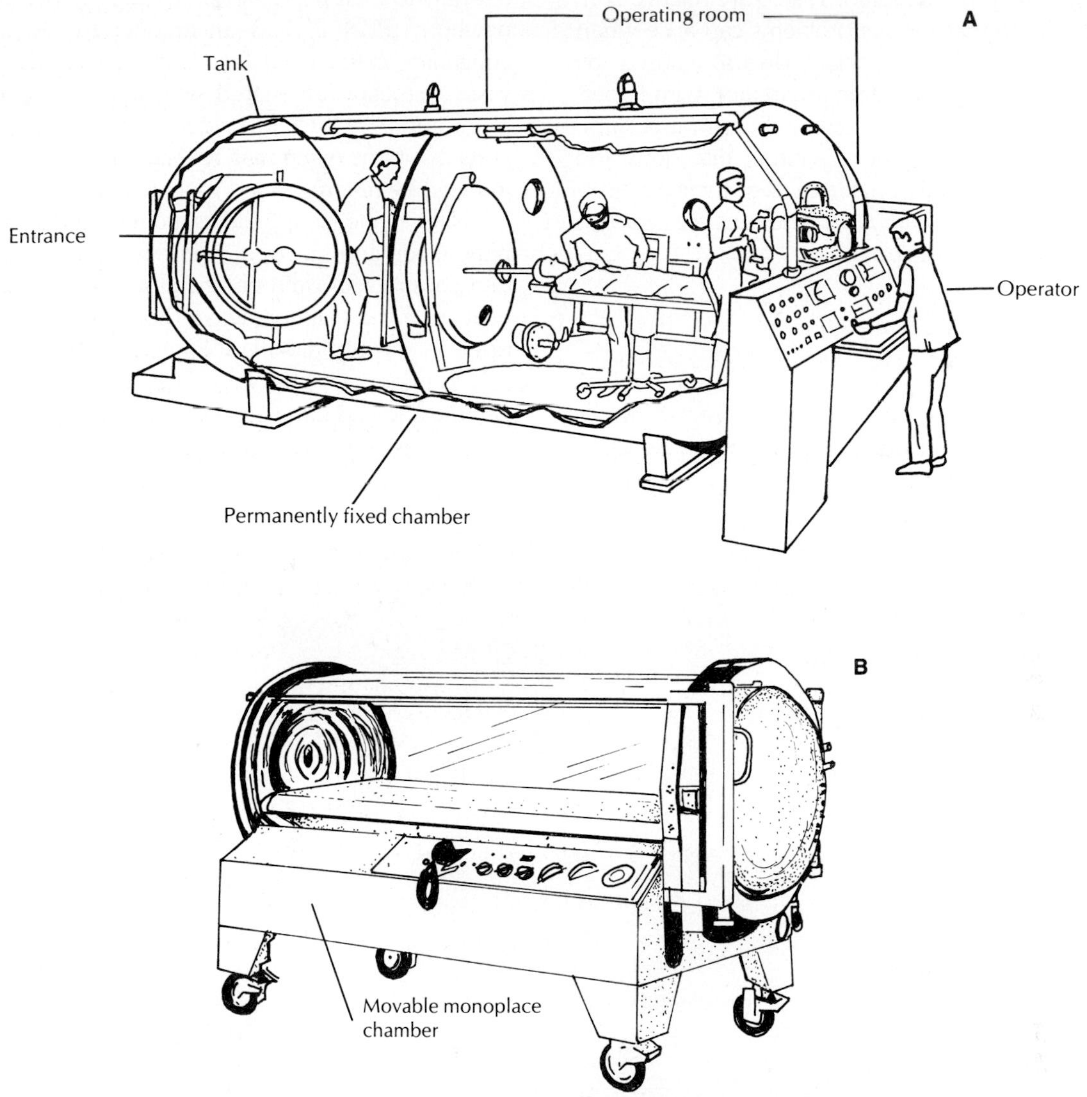

Figure 3-28 Schematics of a multiplace (**A**) and a monoplace (**B**) hyperbaric oxygen chamber. (From Scanlan CL, Wilkins RL, and Stoller JK: Egan's fundamentals of respiratory care, ed 7, St Louis, 1999, Mosby.)

BOX 3-6

Indications for Hyperbaric Oxygen Therapy

Air embolism
Carbon monoxide poisoning
Cyanide poisoning
Decompression sickness
Gas gangrene
Refractory anaerobic infections
Refractory osteomyelitis
Skin grafts
Thermal burns
Wound healing

BOX 3-7

Contraindications for Hyperbaric Oxygen Therapy

Congenital spherocytosis
High fevers
Hypercapnia (>60 torr)
Obstructive airway disease
Optic neuritis
Pneumothorax
Seizure disorders
Sinusitis
Upper respiratory infections
Viral infections

From Kindall EP: Clinical hyperbaric oxygen therapy. In Bennett P and Elliott D, editors: Physiology and medicine of diving, ed 4, Phildelphia, 1993, Saunders.

consequences. The other conditions listed are relative contraindications. Note that serious problems can arise when patients with obstructive bronchial disease caused by asthma, bronchitis, or emphysema are treated with hyperbaric therapy. Gas trapping can result in barotrauma. Similarly, patients who have upper respiratory infections and nasal congestion are usually unable to clear their ears during compression and decompression and thus are prone to eardrum rupture during treatment.

Nitric Oxide Therapy

As discussed in Chapter 2, nitric oxide has been shown to be a potent pulmonary vasodilator. It has been used successfully to treat persistent pulmonary hypertension of the newborn (PPHN),[34] as an adjunct to the treatment of congenital cardiac defects,[35] and to reverse pulmonary vasoconstriction associated with adult respiratory distress syndrome (ARDS).[36,37] Evidence from animal studies suggests that nitric oxide may reverse the bronchoconstriction induced by histamine and methacholine.

Nitric oxide is supplied as a compressed gas mixture of nitric oxide and nitrogen (minimum purity 99%) in cylinders constructed of aluminum alloy.[38] It is supplied this way because it is a highly reactive molecule that is rapidly oxidized to nitrogen dioxide (NO_2) in the presence of oxygen and to nitric acid (HNO_3) in the presence of water. Nitrogen dioxide and nitric acid are toxic if inhaled. In low concentrations, they can cause a chemical pneumonitis; higher

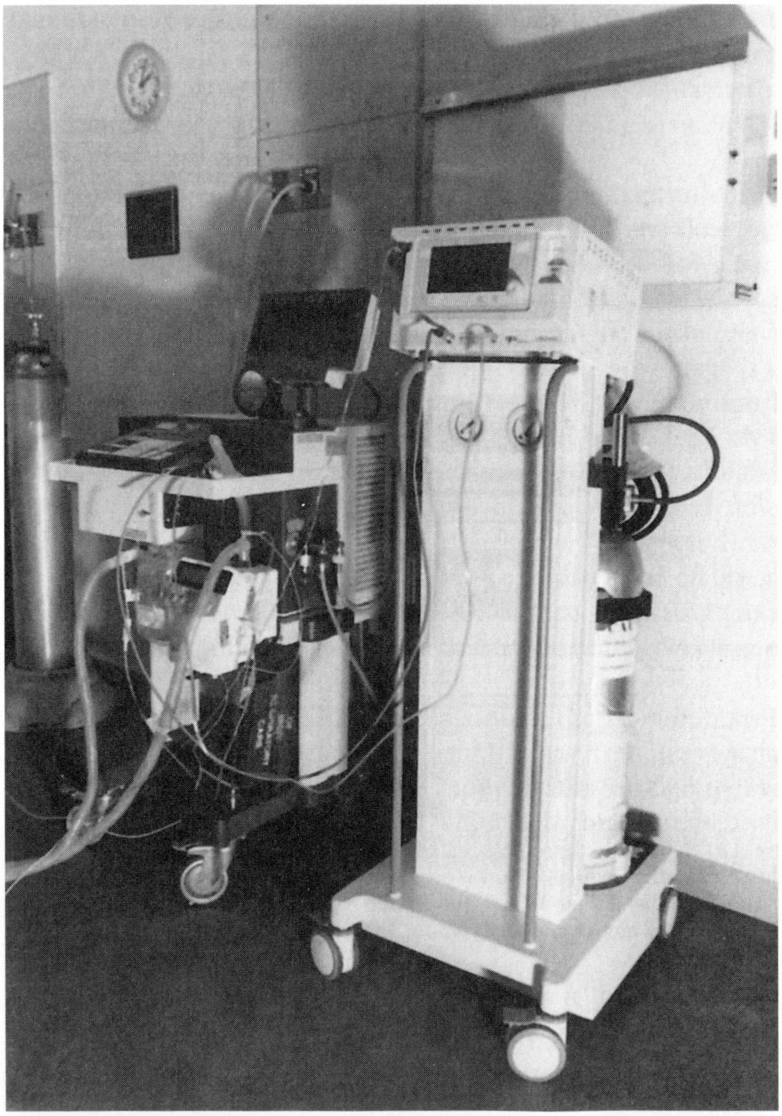

Figure 3-29 Commercially available nitric oxide delivery system. (From Hess D, Ritz R, and Branson RD: Delivery systems for inhaled nitric oxide, Respir Care Clin North Am 3(3):371, 1997.)

concentrations can cause pulmonary edema, which can ultimately lead to death.

The therapeutic dose of nitric oxide is between 2 and 80 parts per million (ppm).[39] Figure 3-29 is a commercially available nitric oxide delivery system manufactured by Ohmeda. The Ohmeda I-NOvent delivery system is designed for use with most conventional critical-care ventilators and can be adapted for use with both adult and pediatric ventilators. Figure 3-30 illustrates the principle of operation.[38] An injection module that consists of a sensor and a gas injection tube is inserted into the inspiratory circuit at the ventilator outlet. Flow in the ventilator circuit is measured, and nitric oxide is injected proportional to the flow to provide the desired dose. The system includes sensors for monitoring oxygen, nitric oxide, and nitrogen dioxide. Gas is sampled downstream of the injection point near the Y-piece in the inspiratory circuit. The gas concentrations are measured with electrochemical cells that are calibrated at regular intervals by the user.[38] A number of alarm systems are available to alert staff members when problems arise, including alarms for high and low nitric oxide, high nitrogen dioxide, as well as high and low oxygen. Other alarms can be set to notify the user when source gas pressure is lost, the electrochemical cells fail, and calibration is required.[38]

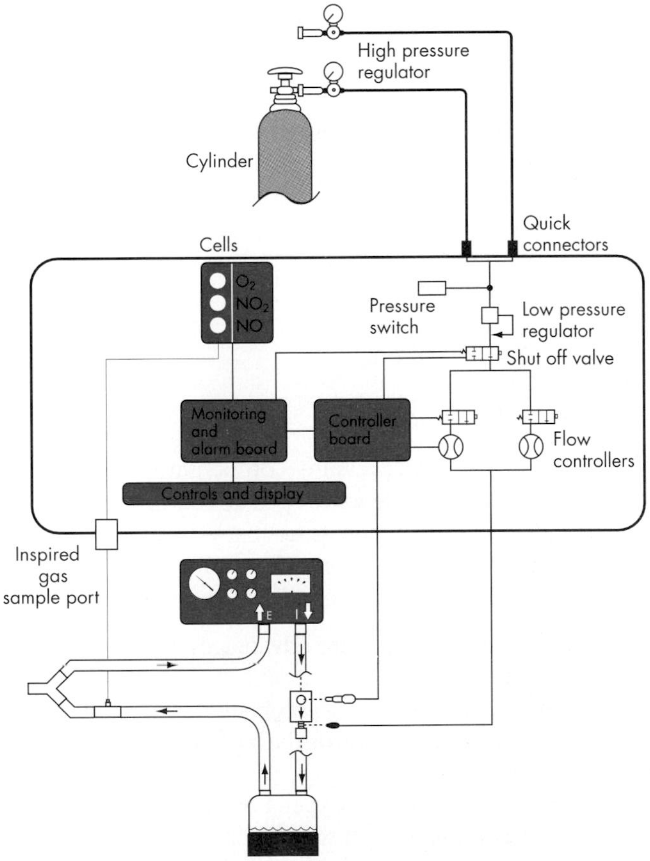

Figure 3-30 Schematic illustrating the principle of operation of the Ohmeda I-NOvent delivery system. (See text for description.) (Redrawn from Hess D, Ritz R, and Branson RD: Inhaled nitric oxide I, Respir Care Clin North Am 3(3):398, 1997.)

Helium-Oxygen (Heliox) Therapy

Helium-oxygen (**heliox**) mixtures have been used on a limited basis to treat patients with airway obstruction.[40-42] Specifically, heliox has been used to manage asthmatic patients with acute respiratory failure, to administer anesthetic gases to patients with small-diameter endotracheal tubes, to treat postextubation stridor in pediatric trauma patients, as an adjunct in the treatment of pediatric patients with refractory croup, and to provide ventilatory support for patients with severe airway obstruction due to chronic bronchitis and emphysema.[43-47]

As stated in Chapter 2, the benefit of breathing heliox is related to its lower density when compared with pure oxygen or air. Remember that the density of a 80%:20% (helium:oxygen) mixture is 0.43 g/L, and that 100% oxygen has a density of 1.43 g/L. Thus an 80%:20% mixture is 1.8 times less dense than 100% oxygen. The lower density promotes laminar flow and reduces the amount of turbulent flow. This relationship is important to remember when administering heliox because the actual flow rate of gas delivered will be approximately 1.8 times greater than the set flow.

Heliox mixtures are supplied in compressed gas cylinders. Two concentrations are generally available: an 80%:20% (helium:oxygen) mixture and a 70%:30% mixture (density = 0.554 g/L). Heliox is usually administered to intubated patients with an intermittent positive pressure device. For nonintubated patients, a well-fitted, simple oxygen mask or a nonrebreathing mask attached to a reservoir bag should be used. The flow rate of gas should be high enough to prevent the reservoir bag from collapsing during inspiration. Nasal cannulas are ineffective for delivering heliox because of leakage. Large-volume enclosures, such as hoods, are also unsatisfactory because helium tends to concentrate at the top of these devices.

It is important to monitor the fractional concentration of oxygen delivered to the patient when administering a heliox mixture. In some cases, commercial cylinders containing helium and oxygen may be "unmixed" (i.e., because of the difference in densities between helium and oxygen, a layering effect can occur). If a sufficient amount of oxygen is not mixed with the helium being breathed by the patient, hypoxemia can result.[48] (Box 3-8 presents a problem-solving scenario involving heliox therapy.)

Carbon Dioxide-Oxygen (Carbogen) Therapy

Carbon dioxide-oxygen mixtures (**carbogen**) are used to treat hiccoughs and carbon monoxide poisoning, as a

BOX 3-8

Decision Making & Problem Solving

You are the therapist on-call when an asthmatic patient is admitted to the emergency department of the hospital. The attending physician requests that you administer heliox containing 30% oxygen to the patient. While administering the gas from a cylinder labeled 70%:30% (helium:oxygen), the patient becomes progressively more dyspneic and cyanotic. What should you do?

See Appendix A for the answer.

BOX 3-9

Clinical Manifestations of Carbon Dioxide Toxicity*

Extrasystole (premature ventricular contractions)
Flushed skin
Full and bounding pulse
Hypertension
Muscle twitching

*Note that hypercapnia cannot be reliably diagnosed on clinical examination only. Arterial blood gases (measurement of partial pressure of arterial carbon dioxide) should be determined in case of doubt.[46]

stimulant/depressant of ventilation, and to prevent the complete washout of carbon dioxide during cardiopulmonary bypass. The frequency of this procedure is limited due to the adverse effects associated with breathing elevated concentrations of carbon dioxide. Box 3-9 lists the clinical manifestations of carbon dioxide toxicity.

Carbogen is supplied in compressed-gas cylinders as either 5%:95% (carbon dioxide:oxygen) or as 7%:93% (carbon dioxide:oxygen). It can be administered to patients with a nonrebreathing mask connected to a reservoir bag. The mask should fit snugly on the patient's face, and the flow rate of gas should be high enough to prevent the bag from collapsing when the patient inhales.

To prevent adverse reactions when administering this type of therapy, it is essential to monitor pulse, blood pressure, and respiration as well as the patient's mental status. Pulse, arterial blood pressure, and minute volume normally increase as the patient breathes carbogen, but the rapidity and level of these changes depend on the concentration of the mixture. Thus changes will occur faster and the effects will be greater if the patient breathes a 7%:93% (carbon dioxide:oxygen) mixture when compared with a 5%:95% mixture. The treatment should be stopped immediately if any of the monitored parameters increase or decrease abruptly or significantly.

Summary

Medical gas therapy is a major responsibility of respiratory care practitioners. The appropriate use of each of the modalities discussed in this chapter requires a knowledge of the operational theories of the devices used to administer medical gases, as well as an understanding of the indications and contraindications for each type of therapy. The guidelines for administering oxygen are well-established, but heliox, nitric oxide, and hyperbaric oxygen therapy are relatively new techniques that may provide alternative strategies for the treatment of hypoxia. Hyperbaric oxygen therapy has been used quite effectively to treat decompression sickness and other diving disorders. Many studies have demonstrated that it may also be an effective treatment for carbon monoxide and cyanide poisoning, as well as a means of preventing tissue necrosis in certain cases.

Review Questions

See Appendix A for answers.

1. Describe an easy method for determining the number of stages in a multistage regulator.
2. Which of the following devices are considered to be high-flow oxygen delivery systems?
   I. Nasal cannula
   II. Nasal catheter
   III. Air-entrainment mask
   IV. Partial-rebreathing mask
   a. I and II only
   b. I, II, and III only
   c. III only
   d. I, II, III, and IV
3. True or False? Back-pressure–compensated flowmeters have their needle valves positioned upstream of the indicator tube, whereas nonback-pressure–compensated flowmeters have their needle valves positioned downstream of the indicator tube.
4. Which of the following are advantages of using TTO therapy catheters?
   I. They limit the patient's mobility.
   II. It is difficult to control the FiO_2 delivered to the patient.
   III. They require lower oxygen flows to achieve a given FiO_2 compared with standard nasal cannulas.
   IV. They are less obtrusive (i.e., more cosmetically pleasing) than nasal cannulas.
   a. I and III only
   b. II and III only
   c. III and IV only
   d. II, III, and IV only

5. What is the air:oxygen entrainment ratio for delivering 40% oxygen through an oxygen adder?
   a. 1:1
   b. 1:2
   c. 1:3
   d. 3:1

6. Studies have shown that mustache and pendant cannulas can reduce the cost of oxygen therapy by as much as:
   a. 10%
   b. 30%
   c. 50%
   d. 80%

7. What is the approximate partial pressure of inspired oxygen of room air if the barometric pressure is raised to 2 atm?
   a. 150 torr
   b. 300 torr
   c. 1200 torr
   d. 1520 torr

8. List five indications and five contraindications for hyperbaric oxygen therapy.

9. Administering heliox can be an effective form of therapy in which of the following situations?
   I. Managing postextubation stridor in pediatric trauma patients
   II. Providing ventilatory support for patients with severe airway obstruction due to chronic bronchitis and emphysema
   III. Administering anesthetic gases to patients with small-diameter endotracheal tubes
   IV. Delivering oxygen therapy to asthmatic children
   a. I and II only
   b. I and III only
   c. I, II, and III only
   d. I, II, III, and IV

10. Which of the following is an indication for delivering nitric oxide therapy?
   I. It has been used successfully to treat PPHN
   II. It can be used as an adjunct to the treatment of congenital cardiac defects
   III. It can be used to reverse pulmonary vasoconstriction associated with ARDS
   IV. It can be used to treat refractory croup
   a. I and III only
   b. II and IV only
   c. I, II, and III only
   d. I, II, III, and IV

11. Helium is approximately 1.8 times less dense than oxygen. The gas flow delivered to a patient receiving an 80%:20% (helium:oxygen) mixture is indicated on the standard oxygen flowmeter as 10 L/min. What is the actual gas flow being delivered to the patient?

12. When carbogen is being administered, which of the following vital signs should be monitored?
   I. Pulse
   II. Blood pressure
   III. Respirations
   IV. The patient's mental status
   a. I and II only
   b. I and III only
   c. I, III, and IV only
   d. I, II, III, and IV

13. What are the clinical manifestations of carbon dioxide toxicity?

References

1. Ward JJ: Equipment for mixed gas and oxygen therapy. In Barnes TA, editor: Core textbook of respiratory care practice, ed 2, St Louis, 1994, Mosby.
2. American Association for Respiratory Care: Clinical practice guideline: oxygen therapy in the acute care hospital, Respir Care 36:1306, 1991.
3. American Association for Respiratory Care: Clinical practice guideline: oxygen therapy in the home or extended care facility, Respir Care 37:918, 1992.
4. Leigh JM: The evolution of oxygen therapy apparatus, Anesthesiology 29:462, 1974.
5. Shapiro BA, et al: Clinical application of respiratory care, 4 ed, St Louis, 1991, Mosby.
6. Eisenberg L: History of inhalation therapy equipment. In International Anesthesiology Clinic: Ventilators and inhalation therapy, Boston, 1966, Little, Brown.
7. Vain NE, et al: Regulation of oxygen concentrations delivered to infants by nasal cannulas, Am J Dis Child 143:1458, 1989.
8. Heimlich HJ: Respiratory rehabilitation with a transtracheal oxygen system, Ann Otol Rhinol Laryngol 91:643, 1982.
9. Wyka K and Scanlan CL: Respiratory home care. In Scanlan CL, Spearman CB, and Sheldon RL, editors: Egan's fundamentals of respiratory care, 6 ed, St Louis, 1995, Mosby.
10. Johnson JT, et al: Transtracheal delivery of oxygen: efficacy and safety for long-term continuous therapy, Ann Oto Rhinol Laryngol 100:108, 1991.
11. Tieb BL and Lewis MI: Oxygen conservation and oxygen conserving devices, Chest 92(2):263, 1987.
12. Shigeoka JW and Bonnekat, HW: The current status of oxygen-conserving devices, Respir Care 30(10):833, 1985.
13. Boothby VM, Lovelace WR, and Bulbulian AH: I. Oxygen administration: the value of high concentration of oxygen for therapy, II. Oxygen for therapy and aviation: an apparatus for the administration of oxygen or oxygen and helium by inhalation. III. Design and construction of the masks for oxygen inhalation apparatus, Proc Mayo Clinic 13:641, 1938.
14. Kacmarek RM: Methods of oxygen delivery in the hospital, Prob Respir Care 3:563, 1990.
15. Barach AL and Eckman, BS: A physiologically controlled oxygen mask apparatus, Anesthesiology 2:421, 1941.
16. Barach AL: Symposium: inhalation therapy historical background, Anesthesiology 23:407, 1962.

17. Campbell EJM: A method of controlling oxygen administration which reduces the risk of carbon dioxide retention, Lancet 2:12, 1960.
18. Scacci R: Air entrainment masks: jet mixing is how they work; the Bernoulli andVenturi principles are how they don't, Respir Care 24:928, 1979.
19. Cohen JL, Demers RR, and Sakland M: Air entrainment masks: a performance evaluation, Respir Care 22:279, 1977.
20. McPherson S: Respiratory care equipment, 5 ed, St Louis, 1995, Mosby.
21. Hill SL, et al: Fixed performance oxygen masks: an evaluation, BMJ 288:1361, 1984.
22. Cox D and Gilbe C: Fixed performance oxygen masks, Anesthesiology 36:958, 1981.
23. Campbell EJM and Minty KB: Controlled oxygen at 60% concentration, Lancet 2:1199, 1976.
24. Fourst GN, et al: Shortcomings of using two jet nebulizers in tandem with an aerosol face mask, Chest 99:1346, 1991.
25. Kuo CD, Lin SE, and Wang JH: Aerosol, humidity, and oxygen levels, Chest 99:1325, 1991.
26. Beckham RW and Mishoe SC: Sound levels inside incubators and oxygen hoods used with nebulizers and humidifiers, Respir Care 27:33, 1982.
27. Davis JC and Hunt TK, editors: Hyperbaric oxygen therapy, Bethesda, Md., 1977, Undersea Medical Society, Inc.
28. Kindall EP: Clinical hyperbaric oxygen therapy. In Bennett P and Elliott D, editors: The physiology and medicine of diving, 4 ed, Philadelphia, 1993, Saunders.
29. Moon RE and Camporesi EM: Clinical applications of hyperbaric oxygen therapy, Prob Resp Care 4:176, 1991.
30. Gallagher TJ, Smith RA, and Bell GC: Evaluation of mechanical ventilators in a hyperbaric environment, Space Environ Med 49:375, 1978.
31. Weaver LK: Hyperbaric treatment of respiratory emergencies, Respir Care 37(7):720, 1992.
32. NHLBI workshop summary: Hyperbaric oxygenation therapy, Am Rev Resp Dis 144(6):1414, 1991.
33. Myers RAM, et al: Value of hyperbaric oxygen in suspected carbon monoxide poisoning, JAMA 246:2478, 1981.
34. Craig J and Mullins D: Nitric oxide inhalation in infants and children: physiologic and clinical implications, Am J Crit Care 4(6):43, 1995.
35. Roberts JD, Lang P, and Bigatello LM:, Circulation 87:447, 1993.
36. Bone RC: A new therapy for the adult respiratory distress syndrome, N Engl J Med 328(6):431, 1993.
37. Bigatello LM, et al: Prolonged inhalation of low concentrations of nitric oxide in patients with severe adult respiratory distress syndrome: effects on pulmonary hemodynamics and oxygenation, Anesthesiology 80(4):761, 1994.
38. Brown RH, Zerhouni EA, and Hirshman C: Reversal of bronchoconstriction by inhaled nitric oxide: histamine versus methacholine, Am J Resp Crit Care Med 150:233, 1994.
39. Howder CL: Cardiopulmonary pharmacology, 2 ed, Baltimore, 1996, Williams & Wilkins.
40. Hess D, Ritz R, and Branson RD: Delivery systems for inhaled nitric oxide, Resp Care Clin North Am, 3(3):371, 1997.
41. Motley HL: Helium-oxygen therapy, Respir Care 18:668, 1973.
42. Curtis JL, et al: Helium-oxygen gas therapy: use and availability for the emergency treatment of inoperative airway obstruction, Chest 90(3):455, 1986.
43. Scanlan CL and Thalken R: Medical gas therapy. In Scanlan CL, Spearman CB, and Sheldon RL, editors: Egan's fundamentals of respiratory care, 6 ed, St Louis, 1995, Mosby.
44. Stillwell PC, et al: Effectiveness of open-circuit and oxyhood delivery of helium-oxygen, Chest 95(6):1222, 1989.
45. Skrinskas GJ, Hyland RH, and Hutcheon MA: Using helium-oxygen mixtures in the management of acute upper airway obstruction, Can Med Assoc J 128:555, 1983.
46. Kemper KJ, et al: Helium-oxygen mixtures in the treatment of postextubation stridor in pediatric patients, Crit Care Med 19(3):356, 1991.
47. Nelson DS and McClellan L: Helium-oxygen mixtures as adjunctive support for refractory viral croup, Ohio State Med J 78(10):729, 1982.
48. Emergency Care Research Institute: Cylinders with unmixed helium-oxygen, Health Devices 19(4):146, 1990.

Internet Resources

1. American Association for Respiratory Care (Clinical Practice Guidelines):
   http://www.aarc.org
2. American Lung Association:
   http://www.lungusa.org
3. Medexplorer (Search engine for medicine):
   http://www.medexplorer.com
4. RT Corner (web site for respiratory therapy students):
   http://www.rtcorner.com
5. Joint Commission on Accreditation of Healthcare Organizations:
   http://www.jcaho.org
6. Global Anesthesiology Server Network:
   http://gasnet.med.yale.edu
7. Nellcor-Puritan Bennett:
   http://www.nellcorpb.com
8. Virtual Hospital:
   http://www.vh.org
9. The American College of Hyperbaric Medicine:
   http://www.hyperbaricmedicine.org
10. The Undersea and Hyperbaric Medical Society:
    http://www.uhms.org
11. History of Oxygen Therapy (L. Martin, MD):
    http://www.mtsinai.org/pulmonary/papers/ox-hist/ox-hist-intro.html
12. Respiratory on the Web (100 sites of interest to respiratory care professionals):
    http://wwww.xmission.com/~gastown/herpmed/respi.htm

CHAPTER 4

CHAPTER OUTLINE

Humidity
- Body Humidity and Deficit
- Maintaining and Monitoring Humidification

Aerosol Therapy
- Aerosol Delivery

KEY TERMS

Absolute Humidity
Aerosol
Aerosol Mask
Brownian Movement
BTPS
Bubble Humidifier
Cascade Humidifier
Chamber
Condensation
Dry Powder Inhaler (DPI)
Evaporation
Geometric Standard Deviation (GSD)
Heat and Moisture Exchangers (HMEs)
Heated Wire
Humidity
Humidity Deficit
Hygroscopic
Inertial Impaction
Jet Nebulizer
Kinetic Activity
Large-Volume Nebulizer (LVN)
Mass Median Aerodynamic Diameter (MMAD)
Metered Dose Inhaler (MDI)
Percent Body Humidity
Relative Humidity
Sedimentation
Small-Volume Nebulizer (SVN)
Spacer
Wick Humidifier

Humidity and Aerosol Therapy

Dennis R. Wissing

CHAPTER LEARNING OBJECTIVES

Upon completion of this chapter, the reader should be able to:

1. Define the three types of humidity.
2. Define the terms *evaporation, aerosol,* and *humidity deficit.*
3. Describe the natural physiologic humidification process.
4. Identify indications for humidity therapy.
5. Describe factors that affect humidification of a gas.
6. Compare low-flow and high-flow humidifiers.
7. Explain the importance of monitoring and maintaining humidity therapy.
8. Describe the physical characteristics of an aerosol.
9. Discuss factors that influence aerosol deposition.
10. Determine the optimal technique for administering aerosol: small volume nebulizer, large volume nebulizer, metered dose inhaler, or dry powder inhaler.
11. Describe the therapeutic indications for aerosol therapy.
12. Explain how pneumatic aerosol generators work to produce an aerosol.
13. Describe how ultrasonic nebulizers work.
14. Discuss the clinical considerations for aerosol therapy.
15. Determine special considerations for administering aerosol therapy.

To safely and effectively administer **humidity** and **aerosol** therapy, it is necessary to understand the rationale and technical considerations, as well as the hazards and limitations of such therapy. Therefore this chapter explores the various devices used to deliver humidity and aerosol, as well as the hazards and precautions associated with each. How humidity and aerosols may be used in various clinical situations during mechanical ventilation, including routine and critical care of infants and pediatric and adult patients, is also discussed.

HUMIDITY

Humidity is water that exists as individual molecules in the vaporous or gaseous state. Although it may not be obvious, these molecules are present in air that we breathe. Vapor is the presence of individual free molecules of a substance that exist below its critical temperature; so humidity is often described as water vapor. Vapor exerts a pressure as a result of the random, constant movement of water molecules. This pressure, called water-vapor pressure (P_{H2O}), varies with the temperature of the gas. That is, as gas temperature increases, water-vapor pressure increases because gas molecules move faster, increasing molecular collisions and bombardment. This principle is illustrated in Figure 4-1. As temperature increases, the **kinetic activity** of the water molecules also increases, resulting in an increase in pressure. Once sufficient kinetic activity is reached, molecules leave the liquid state and enter a vaporous state. This occurs at the boiling point of a substance, which can be defined as the temperature at which the pressure exerted by a substance's molecular activity equals the atmospheric pressure. Critical temperature is defined as the temperature at which a substance's kinetic energy is so high that the substance can only exist as a true gas. Above this temperature, no amount of applied pressure can convert the substance (e.g., water) back to a liquid. Therefore humidity is not a true gas because our atmosphere is at a temperature below the critical temperature of water (374° C); although the terms *gas* and *vapor* are often used interchangeably.

As discussed in Chapter 1, vaporization is the result of water changing from a liquid to a vapor, and can result from boiling or **evaporation.** As water is heated to its boiling point and molecules leave the liquid state and become vapor, water vapor is produced. The boiling point is influenced by the pressure above the water surface. If this pressure increases, the boiling point increases. Likewise, if this pressure decreases, the boiling point decreases. The energy required to vaporize a liquid is called the latent heat of vaporization. Vaporization can also result from evaporation, which occurs when a liquid changes to a vapor without reaching its boiling point. Evaporation occurs when liquid molecules near the surface contain enough kinetic energy to break free and enter a vapor state, reducing the volume of the liquid. For example, when a pan of water is left out and exposed to room air, water loss results. Humidity can be measured as **absolute** or **relative humidity.** Absolute humidity is the actual content or weight of water present in a given volume of gas and may be expressed as either grams per cubic meter (g/m^3) or milligrams per liter (mg/L).

The term *content* is often substituted for *absolute humidity,* which is the ratio of the actual content or weight of the water present in a gas sample relative to the sample's capacity to hold water at that temperature. In other words, relative humidity is a comparison of how much water a gas sample is actually holding with the maximum amount that the gas can hold at a given temperature. Relative humidity is calculated by dividing the amount of water in the gas (content) by the amount of water that the gas can hold at that temperature (capacity). This ratio is expressed as a per-

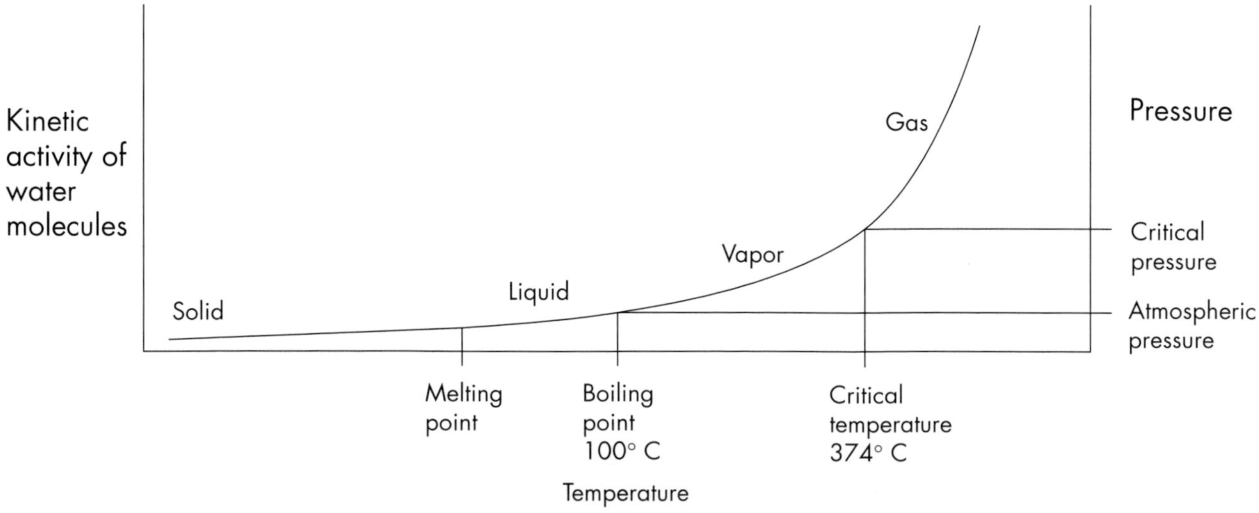

Figure 4-1 The relationship between temperature, pressure, and kinetic activity of water molecules.

BOX 4-1

Calculating Relative Humidity

The actual water content (absolute humidity) of a sample of room air is measured with a hygrometer and is found to be 12 mg/L. If the room air temperature is 20° C (68° F), what is the relative humidity?

Step 1

Refer to Table 4-1, locate 20°, and note the water content. This refers to the maximum amount of water a gas sample at this temperature can hold, which is 17.30 mg/L.

Step 2

Relative humidity is the ratio of what the gas sample is *actually* holding to what the gas sample can hold when saturated with water vapor. To calculate relative humidity, divide the actual content by the capacity:

$$\frac{\text{measured humidity (content)}}{\text{water capacity}} \times 100 = \text{relative humidity}$$

$$\frac{12 \text{ mg/L}}{17.30 \text{ mg/L}} = 69\%$$

Step 3

Interpret the answer. In this case, the room air is holding 69% of what it is capable of holding at 20° C.

TABLE 4-1

Absolute humidity and water vapor pressure at various temperatures when the gas is saturated with water

Temperature (° C)	Absolute humidity (mg/L)	Water vapor pressure (Torr)
19	16.3	16.5
20	17.3	17.5
21	18.4	18.6
22	19.4	19.8
23	20.6	21.0
24	21.8	22.3
25	23.0	23.7
26	24.4	25.1
27	25.8	26.7
28	27.2	28.3
29	28.8	29.9
30	30.4	31.7
31	32.0	33.6
32	33.8	35.5
33	35.6	37.6
34	37.6	39.8
35	39.6	42.0
36	41.7	44.4
37	**43.9**	**46.9**
38	46.2	49.5
39	48.6	52.3
40	51.1	55.1
41	53.7	58.1

centage and can be calculated using humidity measurements of weight (mg/L) or partial pressure (PH_2O). Box 4-1 shows an example of how to calculate relative humidity.

When the amount of water that a gas contains is equal to the gas's capacity, the relative humidity is 100%. When a gas is at capacity (i.e., it contains the maximum amount of water vapor that it can hold at a given temperature), it is described as saturated (i.e., content equals capacity). The term *saturation* is similar to *water-vapor capacity,* which refers to a gas at its maximum partial pressure of water vapor. Table 4-1 shows the relationship between partial pressure of water vapor, temperature, and content. It is important to recognize that a gas exerts a partial pressure of water vapor of 47 torr at 37° C and contains 43.9 mg of water per liter of gas. These values are found in gas in the lower respiratory track as a result of an effective upper and lower airway conditioning process for incoming gas from a wide range of ambient conditions. If absolute humidity is held constant, increasing the temperature of the gas will decrease relative humidity because the higher the gas temperature, the greater the gas's capacity to hold water. Likewise, a decrease in temperature will decrease the gas's capacity to hold water, and the relative humidity will remain at 100%. This phenomenon is often encountered by respiratory care practitioners during heated humidity therapy. When heated humidity is delivered to a patient via large-bore (diameter) corrugated tubing, ambient temperature can cool the gas within the tubing; the absolute humidity remains unchanged, the gas temperature decreases the gas's capacity to hold water, so water vapor is squeezed out of the gas. This excess water, or **condensation,** can accumulate in the delivery tubing and must be removed to eliminate the possibility of the water becoming an obstruction in the gas delivery tube, disrupting gas and humidity delivery to the patient (Figure 4-2).

Percent Body Humidity (% BH) and Humidity Deficit

Percent body humidity (% BH), which is the maximum amount of water that can be held by a gas at body temperature, is often used when discussing relative humidity. Specifically, % BH is gas at **BTPS,** which is defined as a gas at body temperature at the pressure to which the patient is exposed (e.g., atmospheric) and 100% saturated with water vapor. Under normal physiologic conditions, % BH is 43.9 mg/L (see Table 4-1).

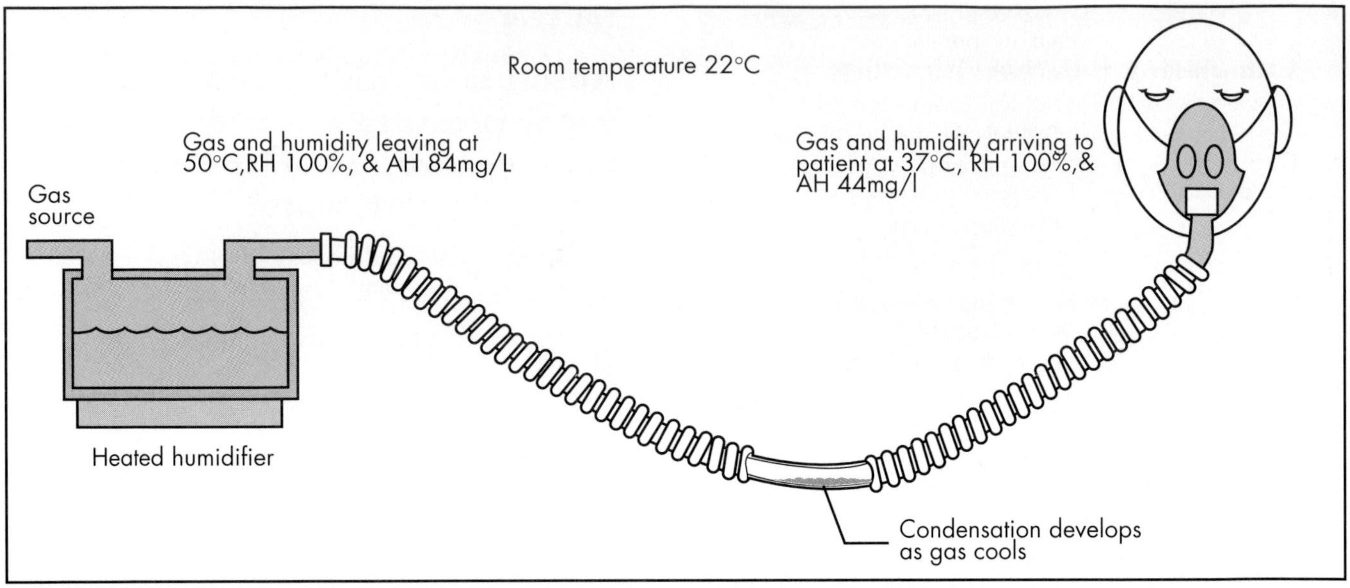

Figure 4-2 Condensation can develop in the gas delivery tube as heated humidity is cooled by ambient conditions. As the temperature of the gas cools, it can hold less water vapor; so excess water leaves the gas and accumulates in gravity-dependent loops of the delivery tubing.

A **humidity deficit** is the difference between the amount of water vapor inspired and water vapor contained in the gas in the lungs. In other words, humidity deficit is the difference between % BH and actual ambient humidity. Under most conditions, the upper airway can eliminate a humidity deficit over a wide range of ambient temperatures and humidity levels. Figure 4-3 shows an example of the humidity deficit of a nonintubated patient spontaneously breathing room air. A humidity deficit becomes clinically significant when the deficit is large and maintained for an extended period of time. A patient breathing a gas that contains little or no humidity may experience pathological changes in the airways, including drying or retention of secretions, airway plugging, and increased incidence of infection. Most spontaneously breathing, nonintubated patients can adequately humidify inspired gas. However, these pathologic changes can occur during other conditions. For example, when the upper airway is bypassed by an artificial airway, there may be systemic dehydration; or when the patient is breathing low-humidity gas and has a high minute volume of respiration. So that the potential danger of a large humidity deficit and the importance of proper humidification of an anhydrous medical gas are fully understood, a brief review of the physiology of natural humidification is provided.

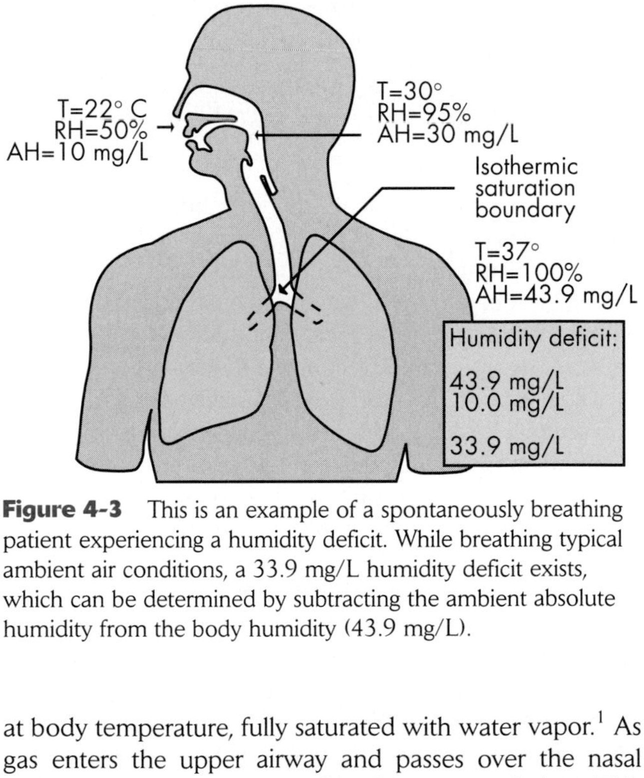

Figure 4-3 This is an example of a spontaneously breathing patient experiencing a humidity deficit. While breathing typical ambient air conditions, a 33.9 mg/L humidity deficit exists, which can be determined by subtracting the ambient absolute humidity from the body humidity (43.9 mg/L).

Physiologic Humidification

The upper and lower respiratory tracts normally provide an effective system for conditioning inspired gas. Besides filtering foreign particles and microbes, the upper airways also warm and humidify inspired gas so that gas traveling beyond the carina enters the lower airways and the alveoli at body temperature, fully saturated with water vapor.[1] As gas enters the upper airway and passes over the nasal turbinates and conchae, gas flow becomes turbulent. This turbulence increases the number of gas molecules that come in contact with the nasal mucosa, allowing incoming gas to be more efficiently warmed. This process, turbulent convection, is an important aspect of normal humidification. As inspired gas is warmed, water is transferred to the incoming gas by evaporation from the mucosa.[2] Therefore as it flows through the upper airways as a result of inspired gases cooling the nasal mucosa, the inspired gas is humidified and warmed through evaporation and convection. This heat energy (previously defined as the latent heat of vaporization) remains in the water vapor until it is released during expiration. As inspiration continues, humidification and warming occur, the mucosa cools, and the incoming gas reaches the isothermic saturation boundary (ISB). This boundary is the point at which inspired gas reaches body humidity (at BTPS) and is normally located just below the carina (See Figure 4-3).[3,4]

During exhalation, heat and humidity are transferred back to the nasal mucosa. As gas exits the lower respiratory tract, heat is transferred back to the mucosa by convection. As the expired gas is cooled by this heat loss, the gas's capacity to hold water decreases, and water is released (condensation) onto the airway lining. Thus as expiration occurs, the airway mucosal lining is rewarmed and rehydrated in preparation for the next inspiration. Although some studies report a difference between the gas-conditioning effects of nose vs. mouth breathing, the clinical significance of these differences is minimal. Data suggest that the upper airway can efficiently condition inspired gases from either nasal or mouth breathing.[5,6] As stated previously, the upper airway is an efficient gas conditioner, despite wide fluctuation of ambient temperature and humidity. As ambient temperature increases above body temperature, blood flow to the turbinates increases and heat is lost from the nasal mucosa.[7] At extremely cold temperatures, the upper airway remains capable of providing the lower airways and alveoli with gas at BTPS.

Clinical Indications for Humidity Therapy

Respiratory care practitioners administer medical gases to a wide variety of patients, from those who are spontaneously breathing (with or without an artificial airway in place) to those who are being mechanically ventilated. To assure effective therapy, an understanding of the indications for humidity therapy is necessary.

Breathing dry or inadequately humidified gas can shift the isothermic saturation boundary farther down the lung, compromising the airway's ability to warm and humidify inspired gas. The boundary may move farther into the peripheral airways with endotracheal intubation, large tidal volumes, or inspiration of a cold gas. If the ISB shifts downward, the airway mucosa is at risk for altered cilia function, a decrease in mucus rheology (flow), mucous membrane dehydration, and retention of secretions.[6] Such alterations of mucosal structure may lead to stagnation of secretions, which may lead to partial or complete airway obstruction and increased incidence of infection. If the patient has pulmonary disease, administration of a dry or poorly humidified gas may exacerbate the existing disease and further compromise respiratory function. Such patients may experience partial to complete airway obstruction from mucus plugging and atelectasis and have the potential for ventilatory failure. Clinical signs and symptoms of inadequate humidification and mucosal damage are listed in Box 4-2.

BOX 4-2

Clinical Signs and Symptoms of Inadequate Airway Humidification

Atelectasis
Dry, nonproductive cough
Increased airway resistance
Increased incidence of infection
Increased work of breathing
Substernal pain
Thick, dehydrated secretions

The goal of humidity therapy is to minimize or eliminate a humidity deficit while the patient is breathing a dry medical gas. Medical gases delivered from a cylinder or central-supply system are delivered at 0% relative humidity. The amount of humidification provided depends on the type of gas flow system used and the gas's entry point into the respiratory system.

Gas flow systems can be categorized as either low-flow or high-flow. A low-flow gas system provides a gas flow lower than the patient's inspiratory needs, whereas a high-flow gas system meets the patient's gas flow needs. In other words, high-flow systems provide all the gas the patient inspires. Gas from a low-flow system can be humidified, but the patient supplements this humidity with ambient water vapor. An example of a low-flow gas system is a **bubble humidifier** (Figure 4-4). As oxygen leaves this device, it is humidified to about 40% to 50% relative humidity. As the patient inspires, humidified gas is obtained from the bubble humidifier and ambient air. As the gas enters the respiratory system, it is further humidified by the airway (as previous described) and reaches BTPS at the isothermic saturation boundary. With low-flow systems, supplemental humidity may increase patient comfort by minimizing drying of the nasal and oral cavities. Recent respiratory care trends include the omission of humidity for dry gases provided to the patient at gas flow rates lower than 4 L/min. Recent data suggest that it is safe to omit supplemental humidity at these flows[8]; however, respiratory care practitioners should exercise clinical judgment as to when supplemental humidity should be omitted with medical gas delivery from a low-flow system.[9] High-flow gas systems, such as a mechanical ventilator or a properly applied nonrebreathing oxygen mask, provide the entire gas flow to the patient, so adequate humidity must be provided. Official standards for humidity have been established by the American Association for Respiratory Care (AARC).[10] These standards include providing a minimum of 30 mg/L of water at 31° to 35° C with 80% to 100% relative humidity to the airway when the patient is breathing gas through a

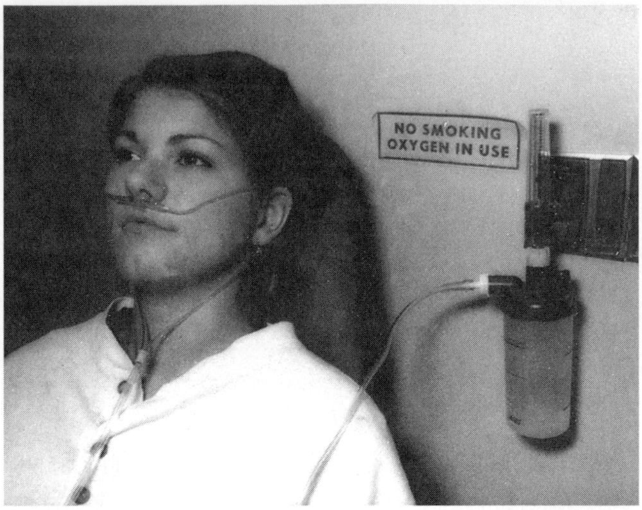

Figure 4-4 A bubble humidifier is a common example of a low-flow humidifier. It humidifies the gas traveling to the patient via nasal cannula to about 40% to 50% of the relative humidity.

> **BOX 4-3**
>
> **Humidity Requirements for Gas Delivery at Various Sites in the Upper and Lower Airway**
>
> **Gas Delivered to:**
>
> **The Nose or Mouth**
> 50% relative humidity with an absolute humidity level of 10 mg/L at 22° C
>
> **The Hypopharynx**
> 95% relative humidity with an absolute humidity level of 28 to 34 mg/L at 29° to 32° C
>
> **The Mid-Trachea**
> 100% relative humidity with an absolute humidity level of 36 to 40 mg/L at 31° to 35° C

high-flow gas system and the upper airway is by-passed with an artificial airway (e.g., endotracheal or tracheostomy tube). Humidity at this level can prevent mucosal damage and inspissation or thickening of airway secretions.

It is recommended that the humidity output of any medical gas delivery system match the normal gas conditions at its entry point into the respiratory tract.[9] Box 4-3 lists the humidity and temperature requirements for gases delivered to various points in the respiratory tract.

Factors that Influence Humidifier Efficiency

Humidity therapy should include either supplying enough water vapor to a dry medical gas to make it equal to ambient conditions in terms of relative humidity and temperature, or providing heated humidity close to body temperature and at 80% to 100% relative humidity when gas is delivered to a bypassed upper airway. Respiratory care practitioners can choose from a variety of devices to provide humidity therapy. The effectiveness of each type of humidification device depends upon the temperature of the gas being delivered, the ratio of the available water surface area to the gas, and the length of time the gas is exposed to water.

Temperature. As mentioned earlier, the higher the temperature of a gas, the more water vapor it can hold. This fundamental concept plays an important role in meeting a patient's humidity needs because heating the humidifier increases the water-carrying capacity of the humidified gas. It is important to recognize that humidified gas delivered to an artificial airway (via endotracheal or tracheostomy tube) must be between 31° and 35° C with a minimum of 30 mg/L of absolute humidity.[10] Therefore appropriate temperature monitoring at the interface of the patient and the humidifying device is necessary to ensure that temperature and gas humidity levels are within the recommended ranges to avoid mucosal or thermal injury (either because of inadequate humidification and temperature or overheated gas).

Unheated humidifiers are less efficient than heated humidifiers because during operation, an unheated humidifier can lose water temperature in its reservoir as gas flows through it.[11] For example, the temperature of the water reservoir of an unheated bubble humidifier with oxygen flowing through it can decrease to 10° C below room temperature. Even though the gas leaving the unit contains high relative humidity, as it travels to the patient it warms and the relative humidity decreases. Once the gas enters the respiratory tract, relative humidity will only be about 30% to 40%.

Surface Area and Time. The greater the ratio of water-surface contact to gas volume, and the longer that the gas is exposed to water, the greater the opportunity for humidification. That is, the greater the water-surface area and the longer the gas is in contact with water, the better the humidification. As gas flows through water, gas molecules are humidified. Typically, during humidity therapy, gas bubbles through or flows across a water reservoir as it travels to the patient. The water-surface area is governed by the amount of water the gas molecules are exposed to, the depth of the water, and the size of the gas bubbles. The larger the surface area and the greater the depth of the reservoir, the smaller the bubbles, and the longer the gas travels (i.e., a slow gas-flow rate) through the water, the greater the humidification.

As will be described later in this chapter, humidifiers may use either a large water reservoir for gas to flow through (e.g., bubble humidifier) or an adsorbent material or wick to increase gas-to-water contact.

BOX 4-4

Types of Humidifiers

Low-Flow Humidifiers

Bubble humidifiers
Simple diffuser humidifiers

High-Flow Humidifiers

Cascade type of humidifiers
Heat and moisture exchangers
Vapor-phase humidifiers
Wick type of humidifiers

Humidity-Generating Equipment

Humidifiers can be divided into two categories: low-flow and high-flow. Low-flow humidifiers provide gas and humidity below the inspiratory gas flow needs of the patient, and high-flow humidifiers provide all of the inspiratory gas and humidity flow to the patient. Box 4-4 lists common devices used for each of these categories.

Low-flow Humidifiers. Low-flow humidifiers are typically classified as bubble type of humidifiers or as bubble-diffuser type of humidifiers. These devices employ a unique physical principle that allows water and gas to come into contact with each other.

Bubble Type of Humidifiers. Of the simple humidifiers, bubble type of humidifiers are the most widely used devices for humidifying medical gases. Such humidifiers include a water reservoir, a diameter index safety system (DISS) connector for attachment to a gas source (e.g., a flowmetering device), a capillary tube that is submerged into the water reservoir, and an outlet for attachment of a delivery device (e.g., an oxygen cannula or mask) (Figure 4-5). A dry gas such as oxygen enters the humidifier through a DISS connector, travels down a capillary type of tube, and exits the tip, breaking up into many small bubbles. Humidification of gas within the bubbles occurs as they rise to the water surface. Once at the surface, the gas bubbles burst, and their water-vapor content is released. The humidifier may also employ a diffuser tip at the distal end of the gas capillary tube to enhance the creation of small gas bubbles. Bubble size is governed by the design of the gas outlet at the bottom of the capillary tube. Some devices have an open lumen, but others employ a diffuser of plastic foam, porous metal, or mesh (Figure 4-6). Diffuser type of humidifiers are more efficient than capillary tube type of humidifiers because the diffuser creates more small bubbles, allowing a greater surface area for gas and water interaction.[8]

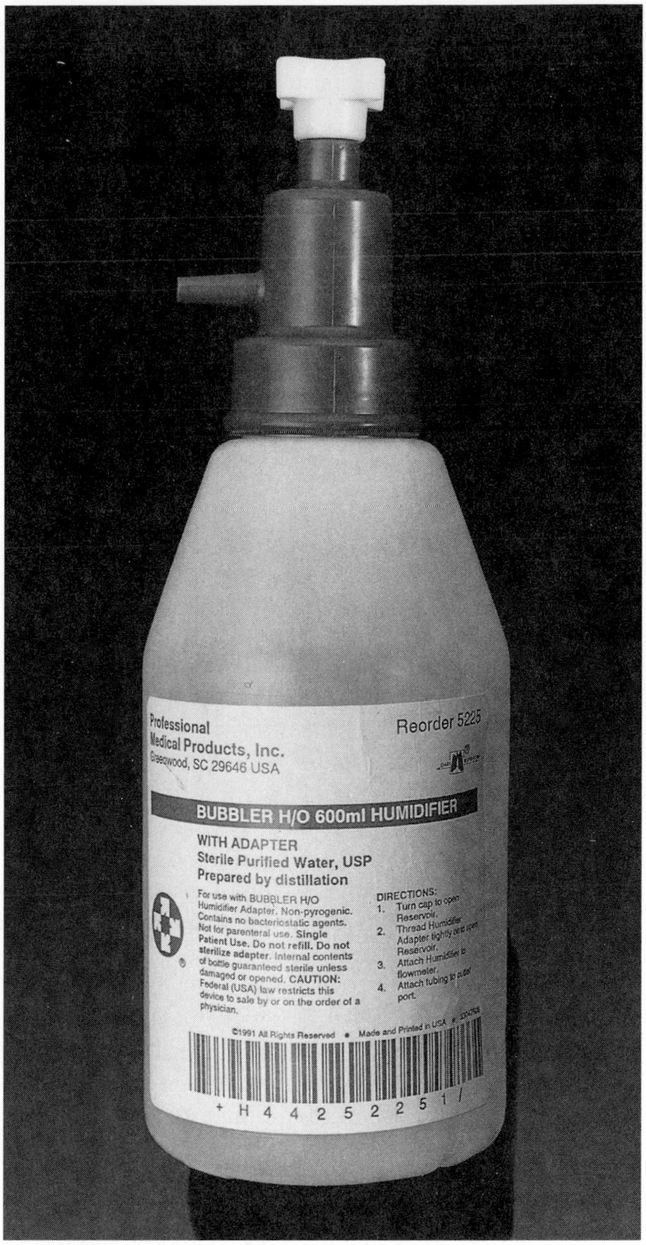

Figure 4-5 A bubble humidifier.

As with other humidifiers, the efficiency of the bubble type of humidifiers depends upon the surface area of the water and gas, the time available for bubbles to remain in contact with the water, and the size of the bubbles. These factors are influenced by the gas flow through the unit (i.e., the faster the gas flow rate, the less time for bubbles and water to stay in contact), the water reservoir level (i.e., the deeper the water, the longer the contact), and the ambient temperature (i.e., the greater the ambient temperature, the lower the relative humidity leaving the device). Bubble humidifiers are more efficient with gas flows of 5 L/min or less. At these flows, absolute humidity is about 10 to 20 mg/L, and relative humidity is 30% to 40% at 37° C.[6,12] At gas flow rates above 5 L/min, delivered humidity decreases

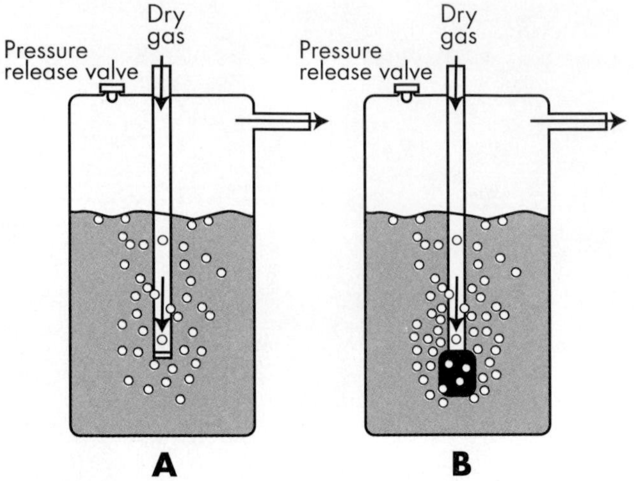

Figure 4-6 Two different types of bubble humidifier capillary tube openings: **A,** An open lumen; **B,** diffuser type of end.

because of the reduced temperature of the reservoir and the shorter bubble-to-water contact time.

There are several technical problems with bubble type of humidifiers that should be considered. For example, they can transport water-bred microbes from the unit to the patient when used with high gas flows. At high gas flows an aerosol is created; if microbes are present in the humidifier or delivery tube, water droplets can become contaminated and, if passed onto the patient, an increased opportunity for airway contamination exists.

Another problem that may arise with bubble type of humidifiers is the possibility of pressure building up within the humidifier itself. This can occur if the small-bore tubing used to deliver the medical gas becomes kinked or obstructed. If this happens, pressure builds and can possibly rupture the device. To prevent this from occurring, bubble humidifiers use a pressure-relief valve that sounds an audible alarm when pressure builds up within the unit. The valve can be gravity-operated or spring-loaded and will remain open if the pressure in the unit exceeds 2 psi. Once the pressure-relief alarm sounds, corrective actions must be taken to restore medical gas delivery to the patient. Also, maintenance of the water level within the humidifier is critical. Bubble type of humidifiers can be purchased either prefilled (disposable) by the manufacturer as intended for single-patient use or nonfilled and permanent (nondisposable). The permanent humidifiers must be filled with sterile water, the level of which must be monitored and maintained; these units must be disinfected or sterilized between patients.

High-flow Humidifiers. High flow humidifiers provide water vapor to the entire gas flow inspired by the patient and include the cascade, vapor-phase, and wick type of humidifiers, as well as **heat and moisture exchangers (HMEs).** These high-flow humidifiers are commonly used with mechanical ventilation.

Patients receiving mechanical ventilatory support usually require an artificial airway. These airways include endotracheal and tracheostomy tubes, which bypass the patient's natural ability to warm and humidify inspired gases. When an artificial airway is in place, supplemental humidity and heat must be provided to ensure that the gas delivered to the patient contains at least 30 mg/L of water and is at 31° to 35° C. Heated humidity is typically required to prevent hypothermia, dehydration of airway secretions, destruction of airway epithelium, and atelectasis.[8,9,13,14]

Four types of humidifiers are commonly used when an artificial airway is in place: cascade, wick, or vapor-phase type of humidifiers and HMEs. Each of these humidifiers will be discussed.

Cascade Humidifiers. Since the early 1960s, the Nellcor Puritan Bennett cascade humidifier, which can provide 100% humidity within a range of desired temperatures, has been a popular means of providing humidity therapy (Figure 4-7). It is basically an advanced bubble type of humidifier used with mechanical ventilation to ensure that gases are delivered to the patient at or near body humidity with high gas flow rates. Gas enters the cascade and travels down a tubelike structure called a tower. Once it reaches the end of the tower, it moves upward through a sheet of plastic that resembles a grid containing many square holes, which produce small bubbles of humidified gas. Many of these bubbles dissipate into water vapor and are carried from the humidifier into the patient's delivery circuit. Water is unable to flow backward through the cascade because there is a one-way valve at the bottom of the tower. Additionally, a small opening on the tower wall above the water line allows the patient's spontaneous effort to be sensed by whatever device is attached to the inlet port of the cascade (e.g., mechanical ventilator).

A heating element in the water reservoir of a cascade type of humidifier heats the water and allows the gas to be warmed before it leaves the unit. The actual electrical heating element is not in direct contact with the water, but is inserted in one of two metal sleeves, which protect the heating element from direct contact with the water, minimizing electrical hazards. Once properly secured, the lid allows a switch underneath it to be depressed to turn on the heating element, which functions as long as the lid to the cascade is properly secure. A thermostat that monitors and helps regulate water temperature by adjusting the heating element temperature is located in the other sleeve. The temperature-control module permits the operator to manually control the temperature of the gas leaving the unit. This temperature does not reflect the actual gas temperature delivered to the patient's airway because as gas travels from the humidifier outlet to the patient, ambient conditions can cool the gas. An auxiliary

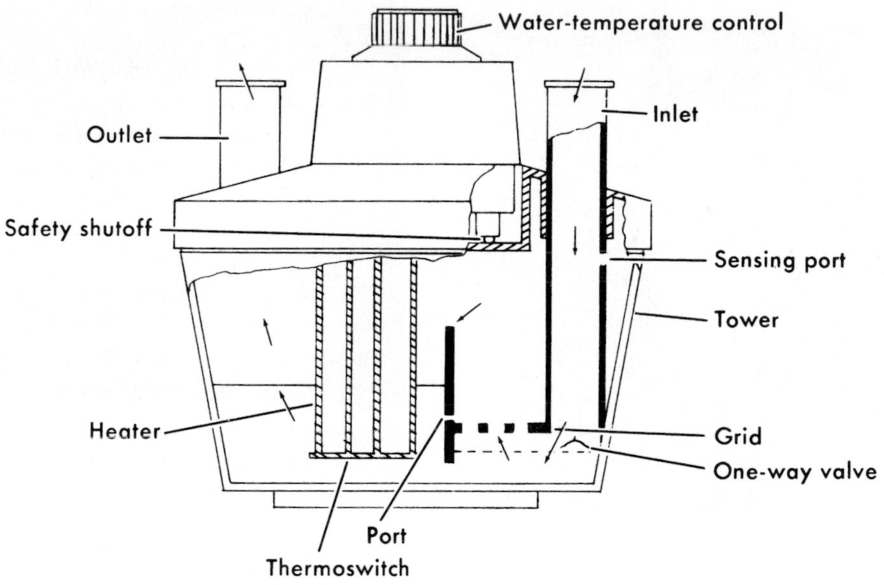

Figure 4-7 The Nellcor Puritan Bennett Cascade Humidifier.

thermometer probe is placed near the patient's airway where inhaled gas temperature can be monitored and the humidifier's temperature-control setting can be adjusted to provide the desired gas temperature. The temperature-control mechanism is color-coded to represent low, medium, and high temperature settings. Despite these markings, respiratory care practitioners must judiciously monitor gas temperatures to avoid humidity deficits or thermal injuries to patient airways.

Nellcor Puritan Bennett manufactures an advanced model of a cascade type of humidifier, the Cascade II, which has a servo-controller that maintains the temperature of the gas leaving the humidifier at a set level. A proximal temperature probe is placed near the patient's airway to measure gas temperature, which in turn provides signals the Cascade II to allow the unit to self-regulate its reservoir temperature to the preset value.

There are two technical considerations of using cascade type of humidifiers. First, the water reservoir or container should always be correctly aligned with the humidifier lid so the seal is secure. Failure to secure a proper fit can result in a leak that may compromise gas delivery to the patient. Other sources of leaks include rupture of the large "O" ring found in the lid and the red "O" ring on the heater well. Also, an external, continuous water-feed system can be attached to help maintain the water level in the water reservoir. If a continuous water-feed system is not used, the water level must be monitored and the bottle manually filled with sterile water as needed. Caution must be exercised during filling so that the reservoir is not contaminated.

Wick Humidifiers. The next category of high-flow humidifiers are **wick humidifiers,** which employ a cylinder-shaped absorbent paper or sponge that draws water from a reservoir using capillary action. As gas passes through the humidifier, it encounters the large surface area of the wick. Evaporation of water from the wick increases the relative humidity of the gas. Heating the unit allows wick humidifiers to provide up to 100% relative humidity at body temperature. Most wick type of humidifiers offer **heated wire** technology as an option, which (as discussed later in this chapter) provides heat to the gas-delivery circuit in attempts to maintain desired gas humidity and temperatures as gas travels to the patient. Examples of models that are marketed as using the wick principle include the Bird Wick Humidifier, the Hudson RCI Conchapak Humidifier, the Fisher and Paykel Dual Servo Humidifier, the Bear VH-820 Humidifier, and Travenol Laboratory's HCL 37-S Humidifier.

The Bird Wick Humidifier (Figure 4-8) is a heated wick humidifier that contains an internal heated wick (an absorbent, blotting type of paper), which is saturated with water it absorbs from a reservoir at the bottom of the unit. Gas entering the inlet port via large-bore, corrugated tubing is directed down, toward a cylindrical **chamber** containing the wick. As the gas flows across the wet, heated wick, water evaporates, saturating the gas that leaves the unit. A constant water level is maintained within the humidifier by a reservoir-feed system connected to the top of the unit (not shown in Figure 4-8). A float mechanism allows water to periodically enter during operation to replace the evaporated water.

A control knob calibrated in reference numbers (from low [0] to high [9]) adjusts the temperature within the unit. An external probe allows gas temperature at a selected site (e.g., at the patient's airway) to be monitored but does not control the heater temperature unless the probe detects a temperature higher than 40° C. If the heater temperature exceeds 40° C, an alarm sounds, and the unit shuts off

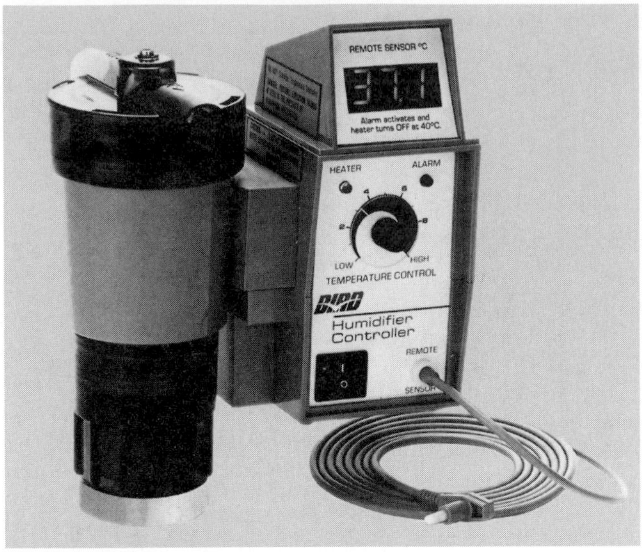

Figure 4-8 The Bird Wick Humidifier. (Courtesy Bird Products Corp., Palm Springs, Calif.)

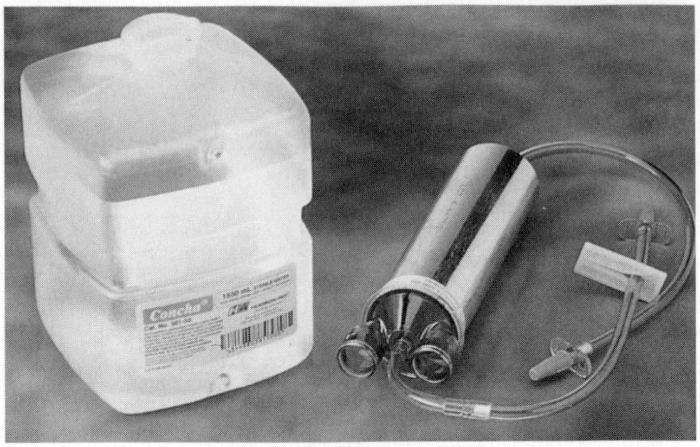

Figure 4-9 The Hudson RCI Conchacolumn. (Courtesy Hudson Respiratory Care, Inc, Temecula, Calif.)

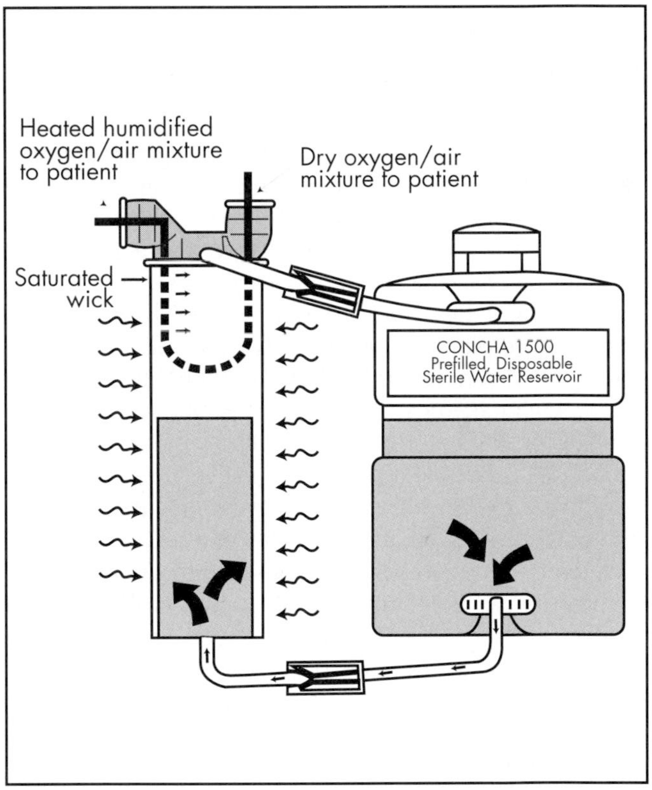

Figure 4-10 The Hudson RCI Conchacolumn and water reservoir assembly. (Redrawn from Hudson Respiratory Care, Inc, Temecula, Calif.)

until the gas temperature cools to below 40° C. The measured temperature is digitally displayed for easy viewing.

The Bird Wick Humidifier provides humidity levels of over 90% of relative humidity at body temperature with high gas-flow rates. The unit can adequately humidify both continuous and intermittent gas flow because it has low resistance to gas flow. It may be used with gas-entrainment devices to provide oxygen-controlled, high gas flow during various types of medical gas therapy.

Another wick type of humidifier is the Conchapak, which is available in a variety of humidification systems with options for adult, pediatric, and neonatal use, heated wire technology, and servo-controlled heating elements.

The Conchapak system has three main components: (1) the servo-controlled heated humidifier (Conchatherm) with or without a heated wire circuit; (2) a humidification column (Conchacolumn); and (3) a sterile water reservoir (Concha sterile water). Hudson provides several different heater units and two unique Conchacolumn designs. The various models available from Hudson include the Conchatherm Heater, the Conchatherm III Plus Heater (16 and 21 volt), the Conchatherm III Humidifier Heater, the Conchatherm IV Heater Humidifier, the pediatric Conchatherm Heater, and the Hi-Flow Conchatherm Heater.

Conchatherm heated humidifiers have a cylindrical heating element (Conchacolumn) that provides a large heating surface area (Figure 4-9). It is made of aluminum with an absorbent paper or wick lining that fits inside and is surrounded by a heating element that maintains an adequate level of heat to ensure that proximal gas temperatures remain at a set level. A side-by-side sterile water reservoir fills the Conchacolumn using a gravity-feed system. A 1650 mL, closed system reservoir continuously feeds the bottom of the column to ensure continuous humidification (Figure 4-10). As the wick is heated and absorbs water, incoming gas is humidified. Gas flow from a mechanical ventilator or gas-flow device enters the top of the column and encounters a heated environment within the chamber. As gas circulates within the column, the heated wick saturates the gas to or near 100% body humidity (based on column temperature).

The Conchatherm III Plus humidifier can be used with or without a heated wire circuit (Figure 4-11). The operator chooses to employ either an intracircuit, heated wire to

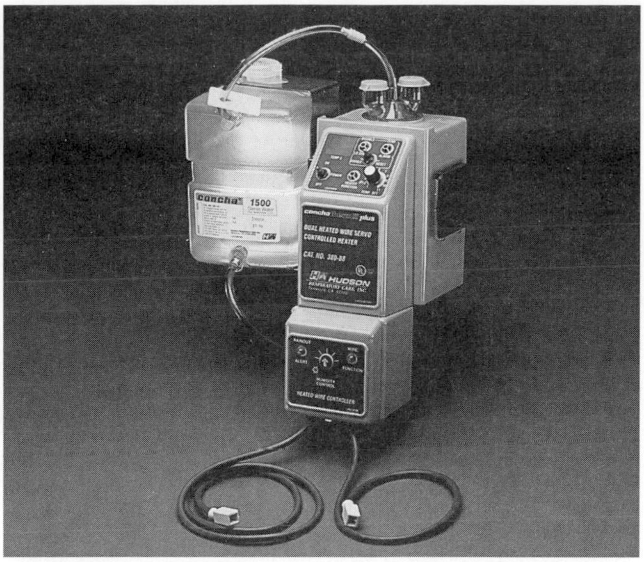

Figure 4-11 The Hudson RCI Conchatherm III Plus Humidifier. (Courtesy Hudson Respiratory Care, Inc, Temecula, Calif.)

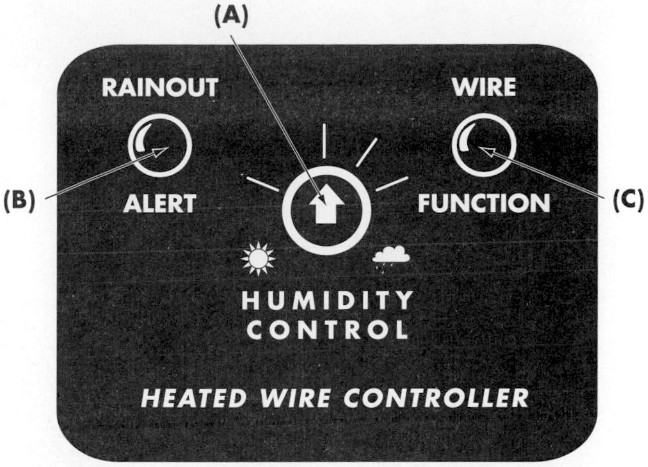

Figure 4-12 The Hudson RCI Conchatherm III Plus Humidifier heated wire control panel. *A,* Humidity control to adjust the temperature gradient between humidifier and patient. *B,* Rain out alert for showing the operator that the desired temperature gradient is not being achieved. *C,* Wire function light to alert the operator when power is available for the heated wire circuit. (Courtesy Hudson Respiratory Care, Inc, Temecula, Calif.)

warm the gas or a conventional circuit with an attached proximal probe to measure the gas temperature delivered to the patient's airway. The servo-controlled heater monitors the heat output of the humidifier. The heated wire controller unit (Figure 4-12) regulates the temperature within the breathing circuit to minimize condensation. Use of the heated wire option with the Conchatherm III Plus humidifier allows the operator to control the temperature gradient between the humidifier and the patient. This unit also provides audio and visual alerts to inform the operator when the gradient is not being achieved and an indicator light to show that the wire is being powered. The humidity control adjusts the temperature gradient between the humidifier and the proximal airway or the patient-end of the heated wire circuit and can create a temperature difference up to 30° C between the patient and the heater. Adjusting this temperature gradient allows respiratory care practitioners to compensate for ventilatory gas circuit conditions and ambient variables because this gradient controls the delivered relative humidity. If no gradient occurs, gas temperature will be constant throughout the length of the gas delivery circuit. If the heater temperature is set 3° C cooler than the patient-end of the circuit (i.e., positive temperature gradient), additional heat is supplied to the gas-delivery circuit. Notice that this setting will potentially deliver less humidity to the patient with less condensation developing in the delivery circuit. With a cooler heater temperature setting, such as with other types of heated humidifiers, a humidity deficit may occur, depending upon the operating temperature, the patient's ventilatory parameters, and the airway status (e.g., dehydration). If the humidity control setting is set to allow the heater to be up to 3° C warmer than the patient-end of the circuit (i.e., negative temperature gradient), increased humidity can be delivered. However, this situation may increase the potential for condensation within the gas-delivery circuit.

If a heated wire is not used with the gas circuit tubing, the heated wire controller is automatically disabled, and the heater performs as a conventional wick humidifier. In this case, a temperature probe may be placed at an appropriate location (e.g., proximal airway) and used to measure the gas temperature leaving the humidifier; a LED readout alerts the user of the gas temperature being delivered. The Conchatherm III Plus humidifier can be used with mechanical ventilators, oxygen diluters or blenders, adjustable nebulizer adapters for aerosol therapy, or nonflammable anesthesia gases. This humidifier includes a self-contained water reservoir; audio-visual alarms; a condensation, or rain out, alarm; and probes for adult, pediatric, and neonatal gas circuits.

The Conchatherm IV Heater Humidifier (Figure 4-13) for adult or neonatal humidification offers microprocessor technology and uses an interactive control algorithm that provides stable proximal airway temperature and a heated wire function (when used). The LED airway temperature display provides the temperature of gas at the proximal airway or column in whole degrees centigrade. This humidifier provides a 20-minute pause mode to allow time for ventilator circuit changes or delivery of nebulized medications. An advanced alarm package includes tracking alarms for delivered gas temperature, high and low temperatures, probe status, and heated wire disconnects. A unique feature of the Conchatherm IV Heater Humidifier is the bar graph

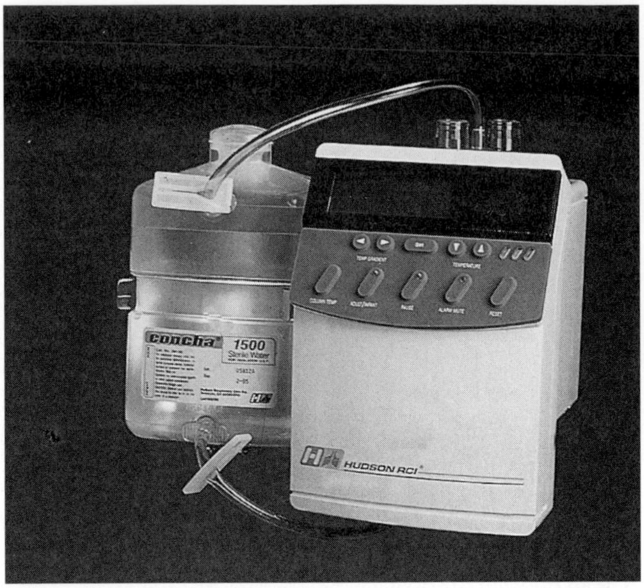

Figure 4-13 The Hudson RCI Conchatherm IV Heater Humidifier. (Courtesy Hudson Respiratory Care, Inc, Temecula, Calif.)

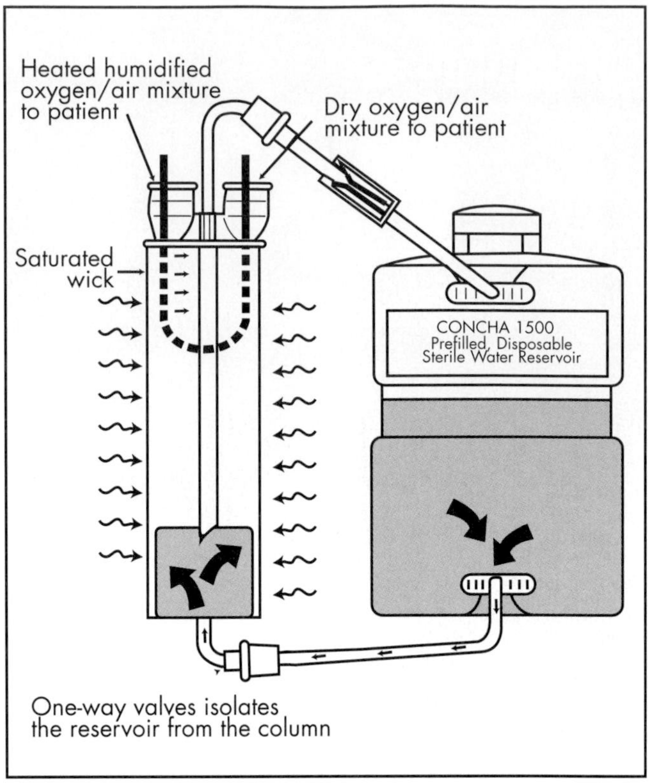

Figure 4-14 The low-compliance Conchacolumn with water reservoir assembly. (Redrawn from Hudson Respiratory Care, Inc, Temecula, Calif.)

on the front panel showing the difference in gas temperature (temperature gradient) between the Conchacolumn outlet and the patient's proximal airway when the unit is used with a heated wire circuit. During operation, the bar graph displays the actual temperature gradient in the heated wire. Other features of the Conchatherm IV Heater Humidifier include digital temperature selection; adjustable heater-to-patient temperature gradient for control of humidity and condensation; a fixed, high-temperature alarm at 40° C; LCD alarm prompters; and continuous, self-diagnostic evaluations of hardware and software functions.

The humidifiers just discussed use the Conchacolumn to provide humidification. Fluid transferred from the reservoir to the Conchacolumn varies during the ventilatory cycle, depending on the mechanical ventilator settings. Fluid transfer is influenced by several factors, such as peak airway pressure, low respiratory rate, reduced water volume in the water reservoir, increased inspiratory:expiratory ratios, and square pressure waveforms.

The Conchacolumn is available in standard- and low-compliance configurations. The compliance changes are usually not significant for adults on mechanical ventilation; however, changes in compliance are clinically significant for neonatal and pediatric patients on pressure-cycled ventilation. With the smaller tidal volumes associated with neonatal mechanical ventilation, an increase in humidifier compliance can result in a decrease in the actual delivered tidal volume. The compliance of the humidification system is a product of the Conchacolumn compliance and the amount of fluid in both the column and reservoir.[15]

It is important to note that as the water level in the column falls, the system's compressible volume increases and compliance changes. In clinical situations where internal circuit or humidifier compliance must remain constant (e.g., with neonatal patients), a low-compliance Conchacolumn is available and should be used. The low-compliance column contains a beveled sensing tube to control the water level in the column and thus the amount of gas allowed above the water reservoir or column (Figure 4-14). This sensing tube stops gas flow to the reservoir if the column water level is above the bevel of the tube. A one-way valve in the upper reservoir tube allows flow into the reservoir and restricts flow back out, thus preventing the reservoir pressure from being vented back into the column during the expiratory phase of mechanical ventilation. A one-way valve in the lower reservoir tube prevents water flow from the column back into the reservoir during the inspiratory phase of mechanical ventilation.[15]

Fisher and Paykel humidifiers are wick humidifiers that may be used for both adult and neonatal high-flow gas humidification (Figure 4-15). The servo-controlled MR 600 and 730 humidifiers have inlets, outlets, a wick, and a heating element. Disposable and reusable humidification chambers are available in sizes for both adults and neonatal patients. A limited water autofeed system is available with the MR 600 and MR 730 models to maintain water in the reservoir chamber. Temperature is regulated with a dual servo-controlled heater with a range of 30° to 39° C, and the MR

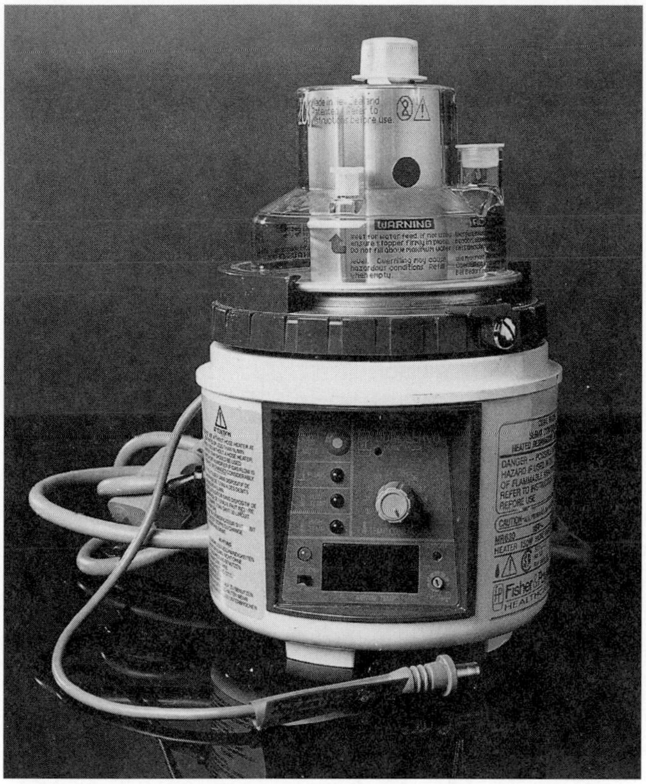

Figure 4-15 The Fisher Paykel MR-730 heated humidifier.

730 has a heated wire option. Various alarms are included in these humidifiers, including high- and low-temperature alarms, a probe disconnect alarm, a heated wire disconnect alarm, and a 3-minute alarm silence option.

Another example of a heated wick humidification system is Travenol Laboratory's HCL 3, which employs a microprocessor system to monitor and control gas temperature, regulate the water-feed system, and operate alarms. Similar to other high-flow humidifiers, this unit produces 100% relative humidity at body temperature by heating and vaporizing water. The HCL 3 employs a disposable humidity chamber that includes an absorbent wick, inlet and outlet adapters, and a water-feed system. The heating element is controlled by a microprocessor to maintain servo-control over gas temperature and the alarm system. A pinch valve provides continuous water feeding to the humidity chamber.

The Bear VH-820 is a wick type of humidifier that can be used for patients of any age (Figure 4-16). It has a spiral chamber, which increases both water surface area and the time gas is exposed to the water surface within the chamber. Gas entering the unit passes over a heating rod before entering the spiral chamber. A microprocessor monitors and servo-controls three positions for the temperature probe: (1) the heating rod, (2) the proximal airway, and (3) the humidifier outlet. A water-feed system relies upon a sensing system that controls a pinch valve, which maintains automatic water filling to the humidity chamber. As

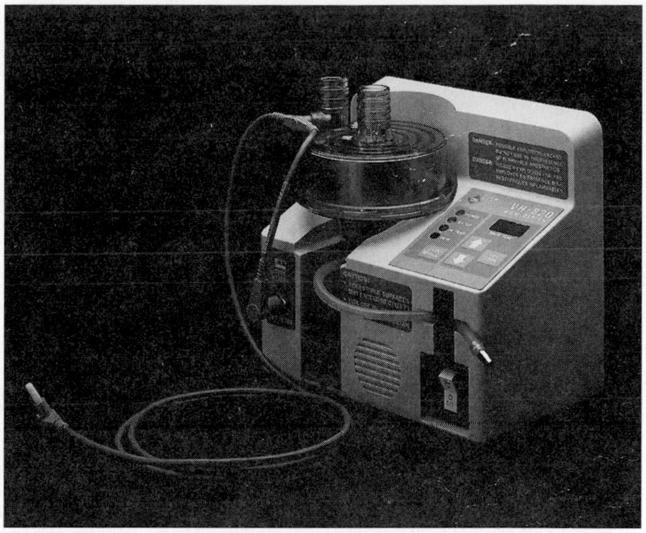

Figure 4-16 The Bear VH-820 heated humidifier. (Courtesy Bear Medical Systems, Inc., Riverside, Calif.)

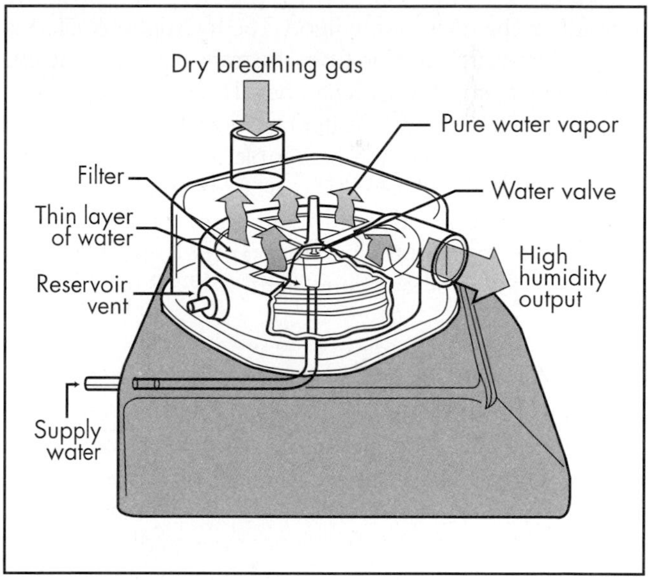

Figure 4-17 The Inspiron Vapor-Phase heated humidifier. (Courtesy of Inspiron, RSP, Irvine, Calif.)

the water level drops below 1 mm, a valve opens and water flows into the chamber, returning the water level to the proper operating level. A gravity-dependent bag or water bottle reservoir allows water to flow into the chamber as necessary.

The Inspiron Vapor-Phase humidifier is a nonservo–controlled humidifier that uses a hydrophobic filter between its liquid and gas chambers (Figure 4-17). This filter allows only water vapor to pass through it; it is impermeable to bulk liquid. A heater raises the temperature of the water underneath the filter, causing rapid evaporation to occur. As warmed water vaporizes and moves across the filter, incoming gas is warmed and humidified to body humidity. Because bulk liquid cannot enter the gas chamber, the

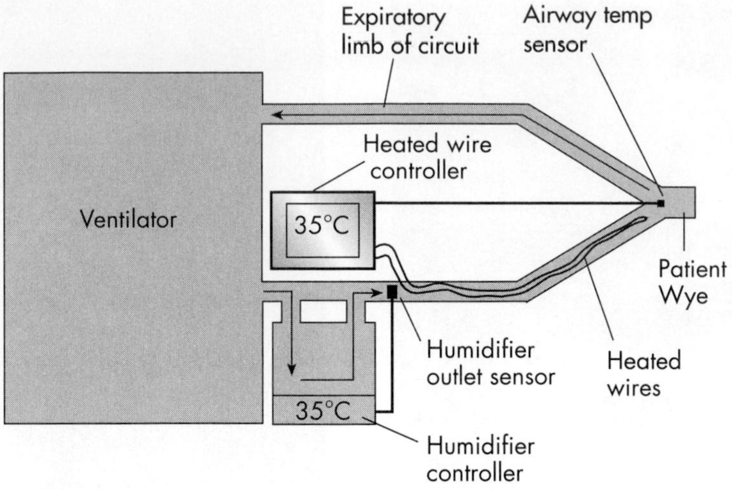

Figure 4-18 A heated wire circuit in the inspiratory limb of the gas delivery tube. (From Scanlan CL, Wilkins RL, and Stoller JK: Egan's Fundamentals of Respiratory Care, ed 7, St Louis, 1999, Mosby.)

humidifier chamber cannot flood. The hydrophobic filter offers a degree of protection from the transmission of bacteria from the water to the gas chamber. The water-feed system consists of a free-standing water reservoir that uses gravity to allow water to flow to the heater plate. An operating temperature range of 30° to 39° C can be achieved; if the chamber temperature exceeds 40° C, an alarm sounds, requiring the operator to adjust temperature. There is also a low-temperature alarm, a probe failure alarm, and a 2-minute alarm silence option.

Heated Wire Circuits

An adjunct to the humidification system often employed to minimize circuit condensation is a heated wire circuit (Figure 4-18). This device is a wirelike structure placed in the lumen of the gas delivery circuit (e.g., ventilator circuit) to maintain a desired gas or temperature gradient throughout the length of the circuit. By maintaining gas temperature at body temperature, condensation (or rain out) can be minimized. Respiratory care practitioners can choose to provide a heated wire to both the inspiratory and expiratory limbs of the mechanical ventilator circuit or only to the inspiratory side of the circuit. The heated wire system maintains both the temperature within the circuit and the temperature of the heated humidifier, so as gas flows to the patient, gas temperature is maintained at or near body temperature. If the inspiratory limb does not have a heated wire, a water trap may be used to collect condensation (Figure 4-19).

Heated wire systems are advantageous because they decrease the labor necessary to maintain the medical gas delivery circuit (e.g., less drain time is required for respiratory care practitioners to remove condensation from the circuit); and they may reduce nosocomial infections resulting from aspiration or lavage of contaminated condensate from circuit movement, and they provide increased absolute humidity.[16] However, heated wire systems may actually decrease relative humidity, resulting in possible inspissation of secretions. As gas leaves the humidifier with a fixed water content and the temperature increases as a result of the heated wire, relative humidity decreases. Studies suggest that relative humidity may be the dominant factor in drying or thinning of airway secretions in the upper airway, and the use of heated wire circuits may contribute to drying of airway secretions.[16]

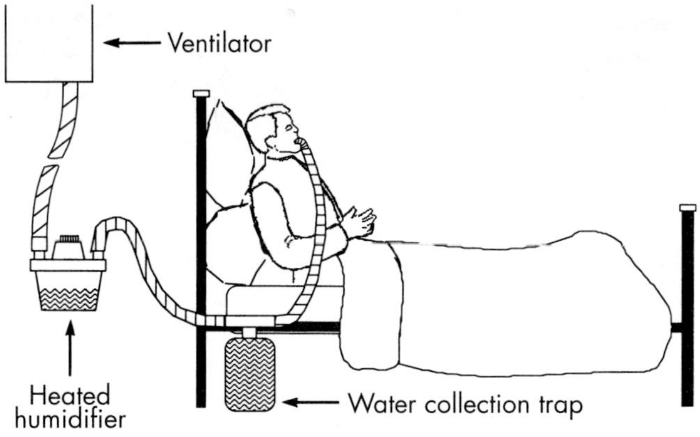

Figure 4-19 Placement of a water trap in a gravity-dependent loop of the heated humidity delivery tube.

Technical Considerations with Using Humidifiers

Respiratory care practitioners should be aware of important considerations when using heated humidifiers, such as maintaining an adequate water supply (i.e., replacing the water reservoir with full units as needed), keeping the water at the proper level, and ensuring tight fittings of the temperature probe connection underneath the heated-wire controller. In addition, monitoring operating and gas output temperatures are vital. If a heated wire is not used, condensation that gathers within the gas delivery circuit must be removed.

Heat and Moisture Exchangers

An alternative to conventional humidification systems is the use of a heat and moisture exchanger (HME), which is commonly referred to as an artificial nose. HMEs can humidify and warm incoming gases in certain patients receiving mechanical ventilation. HMEs function similarly to the upper airway by capturing exhaled heat and moisture and using it to heat and humidify the next inhaled or delivered breath. However, these passive, disposable humidifiers do not add heat or water to the patient's airway. There are many models of HME type of devices available; most have an internal volume of 10 to 98 mL, weigh within the range of 9 to 47 g, and provide a humidity output of 10 to 31 mg/L at a temperature of 30° C.

HMEs are best suited for patients undergoing short-term mechanical ventilation (i.e., 96 hours or less), with minute volumes less than 10 L/min, limited secretions, and a normal body temperature.[10] Several physical characteristics influence the overall effectiveness of HME type of humidifiers, including the temperature and humidity levels of the inspired gas, the gas flow through the unit (e.g., faster flows decrease effectiveness), the internal surface area the gas encounters, the dead space volume of the unit, and the outer casing. An ideal HME has low structural compliance and minimal dead space and is lightweight. An HME should also have standard inlet and outlet connections, offer little resistance to gas flow, and operate at at least 70% of efficiency.[6] HME efficiency is influenced by the size of the tidal volume, the inspiratory gas flow rate, and the fraction of inspired oxygen (FiO_2). As each of these factors increases, the overall efficiency of the HME decreases. It has been recommended that clinical use of HMEs be limited to 5 days or less.[17]

HME type of humidifiers reduce the accumulation of condensation in the mechanical ventilator gas delivery circuit and may act as a barrier to microbes, thus decreasing the incidence of nosocomial infection. The actual effect of HMEs on infection rates associated with mechanical ventilation remains controversial, and several studies report mixed results. However, studies comparing HMEs to conventional heated humidifiers suggest that HMEs may not be a significant factor in nosocomial infections in patients receiving mechanical ventilation.[17]

Generally, there are four types of HMEs that can be used for short term humidity therapy: (1) simple HMEs, (2) heat and moisture exchanging filters, (3) **hygroscopic** condensor humidifiers, and (4) hygroscopic condenser humidifiers with filters.

The simplest HMEs often use layered aluminum with or without a fibrous coating. The use of aluminum casing allows temperatures to be exchanged quickly during gas

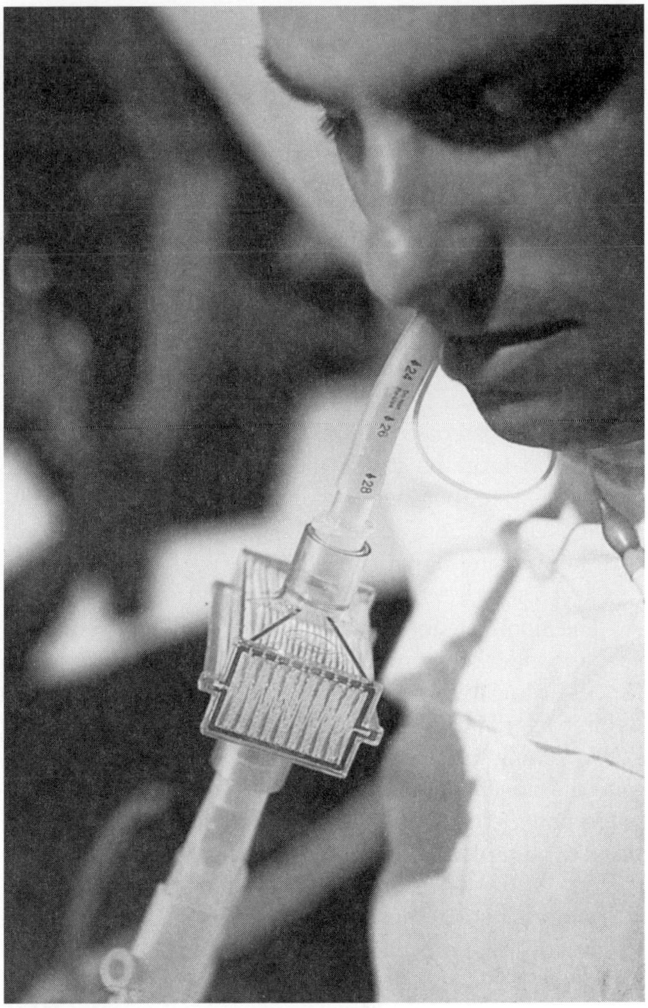

Figure 4-20 The Pall BB-100F HME Filter. (Courtesy Pall Medical, Ann Arbor, Mich.)

movement, with moisture accumulating on the aluminum layers. As the patient exhales, heat and moisture are captured by the HME. Then during the inspiration that follows, the captured heat and moisture humidifies inspired gases. These HMEs are the least efficient for providing humidity.[18]

The second type of HMEs are heat and moisture exchanging filters (HMEFs). Pall Medical Products' BB-100F Heat and Moisture Exchanger Filter (Figure 4-20) is both an HME and a bacterial filter and can provide up to 30 mg of water at a tidal volume of 800 mL and 30° C, with no added work of breathing. In addition, the Pall HMEF is more than 99.999% effective in filtering bacteria and viruses. The internal component responsible for heat and moisture exchange is a hydrophobic, pleated ceramic filter that repels water particles but traps heat and water vapor. Pall also produces a small-volume HMEF with a carbon dioxide monitoring port for anesthesic. This HMEF conserves patient heat and humidity, allows for sampling of expired carbon dioxide, and is greater than 99.999% effective in removing the bacteria and viruses that enter the unit.

The next type of HME is the hygroscopic condenser humidifier (HCH), which is constructed of a low-thermal conductive material (e.g., corrugated paper, wool, or foam) that has been coated with a hygroscopic chemical (calcium chloride or lithium chloride). This special hygroscopic coating increases the retention of exhaled moisture, thus reducing the relative humidity of the expired gas, which results in better humidification of inspired gas when compared with simple HMEs. HCHs capture water particles during expiration as a result of the cool surface area of the condenser element. These water particles become attached to the hygroscopic chemical coating and remain in a liquid state. As inspired gas enters the HCH, water molecules are released from the condensing material to humidify the incoming gas. Most HCH models on the market are capable of providing up to 30 mg of water per liter of gas. Figure 4-21 shows the Hygrolife Mallinckrodt Medical HCH, which provides 30 mg of water per liter of gas at an 800 mL tidal volume and offers low resistance to gas flows up to 90 L/min.

The final category of HME type of devices is hygroscopic condenser humidifiers with filters (HCHFs), which function similarly to the HCHs just described but contain a thin bacterial filter between the condensing material and the incoming gas. Figure 4-22 shows the Gibeck Humid-Vent Compact Filter HCHF, which is composed of corrugated paper coated with calcium chloride and can provide up to 30 mg of water per liter of gas at 30° C.

Technical Considerations for HME Type of Humidifers. Respiratory care practitioners must be aware of the technical considerations and contraindications of using HME type of humidifiers. Contraindications for the use of HME type of humidifiers are listed in Box 4-5. When used during clinical situations, HMEs may aggravate existing pulmonary problems by dehydrating lung secretions. HME use is contraindicated when expired gases do not travel through the HME device (e.g., endotracheal tube cuff leak), when a heated humidifier or **small-volume nebulizer** is part of the ventilation system, and when there are leaks around the inlet or outlet ports. In addition, the dead space volume of HMEs limits their use with neonatal and pediatric patients.

Maintaining and Monitoring Humidification

Mechanical ventilators provide machine-generated gas flow via a circuit to inflate the lungs. With the exception of noninvasive mechanical ventilation (see Chapter 14), patients on mechanical ventilators will have either an endotracheal or tracheostomy tube in place, which bypass the natural mechanism for conditioning incoming gas. The application of dry medical gases is associated with heat loss, dehydration of the airway lining, epithelial damage, destruction of cilia, disruption of pseudostratified columnar and cuboidal epithelial cells, desquamation of cells, mucosal ulceration, and impaired mucocillary transport of secretions.[4] Consequences of the above include secretion retention, atelectasis, and increased incidence of infection. Damage from breathing dry or poorly humidified gas through an artificial airway is proportional to the duration of breathing such a gas mixture.[14] Damaged cilia require several days for repair, and it takes several weeks for the epithelial lining to return to full thickness.[19] With an artificial airway in place, the isothermic saturation boundary can shift distally, altering pulmonary mechanics. Altered mechanics may include a decrease in functional residual capacity and lung compliance and hypoxemia.[20-22]

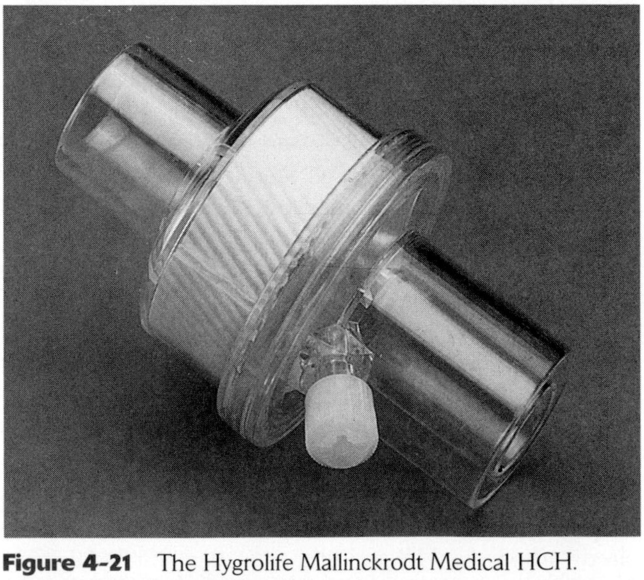

Figure 4-21 The Hygrolife Mallinckrodt Medical HCH. (Courtesy Mallinckrodt Inc, St Louis)

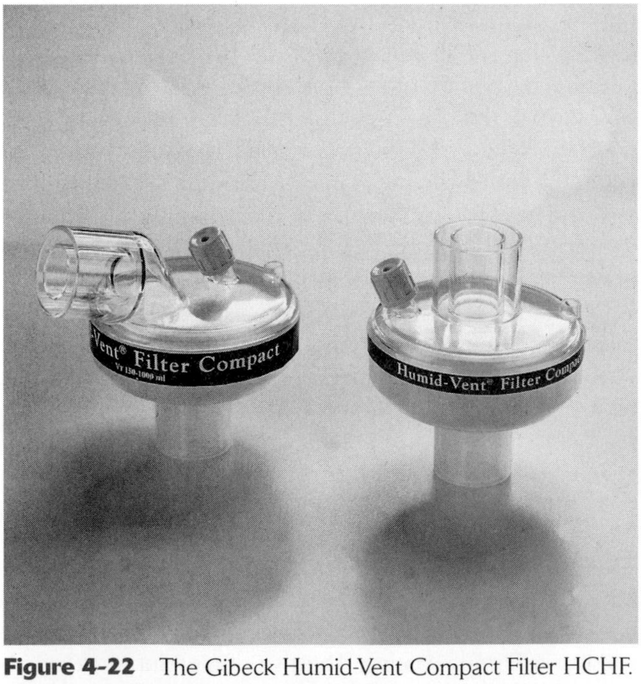

Figure 4-22 The Gibeck Humid-Vent Compact Filter HCHF. (Courtesy Gibeck, Inc., Temecula, Calif.)

BOX 4-5

Contraindications for Using an HME

Increased volume of secretions
Thick, dehydrated secretions
Hypothermia
Large tidal volumes (>1000 mL)
During aerosol therapy
Small tidal volume with large-volume HME devices
With heated humidification
Airway leaks around artificial airway

Similarly to insufficient humidification, there are consequences for overhumidification and overheating. Under normal conditions, heat and moisture exchange occurs within the upper airway via a dynamic equilibrium. The loss and gain of heat and humidity are governed by the physiologic process previously described. This normal equilibrium may be disturbed with the delivery of excess heat and moisture to the airways.

Delivery of gas above body temperature can cause thermal damage to mucosal lining, pulmonary edema, and airway stricture formation. Changes in cilia structure and function have been reported, such as degeneration and adhesion of cilia in smaller airways.[23] In addition, there may be an increase in airway secretions from a decrease in evaporation, which can lead to condensation that may obstruct the airway, leading to atelectasis or an increase in airway resistance.[10] Overhumidification, just as with under humidification, may alter lung mechanics by decreasing functional residual capacity and causing hypoxemia and loss of lung compliance.[21] These changes result from atelectasis and intrapulmonary shunting. Excessive humidification may alter or remove surfactant, further encouraging alveolar collapse. Surfactant changes are more prominent with overhydration than underhydration.[23] Some authors report that hyperthermia may occur because the lungs are unable to discard heat.[4,24] In addition, overhumidification may increase body fluids due to the decrease in insensible water loss from the lungs.[4] This is important to note when providing heated humidity therapy to neonates.

In addition to the physiologic hazards and complications of humidifying the respiratory system, there are technical considerations of humidity therapy that are hazardous. These include the potential for electric shock from heated humidifiers, melting of the circuit by heated wire circuits (possibly burning the patient), increased resistive work while breathing through the humidifier, inadvertent tracheal lavage from unintentional overfilling of the humidifier, and displacement of a condensate bolus. Condensation tends to accumulate within gravity-dependent loops in the gas-delivery circuit while the gas cools as it is delivered to the patient. This condensation can build up and be inadvertently emptied into the patient's airway during patient gas-circuit manipulation (e.g., during routine patient care). Boluses of condensation fluid in the circuit can increase the work of breathing by interfering with the sensing mechanism of the mechanical ventilator or decreasing the diameter of the gas delivery circuit. Under these conditions, the patient must breathe around the bolus to obtain an assisted or spontaneous breath from a mechanical ventilator. This patient-ventilator dysynchrony can result in altered pulmonary mechanics and an increase in the work of breathing.[10]

Monitoring the humidification device requires the respiratory care practitioner to frequently inspect the unit. Monitoring and maintenance include checking humidifier and proximal airway temperature to ensure appropriate gas temperatures, removing condensate from loops in the circuit (water traps or heated wires may be used to minimize fluid accumulation), and maintaining alarm settings to be alerted to gas temperature below 31° C or above 40° C (as discussed previously, the recommended range for proximal airway gas temperatures is 31° to 35° C). An increase in intrahumidifier temperature is common when the unit is turned on and there is an absence of gas flowing through it. This can occur, for example, when servo-controlled units are allowed to warm up without gas flowing through the circuit and without a temperature probe inserted into the proximal airway of the ventilator circuit. Non-servo–controlled units can exceed gas temperatures if the thermostat setting is too high.[6] Elevated intrahumidifier temperatures can result in the delivery of excessive gas temperature to the patient upon initial gas flow through the unit.

Additional monitoring includes maintaining humidifier water reservoir level to ensure a water source for humidification. If an HME is substituted for a heated humidifier, it should be inspected regularly for partial or complete obstruction by airway secretions.[10]

Respiratory care practitioners must document and record the function of the humidification device and the results of therapy. The patient's medical records should include documentation of humidifier settings, proximal airway gas temperature or inspired gas temperature, alarm settings, water level and function of the automatic water feed system, and quantity and quality of airway secretions.[10]

AEROSOL THERAPY

Aerosols are widely used in the care and treatment of patients with pulmonary disease and play a significant role in respiratory care. This section will address aerosol characteristics, factors that effect deposition, aerosol generation, and hazards of aerosol therapy.

An aerosol is a solid or liquid particle suspended in a gas. Aerosol particles range from submicroscopic to macroscopic

BOX 4-6

Clinical Practice Guidelines

Selection of an Aerosol Delivery Device

Description

The device selected for administration of pharmacologically active aerosol to the lower airway should produce particles with an MMAD of 2 to 5 μ. These devices include MDIs, MDIs with accessory devices (e.g., spacers), DPIs, SVNs, LVNs, and ultrasonic nebulizers (USN). Note that this guideline does not address bland aerosol administration and sputum induction.

Indications

The need to deliver aerosolized medications, such as beta adrenergic agents, anticholinergic agents (antimuscarinic), antiinflammatory agents (e.g., corticosteroids), mediator-modifying compounds (e.g., cromolyn sodium), and mucokinetics, to the lower airways.

Contraindications

There are no contraindications to the administration of aerosols by inhalation, although there may be contraindications related to the substances being delivered. Consult the package inserts for product-specific contraindications.

Hazards and Complications

1. Malfunction of device and/or improper technique may result in the delivery of an incorrect dose of medication.
2. Complications of specific pharmacologic agents may occur.
3. Cardiotoxic effects of freon have been reported as idiosyncratic responses that may be a problem with excessive MDI use.
4. Freon may harm the environment by its effect on the ozone layer.
5. Repeated exposure to aerosols has been reported to produce asthmatic symptoms in some caregivers.

Monitoring

1. Device performance
2. Device application technique
3. Patient response, including changes in vital signs

Infection Control

1. Standard precautions for body substance isolation must be used.
2. SVNs and LVNs are for single-patient use or should be subjected to high-level disinfection between patients.
3. Published data establishing a safe-use period for SVNs and LVNs are lacking; however SVNs and LVNs should probably be changed or subjected to high-level disinfection at about 24-hour intervals.
4. Medications should be handled aseptically. Medications from multidose sources in acute-care facilities must be handled aseptically and discarded after 24 hours, unless manufacturer recommendations specifically state that medications may be stored longer than 24 hours. Tap water should not be used as a diluent.
5. MDI accessory devices are only for single-patient use. There are no documented concerns with contamination of medication in MDI canisters. Cleaning of accessory devices is based on aesthetic criteria.

For a complete copy of this guideline, see Respir Care 37:891, 1992.

(readily visible with the naked eye) and, unlike humidity, they can be measured and counted. Common, nonmedical aerosols include dust, fumes from chemical reactions, smoke from the combustion of various materials, mists and fog from condensation (mists are considered larger than fog particles), and smog and haze, which are broad terms describing atmospheric aerosols from natural and artificial processes. Other examples of aerosols include tobacco smoke, viruses, pollen, and fungal spores.

The human respiratory system has developed an elaborate mechanism for defending itself from most inspired aerosols—both therapeutic and nontherapeutic. This section focuses on therapeutic or medical aerosols, including bland and medicated aerosols, administered to patients with a variety of symptoms associated with pulmonary disease. This section addresses aerosol characteristics, generation of aerosol, and clinical use of aerosol in a variety of settings. Respiratory care practitioners should carefully select the appropriate aerosol and method of delivery to optimize care of patients with pulmonary disease.

Aerosol therapy may be divided into three broad categories as described by the AARC Clinical Practice Guidelines[25-27]: (1) delivery of bland aerosol, (2) delivery of aerosol to the upper airway, and (3) delivery of medicated aerosol. Each type of aerosol therapy has distinct indications, clinical uses, and hazards. In most cases, they have a common means of generation, but delivery methods can be unique to a particular medical or bland aerosol (Box 4-6 to Box 4-8).

Bland aerosols include sterile water and hypotonic, hypertonic, and isotonic saline.[28] Bland aerosols are commonly used in the care of patients in hospitals or at home. Aerosolization of cool, sterile saline or water is primarily indicated for upper airway administration. Use of hypotonic or hypertonic sterile saline is indicated for inducing a cough and expectoration of sputum for obtaining specimens for microbiologic evaluation.

BOX 4-7

Clinical Practice Guidelines

Bland Aerosol Administration

Description

For purposes of this guideline, bland aerosol administration includes the delivery of sterile water or hypotonic, isotonic, or hypertonic saline in aerosol form. Bland aerosol administration may be accompanied by oxygen administration.

Indications

Cool, bland aerosol therapy is primarily indicated for upper airway administration; therefore an MMAD greater than or equal to 5 μ is desirable. The use of hypo- and hypertonic saline is primarily indicated for inducing sputum specimens; therefore an MMAD of 1 to 5 μ is desirable. Heated bland aerosol is primarily indicated for minimizing humidity deficit when the upper airway has been bypassed; therefore an MMAD of 2 to 10 μ is desirable. Specific indications include:

1. The presence of upper airway edema (cool bland aerosol)
2. Laryngotracheobronchitis (LTB)
3. Subglottic edema
4. Postextubation edema
5. Postoperative management of the upper airway
6. Bypassed upper airway
7. Need for sputum specimens

Contraindications

1. Bronchoconstriction
2. History of airway hyperresponsiveness

Hazards and Complications

1. Wheezing or bronchospasm
2. Bronchoconstriction when artificial airway is employed
3. Infection
4. Overhydration
5. Patient discomfort
6. Caregiver exposure to droplet nuclei of *Mycobacterium tuberculosis* or other airborne contagion produced as a consequence of coughing, particularly during sputum induction

Assessment of Need

The presence of one or more of the following may be an indication for administration of a water or isotonic or hypotonic saline aerosol:

1. Stridor
2. Brassy, croup-like cough
3. Hoarseness after extubation
4. Diagnosis of LTB or croup
5. Clinical history suggesting upper airway irritation and increased work of breathing (e.g., smoke inhalation)
6. Patient discomfort associated with airway instrumentation or insult
7. Need for sputum induction (e.g., for diagnosis of *Pneumocystis carinii* pneumonia or tuberculosis)

Assessment of Outcome

The desired outcomes for the administration of water, hypotonic, or isotonic saline include:

1. Decreased work of breathing
2. Improved vital signs
3. Decreased stridor
4. Decreased dyspnea
5. Improved arterial blood gas values
6. Improved oxygen saturation as indicated by pulse oximetry (SpO_2)

The desired outcome for the administration of hypertonic saline is a sputum sample adequate for analysis.

Monitoring

The extent of patient monitoring should be determined by the stability and severity of the patient's condition. Monitoring may include:

1. Subjective patient responses of pain, discomfort, dyspnea, or restlessness
2. Heart rate and rhythm
3. Blood pressure
4. Respiratory rate, as well as the breathing pattern and use of accessory respiratory muscles
5. Breath sounds
6. Sputum production quantity, color, consistency, and odor
7. Pulse oximetry (if hypoxemia is suspected)

For a copy of the complete guideline, see Respir Care 38(11):1196, 1993.

Use of cool, bland aerosol is indicated when there is upper airway edema. Cool aerosol, when applied to the airway mucosa, can result in vasoconstriction, thereby reducing mucosal edema. Indications for cool, bland aerosol include stridor, laryngotracheobronchitis, subglottic edema, postextubation edema, hoarseness, and postoperative care of the upper airway (i.e., discomfort associated with bronchoscopy or other invasive instrumentation of the upper airway).[28,29]

Heated aerosol therapy is only recommended when there is a need to decrease a humidity deficit (i.e., when dry gas is delivered to the lungs and the upper airway has been bypassed by an artificial airway). The delivery of heated aerosol by **aerosol mask** to a spontaneously breathing

BOX 4-8

Clinical Practice Guidelines

Selection of a Device for Aerosol Delivery to the Lung Parenchyma

Description

A device selected for administration of pharmacologically active aerosol to the lung parenchyma should produce particle sizes with an MMAD of 1 to 3 μ. Such devices include ultrasonic nebulizers, some LVNs (e.g., the SPAG unit, which is only intended for ribavirin delivery), and some SVNs (e.g., the Circulaire, RespirGard II, and Pari IS 2).

Indications

The indication for selecting a suitable device is the need to deliver a topical medication (in aerosol form) with a site of action in the lung parenchyma or that is intended for systemic absorption. Such medications may include antibiotics, antivirals, antifungals, surfactants, and enzymes.

Contraindications

There are no contraindications to choosing an appropriate device for parenchymal deposition. Contraindications related to the substances being delivered may exist. Consult the package insert for product-specific contraindications to medication delivery.

Hazards and Complications

1. Device malfunction and/or improper technique may result in delivery of incorrect medication doses.
2. For mechanically ventilated patients, the nebulizer design and the characteristics of the medication may affect ventilator function (e.g., filter obstruction, altered tidal volume, decreased trigger sensitivity) and medication deposition.
3. Aerosols may cause bronchospasm or airway irritation, and complications related to specific pharmacologic agents can occur.
4. Exposure to medication should be limited to the patient for whom it has been ordered. Nebulized medication that is released into the atmosphere from the nebulizer or the patient may affect health-care providers and others near the treatment. For example, there has been increased awareness of the possible health effects of aerosols such as ribavirin and pentamidine. Anecdotal reports associate symptoms such as conjunctivitis, decreased tolerance of contact lenses, headaches, bronchospasm, shortness of breath, and rashes in health-care workers exposed to secondhand aerosols. Similar concerns have been expressed concerning health-care workers who are pregnant or are planning to be pregnant within 8 weeks of administration. The potential exposure effects of aerosolized antibiotics (which may contribute to the development of resistant organisms), steroids, and bronchodilators are less often discussed. Because the data regarding adverse health effects on health-care workers and those casually exposed are incomplete, it is wise to minimize exposure in all situations.
5. The Centers for Disease Control and Prevention recommend that:
   a. Warning signs should be posted in an easy-to-see location to apprise all who enter the treatment area of the potential hazards of exposure. Accidental exposures should be documented and reported according to accepted standards.
   b. Staff members who administer medications understand the inherent risks of the medication and the procedures for safely disposing of hazardous wastes. Department administrators should screen staff for adverse effects of aerosol exposure and provide alternative assignments for staff at high risk of adverse effects of exposure (e.g., pregnant women or those with demonstrated sensitivity to the specific agent).
   c. Filters or filtered scavenger systems be used to remove aerosols that cannot be contained.
   d. There be booths or stalls for sputum induction and aerosolized medication administration in areas where multiple patients are treated. Booths or stalls should be designed to provide adequate air flow to draw aerosol and droplet nuclei from the patient and into an appropriate filtration system with exhaust directed to an appropriate outside vent. Note that filters, nebulizers, and other contaminated components of the aerosol delivery system used with suspect agents (e.g., pentamidine and ribavirin) should be handled as hazardous waste. If scavenger systems or specially designed booths are not available, clinicians administering these treatments should wear personal protection devices to reduce exposure to the medication residues and body substances. These devices may include fitted respirator masks, goggles, gloves, gowns, and splatter shields.

Monitoring

1. Device and scavenging system performance
2. Device application technique
3. Patient response

For a copy of the complete Clinical Practice Guideline see Respir Care 41(7):647, 1996.

patient has not been shown to be effective in promoting secretion hydration and expectoration and, as a result, it is not a very common treatment modality.

Contrary to popular belief, the efficacy of using bland aerosol to improve mucus flow or expectoration has not been established. Studies indicate that the physical properties of mucus are only minimally affected by the addition of a bland aerosol.[1,26,28-30] Furthermore, the use of bland aerosol for humidification of the lower airway when the upper airway has been bypassed (i.e., artificial airway) is not as effective as a heated humidifier or HME type of humidifier.[26] Several reasons cited for this finding include difficulty in maintaining the temperature of the aerosol and carrier gas, possible irritation from the aerosol inducing bronchoconstriction, and the risk of cross-contamination. Aerosol particles are capable of transporting microbes, thus becoming a potential source of nosocomial infections.[8]

Medicated aerosol delivery to the upper airway is indicated for upper airway edema and inflammation (e.g., treatment of inflammation associated with laryngotracheobronchitis) when topical anesthesia is required (e.g., to control pain and gagging during placement of invasive upper airway instrumentation) or in the presence of rhinitis (e.g., for relief of seasonal allergy). The administration of a vasoactive aerosol (e.g., steroids, sympathomimetic nose sprays) to the upper airway—especially the nasopharynx—can be effective to decrease nasal congestion and edema associated with allergy or infection. Such agents successfully diminish symptoms such as rhinorrhea, sneezing, and watery discharge.

Medicated aerosol delivery to the lower airway has become the predominant form of medicated aerosol therapy. Inhalation of medicated aerosol allows for rapid onset of effects, is less toxic, and results in fewer side effects than if delivered by mouth or intravenously.[31] The delivery of medicated aerosol focuses on depositing the aerosol of a sufficient dose and at a desired location to produce optimal results. Overall aerosol deposition at specific locations depends upon several factors such as size of the aerosol particle, breathing pattern, and other physical characteristics that will be discussed.

Box 4-9 lists both the diagnostic and therapeutic uses of aerosols. Respiratory care practitioners should be familiar with the generation, delivery, and hazards of aerosol therapy.

BOX 4-9

Common Uses of Nonmedicated and Medicated Aerosols

Nonmedicated Aerosols

Bland Aerosols

Reduce upper airway edema
Induce sputum
Humidify dry medical gases

Hypertonic Saline or Sterile Water

Induce sputum induction

Medicated Aerosols

Sympathomimetic bronchodilators
Antimuscarinic bronchodilators
Mucokinetic agents
Surface-active agents
Antitussive agents
Antimicrobial agents
Glucocorticoids
Antiallergic agents
Local anesthetics
Diagnostic aerosols (for ventilation scans, inhalation challenge for assessing airway response, and dosimetry)

Aerosol Delivery

The following sections describe the principles of operation, use, and clinical consideration for aerosol delivery devices. These devices include small- and large-volume nebulizers, **metered dose inhalers (MDIs), dry powder inhalers (DPIs),** and ultrasonic nebulizers. The use of large container and chamberlike devices to deliver aerosol, as well as aerosol delivery under special situations (i.e., the delivery of ribavirin) will be discussed later.

Clinical Advantages of Aerosol Delivery

Routes for administration of respiratory drugs include enteral, parenteral, topical, and inhalational. For aerosols, inhalation is preferred because it has several advantages. Deposition of aerosols directly onto the respiratory mucosa is a form of topical administration, allowing a drug to be directly administered to the desired location. Aerosolization of medication allows for a high concentration of the drug to be directly deposited onto the mucosa with local therapeutic effects optimized and side-effects minimized. Because of the large surface area of the lung (70 to 80 m^2), absorption and onset of action for aerosolized drugs are rapid. Administration of drugs such as sympathomimetics, anticholinergics, and steroids via inhalation results in fewer side-effects than if given systemically.[32] Additionally, gastric, intestinal, and hepatic enzymes are avoided when drugs are given by inhalation so that drug breakdown is less likely to occur.

Aerosol Physics

The depth and effectiveness of an aerosol delivered to the lungs depends upon multiple factors, including the size and physical characteristics of the aerosol particles, the amount of aerosol produced, the anatomy and geometry of the airways, and the ventilatory pattern. Respiratory care practitioners should be aware of these factors to provide optimal therapy by choosing an appropriate delivery device, educating the patient in aerosol use, and assuring an effective ventilatory pattern.

Respiratory care practitioners often attempt to deliver an aerosol to specific locations in the respiratory tract. The size of the aerosol particles is a major determinant in the therapeutic and diagnostic effectiveness within the respiratory system. Therapeutic and diagnostic aerosols are generally heterodispersed; that is, they are composed of a wide range of particle sizes and shapes. Monodispersed aerosols have a narrow range of diameters and are used during special application of aerosol therapy, such as delivery of ribavirin or pentamidine therapy.[33] Terms to describe aerosol particles include: aerosol volume, particle surface area, **mass median aerodynamic diameter (MMAD),** and **geometric standard deviation (GSD).** Of these measurements, MMAD is the most common measurement used to describe aerosol particles.

Aerosol Volume. As an aerosol is produced and delivered to the respiratory tract, its density may remain constant. Under this condition, aerosol volume is a product of aerosol particle size. The larger the particle size, the larger the volume of the aerosol. The volume of an aerosol particle is directly proportional to the cube of its radius (in inches):

$$\text{Aerosol volume} = 4/3 \times \pi \times (\text{radius}^3)$$

Clinical use of this principle may be appreciated by comparing many small particles with larger particles. Many smaller particles must be administered to the same area of the lung to equal the volume of a few larger ones. Particles that are less than 1 μm have little mass and volume often fail to get deposited in the lung and are usually exhaled. In contrast, particles with larger fluid volume may fail to enter the lower respiratory tract because the upper respiratory tract tends to filter them, thus prohibiting particles larger than 5 μm from entering the lower respiratory tract.

Particle Surface Area. Particle surface area is a function of its diameter (the greater the diameter of an aerosol particle, the greater its surface area), which can be illustrated with the following equation:

$$\text{Particle surface area} = \pi \times (\text{diameter})^2$$

The ratio of surface area to volume increases as particles become smaller and their inertia becomes less. Thus smaller particles are less likely to be deposited by direct impact in the airway and settle more slowly during breath holding.[33]

Mass Median Aerodynamic Diameter. The Mass Median Aerodynamic Diameter (MMAD) is the diameter that divides the range of particle size in half (i.e., 50% of the particles are smaller than the MMAD and 50% are larger).[34] Aerosol particles of equal MMAD have similar deposition patterns in the lung, regardless of their actual size and composition. The concept of MMAD is based on the idea that aerosol particles are created and dispersed in a range of sizes that mimic a typical bell-shaped probability distribution.

Geometric Standard Deviation. The geometric standard deviation (GSD), on the other hand, is a measure of how particle diameters vary. The higher the GSD, the wider the range of particle sizes that are present. As the GSD increases, the MMAD increases because larger particles carry a greater mass,[8] which may reduce the amount of aerosol deposited in the lower airway because a greater portion of larger particles are filtered out of the upper airway.

Depth of Penetration. The depth of penetration of an aerosol particle is inversely proportional to particle size. Most therapeutic aerosols have an MMAD from 1 to 10 μm,[33] and aerosols within this range—depending on their size—are deposited in the upper and lower airways. Although particles with a MMAD less than 5 μm tend to get deposited in the lung, most particles greater than 5 μm are trapped in the upper airway. Aerosols with a MMAD of 0.5 to 2.0 μm are generally targeted for delivery into the lower lung—some as far as the 10th generation of the airway. Particles with MMADs of less than 1 μm are so light and stable that many are not deposited. Even if these small particles remain in the lung, they carry little volume, and their effects are minimal. Table 4-2 shows the approximate location of aerosol particle deposition based on size.

Aerosol Deposition. The goal of aerosol delivery is to deposit a therapeutic or diagnostic aerosol at a certain location within the respiratory tract, but many factors influence aerosol deposition. Such factors include **inertial impaction,** gravity or **sedimentation,** the kinetic activity of the particles, the physical nature of particles, the temperature and humidity of the carrier gas, the patient's ventilatory pattern, and the physical characteristics of the patient's airway.

TABLE 4-2

Particle size and deposition site

Particle size (μm)	Deposition site
>100	do not enter respiratory tract
5-100	mouth, nose, and upper airway
2-5	bronchi and bronchioles
0.5-2	can enter alveoli
<0.5	stable and tend not to become deposited

Inertial Impaction. As a person inspires, gas flow changes direction and inertial impaction can occur, resulting in aerosol deposition on the mucosal lining of the upper and lower respiratory airways. Inertial impaction of particles occurs when gas flow changes direction and some of the particles continue moving forward and collide with the mucosal lining (Figure 4-23). Another factor that encourages aerosol impaction is gas flow rate. High inspiratory gas flows (> 1 L/sec) can enhance inertial impaction and cause some particles to impact on the epithelial lining of the upper airway and posterior aspects of the pharynx. It is important, therefore, to use low inspiratory gas flows (<1 L/sec) to ensure effective aerosol therapy; this can be accomplished by instructing the patient to inhale slowly.

Gravity or Sedimentation. As was already mentioned, the larger the particle, the more likely it will become unstable, fall out of the carrier gas, and be deposited. Small particles (in the 1 to 5 μm range) are deposited by sedimentation due to gravity.[35] The actual sedimentation of a particle is governed by Stokes's Law, which states that the sedimentation rate of a particle nearly equals the particle's density multiplied by the square of it's diameter. In other words, as particles become larger, gravity has a greater effect on them, and they are more likely to settle out of suspension. Therefore larger particles are less stable and are deposited before smaller particles.

One factor that opposes gravity and tends to keep particles in suspension is gas density. Note that a suspension of particles in a gas occurs when gas molecules randomly strike the sides of aerosol particles and keep them "floating" in the gas. The denser the gas, the greater the effects of this bombardment because particles are more likely to remain suspended and be transported by the carrier gas than to settle from gravity. On the other hand, the lighter the gas, the less likely it can transport particles. This principle may be better understood by comparing helium with air as a carrier gas for an aerosol. Because helium molecules are smaller than air molecules, aerosol particles are more influenced by gravity than by the molecular collision with the helium carrier gas. Gravity tends to pull particles out of the gas stream, so helium and oxygen mixtures are poor carriers of aerosol particles.

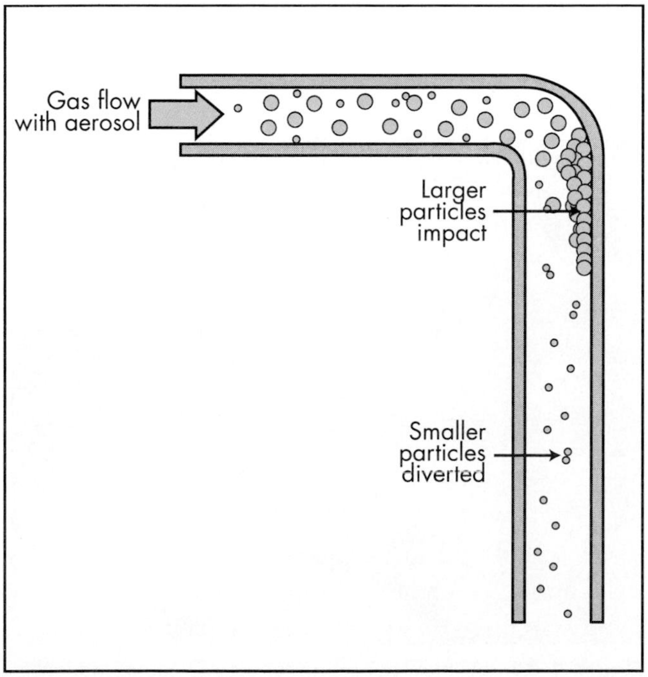

Figure 4-23 Inertial impaction of aerosol particles.

Kinetic Activity. All molecules are continually in motion, colliding with each other and their environment. This phenomenon, kinetic activity, can be seen with submicronic aerosol particles that are less than 1 μm. The random movement of these small particles is called **Brownian movement** (or diffusion). As particles decrease in size, Brownian movement increases. Another way of describing this phenomenon is that the smaller the aerosol particle, the closer it approaches the size of the gas molecules impacting it, thus becoming more susceptible to the Brownian forces. Notice that a particle must be submicroscopic before aerosol deposition is significantly enhanced by kinetic activity. Particles less than 1 μm in diameter are the most stable and tend to be inhaled and exhaled without being deposited on the airway surface. The effects of gravity and kinetic activity on particles in this size range tend to cancel each other. Therefore as aerosol particles increase in size above 1 μm, gravity begins to exert a greater force, affecting particle stability.

Physical Nature of the Particle. The physical nature, or tonicity, of the aerosol particle can also influence deposition. Aerosol particles can either become smaller or increase in size as they travel through the respiratory system. Particles that increase in size within the lungs are called hygroscopic particles. Such particles tend to absorb water and grow in size. As they absorb water and collide with adjacent particles, they consolidate and drop out of the gas stream, which is a key factor to consider when administering solid particles of medication. Hygroscopic tendencies are influenced by the liquid substance (e.g., medication) itself, the tonicity of the particle, the ambient humidity, and the gas temperature, which is discussed in the following section. Hypertonic aerosols have a greater tonicity than body fluids so they tend to absorb water, increase in size, and become unstable earlier than hypotonic aerosols. However, hypotonic aerosols tend to evaporate, decrease in size, and travel further into the respiratory tract. Isotonic aerosol particles have the same tonicity as body fluids and are not likely to change their dimensions.

A clinical example of the principle of tonicity is seen when hypertonic saline aerosol is delivered to enhance expectoration. Hypertonic aerosols are often administered to obtain a sputum sample for microbiological examination because inhalation of a hypertonic aerosol causes larger particles to deposit in the larger airways, thus promoting cough and expectoration.

Temperature and Humidity. The temperature and humidity of the carrier gas also influence aerosol particle size. Particles can either evaporate and get smaller or increase in size, depending on the water content and humidity level of the gas around them. An aerosol that is cooler than room temperature will warm as it travels to the patient via the delivery circuit. As the aerosol warms, particles evaporate and become smaller, so there is potential for deeper deposition in the airways. Heated aerosol cools as it travels to the patient, so particles tend to coalesce and thus become larger, which encourages deposition in the larger airways.[11] When cool aerosol particles are placed in warm, humidified gas (e.g., gas in the respiratory system), they tend to grow as humidity coalesces them. Again, as these particles grow, they are deposited higher in the airway. Dry aerosols (e.g., powdered bronchodilators) tend to clump or aggregate in high humidity environments, thereby reducing their delivered doses.

Ventilatory Pattern and Characteristics of the Patient's Airway. Ventilatory pattern is the most important factor that can be controlled by both the patient and the person administering the aerosol treatment. The ventilatory pattern is influenced by inspiratory gas flow, respiratory rate, and inspiratory pause. High inspiratory gas flow tends to deposit aerosol particles in the upper airways because of inertial impaction. When an aerosol is inhaled at a flow rate higher than 1 L/sec, gas turbulence encourages larger particles to be deposited onto the upper airway lining. Deeper deposition of aerosol particles occurs with slower inspiratory flow. Flow rates lower than 0.5 L/sec result in laminar flow, increasing the chances for deeper deposition.[33] Normal spontaneous inspiratory flows are about 0.5 L/sec (30 L/min).

Tachypnea increases inspiratory flows, which reduces the time the aerosol particle is in the lung and leaves fewer opportunities for deposition.[8] Slower respiratory rates afford the patient improved deposition by allowing more time for aerosol particles to become unstable and fall out of the carrier gas. Slower respiratory rates combined with a breath hold at the end of inspiration have been effective in promoting deeper aerosol deposition.[1,8,33,35] An inspiratory hold of 4 to 10 seconds promotes aerosol deposition. During breath holding, particles have more time to decrease their forward velocity, thus increasing aerosol deposition.

The influence of tidal volume is less predictable. Although larger tidal volumes take in greater amounts of aerosol, the relationship between tidal volume and actual aerosol deposition has not been demonstrated in clinical studies. In a review of the literature, tidal volume was not found to be an important factor in aerosol deposition.[1]

Airway caliber is another factor that influences aerosol deposition. As the caliber of the airway decreases due to bronchoconstriction, edema, or secretions, aerosol deposition is more likely to occur in the upper airway or larger bronchi. Reduced airway diameter may require greater dosages of medicated aerosols to achieve desired effects. Sometimes secretion removal (e.g., airway aspiration or suctioning) can better prepare the respiratory tract for aerosol therapy.

Mouth breathing enhances aerosol deposition in the lower airways more than nose breathing because the nasal cavity can filter out aerosol particles larger than 5 to10 μm in diameter.[8] Furthermore, aerosol deposition (especially medicated aerosols) by mouthpiece is better than by mask. Patients with an increased work of breathing tend to breathe through their mouth in an attempt to decrease resistance to inspiratory flow. Under these conditions, a medicated aerosol should be administered by mouthpiece or MDI whenever possible. Current guidelines recommend that patients under 3 years of age should receive aerosol by mask, and patients over 3 years should receive it by mouthpiece.[27] Other options recommended include using only MDIs (not nebulizers) for children over 4 years of age.[36]

Although this is not supported by research data, patients who cannot tolerate an aerosol mask may benefit from using a blow-by apparatus (Figure 4-24). A blow-by device allows the aerosol spray to be directed right into the patient's oral cavity to promote particle deposition. Note that if the a blow-by method is used without close monitoring, aerosol may be directed toward the nasal passages, compromising aerosol deposition. Aerosol by mask or blow-by device may have similar results in infants because they breathe primarily through their noses. Unfortunately, few controlled studies of nebulized aerosols administered to infants have been completed. For this age group, aerosol therapy is further compromised because of the nonstandardized doses of bronchoactive drugs. Because of the

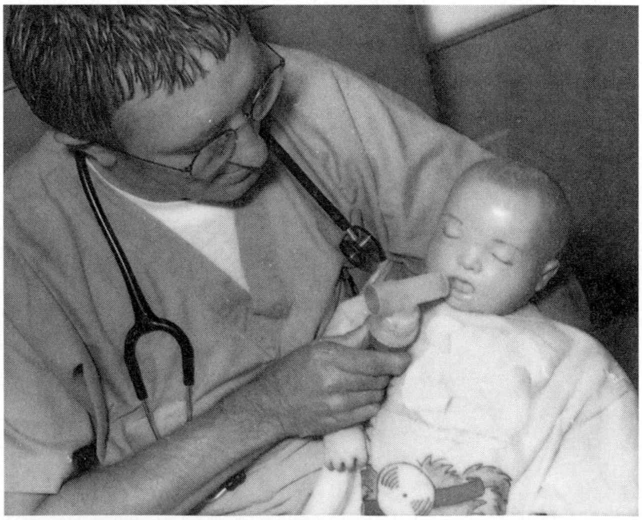

Figure 4-24 A "blow-by" set-up for aerosol administration.

small tidal volumes of infants and the anatomy of their upper airways, doses recommended for older children or adults cannot be used for infants. Very young children and infants may require relatively higher medication doses to achieve effective results.[36]

Therapeutic Use of Aerosol

Aerosols are administered for various reasons, including for therapeutic and diagnostic effects (see Table 4-6). Major aerosol treatments include bronchodilators, antiinflammatory drugs, antimicrobials, anticholinergics, local anesthetics, and bland aerosols. Safe and effective administration of these treatments requires careful selection of the delivery method and monitoring of patient response. In addition, teaching the patient the proper technique for inspiration during an aerosol treatment is the single most important variable that respiratory care practitioners can influence. Optimal patient ventilatory pattern, selection of the appropriate aerosol generator, and administration of the correct aerosol solution allows aerosol therapy to remain one of the most effective respiratory care modalities for preventing and treating pulmonary disease.

The following section discusses aerosol generation and equipment, operation, clinical use, and limitations and emphasizes the commonly used aerosol devices including small and large aerosol generators, MDIs, environmental aerosol units, and special administration of selected aerosols (e.g., pentamidine, ribavirin).

Methods of Aerosol Generation

Aerosols are produced by devices called nebulizers, the most common type of which is the **jet nebulizer.** Jet nebulizers—regardless of reservoir size—use the Bernoulli Principle to produce an aerosol. This principle is based on a decrease in lateral wall pressure to shatter fluid particles into an aerosol at a point where gas flow exits a constriction. When the lateral pressure that surrounds the gas stream decreases below atmospheric pressure, fluid is drawn up a capillary tube (Figure 4-25). When the fluid reaches the gas stream, it is shattered into small particles, which may encounter baffles. (A baffle reduces aerosol particle size.) Baffles include the fluid surface, sides of the aerosol generator, or structures deliberately placed in the front of the gas stream, such as a plastic ball or a flat device (Figure 4-26). Actually, any object in the path of the aerosol particle can be a baffle, just as can any right-angle bend of the tubing carrying the aerosol. When a large, heavy, aerosol particle hits a baffle, its weight and interrupted forward motion cause it to drop back into the fluid reservoir. Baffles prevent larger particles from being delivered to the patient, so a more uniform aerosol size can be generated. Without baffles, larger particles are delivered. Nebulizers without a baffle are called atomizers. Because atomizers produce a wide range of particles, they are not commonly used in respiratory care. However, atomizers may be used in clinical conditions that require large aerosol particles to be applied to the upper airway. Such situations include administration of topical anesthetics or decongestants to the pharynx and nasal passages for insertion of invasive devices such as bronchoscopes, endotracheal tubes, suction catheters, and nasopharyngeal airways.

Classification of Pneumatic Aerosol Generators

Jet nebulizers require compressed gas to generate an aerosol and therefore are considered pneumatic aerosol generators. These types of nebulizers are generally classified as either small-volume nebulizers (SVNs), MDIs, or large-volume nebulizers (LVNs).

Small-Volume Nebulizers (SVN). One of the first medical nebulizers was the DeVilbliss hand-held type, which incorporated a flexible bulb that when squeezed produced gas flow to a jet, which drew the medication into the gas stream and shattered it into an aerosol (Figure 4-27). Since the development of hand-held, squeeze type of nebulizers, manufacturers have created a variety of SVNs that are employed with gas flow circuits used for intermittent positive-pressure breathing (IPPB) therapy, mechanical ventilation, or as hand-held nebulizers powered by low-flow oxygen or compressed air.

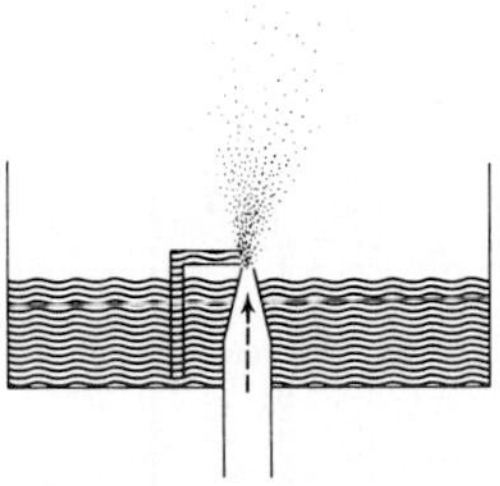

Figure 4-25 The *Bernoulli Principle* used by jet nebulizers to produce an aerosol. (Modified from Cushing IE, Miller WF: Nebulization therapy. In Safar P, Respiratory therapy, Philadelphia, 1965, FA Davis Co.)

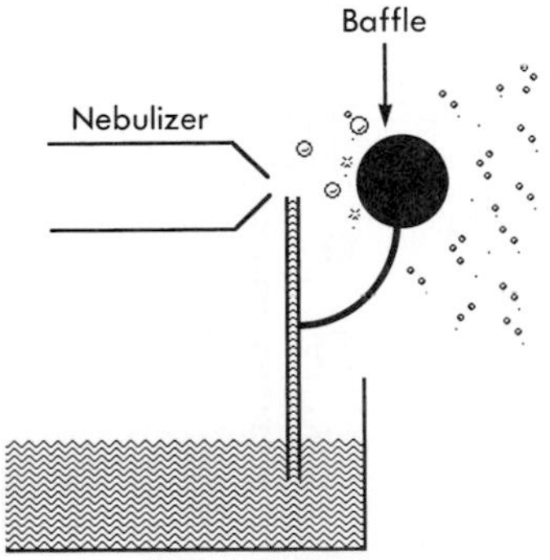

Figure 4-26 Use of a baffle for producing smaller aerosol particles.

All SVNs used with IPPB therapy or mechanical ventilation are classified as either sidestream nebulizers, in which the aerosol is injected into the gas stream, or as mainstream nebulizers, in which the main flow of gas actually passes through the aerosol generator (Figure 4-28). Several nebulizers with the newer disposable circuits for IPPB or mechanical ventilation can be adapted to either mainstream or sidestream placement, depending on the therapeutic indication or need.

Hand-held nebulizers are a popular version of SVN used to administer medicated aerosols (Figure 4-29). Since the late 1970s, they have become a common modality for providing medicated aerosol to patients for the prevention and treatment of pulmonary disease. As a result of the popularity of SVNs, a variety of models are now available, each with its own characteristics, features, and varying aerosol output. Despite differences in the SVNs available, studies have failed to demonstrate the differences in clinical response based on SVN design.[8]

SVNs employ a jet, which uses the Bernoulli principle, as previously discussed. A high-pressure gas is passed through a constriction, adjacent to which is the open end of a capillary tube. The other end of the tube is immersed in the fluid (e.g., medication), and as gas exits the constriction, its forward velocity increases, and the surrounding pressure (i.e., lateral wall pressure) decreases. Liquid is drawn by the subatmospheric pressure and allowed to be shattered by the gas stream. The gas flow and aerosol are allowed to exit the unit via a large-bore outlet, where an adapter fits to accommodate various devices such as a mouthpiece, mask, or gas circuit to a mechanical ventilator. A common SVN set-

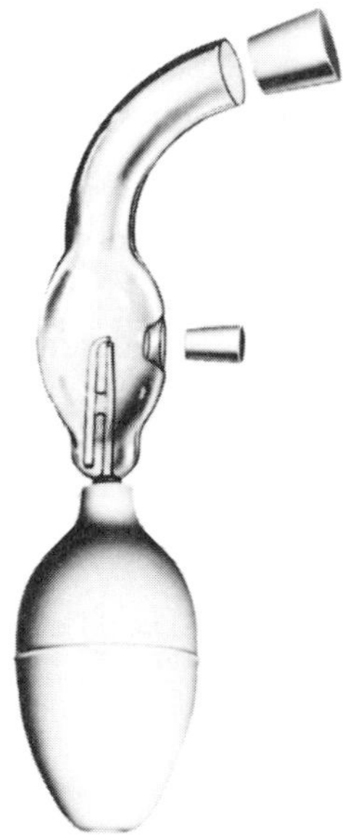

Figure 4-27 The original hand-held bulb type of nebulizer manufactured by DeVilbliss. (Courtesy Sunrise Medical Home Healthcare, Longmount, Colo.)

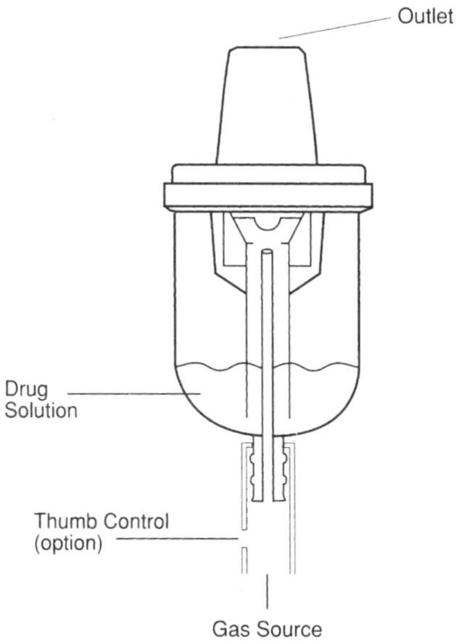

Figure 4-29 A hand-held or small volume nebulizer used for generating aerosol. (Redrawn from Rau JL Jr: Respiratory care pharmacology, ed 5, St. Louis, 1998, Mosby.)

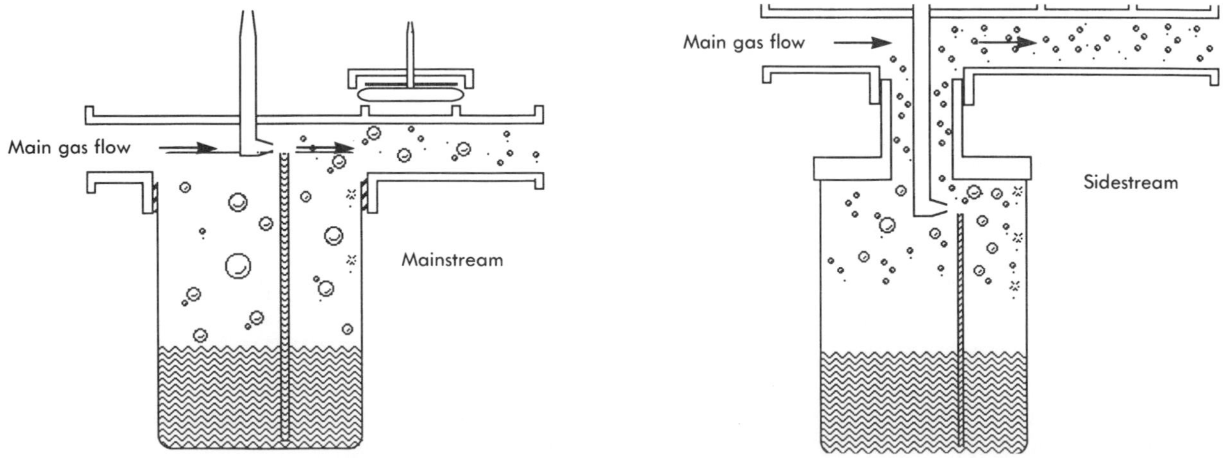

Figure 4-28 Mainstream and sidestream nebulizers.

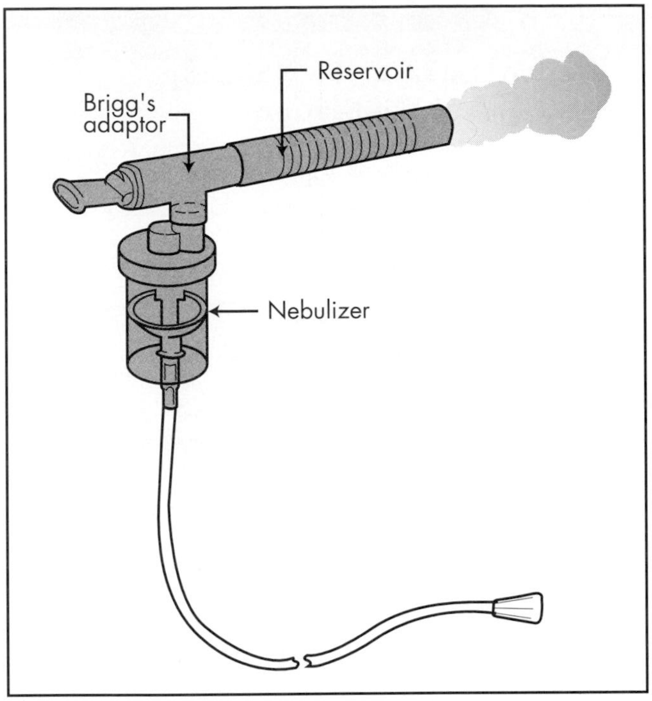

Figure 4-30 A common set-up for an SVN using a Brigg's adapter, reservoir, and mouthpiece.

up is the T-piece (Brigg's adapter) with a mouthpiece and a 50 mL reservoir (Figure 4-30). A reservoir retains additional aerosol for increased deposition. Hand-held SVNs require a gas source, which is usually a portable compressor or flowmeter, to provide flow to generate an aerosol. Typical gas flow rates used with SVNs are 6 to 8 L/min.

SVN performance is related to the amount of liquid in the unit, the dead space within the unit, and the gas flow rate. Typical SVNs provide more aerosol when the nebulizer volume is 4 mL (instead of 2 mL) and when the gas flow rate is from 6 to 8 L/min.[8] As gas flow through the SVN increases, particle size decreases. Fluid nebulized within the SVN usually consists of a medication and diluent (e.g., sterile saline or water). As the fluid level decreases (as a result of nebulizing), the diluent evaporates and the medication concentration increases. The dead space or residual volume is the amount of fluid remaining in the SVN at the point when the nebulizer no longer generates an aerosol, which may vary from model to model. A typical dead space volume ranges from 0.5 to 1 mL. As dead space volume increases, less medication is delivered, so the overall efficiency of the unit decreases. It is common to flick the sides of the SVN or shake the unit when it begins to sputter to encourage larger fluid particles adhering to the inside wall of the unit to return to the small fluid reservoir and be nebulized. This action can increase the actual amount of medication delivered. Most SVNs produce a total fluid output of 0.1 to 0.5 mL/min, and a total fluid volume typically placed in an SVN for therapy is 3 to 4 mL. Gas flow rates through the nebulizer are optimal at 6 to 8 L/min, which produces clinically useful aerosol particles. The average aerosol particle MMAD from an SVN is 1 to 5 μm.[33] Above gas flow rates of 8 L/min, treatment time decreases and less medication may actually enter the patient's airway. Gas flow rates below 6 L/min extend treatment time beyond patient tolerance, resulting in the treatment possibly being turned off before all the medication is nebulized. Even with optimal operation and patient technique, SVNs only provide about 10% of the intended medication to the lower airways. Most of the medication (including diluent) is exhaled or remains as dead space volume (Box 4-10).

> **BOX 4-10**
>
> **Decision Making & Problem Solving**
>
> You are called to the emergency department to deliver a medicated aerosol to a 4-year old child, who is alert but restless and complains of shortness of breath. The child's mother says that the child has had several "asthma attacks" since 1 year of age but that all have been mild and this is the first visit to a hospital. The emergency room physician asks you to suggest an appropriate aerosol device. What do you recommend?
>
> See Appendix A for thc answer.

The brand or model of SVN, the gas flow rate at which it is operated, and the type of medication affect the unit's overall effectiveness. Most SVNs must remain upright to function, but others can function in a variety of positions. The patient's ability to correctly assemble and operate the SVN should be a major factor when selecting brand and model. The intent of the therapy should also influence the type of SVN used. For example, to treat a lung infection, the smaller particles generated by Marquest's Respirgard II SVN penetrate more deeply into the lung parenchyma. For home therapy, however, a durable SVN that is easy to clean and maintain should be considered (Box 4-11).

Other specialty nebulizers, such as the Vortran HEART and the ICN SPAG-2 units (described later in this chapter), may be used to create more uniform particle sizes. Furthermore, a finger control can be used to create nebulization during inspiration, increase the medication delivered, and reduce waste (Figure 4-31). Although it is popular to use an SVN without finger control, continuous nebulization during both inspiration and expiration results in significant waste of the medication.

Use of a SVN during mechanical ventilation is one method to provide various medications to the lungs of intubated patients. SVN use during neonatal mechanical ventilation has significantly decreased over the past several years. Because of the addition of gas flow from the SVN (if an auxiliary gas source is used instead of nebulizer function from the ventilator) and the potential for an increase in airway

BOX 4-11

Decision Making & Problem Solving

A physician requests that you administer an aerosolized antibiotic to a patient with pneumonia. What device could you use, and what MMAD is appropriate?

See Appendix A for the answer.

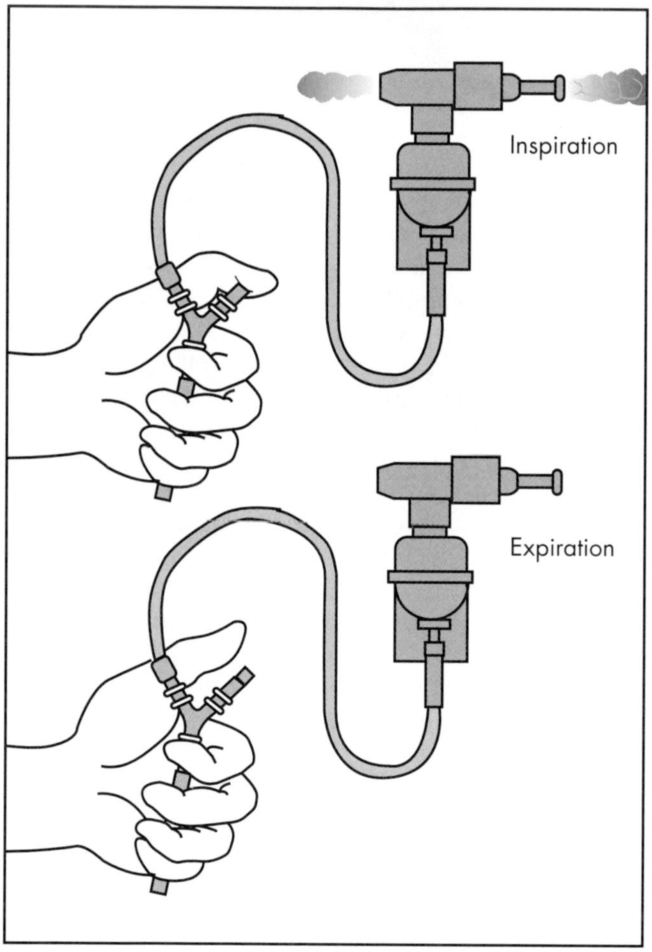

Figure 4-31 Use of a finger control to control aerosol production during inspiration and expiration.

pressures, neonatal SVN therapy has been replaced with alternative methods (i.e., use of a MDIs, reservoirs, and self-inflating bags). This set-up allows medicated aerosol to be artificially ventilated into the patient's artificial airway.

There are several factors that influence aerosol delivery through the gas delivery circuit and artificial airway that need to be noted, including a baffling effect of the ventilator circuit and artificial airway, and the increased inertial impaction of aerosol particles during high inspiratory gas flow. These factors can decrease deposition of medication in the lung. Several studies demonstrate that only about 1% to 3% of the drug is deposited during mechanical ventilation.[37-40]

BOX 4-12

Proper Use of an SVN during Mechanical Ventilation

1. Determine need for therapy.
2. Establish appropriate dose of medication.
3. Assemble the SVN.
4. Place the SVN securely in inspiratory limb of ventilator circuit.
5. Attach a gas source (from either a mechanical ventilator or a flow-metering device) of 6 to 8 L/min to the SVN.
6. Adjust ventilatory parameters (e.g., tidal volume, pressure-limit) to accommodate the excess gas flow from the SVN.
7. Turn off ventilator flow-by or continuous gas flow during SVN therapy.
8. Tap the side of the SVN as needed to nebulize the entire volume of liquid.
9. At the completion of treatment, remove and disassemble SVN and rinse it with *sterile* water or allow it to air dry.
10. Return ventilatory parameters to pretreatment settings.
11. Replace the SVN daily or as indicated.

In addition to adjusting the medication dose as necessary for delivery to intubated, mechanically ventilated patients, SVN placement is a key to providing effective therapy. Studies have shown that placing the SVN in the inspiratory limb at the manifold of the ventilator circuit about 18 inches from the patient's airway is optimal. The least effective location for an SVN is between the patient and wye connector of the ventilatory circuit.[8] If an SVN provides continuous nebulization, medicated aerosol can be wasted during the expiratory phase of ventilation, but this can be avoided by using intermittent SVN aerosolization during mechanical ventilation. Box 4-12 summarizes the correct method of SVN use during mechanical ventilation.

Metered Dose Inhalers. MDIs are available for delivering various medications, including but not limited to, bronchodilators and antiinflammatory and anticholinergic drugs. The MDI was originally manufactured by Riker Laboratories, which is now 3M Pharmaceuticals, in 1956. MDI therapy has developed into a reliable, efficient, and safe method of providing medicated aerosol to the respiratory tract.[32] Effectiveness and portability make MDI therapy an important aspect of caring for patients with pulmonary disease. Although MDIs can be effective, patient instruction and proper use are paramount to optimal delivery. According to the 1994 National Health Interview Survey, 40 million patients use MDIs. With such widespread use, providing patients education in proper MDI use and assessing MDI effectiveness are major tasks of respiratory care practitioners. Despite the simple ap-

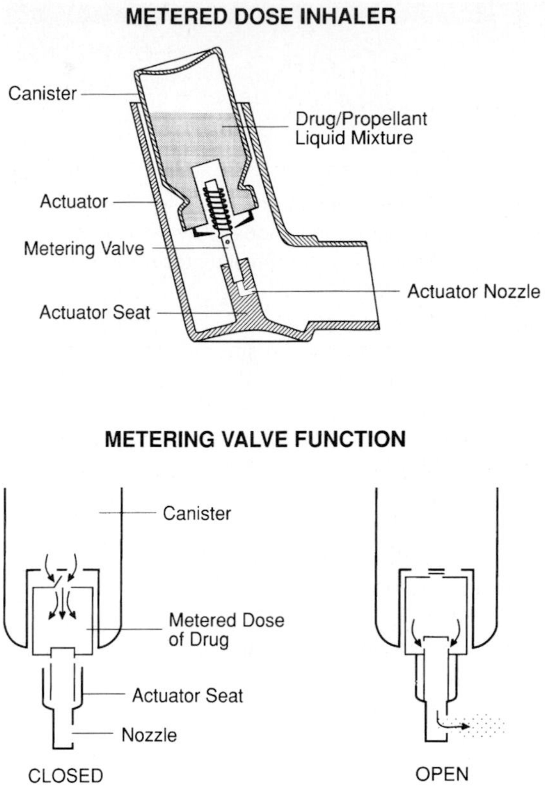

Figure 4-32 A metered dose inhaler. (Redrawn from Rau JL Jr: Respiratory care pharmacology, ed 5, St Louis, 1998, Mosby.)

pearance of MDIs and their ease in generating an aerosol puff, studies report that most patients do not use them correctly, resulting in suboptimal therapy.[32,41]

MDIs (Figure 4-32) are small, pressurized canisters with a mouthpiece that employ pressurized gas propellants. The canisters contain from 80 to 300 doses of a medication, either in liquid or powder form. When the cannister is inverted, placed in its mouthpiece adapter, and then depressed, an aerosolized dose of medication is released. Before January 1996, MDIs used a mixture of two or three chlorofluorocarbon (CFC) propellants with crystals of the medication in suspension. There has since been a total worldwide ban on CFC use, and although medical aerosols are exempt from this ban until the year 2000, many MDI manufacturers are now using alternative CFCs or other propellants, such as hydrofluoroalkanes (HFAs).[33] Studies indicate that HFAs have limited impact on the environment and are safe for use in MDIs.[32]

MDIs contain vapor pressure from 300 to 500 kPa at 20° C. Each time an MDI is actuated, a measured amount of propellant carrying medication crystals is delivered. As the propellant emerges from the MDI, its high vapor pressure causes rapid evaporation and dissipation, while the medication is aerosolized and delivered to the patient's open airway. The forward velocity of the aerosol leaving the MDI is rapid while it is traveling in a forward stream, resulting in a significant amount of medication being deposited in the oropharynx because of inertial impaction. It is estimated that an average of only 10% of the actual medication that leaves the MDI enters the lower respiratory tract.[42]

The size of the aerosol particle produced by the MDI is influenced, in part, by the type of drug and the propellant. The temperature of the propellant also influences aerosol size. If the MDI is placed in a cool environment and the cannister becomes cooler than room temperature, vapor pressure within the cannister decreases, producing larger aerosol particles. In other words, the cooler the MDI becomes, the larger the particles released from it. Studies indicate that deeper deposition and smaller particle MMADs occur when cannister contents are at 37° C.[43] Patients should be instructed to maintain the MDI at a warmer temperature in colder climates to preserve its effectiveness.[44] This may be accomplished by having patients carry the MDI close to their skin or place it in a pocket of clothing near body heat. In addition, proper MDI preparation before use preserves the intended dosage of medication that leaves the unit when the cannister is depressed and the aerosol is produced. Shaking the cannister prior to use allows the medication and propellant to mix. If an MDI has been not used for several days, the first several puffs may contain suboptimal medication levels, so the patient should be advised to actuate the unit two to three times after shaking it before actually inspiring the aerosol.

Successful delivery of medication with an MDI depends on the patient's ability to (1) coordinate the actuation of the MDI at the appropriate time during inspiration, (2) create a slow inspiratory gas flow, and (3) hold their breath for 4 to 10 seconds at end-inspiration. Actuating the MDI late or at the end of inspiration, or stopping inhalation when the cold blast of propellant hits the back of the throat (cold-freon effect) decreases deposition and results in suboptimal therapy. Studies show that inertial impaction of the MDI aerosol decreases if the patient places the mouthpiece 4 cm from an open mouth before actuating the MDI.[1] If the patient is unable to aim the MDI mist at the opened mouth, the MDI mouthpiece should be placed in the entrance to the mouth, or an auxiliary device (discussed later in this chapter) should be used.

Even if the patient demonstrates the correct MDI technique after initial instruction, a follow-up assessment is usually necessary. Patients tend to alter technique over time (e.g., increase inspiratory flow, or poorly coordinate inspiration with MDI actualization), thus compromising MDI effectiveness. This is especially true for pediatric and elderly patients.

Another factor that can affect the delivery of the medication is the time between actuations of the MDI. The initial inspiration of the medication, especially a bronchodilator, increases airway caliber and improves mucus flow. Once this happens, subsequent inspirations from the MDI can be more effective, so it is best to wait from 3 to 10 minutes between actuations.[45] If this length of time is impractical for a

BOX 4-13

Optimal Technique for MDI Use

Without an Accessory Device

1. Determine the need for therapy.
2. Determine number of actuations to be provided.
3. Assemble the MDI and inspect the actuator mouthpiece for foreign matter.
4. Shake the cannister vigorously.
5. If it has been more than 24 hours since last use, actuate one puff into the air while holding the MDI upside down.
6. The patient places the MDI mouthpiece 4 cm from open mouth.
7. Following a normal exhalation, the patient inspires slowly (<60 L/sec) while depressing the MDI cannister.
8. The patient continues inspiration until total lung capacity is reached.
9. At the end of inspiration, the breath is held for 5 to 10 seconds.
10. Wait 1 to 2 minutes between puffs from the MDI.

With an Accessory Device (i.e., holding chamber or spacer)

1. Determine the need for therapy.
2. Determine the number of actuations to be provided.
3. Assemble the MDI and inspect the actuator mouthpiece for foreign matter.
4. Shake the cannister vigorously.
5. If it has been more than 24 hours since the last use, deliver one puff into the air while holding the MDI upside down.
6. Attach accessory device to the MDI.
   a. Place MDI mouthpiece into accessory device.
   b. Place valve stem into MDI cannister holding orifice on accessory device.
7. If using mask, attach it to the accessory device.
8. The patient inspires slowly (<60 L/sec) and the MDI is actuated.
9. The patient continues inspiration until total lung capacity.
10. Wait 1 to 2 minutes between puffs from the MDI.

particular patient situation (e.g., in cases of severe asthma), waiting at least 1 minute between MDI inhalations is minimal. These guidelines also apply to MDI therapy during mechanical ventilation. With the delivery of MDI medication into the gas delivery circuit with mechanical ventilation, waiting 3 to 10 minutes between breaths enhances the effectiveness of the aerosol. Box 4-13 outlines the correct procedure for MDI use (with and without an auxiliary device).

Accessories to Enhance Aerosol Deposition from an MDI. There are several problems associated with coordinating MDI use with inspiration. In addition, handling the unit may be difficult for some patients, especially the elderly, younger patients, and the physically challenged. Even if the patient can handle and actuate the MDI, it is often difficult to coordinate the aerosol with inspiration. The cold-freon effect mentioned earlier may also compromise delivery of medication. Respiratory care practitioners should evaluate each patient's ability to use an MDI and should implement an auxiliary device designed to enhance medication delivery if a patient is unable to correctly perform therapy. Such devices include **spacers** and chambers, spring-loaded actuators, and devices to help the patient depress the cannister to initiate an aerosol puff from the MDI.

There are many spacers and chambers available to be attached to an MDI. (Figure 4-33 shows examples of these devices.) Spacers and chambers may be rigid or collapsible, based on the model and manufacturer. The goals with these auxiliary devices are as follows: (1) to reduce the velocity of the propelled aerosol from the MDI, (2) to decrease inertial impaction, (3) to minimize oropharyngeal deposition of the aerosol, and (4) to improve the synchronization of the patient inspiration and generation of the MDI puff. Studies indicate that use of these devices may increase drug deposition in the lung.[46]

Spacers and chambers act as partial reservoirs for medication. Chambers differ from spacers by employing a one-way valve to hold aerosol particles in the unit until inspiration occurs. Chambers are effective for patients who have problems coordinating inspiration with activation of the MDI.

Spacers and chambers increase the distance for MDI aerosol to travel, which allows time for evaporation, thus reducing aerosol particle size. The larger the volume of the spacer or chamber, the more likely particles will shrink. These devices also reduce the chance of inertial impaction on inspiration by slowing the aerosol's forward velocity. (This chance decreases independently of spacer or chamber size or shape.)

Those who benefit from spacer or chamber use include young children (who cannot coordinate breathing with MDI use), patients in severe respiratory distress, or any patient who has difficulty coordinating MDI puffs with inspiration. Some spacers and chambers emit a whistling alarm if the patient inspires too quickly. This audio feedback encourages patients to maintain an appropriate, slow inspiratory flow.

Monaghan Medical Corporation's AeroVent, shown in Figure 4-34, is one of several reservoirs available that is specially designed for MDIs used with gas delivery circuits for mechanical ventilation and allows improved aerosol deposition to intubated patients. With the AeroVent, the MDI is actuated 1 to 2 seconds before the inspiratory gas arrives

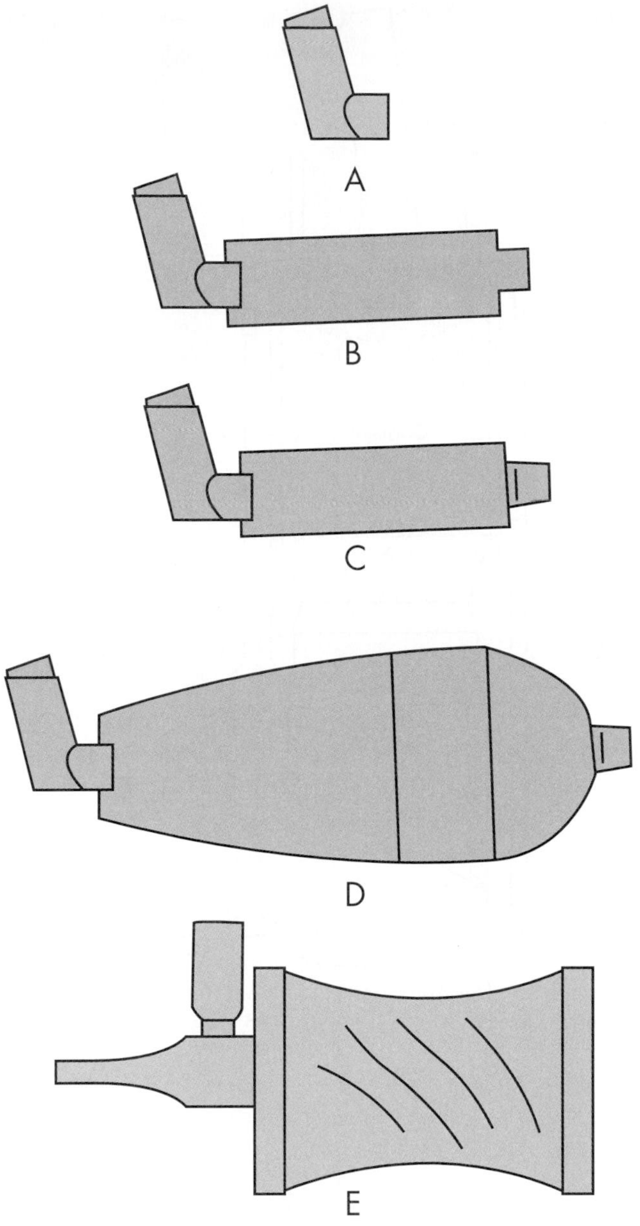

Figure 4-33 Common shapes for reservoirs and chambers used with MDIs: **A,** MDI; **B,** elongated reservoir; **C,** elongated chamber; **D,** pear-shaped chamber; and **E,** collapsible reservoir.

from the mechanical ventilator. An example of a holding chamber for spontaneously breathing older children and adults is Monaghan's AeroChamber (Figure 4-35). The AeroChamber is also available with a mask for administering medication to small children and infants (Figure 4-36).

Additional devices aimed at improving MDI therapy include actuator aids, such as a spring-loaded Autohaler (3M Pharmaceuticals), which requires an inspiratory effort to actuate the MDI (Figure 4-37). When the patient flips up a lever on top of the MDI during an inspiratory effort, a spring-loaded response allows aerosol to leave the MDI. This device helps the patient to get the MDI to release its medication but does not aid in controlling the aerosol once it leaves the MDI.

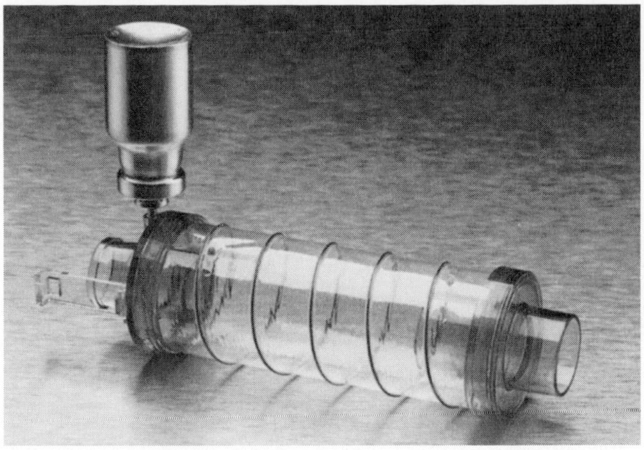

Figure 4-34 The AeroVent reservoir for use with MDIs and gas flow circuits. (Courtesy Monaghan Medical Corporation, Plattsburgh, NY)

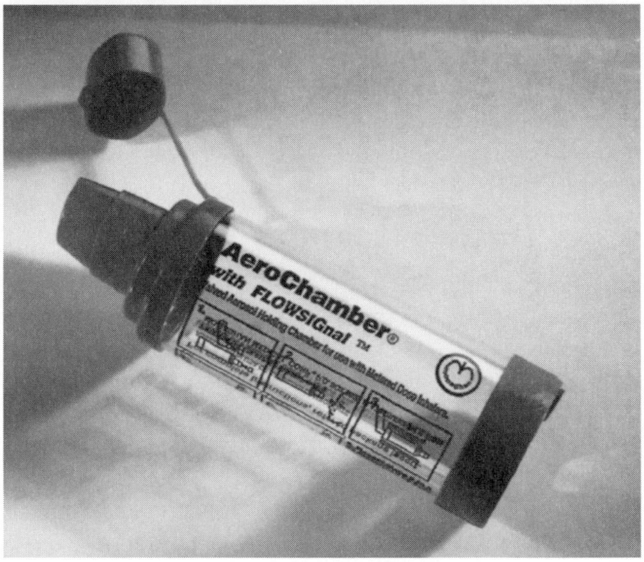

Figure 4-35 The AeroChamber for use with an MDI. (Courtesy Monaghan Medical Corporation, Plattsburgh, NY)

The Vent-Ease device allows patients with muscular or hand coordination difficulties to actuate the MDI (Figure 4-38). The Vent-Ease allows the MDI to be placed within it, and once the extension arm is pressed, the MDI releases its medication. This device aids in MDI actualization and does not effect drug delivery.

Dry Powder Inhalers. DPIs are an alternate method for delivering various medications, such as bronchodilators and antiallergic agents. They are practical, small, portable, and do not use CFCs or require a pressurized gas source. DPIs are breath-actuated, so there is no need to coordinate actuation and inspiration. DPIs may better serve patients who have difficulty using MDIs.

There are several DPIs on the market for treatment of pulmonary disease. Glaxo's Rotohaler (Figure 4-39) provides

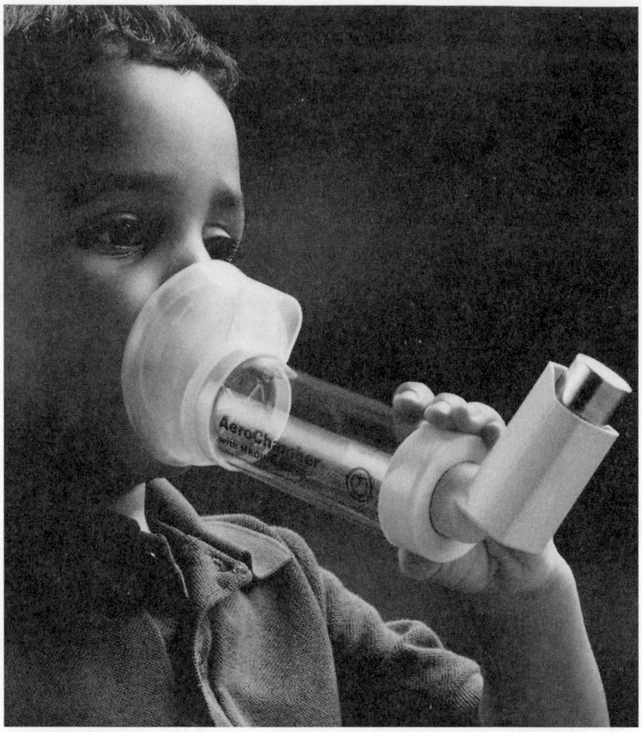

Figure 4-36 The AeroChamber with mask for use with an MDI. (Courtesy Monaghan Medical Corporation, Plattsburgh, NY)

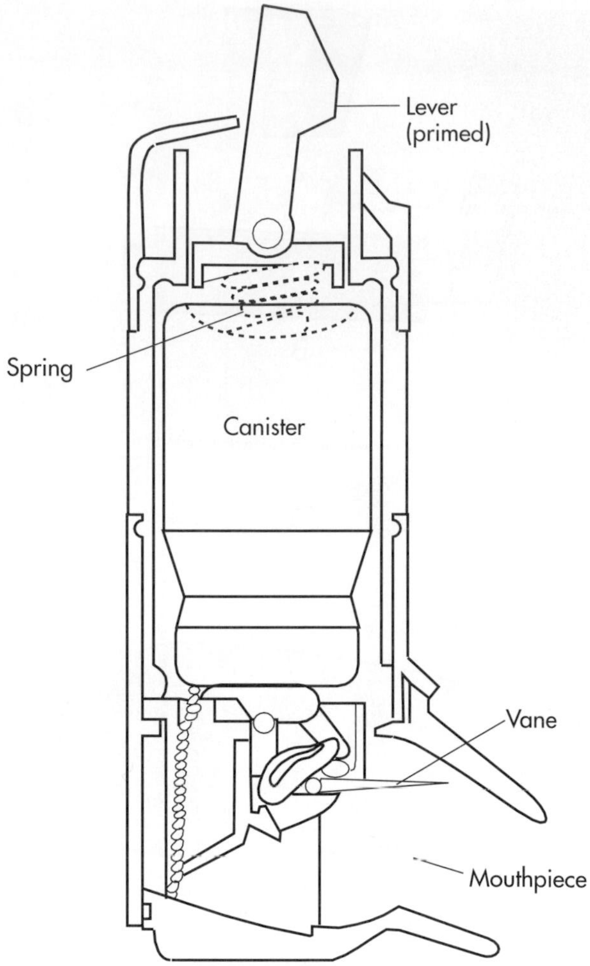

Figure 4-37 The Autohaler MDI. (From Rau JL Jr: Respiratory care pharmacology, ed 5, St Louis, 1998, Mosby.)

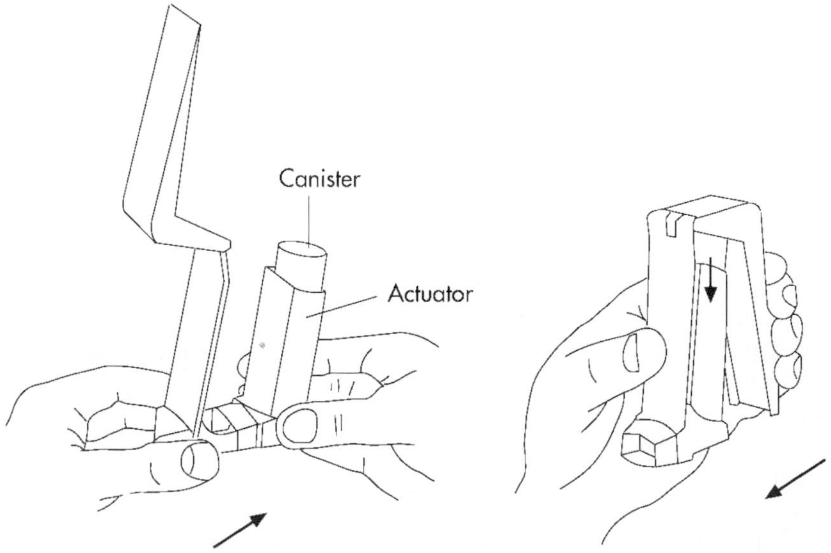

Figure 4-38 The Vent-Ease MDI adapter. (From Rau JL Jr: Respiratory care pharmacology, ed 5, St Louis, 1998, Mosby.)

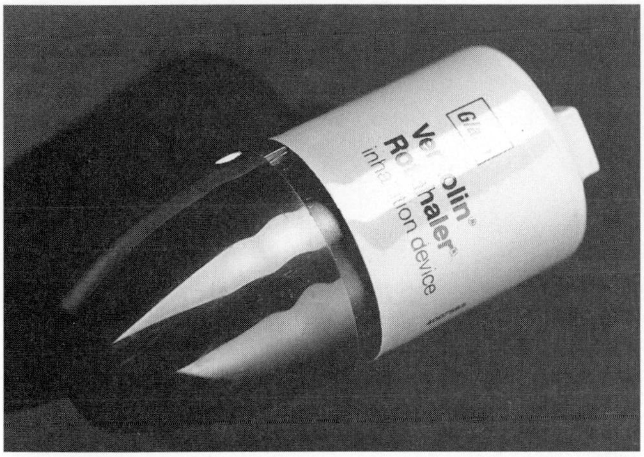

Figure 4-39 The Rotohaler.

BOX 4-14

Optimal Technique for DPI Use

1. Determine the need for therapy.
2. Determine the dose of medication to be delivered.
3. Assemble the DPI and inspect the actuator mouthpiece for foreign matter.
4. Load the medication.
5. The patient exhales to normal end-expiration.
6. The DPI mouthpiece is placed in the patient's mouth and lips are closed.
7. The patient inspires rapidly (>1 L/sec).
8. The procedure is repeated until the medication is gone.

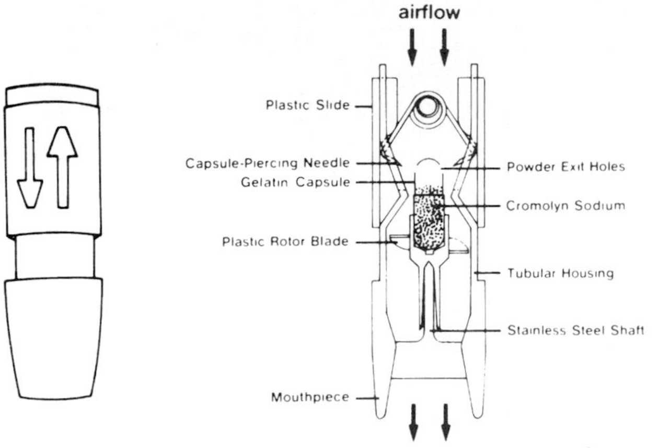

Figure 4-40 The Spinhaler for cromolyn sodium administration. (From Rau JL Jr: Respiratory care pharmacology, ed 5, St Louis, 1998, Mosby.)

a powdered form of albuterol or beclomethasone, and the Fisons Spinhaler (Figure 4-40) is for delivery of cromolyn sodium. These devices require a gelatin capsule containing the powder to be placed in the unit to prepare it for inhalation. The delivery device opens the capsule for the drug to be released. Once the capsule is broken and the powdered medication is ready to be inhaled, the patient must be able to generate sufficient inspiratory flow or the medication will not be delivered to the lung.

Newer DPIs for delivering terbutaline sulfate (e.g., Astra's Turbuhaler), budesonide (e.g., Astra's Pulmicort Turbuhaler), or albuterol (e.g., Glaxo's Diskhaler) are available. The Diskhaler provides a Rotadisk that includes multidoses of the bronchodilator or corticosteroid. Newer DPIs allow patients to see the number of doses remaining and the tools to keep the unit free of dust and other contaminants. Box 4-14 describes the proper technique for DPIs. Respiratory therapists should give special attention to fast inspiratory flow rates (i.e., >1 L/sec) when inhaling from DPIs.

DPIs contain drugs that are either spheronized into agglomerates or mixed with a coarse lactose carrier. Some powdered forms of medications are water soluble so are affected by humidity. If humidified, the powder clumps, compromising delivery. This characteristic of DPIs prohibits them from being used with mechanical ventilation.

Large Volume Nebulizers. A variety of nebulizers are available to provide long-term nebulization of solutions, some of which are bland aerosols, bronchodilators, and mucolytics, as well as other medications (e.g., lidocaine). The LVNs available are either pneumatically or electrically powered. Pneumatically powered units are classified as entrainment nebulizers, and electrically powered units are ultrasonic nebulizers, both of which will be discussed along with indications for use, methods of operation, and maintenance.

LVNs can be used to provide long-term nonmedicated and medicated aerosol therapy, but most are used to deliver nonmedicated or bland aerosols (i.e., sterile water or saline). Nonmedicated aerosols are typically delivered to the upper airway to decrease the chances of edema or humidity deficit. As discussed previously, cold-nebulized bland aerosols can result in vasoconstriction of the upper airway, thus reducing mucosal edema. In addition, cold aerosols, especially sterile water, can induce cough and expectoration for obtaining sputum for microbiologic inspection. Heated bland aerosols may be administered with medical gases to patients who have artificial airways in place. Long-term bland aerosols can be delivered by several types of masks (i.e., facial, tracheostomy, and face tent) (Figure 4-41 and Box 4-15), but an aerosol mask is the most common means of bland aerosol therapy.

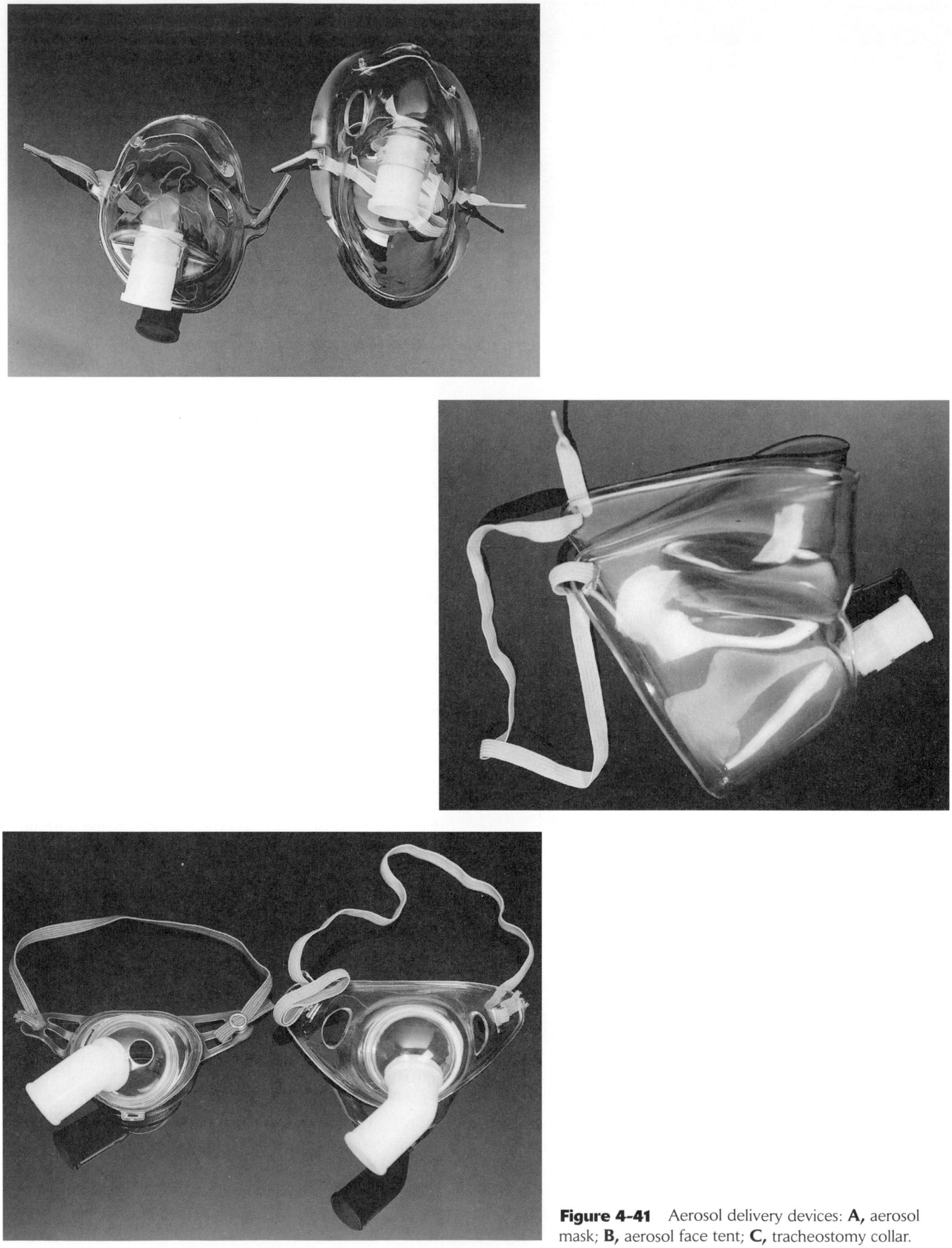

Figure 4-41 Aerosol delivery devices: **A,** aerosol mask; **B,** aerosol face tent; **C,** tracheostomy collar.

BOX 4-15

Decision Making & Problem Solving

A patient is receiving CPAP via an endotracheal tube. What type of humidifying device is appropriate for this patient?

See Appendix A for the answer.

The use of bland aerosols, whether from pneumatic or electric aerosol generators, has not been shown as an effective means of hydrating secretions or improving mucus flow. Instead, data support the use of parenteral and intravenous fluids to better hydrate the respiratory tract mucosal lining.[1,8] The potential limitations of bland aerosol therapy require respiratory care practitioners to be selective in its use.

Aggressive care of patients with bronchospasm may include frequent or continuous delivery of aerosolized bronchodilators. Continuous delivery of a bronchoactive drugs via LVNs has become a common modality of caring for patient airways.[47,48] LVNs work well for the continuous delivery of bronchodilator solutions (e.g., adrenergic and anticholinergic agents) because they have larger reservoirs for the medication. Special pneumatic nebulizer designs allow titrated doses and optimal aerosol particle size to be delivered to patients via mouthpiece or mask or by mechanical ventilation. Vortran's High Output Extended Aerosol Respiratory Therapy (HEART) nebulizer (standard or mini unit) is an example of an LVN designed to deliver continuous therapy. It has a 240 mL solution reservoir and generates particles between 2.2 and 3.2 μm MMAD. Ultrasonic nebulizers, which are discussed later in this chapter, are another method for aggressive administration of a bronchoactive drugs. They allow respiratory care practitioners to provide bronchoactive drugs quickly and at effective particle sizes.

Pneumatic Jet LVNs. These units provide large reservoirs for bland aerosols and have a provision for air entrainment. The Puritan All-Purpose nebulizer (Figure 4-42) incorporates the jet venturi principle to entrain fluid, a pressure-relief valve, and an optional immersion heater to provide heated aerosol. When operated with oxygen, these aerosol generators can provide a range of oxygen percentages. Older units provide a fixed oxygen percentage at three settings: 100%, 70%, and 40% oxygen, but newer units also offer a 35% option. A jet Venturi allows the entrainment of room air to mix with the oxygen flowing through the unit. This mixing occurs at a fixed ratio of air:oxygen for each oxygen percentage setting. The use of fixed oxygen percentages allows the total gas flow from the unit to the patient to be predicted. Table 4-3 lists total gas flows for two oxygen percentage settings with various flowmeter settings from the Puritan All-Purpose Nebulizer.

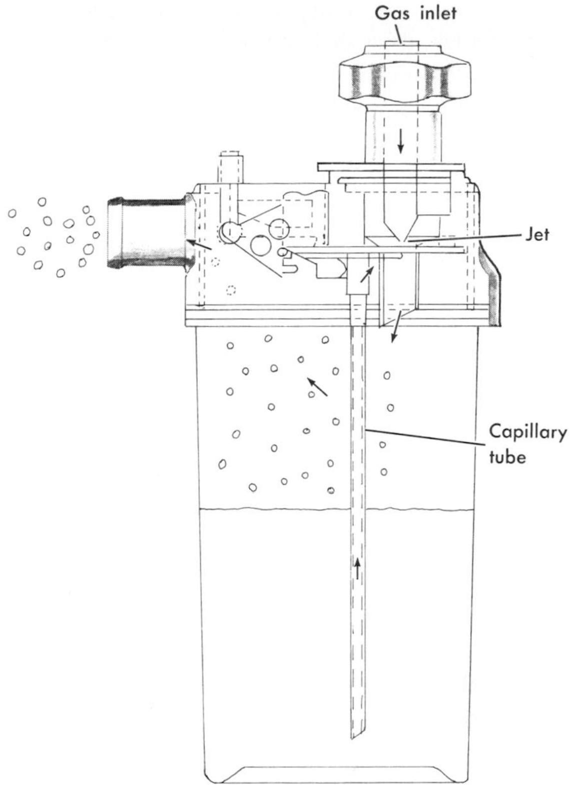

Figure 4-42 The Puritan All-Purpose Nebulizer. (Courtesy Nellcor Puritan Bennett, Mallinckrodt, St. Louis.)

TABLE 4-3

Gas flow from Puritan All-Purpose Nebulizer*

Total unrestricted gas flow from nebulizer (L/min)

Diluted to 40% oxygen concentration	70% oxygen concentration	Flowmeter setting at concentration (L/min)
4	1.6	1
8	3.2	2
12	4.8	3
16	6.4	4
20	8.0	5
24	9.6	6
28	11.2	7
32	12.8	8
36	14.4	9
40	16.0	10
44	17.6	11
48	19.2	12

Courtesy Nellcor Puritan Bennett, Pleasanton, Calif.

*Total gas flow from nebulizer should exceed patient's peak inspiratory flow rate (average 25 to 30 L/min) to achieve maximal aerosol density and stable inspired oxygen concentrations. For accurate flow setting, use a pressure-compensated flowmeter. Newer All-Purpose models have a 35% oxygen setting.

Although there are many permanent aerosol generators on the market, they all share several features, such as drawing fluid from a reservoir and including a jet for air entrainment. Additionally, all units have optional heating elements for producing heated aerosol (see the following section). Nondisposable LVNs must be cleaned and sterilized between patients.

Although still available, nondisposable LVNs have become less popular in recent years because disposable units are more cost-effective. Respiratory care practitioners should choose the type of device that best meets patient needs.

Heated LVNs. Heated aerosol can be administered via several types of heaters (Figure 4-43). The Puritan All-Purpose and the Ohio Deluxe nebulizers can employ an immersion type of heater, which consists of a heating rod that is inserted through a port in the top of the nebulizer and extends into the fluid reservoir. Notice that the immersion heater does not allow temperature to be regulated, so it must be monitored. Also, because the unit is inserted in the solution going to the patient, it must be sterile before use to avoid microbial contamination of the liquid. The immersion heater must be assessed for electrical safety to minimize the chance of electrical shock to the patient or operator during use.

Another option for heated aerosol includes a wraparound, or yolk collar heater (i.e., doughnut heater; see Figure 4-43). The wraparound heater is placed around the fluid reservoir and plugged into an electrical outlet. The collar type of heater works with a maximum temperature of 80° to 85° F. Like the immersion and nonimmersion heaters already discussed, these units typically do not allow the user to vary operating temperatures and will continue to heat, even if the water level is low or absent, increasing the potential for thermal injury. Conversely, the heating element may stop working and fail to heat without warning, so to ensure proper function the unit should be monitored.

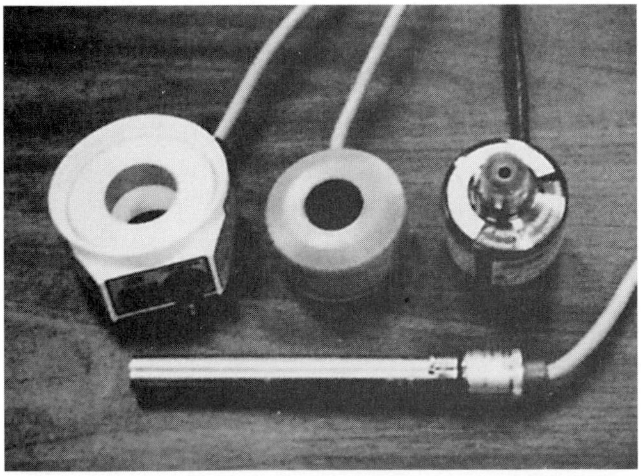

Figure 4-43 Heaters for use with LVNs. (From Scanlan CL, Wilkins RL, and Stoller JK: Egan's Fundamentals of Respiratory Care, ed 7, St Louis, 1999, Mosby.)

Several nebulizers provide heated aerosol by heating the liquid as it passes through a capillary system. With these devices, the solution to be nebulized in the reservoir does not need to be heated before nebulization. The liquid is heated in smaller amounts right before nebulization. This system allows for a shorter warm-up time than the other types of heaters already discussed. This heating method is found with the Chemetron Heated Nebulizer as well as with several nebulizer models provided by Hudson RCI that are discussed later in this chapter.

Other options for heating aerosols include the servo-control heaters provided by Professional Medical Products' Seamless (Dart) nebulizer, which allows automatic gas and aerosol temperature to be adjusted as it self-monitors gas flow temperature. Continuous temperature feedback with an automatic shut-off safeguards against overheating and thermal injury. The ThermaGard Heater is used exclusively with Hudson RCI's Variable Concentration Large Volume Nebulizer, which provides continuous, heated aerosol with adjustable temperature settings. The ThermaGard Heater includes a nonreversing thermal fuse to prevent overheating if the control circuit fails and a push-to-turn temperature adjustment to prevent accidental temperature setting changes.

Medical Molding Corporation's Misty Ox Hi-Fi high-flow nebulizer, which is discussed later in this chapter, uses a Turboheater (3M Pharmaceuticals) to heat gas and aerosol and attaches between the reservoir bottle and the nebulizer manifold (i.e., jet assembly). Gas leaves the nebulizer and flows through the heater, where it is warmed before being delivered to the patient. A similar heater, Hudson RCI's AQUATHERM III External Adjustable Electronic Heater, attaches to the nebulizer to heat the aerosol. An adjustable temperature control allows a range of output temperatures (Figure 4-44). Hudson RCI also provides a collar type of heater, the AQUATHERM External Heater, which provides an output temperature from 35° to 38° C at 8 L/min gas flow with full air entrainment (Figure 4-45 and Box 4-16).

Like humidifiers, the output of aerosol generators depends on several factors, including the length of delivery tubing, the total gas flow of carrier gases, the room temperature, and the solution level in the reservoir. For example, the longer the delivery tube, the cooler the gas being delivered becomes; or the faster the gas flow rate, the greater the tendency for gas and aerosol temperature decreases. In contrast, the lower the solution level, the greater the potential of gas and aerosol temperature increases. As the carrier gas temperature decreases en route to the patient, condensation can occur, creating a fluid bolus in the delivery circuit that can obstruct gas flow and alter the delivered oxygen concentration, creating a partial obstruction, which results in back pressure against the jet. This decreases air entrainment and increases the delivered oxygen

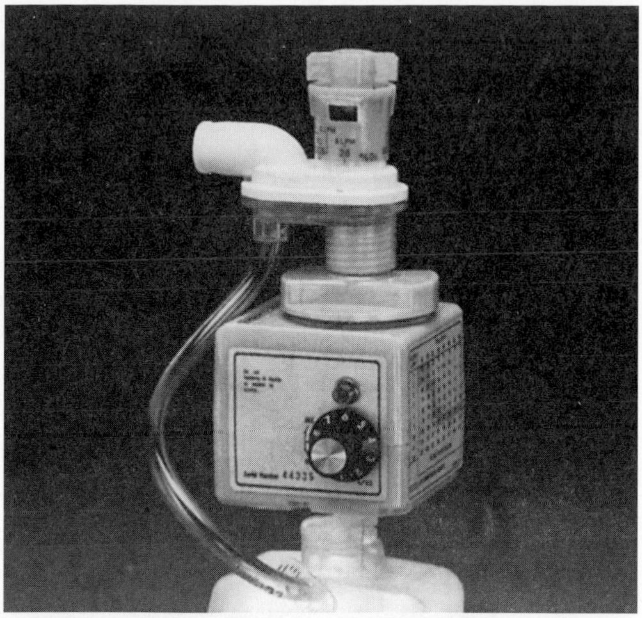

Figure 4-44 The Aquatherm III External Adjustable Electronic Heater. (Courtesy Hudson Respiratory Care, Inc, Temecula, Calif.)

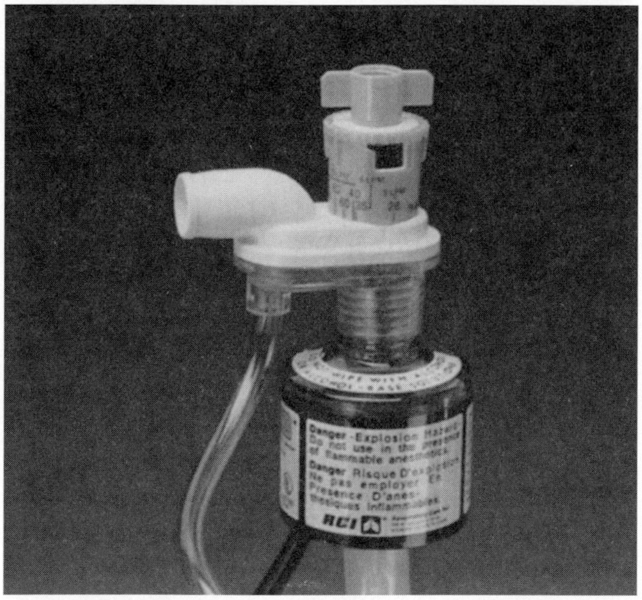

Figure 4-45 The Aquatherm External Heater. (Courtesy Hudson Respiratory Care, Inc, Temecula, Calif.)

percentage. This problem can be avoided by intermittently monitoring the aerosol delivery tube for patency.

Disposable LVNs. It has become common to provide a variety of therapies using disposable, single-patient–use devices. Disposable LVNs also work by the principle of air entrainment, and there are many available for patient use. The following discussion highlights a sampling of the units on the market.

BOX 4-16

Decision Making & Problem Solving

Following abdominal surgery, a 50-year old man is brought to the recovery room and started on a aerosol mask at an FiO_2 of 0.50. While performing your initial assessment of this patient, you notice that his respiratory rate is 20 breaths per minute and he shows signs of respiratory distress. You also note that during inspiration, the aerosol stops flowing from the mask. How would you remedy this situation to ensure the patient 50% oxygen?

See Appendix A for the answer.

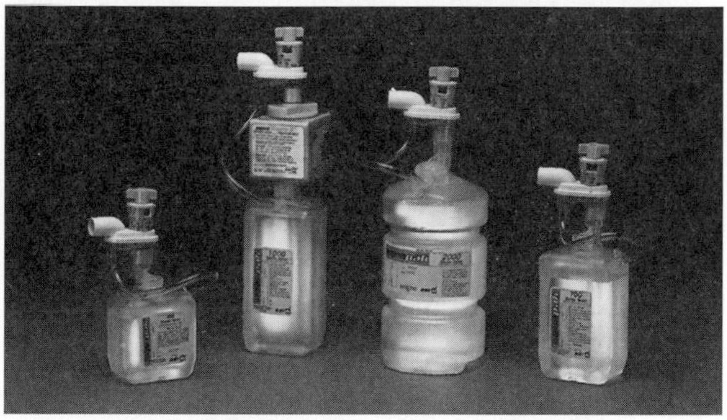

Figure 4-46 Hudson RCI LVNs. (Courtesy Hudson Respiratory Care, Inc, Temecula, Calif.)

Practitioners have a choice of either refillable or prefilled disposable nebulizers. Hudson RCI's disposable LVNs provide large reservoirs with an oxygen percentage range from 28% to 98% (Figure 4-46). Tables 4-4 and 4-5 provide data on the performance of Hudson RCI's disposable LVN and also list the aerosol particle size and humidity output at various gas flows and oxygen concentrations. As with other refillable units, the Hudson disposable unit requires monitoring of the fluid level and is designed for single-patient use.

Prefilled units must be replaced with a new unit before the fluid reservoir reaches a level where aerosol output is no longer acceptable. The Hudson RCI Prefilled Precision Nebulizer (Figure 4-47) is an example of a prefilled nebulizer that generates high aerosol output and aerosol particles in an effective range of 5 μm or less. The Hudson RCI prefilled nebulizer passes aerosol through an offset baffling chamber within the jet assembly where large particles are coalesced and returned to the reservoir. The return tube helps preserve usable water in the reservoir, thus allowing water to be used more times than in other pneumatic nebulizers with similarly sized fluid reservoirs. Because the baffles are efficient, the particles released from the unit are so small that the mist is difficult to see. This unit uses two types of jet manifolds or assemblies. The standard Venturi style of entrainment manifold attaches to the prefilled reservoir with a self-sealing puncture pin, allowing the operator to adjust the diluter ring or entrainment ring for oxygen concentrations from 28% to 98%. The Hudson RCI Critical Care Nebulizer Adapter is an upgrade from the previous jet attachment that also attaches to the reservoir with a self-sealing puncture pin and provides oxygen concentrations from 33% to 98%. Markings on the adjustable entrainment ring are 33%, 35%, 40%, 50%, 60%, 80%, and 98%. This unit has a special baffling system that reduces the noise associated with nebulization. The screw-on, puncture pin design provides a closed system that may decrease the possibility of microbial contamination of the fluid within the unit.

Average outputs from most disposable pneumatic nebulizers are about 1 to 2 mL of fluid per minute. Prefilled units typically have reservoir capacities ranging from 400 to 2200 mL. Table 4-6 provides air and oxygen entrainment ratios and the total gas flow associated with entrainment type of nebulizers (nondisposable and disposable units).

Several models of pneumatic nebulizers can provide high gas flows at high oxygen concentrations. For example, the Misty Ox Hi-Fi Nebulizer can produce up to 42 L/min with an oxygen concentration of 96% (Table 4-7) and offers a range of oxygen concentrations from 60% to 96%.[12]

The Misty Ox Gas Injector Nebulizer is a specially designed pneumatic (nonentrainment) nebulizer capable of high gas flows. It can provide FiO_2s from 0.21 to 1.0 at gas flow rates >100 L/min. This high gas flow nebulizer does not depend on entrainment ports to increase the total gas flow or oxygen concentrations to the patient. To produce high gas flow, this unit uses two flowmeters: one operates the jet and can produce up to 40 L/min, and the other

TABLE 4-4

Aerosol particle sizes associated with Hudson RCI disposable nebulizers at different oxygen flows

Flow rate (L/min)	FiO_2 (%)	Mean diameter (μm) unheated	Mean diameter (μm) heated*
5	28	2.3	1.7
8	35	1.7	1.5
10	40	1.6	1.5
10	60	1.6	1.6
10	80	1.7	1.7
10	98	1.8	1.8
10	98	1.8	1.8

*ThermaGard Heater set at a maximum temperature setting.

TABLE 4-5

Aerosol output of Hudson RCI disposable nebulizers at different oxygen flows

Flow rate (L/min)	FiO_2 (%)	Total output (mL/hour)*	Delivered to patient (mL/hour)†
5	28	36.16	34.06
10	40	45.04	43.03
10	60	31.04	30.68
10	98	24.96	24.30

*Measures nebulizer outlet.
†Measures at the end of a 72" length of 22-mm tubing.

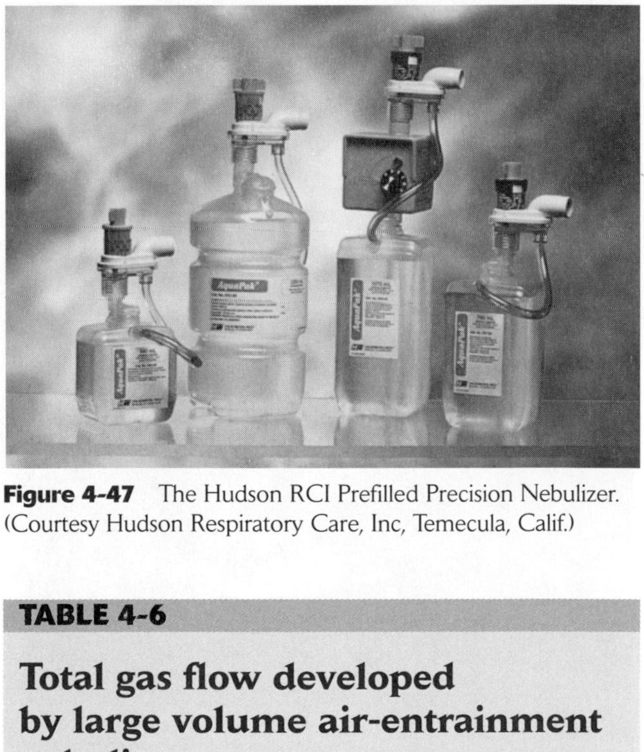

Figure 4-47 The Hudson RCI Prefilled Precision Nebulizer. (Courtesy Hudson Respiratory Care, Inc, Temecula, Calif.)

TABLE 4-6

Total gas flow developed by large volume air-entrainment nebulizers

		Total flow	
FiO_2	Air:oxygen	10 L/minute	15 L/minute
0.24	25:1	260	390
0.30	8.0:1	90	135
0.35	4.6:1	46	69
0.40	3.2:1	32	48
0.60	1.0:1	20	30
0.70	0.6:1	16	24
0.80	0.34:1	13.4	20
0.9	0.14:1	11	16
1.0	0:1	10	15

feeds into the side of the jet manifold with similar flow rates. This unit can generate over 80 L/min with stable oxygen concentrations.[8] An advantage of this design is that back pressure from other devices will not alter oxygen concentrations.

Ultrasonic Nebulizers. Since their introduction in the 1960s, ultrasonic nebulizers have become an alternative means of providing aerosol. The basic principle of ultrasonic nebulizers is that electric current produces sound waves, which are used to break up fluid into aerosol particles. An electric charge (at a high frequency of vibrations) is applied intermittently to a transducer that has a piezoelectric quality (i.e., the ability to change shape when a charge is applied to it). The electric current creates vibrations at the same frequency as the electric charge applied to the piezoelectric transducer. These ultrasonic vibrations travel through the fluid to the surface, where they produce an aerosol (Figure 4-48).

Ultrasonic nebulizers can employ transducers in various configurations. The transducer is placed within a couplant chamber, which contains tap or sterile water (see Figure 4-48) that serves two purposes: (1) it helps absorb mechanical heat produced by the transducer and (2) acts as a medium for the sound waves to be transferred to a prefilled or refillable container that holds the solution to be nebulized. (Couplant must not contain distilled water because of the need for electrolytes to transfer the ultrasonic waves.) The frequency of the electrical energy supplied to the transducer is typically 1.35 megahertz (Mhz). When this frequency is matched with a transducer that can react optimally to it, a vibration at the same frequency is produced. *The frequency determines the particle size of the solution to be nebulized.* The amplitude or strength of the sound waves determines the aerosol output. As amplitude is increased with an adjustable dial, aerosol output increases. (Amplitude is adjusted to meet the patient's inspiratory needs.) Most ultrasonic nebulizers have been constructed so that their particle size range is from 1 to

TABLE 4-7

Total flow rates provided by the Misty Ox Hi-Fi Nebulizer

Entrainment setting	Oxygen flow (L/minute)	Total flow (L/minute)
60%	20-30	40-61
65%	30-40	54-72
75%	30-40	44-58
85%	30-40	37-49
96%	40	42

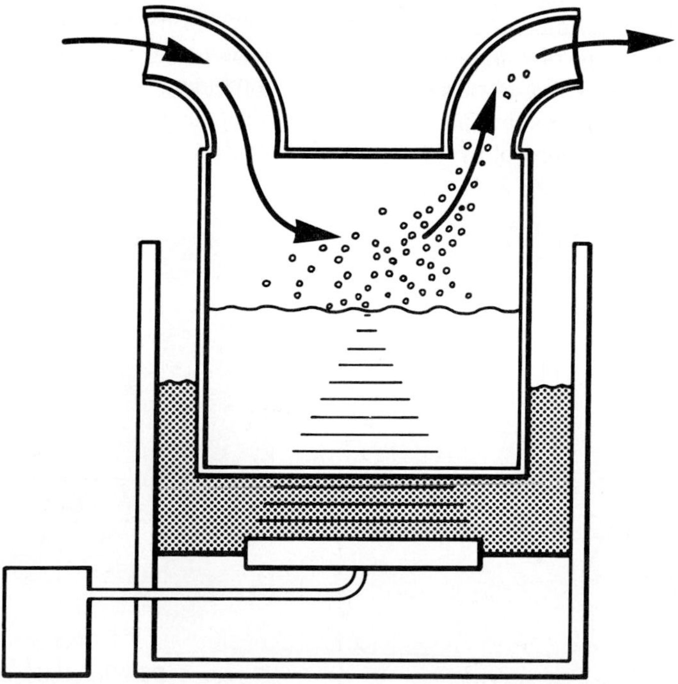

Figure 4-48 The ultrasonic nebulizer. Aerosol is produced when high-frequency sound waves are produced by a transducer and transmitted to the nebulizer compartment, where fluid is broken up into an aerosol. A gas source (e.g., fan) is used to move the aerosol out of the unit. (From Barnes TA: Core textbook for respiratory care practice, ed 2, St Louis, 1994, Mosby.)

10 mm, with a mean size of 3 μm. Fluid output averages are higher than those from pneumatic nebulizers (up to 6 mL/minute). A gas flow source is required to transfer aerosol to the patient; most ultrasonic nebulizers use a fan for this purpose. Supplemental oxygen can be delivered to the unit to provide a range of oxygen concentrations.

Various manufacturers produce ultrasonic nebulizers, such as DeVilbiss (model 800-65 and the 900-35 series), Mistogen (models 142 and 143), Nellcor Puritan Bennett (model US-1), and Monaghan (models 650, 670, and 675). Each manufacturer uses a different shaped transducer. Several versions of SVNs that use the ultrasonic nebulizer principle are also available and can be used to nebulize bronchoactive medications at home. In addition, ultrasonic room humidifiers are available.

Total Flow and FiO_2. As previously defined, to be classified as a high gas-flow system, the total gas and aerosol output from a pneumatic nebulizer must exceed the patient's inspiratory flow and tidal volume to ensure a fixed oxygen concentration. If the unit fails to provide a total gas flow greater than the patient's inspiratory flow, the delivered oxygen concentration decreases. The reduction in oxygen concentration results from the patient taking in additional room air to meet inspiratory flow needs, which dilutes the gas flow from the LVN and lowers the oxygen concentration. During respiratory distress, peak inspiratory flows can increase substantially, so the total nebulizer output must be assessed. This may be accomplished by adjusting oxygen flow through the flowmeter to ensure continuous flow of aerosol from the large openings on the side of the aerosol mask or at the reservoir-end of an aerosol T-piece set up during inspiration and expiration. If a mist is not drifting from the device (e.g., aerosol mask) during inspiration, the patient is inspiring room air and the FiO_2 will decrease (from the dilution effect of the room air). Figure 4-49 shows a typical set-up for delivering aerosol to a spontaneously breathing patient, and Table 4-6 lists the total gas flows associated with a variety of oxygen concentrations and flow rates. Notice that these gas flows are based on fixed air:oxygen entrainment ratios. In other words, for every liter of oxygen that enters the nebulizer jet, a fixed amount of room air is entrained. Air dilution at the aerosol production site of the nebulizers increases aerosol output (in milliliters per hour) and increases total gas flow to the patient. When adjusting the entrainment ring from a high to a lower oxygen concentration, the total gas flow from the device increases for any flowmeter setting. For example, setting the oxygen flowmeter at 10 L/min and the air-entrainment ring to 60% will make the total flow 20 L/min. Decreasing the oxygen concentration to 40% and leaving the flowmeter at 10 L/min will produce a total gas flow of 32 L/min. In addition, as the oxygen concentration from the unit decreases, the aerosol density or amount of aerosol per liter of gas decreases with increased air entrainment.

The actual number of aerosol particles produced at the jet for any given flowmeter setting is fixed, but the number of particles that actually leave the nebulizer is a product of the gas flow. As gas flow increases, more particles are carried out of the unit. There are several ways that high gas flows may be provided to meet the inspiratory demands of a patient with an increased minute volume or inspiratory flow. For example, the high output nebulizers already discussed may be used to ensure high aerosol outputs, but combining several pneumatic nebulizers (attached via a Brigg's adapter) set at the same FiO_2 will also provide an increased gas flow (Figure 4-50). Extending the size of the

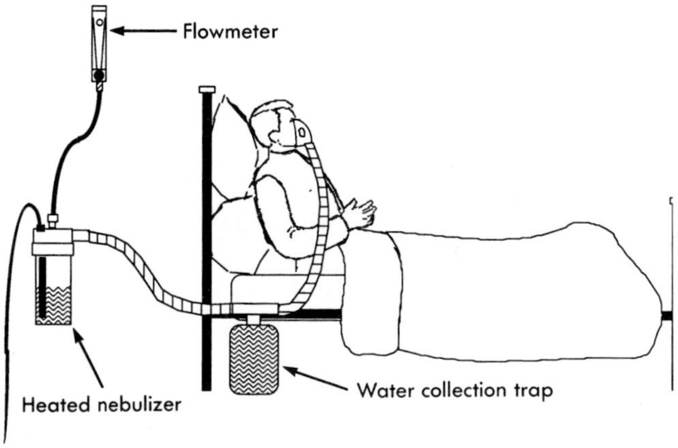

Figure 4-49 A typical set-up for a large volume nebulizer; a water collection bag may be placed in a gravity-dependent loop to collect condensation.

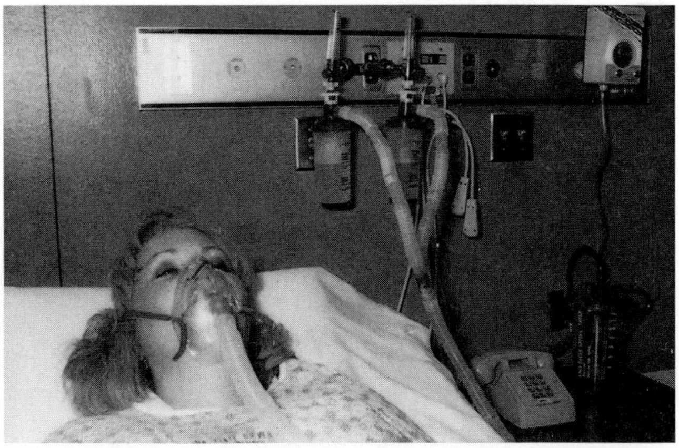

Figure 4-50 To produce high aerosol gas flow, two LVNs are set up, and their delivery tubes are attached via Brigg's adapter to a common delivery device, such as an aerosol mask or a face tent. If both LVNs have the same oxygen and air-entrainment settings and a high-flow gas system is established, then the desired delivered oxygen percentage can be provided.

reservoir space of an aerosol mask by placing a 50 mL corrugated tube in each of the side ports of the aerosol mask (Figure 4-51) will also increase the amount of gas available to the patient. By adding these tubes, additional aerosol may be trapped, increasing the gas and aerosol available to the patient. However, lack of research on this method lends concern to its appropriateness for clinical use.

Special Considerations for Aerosol Therapy

There are special situations when a patient may require a unique method of aerosol delivery such as pediatric aerosol tent enclosures, the delivery of toxic medications (e.g., ribavirin), or methods to control environmental contamination.

For years, infants and pediatric patients with upper airway edema (e.g., croup or laryngotracheobronchitis) have been placed in tents designed to contain gas flow and aerosol for the patient to inhale. These containment units provide a cool, dense aerosol and have been effective in the treatment of upper airway edema. The atmosphere within the tent is continuously flushed out to prevent accumulation of exhaled carbon dioxide. In addition, carbon dioxide may leave the tent by diffusion through the plastic canopy and the space between the tent and bed. A cooling source is necessary to keep the intratent temperature at a comfortable level. The gas directed into the tent can be cooled with a refrigerator unit like the one shown in Figure 4-52. Aerosol containment devices, like the Ohmeda aerosol tent, allow the child to be placed directly in the tent, providing aerosol and an increased oxygen concentration (if the unit is operated by compressed oxygen). The circulating fan in the tent allows gas to be circulated and cooled. Unit maintenance requires the water reservoir to be monitored, the condensation from the refrigerator drain bottle to be emptied, and the oxygen concentration within the tent to be analyzed to ensure it is appropriate.

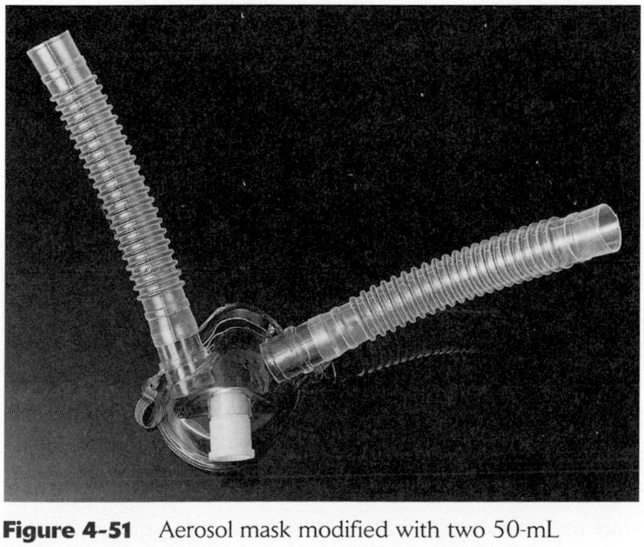

Figure 4-51 Aerosol mask modified with two 50-mL reservoir tubes, which act as possible reservoirs for gas and aerosol.

Patients receiving ribavirin (Virazole) to treat infections from respiratory syncytial virus (RSV) require a special aerosol-generating device called a small-particle aerosol generator (SPAG). ICN Pharmaceutical's SPAG-2 (Figure 4-53) is a jet type of nebulizer specifically for delivering ribavirin. SPAG units employ a drying chamber with a separate flow control to control aerosol particle size, which is 1.2 to 1.4 μm. The SPAG-2 reduces the gas source pressure from 50 to 26 psig and has an adjustable pressure regulator. The regulator has two flowmeters: one to control gas flow into the nebulizer, and the other to feed the drying chamber. As aerosol is generated in the nebulizer, which is in the reservoir chamber, it enters a long, cylindrical drying chamber. The dry flow of gas from the second flowmeter allows aerosol particles to evaporate and reduces the MMAD of the particles going to the patient. The SPAG-2 nebulizer and drying chamber require specific flow rates from the two flowmeters; the nebulizer gas flow rate should be 7 L/min, and the total gas flow from both flowmeters should not to be less than 15 L/min. The SPAG-2 is designed for administering ribavirin via a hood-like chamber or tent. If allowed to escape and enter the room, aerosolized ribavirin can be harmful to caregivers. Ribavirin may cause bronchoconstriction, rash, conjunctivitis, and can be toxic,[12] so caregivers and women who are either pregnant or breast feeding should especially take precautions to avoid aerosolized ribavirin. Such precautions include placing the patient in a private room with negative pressure ventilation (with a total-room gas exchange at least 6 times per hour) and wearing a High-Efficiency Particle Air (HEPA) mask, gloves, gown, and goggles when administering ribavirin.

The SPAG-2 may be used with gas-delivery circuits and mechanical ventilation. Although drug manufacturers do not recommend aerosolizing ribavirin into a gas circuit associated with mechanical ventilation, it has been shown to

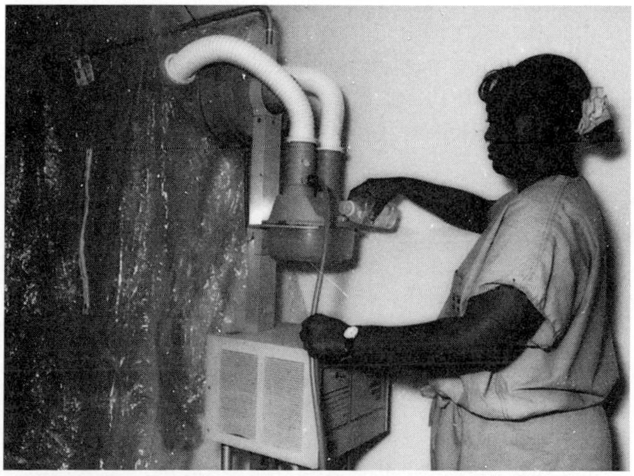

Figure 4-52 An aerosol tent.

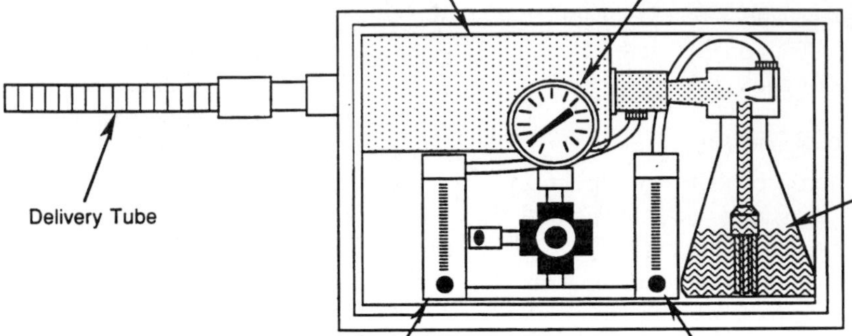

Figure 4-53 A SPAG unit.

be effective when provided to patients with RSV and artificial airways who are receiving mechanical ventilation.[8] However, the ventilator expiratory valve should be protected by filters placed in the expiratory limb of the gas circuit to trap escaping medication. These filters must be changed frequently to avoid increased resistance to expiratory flow.

Hazards of Aerosol Therapy

Hazards associated with aerosol therapy include infection, bronchospasm, overhydration, airway thermal injury, and airway obstruction from swollen mucus. This section will briefly address each of these concerns.

Aerosol particles can cross-contaminate the nebulizer, and thus the patient, and the person providing the therapy. Microbes in the solution to be nebulized can be transported via airborne aerosol to the patient and result in nosocomial infection. Guidelines for the care of aerosol generators often change over time, so respiratory care practitioners should remain aware of current recommendations. The recent guidelines of the Centers for Disease Control (CDC) recommend that humidifiers and aerosol generators be filled with sterile fluids (not tap or distilled water), which should be changed or replaced every 24 hours.[8]

Secondhand exposure to escaped aerosolized toxic medications or microbes exhaled by the patient has become a concern for all caregivers, but especially for respiratory care practitioners. Contaminated aerosol particles exhaled by patients may become airborne and hazardous to people nearby. This is especially a concern during sputum induction. In addition to exhaled microbes, there are several drugs that can be toxic to health care personnel. Currently, the two drugs that are the greatest risk to practitioners are pentamidine and ribavirin, which have been shown to cause conjunctivitis, headaches, bronchospasm, and rashes to caregivers exposed to them (Box 4-17). Patients who have respiratory tract infections or are receiving potentially toxic medications can be placed in an environmental chamber to reduce caregiver risk. This type of booth (Figure 4-54) provides containment of aerosol during therapy and reduces the risk of secondhand inhalation of aerosol and microbes. These units are cleaned between patients and located in a room with negative ventilation. In addition, these boothlike chambers contain HEPA filtering.

> **BOX 4-17**
>
> **Decision Making & Problem Solving**
>
> You are administering aerosolized pentamidine to a patient at home. What protective measures should you use?
>
> See Appendix A for the answer.

Studies have shown that patients with reactive airway disease (e.g., asthma) may experience bronchoconstriction while inhaling bland aerosols, experiencing an increase in airway resistance and work of breathing.[1] This effect of inhaling aerosol tends to be more common with cool than with heated aerosols, and appropriate administration of a bronchodilator before providing bland aerosol may be indicated. Furthermore, aerosolized mucolytics can induce bronchospasm in some patients, so it is standard practice to provide a bronchodilator with aerosolized mucolytics in addition to assessing patient response.

Long-term continuous administration of bland aerosol may result in overhydration of the patient, which is a more serious consideration with aerosol delivery to infants. Excess water can cause overhydration, and excess aerosolized

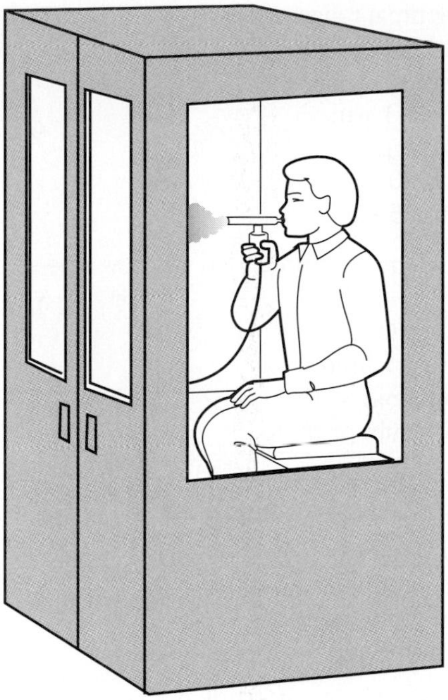

Figure 4-54 An environmental chamber for aerosol delivery to patients.

saline may alter electrolyte concentration, leading to hypernatremia. Although most data published about the potential for overhydration with long-term aerosol (e.g., 72 hours or more) are from canine models, it may be prudent to be cautious when administering bland aerosol. Knowing the narrow use of bland aerosols (e.g., treatment of upper airway edema or sputum induction), aerosol therapy should be clinically applied when the indication is clear and patient monitoring by knowledgeable practitioners is available.

Delivering aerosols to patients with an ineffective cough may result in partial or complete airway obstruction, which occurs when the inhaled aerosol mobilizes secretions that are not properly expectorated. In addition, some secretions swell when exposed to aerosol, becoming an obstruction—especially in patients with diminished cough effort or ability. Appropriate bronchial hygiene techniques and other respiratory care modalities may be necessary with aerosol therapy.

Summary

Supplemental humidity and aerosols are fundamental components of respiratory care. Each type of therapy has a unique set of indications, delivery methods, and hazards. Humidity is water in a vapor state and can be subdivided into absolute humidity, relative humidity, and body humidity states. Under normal physiologic conditions, adequate humidification of inspired atmospheric gases occurs as gas flows through the upper airways. When patients inspire a medical gas through an artificial airway or experience a large humidity deficit by inspiring dry gases, supplemental humidity must be provided. Failure to provide adequate humidity to the lungs can result in drying of secretions and damage to the airway mucosa.

Humidifiers can be classified as either low- or high-flow. A low-flow humidifier does not provide all of the patient's required humidity; additional humidity is entrained from room air. In contrast, a high-flow humidifier can provide saturated gas near or at body temperature. Bubble humidifiers are examples of low-flow humidifiers; wick humidifiers and HMEs are examples of high-flow humidifiers.

An aerosol is composed of particles suspended in a gas. Aerosols used in respiratory care include bland and medicated aerosols. Bland aerosols are used to humidify medical gas or reduce upper airway edema. Medicated aerosols deliver pharmacologic agents to treat respiratory diseases. Respiratory therapists should be aware of the physical principles governing aerosol particle deposition in the lungs to be able to provide optimal aerosol therapy. Such principles include aerosol particle size, inertial impaction, kinetic activity, physical nature of the particle, temperature and humidity of the delivery gas, and ventilatory pattern.

Aerosols can be delivered by small- and large-volume nebulizers, MDIs, and ultrasonic nebulizers. More specialized aerosol generators include SPAG units and high-flow jet nebulizers. Recent advances in MDI design, including reservoirs or spacers, have made them one of the more popular ways to deliver aerosols. The most common hazards of aerosol therapy include overhydration, mucus swelling, cross-contamination, and bronchoconstriction.

Judicious selection of the type of humidity and aerosol therapy to be used, along with the most appropriate mode of delivery can significantly affect patient outcomes. The effectiveness of the therapy can be monitored by carefully assessing the patient's response (in subjective answers or objective measures [e.g., cardiopulmonary status]) to the treatment.

Review Questions

See Appendix A for answers.

1. As gas temperature increases, its capacity to hold water will:
   a. increase
   b. decrease
   c. remain unchanged
2. If the temperature of a saturated gas decreases, which of the following will occur?
   a. condensation develops
   b. absolute humidity increases
   c. relative humidity decreases
   d. water-vapor pressure increases

3. With an artificial airway in place, what should be the minimal level of absolute humidity provided to the patient's airways?
   a. 10 mg/L
   b. 20 mg/L
   c. 30 mg/L
   d. 40 mg/L

4. As oxygen leaves a bubble humidifier, it is near or at 100% relative humidity. As it reaches the patient, what is its approximate relative humidity?
   a. 10 to 20 mg/L
   b. 44 mg/L
   c. 47 torr
   d. 100%

5. Based on the AARC Clinical Practice Guideline, the temperature of medical gas delivered through an artificial airway should be:
   a. 30° C
   b. 31° to 35° C
   c. 36° to 42° C
   d. 37° C

6. As aerosol leaves a heated jet nebulizer and travels to the patient through large-bore corrugated tubing, which of the following can occur?
   a. relative humidity of the delivered aerosol decreases
   b. an increase in absolute humidity is provided to the patient
   c. condensation occurs and can obstruct the aerosol delivery tube
   d. aerosol evaporates, and only humidified gas reaches the patient

7. Which of the following is a contraindication for an HME?
   a. minute volume greater than 10 L/min
   b. minimal secretions
   c. small tidal volumes
   d. short-term mechanical ventilation

8. Application of an HME device should be limited to how long?
   a. 96 hours
   b. 120 hours
   c. 20 days
   d. 30 days

9. Name four types of HME devices.

10. Which of the following will result in increased aerosol deposition?
    a. large tidal volume
    b. slow inspiratory flow rate
    c. decrease in expiratory peak flow
    d. short expiratory times

11. The optimal range of aerosol particle sizes inspired for general deposition through the upper and lower airways is:
    a. 0.1 to 1 μm
    b. 1 to 5 μm
    c. 3 to 10 μm
    d. 5 to 15 μm

12. What is the recommended gas flow rate to operate an SVN?
    a. 1 L/min
    b. 6 to 8 L/min
    c. 10 L/min
    d. 15 L/min or more

13. What is the most important factor influencing aerosol deposition from an MDI?
    a. tidal volume
    b. inspiratory flow rate
    c. respiratory rate
    d. breath hold

14. While inhaling from a DPI, the patient should be instructed to:
    a. breathe in slowly
    b. breathe in quickly
    c. breathe in normally
    d. breathe in deeply and slowly

15. An increase in which of the following can occur if condensation is allowed to accumulate in the large-bore aerosol delivery tubing?
    a. gas flow to the patient
    b. absolute humidity delivered to the patient
    c. FiO_2
    d. total aerosol delivered

References

1. Wissing DR, Boggs PB, and George RB: Use of respiratory care procedures in the management of hospitalized asthmatics, Ann Allergy 61:407, 1988.
2. Walker JEC, et al: Heat and water exchange in the respiratory tract, Am J Med 30:259, 1961.
3. Dery R: The evolution of heat and moisture in the respiratory tract during anesthesia with a non-rebreathing system, Can J Anesth 20:296, 1973.
4. Shelley MP, Lloyd GM, and Park GR: A review of the mechanisms and the methods of humidification of inspired gases, Intensive Care Med 14:1, 1988.
5. Primiano FP Jr, Montague FW Jr, and Saidel GM: Measurement system for water vapor and temperature dynamics, J Appl Physio 56:1679, 1984.
6. Eubanks DH and Bone RC: Principles and applications of cardiorespiratory care equipment, St Louis, 1994, Mosby.
7. Cohen N and Fink J: Humidity and aerosols. In Eubanks DH and Bone RC, editors: Principles and applications of cardiorespiratory care equipment, St Louis, 1994, Mosby.

8. Fink J: Humidity and aerosol therapy. In Spearman C and Sheldon RL, editors: Egan's fundamentals of respiratory care, St Louis, 1995, Mosby.
9. Chatburn RL and Primiano FP: A rational basis for humidity therapy, Respir Care, 32:249, 1987.
10. American Association for Respiratory Care: Clinical practice guideline: humidification during mechanical ventilation, Respir Care, 37:887, 1992.
11. Eubanks DH and Bone RC: Comprehensive respiratory care: a learning system, ed 2, St Louis, 1990, Mosby.
12. White GC: Equipment theory for respiratory care, ed 2, New York, 1996, Delmar.
13. Dahlby RW: Effect of breathing dry air on structure and function of airways, J Appl Physio 61: 312, 1986.
14. Marfatia S, Donahoe PK, and Hendren WH: Effect of dry and humidified gases on the respiratory epithelium in rabbits, J Ped Surg 10:583, 1975.
15. Hudson RCI: Conchatherm III Plus operating manual, Temecula, Calif, 1991, Hudson RCI.
16. Miyao H, et al: Consideration of the international standard for airway humidification using simulated secretions in an artificial airway, Respir Care 41:43, 1996.
17. Branson RD and Davis D Jr: Evaluation of 21 passive humidifiers according to the ISO 9360 standard: moisture output, dead space, and flow resistance, Respir Care, 41:736, 1996.
18. Branson RD, Hess DR, and Chatburn RL: Respiratory care equipment, Philadelphia, 1995, Lippincott.
19. Chalon J, Loew DA, and Malebranche J: Effects of dry anesthetic gases on tracheobronchial ciliated epithelium, Anesthesiol 37(3):338, 1972.
20. Fonkalsrud EW, et al: A comparative study of the effects of dry vs. humidified ventilation on canine lungs, Surgery 78:373, 1975.
21. Noguchi H, Takumi Y, and Aochi O: A study of humidification in tracheostomized dogs, Br J Anaesth 45:844, 1973.
22. Rashad K, et al: Effect of humidification on anesthetic gases and static compliance, Anesth Analg 40:127, 1967.
23. Tsuda T, et al: Optimum humidification of air administered to a tracheostomy in dogs, Br J Anaesth 49:965, 1977.
24. Klein EF and Graves SA: "Hot pot" tracheitis, Chest 65:225, 1974.
25. American Association for Respiratory Care: Clinical practice guideline: selection of aerosol delivery device, Respir Care 37:891, 1992.
26. American Association for Respiratory Care: Clinical practice guideline: bland aerosol administration, Respir Care 38:1196, 1993.
27. American Association for Respiratory Care: Clinical practice guideline: delivery of aerosols to the upper airway, Respir Care, 39:803, 1994.
28. Wanner A and Rao A: Clinical indications for and effects of bland, mucolytic, and antimicrobial aerosols, Am Rev Respir Dis 122(5):79, 1980.
29. Brain J: Aerosol and humidity therapy, Am Rev Respir Dis 122:17, 1980.
30. Dulfano MJ, Adler K, and Wooten O: Physical properties of sputum, IV, effects of 100% humidity and water mist. Am Rev Resp Dis 107:130, 1973.
31. Svedmyr N: Clinical advantages of the aerosol route of drug administration, Respir Care 36:922, 1991.
32. Cottrell GP and Surkin HB: Pharmacology for respiratory care practitioners, Philadelphia, 1995, FA Davis Co.
33. Ward JJ, Hess D, and Helmholz HF Jr: Humidity and aerosol therapy. In Burton GG, Hodgkin JE, and Ward JJ, editors: Respiratory care: a guide to clinical practice, New York, 1997, Lippincott.
34. Dolovich M: Clinical aspects of aerosol therapy, Respir Care 36:931, 1991.
35. Newhouse M and Dolovich M: Aerosol therapy of asthma: principles and applications, Respiration 50(suppl 2):123, 1986.
36. Pedersen S: Choice of inhalation in paediatrics, Eur Respir Rev 18:85, 1994.
37. Alvine GG, Rodgers P, and Fitzsimmons KM: Disposable jet nebulizers: how reliable are they? Chest, 101:316, 1992.
38. Dahlback M, et al: Controlled aerosol delivery during mechanical ventilation, J Aerosol Med, 4:339, 1989.
39. Fuller HD, et al: Pressurized aerosol versus jet aerosol delivery to mechanically ventilated patients: comparison of dose to the lungs, Am Rev Respir Dis, 141:440, 1990.
40. McIntyre NR, et al: Aerosol delivery in intubated, mechanically ventilated patients, Crit Care Med, 13:81, 1985.
41. DeBlaquiere P, et al: Use and misuse of metered-dose inhalers by patients with chronic lung disease, Am Rev Respir Dis 140:910, 1989.
42. Newman SP: Aerosol generators and delivery systems, Respir Care 36:939, 1991.
43. Wilson AF, Muki DS, and Ahdout JJ: Effect of canister temperature on performance of metered dose inhalers. Am Rev Respir Dis, 1991. 143: p. 1034.
44. Lewis, RA and JS Fleming, Fractional deposition from a jet nebulizer: How it differs from a metered dose inhaler, Br J Dis Chest 79:361, 1985.
45. Kacmarek RM and Hess D: The interface between the patient and aerosol generator, Respir Care 36:952, 1991.
46. Konig P: Spacer devices used with metered dose inhalers: breakthrough or gimmick? Chest 88:276, 1985.
47. Moler FW, Hurwitz ME, and Custer JR: Improvement in clinical asthma score and $PaCO_2$ in children with severe asthma treated with continuously nebulized terbutaline, J Allergy Clin Immunol 81:1101, 1988.
48. Portnoy SN, Mercedes GA, and Willsie-Ediger S: Continuous nebulization for status asthmatics, Ann Allergy 69:71, 1992.

Internet Resources

1. American Association for Respiratory Care: http://www.aarc.org
2. National Board for Respiratory Care: http://www.nbrc.org
3. Healthcare Education, Learning and Information Exchange (GlaxoWellcome): http://www.helix.com
4. Medical Sciences Bulletin Respiratory Drug Reviews: http://www.pharminfo.com/pubs/msb/msbresp.html
5. Virtual Hospital (University of Iowa): http://www.vh.org/Welcome/Welcome.html

6. Centers for Disease Control: http://www.cdc.gov
7. Resources for students in the medical sciences: http://medicalstudent.com
8. United Staes Pharmacopeia Drug Information: http://www.healthanswers.com/health_answers/usp_drug_search/frames333.htm
9. Virtual Autopsy (Leicester University): http://www.ie.ac.uk/pathology/teach/VA/titlpag1.html

CHAPTER 5

CHAPTER OUTLINE

KEY TERMS

Berman Airway
Combitube
Double Lumen Endotracheal Tube (DLET)
Endotracheal Tube (ET)
French Sizes
Guedel Airway
Laryngeal Mask Airway (LMA)
Laryngoscope
Luer-Loc
Lukens Sputum trap
Macintosh Blade
Miller Blade
Nasopharyngeal Airway
Nasotracheal Intubation
Oropharyngeal Airway
Sniffer's Position
Translaryngeal Intubation

Artificial Airways

Charles G. Durbin, Jr.

CHAPTER LEARNING OBJECTIVES

Upon completion of this chapter, the reader should be able to:

1. Describe ways to displace the tongue to improve gas exchange in unconscious patients.
2. List several complications from improper placement of oral and nasopharyngeal airways.
3. Describe how to place the laryngeal mask airway and the Combitube (Sheridan Catheter Corp.) in unconscious patients.
4. List the appropriate sequence of steps to insert an endotracheal tube in patients with compromised airways.
5. Identify at least three ways to confirm that an endotracheal tube lies in the trachea.
6. List the equipment necessary to perform invasive ventilation (transtracheal or surgical airway) and describe a procedure for airway entry.
7. List the complications related to invasive airway access and the treatment of each.
8. Review the equipment and steps necessary for obtaining sputum samples from patients with tracheostomy tubes.
9. Describe three ways to wean patients from tracheostomy tubes.
10. List three methods to allow patients with tracheostomy tubes to speak.
11. Identify the airway risks facing intubated patients and identify strategies and equipment for the prevention of each.

One of the most dramatic and rapidly fatal medical emergencies occurs when a person loses the ability to breathe spontaneously. This can be caused by upper airway obstruction, as with foreign body aspiration; lower airway obstruction, as with severe bronchospasm or a tension pneumothorax; or from an altered respiratory drive, as with depressant drug overdose or following a stroke. Failure to restore adequate respiratory gas exchange can result in hypoxic brain injury or death within minutes. These serious consequences have led to universal acceptance of the "ABCs of resuscitation" (Airway, Breathing, and Circulation) with establishment of an adequate airway as the first and highest priority.

This chapter reviews the devices and techniques used to establish and maintain a patent upper airway, including tongue-displacement devices and ETs and TTs. Table 5-1 briefly describes some of these devices. Additional equipment used for patients with artificial airways, as well as some of the risks and problems encountered in their use will be described. A variety of devices and pieces of equipment have been developed over the years with some only fitting a small, clinical niche. Many airway devices have passed into history, never gaining widespread popularity. Only devices with a significant following are described in detail here.

Securing a Patent Upper Airway—Displacing the Tongue

Simple maneuvers are often effective to restore breathing to patients with obstructed airways. In the supine position, when the pharyngeal and tongue muscles lose tone, the tongue falls backward, possibly occluding the pharynx. Elevating and extending the head advances the jaw and moves the tongue forward, maybe opening a closed air-

TABLE 5-1

Devices and techniques used to establish and maintain a patent upper airway

Device or maneuver	Description	Concerns and contraindications
Extreme extension, or "Sniffer's position"	Extension of the occiput with flexion of the lower cervical spine	Unstable cervical spine
Jaw thrust or chin lift	Anterior displacement of the mandible with or without dislocation of the tempromandibular joints	Tempromandibular joint disease or a fractured mandible
Orophrangeal airways	Rigid, curved device with an air passage, placed through the mouth with end resting distal to the tongue above the glottic opening	Gagging or vomiting, improper size, incorrect placement
Nasopharyngeal airways	Soft or semi-rigid hollow tube placed through the nares, the tip lying distal to the tongue above the glottic opening	Gagging or vomiting (usually better tolerated in noncomatose patients); posterior pharyngeal wall dissection; severe bleeding
Laryngeal mask airways	Custom-formed, soft mask with a hollow tube fitting into the pyriform sinuses directly above the larynx	Confirmation of correct placement difficult, mask may fold, epiglottis may obstruct laryngeal opening, trachea not protected from aspiration
Endotracheal tubes	Semi-rigid, hollow tube placed into the trachea with or without an inflatable cuff	Usually requires special devices (e.g., laryngoscope) and technical skill for consistent correct placement, tracheal placement must be objectively confirmed, and esophageal placement and ET displacement avoided
Transtracheal invasive airway	Emergent, direct entry into the trachea below the larynx by a large-bore needle, or surgical incision with ET	Hypoxia, bleeding, nerve or esophageal injury, failure to establish an airway, gas dissection
Tracheostomy tubes	A hollow tube, with or without a cuff, electively inserted directly into the trachea through a surgical incision or with a wire-guided progressive dilation technique	Hypoxia, bleeding, nerve or esophageal injury, failure to establish the airway due to nontracheal placement, displacement

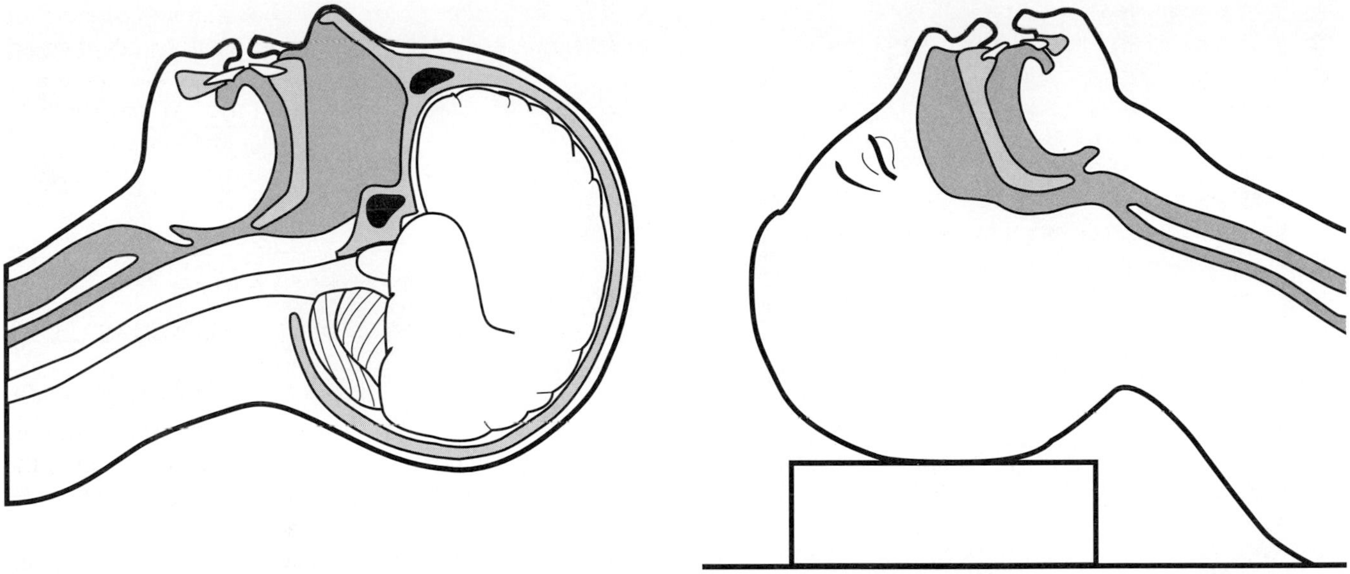

Figure 5-1 "Sniffer's position," the optimal position for opening the upper airway, can be obtained by supporting the occiput of the head on a solid surface and extending the head. This is also the optimal position for oral intubation using a curved laryngoscope blade.

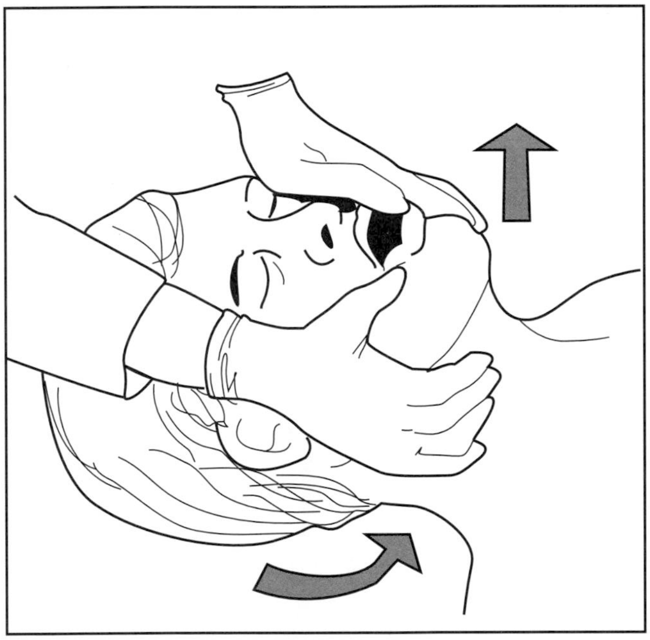

Figure 5-2 The index fingers of both hands are used to perform a jaw thrust, which displaces the temporomandibular joints anteriorly, achieving a patent airway without neck extension. This is particularly useful for patients with cervical injuries.

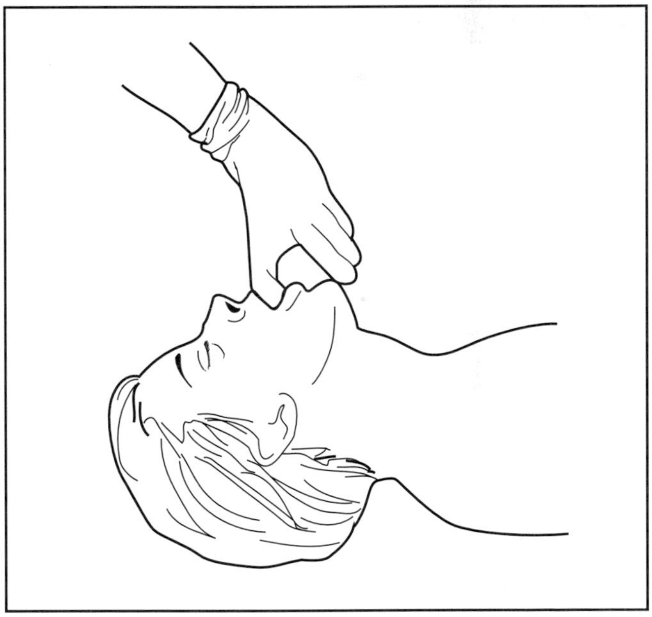

Figure 5-3 A chin lift is another method for opening the upper airway by moving the tongue anteriorly and can be successful without extending the cervical spine.

way. This so-called "sniffer's position," shown in Figure 5-1, opens the upper airway and places the long axes of the mouth, pharynx, and larynx in close alignment. This head position is also optimal for endotracheal intubation with direct vision. By forcing the jaw anteriorly with a jaw thrust or a chin lift maneuver (Figures 5-2 and 5-3), the tongue is moved farther from the hard and soft palates, so a patent upper airway may be achieved. In some patients, these simple manual maneuvers are ineffective for opening air passages past an obstructing tongue, so mechanical devices must be used.

The most common device for this purpose is the oral pharyngeal airway. A **Guedel airway** consists of a hollow, central channel for air passage, a buccal flange, a bite portion, and a curved portion that follows the contour of the hard palate. The airway must extend past the posterior part of the tongue to allow air to pass. A **Berman airway** is shaped similarly to the Guedel airway but has a different

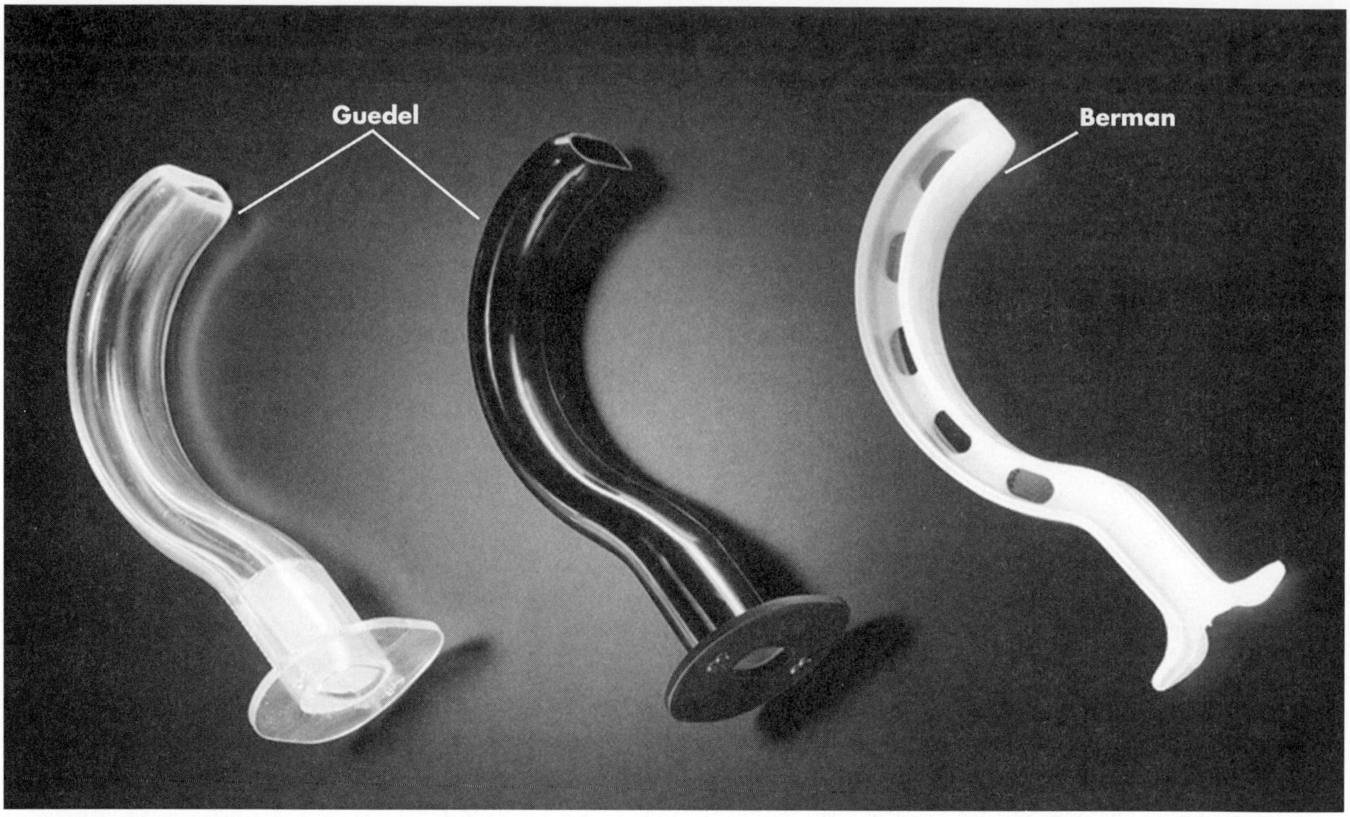

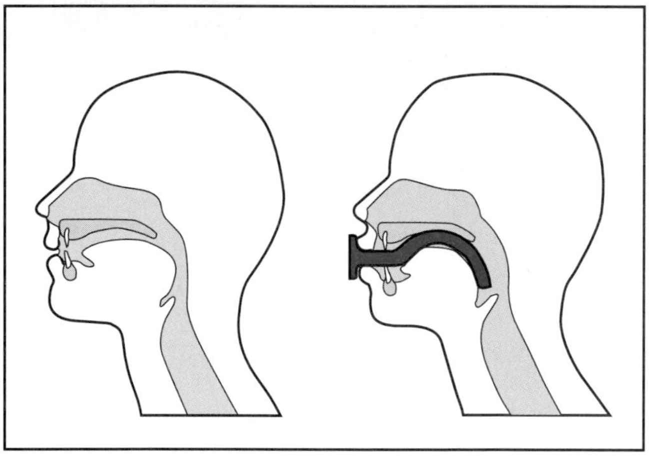

Figure 5-4 Guedel and Berman airways are upper airway devices used to provide air passage distal to an obstructing tongue. (Courtesy Allegiance Medical Care, McGraw Park, Ill.)

cross-section profile without a protected central channel (Figure 5-4). Available in a variety of lengths, the American National Standards Institute (ANSI) standard for oral airways is that the size is the "nominal" length in millimeters. This measurement convention is shown in Figure 5-5. Because jaw sizes differ markedly among individuals, the correct-size oropharyngeal airway can be estimated as one that reaches from the angle of the jaw or the earlobe to the lips. *It is safer to choose an airway that is too large rather than one even slightly too small.* This is because the tongue will not be bypassed by an airway that is too short, so no air will pass into the lungs. If the airway is too long, the excess

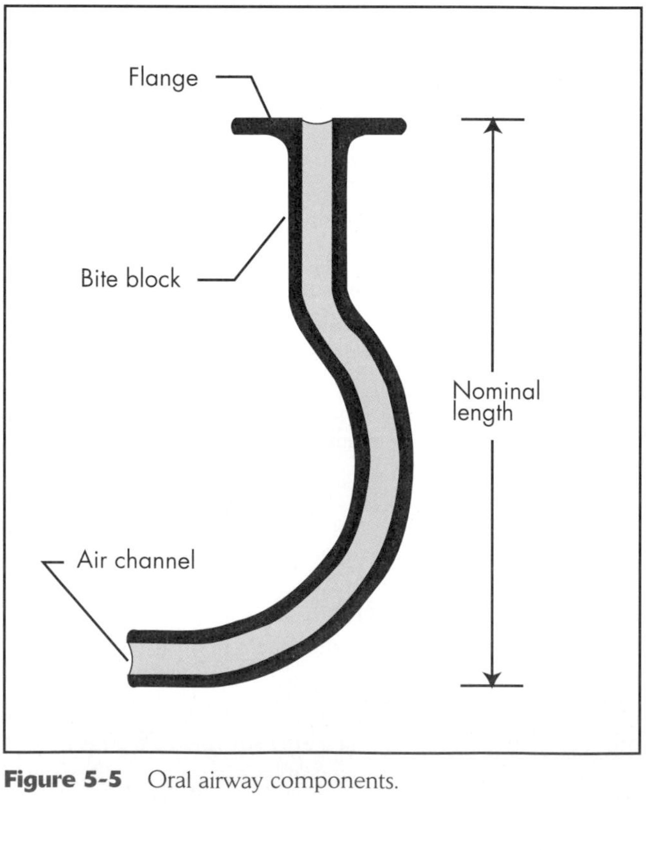

Figure 5-5 Oral airway components.

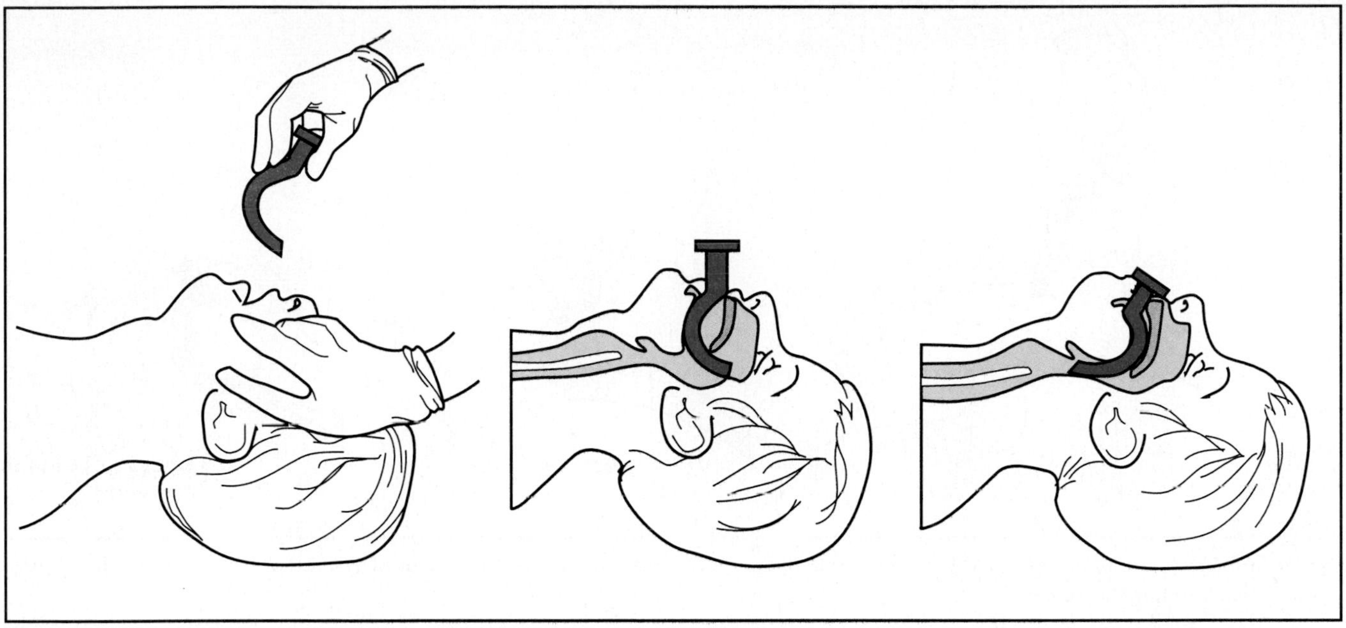

Figure 5-6 Antianatomical insertion of an oral airway.

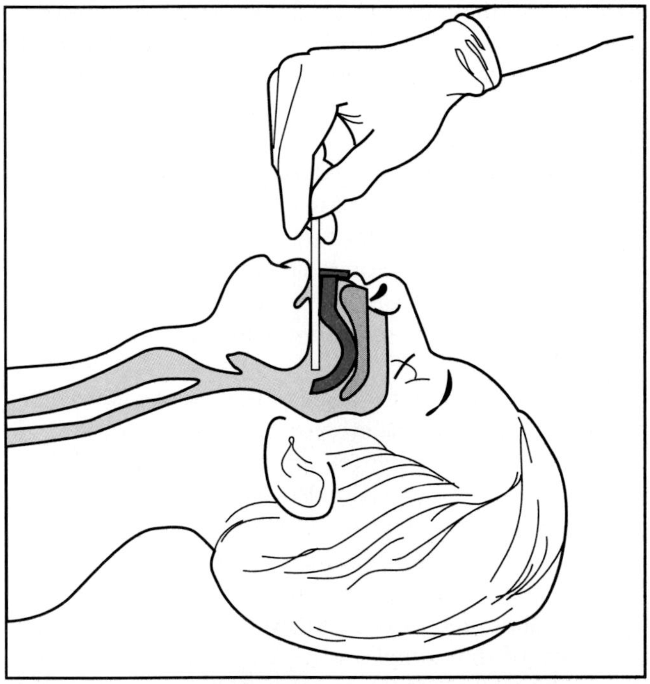

Figure 5-7 Anatomical insertion of an oral airway with a tongue blade.

length will protrude from the mouth, but the air passage will be patent.

An oropharyngeal airway may be inserted into an unconscious person in several ways. Using a tongue blade or gloved fingers the mouth can be opened and the airway inserted following the curve of the hard palate and seated with the tip past the back of the tongue. Getting the tip past the flaccid tongue is sometimes difficult, but it is essential for success. To reduce the likelihood of the airway tip getting hung up on the back of the tongue, the airway should be inserted upside down with the tip riding along the hard palate until past the tongue, when it should be rotated 180 degrees. A modification of this technique that may be less traumatic to the palate is to insert the airway rotated 90 degrees from the side of the mouth, using it like a tongue blade to move the tongue out of the way, and then rotate it back 90 degrees to seat it. These insertion techniques are illustrated in Figures 5-6, 5-7, and 5-8.

Correct size and proper seating are essential to creating an open air passage with an oropharyngeal airway. An important sign that the distal airway tip may not have passed the back of the tongue is if the flange protrudes from the patient's mouth. If attempts to push the airway farther in just bounce it back out, it is probably catching on the back of the tongue and should be removed and replaced immediately using one of the above described methods. An alternative technique for seating an airway that has failed to pass the tongue is to perform a jaw thrust and push (with the thumbs) the airway in past the anteriorly displaced tongue. This is shown in Figure 5-9.

Specialized oral airways, some of which are shown in Figure 5-10, have been developed to allow blind and fiberoptic-directed endotracheal intubation. The simplest of these is a hollow, bite block that protects the endoscope from damage if the patient reflexively bites down during the procedure. Airways that facilitate intubation either have open channels or are split devices that can be removed leaving the ET or fiberoptic device in place.

NASOPHARYNGEAL AIRWAYS

Oropharyngeal airways are contraindicated in patients who retain airway protective reflexes because gagging or

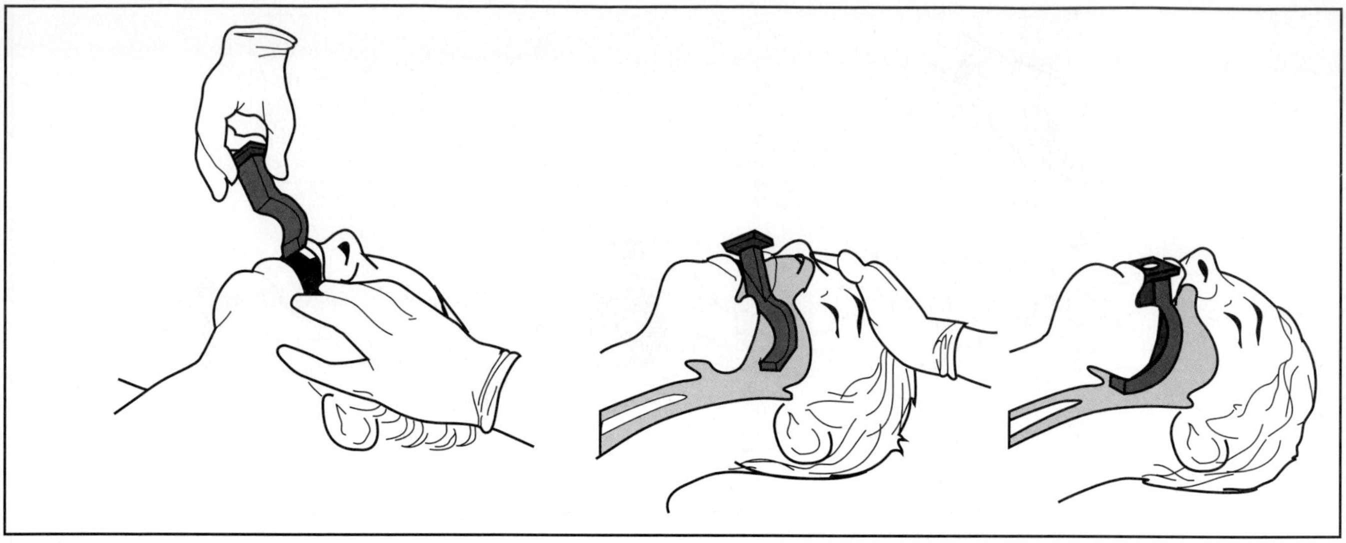

Figure 5-8 Insertion of an oral airway from the side of the mouth. The airway itself can be used as a tongue blade to displace the tongue while inserting the airway.

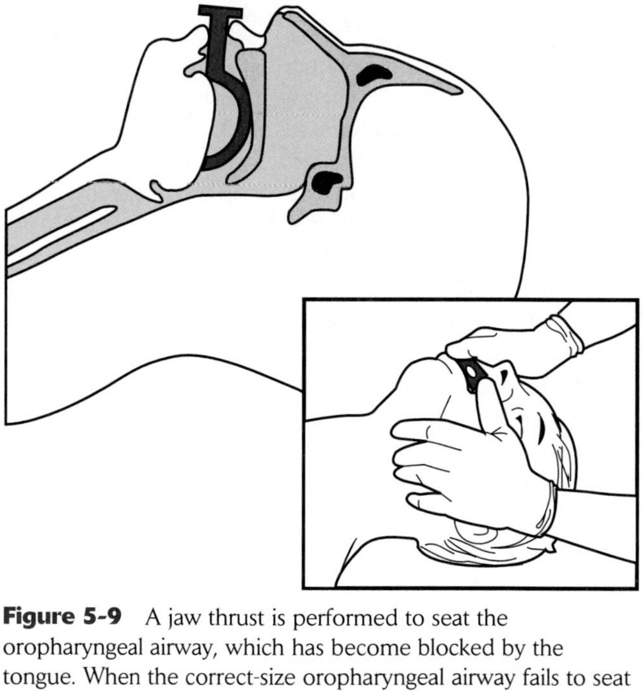

Figure 5-9 A jaw thrust is performed to seat the oropharyngeal airway, which has become blocked by the tongue. When the correct-size oropharyngeal airway fails to seat properly and protrudes from the mouth, performing a jaw thrust and using the thumbs to insert the airway will provide proper placement.

vomiting may result. Such airways can cause dental damage if the patient forcibly bites the hard plastic or metal airway. If the patient struggles to extrude the airway, attempts at insertion should be abandoned, and an improved head position or a nasopharyngeal airway should be used to open the upper airway. **Nasopharyngeal airways,** which are also called nasal trumpets or nasal airways, are better tolerated in semi-awake patients who retain some airway protective reflexes.

Nasopharyngeal airways resemble shortened, uncuffed endotracheal tubes and are made of soft latex or polyethylene. The end is flared to prevent airway loss through the nose. The ANSI sizing system gives the internal diameter in millimeters, although **French sizes** (i.e., the external circumference in millimeters) are also frequently used. The critical size, however, is related to the airway length, which must be long enough to pass to a position beyond the tongue base. Each manufacturer uses a different length: diameter ratio, so the proper airway for a certain patient may be a matter of trial and error. The correct length of the nasopharyngeal airway can be estimated by positioning the airway along the side of the head. For proper function, the tip should extend past the angle of the jaw. An airway that is too long may enter the esophagus and not provide an air passage. Unlike oropharyngeal airways, nasopharyngeal airways that are too short will not make a bad airway worse, they just will not improve the problem.

Nasal bleeding can complicate insertion of the nasopharyngeal airway. Correct insertion technique, generous lubrication, and vasoconstrictive agents can reduce the frequency of this complication. A mixture of local anesthetic solution (i.e., 4% lidocaine) and phenylephrine (Neo-Synephrine) or oxymetazoline (Afrin) is effective in this regard. Previously, cocaine hydrochloride was used for this purpose, but the hypertensive risks and the concern over dispensing a controlled substance led to its abandonment. In emergency situations, the airway should only be well-lubricated to avoid having to wait for drug effects to occur.

The airway is inserted parallel to the floor of the nasal pharynx and slightly medially (Figure 5-11). Mistakenly, it is often attempted to insert the airway "up the nose" (parallel to the long axis of the nose), which increases the likelihood of bleeding and fails to secure placement. The nasal

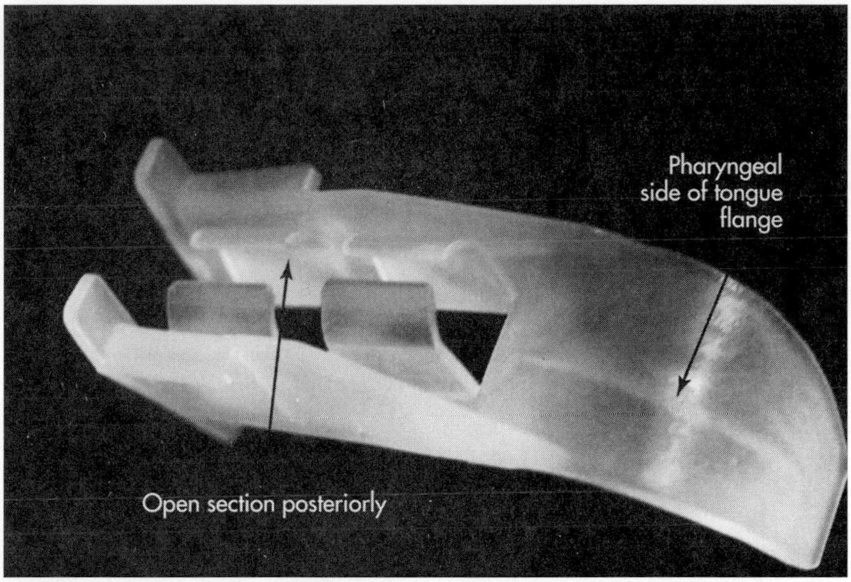

Figure 5-10 Intubating airways can be used to support and direct a fiberoptic bronchoscope and ET into the trachea with direct vision. The incomplete channel allows separation of the scope from the airway after tracheal intubation. (From Benumof JL: Airway management: principles and practice, St Louis, 1996, Mosby.)

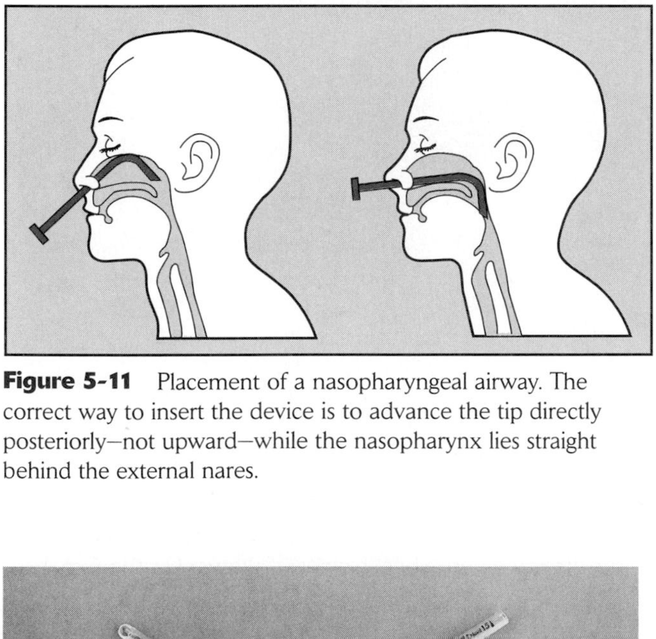

Figure 5-11 Placement of a nasopharyngeal airway. The correct way to insert the device is to advance the tip directly posteriorly—not upward—while the nasopharynx lies straight behind the external nares.

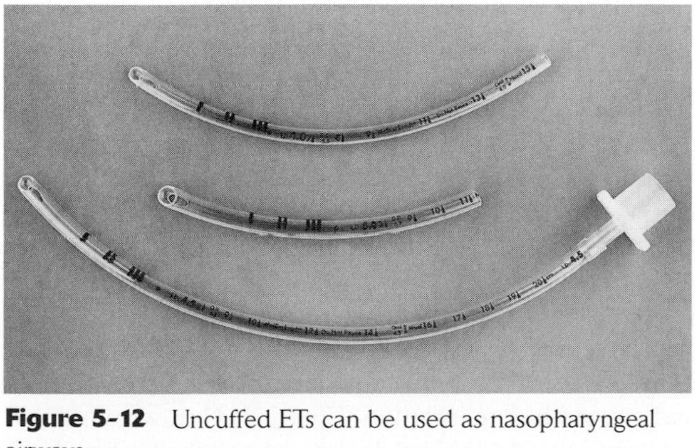

Figure 5-12 Uncuffed ETs can be used as nasopharyngeal airways.

pharyngeal opening is usually directly posterior to the anterior nares. The size of the external nares is unrelated to the room between the nasal turbinates. If undue resistance is met on one side of airway insertion, it should be attempted on the other side. Softer airways are less likely to cause bleeding and will conform to a distorted passageway as they pass through a narrow nasal channel. They are also more likely to obstruct or disallow passage of a suction catheter. The airway should be inserted with gentle, continuous pressure unless significant resistance is encountered. A airway that is smaller in diameter may be used if a larger one cannot be inserted. If only a small airway can be passed through the external nasal passage, it may not function because of its concomitant short length.

Uncuffed ETs can be used as nasopharyngeal airways (Figure 5-12). Tube length can be customized to fit individual patient anatomy. A long, thin tube can be created by trimming the tube to proper length. The tube connector can be used to prevent the tube from disappearing into the nose; however, the friction fit may be inadequate to prevent accidental separation. Also, the connector's internal diameter is smaller than the tube and may prevent suction catheter passage and limit gas flow rates during ventilation. Leaving extra length so that the tube can be taped at the correct distance is another solution, but it may reduce the efficiency of mask ventilation. Cut endotracheal tubes for nasopharyngeal airways are often used for infants and children. Movement can be prevented by placing a safety pin through the side of the tube, avoiding compromise of the center lumen with the tube secured with tape (Figure 5-13).

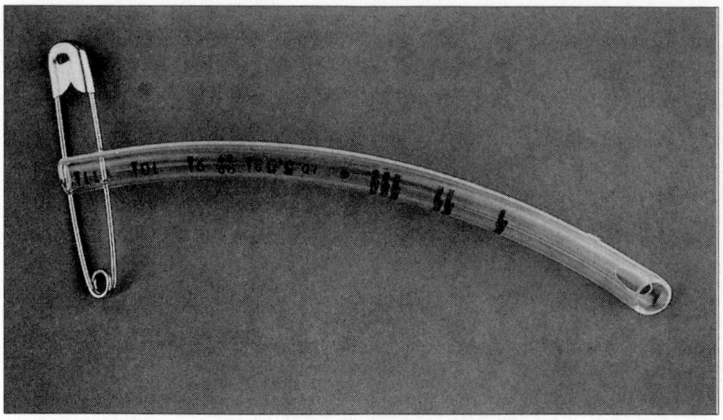

Figure 5-13 Use of a safety pin to help secure a custom-cut ET used as a nasopharyngeal airway.

As mentioned above, nasal bleeding is a real concern, so nasopharyngeal airways should be used with caution in patients prone to uncontrollable bleeding. If bleeding occurs, use vasoconstrictors and tamponade the source (by leaving the device in place), although significant hemorrhage may necessitate a transfusion. A relative contraindication for nasopharyngeal airway use is a basal skull fracture. Penetration of the brain by the airway is possible, although unlikely, so this risk must be weighed against the urgency of the airway need and the failure of other techniques. Sinus infection is a longer-term risk of nasopharyngeal tube placement.

As with oral airways, fiberoptic or blind tracheal entry can be facilitated with a nasopharyngeal airway. Removal of the device after intubation is more difficult because split devices are not commercially available. Nasopharyngeal airways are useful for protecting the nose from trauma during blind nasotracheal suctioning. Once securely in place, they are usually well-tolerated—even in individuals who are awake.

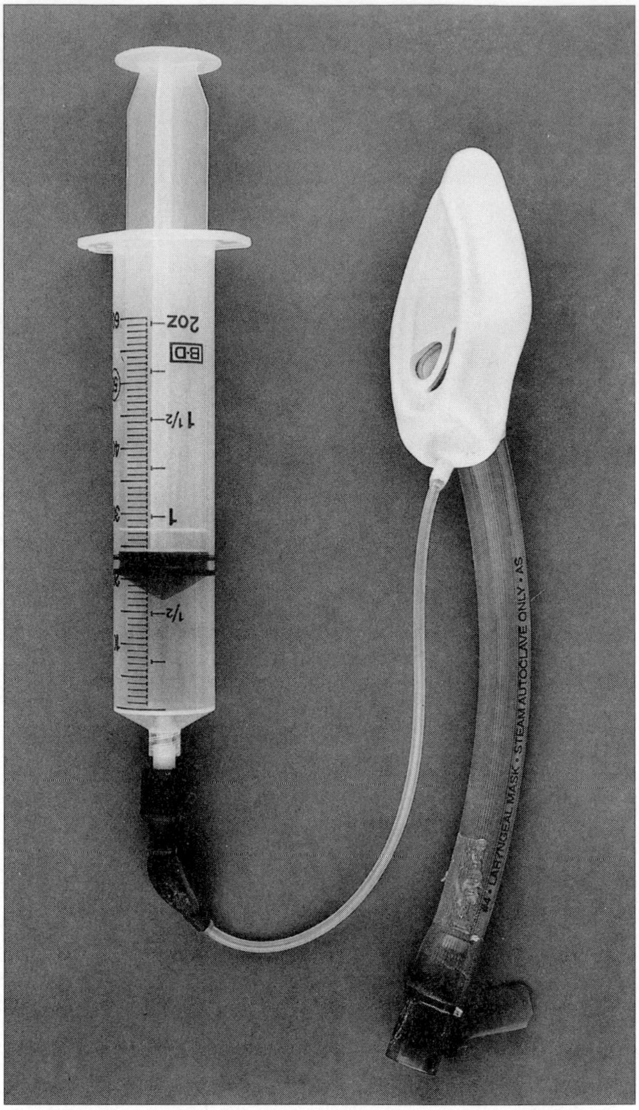

Figure 5-14 For correct LMA insertion, the cuff should be completely deflated with the mask forming an upward, open-bowl configuration. This minimizes risk of oral damage and helps prevent the mask from folding over during insertion.

Laryngeal Mask Airway (LMA)

Recently becoming popular, this "mask on a tube" is designed to form a low-pressure seal in the laryngeal inlet by means of an inflated cuff. It is placed blindly and bypasses the upper airway structures. Its tip rests against the upper esophageal sphincter (cricopharyngeus muscle), and the cuff seats laterally in the pyriform fossa. It is equipped with a standard 15-mm slip fitting, and positive-pressure ventilation can be delivered. Pressures exceeding 20 cm of water usually result in ventilation volume loss and gas leakage around the cuff. This device does not replace endotracheal intubation because the lung is not protected from aspiration, although the quantity of aspirated material may be reduced. The LMA is a useful emergency airway device for several reasons: (1) insertion is simple and easy to teach and learn; (2) it provides a patent airway that is usually superior to that from an oral or nasopharyngeal device; (3) it does not require airway manipulation or extreme head positioning; and (4) once in place it frees the users' hands for other tasks. Its major drawbacks are as follows: (1) the expense; reusable models are handmade from silicone rubber and cost about $200, and disposable models cost about $36; (2) choosing the correct size is difficult because the larynx is not seen, so standard sizes are used but may not fit correctly, requiring a different-sized replacement; and (3) aspiration is not prevented. Sizes for neonates (size 1); children (sizes 2 and 2 1/2); and small, normal, and large adults (sizes 3,4, and 5) are available in the reusable form, but only adult sizes (3, 4, and 5) are available as single-use devices.

The cuff is inflated and examined for discoloration and its ability to maintain inflation, then it is deflated completely and everted before insertion (Figure 5-14). A water-soluble lubricant is used to help slide the cuff past the hard and soft palates. The insertion technique is shown in Figure 5-15. A

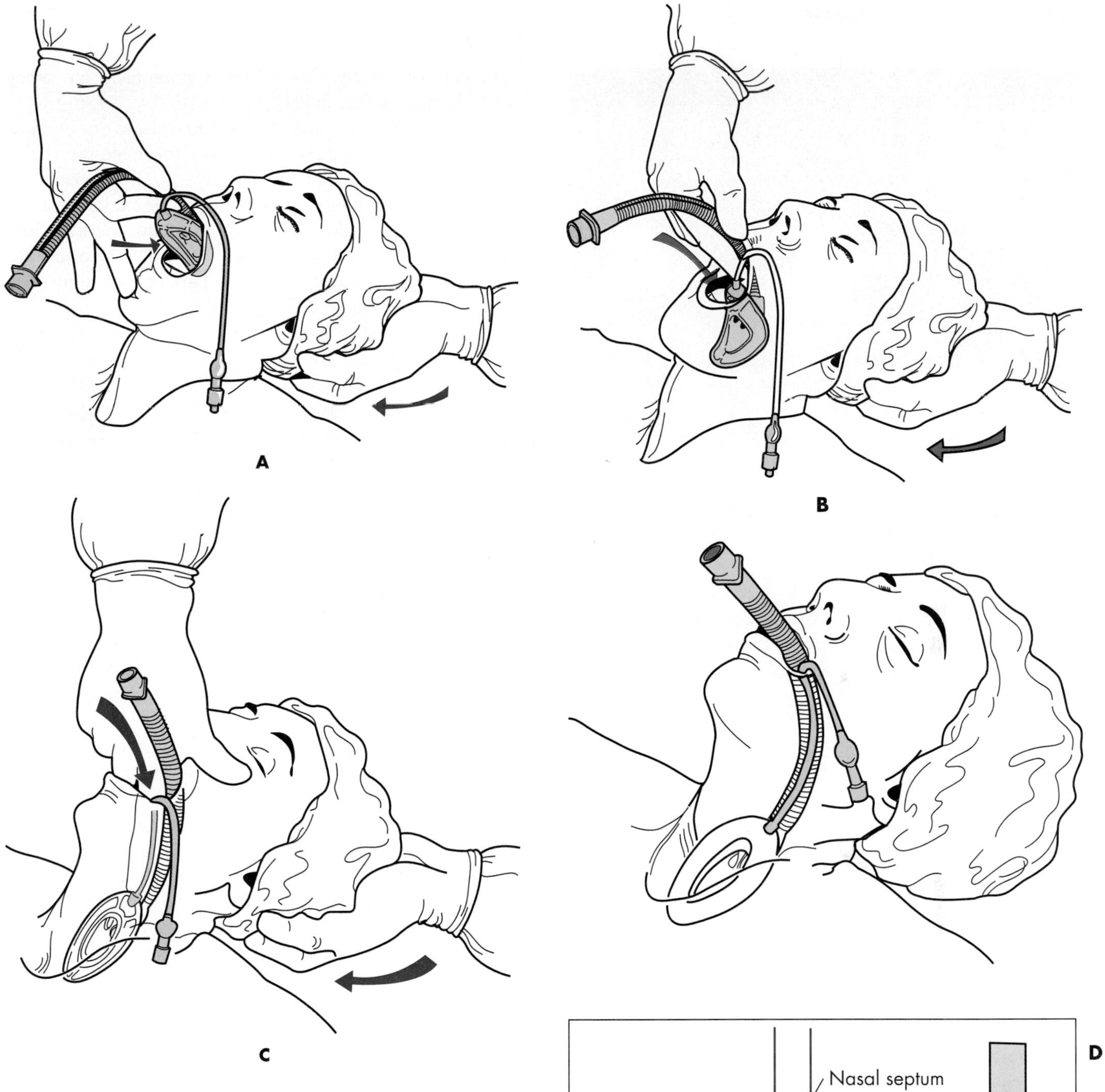

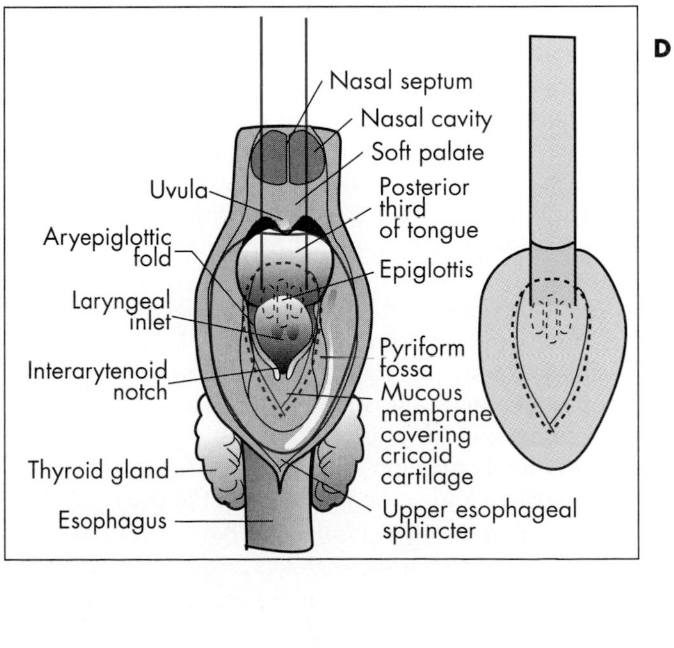

Figure 5-15 **A,** The LMA is held like a pencil and inserted into the open mouth with only the slightest neck extension. **B,** The LMA is directed posterior and down to the oropharynx. **C,** The LMA is advanced with the opposite hand and guided into the posterior pharynx. **D,** The final location of the LMA after correct placement. (Redrawn from Gensia Automedics, San Diego, Brain Medical Limited, 1992.)

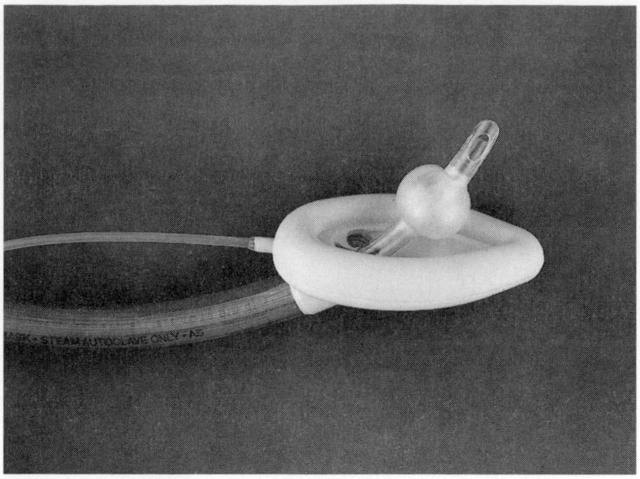

Figure 5-16 A small, cuffed ET can be passed through an LMA and will frequently enter directly into the trachea. A fiberoptic endoscope can be used to confirm and direct intubation through the LMA if blind placement fails.

black line along the length of the tube marks the center of the device and is used to prevent twisting on placement. The head may be extended and a finger used to guide the deflated cuff past the tongue and pharynx. The tube is held in place with the other hand while the guiding fingers are withdrawn. The tube is then advanced until it is fully seated, and resistance to further insertion is felt. The cuff is inflated and if it is seated correctly in the pyriform sinuses, the tube will move back about 1 cm out of the mouth. If the mask is too small, it may pass down the esophagus, and no backward movement will occur on cuff inflation. The final test of correct placement is that adequate breath sounds are present over both lung fields and not over the stomach with positive-pressure ventilation. If ventilation fails, the head position may be altered (further extension is usually helpful), the LMA inserted farther, or the device removed and reinserted. A size change may also be necessary. Once the device is properly placed and a patent airway obtained, the tube is secured with tape; then either spontaneous or positive-pressure ventilation can be used. Attention must still to be paid to the airway when it is secured with the LMA because loss of airway patency, which can be due to device dislodgment or twisting, foreign body aspiration, or LMA obstruction, has been reported.

Blind (or fiberoptic) intubation with a cuffed endotracheal tube can be performed through an LMA to establish a definitive or secure airway, as shown in Figure 5-16. Occasionally the epiglottis is trapped under the LMA (it usually lies on top of the mask cuff), but this seems to have little effect on its function. The LMA is of particular use in patients with a known or anticipated difficult airway. Pregnant and obese patients predictably have improved ventilation with an LMA when compared with other upper airway control devices. The LMA is potentially life-saving when intubation has failed.

LMA use is becoming widespread outside of operating rooms because it is easier to master the necessary LMA skills than those needed for effective mask ventilation or endotracheal intubation. Emergency personnel are reporting excellent results in field trials. Infant and pediatric use is especially encouraging because the skills necessary for other airway techniques for these patients are difficult to learn and maintain.

After use, LMAs should be mechanically washed with a mild soap solution and autoclaved at 134° C or less. The cuff must be completely evacuated or it will rupture during the sterilization process. Glutaraldehyde should not be used because it is quite toxic to the laryngeal mucosa. LMAs may be resterilized 100 to 200 times, but marked discoloration or failure of the pilot tube and cuff to hold pressure are indications that the tube should be discarded.

Combitube

The **Combitube** is a double-lumen device designed to provide a patent upper airway when inserted blindly in comatose patients with airway difficulties or after failed intubation. It has two cuffs designed to seal in the esophagus and the pharynx (Figure 5-17). The tube is lubricated and inserted through the mouth, following the contour to the pharynx. Insertion continues until the depth marks reach the lips or significant resistance is encountered. The cuffs are then inflated, the esophageal cuff with 15 mL and the pharyngeal cuff with 100 mL. The esophageal lumen may occasionally enter the trachea, and because it has an opening at its end, it can be used as a conventional ET. Ventilation is normally provided through the other lumen, which opens in a series of holes into the hypopharynx. The esophageal cuff affords some protection from regurgitation, but as with the LMA, the Combitube is not considered a secure airway device. A nasogastric tube can be inserted through the esophageal lumen into the stomach for decompression, unfortunately only one size (for average adults) is available.

Endotracheal Tubes

The definitive device for airway management is a cuffed ET. ETs allow ventilation with high levels of positive pressure, provide direct access to the lower airway for secretion removal and drug delivery, prevent aspiration of foreign material into the lung, and permit bronchoscopic examination of the peripheral airways. Placing an ET requires a high degree of skill and specialized equipment (i.e., **laryngoscopes**), and risks hypoxia and hypercarbia during attempted placement. Prior to ET placement, adequate gas exchange must be established using other airway devices or

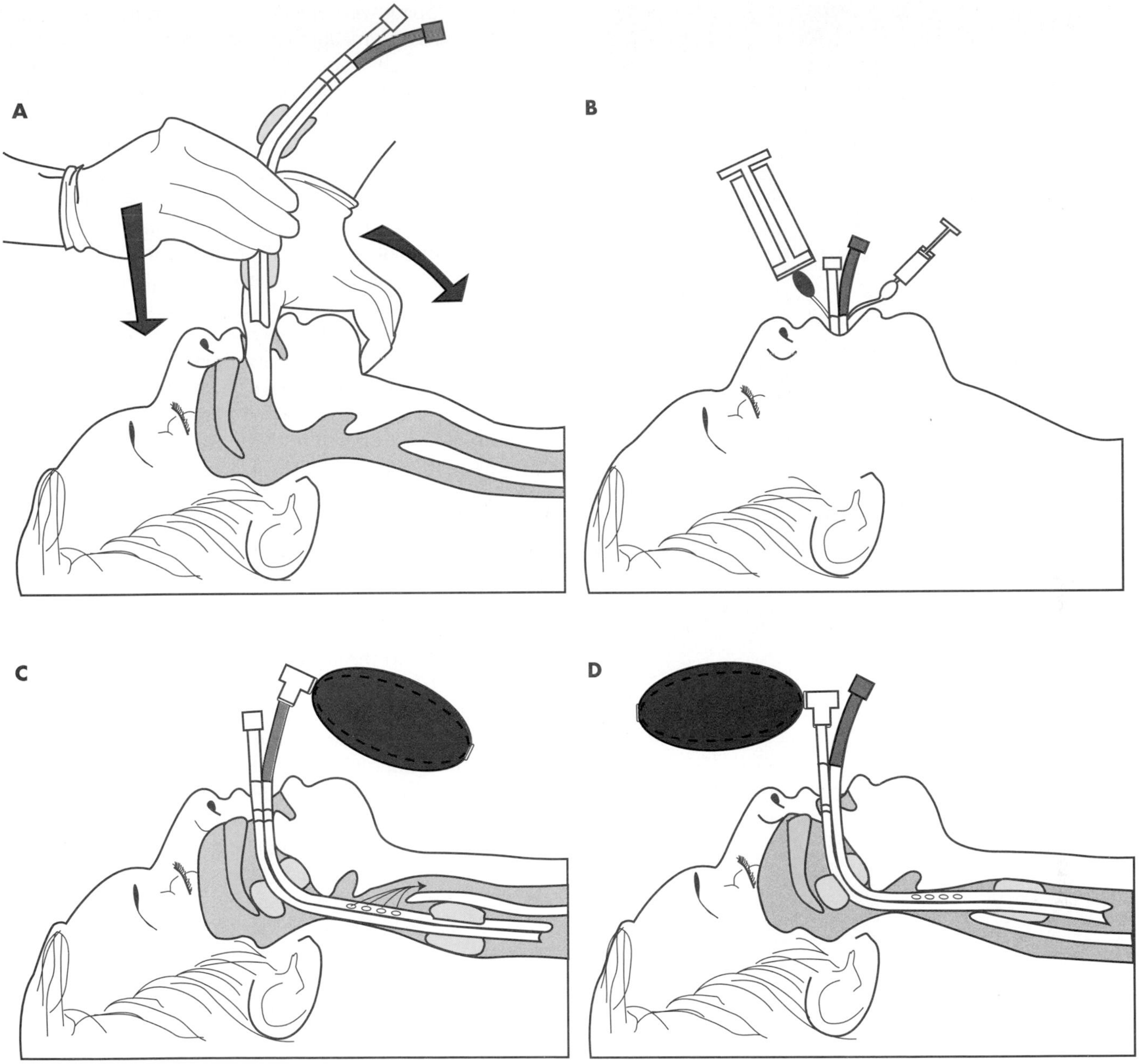

Figure 5-17 The Combitube is inserted with the head in the neutral position (**A**) and both cuffs inflated (**B**). The two possible locations of the distal lumen are shown in C and D.

maneuvers. Intubation may be an urgent procedure but should rarely be performed in a patient without a previously established patent airway and at least reasonable gas exchange. *If a patent airway cannot be established by a simple means, an invasive airway (needle or surgical cricothyrotomy)—not insertion of an ET through the mouth or nose—should be performed quickly.* Therefore endotracheal intubation should be an elective procedure.

The conventional, or Murphy type, of ET consists of a round, plastic tube with a beveled tip, a sidehole (Murphy eye) opposite the bevel, a cuff attached to a pilot balloon with a spring-loaded valve, and a 15-mm standard connector. These components are shown in Figure 5-18. The tube should have distance markers indicated and a radiopaque maker imbedded along its length. The Murphy eye allows gas flow if the bevel tip becomes occluded. ETs lacking Murphy eyes are called Magill type of tubes. ETs are sized by internal diameter (in millimeters), although occasionally French sizes are reported (outer circumference in millimeters). Uncuffed tubes are generally used for children because the smaller lumen necessary to accommodate a cuff would further compromise an airway that is already small in diameter. Also, the narrowest part of an infant's airway is below the larynx at the cricoid ring, and a snug fit at this

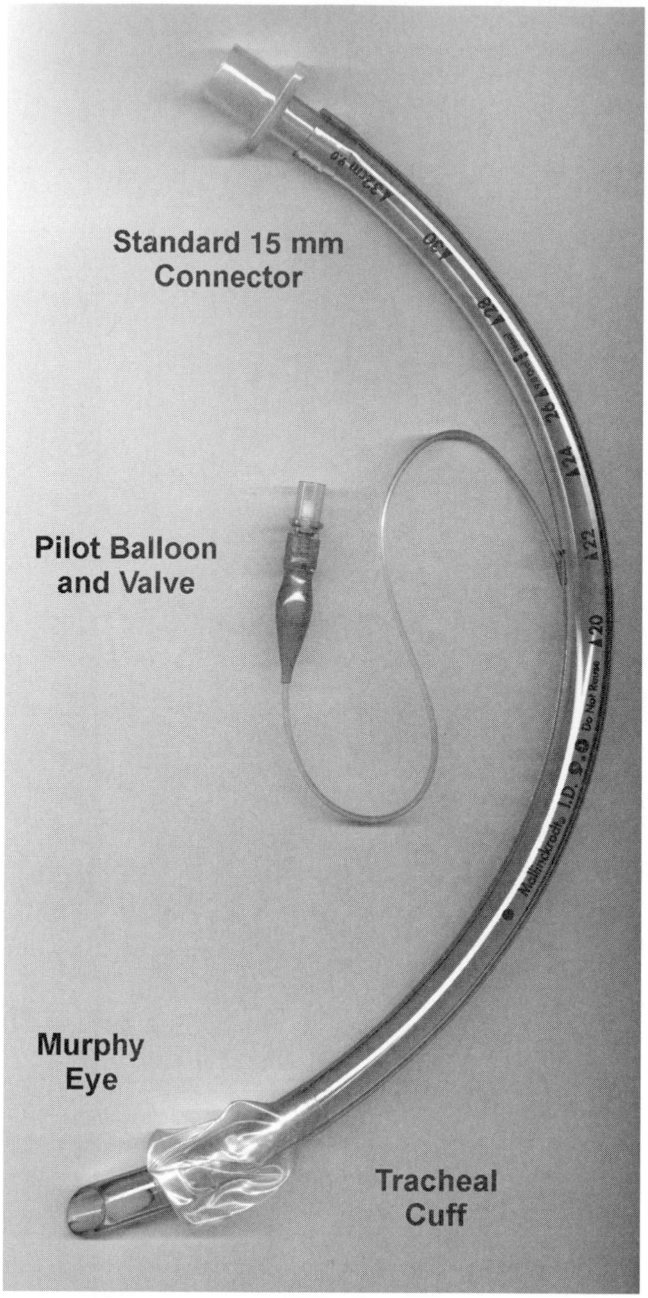

Figure 5-18 The components of a cuffed ET.

level will permit positive-pressure ventilation. The correct-size tube for an infant or child can only be determined during actual intubation; a tube that will not pass easily down the trachea should be changed for a smaller diameter tube. To avoid post-intubation croup or subglottic stenosis, an air leak at about 20 cm H_2O should be obtained in children intubated with an uncuffed ET.

Many variants of the basic ET design have been developed to solve clinical problems. The plastic tube tends to collapse and obstruct when bent at an angle, which frequently occurs in the posterior pharynx with a nasally placed ET. Spiral wire embedded tubes (Figure 5-19) help prevent this problem, but these tubes are flimsy, do not hold a preformed arch shape, and are often difficult to place in the trachea. Another solution to the bending/kinking problem is the RAE tube (Ring-Adair-Elwin), which has a preformed bend for oral or nasal intubation, as shown in Figures 5-20 and 5-21. Because bend placement is based on tube diameter and "average" patient dimensions, these tubes may not be the correct shape for certain patients and should be used with caution. The Cole tube (Figure 5-22) was developed to allow a larger diameter tube in the upper airway with a tapered tip passing through the vocal cords and cricoid ring in infants. This design would theoretically reduce dead space and improve gas flow; however, the shoulder of the tube may rest on the larynx, and a high incidence of laryngeal complications has been noted with use of this tube.

During laser surgery in the airway, problems with ET fires have been reported. Flexible, corrugated metal tubes without cuffs, foil-wrapped tubes, and water-filled double-cuffed tubes have helped overcome this problem. Several of these devices are shown in Figure 5-23.

Aids to Endotracheal Intubation

The ET is placed through the mouth or nose into the trachea, and the cuff forms a seal against the tracheal wall. Placement of the ET is usually performed using a laryngoscope, which allows direct vision of the larynx and control of the supraglottic structures. Laryngoscopes consist of a handle that also contains batteries and a detachable blade with a light. There are two basic types of laryngoscope blades: straight (**Miller** type) and curved (**Macintosh** type). Laryngoscopy is performed slightly differently with each type of blade. With either blade attached, the handle is held like a hammer in the left hand (although "left handed" models have been made, which are to be held in the right hand) with the blade down and the long axis directed forward (Figure 5-24). The mouth is opened and the blade is inserted along the right side of the tongue. Once past the base of the tongue, the blade is brought back to the midline of the oral cavity, moving the tongue completely to the left. With the straight blade, the epiglottis is identified and hooked with the tip of the blade, the jaw and epiglottis are lifted forward and upward (not rocked backward, causing trauma to the upper teeth), and the light then shines on the larynx and down the trachea. With a curved blade, the epiglottis is identified and the tip inserted above it into the vallecula. With the same forward and upward lifting, the larynx is illuminated, and the ET can be passed into the trachea. The light is farther down toward the tip on straight blades and brightly illuminates the larynx, while the light on curved blades is about midway down the blade and illuminates the pharynx and supraglottic area. The broad flange (Figure 5-25) of the curved blade gives better tongue control and more working room

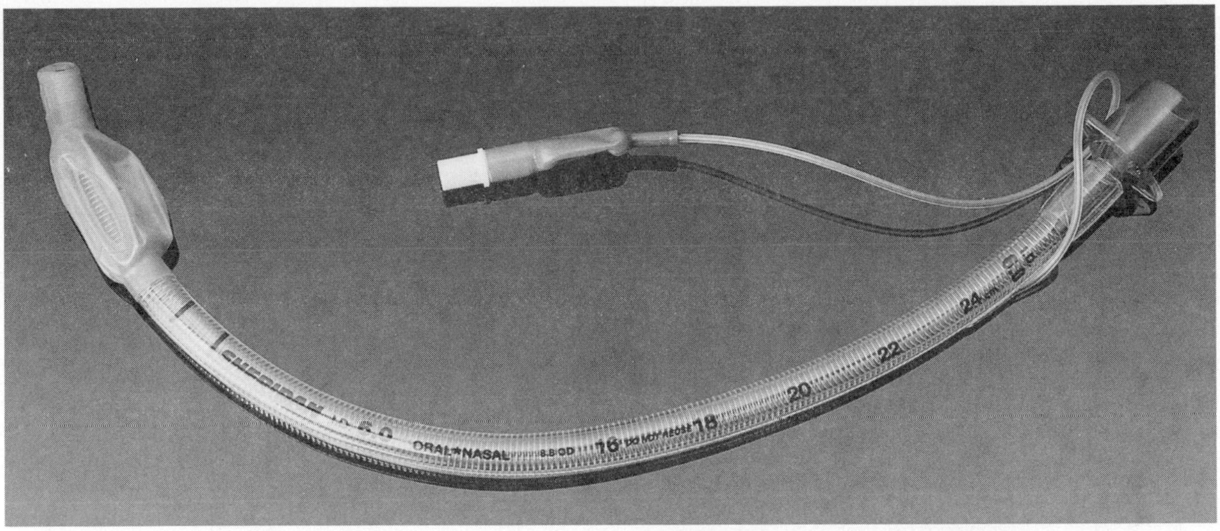

Figure 5-19 Spiral wire-reinforced ET.

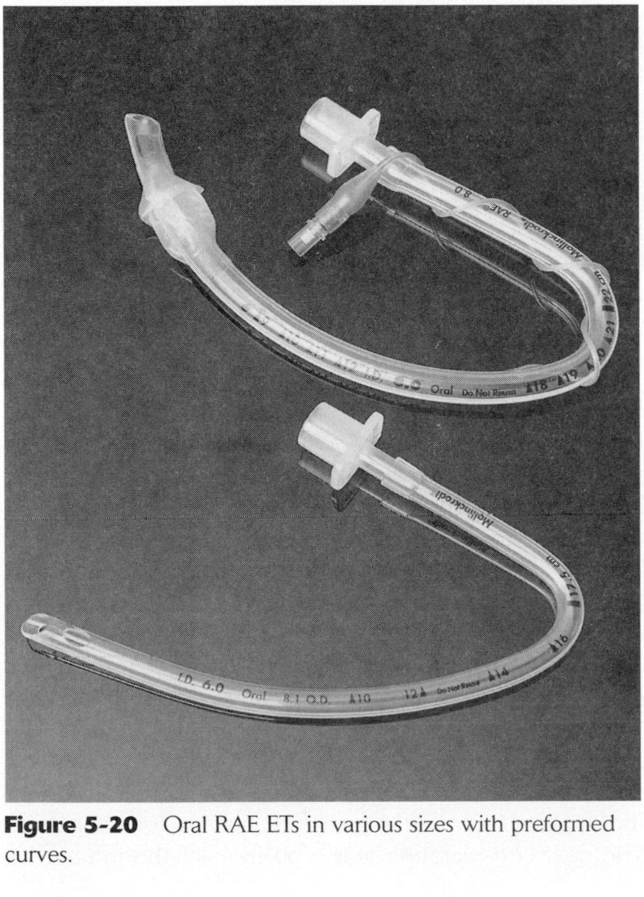

Figure 5-20 Oral RAE ETs in various sizes with preformed curves.

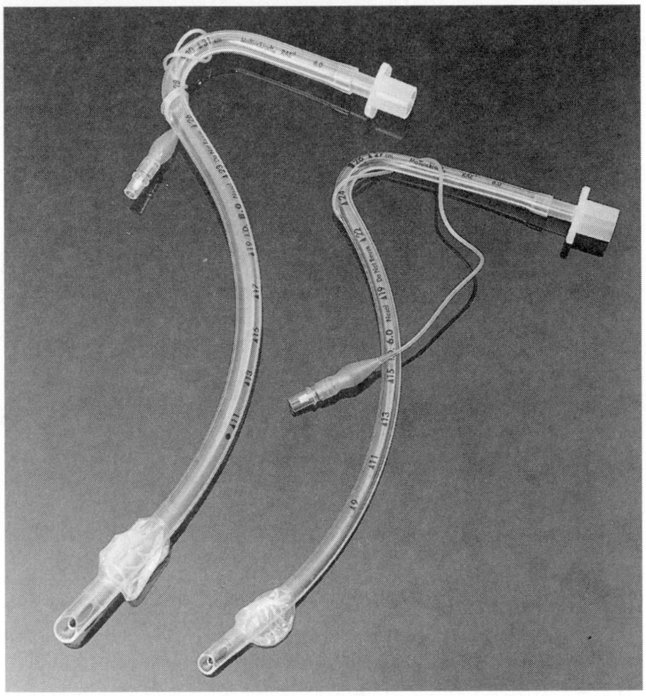

Figure 5-21 Nasal RAE ETs in various sizes with nasal curves.

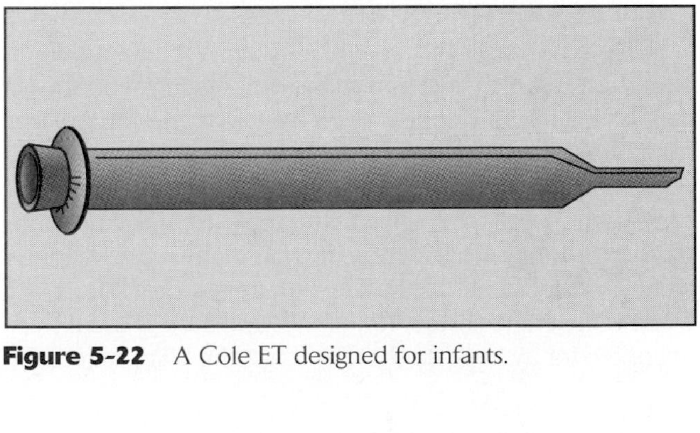

Figure 5-22 A Cole ET designed for infants.

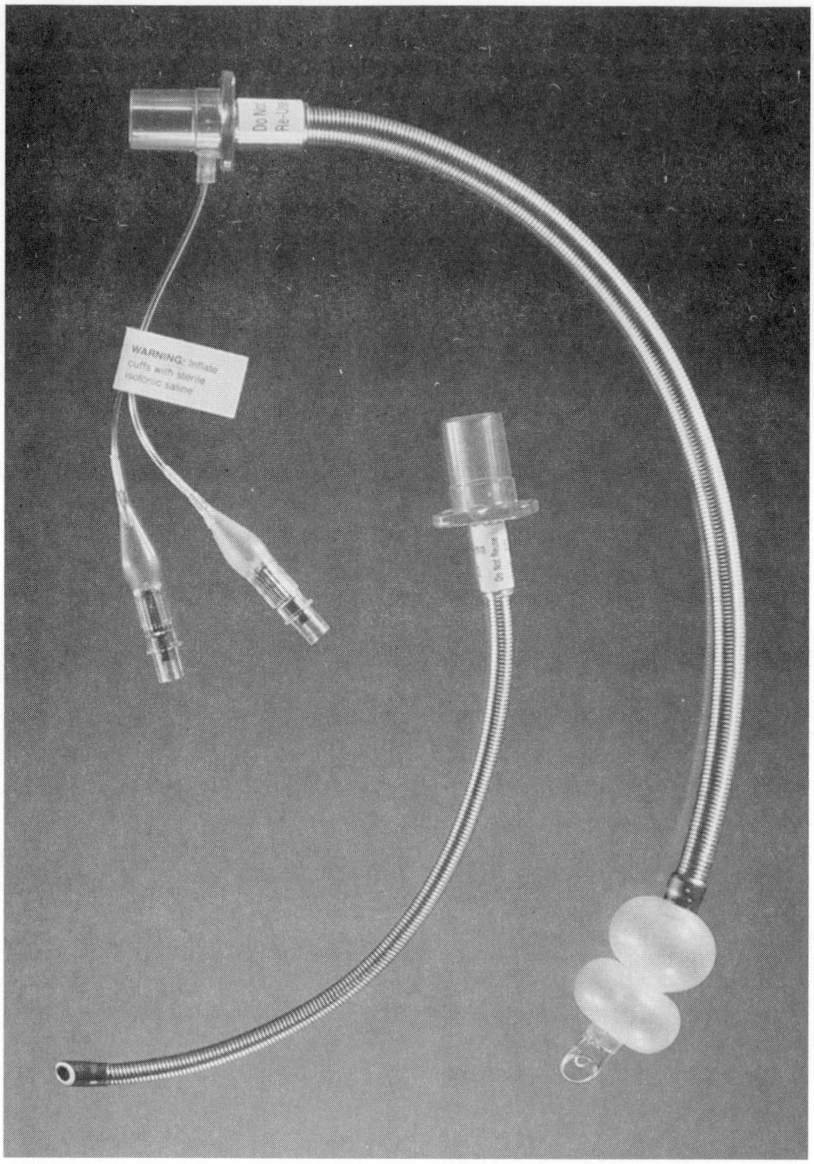

Figure 5-23 Flammable materials cause problems during laser surgery. Metal tubes, foil-wrapped tubes, and water-filled cuffs are some solutions to this problem. (Courtesy Allegiance Medical Care, McGraw Park, Ill.)

for tube insertion than the straight blade. In children, the epiglottis is less rigid than in adults, and often a straight-blade technique (i.e., hooking the epiglottis) is necessary, even if a curved blade is used.

The basic laryngoscope blades have been modified over the years. The size and shape of the flange and the location of the light on the curved blade are common places for innovation. Ports for suction or oxygen insufflation have been added. Straight blades have had modifications of cross-sectional shape to give better tongue control or working room during ET insertion. No standardized size equivalency is represented in blade numbers, but a #0 or #1 blade is generally correct for infants, and a #3 is usually appropriate for average adults. The angle the blade leaves the handle is another area of modification. An acute angle may improve visualization, and an obtuse or offset angle may allow insertion of the blade when pendulous breasts or an orthopedic apparatus is in the way. An angled blade tip, a mirror, or a prism may allow the intubator to see "around the corner" into the larynx. These specialized devices are expensive and require practice to master their use.

Although being able to see the laryngeal structures is useful, a good view does not guarantee ET insertion. Manipulating the ET into the trachea can be facilitated in several ways. The first is proper head position. As shown in Figure 5-1, the **sniffer's position** is ideal for opening up the upper airway and aligning the trachea for intubation. The next consideration is the position of the intubator's

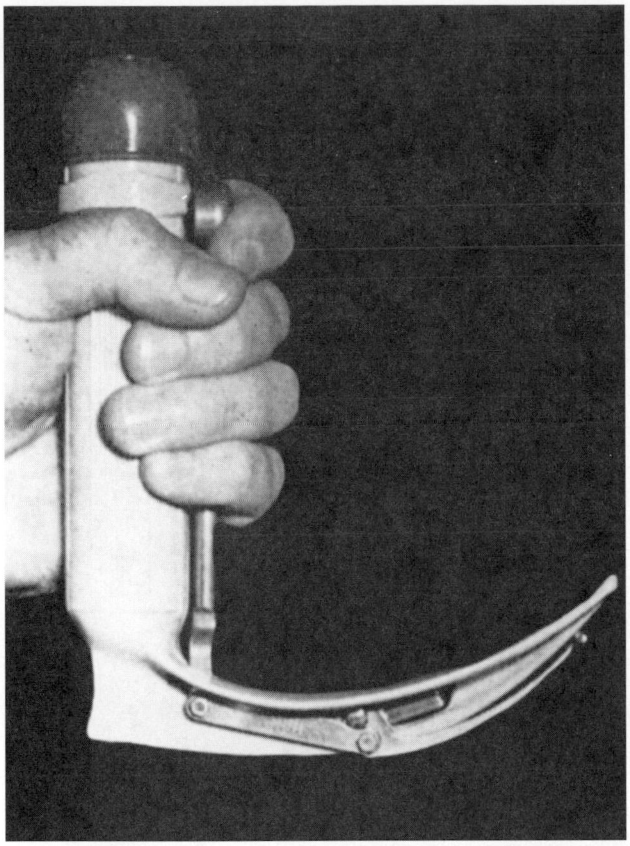

Figure 5-24 The laryngoscope is held like a hammer in the left hand. (From GC Grant: A new laryngoscope, Anesthes Intens Care V(3):263, 1977.)

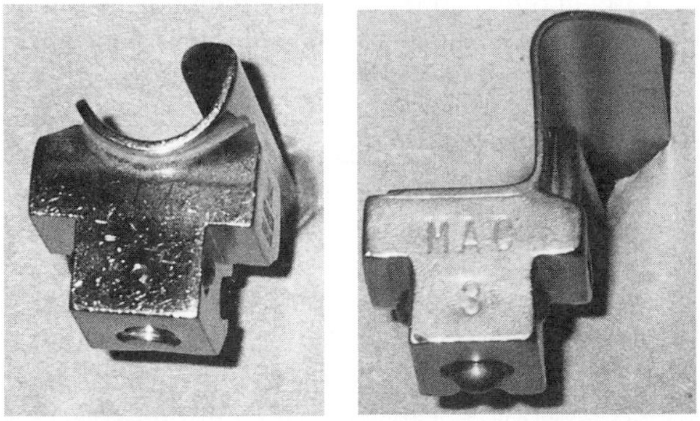

Figure 5-25 Cross-section of straight and curved blades. The broad flange of the curved blade gives better tongue control and working room during intubation.

head. The head should be far enough away from the mouth to allow binocular vision (Figure 5-26, **A** and **B**). In **B,** the intubator is too close to the airway, and depth perception is compromised. In general, if the laryngoscope arm is 45 degrees or more at the elbow, eye distance will be correct. In difficult intubations, the larynx is often described as being anteriorly placed, which means that the laryngeal opening is above the field of vision. A malleable

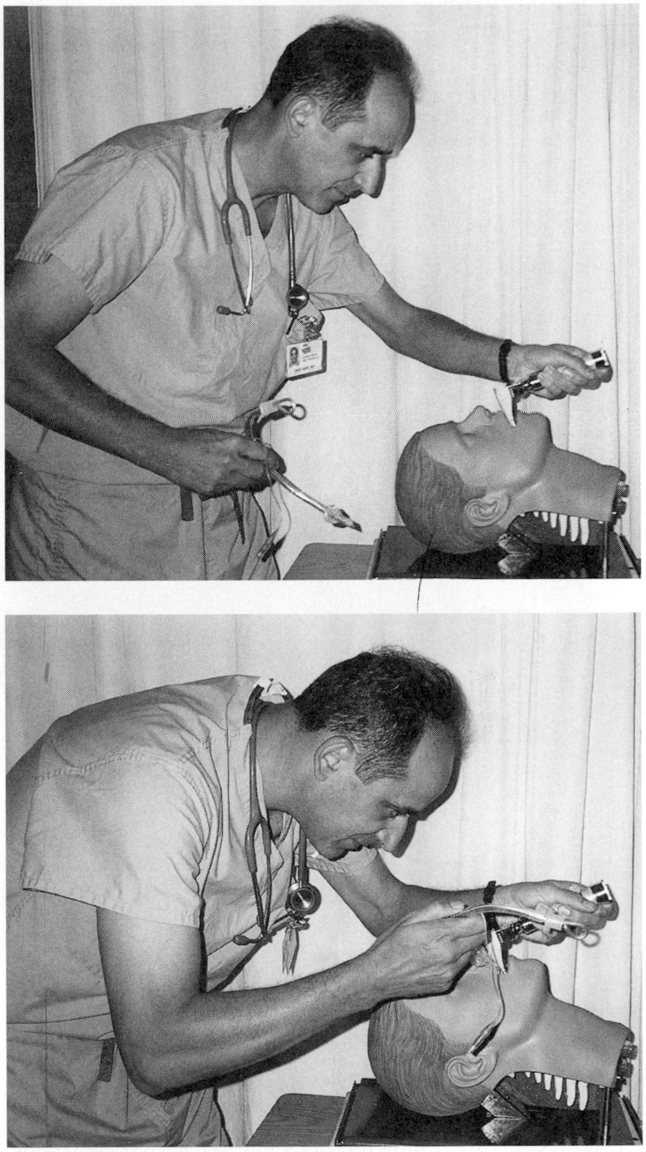

Figure 5-26 **A,** The correct head to trachea distance during intubation allows depth perception to be maintained. **B,** Being too close to the airway does not allow the proper distance to be perceived, so intubation is more difficult.

stylette can be inserted into the ET to provide stiffness and be bent to give the tube an upward hook at its end. This so-called "hockey stick curve" is very useful if the problem is an anterior location of the larynx. Intubation can often be accomplished with this curved tip, even if a direct laryngeal view is not possible. So that it can be easily withdrawn, the stylette should be lubricated before it is placed into the ET. Another solution to controlling the ET tip is the Endotrol Tube (Mallinckrodt Medical, Inc.). With this device, an implanted string with a pull-ring turns the tip anterior when pulled (Figure 5-27). This device is particularly well-suited for blind **nasotracheal intubation.**

When the larynx cannot be seen, it may be possible to pass a rigid stylette blindly into the trachea. The Eschelmann

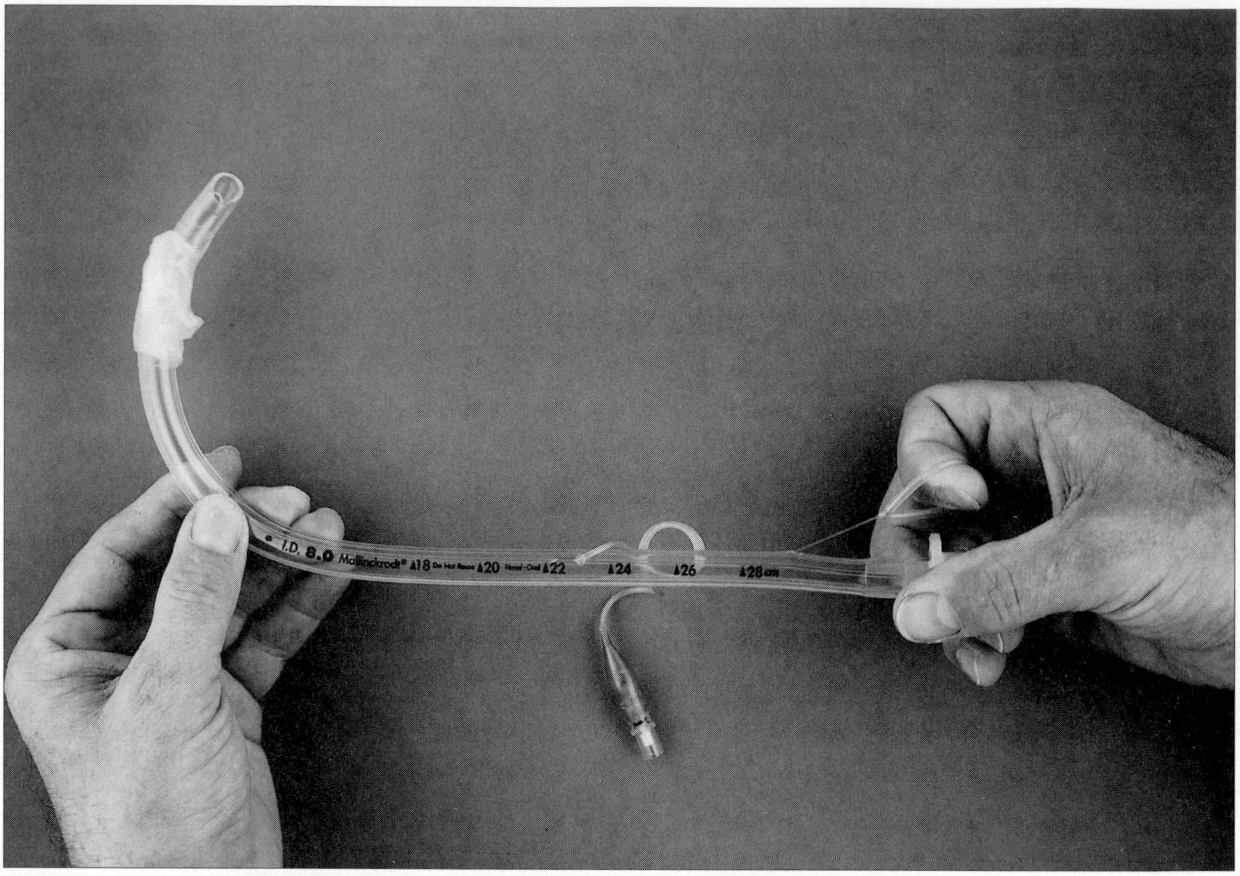

Figure 5-27 The Endotrol Tube has a string that when pulled directs the tip anteriorly during intubation attempts.

stylette or the gum elastic bougie is such a device. A characteristic washboard feeling is obtained when the device is advancing down the trachea over the tracheal rings. An ET can be threaded over the stylette to obtain intubation.

Lighted stylettes can be used to blindly place ETs in spontaneously breathing patients. In a darkened room, the light at a the tip of the ET can be seen through the tissues of the neck. A characteristic V-shaped shadow is seen when the tube is directly in the trachea. The ET is then slid off the stylette into the trachea.

Nasotracheal intubation is usually performed in spontaneously breathing, semiconscious individuals. As with nasopharyngeal airway insertion, a well-lubricated ET is inserted posteriorly, directly through the nasopharynx. Topical local anesthetics and vasoconstrictors should reduce patient discomfort and bleeding. Instead of the sniffing position, a neutral or slightly flexed head position is optimal for blind nasal intubation. Breath sounds or moisture in the tube is used to identify the tip location and the timing of tube advancement. Breath sounds or moisture disappears when the tube enters the esophagus. ETs are placed just above the larynx and rapidly advance 1 to 2 cm during inspiration when the cords are maximally abducted. If tracheal topical anesthesia is not used, a vigorous cough will follow successful tracheal intubation. Turning the head to one side or the other or flexing it further, or pushing the thyroid cartilage posteriorly may lead to success. Use of the fiberoptic bronchoscope may be necessary to complete nasotracheal intubation in some difficult settings. A nasally inserted ET tube can be directed anteriorly into the trachea using a laryngoscope in the mouth and Magill forceps, although care must be taken not to rip the cuff with the sharp teeth of the Magill forceps.

Fiberoptic laryngoscopy allows ET insertion by using the scope as a guide. The ET is threaded over the scope before endoscopy, but the standard ET connector needs to be removed first. Once the airway is entered, the tube can be guided over the scope and into the trachea. This technique can be used for oral or nasal intubation. Skill in fiberoptic examination of the unintubated patient is a prerequisite for this technique (Box 5-1).

Blind oral ET insertion techniques have been described. Using two fingers to retract the epiglottis and direct the tube tip anteriorly can result in proper placement. The Berman intubating airway (Berman II) is an oropharyngeal airway with a hooked end and an open channel for an ET. The ET is placed through the channel while the tip is used to lift the

BOX 5-1

Decision Making & Problem Solving

A 56-year old man who has experienced cardiopulmonary arrest is admitted to the emergency department. Several attempts to insert an ET have not established a definitive and secure airway. What alternative methods could be used to establish a secure airway for this patient?

See Appendix A for answer.

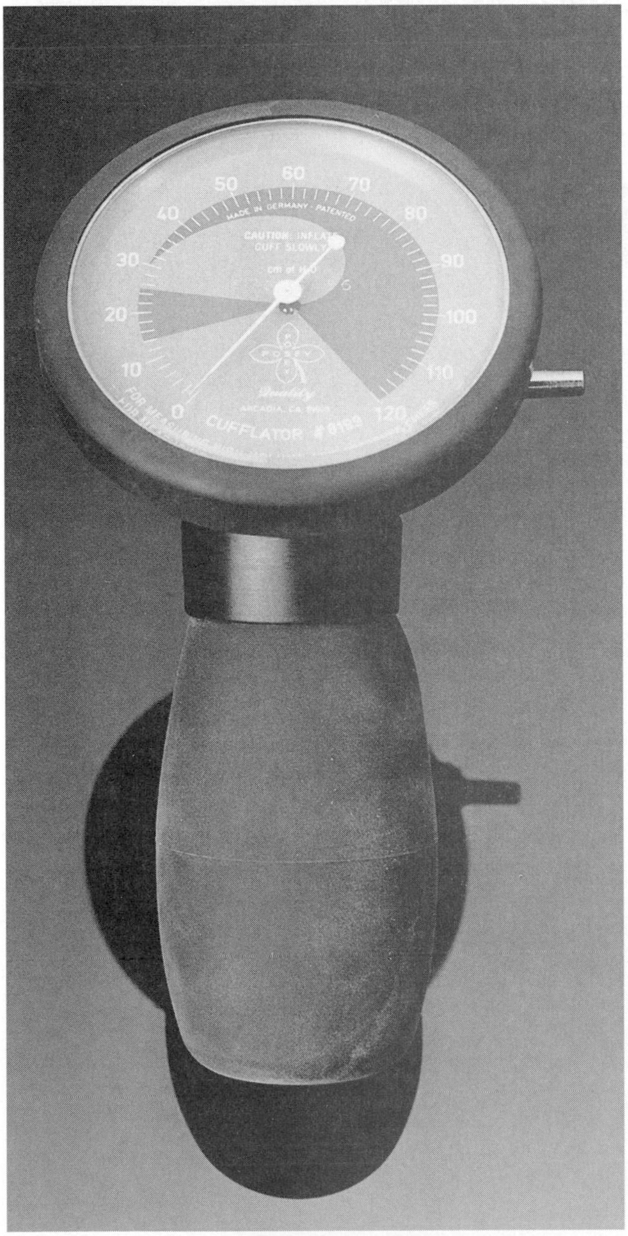

Figure 5-28 A device for measuring ET cuff pressure.

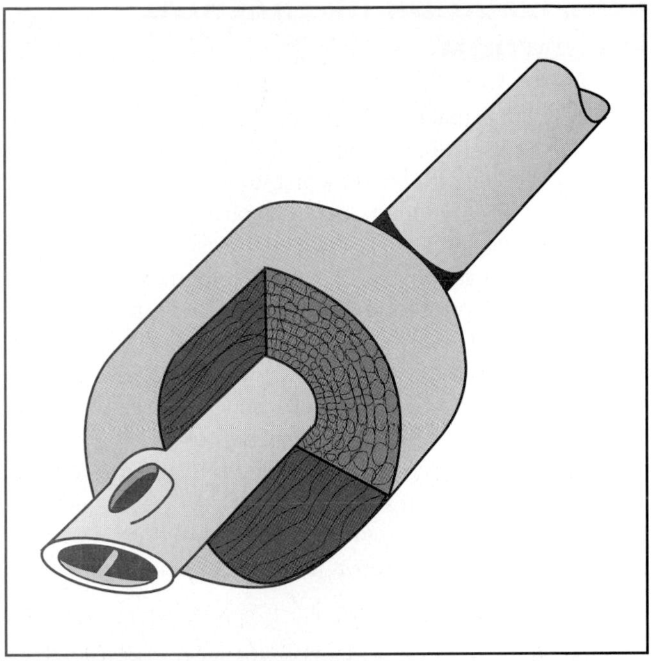

Figure 5-29 An ET tube with a self-inflating, foam-filled cuff.

vallecula. The tube can be passed into the trachea blindly and then dislodged from the open channel of the airway.

Once the ET is in place in the trachea, the cuff can be used to form a seal with the tracheal wall. Usually, air is inflated through the one-way valve in the pilot balloon until a seal forms or high pressure develops. Most ET cuffs are large-volume, low-pressure devices meant to contact a large portion of the tracheal wall with a low pressure. Because of tracheal mucosal blood pressure-flow characteristics, cuff pressure should be below 25 cm Hg to prevent tracheal damage. A manometer for determining and regulating cuff pressure is shown in Figure 5-28. If a manometer is not available, a "just seal" or "minimal seal" technique can be used to minimize the lateral tracheal wall pressure from the inflated cuff. For some patients who require high airway pressure for mechanical ventilation, cuff pressure cannot be kept below 25 cm Hg without significant volume loss. Whatever pressure is needed should be used to guarantee adequate ventilation and protection from aspiration. An alternative to an inflatable cuff is a self-inflating one that is filled with foam (Figure 5-29). Prior to insertion, this type of cuff must be actively deflated and clamped, then the clamp is removed and the cuff is allowed to expand to form a seal. There is no valve in the pilot port of foam-filled cuffs. A common problem with ETs is that they are inserted or migrate too far into the trachea, so the cuff may obstruct a bronchus, or only one lung may be ventilated. Right mainstem intubation is most common, especially in children, because the angle of take-off of the right main bronchus is less than that of the left.

Confirmation of Tracheal Intubation

Objective confirmation of tracheal placement, rather than esophageal intubation, is imperative. This is especially true after intubating with a blind technique. The best way to confirm correct placement is to detect expired carbon dioxide is with a capnograph or a color-change device; however, these devices will not detect carbon dioxide when cardiac output is profoundly depressed (e.g., during chest compressions for cardiac arrest). The esophageal detection device (a rubber bulb attached to the ET) will rapidly reinflate if the ET is in the trachea, but will remain collapsed if the ET is in the esophagus (Figure 5-30). This device does not depend on cardiac function to confirm correct tube placement. False positive and negative results have been reported by this device in obese and pregnant patients. *Auscultation should be performed in at least three areas after intubation.* This examination should evidence bilateral thoracic breath sounds, but no audible sounds over the gastric area. Sounds from esophageal and gastric ventilation can be heard transmitted to the chest. Directly viewing the trachea with a bronchoscope passed through the ET is another way to confirm correct placement. Chest radiography (anterior-posterior view) is useful for confirming the tube depth in the chest relative to the carina—but not the correct location within the trachea. A lateral film can identify tracheal rather than esophageal placement, but the other techniques described give quick feedback of incorrect placement in enough time to prevent disaster (Box 5-2).

Surgical Airway Devices

On rare occasions, the establishment of a patent airway with the previously described techniques (i.e., head posi-

Figure 5-30 Esophageal detection device. (Courtesy ARC Medical, Inc.)

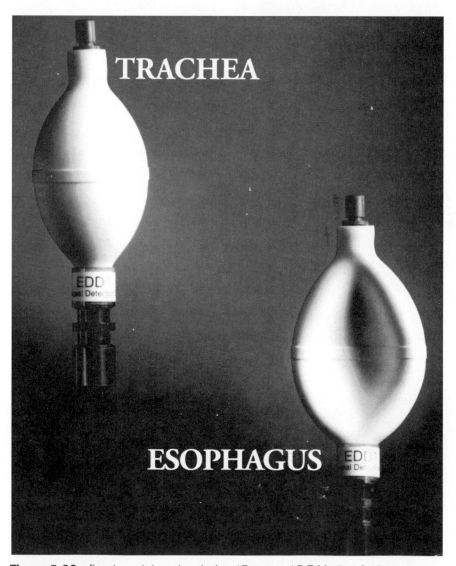

BOX 5-2

Decision Making & Problem Solving

After an emergency intubation of a patient in the surgical intensive care unit (SICU), a capnometer is attached to the ET to confirm its placement. The indicator shows a carbon dioxide level of zero. How would you interpret this finding?

See Appendix A for answer.

tion, oral and nasal airways, LMA, and Combitube) is unsuccessful, and the patient becomes hypoxic. Invasive airway access should be quickly established to prevent death or severe brain injury. In experienced hands, one brief intubation trial may be attempted before transtracheal needle or tube placement in such circumstances. The simplest invasive airway device is a large-bore intravenous catheter inserted percutaneously through the cricothyroid membrane. This easily identified space is between the thyroid cartilage and the cricoid ring. A 14-gauge or larger catheter over a needle intravenous device is attached to a syringe and inserted through the cricothyroid membrane. Continuous aspiration is applied until air returns, then the catheter is passed over the needle into the trachea (Figure 5-31). To provide adequate gas delivery through a tracheal needle, a high-pressure gas source (50 psi) must be used. A pressure interrupter or Saunders valve (Figure 5-32) must be attached to the catheter with a Luer-Lok system to prevent disconnection from the catheter during ventilation. Expiration is passive and occurs through the upper airway. With brief jets of gas, normal ventilation and oxygenation can be maintained with this technique. *To be successful in an emergency, the proper equipment must be assembled and ready for use ahead of time.* Complications of needle-jet ventilation include formation of a false passage, development of subcutaneous emphysema, creation of a pneumothorax, bleeding, failure to ventilate, and damage to neck structures.

A cricothyroidotomy is a surgical incision in the trachea that passes through the cricothryroid membrane. A

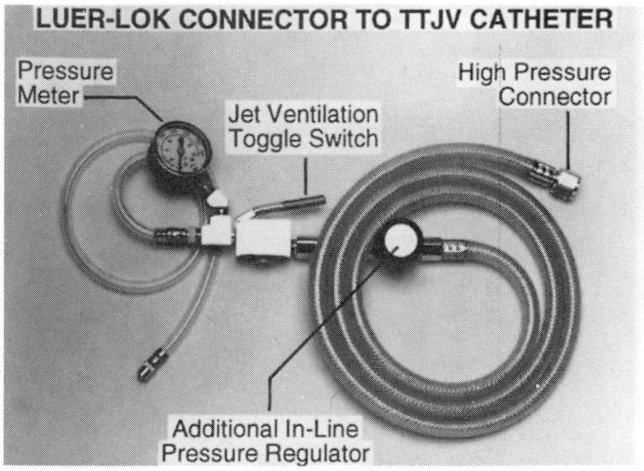

Figure 5-32 A high-pressure jet ventilator system. (From Benumof JL: Airway management: principles and practice, St Louis, 1996, Mosby.)

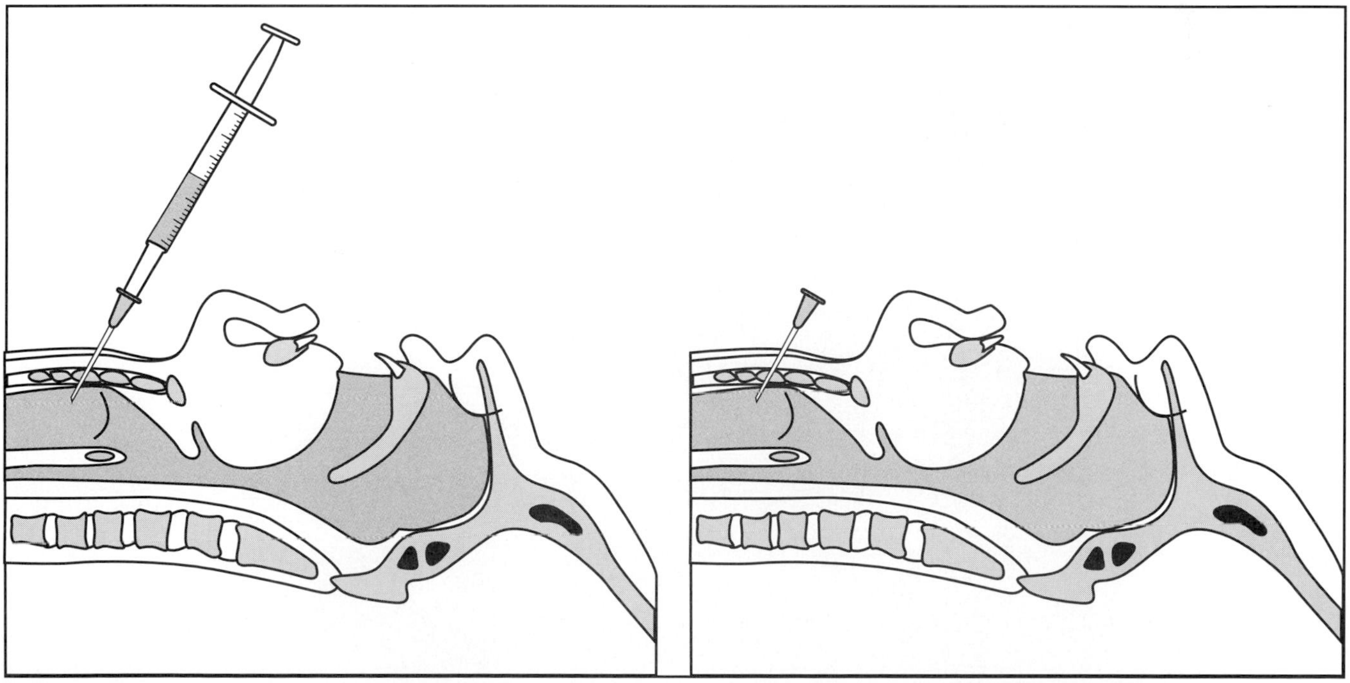

Figure 5-31 Transtracheal jet ventilation can be performed through a large-bore intravenous catheter placed through the cricothyroid membrane.

conventional ET or tracheostomy tube can be placed through the incision. Routine airway equipment can be used to provide ventilation and oxygen delivery with the tube in place. A single, horizontal, slash incision through the skin to the trachea is performed. Bleeding is usually minimal because no large vascular structures lie in the area of the incision. Complications include false placement and failure to provide adequate gas exchange, bleeding, and damage to other neck structures. Subglottic or laryngeal stenosis may be a long-term problem following cricothyroidotomy. Most authorities suggest elective conversion of an emergency cricothyroidotomy to a formal tracheostomy to reduce the likelihood to these dreaded problems.

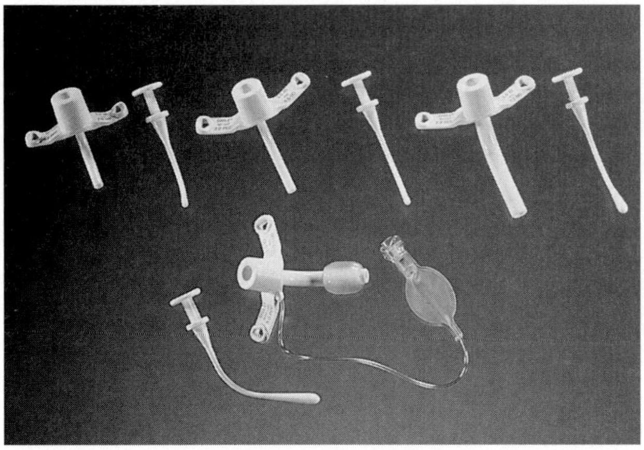

Figure 5-33 A conventional cuffed TT. (Courtesy of Shiley, Mallinckrodt, St Louis.)

TRACHEOSTOMY TUBES

Similar to an ET, a tracheostomy tube (TT) consists of a round, plastic tube—with or without a cuff, pilot balloon, and valve—but with a standard 15-mm connector (Figure 5-33). Metal TTs are occasionally used to maintain a patent stoma, allow for suctioning, or gradually reduce the stoma size. These tubes are rarely equipped with a cuff and need adapters to be mated with standard airway equipment. TTs are bent at a 90 degree angle to fit flat against the skin and lie parallel to the axis of the trachea. Similar to ETs, sizes are assigned as the internal diameter in millimeters, although the use of French sizes is still popular. TTs are generally more rigid than ETs, although more flexible TTs are now available that are less likely to kink and must be carefully selected to fit the patient correctly. TTs typically have a collar that is used to secure the tube. The distance from the collar to the bend, the length of the tube distal to the bend (Figure 5-34), and the size and shape of the cuff vary by manufacturer and may be quite different. Some tubes have movable collars that accommodate different skin-to-tracheal distances. The standard fitting may be part of a removable connector or inner cannula. TTs are usually placed occluded with a blunt, solid obturator that makes passage through the tissues less traumatic and less difficult. The obturator is removed once the tube is in place but should remain with the patient and be conveniently available to reinsert the TT if it is accidentally dislodged. Some surgeons place strong, tagging sutures at the corners of the tracheal incision that can be grasped and pulled forward to expose the tract and facilitate reinserting a displaced TT. *If ventilation is difficult after urgent replacement of a dislodged TT,*

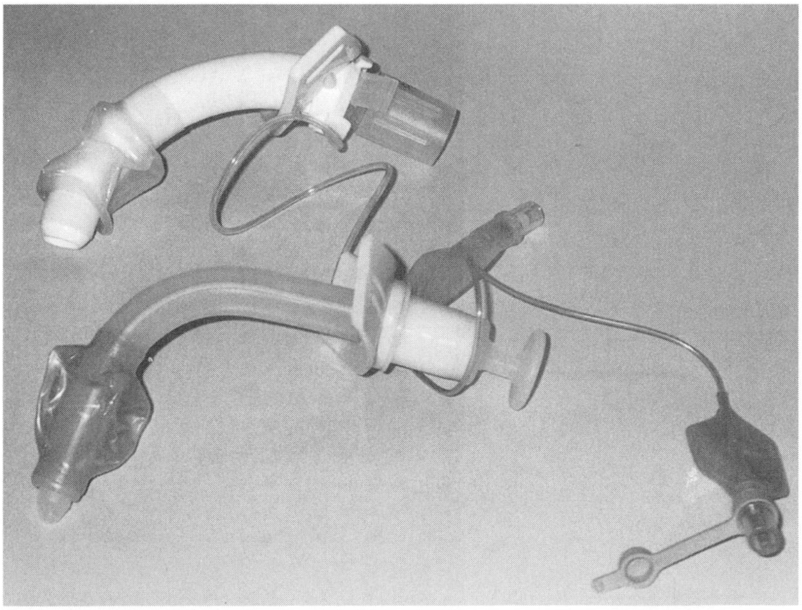

Figure 5-34 TTs come in preformed shapes with lengths that are not standardized.

it may not lie in the trachea, and manual ventilation through the upper airway should be initiated without delay. TT cuffs are various sizes and, like ET cuffs, can cause mucosal ischemia if overpressurized. Cuff pressure monitoring and pressure reduction are a method of reducing complications associated with placement of TTs.

Although modern materials are less toxic than the hard rubber from which ETs and TTs were originally made, these artificial airways can damage the structures through which they pass. Translaryngeal airways can damage the nasal septum, the tongue, and the larynx, as well as the trachea from cuff pressure and tip trauma. TTs can cause damage at cuff and tip locations as well as at the stoma. Severe vocal cord damage and laryngeal stenosis are dreaded complications from **translaryngeal intubation.** They are difficult to treat and may permanently disable the patient. These complications increase with the duration of intubation and the larger diameter of the tube. If the need for tracheal intubation exceeds 2 to 3 weeks in adults, a tracheostomy is usually performed to decrease laryngeal complications. Trauma from the tube cuff or tip can result in tracheal ulcers, cartilage loss, malacia, or rupture, which are complications of both TTs and ETs. Granulation tissue may form at the TT stoma; and after removal of the TT, stenosis at the stomal site may occur in up to 10% of patients. Treatment of these complications is difficult and often requires resecting of tracheal segments or placement of a stent.

With intubation, the patient's ability to speak is lost. This loss of control can lead to psychological stress. Several methods for allowing semi-normal speech with a tracheostomy have been developed. A fenestrated TT is one in which there is a hole in the curved portion of the tube above the cuff that can be used to allow air to pass into the upper airway through the larynx so that normal speech is possible (Figure 5-35). When positive-pressure ventilation is needed, an inner, nonfenestrated cannula can be inserted. A one-way valve attached to the TT will allow inspiration from the TT and exhalation upward through the larynx. Two available devices, the Passy-Muir valve and the Olympic Trach-Talk, are shown in Figures 5-36 and 5-37. These devices can only be used in patients capable of initiating and maintaining spontaneous ventilation. Obviously, without an open upper airway, unobstructed fenestration, or a deflated TT cuff, a lethal, closed system with no portal for exhalation would exist. *When attaching one-way valves to patients with artificial airways, careful observation for immediate problems with exhalation is essential* (Box 5-3). In patients unable to sustain unaided ventilation, an extra port on the TT can be used to provide gas flow through the larynx. The Pitt Speaking TT in Figure 5-38 was designed for this purpose. Speech with it is usually only a whisper. Vibrating devices can be used in the mouth or on the neck to produce audible speech when mouthing words. Restoration of the ability to speak in patients with artificial airways can improve the patient's mood, increase cooperation with caregivers, and accelerate recovery.

Once the need for a TT no longer exists, the patient should be weaned from his tracheostomy. If the tube is simply removed and the stoma covered with an occlusive dressing, the stoma will close in several days. Some clinicians prefer to gradually reduce the TT size every few days until only a small tube is in place. If direct tracheal access—but not ventilation—is needed for a longer time, several devices can be used to keep a stoma patent. A 4-mm, uncuffed metal or silastic TT allows tracheal suctioning and causes very little airway obstruction in most adult patients. If reinsertion of a larger, cuffed tube is later needed, the tract can be easily dilated to accommodate a larger tube. Another device used to maintain a tracheostomy stoma is the Olympic button shown in Figure 5-39. It protrudes slightly into the airway but is usually less obstructive than a small TT. It is usually kept capped or plugged unless airway access is needed; it cannot be effectively used to provide positive-pressure ventilation but can be exchanged for a cuffed TT if necessary.

SPECIALIZED ETs

Occasionally, it is desirable to provide a different kind of ventilatory support to each lung, and specialized ETs that allow independent lung ventilation are available. These tubes were developed for bronchoalveolar lavage (to treat alveolar proteinosis) and performing differential lung function tests before a pneumonectomy. They have been refined and are frequently used to reduce risk during anesthesia for lung resection. Sometimes **double lumen ETs (DLET)** are used outside the operating room to protect the "good" lung from blood contamination in patients with massive hemoptysis. Probably the most common use of these devices outside the operating room is following single lung transplant when the compliance of the native lung

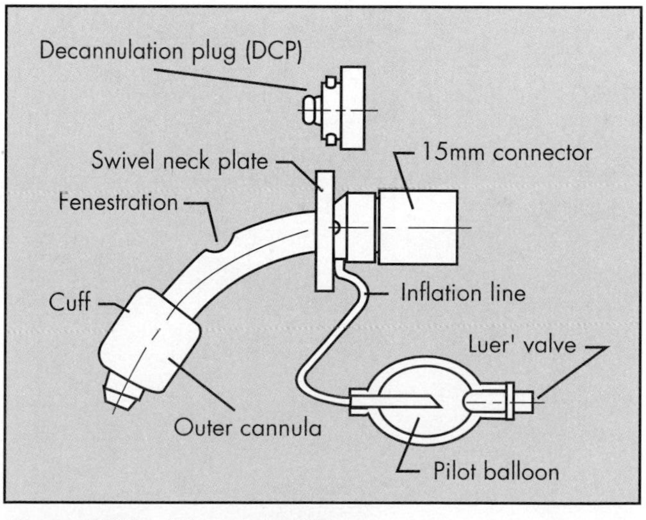

Figure 5-35 A fenestrated TT.

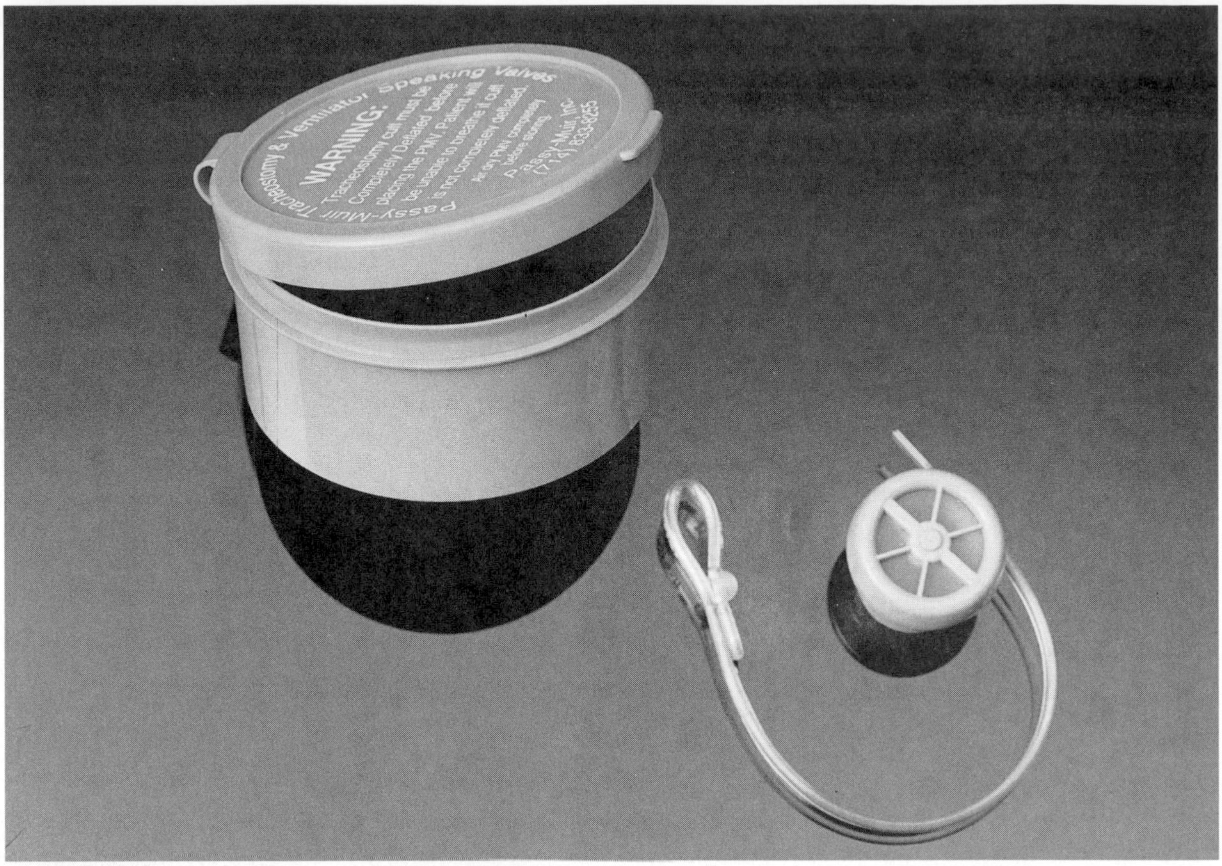

Figure 5-36 A Passy-Muir speaking tracheostomy valve.

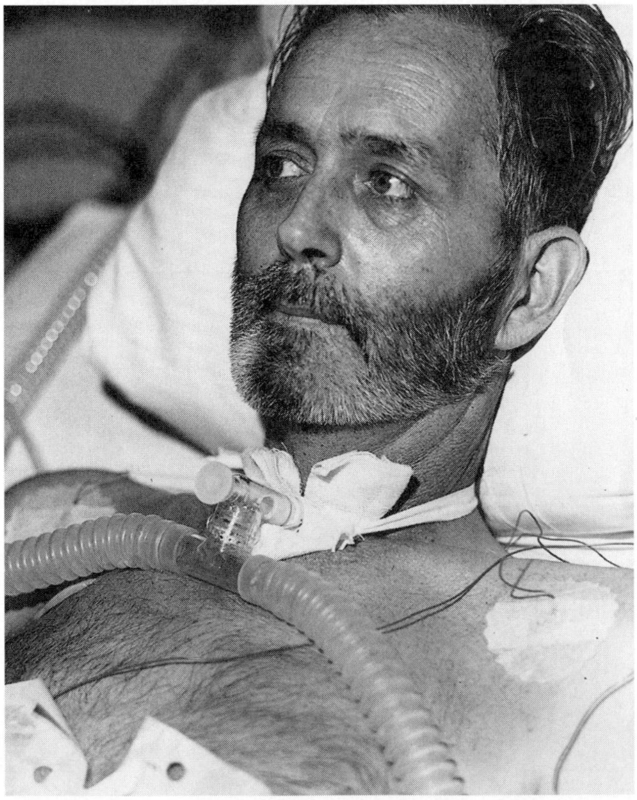

Figure 5-37 An Olympic Trach-Talk speaking device.

BOX 5-3

Decision Making & Problem Solving

A patient has a fenestrated TT in place. To evaluate the patient's ability to move air around the tube and into the upper airway, what procedure should the respiratory therapist perform?

See Appendix A for answer.

and that of the transplanted lung are very different. Two ventilator systems can be used to titrate appropriate support for each lung independently. DLETs consist of two separate, semicircular lumens fused together. At the tip, one lumen terminates in a right or left main bronchial tube with a small cuff. The other terminates in the trachea below the tracheal cuff to provide ventilation to the other lung. Two standard adapters and pilot balloons are present (Figure 5-40).

If possible, only left-sided DLETs should be used. They seat more easily (with less of an acute angle of take-off from the left main bronchus), and the bronchial cuff will not occlude the upper lobe bronchus. The right upper lobe

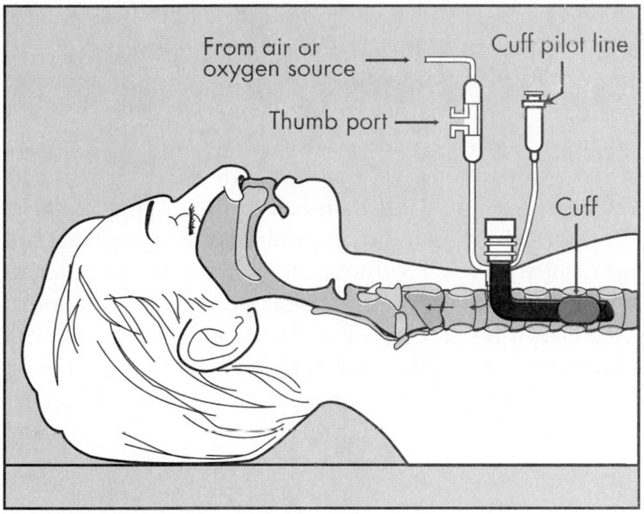

Figure 5-38 A Pittsburgh speaking TT.

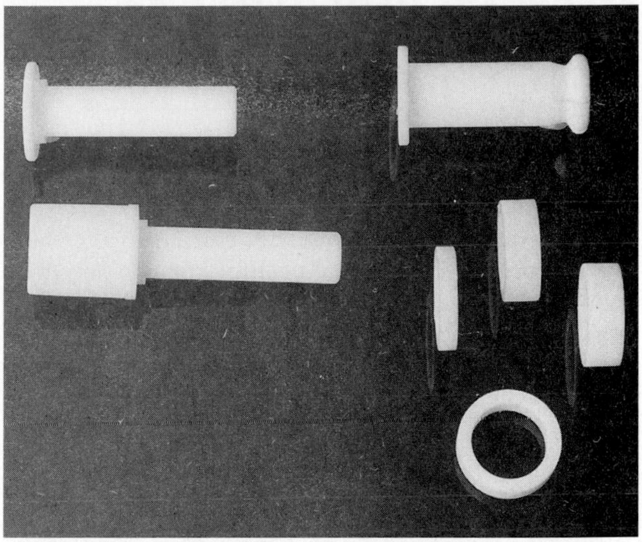

Figure 5-39 An Olympic tracheostomy button.

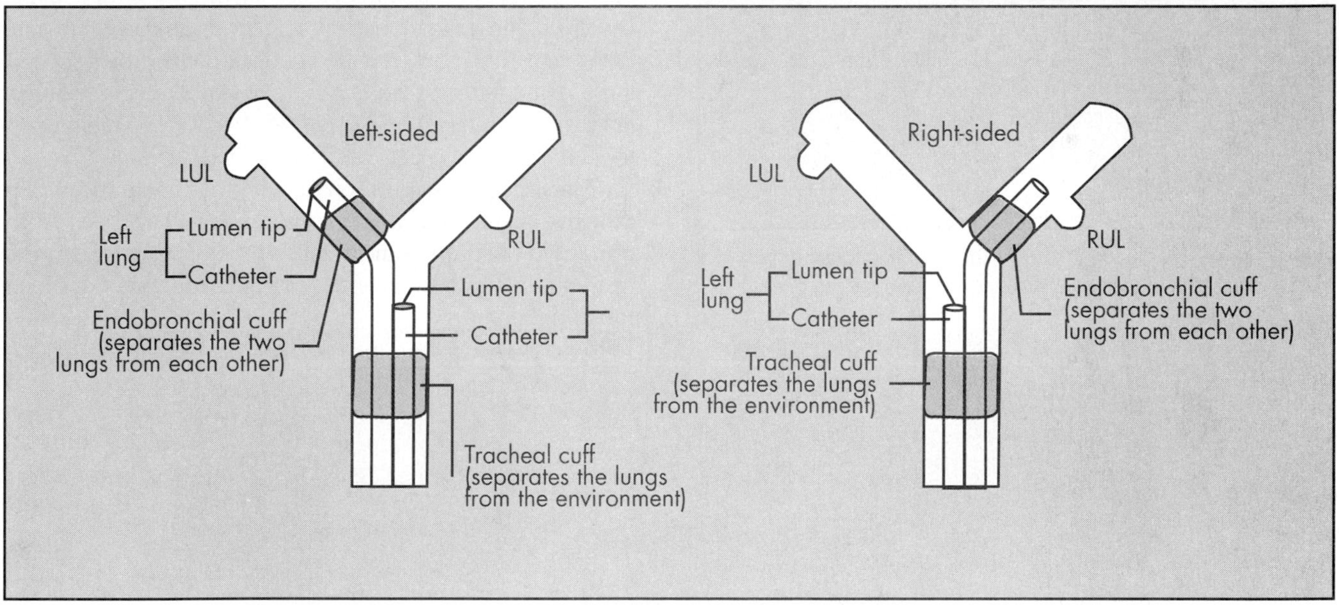

Figure 5-40 A DLET.

bronchial take-off is only 1 to 2 cm from the carina, and it is likely that the bronchial cuff will occlude the upper lobe bronchus if a right-sided tube is placed. A recent modification of right-side cuff design (i.e., placing the cuff diagonally on the bronchial lumen) may decrease this problem (Figure 5-41). Although physical examination with sequential occlusion of individual lumens can be used to confirm proper seating of DLETs, direct visualization with a small fiberoptic bronchoscope passed through the tracheal lumen is a more reliable method of confirming correct placement. The bronchial cuff should be just visible below the carina. Tubes are in French sizes: 35 and 37 are usually used for average women; 39 and 41 for average men. The bronchial cuff should take from 1 to 3 cc of air to seal if the correct-size tube has been chosen and the cuff is properly seated. A high-pressure bronchial seal should be avoided because bronchial stenosis is a devastating injury that may result. Because of their bulk and rigidity, DLETs are often difficult to place through the larynx. Prolonged intubation attempts may be necessary. This is especially true with an airway full of blood in a patient with massive hemoptysis. Although the idea of using a DLET in patients with massive hemoptysis is appealing, the technical issues of placement can be daunting. Other specialized ETs may have distal airway channels. One is the Hi-Lo Jet ET (Mallinckrodt Medical Inc.), in which the additonal lumen can be used for distal airway pressure monitor jet ventilation (Figure 5-42). Another specialized ET has lumens designed for tracheal drug delivery (Figure 5-43).

Equipment Used to Manage Artificial Airways

Intubated patients have their upper airways bypassed. Humidifying and warming inspired gases are primary functions of the upper airway. Active or passive humidification systems should be used in patients using ETs for a prolonged period. Even with these devices, airway secretions may be increased because of tracheal irritation and thickened from inadequate humidification or infection. The ability to cough is severely compromised because the glottis cannot be closed when the patient is intubated. Secretions must be aspirated from the lung in most intubated patients. Suction catheters are illustrated in Figure 5-44. Suction catheters are available in a variety of sizes and designs, but it is generally recommended that the catheter diameter should be less than half of the internal diameter of the artificial airway. It is important to recognize that suction catheters are sized according to the tube's outer diameter (French size). Conversion from inner to outer diameter can be accomplished by multiplying the internal diameter by 3 and then dividing the product by 2. For example, a size 8.0 (inner diameter) TT requires a 12 French catheter.

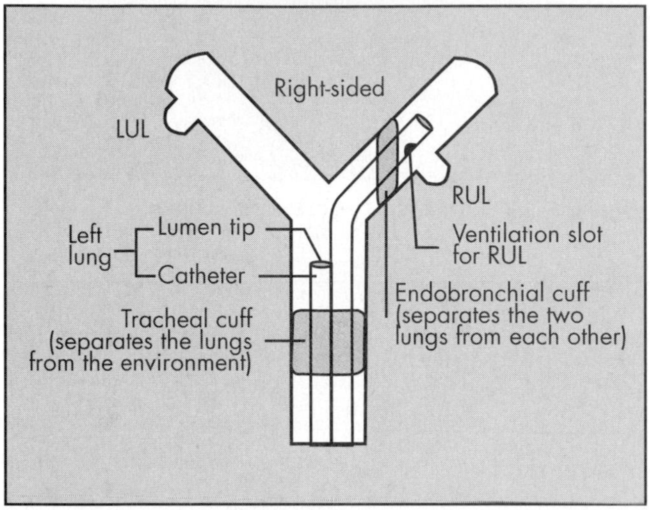

Figure 5-41 A diagonal cuff on the endobronchial lumen may decrease incidence of obstruction of the right upper lobe bronchus.

$$(8.0 \times 3) \div 2 = 12 \text{ Fr}$$

Preoxygenation, sterile preparation, and standard precautions should be used during endotracheal suctioning. Inline closed-system suction devices (Figure 5-45) may reduce caregiver and patient risk of infectious disease exposure, lower costs, and compromise ventilation less during suctioning. Sterile sputum samples can be obtained using a **Lukens sputum trap** (Figure 5-46). Box 5-4 provides a sample protocol for suctioning patients with artificial airways.

Many devices have been developed to help secure ETs. Effective methods of securing these tubes are especially important in children. Judicious use of sedation and physical restraint are important for the comfort and safety of the intubated patient.

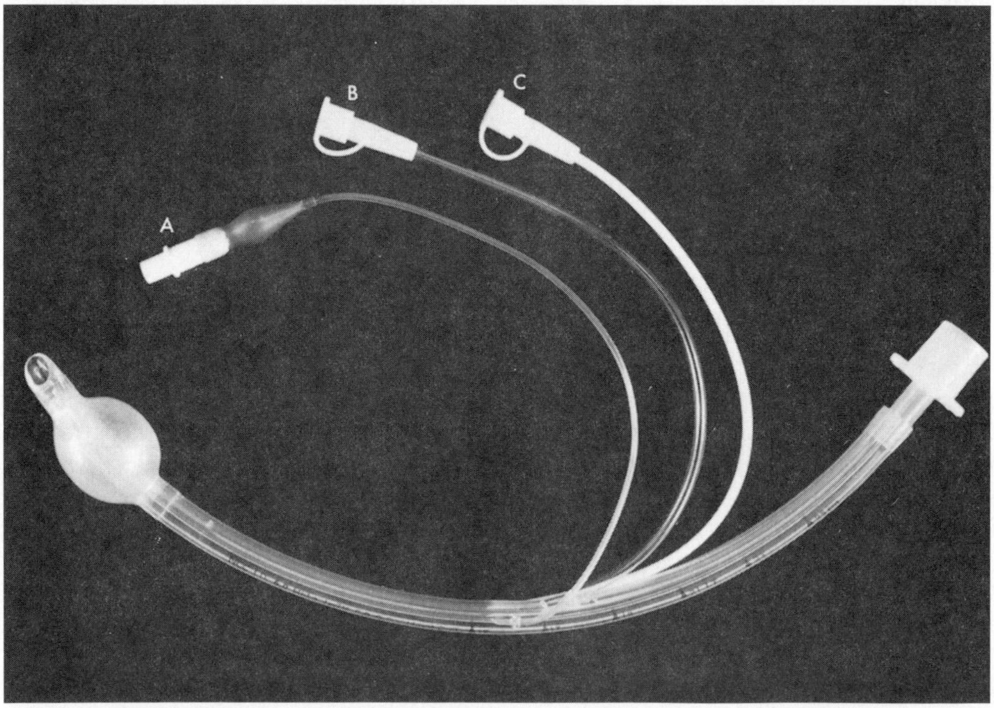

Figure 5-42 An ET with multiple lumens for jet ventilation and airway pressure measurement. (Courtesy Allegiance Medical Care, McGraw Park, Ill.)

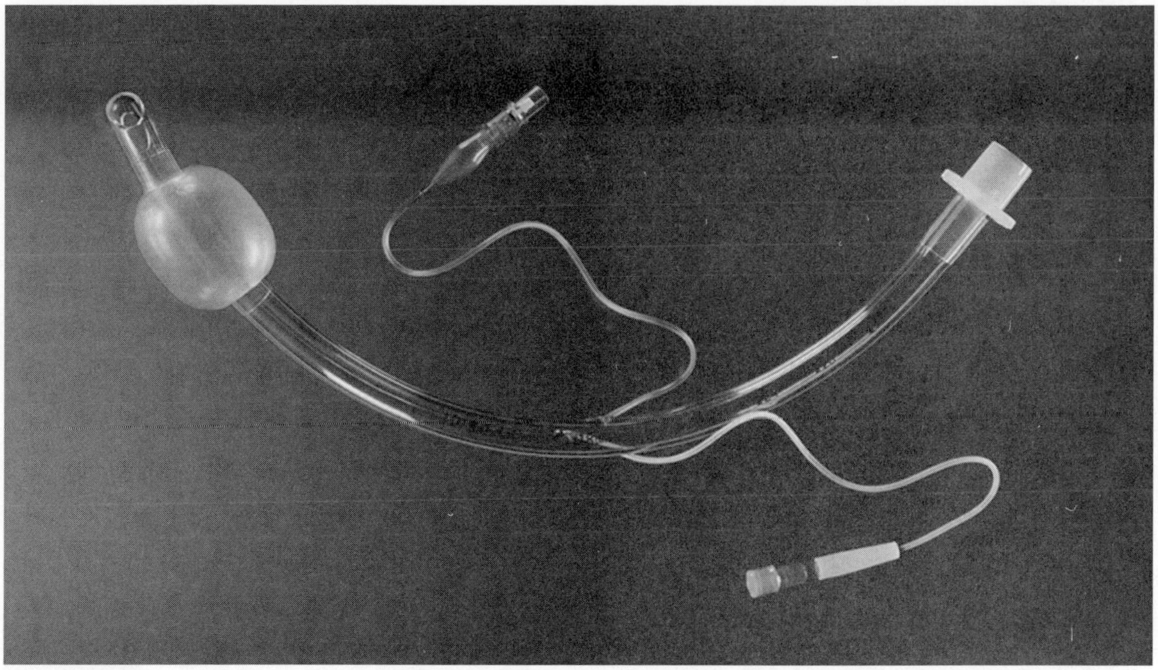

Figure 5-43 An ET with an additional port to be used for instillation of medications. (Courtesy Allegiance Medical Care, McGraw Park, Ill.)

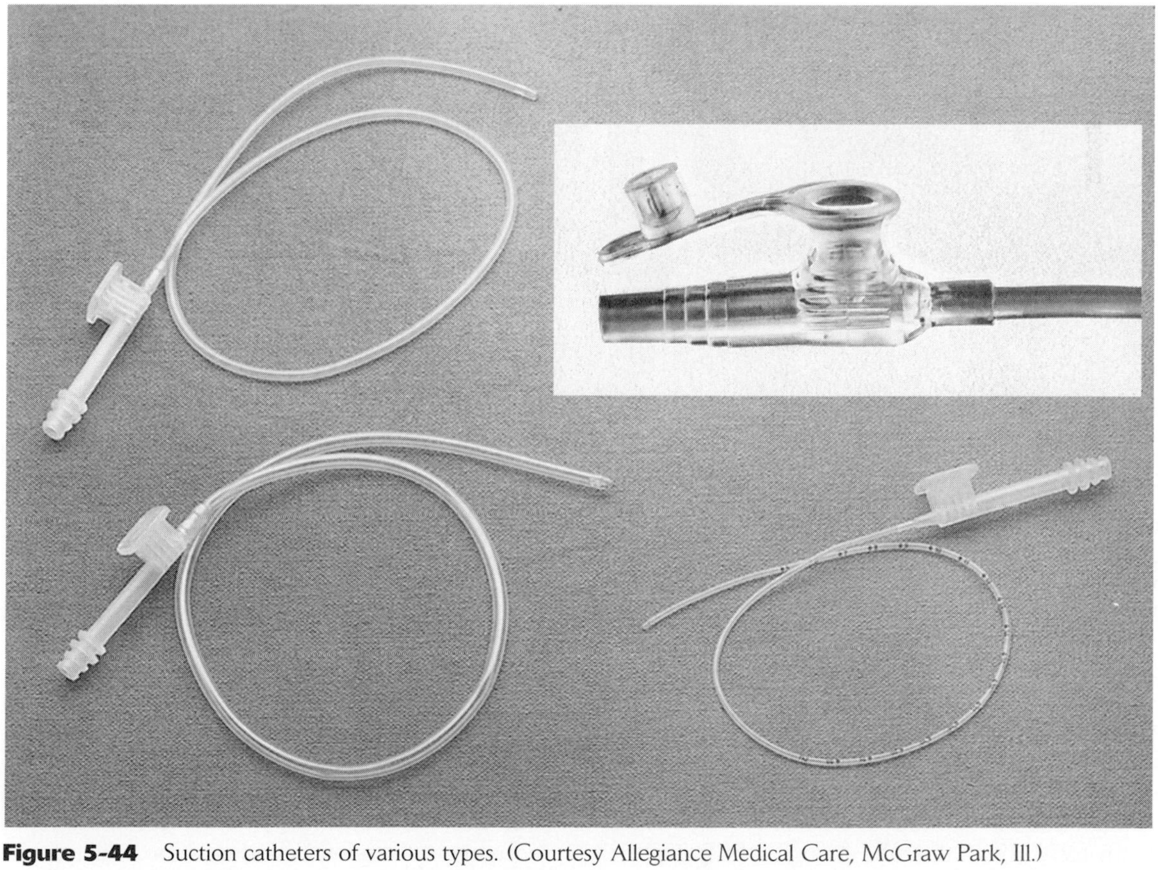

Figure 5-44 Suction catheters of various types. (Courtesy Allegiance Medical Care, McGraw Park, Ill.)

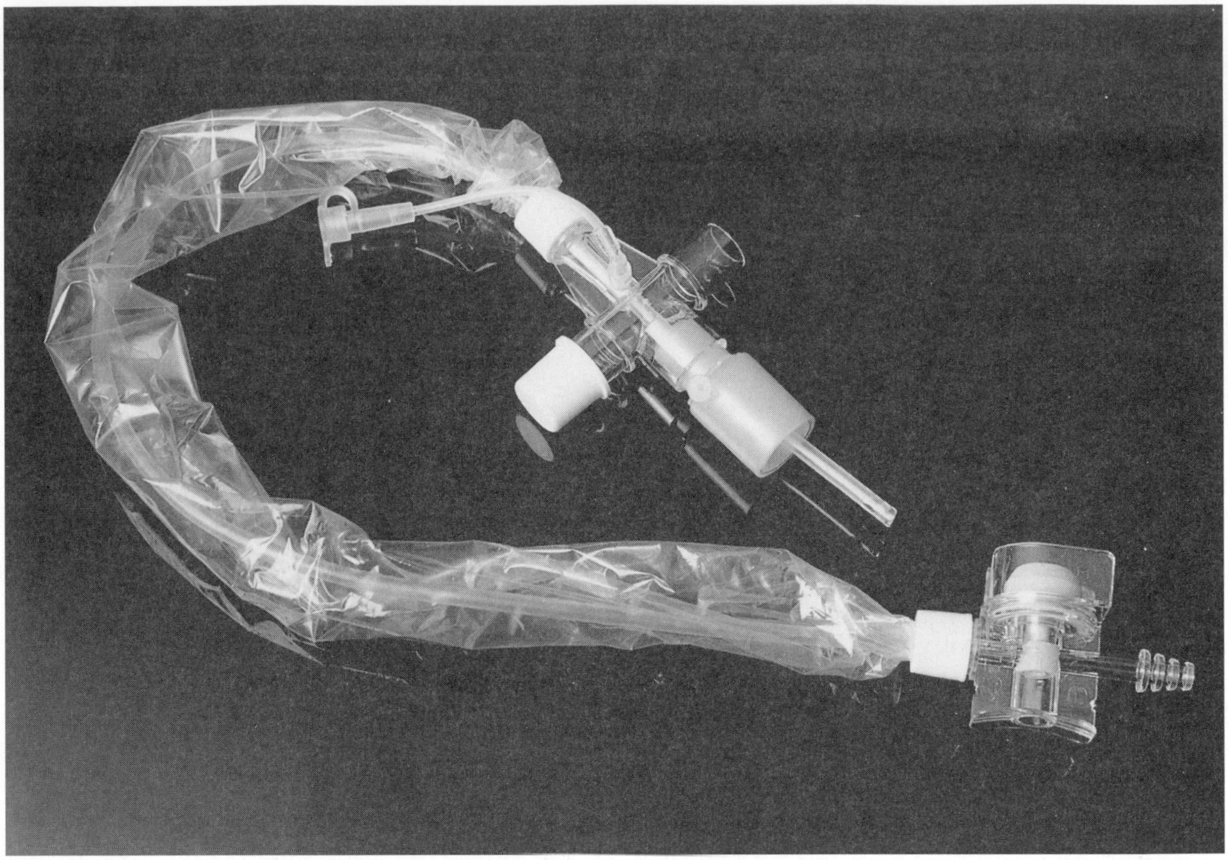

Figure 5-45 A closed-system suction catheter.

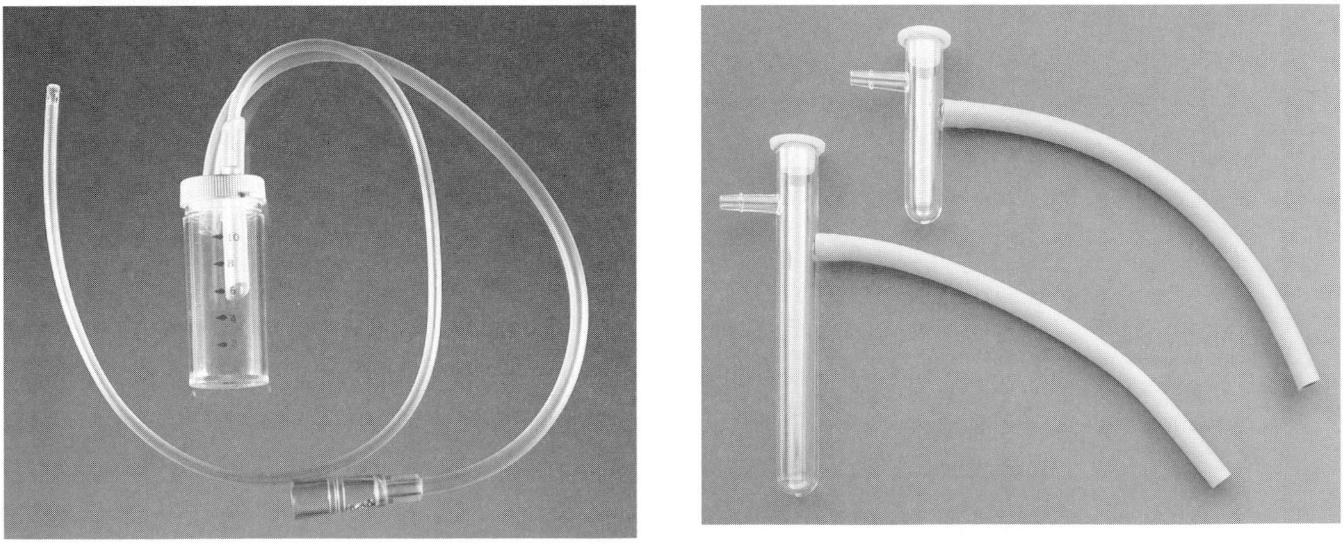

Figure 5-46 Uncontaminated sputum samples may be collected with a Lukens sputum trap. (Courtesy Allegiance Medical Care, McGraw Park, Ill.)

Changing an ET may pose significant risk to critically ill patients. A catheter designed specifically for this purpose is shown in Figure 5-47. The tube changer is inserted through the ET, and the tube is withdrawn and removed. Oxygen can be insufflated through the tube changer during the procedure. A new ET can be slipped over the tube changer and threaded down it into the lung. Occasionally, the new tube catches on the larynx and needs to be gently rotated into position, but this method is not always successful, so equipment for reintubation must be at hand.

BOX 5-4

Protocol for Suctioning Patients with Endotracheal Tubes

1. The following equipment should be available:
   a. Functional vacuum system that can generate pressures from 100 to 150 mm Hg.
   b. Suction catheter and sterile water or saline for instillation.
   c. Protective equipment, including gloves, masks, and eye protection.
   d. Pulse oximeter.
2. Explain the procedure to the patient.
3. Wash your hands with antibacterial soap. Glove both hands and attach the catheter to the vacuum system using aseptic technique.
4. Preoxygenate the patient with 100% oxygen for a minimum of 30 to 60 seconds before suctioning. Note the baseline heart rate, electrocardiogram (ECG) rhythm, and pulse oximeter saturation.
5. Advance the catheter without suctioning until an obstruction is detected. Apply suction and gently withdraw the catheter. Limit the suctioning time to 10 to 15 seconds or less if indicated by ECG and pulse oximeter readings. Instillation of several milliliters (1 to 3 mL) of sterile saline (0.9% NaCl) may help to decrease the viscosity of the secretions in patients with thick tenacious mucus.
6. Allow the patient to rest and provide postsuctioning oxygenation and hyperinflation.
7. Repeat the procedure only as needed. Note that the patient's mouth or trachea should not be suctioned after the nose.

From Ptevak DJ and Ward JJ: Airway management. In Burton GC, Hodgkin JE, and Ward JJ, editors: Respiratory care: a guide to clinical practice, ed 4, Philadelphia, 1997, JB Lippincott.

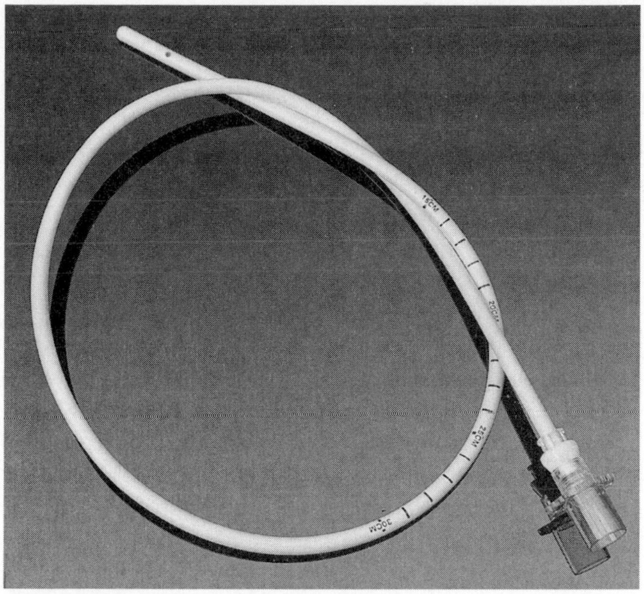

Figure 5-47 An ET tube changer.

A common indication for changing a tube is failure of the cuff to hold pressure. If the pilot balloon remains inflated, and the tube transiently seals when more air is added but quickly develops a leak again, the cuff has probably herniated through the vocal cords. This can be remedied by deflating the cuff completely, advancing the ET 2 to 3 cm, and reinflating the cuff. If the pilot balloon holds pressure while the syringe is attached but deflates when it is disconnected, the pilot-tube valve is probably defective. This can be overcome by inserting a stopcock into the valve, inflating the cuff, and turning the stopcock off toward the cuff. The pilot balloon and valve can be replaced with a blunt needle, and the stopcock inserted into the pilot tube after the balloon has been cut off (Figure 5-48). These methods of valve and pilot balloon repair may save patients the risk and trauma of reintubation.

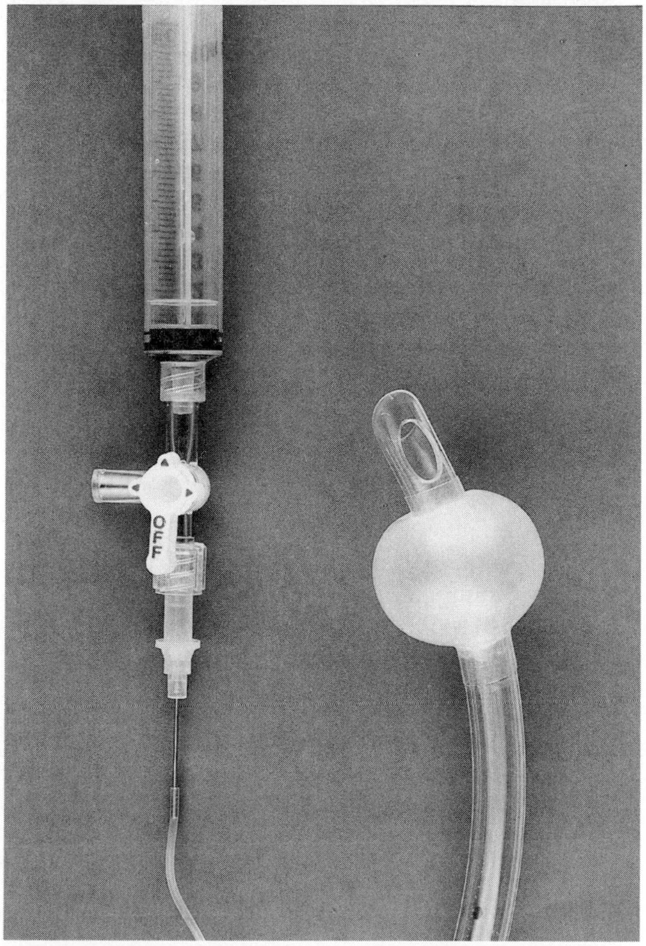

Figure 5-48 If the pilot balloon or pilot balloon valve fails to hold air, the entire assembly may be temporarily replaced by inserting a cut-off 19-gauge needle with a stopcock into the pilot tubing.

Summary

Inadequate gas exchange is an acute emergency. Failure to restore adequate respiratory gas exchange can result in hypoxic brain injury or death within minutes. Various devices, such as oral and nasopharyngeal airways, **laryngeal mask airways,** and Combitube, can be used in emergency situations to improve the patency of the upper airway and permit manual ventilation.

ETs and TTs are definitive devices for airway management, allowing for ventilation with high levels of positive pressure, as well as directing access to the lower airways for secretion removal and drug delivery. These devices also prevent aspiration of foreign materials into the lung, and allow bronchoscopic examination of the peripheral airways. Correct sizing, proper placement, and securing of ETs and TTs are essential for creating and maintaining an open airway.

Providing adequate, routine bronchial hygiene should be a primary concern of respiratory therapists caring for patients with ETs or TTs in place. Proper airway management can reduce caregiver and patient risk of infectious disease exposure and prevent many of the complications associated with artificial airways.

Review Questions

See Appendix A for answers.

1. The most important concern in an unconscious person is:
   a. establishing a patent airway
   b. calling for help
   c. administering oxygen by mask
   d. preventing aspiration
2. The laryngeal mask airway:
   a. is a definitive, secure airway
   b. can be easily inserted in a conscious patient
   c. bypasses upper airway obstructions
   d. can be used to provide positive-pressure ventilation in patients with reduced pulmonary compliance
3. A patient with a foam cuff tracheostomy tube:
   a. should have a syringe to inflate the cuff
   b. will need a stopcock on the pilot balloon to form a tracheal seal
   c. will have the pilot balloon valve "open" to seal the cuff
   d. should have the pilot balloon "tense" to guarantee a good seal
4. Which of the following is the preferred artificial airway for a liver patient who is vomiting blood?
   a. nasotracheal intubation with a cuffed tube
   b. oral intubation with a cuffed tube
   c. laryngeal mask airway
   d. cricothyroidotomy with a cuffed tube
5. A Combitube is placed in an unconscious patient. If breath sounds are clearly heard when ventilating through the pharyngeal lumen with both cuffs inflated, which of the following is true?
   a. a gastric tube should not be passed through the esophageal lumen
   b. the lung is not protected from aspiration
   c. oxygen should be added to the esophageal lumen
   d. more air should be placed in the pharyngeal cuff
6. When placing an appropriately sized oral pharyngeal airway, the flange protrudes out of the mouth. Attempts to insert it result in the device popping back out. This could be caused by:
   a. the airway catching on the back of the tongue
   b. using too small of an airway
   c. a foreign body in the pharynx
   d. false teeth
7. Which of the following is a complication of performing a cricothyroidotomy?
   a. gas embolism syndrome
   b. cervical spinal cord injury
   c. stroke
   d. subcutaneous emphysema
8. The most important concern with blind nasal intubation is:
   a. failure to recognize esophageal intubation
   b. nasal hemorrhage
   c. sinusitis
   d. loss of ability to speak
9. After oral intubation, there is no carbon dioxide during exhalation. This could be due to:
   a. esophageal intubation
   b. cardiac arrest
   c. low cardiac output
   d. all of the above
10. A patient has a 7.0 (inner diameter) TT in the trachea. What size suction tube should be used?
    a. 10 Fr
    b. 12 Fr
    c. 14 Fr
    d. 16 Fr
11. List three methods that can be used to confirm placement of an ET in the trachea rather than the esophagus.
12. A _____ laryngoscope blade should be used when attempting intubation of an average adult.
    a. #0
    b. #1
    c. #3
    d. #6

13. Which of the following are complications associated with TT placement?
    I. Hypoxia
    II. Hemorrhage
    III. Nerve injury
    IV. Gas dissection of the tissues surrounding the tracheotomy site
    a. I and II only
    b. II and III only
    c. I, II, and IV only
    d. I, II, III, and IV

14. Trauma from overinflation of an endotracheal tube cuff can result in:
    I. Tracheal ulcers
    II. Tracheal cartilage loss
    III. Tracheal malacia
    IV. Tracheal rupture
    a. I only
    b. I and II only
    c. II, III, and IV only
    d. I, II, III, and IV

15. The proper ET size for a premature infant is:
    a. 2.5-mm inner diameter
    b. 3.5-mm inner diameter
    c. 4.0-mm inner diameter
    d. 4.5-mm inner diameter

16. A large, adult, male patient has a 7-mm (inner diameter) ET in place and is being mechanically ventilated. Cuff pressures of 35 cm H_2O are required to maintain an adequate cuff seal. Which of the following strategies would you suggest to correct this problem?
    a. lower cuff pressures to no more than 25 cm H2O
    b. change the ET tube to an 8.5-mm (inner diameter) tube
    c. request placement of a TT
    d. periodically deflate and inflate the cuff

17. A patient who has undergone a single lung transplant is to be ventilated with two ventilators connected in tandem. What is the most appropriate type of airway to use?
    a. Magill type of ET
    b. Murphy type of ET
    c. DLET
    d. combination of TT and oral ET

Bibliography

1. Asai T and Morris S: The laryngeal mask airway: its features, effects and role, Can J Anesth 41:930, 1994.
2. Benumof JL and Scheller MS: The importance of transtracheal jet ventilation in the management of the difficult airway, Anesthesiol 71:769, 1989.
3. Burkey B, Esclamado R, and Morganroth M: The role of cricothyroidotomy in airway management, Clin Chest Med 12:561, 1991.
4. Dorsch JA and Dorsch SE: Understanding anesthesia equipment: construction, care and complications, ed 3, Batlimore, 1994, Williams & Wilkins.
5. Hastings RH and Marks JD: Airway management for trauma patients with potential cervical spine injuries, Anesth Analg 73:471, 1991.
6. Josephson GD, et al: Airway obstruction: new modalities in treatment, Med Clin North Am 77:539, 1993.
7. Schwartz DE and Wiener-Kronish JP: Management of the difficult airway, Clin Chest Med 12:483, 1991.
8. Tobias JD: Airway management for pediatric emergencies, Ped Ann 25:317, 1996.
9. Todres ID: Pediatric airway control and ventilation, Ann Em Med 22:440, 1993.
10. Bronson RD, Hess DR, and Chatburn RL: Respiratory care equipment, Philadelphia, 1995, JB Lippincott.

Internet Resources

1. American Association for Respiratory Care
   http://www.aarc.org
2. American Society of Anesthesiologists
   http://www.asahq.org
3. National Library of Medicine (Medline/Grateful Med Services
   http://www.nlm.nih.gov/databases/freemedl.html
4. Airway images from the University of Miami
   http://umdas.med.miami.edu
5. Mallinckrodt Corporation
   http://www.mallinckrodt.com
6. Healthcare Professionals Resources
   http://www.healthanswers.com
7. The Internet Journal of Emergency and Intensive Care Medicine
   http://www.ispub.com/journals/ijeicm.htm
8. The Internet Journal of Pulmonary Medicine
   http://www.ispub.com/journals/ijpm.htm
9. The Internet Journal of Anesthesiology
   http://www.ispub.com/journals/ija.htm

CHAPTER 6

CHAPTER OUTLINE

Lung Expansion Therapy

J. M. Cairo

CHAPTER LEARNING OBJECTIVES

Upon completion of this chapter, the reader should be able to:

1. Compare spring-loaded and diaphragm types of manual resuscitators.
2. Summarize the current standards for manual resuscitators established by the American Society for Testing Materials (ASTM), the International Standards Organization (ISO), the Emergency Care Research Institute (ECRI), and the American Heart Association (AHA).
3. Compare volume-displacement and flow-dependent incentive spirometers.
4. Describe two types of machines used to administer IPPB therapy.
5. State the operational theory of IPV.
6. Discuss how EPAP, CPAP, and PEP therapy are used to mobilize secretions and treat atelectasis.
7. Identify the major components of pneumatically and electrically powered percussors.

KEY TERMS

Bennett Valve
Cardiopulmonary Resuscitation (CPR)
Diluter Regulator
Duckbill Valve
Fishmouth Valve
Flow-Dependent Incentive Spirometers
Gas-Collector Exhalation Valve
High-Frequency Percussive Breaths
Leaf Type of Valve
Magnetic Valve Resistors
Mainstream Nebulizer
Negative End-Expiratory Pressure (NEEP)
Nonrebreathing Valve
PEP Therapy
Phasitron
Sidestream Nebulizer
Spring-Loaded Resistors
Sustained Maximum Inspiration (SMI)
Volume-Displacement Incentive Spirometers
Underwater Seal Resistors
Weighted Ball Resistors

Lung expansion therapy is an integral part of respiratory care. Various strategies and devices have been used to help patients attain and maintain optimal lung volume. The most common strategies include deep breathing exercises, directed coughing, postural drainage, endotracheal suctioning, and medical aerosol.[1] Some of the devices used in lung expansion therapy are incentive spirometers, IPPB devices, and chest wall percussors. Note that manual resuscitators are included in this chapter because they are also commonly used to hyperinflate mechanically ventilated patients before and after suctioning.

The primary indication for lung expansion therapy is to prevent atelectasis.[1,2] If untreated, atelectasis can result in pulmonary shunting, hypoxemia, hypercapnia, and ultimately, respiratory failure. Factors that contribute to the development of atelectasis include retained secretions, altered breathing patterns, pain associated with surgery and trauma, chronic obstructive and restrictive pulmonary diseases, prolonged immobilization in a supine position, and increased intraabdominal pressure.[1]

The most common devices used by respiratory care practitioners to perform lung expansion therapy are described in this chapter. Selection of the appropriate device should be based on the patient's ability to perform the assigned therapy. Continuation of or changes in therapeutic goals should be determined by frequent assessment of patient status through physical assessment and review of laboratory tests.

MANUAL RESUSCITATORS

Manual resuscitators (or resuscitator bags) are portable, hand-held devices that provide a means of delivering posi-

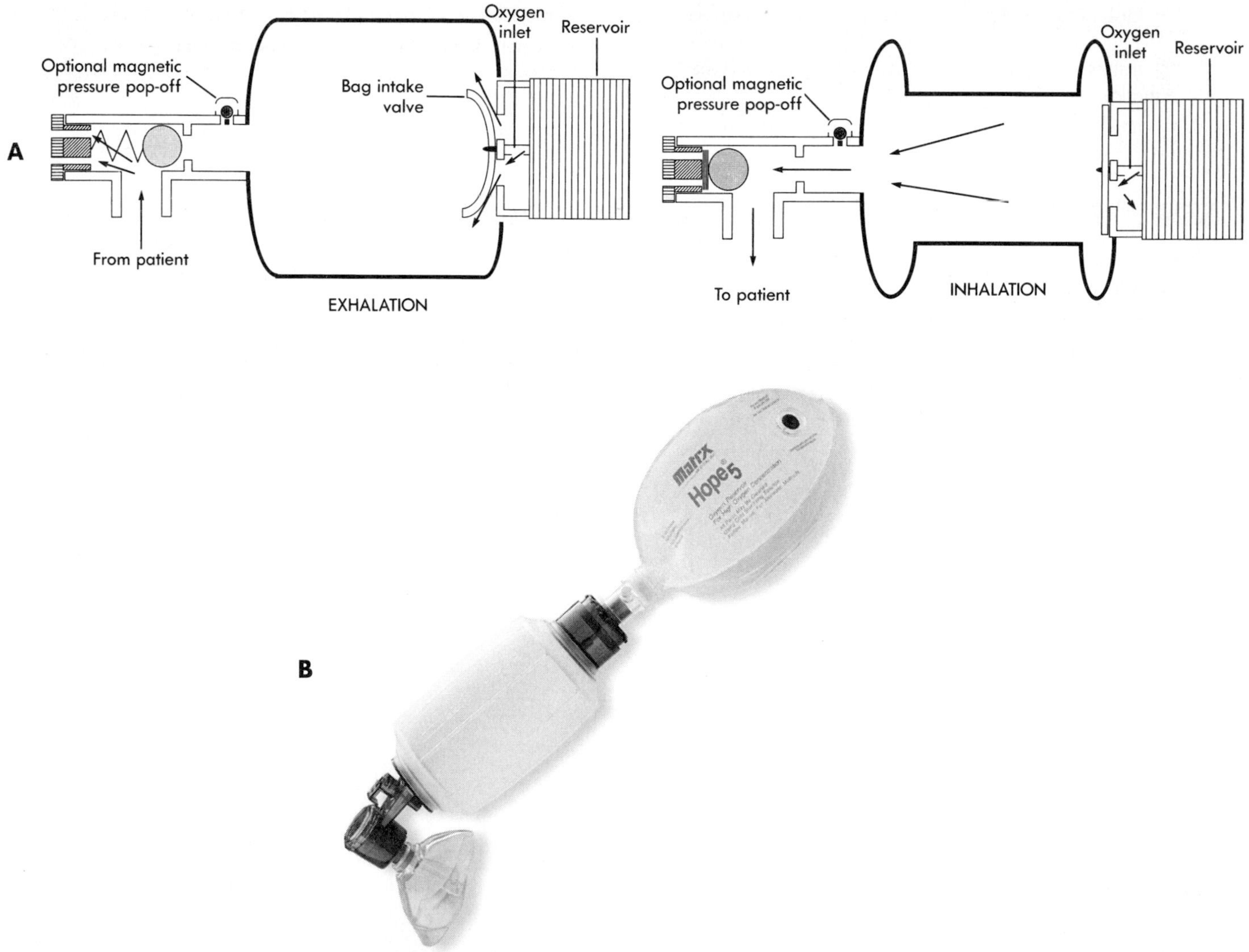

Figure 6-1 **A,** Valves for the Ohio Hope II resuscitator. **B,** The adult model of the Hope II with an oxygen reservoir. (B, Courtesy MDS Matrx, Orchard Park, NY.)

tive pressure to a patient's airway. These devices incorporate a self-inflating bag, an air-intake valve, a nonrebreathing valve mechanism, an oxygen-inlet nipple, and an oxygen reservoir, which may be a tube or a bag.[1,2] Manual resuscitators can deliver room air, oxygen, or air/oxygen mixtures via mask or through an adaptor that attaches directly to a patient's endotracheal tube (ET).

As their name implies, manual resuscitators were originally designed to ventilate patients during **cardiopulmonary resuscitation (CPR),** but they have become an indispensable part of managing mechanically ventilated patients. They can be used to hyperinflate patients with enriched oxygen mixtures before and after suctioning procedures, as well as to ventilate bradypneic or apneic (ventilator-dependent) patients while they are being transported from one area of the hospital to another.

Types of Manual Resuscitators (Bag-Valve Units)

Manual resuscitators are generally classified by the type of **nonrebreathing valve** used.[3] Therefore two classes of resuscitators are usually described: those using a **spring-loaded** mechanism, and those relying on diaphragm valves. Diaphragm valves can be further subdivided into **duckbill** or **fishmouth** and **leaf type of valves.**

Spring-Loaded Valves

Spring-loaded devices use a nonrebreathing valve that consists of a disk or ball attached to a spring. When the operator compresses the self-inflating bag, a spring pushes a disk or ball against the exhalation port, occluding it, and gas is directed to the patient's airway. Once the flow from the bag stops, the exhalation port opens, and gas exhaled by the patient is vented to the atmosphere. Simultaneously, as gas enters the self-inflating bag through the one-way air inlet valve (which is attached to a reservoir), the bag inflates. The air-inlet valve can be attached directly to the nonrebreathing valve or located separately at the bottom of the bag.

The most common examples of this type of manual resuscitator are the early Ambu (Air-Mask-Bag Unit) system, the Ohio Hope II Bag, the Air Viva, and the Vital Signs Stat Blue Resuscitator. Early versions of the Ambu (Air-Mask-Bag) system used a spring-loaded, disk type of nonrebreathing valve that is no longer produced. The Hope II (Figure 6-1) and the Vital Signs Stat Blue (Figure 6-2) resuscitators both rely on the spring-disk type of nonrebreathing valve. Notice that the reservoir of the Hope II resuscitator, which allows for oxygen accumulation and potential delivery of 100% oxygen, is located on the bottom of the self-inflating bag. This reservoir is designed so that the angle of the oxygen inlet valve allows for oxygen flows in excess of 30 L/min to be used without interrupting normal function. The Vital Signs Stat Blue Resuscitator differs from the Ohio Hope II bag because oxygen is drawn in through the neck, where a reservoir is attached.

Diaphragm Valves

Duckbill Valves. This second class of resuscitators incorporates diaphragm type of nonrebreathing valves in place of spring-loaded mechanisms. The Laerdal Silicone Resuscitator, the Laerdal Adult Resuscitator, the Laerdal Infant and Child Resuscitators (Figure 6-3), the Hudson Life Saver II resuscitator (Figure 6-4), and the Life Design Systems (LDS) disposable resuscitators are examples of devices that use the duckbill/diaphragm valves.

The operational principle of these devices is comparable to that of spring-loaded resuscitators. Compression of the bag pushes a diaphragm against the exhalation ports. At the same time, the duckbill valve opens and gas flows to the patient. Once the flow from the bag ceases, the duckbill valve closes, and the diaphragm is pushed away from the exhalation port. Exhaled gas can then exit through the exhalation ports. During reexpansion of the bag, the bag inlet valve allows air and/or oxygen from the reservoir to enter the self-inflating bag. Notice that the inlet valve is a simple, one-way, leaf valve that closes when the bag is compressed to prevent gas leakage. The one-way valve opens when the bag reexpands as a result of subatmospheric pressure within the bag.

Leaf Valves. Resuscitators that use leaf type of valves operate similarly to duckbill resuscitators. As shown in Figure 6-5, when the bag is compressed, a diaphragm swells and occludes the exhalation ports. The leaf valve in the middle of the diaphragm is pushed open, and gas is directed to the

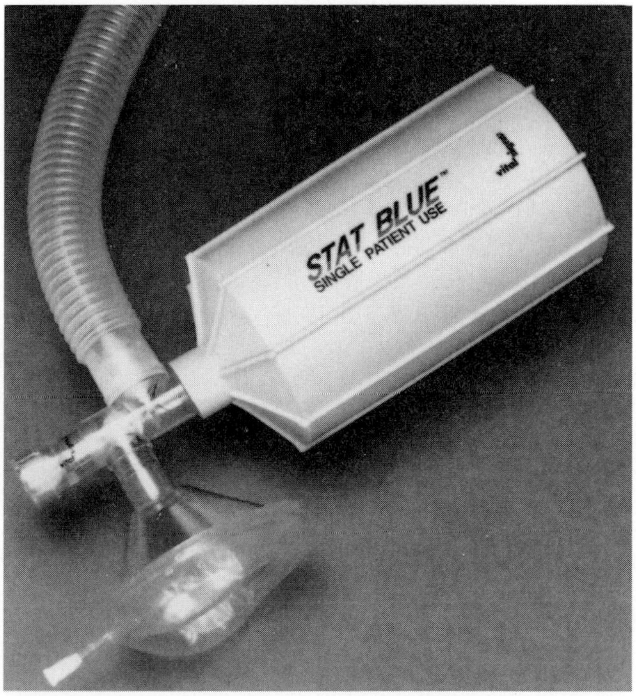

Figure 6-2 Vital Signs Stat Blue Resuscitator. (Courtesy Vital Signs, Totowa, NJ.)

A

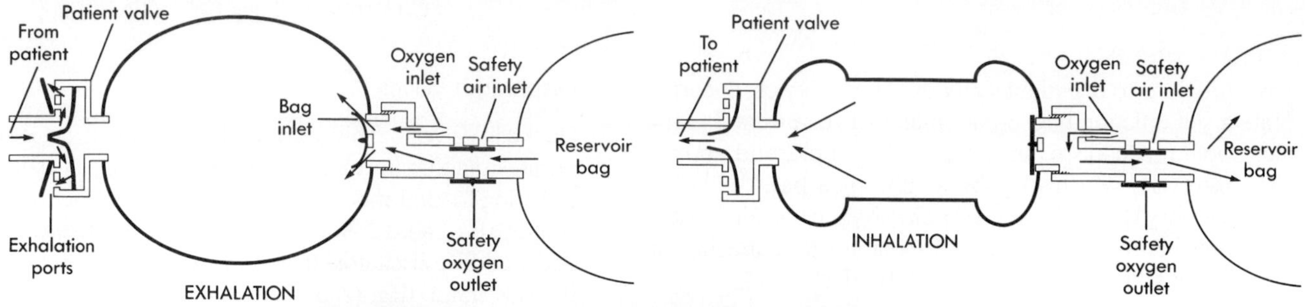

B

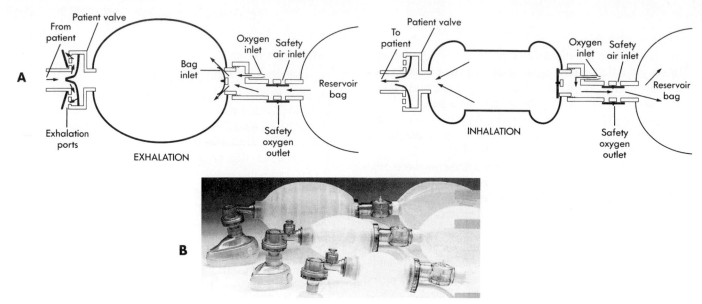

Figure 6-3 **A,** Valves for the adult and child with an oxygen reservoir system for adults. **B,** The Laerdal adult and infant resuscitators with oxygen reservoir systems. (B, courtesy Laerdal Medical Corp., Wappingers Falls, NY.)

A

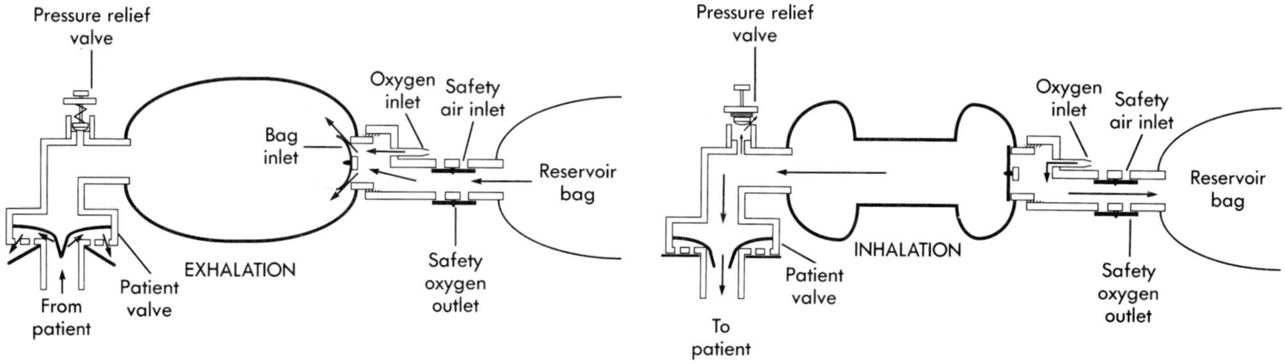

B

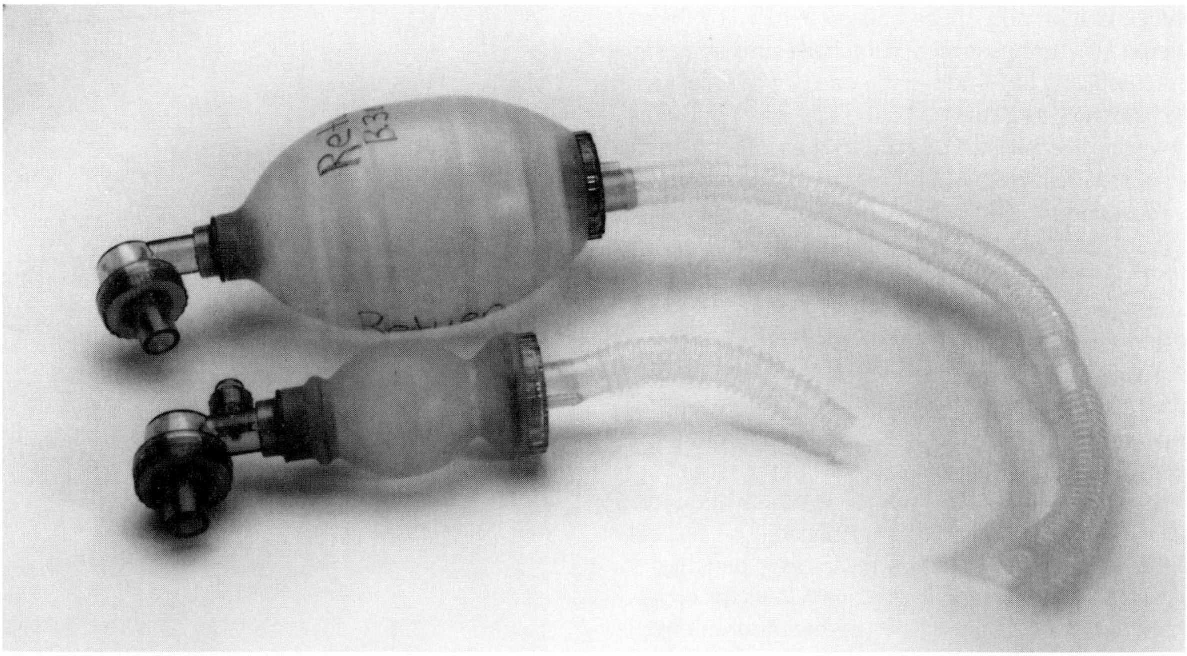

Figure 6-4 **A,** Valves for the Laerdal Child and Infant Resuscitators with oxygen reservoir systems. **B,** Laerdal Silicone Resuscitators with oxygen reservoir systems.

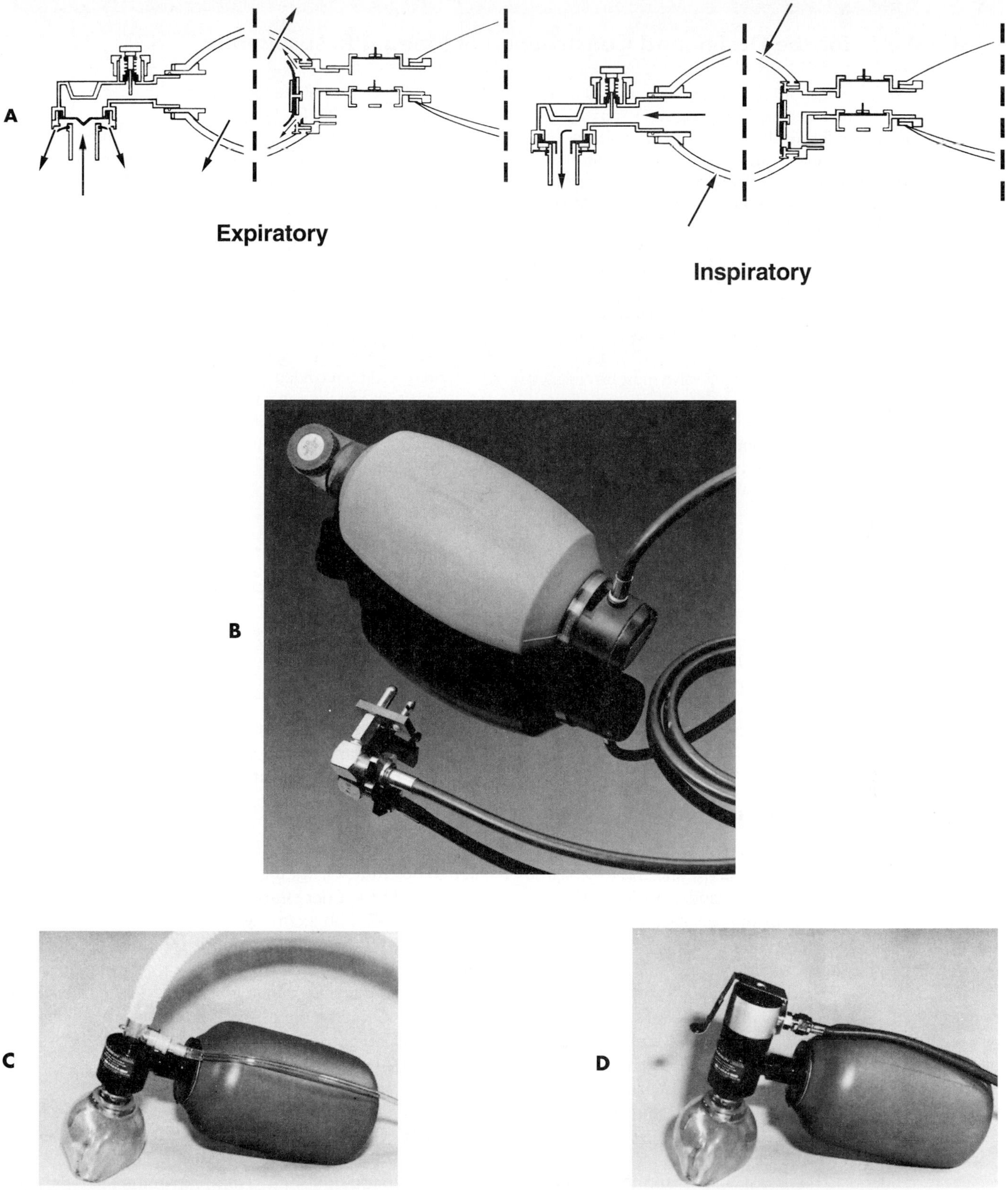

Figure 6-5 **A,** Operations of the leaf and diagram valves for a Hudson manual Resuscitator (as well as for a Robertshaw Bag Resuscitator). (Courtesy Hudson Oxygen Therapy Sales Co, Temecula, Calif.) **B,** Hudson Lifesaver Manual Resuscitator with a manufacturer-supplied reservoir system attached. **C,** A modified reservoir system with 22-mm T-connection used for attaching the oxygen inlet at a right angle to the bag-inlet valve. **D,** Robertshaw Demand Valve attached to the bag inlet for providing 100% oxygen or other source gas to bag.

BOX 6-1

Standards for the Design and Construction of Manual Resuscitators

1. The ASTM and the ISO recommend that manual resuscitators must be capable of delivering an FiO_2 of 0.85 with an oxygen flow of 15 L/min. Recognize that these are minimum requirements and may not be optimal for treating patients during cardiopulmonary resuscitation. It is therefore prudent to choose a device that can deliver $FiO_2s \geq 0.95$.
2. Manual resuscitators must be able to operate at extreme temperatures (−180° to 600° C) and at a relative humidity of 40% to 96%.
3. Adult resuscitators shall deliver a tidal volume of at least 600 mL into a test lung set at a compliance of 0.02 L/cm H_2O and a resistance of 20 cm H_2O/L/sec.
4. The resuscitator's nonrebreathing valve must be designed so that the valve will not jam at oxygen flow rates up to 30 L/min.
5. If the resuscitator valve malfunctions because of foreign obstruction (e.g., vomitus), the valve must be restored to proper function within 20 seconds.
6. Patient connectors of the resuscitator valve must have a 15:22-mm (ID:OD) fitting.
7. Resuscitators used for adults should not have a pressure-limiting system. Bag-valve devices used for children must incorporate a pressure-release valve that limits peak inspiratory pressure to 40 +/− 10 cm H_2O; devices used for infants may incorporate a pressure-release valve that limits peak inspiratory pressure to 40 +/− 5 cm H_2O.
8. When a pressure-limiting system is incorporated into a resuscitator, an override capability must exist that is readily apparent to the operator (i.e., it should be visible that the valve is on or off), and an audible signal should indicate that the gas is being vented. The override mechanism should be provided for times when lung impedance is high and the patient has an ET in place.
9. The resuscitator must be able to operate after being dropped from a height of 1 meter onto a concrete floor.

patient. During exhalation, the bag reexpands, creating a negative pressure that causes the diaphragm to move away from the exhalation ports. The leaf then closes and prevents exhaled gas from leaking into the bag. The bag inlet valve is opened, and the bag reinflates. The Respironics disposable resuscitator, the Hudson Lifesaver, and the Robertshaw Resuscitators are examples of devices that use leaf valves.

Standards for Manual Resuscitators

Standards for the design, construction, and use of manual resuscitators are published by the ASTM and the ISO.[4,5] The ECRI and the AHA also provide standards for the use and evaluation of manual resuscitators, specifically relating to the level and timing of ventilation during CPR.[6] (Box 6-1 summarizes these standards.)

Table 6-1 compares the performance patterns required by the ASTM, ISO, and AHA standard; although it may not be possible to deliver a tidal volume of 800 mL (as specified by the AHA) unless a patient is intubated. Figure 6-6 shows the results of several studies in which investigators measured the average tidal volumes delivered by one-handed compression of the bag.[7-12] It has been suggested that the lower tidal volumes could have resulted from either an inability to maintain an adequate mask seal while ensuring a patent airway, or from gastric expansion. Another consideration is that the operator may be unable to deliver an appropriate tidal volume unless the bag is compressed with both hands. Although manual resuscitators may differ in design, it is generally agreed that ideal manual resuscitators should possess certain characteristics.[13,14,15] Box 6-2 lists the characteristics of ideal manual resuscitators.

Oxygen-Powered Resuscitators

Oxygen-powered resuscitators are pressure-limited devices that work similarly to reducing valves. A typical oxygen-powered resuscitator consists of a demand valve that can be manually operated or patient-triggered.[2] Oxygen-powered resuscitators can deliver 100% oxygen at flows less than 40 L/min. Inspiratory pressures are generally limited to 60 cm H_2O, but the pressure-relief valve may be set to 80 cm H_2O, if necessary.

Figure 6-7 is an example of an oxygen-powered resuscitator. When the manual control actuator is depressed, oxygen enters the device from a 50 psig gas source and flows to the patient through a standard 15:22 mm (inner diameter [ID]:outer diameter [OD]) connector. The connector can be coupled to a mask, an ET, a tracheostomy tube (TT), or an esophageal obturator airway.

INCENTIVE SPIROMETERS

Incentive spirometry (IS) is a lung expansion technique designed to mimic natural sighing or yawning by encouraging patients to take slow, deep breaths.[17] It is a simple and relatively safe method of preventing atelectasis in alert patients who are predisposed to shallow breathing (e.g., pa-

TABLE 6-1

Ventilation patterns specified by standards for FDO_2 and ventilation for bag-valve devices

	Ventilation pattern (mL × cycles/min)*					
Specification	**ASTM[4]**	**ISO[5]**	**AHA[6]**	**O_2 flow (L/min)**	**Compliance L/cm H_2O**	**Resistance cm H_2O/L/sec**
FDO_2						
Adult	600 × 12	600 × 12	800 × 12	15	0.020	20
Child	300 × 20	15/kg × 20	N/A	15	0.010	200
Infant	20 × 60	20 × 60	6–8/kg × 40	15	0.001	400
Ventilation						
Adult	600 × 20	600 × 20	800 × 12		0.020	20
Child 1	300 × 20	15/kg × 20	N/A		0.010	20
Child 2	70 × 30	150 × 25	N/A		0.010	20
Infant 1	70 × 30	20 × 60	6–8/kg × 40		0.010	20
Infant 2	20 × 60	N/A	N/A		0.010	400

*ASTM = American Society for Testing and Materials; ISO = International Standards Organization; AHA = American Heart Association; FDO_2 = fraction of delivered oxygen; N/A = not available.

From Barnes TA: Core textbook of respiratory care practice, ed 2, St Louis, 1994, Mosby.

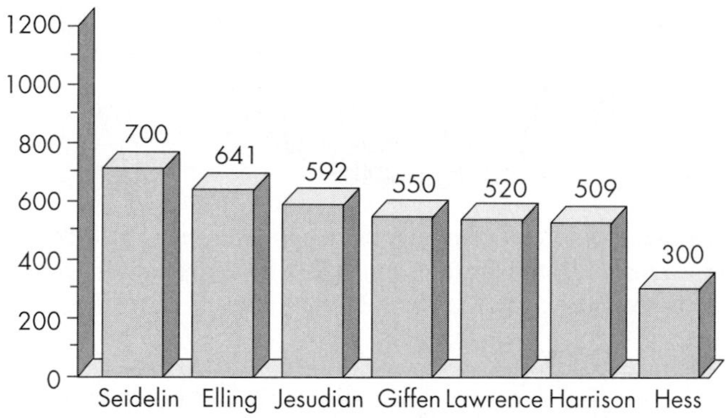

Figure 6-6 Tidal volume by bag-valve-mask devices from published studies. (From Barnes TA: Core textbook of respiratory care practice, ed 2, St Louis, 1994, Mosby.)

tients recovering from thoracic or upper abdominal surgery, chronic obstructive pulmonary distress [COPD] patients recovering from other surgery, patients immobilized or confined to bed). The only contraindication of IS involves patients who are confused, uncooperative, or unable to effectively deep breathe (i.e., vital capacity <10 mL/kg, or inspiratory capacity <1/3 predicted value).[17]

Although commercially produced incentive spirometers have been available for about two decades, the concept of **sustained maximum inspiration (SMI)** has been used since the latter part of the 19th century.[18,19,20] Blow-bottles, blow-gloves, and carbon dioxide-induced hyperventilation are examples of devices and techniques that were used by clinicians before the introduction of incentive spirometers to accomplish the goal of having patients take deep breaths to prevent atelectasis.

The principle of incentive spirometry is based on the idea that the patient is encouraged to achieve a preset volume or flow, which is determined from predicted values or baseline measurements. Commercially available incentive spirometers are classified as either **volume-displacement** or **flow-dependent** devices. With volume-displacement devices, the volume of air that the patient inspires during a sustained maximum inspiration is measured and displayed. In contrast, flow-dependent devices measure the inspiratory flow that the patient achieves during a maximum sustained inspiratory effort. Volume displacement can be derived with these latter devices by multiplying the flow achieved by the amount of time the flow is maintained.

We are not aware of any prospective studies that have demonstrated that incentive spirometry is superior to other hyperexpansion methods relying on natural deep breathing exercises. Indeed, evidence suggests that deep breathing alone—without an incentive spirometer—can be beneficial in preventing or reversing pulmonary complications.[21,22] The advantage of using an incentive spirometer may be related to the fact that patients receive immediate visual feedback about whether they are achieving the prescribed goal (Box 6-3). Furthermore, patients can perform the treatment regimen without the direct supervision of a respiratory therapist once they have demonstrated mastery of the technique, thus providing a cost-effective approach to lung expansion therapy. Box 6-4 summarizes the AARC Clinical Practice Guideline for incentive spirometry.

BOX 6-2

Properties of an Ideal Manual Resuscitator

1. It should be lightweight and held easily in one hand.
2. It should have standard 15:22 mm (ID:OD) patient adaptors.
3. The bag-valve device should be easy to disassemble, clean, and reassemble.
4. It should be constructed of durable materials (e.g., rubber, silicone, or polyvinyl chloride).
5. The nonrebreathing valve should prevent back leaking of patient-exhaled gases into the bag. It should have a low resistance to inspiratory and expiratory airflow and a small dead space volume (<30 mL for adult models). The nonrebreathing valve should be transparent to allow detection of vomitus or any other obstruction.
6. A manual resuscitator should be able to deliver oxygen concentrations of 0.40 when oxygen is available and at least 0.85 when a reservoir is present.
7. The bag construction should allow rapid refill so faster respiratory rates can be achieved as necessary.
8. The volume of the self-inflating bag should be at least twice the volume to be delivered because not all of the bag volume will be delivered when the bag is compressed. For example, adult resuscitators should have a volume of 1600 mL or more to be able to deliver a tidal volume of 800 mL. Resuscitation bags used for children should have a volume of at least 500 mL, and infant bags should hold at least 240 mL.
9. The bag-valve device should allow a positive end expiratory pressure (PEEP) valve and/or spirometer attachments to measure exhaled volumes. It should be equipped with a tap for monitoring airway pressure with an aneroid manometer.
10. Every manual resuscitator should be supplied with a face mask that attaches to the standard patient connector of the resuscitator. The mask should provide an effective seal when applied to the patient's face.

BOX 6-3

Decision Making & Problem Solving

You are asked to assess a 50-year old postoperative woman recovering from abdominal surgery. A physical examination revealed no acute distress, but the patient is having problems clearing secretions. Auscultation of the chest indicates retention of secretions, particularly in the right lower lung; the patient has no history of lung disease. Suggest a therapeutic plan for her.

See Appendix A for the answer.

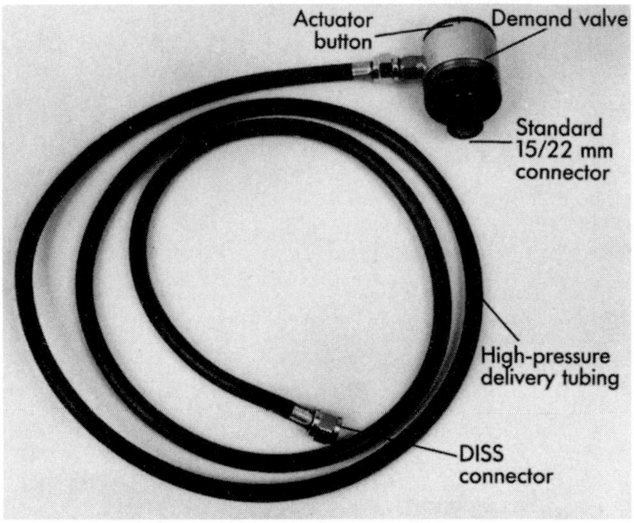

Figure 6-7 Gas-powered resuscitator. (From Scanlan CL, Spearman CB, and Sheldon RL: Egan's fundamentals of respiratory care, ed 7, St Louis, 1998, Mosby.)

Volume-Displacement Devices

Figure 6-8 is a schematic of a prototype of a volume-displacement incentive spirometer. The operational principle is simple: the patients inhale air through a mouthpiece and corrugated tubing attached to a flexible plastic bellows. The volume of air displaced is indicated on a scale, which is located on the device enclosure. Once patients have achieved the maximum volume, they are instructed to hold this volume constant for 3 to 5 seconds. They can then remove the mouthpiece and exhale, while the bellows expand to the starting position. Some authors have suggested that patients should perform a minimum of 5 to 10 breaths per session every hour while awake.[17] Notice that the respiratory therapist does not have to be present for each performance, and patients should be encouraged to perform this therapy independently.

Incentive spirometers used for adult patients typically have a total volume capacity of about 4 L, and those used for children have a volume capacity of about 2 L. DHD Medical Products' Volurex incentive spirometer (Figure 6-9, *A*) is a disposable device that operates similarly to the prototype unit just described. It is slightly more sophisticated, however, in that after the patient inhales, the plastic bellows must be released by the push of a button before it returns to its starting position. Sherwood Medical's Voldyne Exerciser (Figure 6-9, *B*) and DHD's Coach 2300 (Figure 6-9, *C*) and Coach Jr consist of a movable piston in a clear cylinder. As the patient inhales, the piston rises and the inspired volume is indicated on a scale engraved on the side of the cylinder. A flow indicator is also included as a visual aid encouraging the patient to take slow, deep breaths.

Although most incentive spirometers are designed for single-patient use, multiple-use devices are also available. Single-patient devices are usually made of plastic and can

BOX 6-4

Clinical Practice Guidelines

Incentive Spirometry (IS)

Indications

1. Conditions predisposed to the development of pulmonary atelectasis, such as upper-abdominal surgery, thoracic surgery, and surgery in patients with chronic obstructive pulmonary disease (COPD).
2. Pulmonary atelectasis.
3. Restrictive lung defects associated with quadriplegia and/or dysfunctional diaphragm.

Contraindications

1. Patient cannot be instructed or supervised to ensure appropriate use of the device.
2. Patient is unable to deep breathe effectively (e.g., vital capacity <10 mL/kg, or inspiratory capacity is less than one third of that predicted.)

Complications

1. Must be closely supervised or performed as ordered.
2. Inappropriate as the only treatment for major lung collapse or consolidation.
3. Hyperventilation.
4. Barotrauma (emphysematous lungs).
5. Discomfort secondary to inadequate pain control.
6. Hypoxia secondary to interruption of oxygen therapy if face mask or shield is being used.
7. Exacerbation of bronchospasm.
8. Fatigue.

Assessment of Outcome

Absence of or improvement in signs of atelectasis:

a. decreased respiratory rate
b. resolution of fever
c. normal pulse rate
d. no crackles on auscultation, or improvement in previously absent or diminished breath sounds
e. normal chest radiograph
f. improved arterial oxygenation
g. increased vital capacity and peak expiratory flows
h. return of functional residual capacity (FRC) or vital capacity to preoperative values without lung resection
i. improved inspiratory muscle performance

Monitoring

Direct patient supervision is not necessary once that patient has demonstrated mastery of the technique; however preoperative instruction, volume goals, and feedback are essential to optimal performance.

AARC Clinical Practice Guideline: Incentive spirometry, Respir Care 36:1402, 1991.

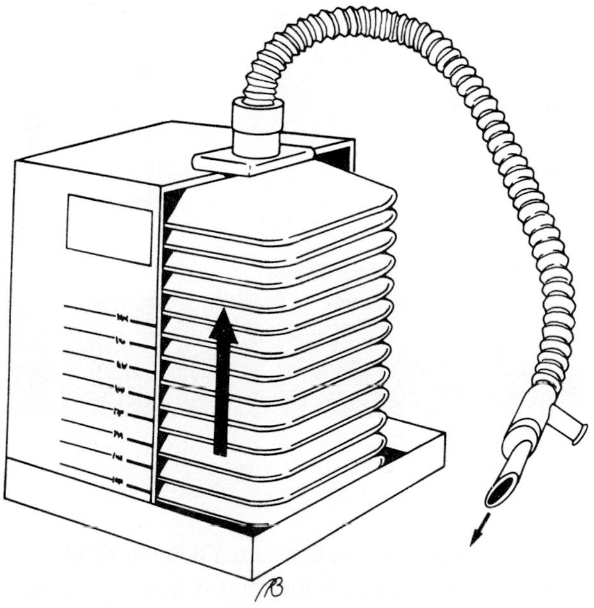

Figure 6-8 A volume-incentive breathing exerciser. (From Eubanks DH and Bone RC: Comprehensive respiratory care, a learning system, ed 2, St Louis, 1990, Mosby. Used by permission.)

be discarded after the patient has completed the course of therapy. (Actually, patients should be encouraged to keep these devices and use them if similar respiratory illnesses are incurred.) Multiple-use incentive spirometers are usually electrically powered devices that use disposable mouthpieces and flow tubes and typically require that a respiratory therapist be available during treatment. The Spirocare incentive spirometer (Figure 6-10) and the TVS incentive spirometer are electrically powered devices that use light indicators as feedback of patient performance. Both units also use disposable mouthpieces that are attached to flowmeters, which measure the flow of air as the patient inhales and then translate it into a volume signal.

Flow-Dependent Devices

Figure 6-11 shows a typical flow-dependent incentive spirometer, which consists of a mouthpiece and corrugated tubing connected to a manifold that is composed of three flow tubes containing lightweight plastic balls. As the patient inhales through the mouthpiece, a negative pressure is created within the tubes, causing them to rise. The device is designed so that the number of balls and the level that the balls rise depends on the flow achieved. At lower flows, the

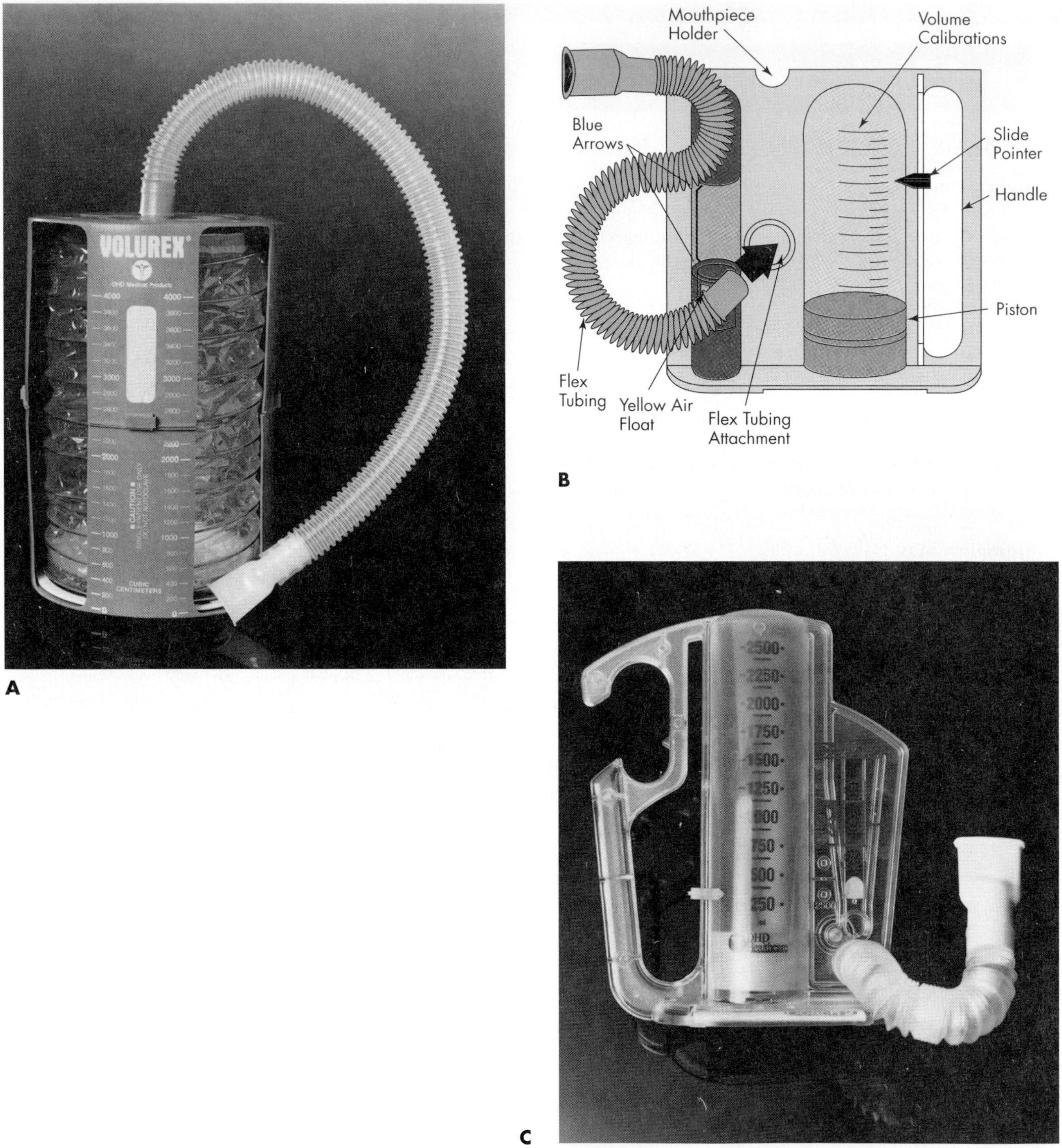

A

B

C

Figure 6-9 **A,** A Volurex incentive spirometer. **B,** A Picture Voldyne Exerciser. (Courtesy Sherwood Medical, St. Louis.) **C,** A DHD Coach 2300.

first ball rises to a level that depends on the magnitude of the flow. As the inspiratory flow increases, the second ball rises, followed by the third ball. The flow achieved by the patient can be estimated based on the manufacturer's specifications. For example, with Sherwood Medical's Triflo incentive spirometer, the patient must achieve a flow of 600 mL/sec to raise the first ball. A flow of 900 mL/sec is required to raise the second ball, and a flow of 1200 mL/sec must be generated to raise the third ball. As with volume-displacement incentive spirometers, it is important that the patient perform a maximum sustained inspiration.

The DHD Respirex incentive spirometer (Figure 6-12) consists of a single tube containing a plastic ball. An adjustable volume selector can be used to vary the patient ef-

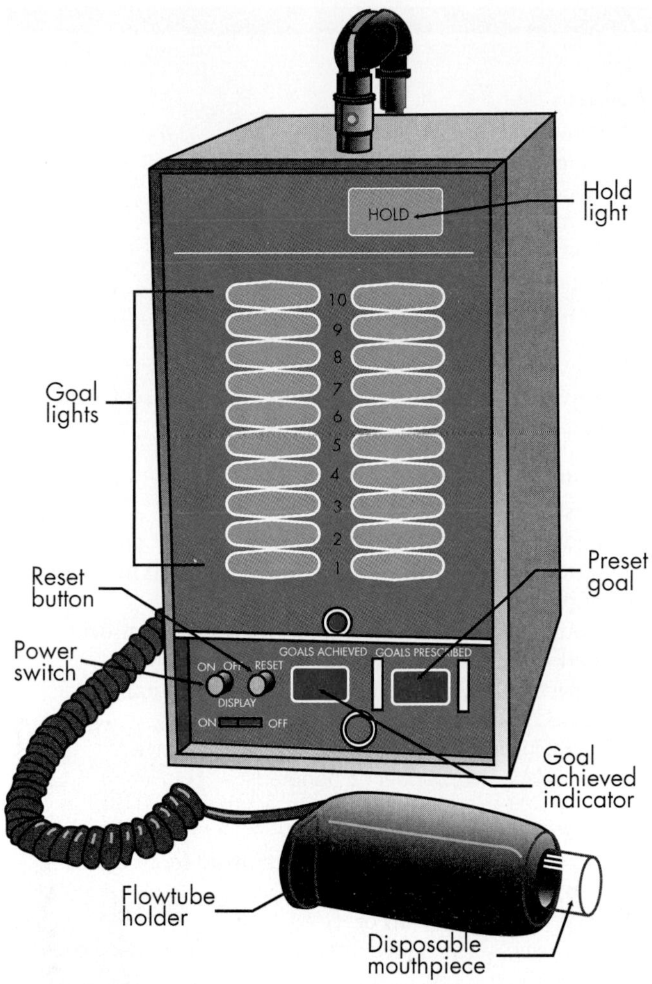

Figure 6-10 Multiple-use, electrically powered incentive spirometer.

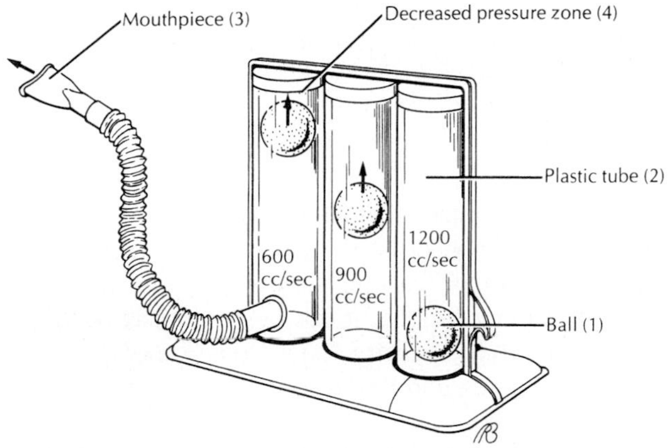

Figure 6-11 A flow-oriented incentive spirometer. (From Eubanks DH and Bone RC: Comprehensive respiratory care, St Louis, 1985, Mosby.)

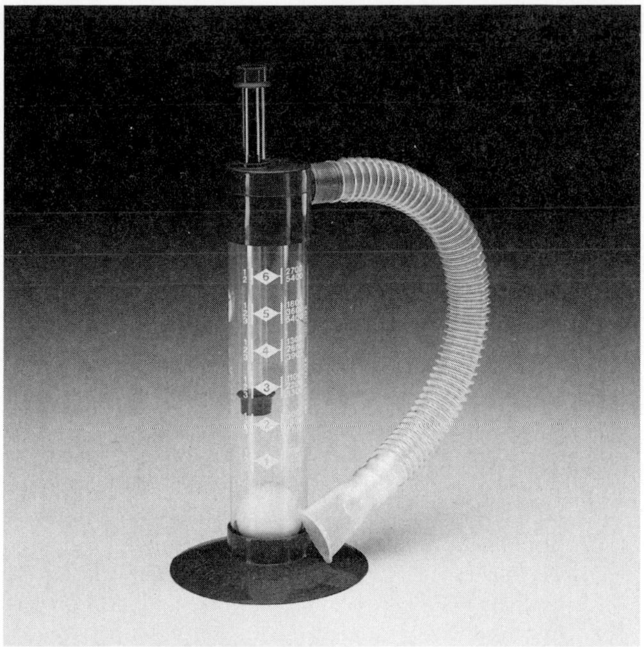

Figure 6-12 A DHD Respirex incentive spirometer. (Courtesy DHD Medical Products.)

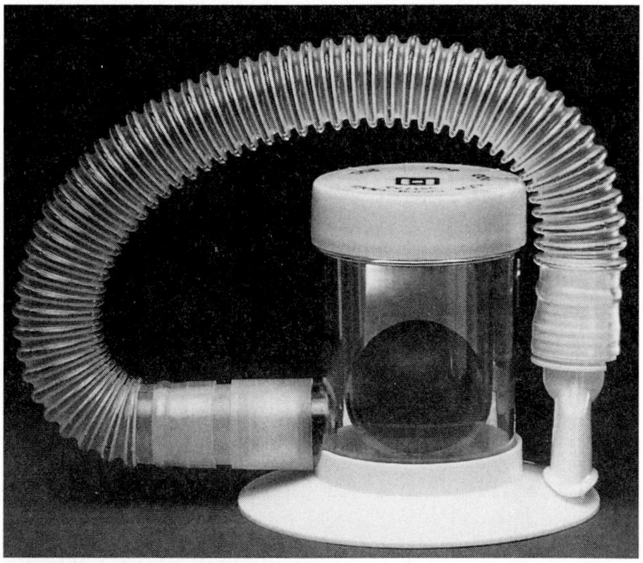

Figure 6-13 A Hudson incentive spirometer. (Courtesy Hudson RCI, Temecula, Calif.)

fort necessary to attain the desired inspiratory capacity. The Intertech incentive spirometer uses a similar design but can also display the number of successful efforts and the maximum flow achieved.[18] The Hudson incentive spirometer (Figure 6-13) uses a different type of design: the patient inhales through a mouthpiece and corrugated tubing connected to a dual-chamber device. The two chambers of this device are arranged in series. The ball in the inner chamber rises when the patient achieves a flow that equals the inspiratory flow selected by the operator. Inspiratory flows vary from 200 mL/second to 1200 mL/second.

BOX 6-5

Clinical Practice Guidelines

Intermittent Positive Pressure Breathing (IPPB)

Indications

1. The need to improve lung expansion, particularly for those patients who demonstrate clinically important atelectasis when other forms of therapy, such as incentive spirometry, CPT, deep breathing exercises, and PAP are unsuccessful. It may also useful for patients who cannot cooperate with standard lung expansion techniques.
2. Inability to adequately clear secretions because of pathology that severely limits the patient's ability to ventilate or cough effectively.
3. As an alternative to endotracheal intubation and continuous ventilatory support for patients requiring short-term ventilatory support.
4. To deliver aerosolized medications to patients fatigued as a result of respiratory muscle weakness. It can also be used to deliver aerosolized medications to patients not able to use an MDI.

Contraindications

1. Elevated intracranial pressure (ICP >15 mm Hg)
2. Hemodynamic instability
3. Recent facial, oral, or skull surgery
4. Tracheoesophageal fistula
5. Recent esophageal surgery
6. Active hemoptysis
7. Nausea
8. Air swallowing
9. Active, untreated tuberculosis
10. Radiographic evidence of bleb
11. Hiccups

Hazards

1. Barotrauma, pneumothorax
2. Hemoptysis
3. Hypocarbia (hypocapnia)
4. Increased airway resistance
5. Gastric distension
6. Impeded venous return
7. $\dot{V}/\dot{Q}$ mismatch
8. Air trapping, auto-PEEP, overdistended alveoli
9. Psychological dependence
10. Impaction of secretions due to inadequate humidification

Assessment of Need

1. Presence of atelectasis
2. Reduced pulmonary function: FVC <70% of predicted; MVV <50% of predicted; or VC <10 mL/ kg of predicted, precluding an effective cough
3. Neuromuscular disorders (e.g., kyphoscoliosis) associated with reduced lung volumes
4. Fatigue or respiratory muscle weakness with impending respiratory failure
5. If effective, the patient preference for a positive-pressure device should be honored

Assessment of Outcomes

1. Tidal volume during IPPB is greater than during spontaneous breathing by at least 25%
2. Increase in $FEV_{1.0}$ or PEF
3. Improved cough with treatment, leading to better clearance of secretions
4. Improvements in chest radiographs
5. Improved breath sounds
6. Favorable patient response

AARC Clinical Practice Guideline: Intermittent positive pressure breathing (IPPB), Respir Care 38:1189, 1993.

Intermittent Positive Pressure Breathing (IPPB) Devices

IPPB is a short-term therapeutic modality that involves the delivery of inspiratory positive pressure to spontaneously breathing patients. Since its introduction in 1947, IPPB has been used for a variety of reasons, including short-term ventilatory support and lung expansion therapy, and as an aid in delivering aerosolized medications.[23] During the past two decades, the effectiveness of IPPB as a therapeutic modality has been questioned rigorously, resulting in a reassessment of the indications for its prescription. In 1993, the AARC produced a Clinical Practice Guideline providing a rational basis for prescribing and administering IPPB treatments (see Box 6-5 for a summary of this guideline).[23] It should be recognized that although IPPB is not the therapy of choice when other less invasive therapies can be used for aerosol delivery or lung expansion in spontaneously breathing patients, it can be potentially beneficial when incentive spirometry, chest physiotherapy, deep breathing exercises, and PAP techniques have been unsuccessful (Box 6-6).[23]

IPPB can be administered with any device that can deliver intermittent positive pressure to the airway (e.g., conventional mechanical ventilators or manual resuscitators), but it is most often performed with specially designed electrically and pneumatically powered ventilators. These specially designed IPPB machines are usually categorized as patient-triggered, pressure-cycled mechanical ventilators. Regardless of the manufacturer, all IPPB machines require a

BOX 6-6

Decision Making & Problem Solving

A 38-year old man is admitted to the hospital from a rehabilitation center with a diagnosis of pneumonia. He has quadriplegia and permanent brain damage as a result of a motor vehicle accident. He also has a permanent tracheostomy but does not require ventilatory support. Current evaluation reveals the following: temperature = 103° F; respiratory rate = 28 breaths/min; heart rate = 100 beats/min; SpO_2 on 30% heated tracheostomy collar is 93%. Copious amounts of thick, green secretions are present, and the patient coughs only when stimulated with suctioning. Crackles are present in both bases. Based on these findings, what form of respiratory care would you recommend?

See Appendix A for answer.

45 to 55 psig gas pressure source, such as a compressed gas cylinder, a bulk air or oxygen system, or an air compressor. Furthermore, they all incorporate control valves that begin inspiration when a negative pressure is generated by the patient and terminate it when a preset pressure is achieved. The amount of negative pressure (i.e., patient effort) required to initiate inspiration depends on the sensitivity of the device, which may be fixed or adjustable. The pressure that must be achieved to end inspiration, and thus initiate exhalation, can typically be adjusted to as high as 60 cm H_2O.[23]

Machines manufactured by Nellcor Puritan Bennett and the Bird Corporation are the most widely used devices for IPPB therapy. A brief description of the most commonly used IPPB units produced by these companies follows.[2]

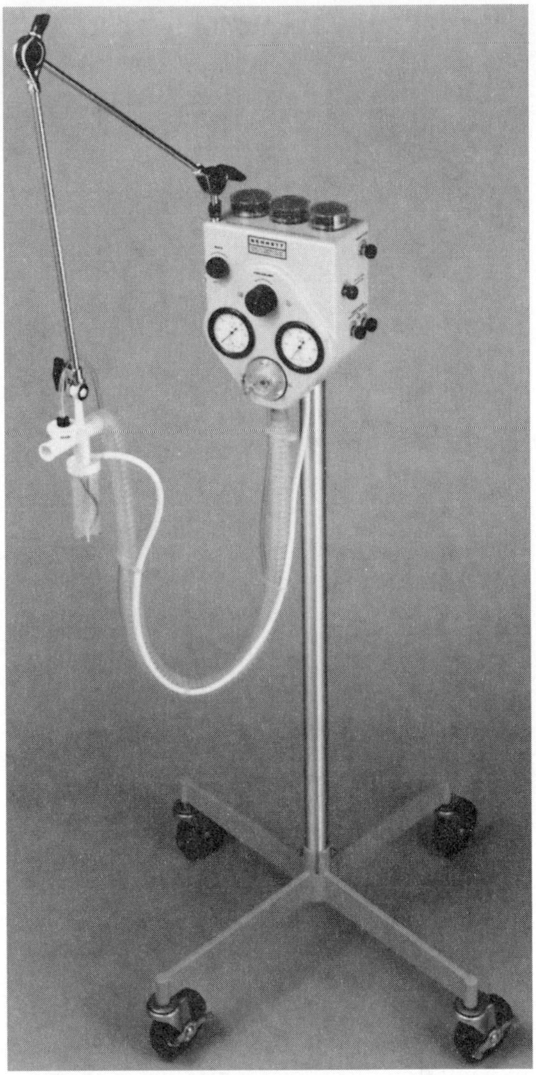

Figure 6-14 A Bennett PR-1 ventilator. (Courtesy Nellcor Puritan Bennett Corp., Pleasanton, Calif.)

Nellcor Puritan Bennett Devices

Nellcor Puritan Bennett manufactures pneumatically and electrically powered IPPB machines. The tank ventilator (TV), the pedestal ventilator (PV), and the pedestal respirator (PR) series are pneumatically powered IPPB machines; the air-powered (AP) series of ventilators are electrically powered. The PR-1 and PR-2 models are the most commonly used pneumatically powered IPPB devices. The AP-4 and AP-5 models are the most commonly used electrically powered IPPB machines.[18,19,20]

Nellcor Puritan Bennett PR Series

The PR-1 (Figure 6-14) and PR-2 (Figure 6-15) ventilators are pneumatically powered devices that can be time- or pressure-triggered, but both are flow cycled and pressure-limited. (Note that time cycling allows these devices to provide controlled, short-term ventilatory support.) They can deliver either 100% source gas or air-diluted source gas.

The PR-2 has adjustable controls for setting the pressure limit and the sensitivity or level of negative pressure that must be achieved to initiate inspiration. It also has controls for adjusting the peak flow, inspiratory and expiratory nebulizer gas flows, and **negative end-expiratory pressure (NEEP).** A terminal flow control is provided for minor leak compensation. In contrast, the PR-1 does not have a peak flow control or the capability of providing NEEP. The PR-1 does not have separate controls for inspiratory and expiratory nebulization; instead, the inspiratory nebulization is a composite of continuous nebulization and the inspiratory nebulizer flow. The PR-1 does not have an expiratory time control.

Gas flow through the PR-2 ventilator is shown in Figure 6-16. (Note that gas flow through the PR-1 is comparable.) Compressed gas from a 50 psig gas source enters the ventilator through a brass filter. It is directed to a diluter regulator, to the nebulizer pressure switch, and to a low-pressure

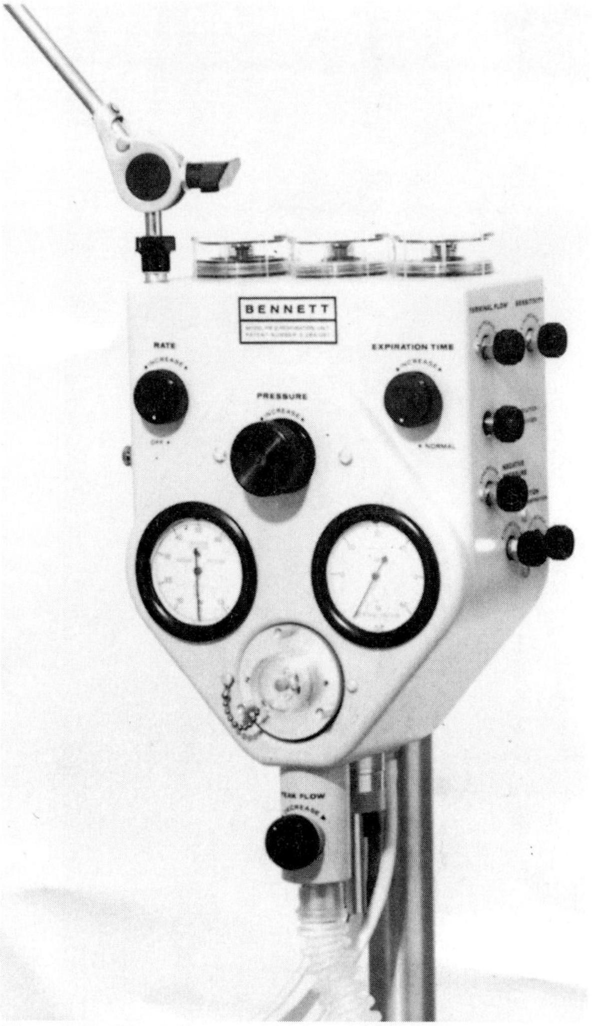

Figure 6-15 A Bennett PR-2 ventilator. (Courtesy Nellcor Puritan Bennett Corp., Pleasanton, Calif.)

regulator. The **diluter regulator** (Figure 6-17) is an adjustable reducing valve that regulates the gas pressure delivered to the patient. It can be set from 0 to 30 cm H_2O using a control knob on the front panel of the machine. Gas flow to nebulizer switch controls the flow of gas to the nebulizer during inspiration and expiration. Nebulizer flow can be adjusted with two knobs on the lower part of the machine's side panel. (Note that the nebulizer is powered by 100% source gas, therefore use of the nebulizer affects the delivered FiO_2 when the PR-2 is set to air-dilution mode.) Gas flow to the nebulizer also controls a Venturi that allows the application of NEEP from 0 to −6 cm H_2O. The NEEP level can be adjusted with a knob just above the inspiratory nebulizer control on the side panel. NEEP was originally proposed as a means of reducing the level of airtrapping experienced by some patients during IPPB. Because it was subsequently found that applying NEEP actually increased the level of airtrapping, this therapeutic mode is no longer used.[19]

From the diluter regulator, gas flows to the **Bennett valve,** which consists of a counter-weighted, hollow drum with attached vanes (Figure 6-18). (It is called a *Bennett valve* for Dr. Ray Bennett who invented it in 1945 for use in high-altitude aircraft breathing apparatuses. After World War II, the valve was adapted for medical applications.[18]) The drum rotates in a special housing on the front and rear jeweled bearings.* As Figure 6-18, *A* shows, the drum vane creates a barrier between atmospheric and circuit pressures. Inspiration is triggered when the patient removes enough volume from the tubing to create a pressure gradient of 0.5 cm H_2O across the valve, thus causing it to rotate counterclockwise (*B*). (Note that the manufacturer presets the sensitivity of the machine at 0.5 cm H_2O, but the sensitivity [or amount of patient effort] that must be exerted to trigger inspiration can be changed by rotating the sensitivity knob counterclockwise.) The sensitivity of this valve is ultimately controlled by gas that flows to the low-pressure regulator mentioned above. Gas flow from the low-pressure regulator is directed to the Bennett valve via a port located just above the upper drum vane. As the sensitivity is increased, the gas flow through the port rotates the drum counterclockwise toward inspiration, making it easier for the patient to trigger the ventilator (i.e., the patient can trigger inspiration with less effort). A small flow of gas from the valve travels out of the exhalation valve line and inflates an exhalation diaphragm, preventing gas from escaping through the exhalation port during the inspiratory phase. Gas, which is directed into the breathing circuit and to the patient, flows through the valve, holding it open. As the pressure proximal to the valve is kept constant, the pressure gradient decreases, allowing gravity to cause a counterweight to slowly rotate the valve clockwise, back toward the closed position (*C*). When the flow through the valve decreases to 1 to 3 L/min, the force of gravity is sufficient to swing the valve completely closed, thus terminating inspiration (*D*). Once the valve is closed, gas flow to the exhalation diaphragm is halted and the diaphragm deflates, allowing gas from the patient circuit to flow into the room.

Notice that the Bennett valve also includes a port (which releases gas from within the drum to atmospheric pressure [exhalation]), a bleed hole (which allows a small leak when the valve opens to prevent it from recoiling or fluttering), and two manometer ports (see Fig 6-18, *A*). One of these manometer ports is for controlling pressure from the diluter regulator, and the other monitors pressure in the patient circuit.

Nellcor Puritan Bennett AP Series

The AP-4 and AP-5 units (Figure 6-19) are electrically powered, pressure-limited ventilators. Unlike the PR series, these devices are only patient triggered, so they can be used for

*It is important to recognize that the bearing and housing have serial numbers that must match. These components are specially machined, and mismatching of the serial numbers or damage to the bearing will impair the function of the valve.[2]

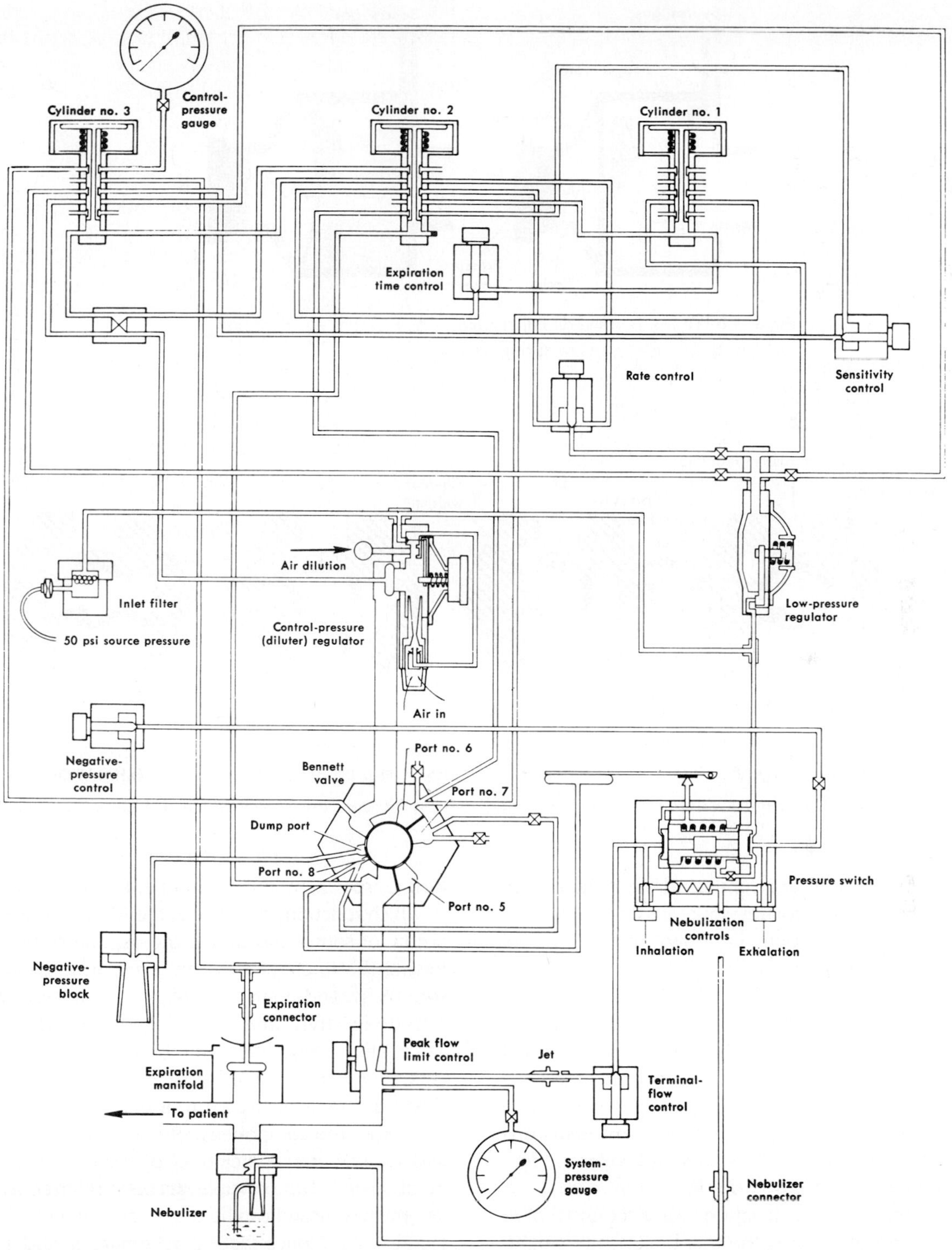

Figure 6-16 A flow schematic of a PR-2 ventilator as shown from behind the device. (Courtesy Nellcor Puritan Bennett Corp., Pleasanton, Calif.)

IPPB therapy but not for providing short-term ventilatory support of apneic patients. As shown in Figure 6-20, air from the unit's compressor passes through a filter and flows to the Venturi jet in the pressure control and then to a needle valve that controls the level of nebulization. The Venturi jet entrains additional air through an intake filter, and there is a spring-disk release valve instead of the diluter regulator of the PR series. When the pressure in the system control unit exceeds that of the spring tension, the pressure pushes the disk to the left, allowing the excess pressure to vent to ambient pressure. Note that the spring tension on the disk, and thus the peak pressure, can be adjusted to values of 0

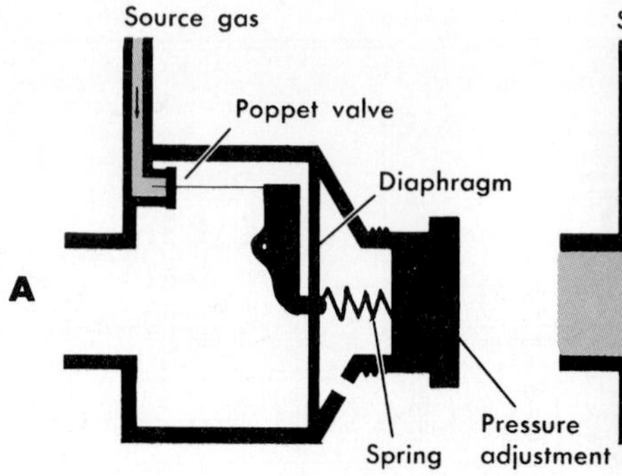

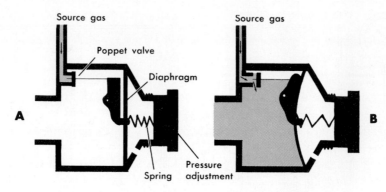

Figure 6-17 A Bennett diluter regulator. **A,** Pressure equals spring tension. **B,** Pressure is below spring tension.

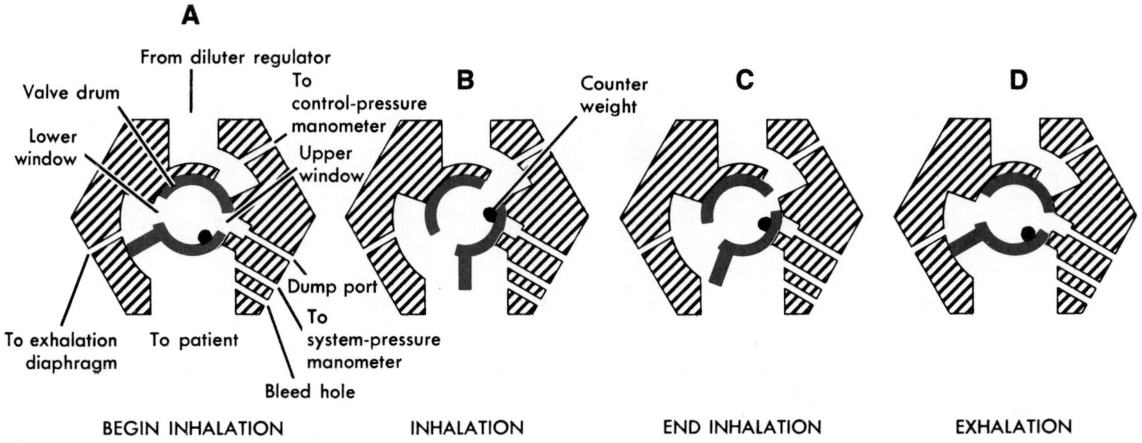

Figure 6-18 The Bennett Valve: a functional diagram. (Courtesy Nellcor Puritan Bennett Corp., Pleasanton, Calif.)

to 30 cm H_2O. With all gas venting through the release valve, the Bennett valve rotates shut, starting exhalation. When the Bennett valve opens, gas flows from the control unit to the patient.

Nellcor Puritan Bennett Circuits

The basic components of the Nellcor Puritan Bennett breathing circuit comprise large-bore corrugated tubing, a nebulizer, and an exhalation valve. As discussed in Chapter 4, two types of nebulizers are available: **mainstream** (Bennett slip/stream; Figure 6-21, *A*) and **sidestream** (Bennett Twin) **nebulizers** (Figure 6-21, *B*).

The Bennett retard exhalation valve consists of a spring that is compressed as the diaphragm nut is tightened (Figure 6-22). When the nut is loosened, the spring pushes the diaphragm closer to the shoulder of the exhalation valve, causing a resistance to expiratory gas flow. The **gas-collector exhalation valve** (Figure 6-23) allows expired gases to be measured through one directional port.

Bird Devices

The prototype Bird ventilator is the Mark 7, which was designed and developed by Forrest M. Bird, founder of the Bird Corporation. Bird subsequently introduced the Mark 8, which functions similarly to the Mark 7, but can provide a flow of source gas during the expiratory phase, thus allowing the operator to apply a negative expiratory pressure. A second generation of Bird ventilators were introduced in the late 1970s and provided additional capabilities. These latter units, however, also used the same ceramic control valve and ambient and pressure compartments as the first generation of Bird ventilators.

Before the components of the various Bird IPPB ventilators are described, their basic operational principle should be discussed. This principle has been referred as *magnetism vs. gas pressure* and can be described using the schematic in Figure 6-24. Notice that the schematic includes a series of boxes. Each box is divided into two compartments by a diaphragm, which has metal clutch plates attached to either side. Permanent magnets, which are aligned with the clutch plates, are located in each compartment. The left compartment is exposed to atmospheric pressure through a port in the lower left corner of box. The pressure on the right side of each box can be varied by moving gas into and out of a port in the lower right corner of the box.

If the two compartments are subjected to atmospheric pressure (Figure 6-24, *A*), there is no pressure difference

A

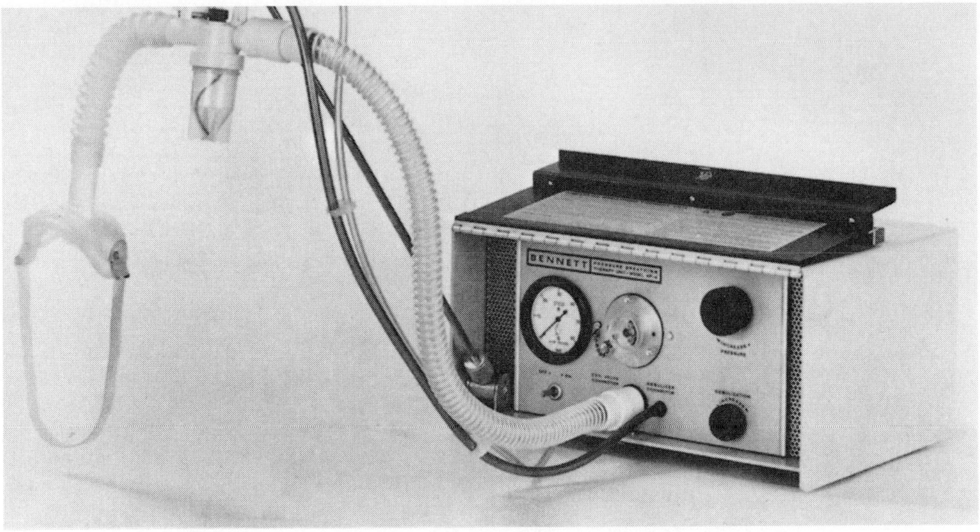

B

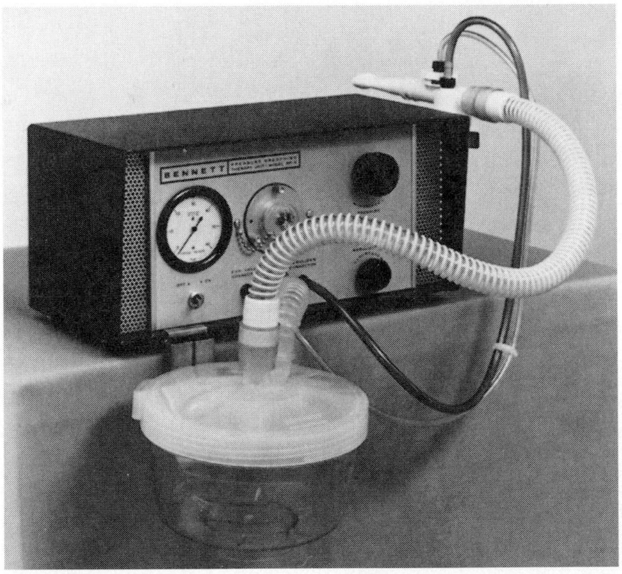

Figure 6-19 **A,** A Bennett AP-4. **B,** A Bennett AP-5. Both units are air compressor-driven ventilators. (Courtesy Nellcor Puritan Bennett Corp., Pleasanton, Calif.)

between them, and the diaphragm remains straight. But when a pressure gradient is created between the right and left compartments, the diaphragm flexes. In *B,* as gas volume is removed from the right compartment, the pressure inside the compartment decreases to below atmospheric, causing the diaphragm and the attached metal plates to flex to the right. The clutch plate on the right is now close to the magnet on the right, and the plate and magnet are attracted to each other. Although the pressure on the right may return to atmospheric pressure (*C*), the diaphragm will remain attracted to the right magnet until sufficient gas volume and pressure are added to the right side to overcome the magnetic attraction (*D*). Once there is sufficient positive pressure to overcome the magnetic attraction, the diaphragm will be pushed to the left where it will remain.

Bird Mark 7 Series

The Mark 7 is a pneumatically powered ventilator, which can be time-, pressure-, or manually triggered and time- or pressure-cycled. Similar to the Nellcor Puritan Bennett PR series, the Mark 7 can be used to provide short-term ventilatory support, but it is primarily used as a means of delivering IPPB therapy.

Figure 6-25 shows the major components of the Bird Mark 7 ventilator. Gas flow through the Mark 7 is shown in Figure 6-26. During inspiration (*A*), negative pressure generated by the patient (along with atmospheric pressure in the left compartment) causes the diaphragm to move toward the right, away from the left compartment. Gas flow is allowed to pass through the ceramic control switch and then splits, traveling in the left side to the Venturi jet and passing to the line powering the nebulizer and exhalation

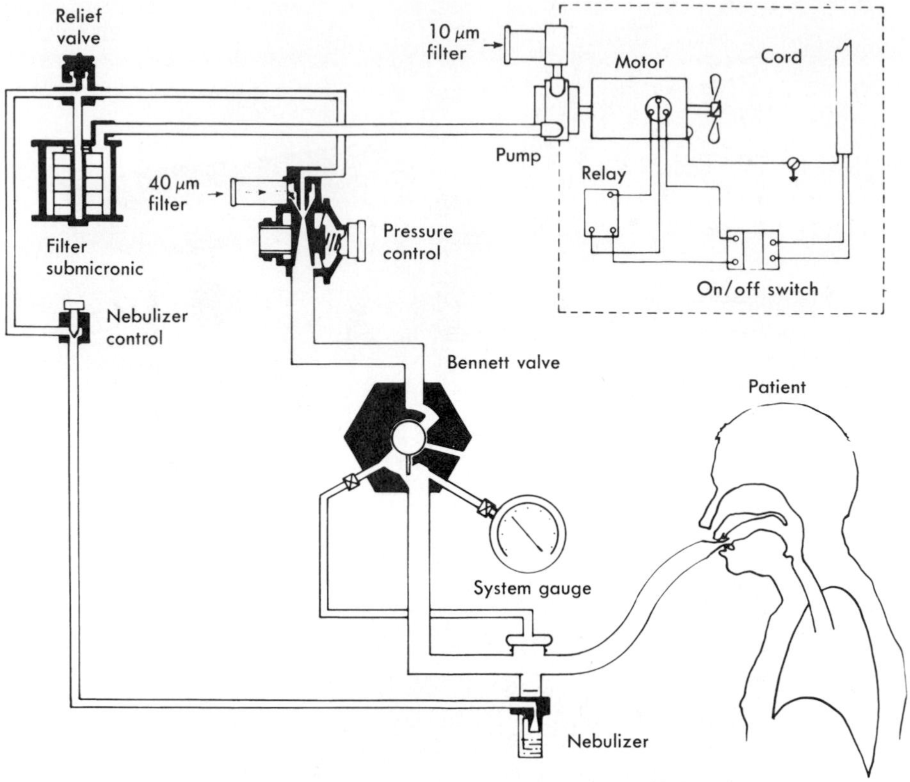

Figure 6-20 A functional diagram of AP series ventilators. (Courtesy Nellcor Puritan Bennett Corp., Pleasanton, Calif.)

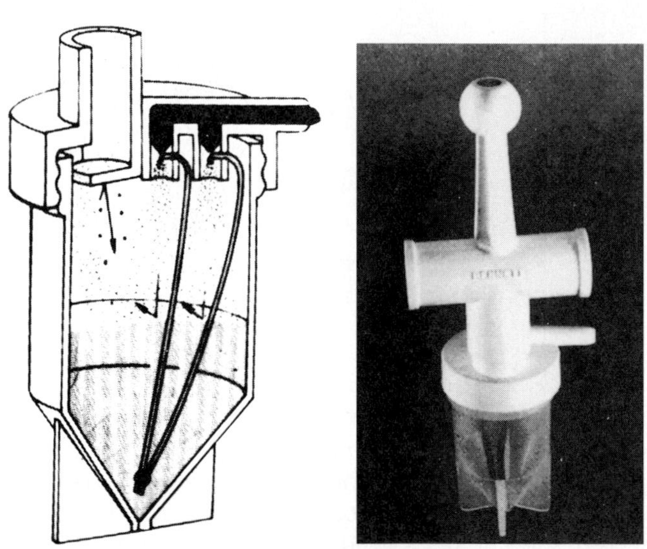

Figure 6-21 A Bennett Twin jet nebulizer. (Courtesy Nellcor Puritan Bennett Corp., Pleasanton, Calif.)

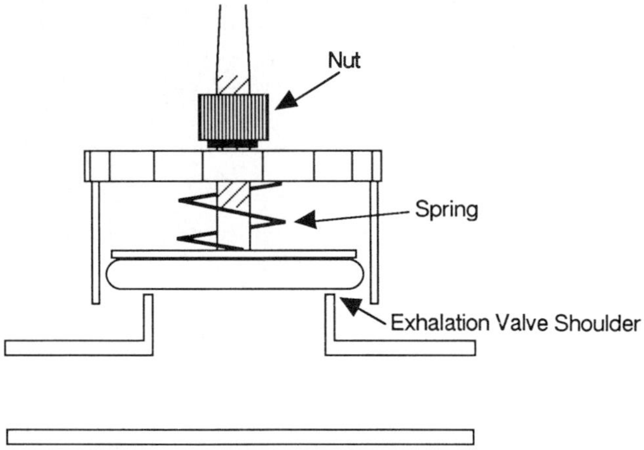

Figure 6-22 A Bennett retard exhalation valve.

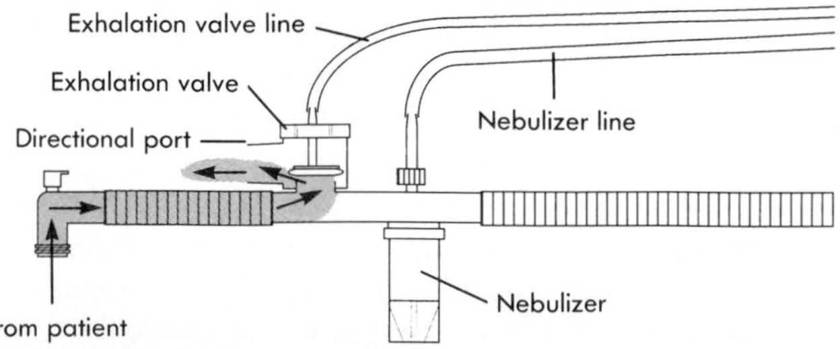

Figure 6-23 A Bennett gas collector exhalation valve.

valve. The Venturi jet then entrains air, and gas moves through the Venturi gate to the patient. This gas then enters the patient's lungs, and the pressure begins to build in the right compartment. Thus at the beginning of inspiration, gas flow into the circuit comes from three sources: (1) the Ven-

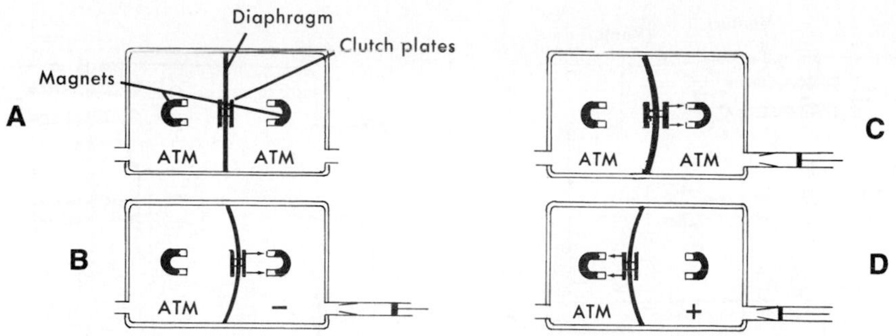

Figure 6-24 Pressure changes across the diaphragm with magnetic force (see text for explanation). *ATM,* Atmospheric pressure. (Modified from Bird Corp., Palm Springs, Calif.)

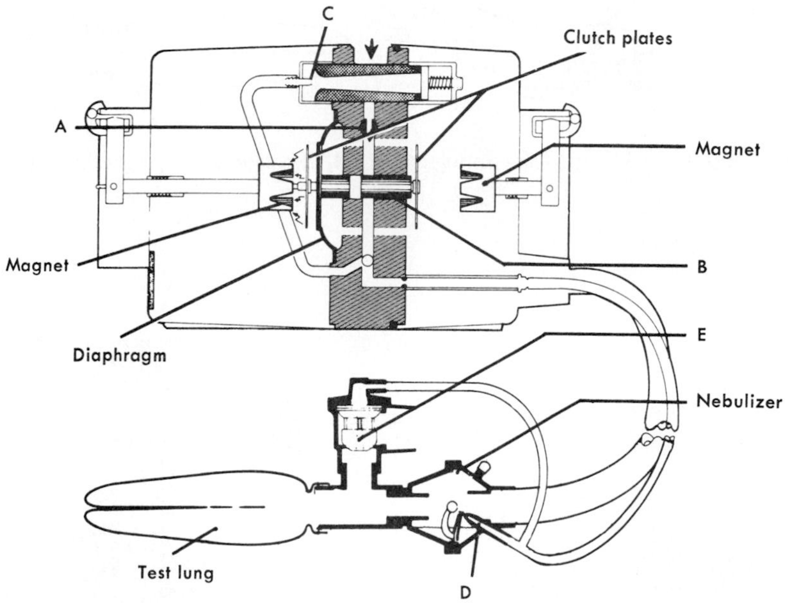

Figure 6-25 Structure of a Bird Mark 7. (Courtesy Bird Corp., Palm Springs, Calif.)

turi, (2) air the Venturi entrains, and (3) the nebulizer jet. As end-inspiration is approached, the pressure in the right compartment equals the forward pressure through the Venturi, and the Venturi gate closes. The gas from the Venturi jet is then forced into the left side of the machine, flushing that compartment with source gas. Once the Venturi gate closes, the only gas flowing into the patient's system during the remainder of inspiration comes from source gas through the nebulizer jet. Eventually, this jet adds enough gas to make the pressure exceed the magnetic attraction of the right (pressure-controlled) magnet. The diaphragm, clutch plate, and ceramic switch are then forced to the left, occluding gas flow into the respirator and starting exhalation. The amount of pressure needed to end inspiration depends on the magnetic attraction between the right clutch plate and the corresponding magnet. Like the left clutch plate and magnet, the amount of attraction is related to the distance between the right plate and its magnet. The distance, and thus the peak inspiratory pressure, can be set with the pressure adjustment lever on the right side of the machine. Because gas is no longer flowing into the flow control valve, the gas in the lines below the ceramic switch exits through the jets. The diaphragm and exhalation valve are now uncharged, and the existing positive pressure in the patient circuit simply pushes the exhalation valve gate open, allowing the patient to exhale passively (*B*).

The Mark 7 contains a pneumatic expiratory timing device that can be used to provide pressure-cycled ventilation. The timer is a pneumatic cartridge with an adjustable leak (Figure 6-27). On inspiration, the cartridge is charged by source gas, which enters via a one-way valve. The gas pushes the diaphragm to the left, depressing the spring and moving the plunger and arm to the left. The leak from the cartridge around the needle valve control is small when

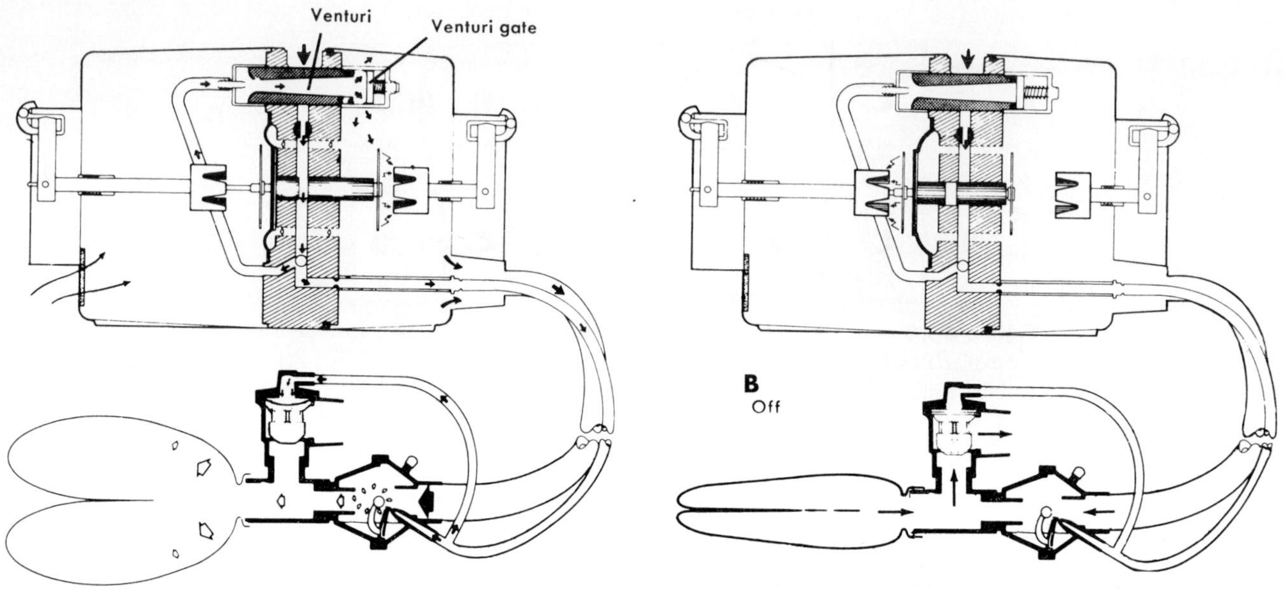

Figure 6-26 **A,** Inhalation. (Courtesy Bird Corp., Palm Springs, Calif.) **B,** Exhalation. (Courtesy Bird Corp., Palm Springs, Calif.)

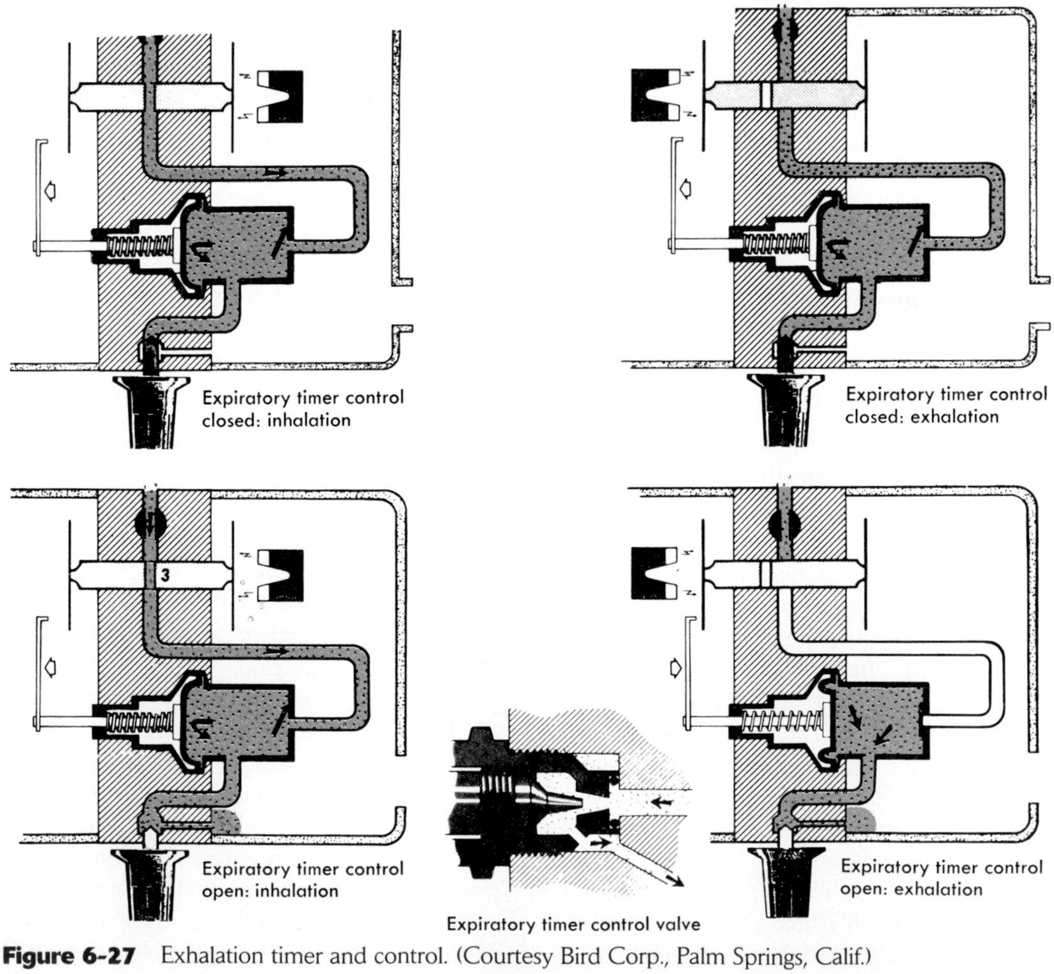

Figure 6-27 Exhalation timer and control. (Courtesy Bird Corp., Palm Springs, Calif.)

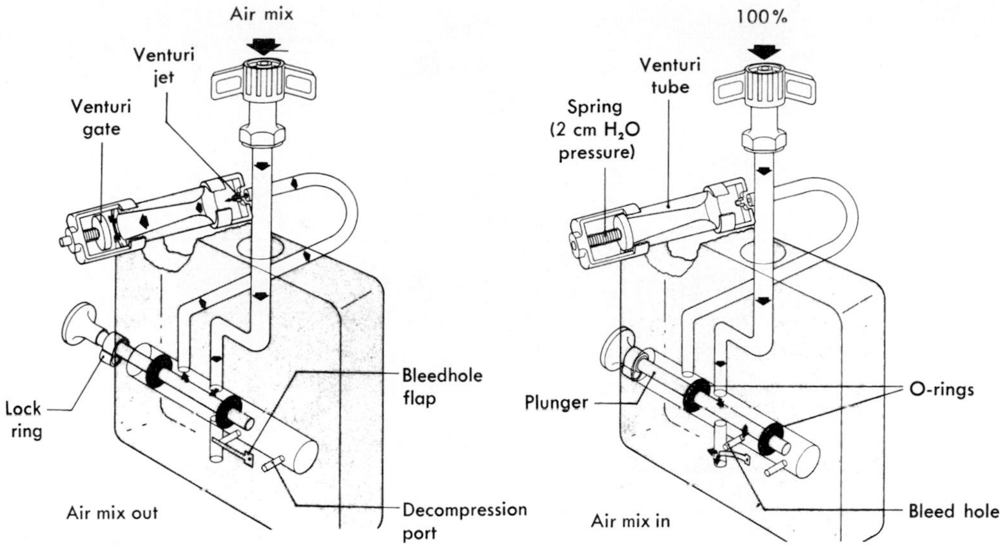

Figure 6-28 Air-Mix control for Bird Mark 7. The schematics show typical patterns for flow and pressure during Air-Mix (*left*) and 100% oxygen (*right*). (Courtesy Bird Corp., Palm Springs, Calif.)

compared with the incoming gas flow. Thus once inspiration has begun, the unit is completely charged until inhalation ends. At end-inspiration, no source gas is supplied to the cartridge, and the one-way entrance valve closes. The only way for gas to leave the cartridge is the leak past the needle valve on the outflow track. As gas leaks out, pressure decreases, and the diaphragm is pushed to the right by the spring. Concurrently, the plunger and its attached arm are moved slowly to the right. Once the arm touches the clutch plate, the clutch plate is pushed away from the magnet, and the ceramic switch is moved into the "on" position. Thus the length of expiratory time is controlled by the needle valve; and the greater the leak past the needle valve, the faster the cartridge will discharge and the shorter the exhalation time.

Notice that directly below the ceramic switch is the air-mix control. As shown in Figure 6-28, it is a two-position switch, allowing for delivery of either an air-mixed gas (varying FiO_2) or a gas with an FiO_2 of 1.0. When this switch is pushed in, the O rings seal the incoming source gas and direct it out the reed-covered bleed hole in the center body, providing a constant flow during the inspiratory phase. When the air-mix control switch is pulled out, the top O ring blocks the bleed hole, and gas is directed to the jet of the air-mix Venturi. The decompression port above the bleed hole allows the plunger to be pushed in without compressing the gas behind it, so functionally it plays no part in the air-mix control. In the air-mix (switch pulled out) setting (Figure 6-28, *A*), source gas is from: (1) the Venturi jet, (2) the air entrained by the Venturi system, and (3) the nebulizer jet. In the air-mix position, the Venturi is activated, producing a descending flow pattern and an irregular pressure waveform that ranges from ascending to rectangular, depending on the compliance and resistance of the patient's respiratory system. In the 100% setting (i.e., switch pushed in; *B*), there are two sources of gas flow throughout inspiration, producing a square-wave or constant flow pattern and an ascending pressure waveform.

Bird Mark 8 Series

The Bird Mark 8 (Figure 6-29) is functionally similar to the Mark 7, but it can provide a constant flow of source gas during the expiratory phase. The knob for adjusting the level of flow is on top of the machine, connected to a needle valve and a flow interrupter switch. The switch is a pneumatic cartridge containing a plunger, spring, and diaphragm. During inspiration, gas flows through the ceramic switch, which charges the cartridge and blocks the flow of 50 psig source gas to the Venturi. During expiration, gas flowing through the Venturi entrains expired gases from the circuit and the patient and directs them out the exhalation valve.

The Bird Mark 8 was originally designed to allow for the application of NEEP. As was already stated, NEEP has been shown to be ineffective in reducing airtrapping and is no longer used.

Bird Mark 10 and 14 Series

The Mark 10 and Mark 14 ventilators are similar to the Mark 7 series, except that they do not have an air-mix control, which means that they can only operate in the air-dilution mode.[20] Additionally, they include a control for providing inspiratory flow acceleration, which can be used to compensate for leaks in the system. The primary difference between the Mark 14 series and the Mark 10 series is that Mark 14 ventilators can produce pressures as high as 200 cm H_2O.[20]

A

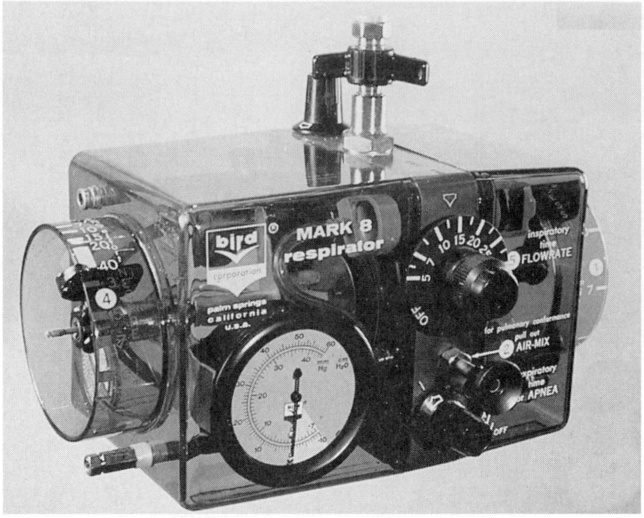

B

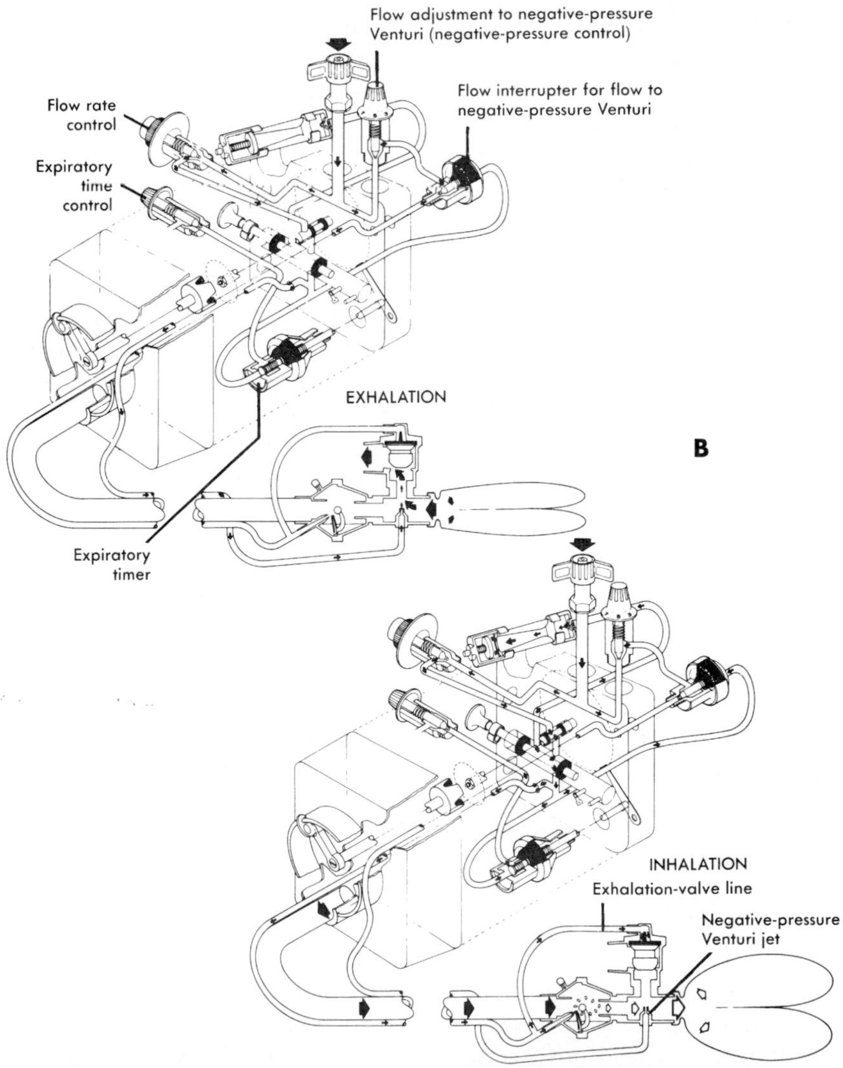

Figure 6-29 ***A,*** Bird Mark 8. ***B,*** Bird Mark 8 flow diagram. (Courtesy Bird Corp., Palm Springs, Calif.)

BOX 6-7

Decision Making & Problem Solving

A 22-year old man previously diagnosed with cystic fibrosis is admitted to the emergency department following a recent history of upper respiratory infection. A physical examination reveals that the patient is alert and cooperative; his respiratory rate is 40 breaths/min. Coarse, wet breath sounds are heard over all lung fields. He reports producing copious amounts of purulent, foul-smelling sputum for the past 3 days. His heart rate is 110 beats/min, and his oral temperature is 102° F. Arterial blood pressure is 150/100; MIP is −50 cm H_2O; and SpO_2 is 90%. Chest radiographs show bilateral pneumonia. The pulmonology resident suggests using IPPB treatments. Do you agree with this suggestion?

See Appendix A for answer.

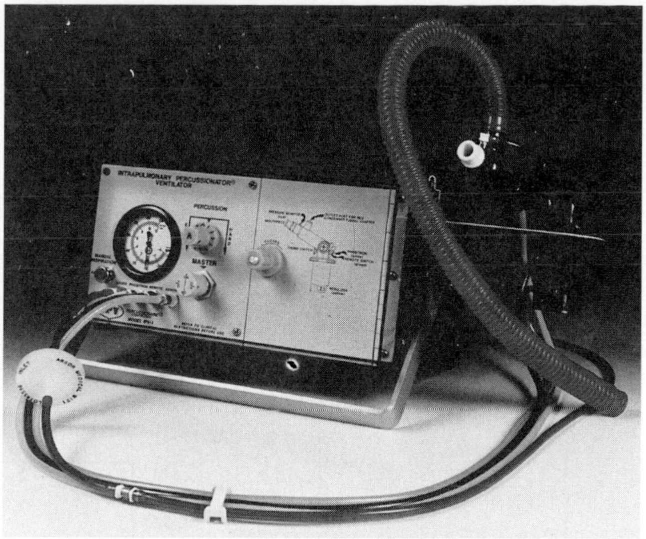

Figure 6-30 A Percussionaire Intrapulmonary Percussive Ventilator (IPV-1). (Courtesy Percussionaire Corp., Sand Point, Ohio.)

Intrapulmonary Percussive Ventilation (IPV)

This relatively new form of IPPB therapy was introduced by Forrest Bird in 1979 as an adjunct technique for mobilizing airway secretions. It involves the delivery of **high-frequency percussive breaths** into the patient's airways instead of applying percussions to the outside of the chest wall as in standard CPT techniques (Box 6-7).[24]

The Percussionaire Intrapulmonary Percussive Ventilator (IPV-1), which is the prototype IPV device, is shown in Figure 6-30. It is manually cycled and can provide pressure- or flow-targeted breaths. Inspiration can be triggered manually by selecting push-button control on the nebulizer (i.e., the patient is typically instructed to trigger inspiration by depressing the button for 5 to 10 seconds). Alternately, the therapist can trigger the percussive cycle by pressing the inspiration button on the control panel. Expiration is manually cycled by releasing the inspiratory control button.

The Percussionaire is powered by a 25 to 50 psi compressed-gas source. Figure 6-31 shows gas flow through the IPV-1 unit.[24] Gas enters the unit and passes through a filter before flowing into a pressure regulator, which reduces the pressure to a value preset by the operator. From there, gas flows to: (1) an oscillator cartridge and a **Phasitron,** which increases and decreases air pressures, (2) a nebulizer, and (3) a remote control. Gas travels from the Phasitron outlet through small-bore tubing to the Phasitron unit, which contains a sliding Venturi (Figure 6-32). The Venturi slides forward during the impact phase, and a burst of air travels into the Venturi orifice, which in turn entrains room air (i.e., for each unit of gas that passes through the Venturi, four units of air are entrained). This enhanced burst of gas then passes through the mouthpiece to the patient. Following the injection phase, the Venturi slides back, and the expiratory valve simultaneously opens, allowing the patient to passively exhale.

The nebulizer receives high-pressure gas from the internal regulator via the small-bore tubing connected to the front of the unit. Air flows through the jet, past the nebulizer, creating an area of reduced pressure that draws medication from the reservoir. A high-pressure gas at the top of the jet meets the stream of medication, creating a mist that is delivered to the circuit. Note that the entrainment post of the Venturi is connected to the nebulizer by large-bore aerosol tubing, thus allowing the patient to receive the mist during the percussive phase of operation.

The Percussionaire can deliver percussive pressures of 25 to 40 cm H_2O at about 100 to 300 cycles per minute, or 1.7 to 5.0 Hz (Figure 6-33).[24] The effectiveness of IPV therapy, compared with that of traditional chest physiotherapy techniques, is still under investigation. It has been suggested that IPV may provide another potentially useful method of improving sputum mobilization in certain patients (e.g., cystic fibrosis, chronic bronchitis)[24]; but although these studies are encouraging, additional studies are needed to more clearly define the appropriate indications and contraindications for IPV therapy. Indeed, as Fink[24] has pointed out, it can only be assumed that the contraindications and hazards for IPV are similar to those of other forms of mechanical ventilation.

Positive Airway Pressure (PAP) Devices

PAP techniques, which include continuous positive airway pressure (CPAP), expiratory positive airway pressure (EPAP),

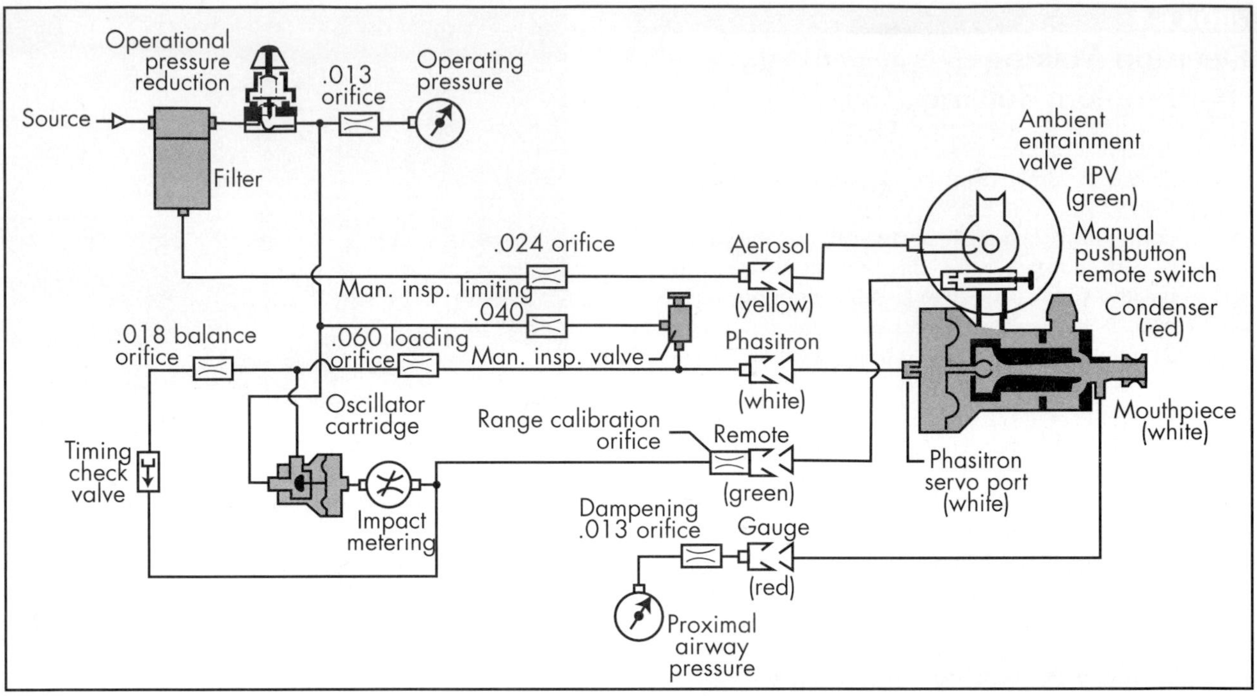

Figure 6-31 Gas flow through the IPV-1. (Courtesy Percussionaire, Palm Springs, Calif.)

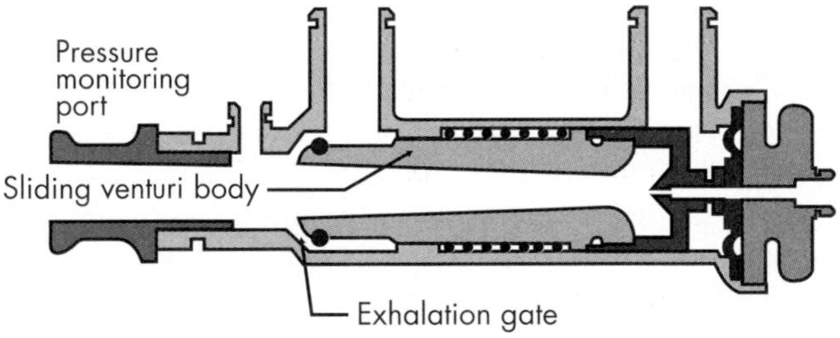

Figure 6-32 A Phasitron unit used in the IPV-1.

and positive expiratory pressure (PEP), are airway adjuncts that can be used to enhance bronchial hygiene therapy by reducing airtrapping in susceptible patients.[25,26] As such, these techniques have been shown to be quite effective in mobilizing retained secretions, preventing or reversing atelectasis, and optimizing the delivery of bronchodilators for patients with cystic fibrosis and chronic bronchitis. The AARC has produced a Clinical Practice Guideline for PAP adjuncts to bronchial hygiene therapy, which should be read before PAP therapy is performed on patients.[26] Box 6-8 summarizes several important points from this guideline.

Continuous Positive Airway Pressure (CPAP)

This form of PAP therapy involves the application of positive pressure to a patient's airways throughout the respiratory cycle (i.e., the airway pressure is consistently maintained between 5 and 20 cm H_2O during both inspiration and expiration). It is accomplished by having the patient breathe from a pressurized circuit that incorporates a threshold resistor in the expiratory limb.

Figure 6-34 shows four types of threshold resistors: **underwater seal resistors, weighted-ball resistors, spring-loaded valve resistors,** and **magnetic valve resistors.**[25] With underwater seal resistors, tubing attached to the expiratory port of the circuit is submerged under a column of water. The level of CPAP is determined by the height of the column. Weighted-ball resistors consist of a specially milled steel ball placed over a calibrated orifice, which is attached directly above the expiratory port of the circuit. It is important that the balls are maintained in a vertical position to ensure consistent pressure.[1] Spring-loaded resistors rely on a spring to hold a disc or diaphragm down over the expiratory port of the circuit. Magnetic valve resistors contain a bar magnet that attracts a ferromagnetic disc seated on the expiratory port of the circuit. The amount of pressure required to separate the disc from the magnet is determined by the distance between them (i.e., the greater the distance between the magnet and the disc, the lower the pressure required to open the expiratory port, and thus the lower the level of CPAP). All of these valves operate on the principle that the level of PAP generated within the circuit depends on the amount of resistance that must be overcome to allow gas to exit the exhalation valve. The main advantage of threshold resistors is that they provide predictable, quantifiable, and constant force during expiration that is independent of the flow achieved by the patient during exhalation.[1]

BOX 6-8

Clinical Practice Guidelines

Use of Positive Airway Pressure Adjuncts to Bronchial Hygiene Therapy

Indications

1. To reduce air trapping in patients with asthma and/or COPD
2. To help mobilize retained secretions in patients with cystic fibrosis and/or chronic bronchitis
3. To prevent or reverse atelectasis
4. To optimize bronchodilator delivery in patients receiving bronchial hygiene therapy

Contraindications

1. Patients unable to tolerate the increased work of breathing (acute asthma, COPD)
2. Intracranial pressure >20 mm Hg
3. Hemodynamic instability
4. Recent facial, oral, or skull surgery
5. Acute sinusitis
6. Epistaxis
7. Esophageal surgery
8. Active hemoptysis
9. Nausea
10. Known or suspected tympanic membrane rupture or other middle ear pathology
11. Untreated pneumothorax

Assessment of Outcome

1. Increased sputum production in patients producing >30 mL/day of sputum without PEP suggests that therapy should be continued
2. Improved breath sounds (i.e., diminished breath sounds change to adventitious breath sounds) that can be auscultated over the larger airways, demonstrating that therapy is indicated
3. Patient response to therapy
4. Changes in vital signs: moderate changes in respiratory rate and/or pulse rate are expected, but bradycardia, tachycardia, an increasingly irregular pulse, or a drop or dramatic increase in blood pressure are indications to stop therapy
5. Changes in arterial blood gases or oxygen saturation should improve as atelectasis resolves

Monitoring

1. Patient response to pain, discomfort, dyspnea, and therapy in general
2. Pulse rate and cardiac rhythm (if electrocardiogram is available)
3. Breathing pattern and rate
4. Sputum production (quantity, color, consistency, and odor)
5. Mental function
6. Cyanosis or pallor
7. Breath sounds
8. Blood pressure
9. Pulse oximetry (if hypoxemia with the procedure has been previously demonstrated or is suspected)
10. Blood gas analysis (if indicated)
11. Intracranial pressure in patients for whom this value is of critical importance

AARC Clinical Practice Guideline: Use of positive airway pressure adjuncts to bronchial hygiene therapy, Respir Care 38:516, 1993.

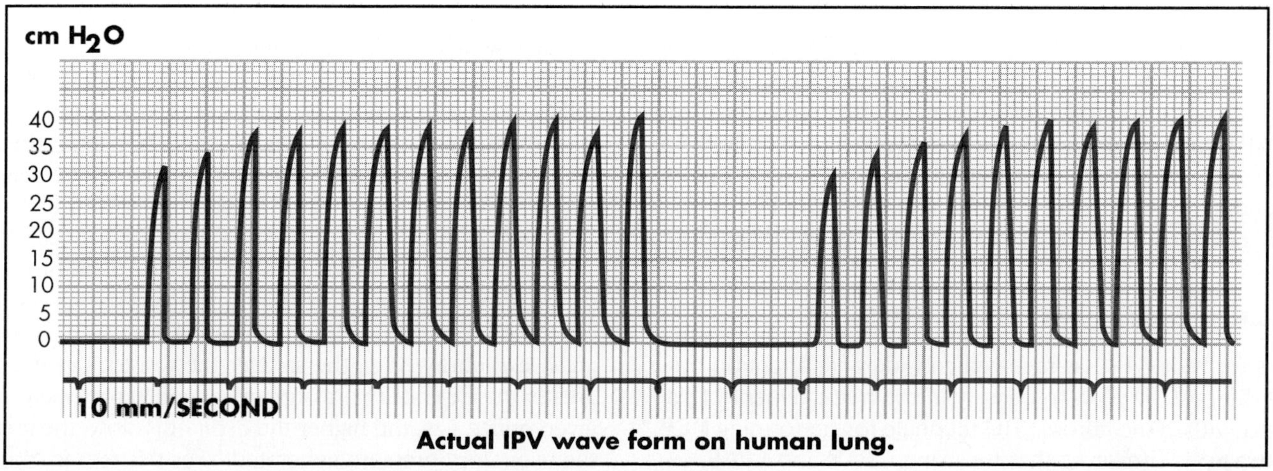

Figure 6-33 A pressure waveform generated during operation of the IPV-1.

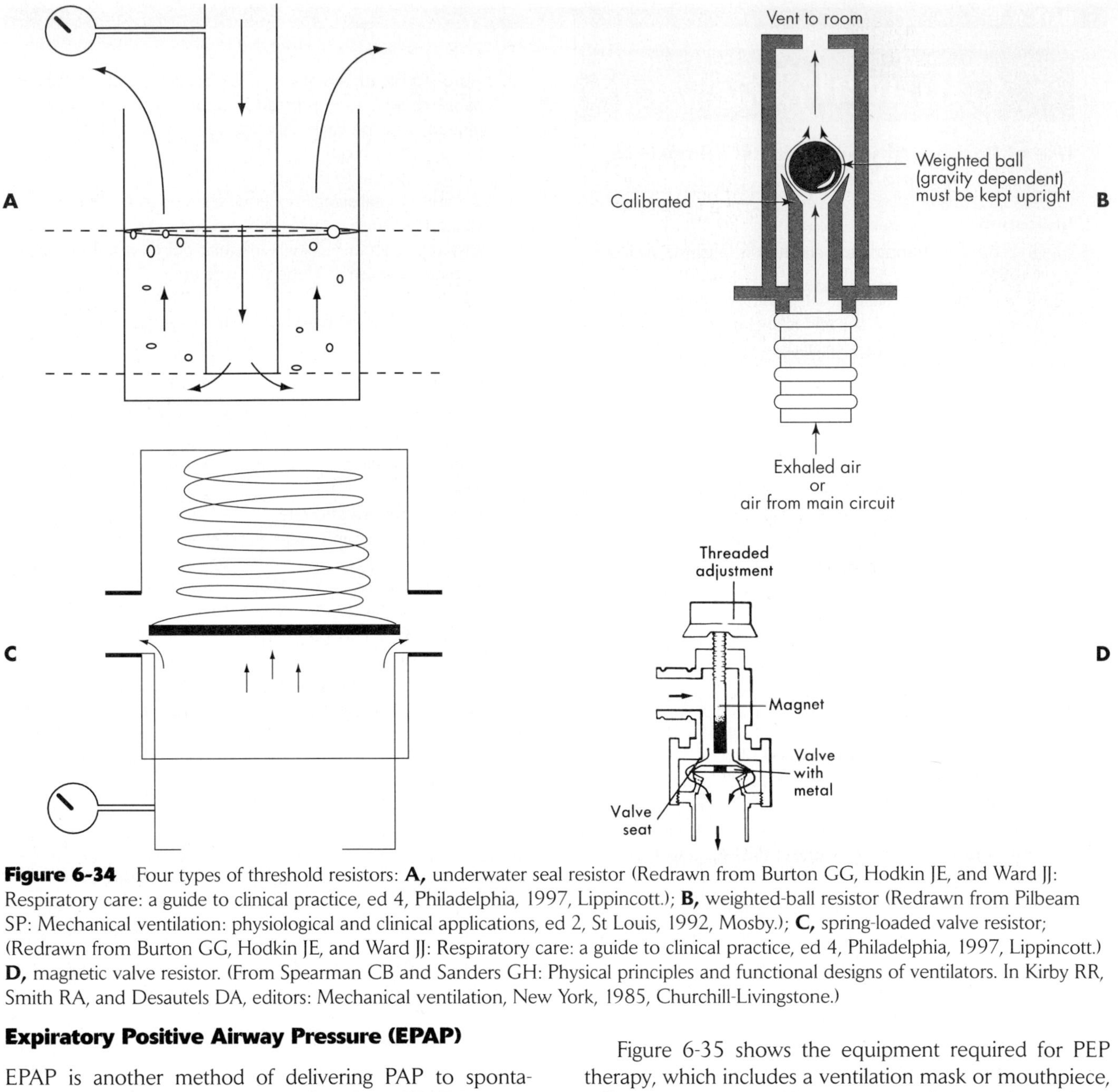

Figure 6-34 Four types of threshold resistors: **A,** underwater seal resistor (Redrawn from Burton GG, Hodkin JE, and Ward JJ: Respiratory care: a guide to clinical practice, ed 4, Philadelphia, 1997, Lippincott.); **B,** weighted-ball resistor (Redrawn from Pilbeam SP: Mechanical ventilation: physiological and clinical applications, ed 2, St Louis, 1992, Mosby.); **C,** spring-loaded valve resistor; (Redrawn from Burton GG, Hodkin JE, and Ward JJ: Respiratory care: a guide to clinical practice, ed 4, Philadelphia, 1997, Lippincott.) **D,** magnetic valve resistor. (From Spearman CB and Sanders GH: Physical principles and functional designs of ventilators. In Kirby RR, Smith RA, and Desautels DA, editors: Mechanical ventilation, New York, 1985, Churchill-Livingstone.)

Expiratory Positive Airway Pressure (EPAP)

EPAP is another method of delivering PAP to spontaneously breathing patients and differs from CPAP because it involves the creation of PAP only during expiration. With EPAP, the patient generates a subatmospheric pressure on inspiration, and then exhales against a threshold expiratory resistance similar to those described for CPAP devices. Airway pressures during EPAP can be set at 10 to 20 cm H_2O.

Positive Expiratory Pressure (PEP)

This form of PAP has received considerable attention during the past 10 years, especially in the management of patients with cystic fibrosis. The rationale for performing **PEP therapy** is similar to that for using CPAP and EPAP, except that PEP seems to be less cumbersome and more manageable for patients.

Figure 6-35 shows the equipment required for PEP therapy, which includes a ventilation mask or mouthpiece, a T-piece assembly with a one-way valve, a series of fixed orifice resistors (or an adjustable orifice resistor), and a pressure manometer.[1,26] Notice that bronchodilator therapy with an MDI or SVN can be performed simultaneously by attaching these devices to the inspiratory port of the mask or mouthpiece.

The amount of PAP generated with the fixed-orifice resistor varies with the size of the orifice and the level of expiratory flow produced by the patient. For example, for any given expiratory flow, the smaller the resistor's orifice, the greater the expiratory pressure generated. Conversely, for a given orifice size, the higher the expiratory flow, the greater the expiratory pressure generated.[1] For this reason, the patient must be encouraged to achieve a flow high enough to maintain expiratory pressure at 10 to 20 cm H_2O.

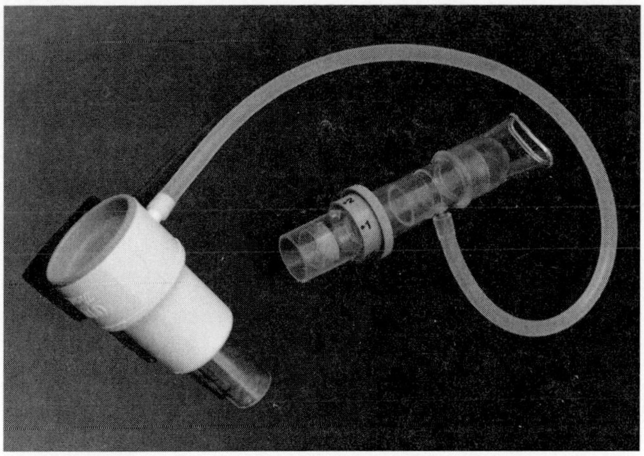

Figure 6-35 Equipment used during PEP therapy.

The procedure for performing PEP therapy is shown in Box 6-9. Several factors should be considered when creating a therapeutic regimen using these devices. The level of resistance chosen should allow the patient to achieve the therapeutic goal of generating PEP of 10 to 20 cm H_2O with an inspiratory:expiratory (I:E) ratio of 1:3 or 1:4. The patient should perform 10 to 20 breaths through the device, then perform a series of two to three huff coughs to clear loosened secretions. This cycle should be repeated 5 to 10 times during a 15- to 20-minute session. Finally, the patient should be encouraged to learn how to self-administer this therapy, though more than one session may be required to ensure patient proficiency in using these devices.

BOX 6-9

Procedure for Performing PEP Therapy

1. The mask is applied tightly but comfortably over the patient's nose and mouth. When a mouthpiece is used, patients are instructed to form a tight seal around the mouthpiece.
2. Patients are instructed to inspire through the one-way valve to a volume that is greater than their normal tidal volume—but not their total lung capacity.
3. At the end of inspiration, patients are encouraged to actively but not forcefully exhale to FRC to achieve an airway pressure of 10 to 20 cm H_2O.
4. Patients should perform 10 to 20 breaths through the device, then perform a series of two to three huff coughs to clear loosened secretions.
5. This cycle should be repeated 5 to 10 times during a 15- to 20-minute session.

CHEST PHYSIOTHERAPY DEVICES

Chest physiotherapy (CPT) is a collection of techniques used to help clear airway secretions, improve the distribution of ventilation, and enhance the efficiency and conditioning of the respiratory muscles.[18] Such techniques include breathing exercises, directed coughing, postural drainage, and chest percussion and vibration.

Percussion and vibration, both of which involve the application of mechanical energy to the chest wall, provide a means of loosening retained secretions from the walls of the tracheobronchial tract. Once loosened, the secretions can be coughed up and expectorated or be removed by suctioning.

Percussion and vibration can be accomplished using either the hands or various mechanical or electrical devices. For this discussion, chest percussors have been divided into three categories: manual percussors, pneumatically powered devices, and electrically powered devices.

Manual Percussors

The traditional method of administering CPT involves cupping the hand (as if scooping water from a basin) and clapping on the patient's chest wall. Although this technique is quite effective in most cases, it can be tiring for the person administering the therapy and somewhat painful for the patient (if performed by someone inexperienced in CPT). As a result of these potential problems, several companies have produced some simple manual percussors that are fairly inexpensive and easy to use. Figure 6-36 shows a typical manual percussor marketed by DHD Medical Products. This device is made of soft vinyl and is formed to the shape of the palm. It is available in neonatal, pediatric, and adult sizes.

Pneumatically Powered Devices

These percussors are powered by a compressed-air or oxygen source that operates at 45 to 55 psig. Although devices may differ in the number of accessories provided, each device usually comprises a high-pressure hose, a body with controls for varying the frequency and force of percussive strokes, and a remote head with a concave applicator. Several common examples of pneumatically powered percussors are the Fluid Flo (Figure 6-37), the Hudson Pediatric, the Mercury MJ, and the Fluid Flo percussors. The Strom PPS3, the Mercury MJ, and the Fluid Flo are designed for pediatric and adult patients. The Fluid Flo is only for adult patients.

Electrically Powered Percussors

Most of these devices are powered by electrical outputs of 110 volts of alternating current, although some units are battery powered. Several of the more common units available in the United States are produced by General Physiotherapy (the Vibramatic/Multimatic, the Flimm Fighter, and the Neo-Cussor), Strom, and Nellcor Puritan Bennett

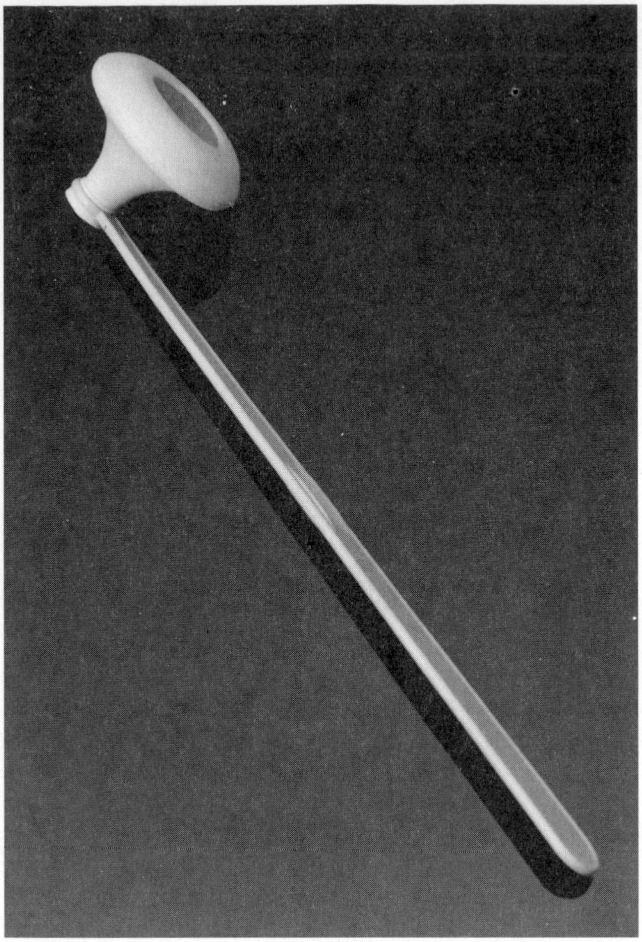

Figure 6-36 A manual percussor.

(Vibrator/Percussor). Most units typically have a variable control switch for setting the frequency of percussions and can be used for both adult and pediatric patients.

Each system, however, has unique features. The Vibramatic/Multimatic (Figure 6-38) produces two directional forces: one produces a stroking action that operates perpendicular to the chest wall to loosen mucus attached to

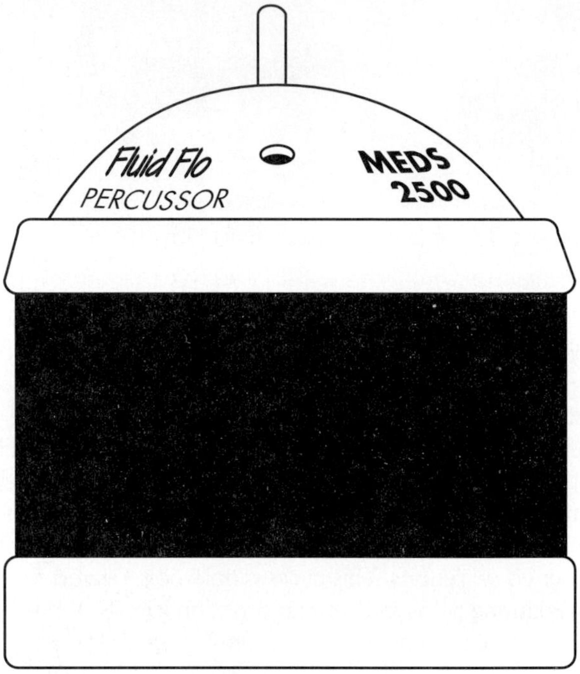

Figure 6-37 A Fluid Flo pneumatic percussor. (Courtesy Med Systems, Inc., San Diego, Calif.)

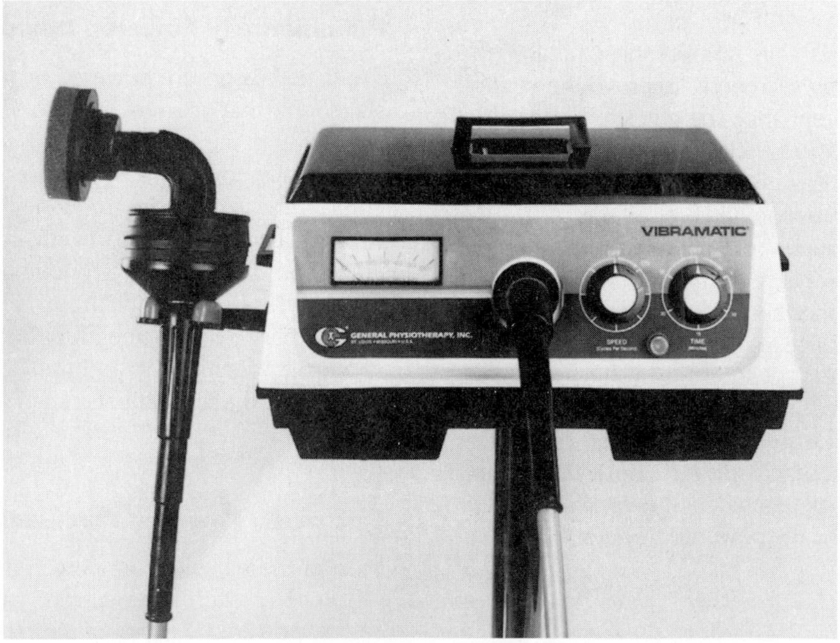

Figure 6-38 A Vibramatic/Multmatic electrically powered percussor. (Courtesy General Physiotherapy, Inc., St Louis)

the tracheobronchial tubes, and the other operates parallel to the chest wall and moves the mucus toward the central airways. The Flimm Fighter is designed primarily for home use–it comes with a foam pad and a Velcro (Velcro USA, Inc., Manchester, NH) belt to allow for self-application of the device.[19] The Neo-Cussor is a battery-operated device that uses a disposable applicator and is specifically designed for use with neonates and pediatric patients. The Nellcor Puritan Bennett Vibrator/Percussor allows for independent control of frequency and stroke intensity.

Summary

The primary indication for lung expansion therapy is to prevent and treat atelectasis. Various strategies and devices are available to accomplish this goal. Incentive spirometry, IPPB, PAP techniques, and CPT have all been shown to be effective lung hyperexpansion methods. Selection of the appropriate device and therapeutic mode should be based on the patient's ability to perform the procedure and on the therapeutic goals. Evaluation of the effectiveness of therapy should be based on history and physical findings, chest radiographs, and a review of laboratory tests (i.e., arterial blood gases).

Review Questions

See Appendix A for answers.

1. What is the primary indication for lung inflation therapy?
   I. Prevent atelectasis
   II. Prevent hypoxemia
   III. Reverse hypercapnia
   IV. Reduce pulmonary shunting
   a. I only
   b. I and II only
   c. II and III only
   d. I, II, III, and IV
2. What is the minimum FiO_2 that a manual resuscitator with a reservoir should deliver according to ASTM and ISO recommendations?
   a. 0.40 with an oxygen flow of 8 L/min
   b. 0.70 with an oxygen flow of 10 L/min
   c. 0.85 with an oxygen flow of 15 L/min
   d. 1.0 with an oxygen flow of 6 L/min
3. Which of the following are standards recommended for the design and construction of manual resuscitators?
   I. Manual resuscitators must be able to operate at relative humidities of 40% to 96%.
   II. Adult resuscitators must deliver a tidal volume of at least 600 mL into a test lung set at a compliance of 0.02 L/cm H_2O.
   III. The resuscitator's nonrebreathing valve must be designed so that the valve will not jam at oxygen flows up to 40 L/min.
   IV. Resuscitators that are used for adults should have a pressure-limiting system.
   a. I only
   b. I and II only
   c. I, II, and III only
   d. I, II, III, and IV
4. Incentive spirometry is indicated for patients who are predisposed to develop atelectasis. List four medical conditions where incentive spirometry is indicated.
5. You are asked to show an adult patient how to properly use a Triflo incentive spirometer. Briefly describe the technique the patient must master to achieve optimum results with this device.
6. Which of these parameters is used to set the therapeutic goal for a patient using a volume-displacement incentive spirometer?
   a. total lung capacity
   b. inspiratory capacity
   c. inspiratory reserve volume
   d. expiratory reserve volume
7. You are asked to suggest a lung inflation therapy for a 55-year old man who is 72 inches tall and weighs 85 kg. He has just undergone a cholecystectomy and his chest radiograph shows right middle lobe atelectasis. He has a 10 pack-per-year history of smoking cigarettes, and his preoperative pulmonary function studies showed that his vital capacity was 20 mL/kg. He is alert and cooperative but complains of some upper abdominal pain when taking a deep breath. What modality would you suggest?
8. Which of the following are contraindications for administering IPPB?
   I. Active hemoptysis
   II. Nausea
   III. Intracranial pressure >15 mm Hg
   IV. Recent esophageal surgery
   a. I and III only
   b. II and III only
   c. I, II, and III only
   d. I, II, III, and IV
9. The AARC Clinical Practice Guideline for IPPB states that this form of therapy is a viable lung expansion technique for patients with reduced lung function. Which of the following findings from a patient suggest that IPPB is warranted?
   I. FVC = 50% predicted
   II. $FEV_{1.0}$ = 70% predicted
   III. MVV <50% predicted
   IV. VC = 15 mL/kg

a. I only
b. IV only
c. II and III only
d. I and III only

10. You can set the tidal volume delivered by a Bennett PR-2 ventilator by adjusting which of these parameters?
a. inspiratory time
b. inspiratory flow
c. peak inspiratory pressure
d. trigger sensitivity

11. What FiO_2 will a patient receive if the air-mix control on the Bird Mark 7 is pushed in?

12. What types of percussive pressure does the Percussionaire IPV device deliver?
a. 10 to 20 cm H_2O
b. 25 to 40 cm H_2O
c. 50 to 100 cm H_2O
d. >200 cm H_2O

13. Name four types of threshold resistors used to administer CPAP.

14. Which of the following are considered positive outcomes to PEP therapy?
I. Increased sputum production
II. Increased respiratory rate
III. Resolution of hypoxemia
IV. Diminished breath sounds become adventitious sounds that can be auscultated over the larger airways
a. I only
b. I and III only
c. II and III only
d. I, III, and IV only

References

1. Fink JB: Volume expansion therapy. In Burton GC, Hodgkin JE, and Ward JJ, editors: Respiratory care, a guide to clinical practice, ed 4, Philadelphia, 1997, Lippincott.
2. McPherson SP: Respiratory care equipment, ed 5, St Louis, 1995, Mosby.
3. Barnes TA and Watson ME: Cardiopulmonary resuscitation and emergency cardiac care. In Barnes TA, editor: Core textbook of respiratory care practice, ed 2, St Louis, 1994, Mosby.
4. Standard specification for performance and safety requirements for resuscitators intended for use with humans, Designation F-920-985, Philadelphia, American Society for Testing and Materials.
5. ISO Technical Committee ISO/TC 121, Anesthetic and Respiratory Equipment: International standard ISO 8382: resuscitators intended for use with humans, Switzerland, 1988, International Organization for Standardization.
6. Emergency Cardiac Care Committee, American Heart Association: Textbook on advanced cardiac care, ed 4, Dallas, 1996, American Heart Association.
7. Eiling R and Plitis J: An evaluation of emergency medical technicians' ability to use manual ventilation devices, Ann Emerg Med 12:765, 1983.
8. Giffen PR and Hope CE: Preliminary evaluation of a prototype tube-valve-mask ventilator for emergency artificial ventilation, Ann Emerg Med 20:262, 1991.
9. Harrison RR, et al: Mouth-to-mask ventilation: a superior method of rescue breathing, Ann Emerg Med 11:74, 1982.
10. Hess D and Baran, C: Ventilatory volumes using mouth-to-mouth, mouth-to-mask, and bag-valve-mask techniques at various resistances and compliances, Respir Care 32:1025, 1987.
11. Jesudian MC, et al.: Bag-valve-mask ventilation two rescuers are better than one: preliminary report, Crit Care Med 13:122, 1985.
12. Seidelin PH, Stolarek IH, and Littlewood DG: Comparison of six methods of emergency ventilation, Lancet 2:1274, 1986.
13. Hess D, Goff G, and Johnson K: The effects of hand size, resuscitator brand, and the use of two hand on volume delivered during adult bag-valve ventilation, Respir Care 34:805, 1989.
14. Barnes TA: Emergency ventilation techniques and related equipment, Respir Care 37:673, 1992.
15. Melker RJ and Banner MJ: Ventilation during CPR: two rescuer standards reappraised, Ann Emerg Med 14:397, 1985.
16. Sainbury DA, Davis R, and Walker MC: Artificial ventilation for cardiopulmonary resuscitation, Med J Aus 141:509, 1984.
17. AARC Clinical Practice Guideline: Incentive spirometry, Respir Care 36:1402, 1991.
18. Scanlan CL, Spearman CB, and Sheldon RL: Egan's fundamentals of respiratory care, ed 5, St Louis, 1990, Mosby.
19. Eubanks DH and Bone RC: Principles and applications of cardiopulmonary care equipment, St Louis, 1994, Mosby.
20. Branson RD, Hess DR, and Chatburn RL: Respiratory care equipment, Philadelphia, 1995, Lippincott.
21. Craven JL, et al: The evaluation of incentive spirometry in the management of postoperative pulmonary complications, Br J Surg 61:793, 1974.
22. Petz TJ: Physiologic effects of IPPB, blow bottles, and incentive spirometry, Curr Rev Respir Ther 1:107, 1979.
23. AARC Clinical Practice Guideline: Intermittent positive pressure breathing (IPPB), Respir Care 38:1189, 1993.
24. Operator's Manual of the Percussionaire Intrapulmonary Percussive Ventilation (IPV-1) unit, Percussionaire Corporation, Palm Beach, Calif.
25. Pilbeam SP: Mechanical ventilation, ed 3, St Louis, 1998, Mosby.
26. AARC Clinical Practice Guideline: Use of positive airway pressure adjuncts to bronchial hygiene therapy, Respir Care 38:516, 1993.

Internet Resources

1. American Association for Respiratory Care: http://www.aarc.org

2. American Society for Testing and Materials: http://www.astm.org
3. American Society of Anesthesiologists: http://www.asahq.org
4. American College of Chest Physicians: http://www.chestnet.org
5. American Thoracic Society: http://www.thoarcic.org
6. National Library of Medicine (Free access to Medline): http://www.nlm.nih.gov/databases/freemedl.html
7. Medweb–Respiratory Medicine Resources: http://www.gen.emory.edu/medweb/medweb.respmed.html
8. Medscape–Respiratory Care: http://www.medscape.com/Home/Topics/RespiratoryCare/RespiratoryCare.html
9. Medical Business Search Engine: http://www.infomedical.com
10. Internet Scientific Publications, L.L.C. On-Line Journals: http://www.ispub.com/journals.htm

CHAPTER 7

CHAPTER OUTLINE

KEY TERMS

Accuracy
Airway Resistance
Alveolar Ventilation
Anemometer
Aneroid Manometer
Auto-PEEP
Bell Factor
Body Plethysmography
Capnogram
Chemiluminescence Monitoring
Closed-Circuit Calorimeters
Dead Space Ventilation
Doppler Effect
Dry-Rolling Seal Spirometer
Electrochemical
Electrochemical Monitoring of Nitrogen Oxides
Electromechanical Transducer
Energy Expenditure
Fleisch Pneumotachometer
Functional Residual Capacity (FRC)
Galvanic Analyzer
Haldane Effect
Indirect Calorimetry
Inert Gas Techniques
Kymograph
Lung and Chest Wall Compliance
Mainstream Capnograph
Metabolic Carts
Minute Ventilation
Monel
Open-Circuit Calorimeters
$P_{0.1}$
Paramagnetic
Peak Flow Meter
Peak Inspiratory Pressure (PIP)
Plateau Pressure
Polarographic Oxygen Analyzers
Pneumotachograph
Precision
Quenching
Residual Volume (RV)
Respiratory System Compliance
Sidestream Capnograph
Stead-Wells Spirometer
Thermal Flowmeter
Thoracic Gas Volume (TGV)
Total Lung Capacity (TLC)
Vital Capacity (VC)
Wheatstone Bridge
Work of Breathing

Assessment of Physiologic Function

J. M. Cairo

CHAPTER LEARNING OBJECTIVES

After reading this chapter, the reader should be able to:

1. Identify three types of volume-collecting spirometers.
2. Explain the operational theory of thermal flowmeters.
3. Name three types of pneumotachometers.
4. Discuss the ATS standards for spirometry.
5. Describe three types of body plethysmographs.
6. Compare the nitrogen washout and the helium dilution techniques for measuring functional residual capacity (FRC) and residual volume.
7. Explain the operational theories of strain gauge, variable inductance, and variable capacitance pressure transducers.
8. Describe various conditions that interfere with the operation of impedance pneumographs.
9. List and describe measured and derived variables that are commonly used to assess respiratory mechanics.
10. Compare the operational principles of the three types of oxygen analyzers used in the clinical setting.
11. Describe two techniques for monitoring nitrogen oxides in the clinical setting.
12. Identify the components of a normal capnogram.
13. Assess an abnormal capnogram and suggest possible pathophysiologic processes that could contribute to the contour of the carbon dioxide waveform.
14. Compare closed-circuit and open-circuit indirect calorimeters.
15. Calculate energy expenditure using measurements obtained during indirect calorimetry.
16. Explain how indirect calorimetry can be used to determine substrate utilization patterns in healthy subjects and in those with cardiopulmonary dysfunctions.

Respiration is the exchange of oxygen and carbon dioxide between an organism and its environment. Normal gas exchange in humans requires efficiently operating chest bellows and lungs, an alveolar-capillary network in which ventilation and blood flow are evenly matched, intact systemic circulation for transporting oxygen from the lungs to the tissues and carbon dioxide from the tissues to the lungs, and integrated neural and chemical control mechanisms that regulate pH, oxygen, and carbon dioxide levels in the blood.[1] If any of these processes fail, hypoxia, hypercapnia, and ultimately respiratory and cardiovascular failure may result.

Advances in microprocessor technology have significantly improved our ability to evaluate patient respiratory function, both in the laboratory and at the bedside. This chapter discusses the devices and techniques commonly used by respiratory care practitioners to assess respiratory system mechanics, gas exchange, and metabolic function of patients with cardiopulmonary disease.

Respiratory System Mechanics

Ventilation is usually the movement of air between the atmosphere and the lungs. Gas flow into and out of the respiratory system is influenced by the pressure gradient that exists between the airway opening and the alveoli and the impedance offered by the lungs and the chest wall. Respiratory muscular effort or the force generated by a mechanical ventilator establishes the pressure gradient between the atmosphere and the alveoli. The impedance to airflow results from the elastic and frictional forces that are offered by the lungs and thorax.[2]

The mechanics of breathing can be assessed by measuring the air volume exchanged during ventilation, the gas flow into and out of the lungs, and the pressure that must be generated to achieve a given volume or flow during breathing. Derived variables (e.g., **airway resistance, lung and chest wall compliance,** and **work of breathing**) can be calculated using the three measurements just mentioned.

The usefulness of respiratory mechanics measurements ultimately depends on the accuracy and precision of the equipment used. **Accuracy** can be explained as how closely a measured value is related to the true (correct) value of the quantity measured. The accuracy of any instrument depends on its linearity and frequency response, its sensitivity to environmental conditions, and how well it is calibrated.[3] Accuracy of mechanics measurements is also influenced by patient cooperation while performing the test. In most cases, patient cooperation depends on a firm understanding of how to perform the test. If the technologist does not properly instruct patients how to perform the test, the results can be severely affected. **Precision** is the expression of an instrument's ability to reproduce a measurement (i.e., repeatability). The precision of a measuring device can be quantified by calculating the standard deviation of repeated measurements made by the device.[3]

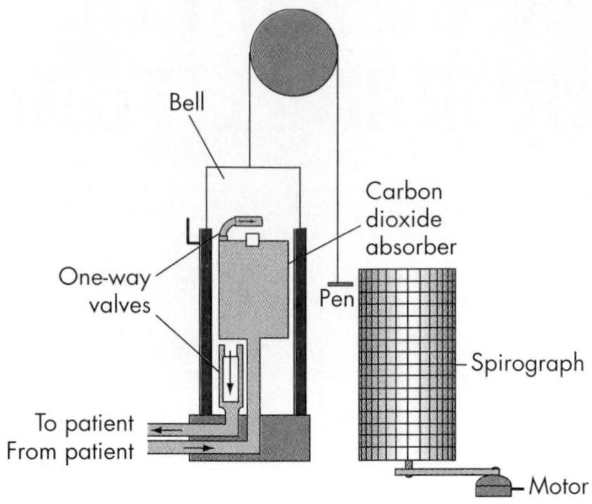

Figure 7-1 Water-sealed spirometer. (Modified from Collins Medical, Inc., Braintree, Mass.)

Volume and Flow Measurements

A spirometer is a device for measuring volume and/or flow changes at the airway opening. Therefore spirometers are generally classified by whether they measure lung-volume changes or airflow. Volume-displacement devices measure lung-volume changes by collecting exhaled gas into an expandable container and noting the amount of displacement that occurs. Typical examples of volume-collecting devices include water-sealed spirometers, bellows spirometers, and **dry-rolling seal spirometers.** Flow-sensing devices measure airflow by using thermal or hot wire anemometers, turbine flowmeters, and differential pressure **pneumotachographs.**

Water-Sealed Spirometers

As Figure 7-1 shows, a water-sealed spirometer consists of a bell that is sealed from the atmosphere by water. The patient is connected to the bell in rebreathing fashion by a breathing circuit, which consists of tubing with one-way valves and a carbon dioxide absorber. The bell, which is made of metal (usually aluminum), is suspended by a chain and pulley mechanism with a weight that counterbalances the weight of the bell.* A pen attached to the chain and pulley mechanism records bell movements on a separate motor-driven rotating drum called a **kymograph.** As patients exhale into the system, the bell moves upward and the attached pen moves proportionately downward on graph paper, creating a **spirogram.** Inhalation causes the

*The counterweight minimizes the effects of gravity acting on the metal bell.

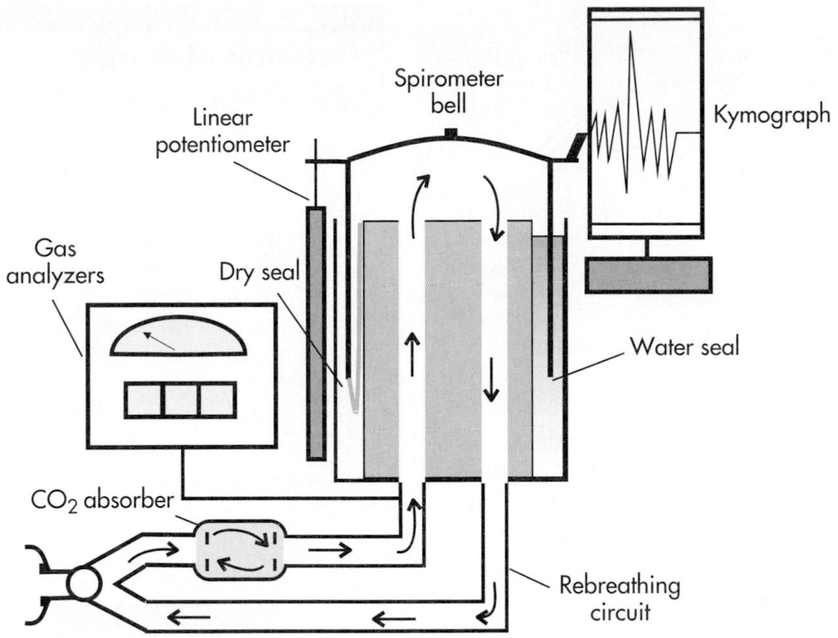

Figure 7-2 **A,** Stead-Wells spirometer. (From Ruppel G: Manual of pulmonary function testing, ed 7, St Louis, 1998, Mosby.)

bell to move downward and the pen to move upward. The rotating drum can move at a constant speed (32, 160, or 1920 mm/min), allowing the operator to measure volume changes relative to time. The slower speeds (32 and 160 mm/min) are used for measuring tidal volume, **minute ventilation** ($\dot{V}_E$), and maximum voluntary ventilation (MVV). The slower speeds are also used for specialized measurements (e.g., the diffusion capacity of carbon monoxide [D_LCO]). The fastest speed (1920 mm/min) is used for recording volume changes during forced vital capacity (FVC) maneuvers.

Two bell sizes are available: 9 L and 13.5 L. The volume of the bell determines how many millimeters the pen moves when a given volume is displaced. For example, a 9 L bell will move 1 mm for every 20.93 mL of gas displaced, and a 13.5 L bell will move 1 mm for every 41.73 mL of gas displaced. (Note that the number of milliliters of gas that must be displaced to cause the kymograph pen to move 1 mm is called the **bell factor.**) The total gas volume displaced during a breath is calculated by multiplying the number of millimeters the pen is displaced on the spirogram by the bell factor for the spirometer.

The **Stead-Wells spirometer** (Figure 7-2) is similar in design to the original Collins water-sealed spirometer, except that a plastic bell is used instead of the metal one, eliminating the need for a counterweight because the bell weighs less. Stead-Wells spirometers show excellent frequency response characteristics, especially when recording rapid breathing maneuvers, such as FVC, timed expiratory volume measurements (e.g., forced expiratory volume in 1 second, or $FEV_{1.0}$), and MVV. Stead-Wells spirometers are available in 7-, 10-, and 14-L bell sizes. The pen recorder for the Stead-Wells spirometer is attached directly to the bell, so as the bell moves upward during exhalation, the pen inscribes on the spirogram in an upward motion. Conversely, the bell and pen move downward during inhalation.

Bellows Spirometers

With this type of spirometer, exhaled gases are collected into an expandable bellows (Figure 7-3). Air entering the bellows causes the free wall of the bellows to move outward, and its displacement is directly related to the volume of air exhaled. Volume changes can be recorded by attaching a pen recorder or a potentiometer to the free wall of the bellows.

The bellows is usually constructed of silicon rubber or plastic, and several different designs are currently available. These designs differ in that the free wall can move horizontally, vertically, and/or diagonally. The frequency response of these devices is good, so they can be used to measure lung-volume changes during rapid breathing maneuvers (e.g., FVC, FEV_1, and MVV).

Dry-Rolling Seal Spirometers

These devices consist of a canister containing a piston that is sealed to it with a rolling diaphragmlike seal. As Figure 7-4 shows, gas entering the cylinder displaces the piston. The large surface area of the piston minimizes the mechanical resistance to movement and gives these devices good frequency response characteristics. A pen recorder

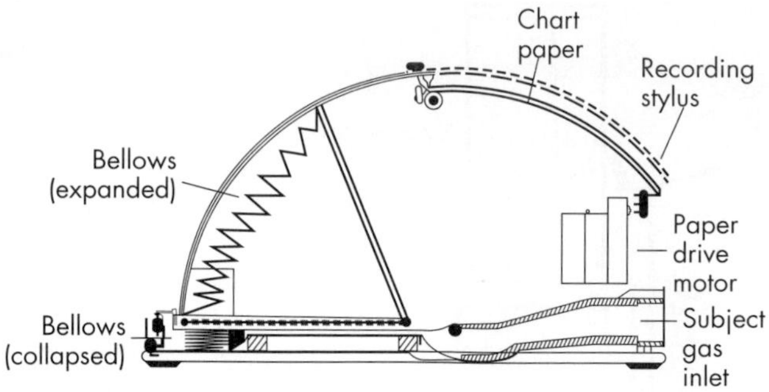

Figure 7-3 Wedge-bellows spirometer. (Modified from Vitalograph, Shawnee Mission, Kan.)

BOX 7-1

Decision Making & Problem Solving

You are asked to perform bedside spirometry on a patient receiving bronchodilator therapy. You connect the mouthpiece to the measuring device (a heated-wire or thermal flowmeter) and instruct the patient to breathe in deeply and exhale forcefully into the mouthpiece. When the patient does this, you notice that the digital display fails to register a reading of estimated volume. What could cause this type of problem?

See Appendix A for the answer.

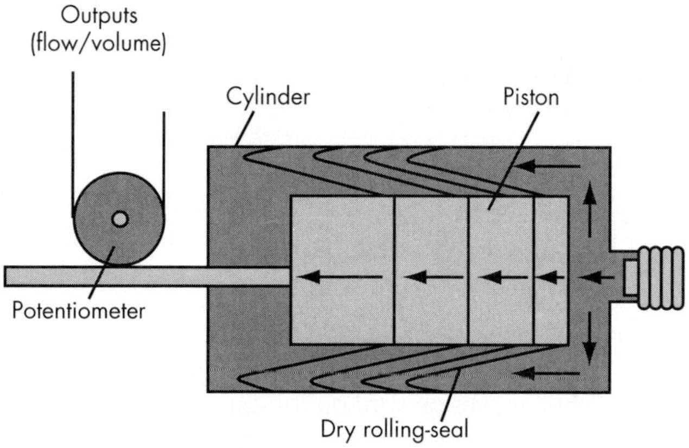

Figure 7-4 Dry-rolling seal spirometer. (From Datex-Ohmeda, Madison, Wis.)

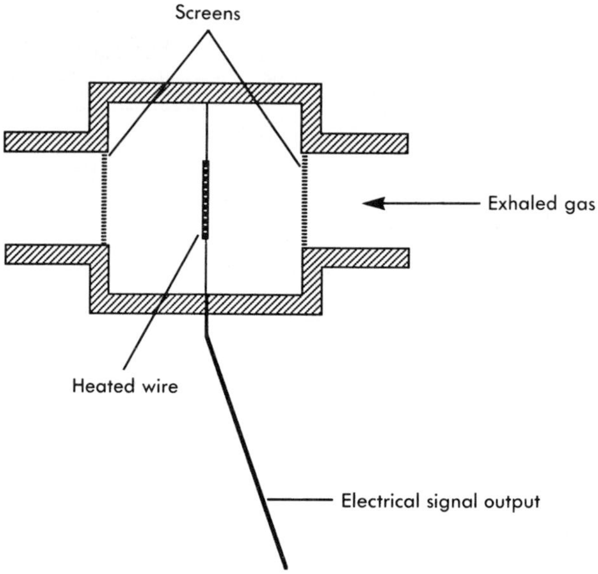

Figure 7-5 Thermal ("hot wire") anemometer.

or potentiometer attached to the cylinder shaft detects the piston's movement and registers the signal on an output display (e.g., graph paper or an oscilloscope).

Thermal Flowmeters

Figure 7-5 is a schematic of a thermal or "hot wire" **anemometer.** These devices use sensors that are temperature-sensitive, resistive elements (e.g., thermistor beads or heated wires). **Thermal flowmeters** operate on the principle that as gas passes over the thermistor bead or the heated wire, the sensor cools and changes its resistance, which in turn is proportional to the gas flow past it.* With thermistor beads, cooling increases resistance, whereas with a heated wire, cooling decreases resistance. Gas flow can be calculated because the amount of power needed to maintain the temperature of the heating element above the ambient temperature is related to the velocity of the gas flow. Actually, the signal is related to the log of the velocity of gas flow, and therefore must be linearized.[3] Thermal flowmeters are unidirectional devices and cannot be used for measuring bidirectional flows during breathing. Box 7-1 presents a decision-making problem involving a thermal flowmeter spirometer.

Turbine Flowmeters

Turbine flowmeters (Figure 7-6) use a rotating vane or turbine to measure gas flow. As gas flows through the device, the vane turns at a rate dependent on the flow rate of the gas. The flow rate can be measured by counting the number of times the vane turns, which can be done mechanically (by linking the vane to a needle attached to a calibrated display) or electronically (by using a light beam that is interrupted each time the vane turns).

Turbine flowmeters, such as hand-held respirometers, are usually accurate for flows between 3 and 300 L/min. They are portable and easy to use, but they are slow to respond to flow changes due to inertia (low frequency re-

*The amount of cooling depends on the gas viscosity and the thermal conductivity of the gas being measured.

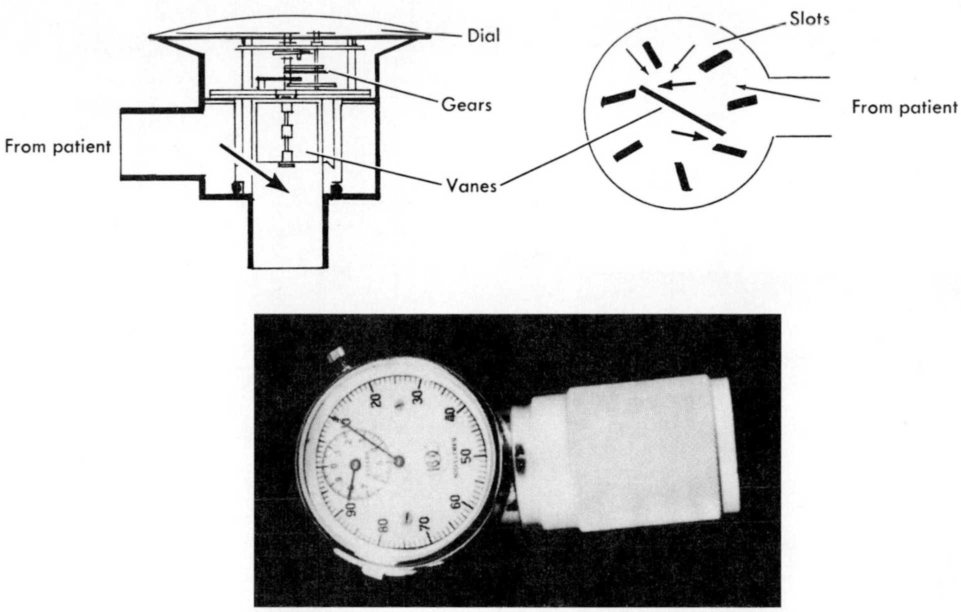

Figure 7-6 Turbine flowmeter.

sponse). Some turbine devices, such as those found in commercially available **metabolic carts** use a bias flow of gas to keep the turbine constantly turning, thus reducing the inertia of the vane.[3] These devices are good for measuring unidirectional flow, but they are inaccurate for measuring bidirectional flows.[2]

Some **peak flow meters** operate by measuring the gas flow against a rotating vane. The operating mechanism consists of a pivoted vane with an attached needle indicator. The rotation of the vane is opposed by air resistance and a calibrated spring. During a forced exhalation, the vane and the indicator needle rotate until the maximum available flow is reached. The indicator needle attached to the vane is spring-loaded, and therefore maintains the measurement of peak expiratory flow (PEF) until it is mechanically reset.

Peak flow meters are typically calibrated in liters per minute. The Wright Peak Flow Meter (Figure 7-7 *A*), designed by B. M. Wright, can measure flows between 60 and 1000 L/min with an accuracy of ±10 L/min. Its reproducibility is within ±2 L/min. Because of its wide range, it can be used to measure peak flows for both pediatric and adult patients. Reusable and disposable mouthpieces are available in pediatric and adult sizes, so these devices can be used for multiple patients.

Increased use of peak flow meters in the management of asthmatics has prompted many medical device manufacturers to market inexpensive peak flow meters that are durable and easy to use (See Figure 7-7 *B*). These expendable units are constructed of plastic and operate with a piston and spring mechanism. Exhaled air pushes against the piston, causing the needle to move on a calibrated scale. Although these devices possess accuracy and reproducibility similar to nonexpendable peak flow meters, they typically operate over a slightly narrower range of flows (80 to 800 L/min).

Pneumotachographs

Several different types of pneumotachographs are shown in Figure 7-8, including a Fleisch type of pneumotachograph, a screen pneumotachograph, a variable orifice pneumotachograph, and an ultrasonic pneumotachograph. All of these devices except the ultrasonic pneumotachograph operate on the principle that gas flow through them is proportional to the pressure drop that occurs as the gas flows across a known resistance. Ultrasonic pneumotachographs rely on the **Doppler effect** to quantify the airflow velocity.

The **Fleisch pneumotachograph** (see Figure 7-8 *A*) uses a bundle of brass capillary tubes arranged parallel to create the known resistance.[4] A differential pressure transducer monitors the pressures before and after the resistance and converts the difference into a flow signal. (With unidirectional flow, a single pressure measurement is required.) A heater is attached to raise the temperature of the entering gas and prevent moisture condensation on the capillary tubes.*

Fleisch pneumotachographs are most accurate when the gas flow is smooth or laminar. Turbulent airflow, which occurs at high flows or with obstructions or bends in the breathing circuit, can adversely affect the accuracy of airflow measurements. Turbulent airflow can also be caused by increases in the gas viscosity. Therefore it is important to compensate for different viscosities either mathematically or by calibrating the instrument with the gas mixture breathed during measurement. For example, room air has

*The accumulation of moisture on the capillary tubes can change their resistance and thus alter the accuracy of the device.

A

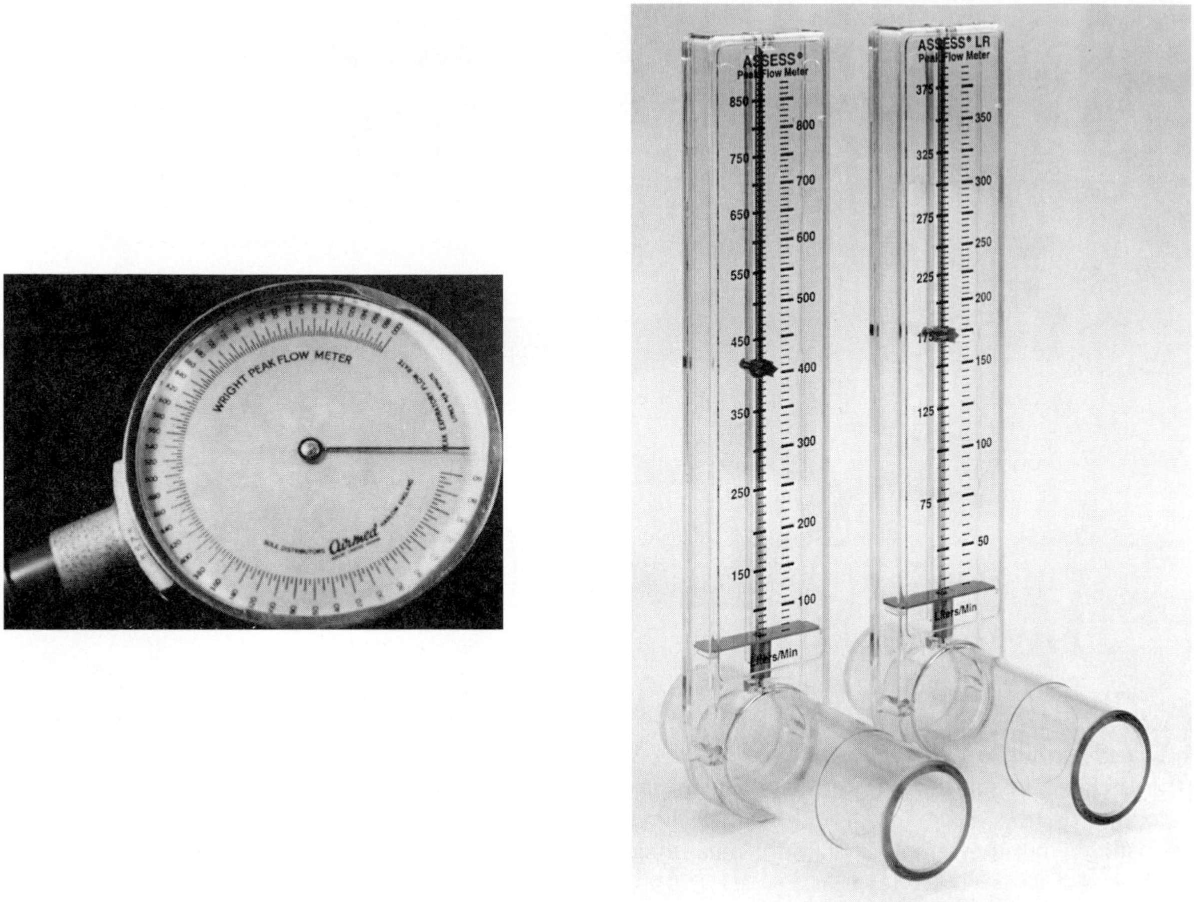

B

Figure 7-7 **A,** Wright Peak Flow Meters; **B,** Commercially available disposable peak flow meter. (***B,*** Courtesy HealthScan/Respironics, Inc, Cedar Grove, NJ. In Ruppel GL: Manual of pulmonary function testing, ed 7, St Louis, 1998, Mosby.)

a viscosity of 184 poise (P), and 100% oxygen has a viscosity of 206 P. A pneumotachograph calibrated with room air will show an error of 12% if it used to measure airflow in a patient breathing 100% oxygen.[5]

Ceramic pneumotachographs are similar in design to Fleisch pneumotachographs, except that they use ceramic material containing a number of parallel channels to create the fixed resistance. The ceramic channels smooth the air flowing through them and provide a constant resistance to airflow. A heating element is incorporated into the design. The temperature of the gas mixture flowing through these devices tends to equilibrate with the temperature of the ceramic material because of the high heat capacity of the ceramic. Additionally, moisture that condenses during breathing tends to be absorbed by the porous ceramic material, rather than occluding the tubes.[5]

Screen pneumotachographs (see Figure 7-8 *B*) use a series of fine-mesh screens to create a fixed resistance. Most of these devices use a stainless-steel (**Monel**) screen with a mesh size of 400 wires/in.[5] When a triple screen configuration is used, the center screen acts as the main resistive element, and the two outer screens smooth the airflow and protect the inner screen from particulate matter.[5] Similar to Fleisch type of devices, a heating element is incorporated to prevent water condensation on the metal screens.

Some screen type of devices use fibrous material, which looks like a paper filter, instead of metal screens to create the known resistance. These devices operate at ambient temperature, and therefore do not require a heating element. The main advantage of using them is that they are inexpensive and disposable, allowing patients to have their own peak flow meter, which reduces the risk of cross-contamination. The disadvantages of using these devices are that they are unidirectional devices, and the accuracy varies by device.[5] Additionally, moisture absorbed by the paper filter can severely affect device accuracy.

Variable orifice pneumotachographs (see Figure 7-8 *C*) are disposable, bidirectional, flow-measuring devices that use a variable area, flexible obstruction for measuring flow as a function of the pressure differential generated by the obstruction. They contain minimum dead space (about 10 mL) and can measure flows from 1.2 to 180 L/min.[2] Although the flow-pressure characteristics of variable orifice pneumotachographs are nonlinear, this discrepancy can be compensated for electronically.

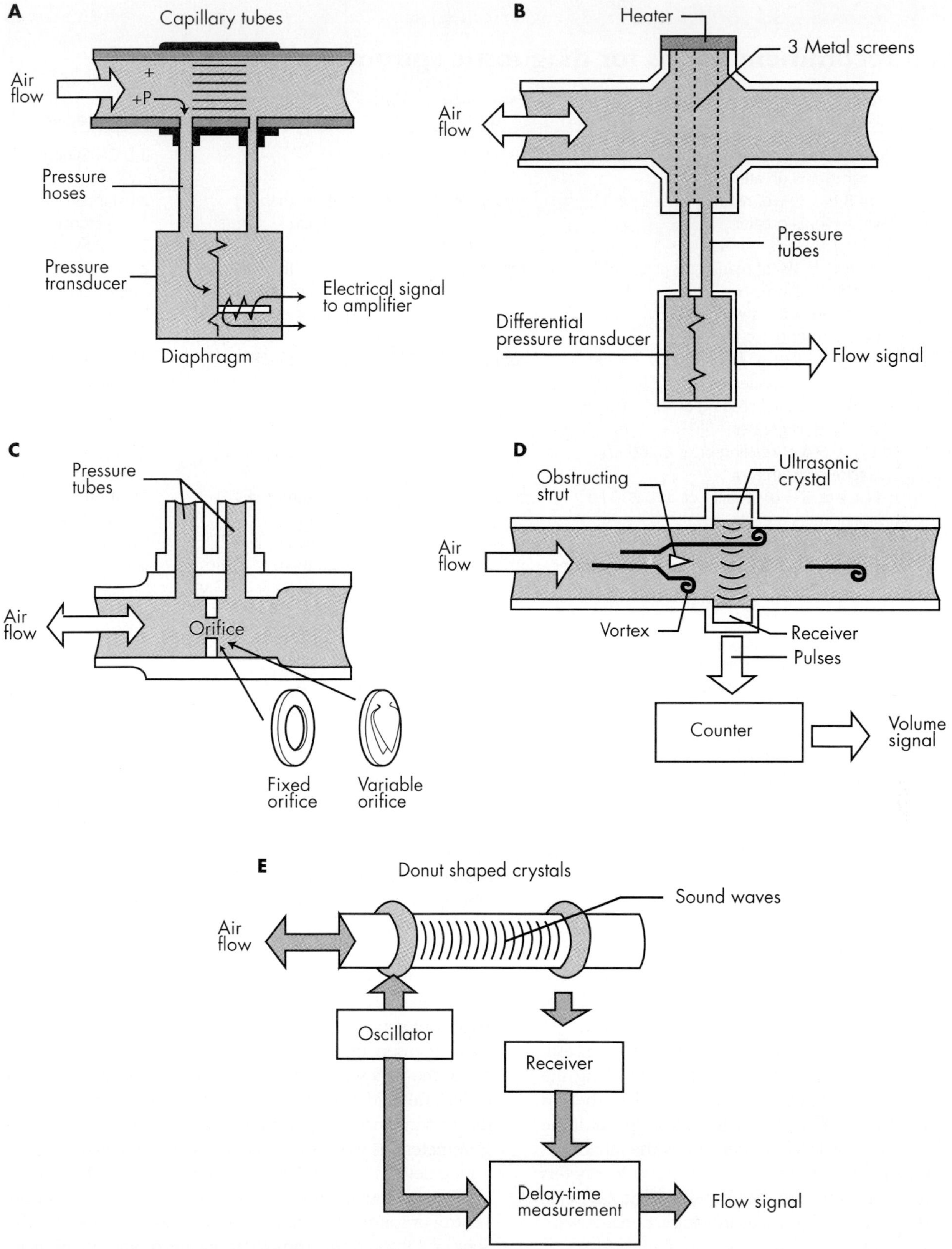

Figure 7-8 Pneumotachographs. **A,** Fleisch type of device; **B,** screen type of device; **C,** variable orifice device; **D,** vortex ultrasonic device; **E,** non-vortex device. (Redrawn from Sullivan WJ, Peters GM, and Enright PL: Pneumotachography: theory and clinical application, Respir Care 29:736, 1984.)

TABLE 7-1

Minimal recommendations for diagnostic spirometry*

Test	Range/accuracy (*BTPS*)	Flow range (*L/s*)	Time (*s*)	Resistance and back pressure	Test signal
VC	0.5 to 8 L ± 3% of reading or ± 0.050 L, whichever is greater	zero to 14	30		3-L Cal Syringe
FVC	0.5 to 8 L ± 3% of reading or ± 0.050 L, whichever is greater	zero to 14	15	Less than 1.5 cm $H_2O/L/s$	24 standard waveforms 3-L Cal Syringe
FEV_1	0.5 to 8 L ± 3% of reading or ± 0.050 L, whichever is greater	zero to 14	1	Less than 1.5 cm $H_2O/L/s$	24 standard waveforms
Time zero	The time point from which all FEV_t measurements are taken			Back extrapolation	
PEF	Accuracy: ± 10% of reading or ± 0.400 L/s, whichever is greater Precision: ± 5% of reading or ± 0.200 L/s, whichever is greater	zero to 14		Same as FEV_1	26 flow standard waveforms
$FEF_{25-75\%}$	7.0 L/s ± 5% of reading or ± 0.200 L/s, whichever is greater	± 14	15	Same as FEV_1	24 standard waveforms
$\dot{V}$	± 14 L/s ± 5% of reading or ± 0.200 L/s, whichever is greater	zero to 14	15	Same as FEV_1	Proof from manufacturer
MVV	250 L/min at V_T of 2 L within ± 10% of reading or ± 15 L/min, whichever is greater	± 14 ± 3%	12 to 15	Pressure less than ± 10 cm H_2O at 2-L TV at 2.0 Hz	Sine wave pump

*Unless specifically stated, precision requirements are the same as the accuracy requirements.

From American Thoracic Society: Standardization of Spirometry, 1994 update, Am Rev Respir Dis 152:1107, 1995.

Vortex ultrasonic flowmeters (see Figure 7-8 *D*) use struts to create a partial obstruction to gas flow. As gases flow past these struts, whirlpools or vortices are produced. The frequency at which these whirlpools are produced is related to gas flow through the struts. An ultrasonic transmitter perpendicular to the flow produces sound waves that are modulated by the frequency of the vortices. The extent of modulation related to actual flow is then determined.[6] Vortex ultrasonic flowmeters are not affected by the viscosity, density, or temperature of the gas being measured. They are unidirectional devices, and therefore cannot measure inspiratory or expiratory flow simultaneously.[2]

Non-vortex ultrasonic flowmeters (see Figure 7-8 *E*) estimate airflow by projecting pulsed sound waves along the longitudinal axis of the flowmeter (i.e., parallel to the gas flow instead of across it). The theory is that the speed of the ultrasonic wave transmission is influenced by the rate of gas flow through the device.[4] Non-vortex ultrasonic flowmeters are not affected by moisture or the viscosity of the gas being breathed, and can be used to measure bidirectional flows.

American Thoracic Society (ATS) Standards for Spirometry

In 1979, ATS members met in Snowbird, Utah to discuss standardization of the instruments and techniques used during spirometric testing. A statement was subsequently released providing recommendations for the standardization of spirometry.[7] (Table 7-1 gives a summary of these recommendations.) The central goal of this and another document published in 1987 was to improve performance characteristics of spirometers and decrease variability of laboratory testing.[8] To date, most spirometer manufacturers have complied with the standards suggested by the ATS, and as a result, spirometry results are not only consistent within a laboratory but also between laboratories.

As was just stated, the recommendations of the 1979 ATS Conference and the subsequent document published in 1987 focused on instrumentation. In 1991 and again in 1995, the ATS widened the scope of its recommendations to include guidelines for the selection of reference values, the performance of spirometry, and the quality control of spirometers, as well as minimal recommendations for monitoring devices.[9,10] Guidelines for the selection of reference values, along with guidelines for the calibration and quality control of spirometers, have been presented by the ATS.[9,10] Table 7-2 lists the recommendations for monitoring devices.

The impetus for establishing standards for monitoring devices was the increased use of portable peak flow meters in the management of asthmatic patients. Note that the standards for monitoring devices are different from those recommended for spirometry because they only

TABLE 7-2

Minimal recommendations for monitoring devices

Requirement	FVC & FEV_t (*BTPS*)	PEF (*BTPS*)
Range	High: 0.50 to 8 L Low: 0.5 to 6 L	High: 100 L/min to ≥ 700 L/min but ≤ 850 L/min Low: 60 L/min to ≥ 275 L/min but ≤ 400 L/min
Accuracy	± 5% of reading or ± 0.100 L, whichever is greater	± 10% of reading or ± 20 L/min, whichever is greater
Precision	± 3% of reading or ± 0.050 L, whichever is greater	Intradevice: ≤ 5% of reading or ≤ 10 L/min, whichever is greater Interdevice: ≤ 10% of reading or ≤ 20 L/min, whichever is greater
Linearity	Within 3% over range	Within 5% over range
Graduations	Constant over entire range High: 0.100 L Low: 0.050 L	Constant over entire range High: 20 L/min Low: 10 L/min
Resolution	High: 0.050 L Low: 0.025 L	High: 10 L/min Low: 5 L/min
Resistance	Less than 2.5 cm H_2O/L/s, from zero to 14 L/s	Less than 2.5 cm H_2O/L/s, form zero to 14 L/s
Minimal detectable volume	0.030 L	—
Test Signal	24 standard volume-time waveforms	26 standard flow-time waveforms

High = high range, and low = low range devices.

From American Thoracic Society: Standardization of Spirometry, 1994 Update, Am Rev Respir Dis 152:1107, 1995.

address FVC, FEV_1, and PEF. They also have wider ranges of accuracy (±5% for monitoring devices vs. ±3% for diagnostic spirometry) and a requirement of a 3% precision (or 0.050 mL, whichever is greater). For these reasons, the ATS "does not recommend the use of monitoring devices for diagnostic purposes in the traditional diagnostic setting where one is comparing a measured value with a reference values."[10]

In 1996, the AARC produced a Clinical Practice Guideline for Spirometry,[11] which updates prior ATS statements on spirometry. It includes indications and contraindications, hazards and complications, and limitations of methodology. It also provides recommended times for withholding commonly used bronchodilators before testing when bronchodilator response is to be assessed. A separate statement on assessing patient response to bronchodilator therapy at the point of care is also available.[12]

Measurement of Residual Volume

Vital capacity (VC) and its subdivisions can be measured in the pulmonary function laboratory with any of the aforementioned spirometers. Measurements of **residual volume (RV), functional residual capacity (FRC),** and **total lung capacity (TLC)** are obtained using **body plethysmography** and **inert gas techniques,** such as nitrogen washout and helium dilution.[13,14,15]

Body Plethysmography

A body plethysmograph (or "body box") is a rigidly walled, airtight enclosure, as shown in Figure 7-9. Three types of body plethysmographs are usually described: constant-volume *pressure* plethysmographs, constant-pressure *volume* plethysmographs, and variable pressure and volume *flow* plethysmographs. Pressure type of devices are the most common plethysmographs used. With these devices, the patient sits within the enclosure, which contains a pressure transducer within the wall of the device, and breathes through a mouthpiece connected to an assembly containing an electronic shutter and a differential pressure pneumotachometer. Mouth pressure and box pressure changes measured during tidal breathing and panting maneuvers performed by the patient at the end of a quiet expiration are displayed on an oscilloscope and directed to a microprocessor unit that calculates **thoracic gas volume (TGV)** from empirically derived pressure-volume relationships.[13,14] (Note that the reference pressure-volume relationships are empirically derived using an electronically driven piston to deliver known volumes into the enclosure. Pressure changes associated with a known volume change are recorded in the system's microprocessor and used to calculate the thoracic gas volume.) The microprocessor corrects for variations in ambient temperature and pressure from data entered manually by the technologist.

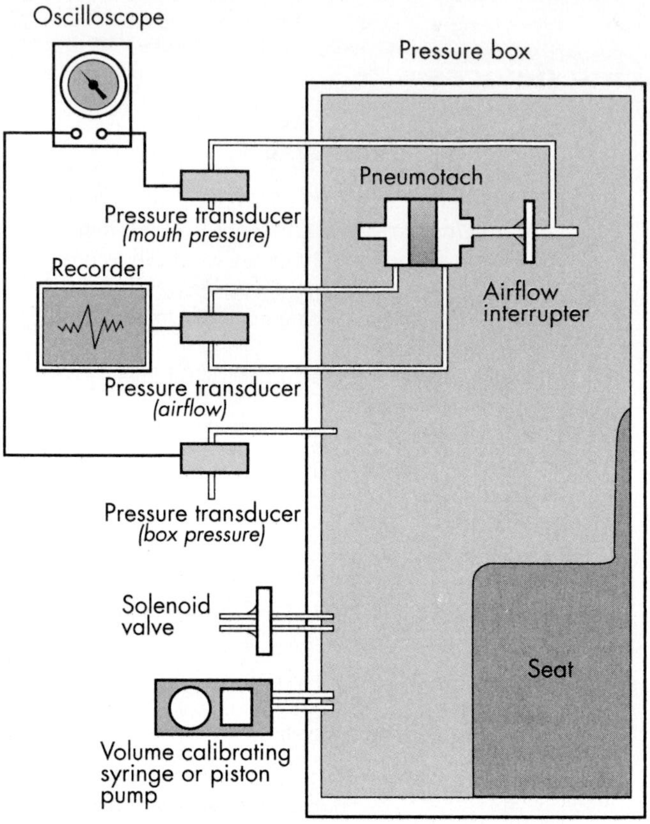

Figure 7-9 Schematic of a constant volume (pressure) plethysmograph. (Redrawn from Miller WF, Scacci R, and Gast LR: Laboratory evaluation of pulmonary function, Philadelphia, 1987, J.B. Lippincott.)

The FRC is calculated using the following relationship:

$$V_{FRC} = \Delta V/\Delta P \times P_B - P_{H2O},$$

where ΔV and ΔP are the box volume and alveolar pressure changes measured during the panting maneuver, P_B is the ambient barometric pressure, and P_{H2O} is the water vapor pressure (assume 47 mm Hg for 37° C). The resultant thoracic gas volume measured at FRC (V_{FRC}) is then corrected for the volume displaced from the box by the patient[14] (see Box 7-2).

Inert Gas Techniques

Nitrogen washout tests are performed using the equipment shown in Figure 7-10, including a spirometer with a rapidly responding nitrogen analyzer, a source of 100% oxygen, a nonrebreathing valve, and the appropriate tubing.[14] The FRC is determined by initiating the test at the end of a quiet expiration. The patient inspires 100% oxygen and exhales into the spirometer through the nonrebreathing valve. The patient continues to breathe the 100% oxygen until the exhaled nitrogen concentration is less than 1.5%. The nitrogen volume present in the lungs at the beginning of the test (i.e., FRC) can be determined by first measuring the total volume of exhaled gas and then multiplying this volume by the percentage of nitrogen in the mixed expired air, which is measured with the nitrogen analyzer.[15] This resultant volume represents the nitrogen volume in the lungs at the beginning of the test. Multiplying this volume by 1.25 allows the lung volume at the beginning of the test to be determined.* Remember that the resultant volume is measured under ambient conditions (ATPS) and must be converted to BTPS by multiplying the ATPS measurement by a correction factor. (See Box 1-5 for the formula for calculating ATPS-BTPS conversions.)

Helium dilution tests can be performed using an apparatus like the one illustrated in Figure 7-11. Note that this type of device contains a spirometer with a thermal conductivity analyzer (for measuring helium), a mixing fan, a source of helium and oxygen, and the appropriate tubing for a rebreathing breathing circuit.[14,15] The FRC is measured while patients breathe into and out of a reservoir containing known concentrations of helium and oxygen. As patients breathe into and out of the system, the added volume of air from the patient's lungs dilutes the helium concentration. The end point of the test is reached when the helium percentage remains steady for 2 minutes, indicating that the helium is equilibrated between the spirometer and the patient's lungs. The FRC volume is calculated as:

$$FRC = (He_{mL}/He_{final}) - (He_{mL}/He_{initial}) - Vrb - Vcorr,$$

where He_{mL} is the number of milliliters of helium added to the system, $He_{initial}$ is the helium concentration at the beginning of the test, He_{final} is the helium concentration at the end of the test, *Vrb* is the apparatus dead space, and *Vcorr* is a correction volume for the amount of helium that is theoretically absorbed by the body, respiratory quotient (RQ) changes, and changes in nitrogen in the circuit.[15]

It is important to recognize that the inert gas techniques can only measure gas volumes in communicating airways (i.e., airways that are open between the mouth and the alveoli), whereas body plethysmography measures all of the volume in the thorax (i.e., thoracic lung volume). Therefore inert gas measurements of FRC for patients with chronic obstructive pulmonary disorder and severe air trapping are lower than FRC (i.e., TGV) measurements from body plethysmography.

Pressure Measurements

In Chapter 1, several simple devices that can be used to measure pressure (e.g., U-shaped tubes and mercury barometers) were described. These devices were effective in measuring constant or slowly changing pressures (e.g., atmospheric pressure) but limited in their ability to measure dynamic pressures. Pressure changes, such as those occur-

*The correction factor of 1.25 is used because the room air that filled the patient's lungs before the test began contains 79% nitrogen.

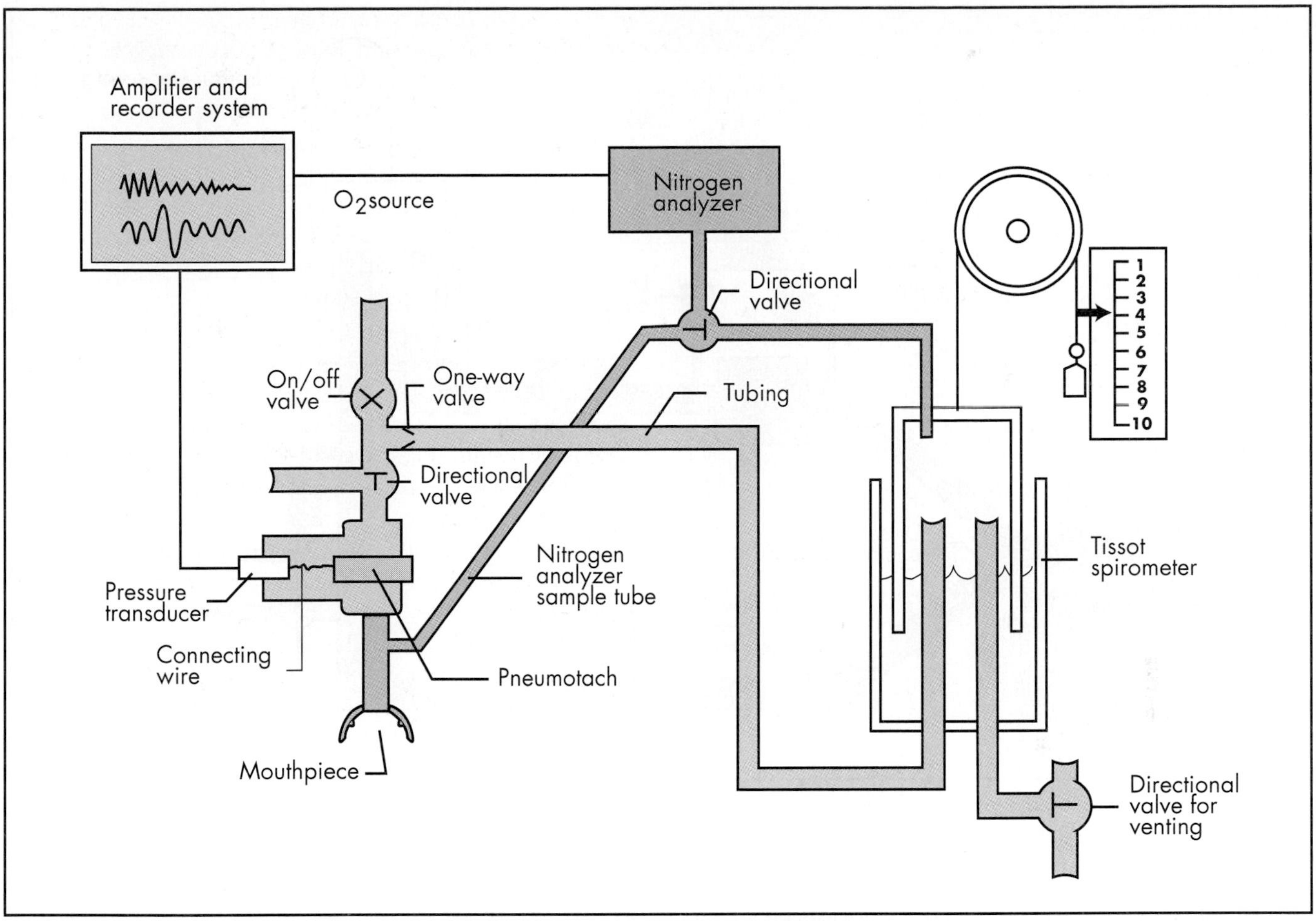

Figure 7-10 Breathing circuit for performing nitrogen washout tests. (Redrawn from Miller WF, Scacci R, and Gast LR: Laboratory evaluation of pulmonary function, Philadelphia, 1987, J.B. Lippincott.)

ring during breathing, can be measured with an aneroid manometer or an **electromechanical transducer.**

An **aneroid manometer** (Figure 7-12) consists of a vacuum chamber with a flexible cover or diaphragm that flexes when pressure is applied to it. This flexing motion is translated into a pressure measurement via a lever system that is attached to a calibrated scale. The Bourdon gauge, which consists of a coiled tube with a needle attached to a calibrated scale by a gear mechanism (see Chapter 1), is a variation of this concept. As the pressure within the Bourdon tube increases, its force tends to straighten the tube, causing the attached needle to become displaced. The amount of displacement is measured on the calibrated scale.

Aneroid manometers are used extensively in mechanical ventilators and as independent units for instantaneous pressure measurements, such as maximum inspiratory and expiratory pressures. The pressure is displayed relative to atmospheric pressure or as gauge pressure (psig). Thus a gauge pressure of 5 mm Hg measured at sea level (1 atmosphere = 760 mm Hg) corresponds to an absolute pressure of 765 mm Hg. Although aneroid manometers can measure a wide range of pressures, their frequency response is low.

Electromechanical transducers are generally classified as strain gauge devices, variable inductance devices, or variable capacitance devices.[3] Strain gauge pressure transducers (Figure 7-13 *A*) use sensors that consist of a metal wire or semiconductor incorporated into a **Wheatstone bridge** circuit. When pressure is applied to the sensor, the wire or semiconductor elongates, causing its electrical resistance to increase. The increased resistance decreases the output voltage by an amount that is proportional to the applied pressure.

The variable inductance transducer (see Figure 7-13 *B*) consists of a stainless steel diaphragm that is positioned between two coils. When the diaphragm is not flexed, the inductance of the two coils is equal. The diaphragm flexes when pressure is applied, changing the inductance between the two coils by an amount that is proportional to the applied pressure. The variable capacitance transducer (see Figure 7-13 *C*) operates similarly to variable inductance devices, except that the diaphragm of the capacitance device constitutes one plate of a capacitor. The other half of the plate is a stationery electrode. Displacement of the diaphragm alters the capacitance of the device and changes the output voltage in a manner that is proportional to the applied pressure.[3]

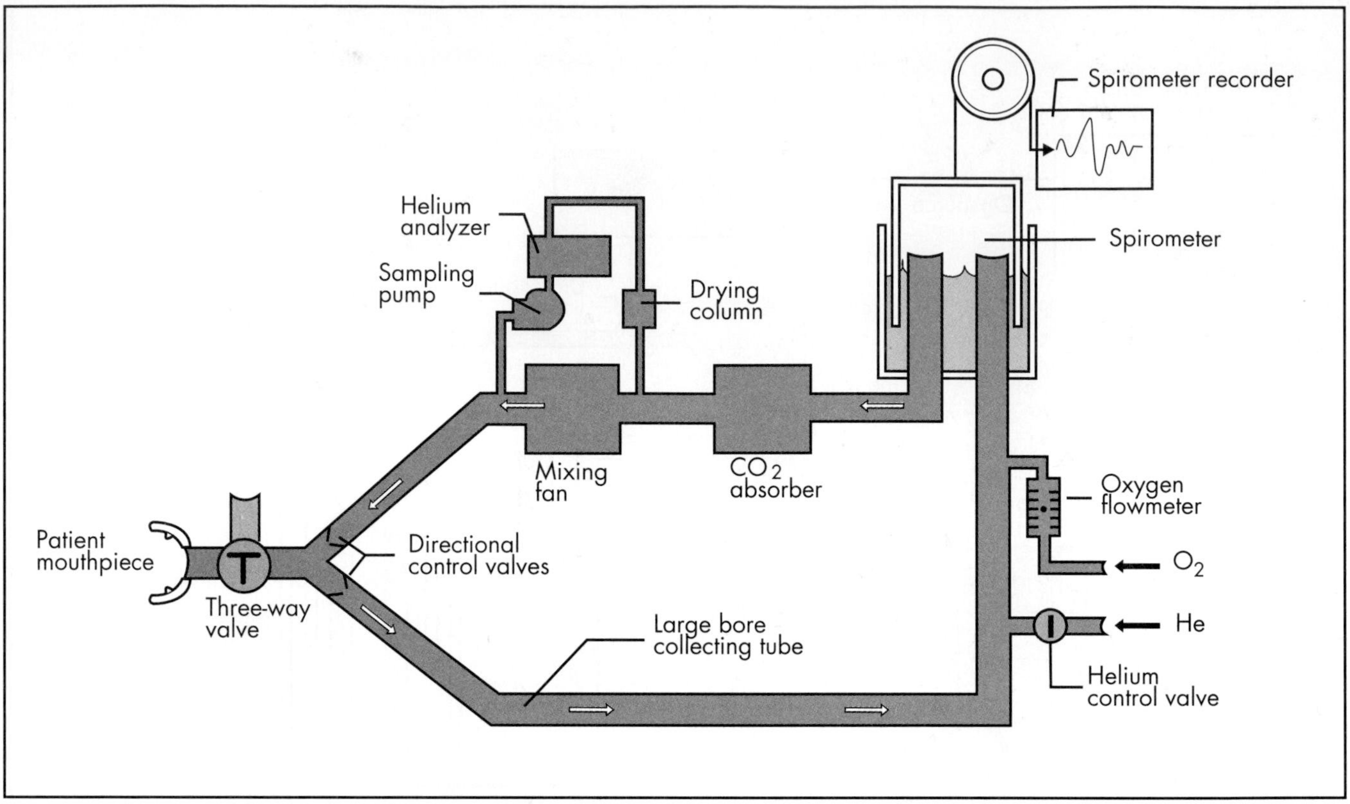

Figure 7-11 Breathing circuit for performing helium dilution tests. (Redrawn from Miller WF, Scacci R, and Gast LR: Laboratory evaluation of pulmonary function, Philadelphia, 1987, J.B. Lippincott.)

BOX 7-2

Decision Making & Problem Solving

Lung volume measurements obtained with a body plethysmograph are an application of what gas law?

See Appendix A for the answer.

Strain gauge and variable inductance pressure transducers are commonly used for measuring respiratory and cardiovascular pressures. These devices respond quickly to pressure changes, and thus have good frequency response characteristics over a wide range of pressures. These devices are usually quite stable, being relatively insensitive to vibration and shock.[3] Variable capacitance transducers are large, bulky, very sensitive to vibration, and have poor frequency response compared with strain gauge and variable inductance types of transducers.

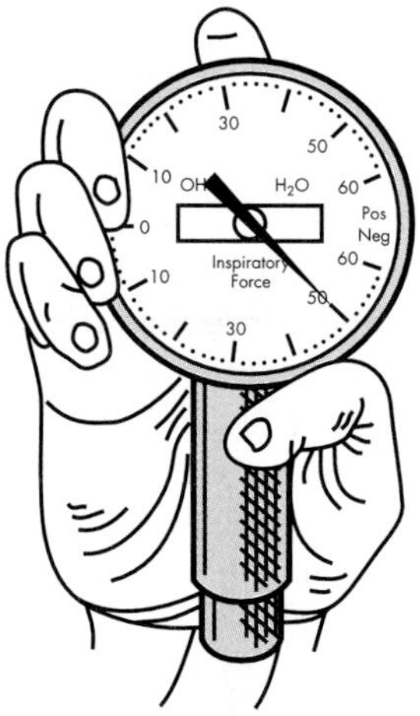

Figure 7-12 Aneroid manometer. (From Pilbeam SP: Mechanical ventilation: physiological and clinical applications, ed 1, St Louis, Multimedia Publishing.)

Bedside Measurement of Respiratory Mechanics

A number of commercial systems are now available for measuring bedside respiratory mechanics, especially during artificial ventilation. These include "stand alone" units, such as Allied Medical's BICORE CP-100 system and Novametrix Medical Systems' Ventrac system, as well as microprocessor units that are incorporated into some of the new ventilators (e.g., Siemens Servo 300 and Drager E4 ventilators).

The BICORE CP-100 Pulmonary Monitor (Figure 7-14) and the Ventrac system use variable orifice pneumotachographs to measure airflow and airway pressures and an electronic transducer attached to a triple-lumen esophageal catheter to measure esophageal pressures (i.e., esophageal pressure~intrapleural pressure). These catheters are multi-

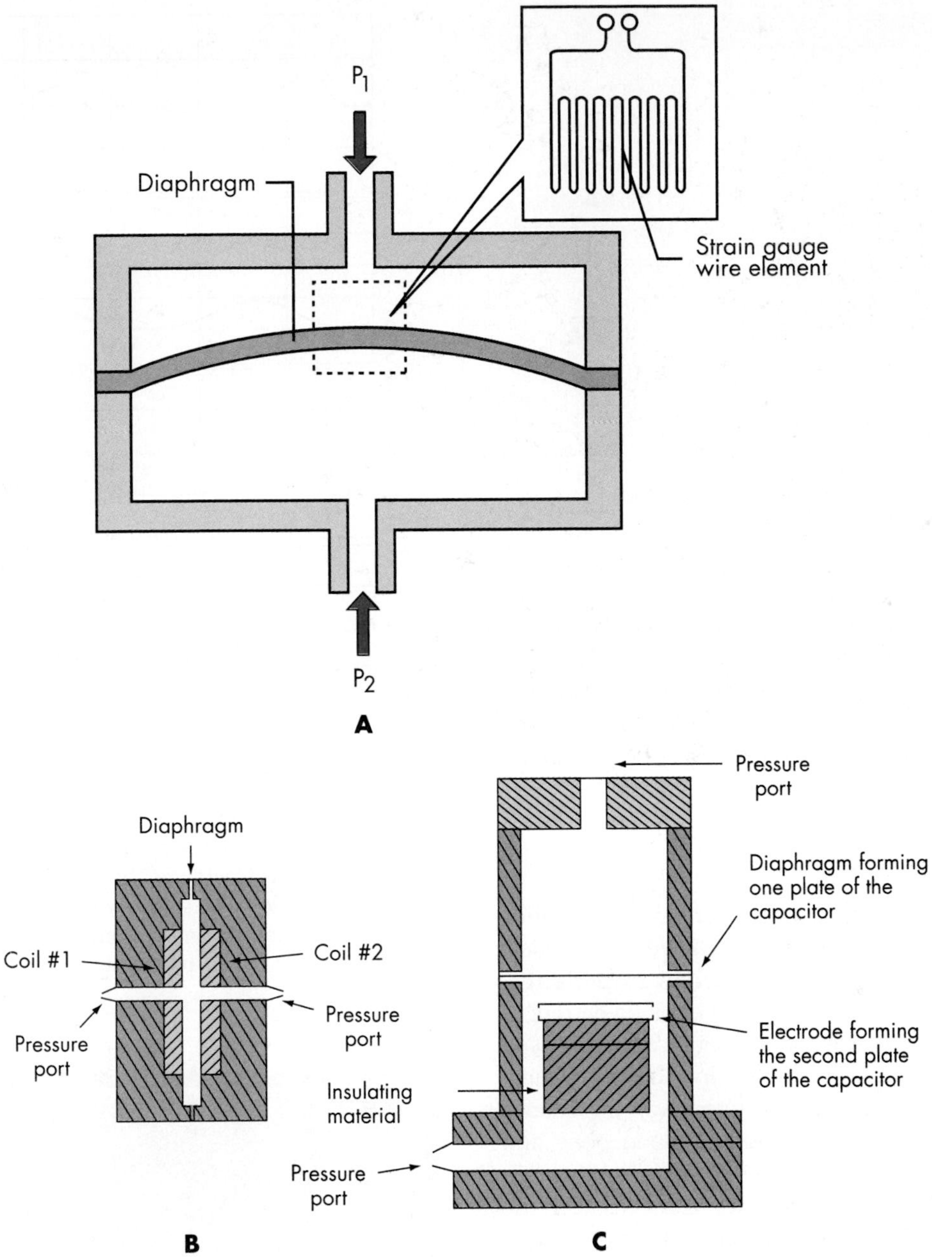

Figure 7-13 Electromechanical transducers. **A,** strain gauge device; **B,** variable inductance device; **C,** variable capacitance device. (B and C courtesy Snow M: Instrumentation. In Clausen JL, editor: Pulmonary function testing guidelines and controversies, New York, 1992, Academic Press.)

functional and may be used for gastric suctioning and feeding. The catheter can be positioned by noting the pressure recorded as the catheter is inserted. Its ideal position is the lower third of the esophagus, which is easily detected because when the catheter enters into the stomach, a positive pressure is recorded. Thus once the pressure becomes positive, the catheter can be correctly positioned by retracting it until the pressure returns to a negative value. The catheter can be anchored to the nose with surgical tape.

Airflow and pressure measurements are relayed to the system's microprocessor and displayed on a cathode ray tube (CRT). The system can display real time tracings of airway pressure, tidal volume, and airflow measured at the mouth (Figure 7-15). The microprocessor unit can also provide flow-volume, pressure-volume, and pressure-flow plots, along with calculations of airway resistance, patient-ventilator compliance, intrinsic or **auto-PEEP, $P_{0.1}$,** and work of breathing. Although both the BICORE CP-100 and Ventrak systems can be used with spontaneously breathing patients, they are almost exclusively used by clinicians to monitor the respiratory system mechanics of mechanically ventilated patients.

As was already mentioned, many of the new ventilators can also provide respiratory mechanics measurements.

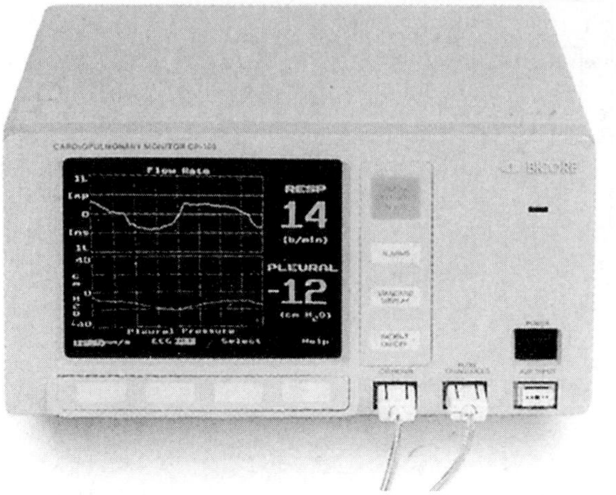

Figure 7-14 The Bicore pulmonary monitor. (Courtesy Bird Products, Palm Springs, Calif.)

These ventilators contain pressure and airflow transducers for measuring airway pressures and airflow, which can be displayed in real time. A microprocessor incorporated into the system's hardware provides calculations of airway resistance, lung compliance, and intrinsic PEEP. (See Chapter 9 for a discussion of intrinsic or auto-PEEP.)

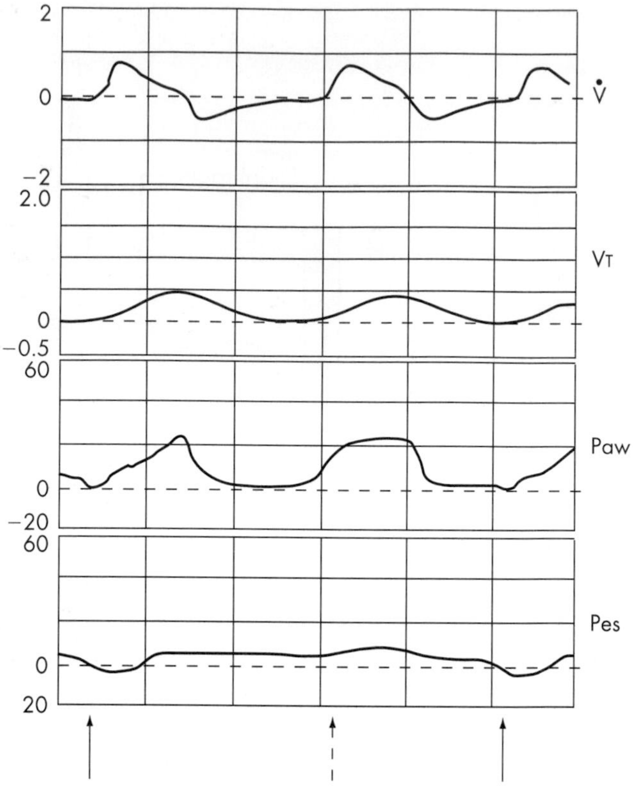

Figure 7-15 Real-time tracings of airway pressure, tidal volume, and airflow at the mouth recorded during mechanical ventilation. (From MacIntyre NR and Gropper C: Monitoring ventilatory function II: respiratory system mechanics and muscle function. In Levine RL and Fromm RE, editors: Critical care monitoring: from prehospital to ICU, St Louis, 1995, Mosby.)

Impedance Plethysmography

These devices estimate lung-volume changes by measuring the changes in electrical impedance between two electrodes placed on the chest wall. **Electrical impedance,** which is opposition to the flow of an alternating current, is determined by the resistance and capacitance of the circuit through which the current must pass. In the case of lung-volume measurements, changes in chest wall impedance are caused by variations in the amount of blood, bone, and tissue present. Thus as the chest wall expands during inspiration, thoracic blood volume increases. Conversely, as the lungs deflate during expiration, thoracic blood volume decreases, and its electrical impedance decrease. Note that the contributions of air to electrical impedance are minimal.

The electrodes used in impedance plethysmography are similar to the standard electrocardiograph electrodes and are placed in the midclavicular line at the level of the manubrium. A constant high-frequency (100 kHz), low-amplitude, electrical current is passed between the two electrodes, and the return voltage is used to calculate the impedance. Variations in impedance measured during the respiratory cycle are demodulated and displayed as a waveform. The respiratory rate is extrapolated from a 4 to 6 breath average.[16]

Impedance pneumography is most often used in home apnea monitoring units, like the one shown in Figure 7-16. Each unit contains adjustable low and high respiratory rate alarms. The sensitivity of the monitor can be adjusted by the operator to avoid false alarms due to changes in impedance caused by movement instead of by changes in respiration.

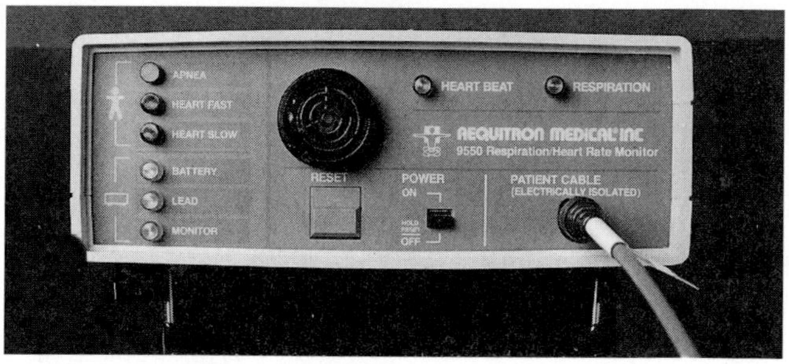

Figure 7-16 Apnea monitor.

Recent evidence suggests that bradycardia and upper airway obstruction may cause these monitors to fail to recognize apnea.[17,18] In the case of bradycardia, cardiac oscillations and intrathoracic blood-volume changes cause an increase in impedance, which is sensed as part of the respiratory cycle. Continued respiratory efforts in the presence of upper airway obstructions are sensed as normal respiratory efforts.

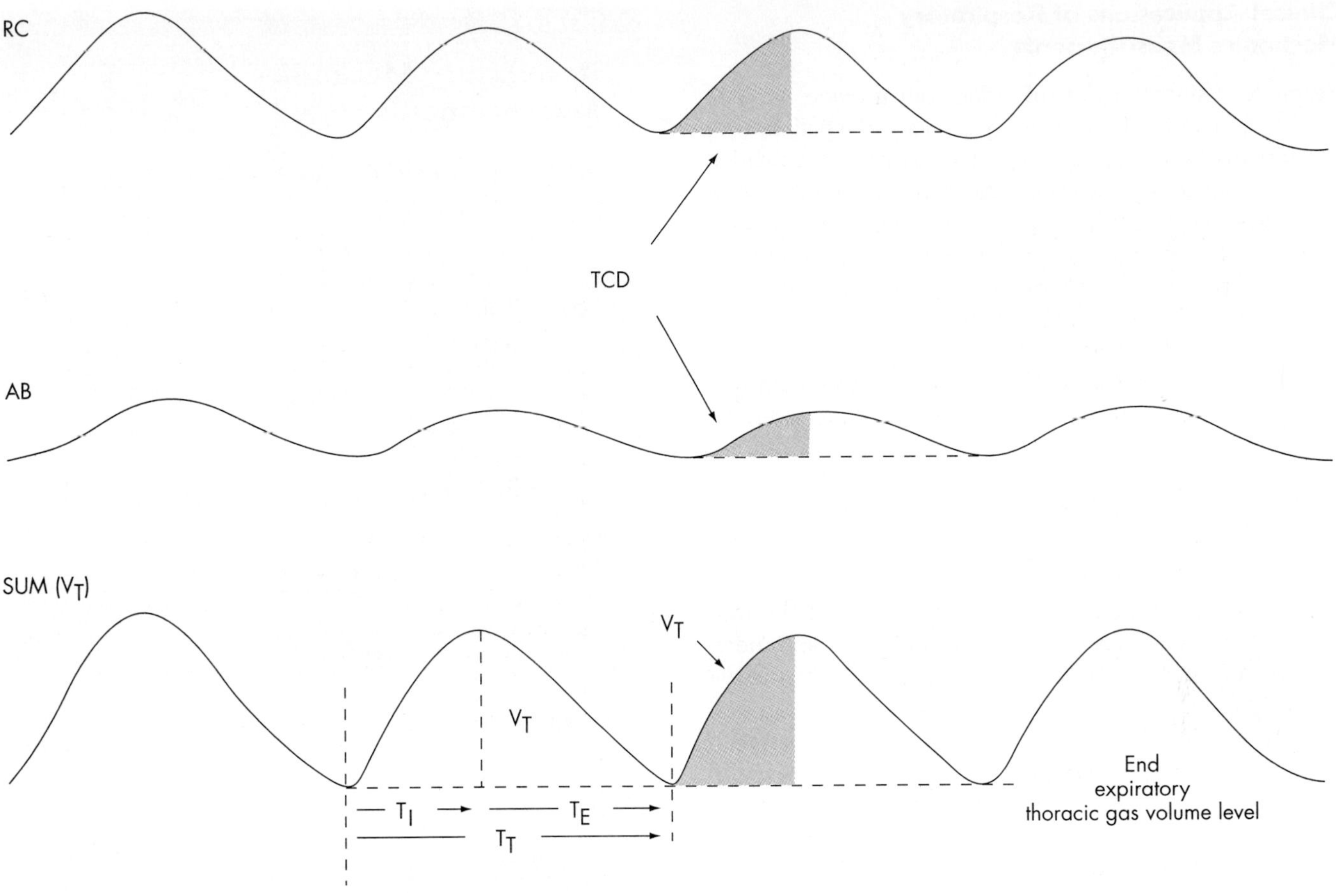

Figure 7-17 Idealized Respiratory inductive plethysmography tracing showing ribcage (*RC*), abdominal (*AB*), and total compartment displacement (*TCD*). Note that RC and AB motions are in synchrony. TCD equals the sum of RC and AB. Inspiratory time (T_I), expiratory time (T_E), and total respiratory times (T_T) are marked on the TCD tracing. (From Branson R and Campbell, RS: Impedance pneumography, apnea monitoring, and respiratory inductive plethysmography. In Kacmarek RM, Hess D, and Stoller JK: Monitoring in respiratory care, St Louis, 1993, Mosby.)

Respiratory Inductive Plethysmography

This technique is based on the principle developed by Konno and Mead[19] that the respiratory system moves with two degrees of freedom. That is, it consists of two moving parts: the rib cage and the abdomen. During inspiration, the rib cage moves outward as the lungs expand in the thorax. Simultaneously, the abdomen is displaced outward by the downward movement of the diaphragm. Because the two compartments are arranged in a series, the sum of the two displacements can be used to calculate the air volume inspired (Figure 7-17).

The respiratory inductive plethysmograph consists of two elastic cloth bands into which insulated polytetrafluoroethylene wire has been sewn in a sinusoidal pattern.[20] One band is placed around the rib cage, and the other is placed around the abdomen. The wires of the two bands are connected to an oscillator, which provides a 20-mV, alternating current voltage at a frequency of 300 kHz. Changes in the cross-sectional diameter of the wire caused by changes in the ribcage or abdominal diameter alter the oscillatory frequencies as a function of changes in self-inductance.[20] The frequency alterations are processed and converted to analog voltages that are then displayed on an oscilloscope or with a pen recorder.

Clinical indices that are most often reported from respiratory inductive plethysmography include tidal volume and respiratory rate. The total compartmental displacement (TCD, or the sum of ribcage plus abdominal movements) can be expressed as TCD/V_T. The percentage of the total displacement (i.e., tidal volume) contributed by ribcage movement is expressed as %RC/V_T.

Respiratory inductive plethysmography has been used extensively in research on respiratory muscle function. It has also been used clinically as a means of monitoring breathing patterns of patients in sleep laboratories, in pulmonary function laboratories, and in intensive care units (ICUs). In the ICU, it has been primarily used to identify uncoordinated thoracoabdominal movements that are associated with respiratory muscle fatigue and/or failure.[20]

Clinical Applications of Respiratory Mechanics Measurements

Respiratory system mechanics data can provide valuable information about the ventilatory capacity of a patient with cardiopulmonary disease. These data are generally divided into two categories: measured and derived variables. Measured variables include lung volumes and capacities, airflow, and airway and intrapleural pressures. Airway resistance, **respiratory system compliance,** and work of breathing are derived variables that can be calculated from volume, flow, and pressure measurements.

Box 7-3 contains a list of some of the more common respiratory mechanics measurements that are used by clinicians.

BOX 7-3

Respiratory Mechanics Measurements

Standard Lung Volumes and Capacities

Tidal volume (TV or V_T)
Inspiratory reserve volume (IRV)
Expiratory reserve volume (ERV)
Residual volume (RV)
Total lung capacity (TLC)
Vital capacity (VC)
Functional residual capacity (FRC)
Inspiratory capacity (IC)

Dynamic Lung Volumes (Flows)

Forced vital capacity (FVC)
Forced expiratory volume in 1 second ($FEV_{1.0}$)
Forced expiratory flow from 25% to 75% of the vital capacity (FEF_{25-75})
Peak expiratory flow (PEF)

Minute Ventilation

Minute volume (MV, $\dot{V}_E$, or $\dot{V}_I$)
Breathing frequency (f_B)

Respiratory Pressures

Maximum inspiratory pressure (MIP)
Maximum expiratory pressure (MEP)
Peak airway inspiratory pressure (PIP)
Plateau pressure ($P_{plateau}$)

Lung Volumes and Airflow

Laboratory measurements of lung volumes focus on the standard subdivisions shown in Figure 7-18. As was already stated, simple spirometers can measure three of the four standard lung volumes (i.e., V_T, IRV, and ERV) and therefore the VC and IC. They can also measure all of the dynamic lung volumes, including FVC, FEV_1, FEF_{25-75}, and peak flows. RV, FRC, and TLC cannot be measured with simple spirometry; they require specialized equipment and procedures, such as body plethysmography and inert gas techniques. Simple spirometry is used as a screening technique, and full lung-volume tests are usually reserved for patients demonstrating abnormal spirometric results.[15] Table 7-3 describes the characteristic lung-volume changes associated with obstructive and restrictive pulmonary disorders; and Box 7-4 presents a case related to lung-volume measurements in COPD patients.

At the bedside, the most commonly measured lung volume is the expired minute volume. In spontaneously breathing patients, the minute volume is usually measured with a hand-held respirometer. For mechanically ventilated patients, minute volume can be measured by attaching a spirometer to the exhalation valve of the ventilator. In most newer ventilators, a flow transducer is incorporated into the system design to give continual updates of tidal and minute volume. (Note that minute volume is calculated based on 5 to 10 breaths and extrapolated to a minute volume value.)

Minute ventilation expresses patient ventilatory needs in liters per minute. It is influenced by the metabolic demands of the tissues and the level of **alveolar ventilation.** For example, elevated minute volumes are associated with increased metabolic rates and/or reductions in effective ventilation (decreased alveolar ventilation or increased **dead space ventilation**).

Monitoring dynamic lung volumes can also alert the clinician to significant changes in a patient's airway resistance. Peak expiratory flow rate (PEF) measurements are routinely monitored at the bedside to assess the effectiveness of bronchodilator therapy. These same devices can be used at home by asthmatic patients to monitor daily variations in airway resistance and thus guide therapeutic interventions.[12] (Box 7-5 summarizes the AARC Clinical Practice Guideline for assessing response to bronchodilator at point of care.)

Airflow measurements during mechanical ventilation can signal changes in the resistance and compliance of the patient-ventilator system. For example, high frequency ripples on the inspiratory flow tracing can indicate turbulent flow caused by secretions in the airway or water in the ventilator circuit.[21] Expiratory flow limitations should be suspected if the decay in expiratory flow is linear instead of exponential.[15]

Airway Pressures

The most common airway pressure measurements made on spontaneously breathing patients are the maximum inspiratory and expiratory pressures (MIP and MEP), **peak inspiratory pressure (PIP),** and static, or plateau, pressure ($P_{plateau}$).

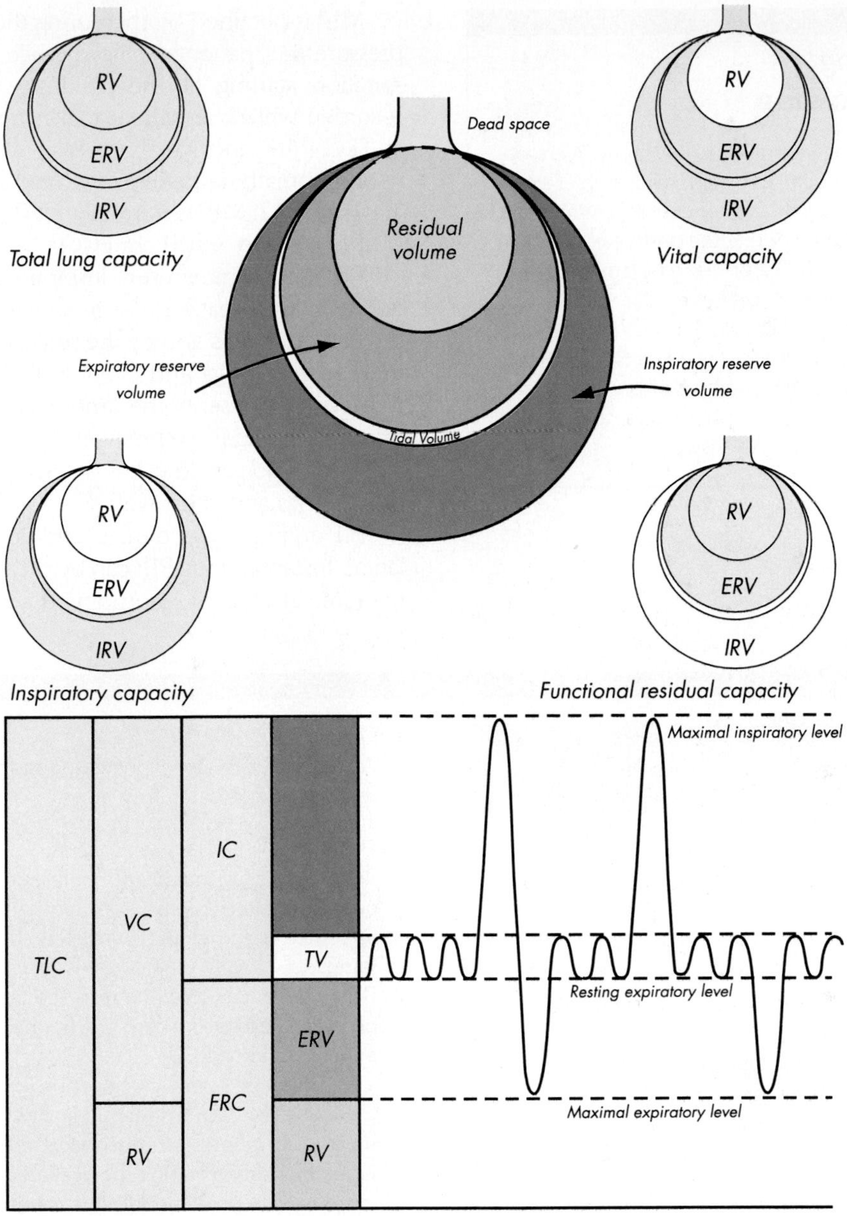

Figure 7-18 Standard lung volumes and capacities. (From Comroe J: The lung, ed 3, Chicago, 1986, Mosby.)

TABLE 7-3

Static and and dynamic lung volume changes associated with obstructive and restrictive pulmonary diseases

	Obstructive pulmonary disease	Restrictive pulmonary disease
TLC	Increased	Decreased
FRC	Increased	Normal or Decreased
VC	Normal or Decreased	Decreased
FEV_1	Decreased	Decreased
FEV_1/VC	Decreased	Normal
FEF_{25-75}	Decreased	Normal
MVV	Decreased	Decreased in severe disease

BOX 7-4

Decision Making & Problem Solving

The following lung volume measurements were obtained from a 65-year old man whose chief complaint is shortness of breath on exertion, which has increased significantly during the past year. He has a 40-pack per year history of cigarette smoking (i.e., he smoked 2 packs of cigarettes per day for 20 years). FVC is 60% of predicted; FEV_1 is 50% of predicted; FEF_{25-75} is 40% of predicted; $FEV_{1.0}/VC$ is 60% of predicted; RV is 140% of predicted; and FRC is 150% of predicted. Interpret these results.

See Appendix A for the answer.

MIP is obtained by measuring the maximum sustained pressure that patients achieve while making a forceful inspiration starting at the residual volume. The MEP is recorded while the patient makes a forceful effort starting at TLC. MIP and MEP are easily obtained from spontaneously breathing patients with an apparatus like the one in Figure 7-12. MIP is normally −60 to −100 cm H_2O, and MEP is +80 to +100 cm H_2O.

PIP is the maximum inspiratory pressure generated during a tidal breath. PIP is influenced by the gas flow into the patient's lungs and by the resistance and compliance of the patient's lungs and chest wall. The static or **plateau pressure** represents the amount of pressure required to maintain the tidal volume within the patient's lungs during a period of no gas flow. It is determined by the compliance of the lungs and chest wall.[21,22]

PIP and $P_{plateau}$ are measured during mechanical ventilation. Instantaneous PIP can be measured with an aneroid manometer that is incorporated into the ventilator (see

BOX 7-5

Clinical Practice Guidelines

Summary of Assessing Response to Bronchodilator Therapy at Point of Care

Indications:

1. To confirm appropriateness of therapy.
2. To individualize patient's dose per treatment and/or frequency of administration.
3. To help determine patient status during acute and long-term pharmacological therapy.
4. To determine a need for change of therapy.

Contraindications

In cases of acute severe distress, some assessment maneuvers may be contraindicated or should be postponed until therapy and supportive measures have been instituted.

Hazards/Complications

Forced exhalations may be associated with bronchoconstriction, airway collapse, and paroxysmal coughing with or without syncope.

Limitations of Methodology

1. Cost and accessibility.
2. Patient inability to perform FVC or PEF maneuvers.
3. Accuracy and reproducibility of peak flow meters vary among models and units, so results from the same device should be compared for consistency and accuracy.
4. The measurement of peak flows is an effort-dependent test. The patient should be encouraged to perform the maneuver vigorously. Three trials are desirable; report the best of the three peak flows measured.
5. An artificial airway will increase resistance and may limit inspiratory and expiratory flows.

Resources

1. Equipment may include portable laboratory spirometer, peak flow meter, stethoscope, and pulse oximeter. Spirometers and peak flow meters should adhere to ATS standards.
2. Personnel performing the tests should be licensed or credentialed respiratory care practitioners or persons with equivalent knowledge.
3. The patient or family caregiver providing maintenance therapy must demonstrate an ability to monitor and measure response to bronchodilator, use proper technique for administrating medication and using the devices, modify doses and frequency as prescribed and instructed in response to adverse reactions or increased severity of symptoms, and appropriately communicate the severity of symptoms to the physician.

Monitoring

The following observations will assist the clinician in assessing the response to bronchodilator therapy:

1. Patient's general appearance, use of accessory muscles, and sputum volume and consistency.
2. Patient's vital signs and measurements of FVC, FEV_1, PEF, and pulse oximetry.
3. In ventilator patients, PIP, $P_{plateau}$, increased inspiratory/expiratory flows (F-V loops), and decreased autoPEEP.

For a copy of the complete text, see Respiratory Care 40(12):1300, 1995.

Chapter 9). PIP can be derived from continuous recordings of airway pressure that can be made during the breathing cycle using a strain-gauge transducer. $P_{plateau}$ is measured during mechanical ventilation by occluding the expiratory valve of the ventilator at the end of a tidal inspiration and noting the new pressure level. Most newer ventilators have a manual control incorporated into the ventilator circuit that operates an inflation-hold shutter valve that closes at the end of inspiration.[21,22]

Figure 7-19 is a tracing that shows the measurement of PIP and $P_{plateau}$. Note that PIP is greater than $P_{plateau}$, but remember that PIP is a dynamic measurement and $P_{plateau}$ is measured under static conditions. The PIP represents the total force that must be applied to overcome the elastic and frictional forces offered by the patient-ventilator system, whereas $P_{plateau}$ represents that portion of the total pressure required to overcome only elastic forces.

Increases in the elastance of the respiratory system (i.e., decreases in compliance of the lung and/or chest wall) increase both PIP and $P_{plateau}$. Elevated airway resistance increases peak airway pressure but does not affect $P_{plateau}$.

Airway Resistance

Airway resistance is the opposition to airflow from nonelastic forces of the lung. It can be calculated by subtracting $P_{plateau}$ from PIP and dividing the resultant pressure by the airflow. Airway resistance averages 2 to 5 cm H_2O/L/second. It is primarily determined by the caliber of the airway (according to Poiseuille's law, a twofold decrease in airway diameter results in a sixteenfold increase in airway resistance). Thus retention of secretions, peribronchiolar edema, and bronchoconstriction associated with asthma result in increased airway resistance. Smoke inhalation can also cause severe bronchoconstriction. Conversely, bronchodilation causes a reduction in airway resistance, such as occurs after the administration of a bronchodilator (see Box 7-5).

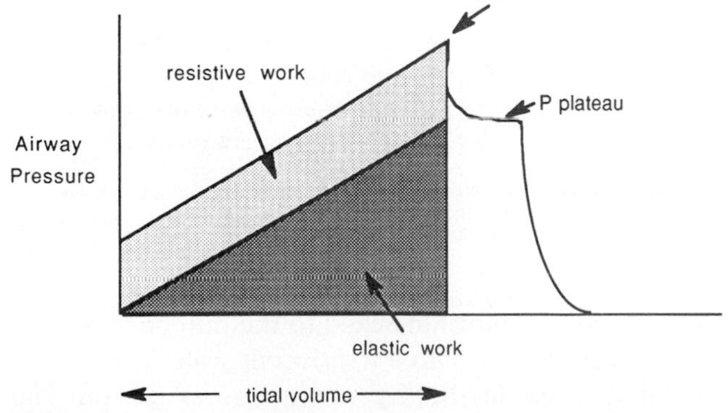

Figure 7-19 Airway pressure tracing showing peak airway pressure and plateau pressure. (From Pilbeam SP: Mechanical ventilation, ed 3, St Louis, 1998, Mosby.)

Respiratory System Compliance

Respiratory system compliance can be simply defined as the distensibility of the lungs and chest wall. Lung-thorax compliance can be determined by dividing the tidal volume by $P_{plateau}$. The normal compliance of the respiratory system averages 0.1 L/cm H_2O.

Pathologic conditions (e.g., pulmonary interstitial fibrosis, atelectasis, and pulmonary vascular engorgement) decrease the compliance of the pulmonary parenchyma, resulting in increases in both $P_{plateau}$ and PIP (i.e., decreasing lung compliance). Conditions such as kyphoscoliosis and myasthenia gravis increase PIP and $P_{plateau}$ by reducing chest wall compliance.[22]

Work of Breathing

In normal healthy individuals, work of breathing only constitutes about 2% to 5% of total oxygen consumption, but this value can rise sharply with a pathologic pulmonary condition. Therefore increases in airway resistance or decreases in respiratory system compliance can lead to considerable increases in work of breathing, and thus oxygen consumption.

Although there is considerable interest in using work of breathing measurements in clinical practice, the technique is somewhat difficult to master and limited in use. Its most practical uses have been in establishing optimum levels of pressure-support ventilation and determining the work of breathing for various forms of ventilatory support.

Table 7-4 summarizes the lung mechanics measurements used to assess patients receiving ventilatory support.

MEASUREMENT OF INSPIRED OXYGEN

Oxygen Analyzers

Three types of analyzers are available for measuring the oxygen concentration in inspired gases: (1) **paramagnetic** analyzers, (2) **electrochemical** analyzers (including **polarographic** and galvanic devices), and (3) electric analyzers.

Paramagnetic Analyzers

The paramagnetic oxygen analyzer was first described by Pauling, Wood, and Sturdivant[23] in 1946 and relies on the fact that oxygen is a paramagnetic gas and the other respired gases (e.g., nitrogen and carbon dioxide) are diamagnetic. Thus the paramagnetic oxygen molecules align themselves with the strongest part of a heterogenous magnetic field. The diamagnetic nitrogen and carbon dioxide molecules are repelled by the magnetic field, so they tend to be found in the weaker part of a magnetic field.

The Beckman D-2 oxygen analyzer is an example of a device that uses the physical principle of paramagnetism to measure oxygen concentration. As Figure 7-20 shows, a glass dumbbell filled with nitrogen is suspended on a quartz string and held in place by two magnets. The

TABLE 7-4

Measurements of lung mechanics used to assess ventilatory function in mechanically ventilated patients

Variable	Description	Measuring technique
Effective compliance (C_{eff})	The reciprocal of the elastic property of the patient-ventilator system (mL/cm H_2O)	Mandatory (i.e., passive inspiration expiration) breath (V_T); end-inspiratory pause of at least 1 sec ($P_{plateau}$); corrected for tubing compression. Calculation: $C_{eff} = V_T/(P_{plateau} - \text{total PEEP})$.
Inspiratory resistance	Inspiratory resistive component of patient-ventilator system impedance (cm $H_2O \times$ sec $\times L^{-1}$)	Mandatory (i.e., passive inspiration and expiration) breath (V_T) with fixed constant flow over fixed time (T_i); end-inspiratory pause as described for C_{eff}. Calculation: $R_I = \frac{P_{peak} - P_{plateau}}{V_T/T_i}$
Expiratory resistance	Expiratory resistive component of the patient-ventilator system (cm $H_2O \times$ sec $\times L^{-1}$)	Mandatory (i.e., passive inspiration and expiration) breath (V_T); end-inspiratory pause as described for C_{eff}. Calculation: $R_E = \frac{P_{plateau} - \text{total } PEEP_{tot}}{\text{Flow at onset of exhalation}}$.
Mean airway pressure	Average airway pressure over a respiratory cycle	Mean airway pressure should be reported over a time period that includes a representative number of machine- and patient-cycled breaths.
Negative inspiratory force (NIF)	Maximal negative inspiratory pressure generated by patient, against closed circuit	One-way valve allowing expiration; expiratory hold of 15 to 20 seconds.
Intrinsic positive end-expiratory pressure (auto-PEEP)	Positive end-expiratory alveolar pressure due to inadequate expiratory time, dynamic airway collapse, or both	Auto-PEEP measurement is clinically important but may be difficult during spontaneous or assisted breathing. It is recommended that the ventilator be equipped with an expiratory hold control to facilitate manual determination of auto-PEEP by airway occlusion as close to the proximal airway as possible; circuit pressures should stabilize during the expiratory hold. Measurement reflects total PEEP but tends to underestimate the intrinsic component because of pressure equilibration in compliant circuitry.

From MacIntyre NR and Gropper C: Monitoring ventilatory function II: respiratory system mechanics and muscle function. In Levine RL and Fromm RE, editors: Critical care monitoring: from prehospital to ICU, St Louis, 1995, Mosby.

dumbbell and the magnets are enclosed within a sample chamber. When oxygen is introduced into this chamber, it is attracted to the magnetic field, which causes the dumbbell to rotate slightly. The amount of rotation depends on the concentration of the oxygen introduced into the chamber. The oxygen concentration can be measured because a mirror attached to the dumbbell reflects a light focused on it onto a translucent scale. The scale is calibrated to display both partial pressures (in mm Hg) and the percent of oxygen concentration.

The following points should be remembered when using these devices: (1) Because these devices do not re-

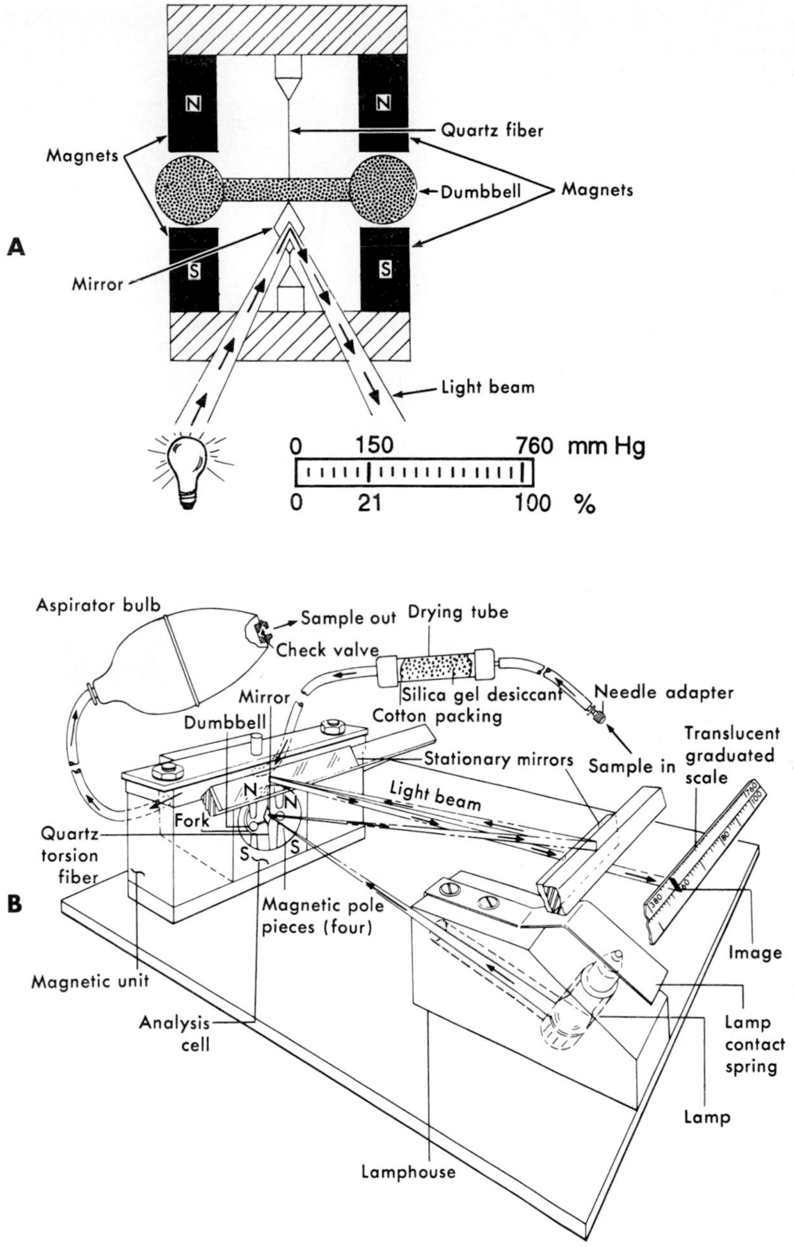

Figure 7-20 **A,** Physical oxygen analyzer (Pauling principle) (Modified from Belleville JW and Weaver CS: Techniques in clinical physiology: a survery of measurements in anesthesiology, New York, 1969, Simon & Schuster, Inc.); **B,** Beckman D-2 analyzer. (Courtesy Beckman Coulter, Fullerton, Calif.)

quire an external power source, they can be used with flammable gases, but an AA battery is required to operate the light bulb. (2) These devices do not consume oxygen during analysis. (3) Displacement of the dumbbell varies with the number of oxygen molecules introduced into the magnetic field; thus the analyzer reading is more closely related to the partial pressure than to the percentage of concentration. Consequently, when these devices are used at high altitudes, the partial pressure of oxygen is reported accurately, but the percentage of concentration is low.[24] This problem can be alleviated by dividing the partial pressure reading by the ambient pressure that is measured separately. (4) Manufacturers calibrate paramagnetic analyzers with dry gases, so it is important to dry the gas sample before analysis by aspirating it through a column of anhydrous cobalt chloride (Silica gel).* (5) Paramagnetic analyzers can only provide intermittent analyses; they cannot continuously measure oxygen concentration.

*These crystals are blue when dry, but become pink when saturated with water vapor.

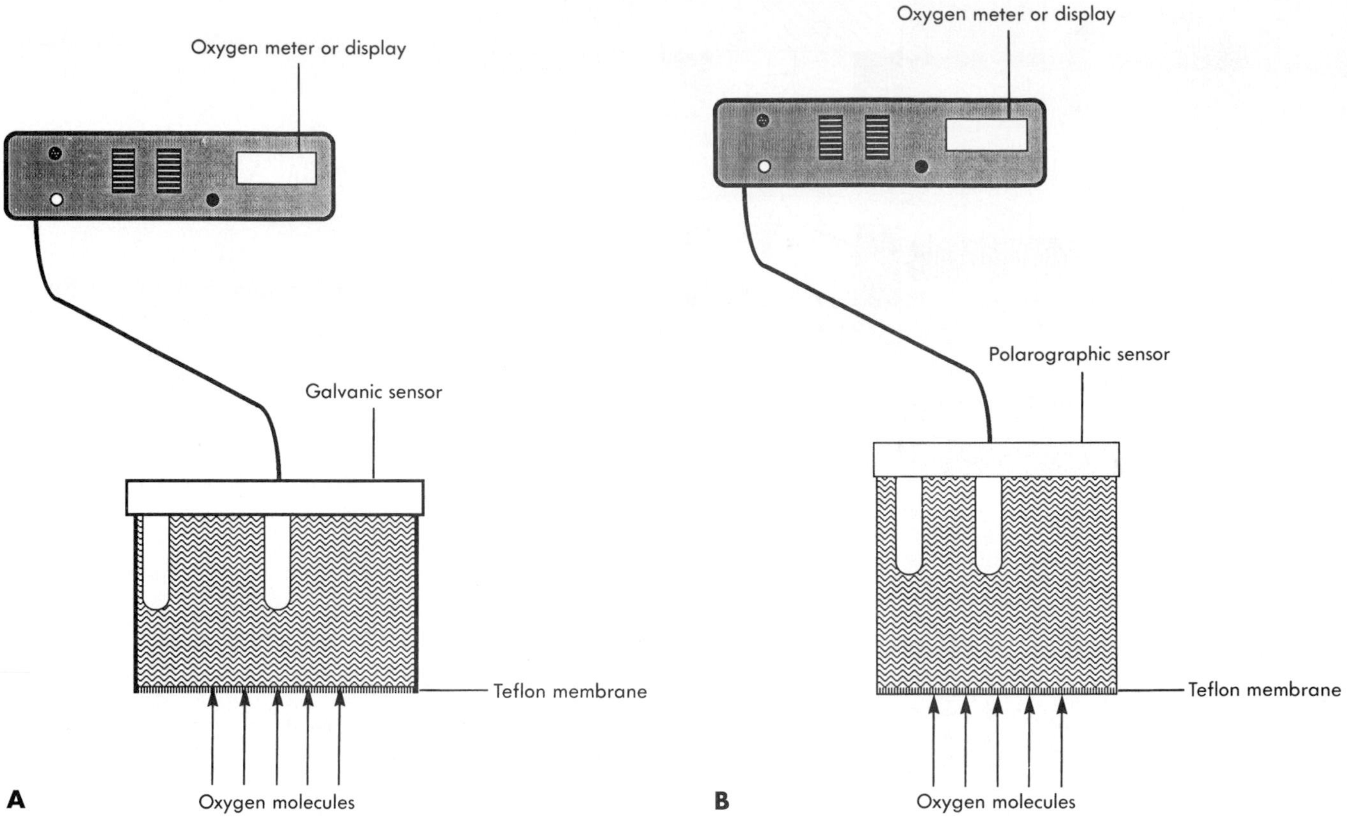

Figure 7-21 Electrochemical oxygen analyzers. **A,** Galvanic device. **B,** Polarographic device.

Electrochemical Analyzers

These are the most commonly used oxygen analyzers. They are generally classified as galvanic or polarographic devices.

Galvanic analyzers use an oxygen-mediated chemical reaction to generate an electrical current. As shown in Figure 7-21 *A,* a gold cathode and a lead anode are immersed in a potassium hydroxide bath. The gas sample to be analyzed is separated from the bath by a semipermeable membrane that is usually made of polytetrafluoroethylene (Teflon). As oxygen diffuses across the membrane into the hydroxide solution, it reacts with water and free electrons from the gold cathode to form hydroxyl ions (OH^-). The OH^- ions diffuse toward the lead (Pb) anode, forming lead oxide (PbO_2), water, and free electrons. The flow of the electrons produces a current that can be measured with an ammeter, and the amount of current flow detected is directly related to oxygen concentration. (Note that galvanic oxygen analyzers do not have to be "turned on." They continually read 21% oxygen when the sensor is exposed to room air, so it is important to keep the sensor capped to prolong its life.)

Polarographic analyzers also use an oxygen-mediated chemical reaction to create current flow, but they differ slightly in design from galvanic type of devices (see Figure 7-21 *B*). Polarographic analyzers contain a platinum cathode and a silver anode immersed in a potassium hydroxide bath. Additionally, they typically use a 9-V battery to polarize the silver anode, resulting in an improved response time because the OH^- ions are attracted to the difference in electrical charge. The reaction formula is basically similar to that of galvanic analyzers, but the reaction time is faster.

Galvanic and polarographic analyzers can be used for intermittent or continuous monitoring of FiO_2 and can be used with flammable gases during anesthesia. Because they respond to changes in partial pressure, readings can be affected by changes in ambient pressure, as may occur during mechanical ventilation or at high altitudes. Although galvanic analyzers have a slower response time than that of polarographic analyzers, they do not require an external power supply, and their electrodes may last longer.

Commercially available galvanic analyzers are available from Teledyne, Hudson, Biomarine, and Ohmeda. Polarographic oxygen analyzers are available from Sensormedics, Hudson-Ventronics, IL, IMI, Teledyne, and Critikon.

Electrical Analyzers

These analyzers operate on the principle of thermal conductivity and use an electronic device called a Wheatstone

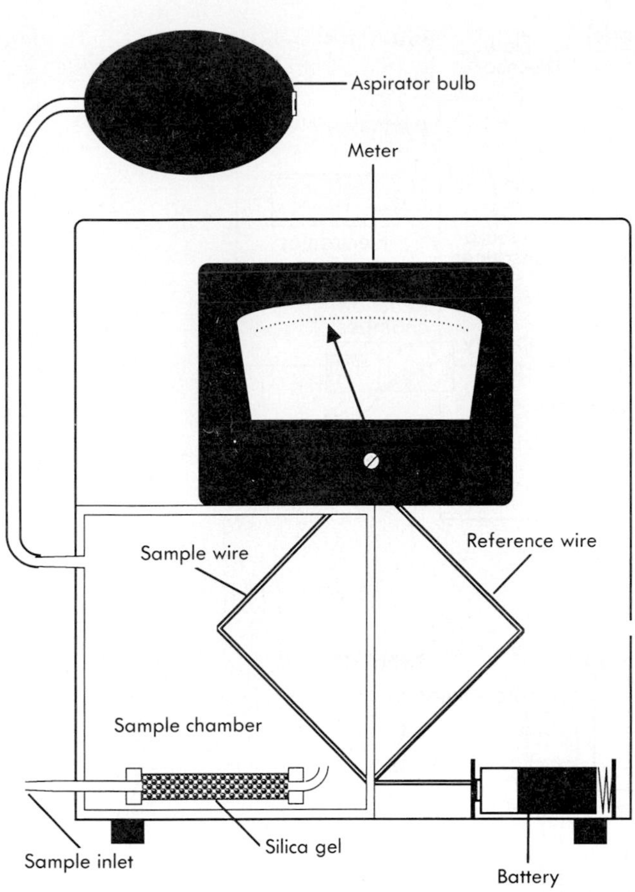

Figure 7-22 Electrical oxygen analyzer showing Wheatstone-bridge circuit.

bridge. Figure 7-22 shows how these devices operate. Two parallel wires receive current flow from an external power source, usually a battery. One of these wires, which serves as the reference, is exposed to room air. The other wire is located in the sample chamber and is exposed to the gas being analyzed. If the sample gas contains a higher oxygen: nitrogen ratio than room air, the sample wire cools, and its resistance decreases because oxygen is a better conductor of heat than nitrogen. Consequently, current flow increases through the sample wire when compared with the reference wire. An ammeter detects the change in current flow and relates it to oxygen concentration.

The primary advantage of using an electrical analyzer is that it compares the oxygen concentration of an unknown gas with ambient air. Therefore it is responsive to changes in the percent of oxygen instead of partial pressure, and it is unaffected by changes in pressure (e.g., those that occur with altitude changes). Several problems can occur when using these devices. For example, the Wheatstone bridge can generate significant amounts of heat and therefore is dangerous to use in the presence of flammable gases. Also, because contaminant gases can dissipate heat at different rates than oxygen and nitrogen, if gases other than oxygen and nitrogen are present, it can lead to erroneous FiO_2s.

MEASUREMENT OF NITROGEN OXIDES

As discussed in Chapter 3, nitric oxide (NO) is a simple, diatomic molecule that can cause vasodilation, macrophage cytotoxicity, and platelet adhesion.[25] It has been used to successfully treat pulmonary hypertension in neonates and to improve gas exchange in critically ill patients.[26,27]

Because of the potential for pulmonary toxicity induced by high levels of NO and nitrogen dioxide (NO_2), it is important to monitor the concentration of these molecules when nitric oxide is used clinically. Body and Hartigan[25] have recently written an excellent review of nitrogen oxide measurement. Two types of monitoring systems are routinely used when administering nitric oxide: **chemiluminescence monitoring** and **electrochemical monitoring.**[26] A brief discussion of each follows.

Chemiluminescence Monitoring

Chemiluminescence monitoring involves the quantification of gas-specific photoemission.[25] Gases sampled by the chemiluminescence monitor react with ozone (O_3) to produce nitrogen dioxide with an electron in an unstable excited state (NO_2*). As this unstable molecule decays to its lower energy (ground) state, photons are emitted with energies in the 600 to 3000 nanometer (nm) wavelength range.[25] Photon emissions are measured by photomultiplier tubes and electronically converted into a displayable signal.

Nitrogen dioxide levels can be measured indirectly by converting NO_2 to NO with a catalytic or chemical converter, and then measuring the NO concentration as described above.[27] Thermal catalytic converters, which are made of stainless steel, operate at temperatures of 600° to 800° C.[25] Chemical converters rely on molybdenum and carbon to convert NO_2 to NO. Although chemical converters must be periodically replenished, they can be used at lower temperatures and are more stable than catalytic converters. They are also less affected by interference from other gases.

The NO_2 concentration is determined by measuring the total concentration of nitrogen oxides and subtracting the NO concentration. Figure 7-23 contains schematics of two different types of commercially available chemiluminescence nitrogen oxide monitors. In *A,* one reaction chamber is used to measure NO and NO_2. This system operates on the principle that the NO_2 converter is switched into the sample line at 10- to 30-second intervals. *B* shows a system that uses two separate chambers for measuring NO and NO_2, with a single photomultiplier tube for measuring the outputs from both chambers.

The accuracy of a chemiluminescence monitor can be altered either by variations in the sample gas composition or by interference with the operation of the photomultiplier tubes.

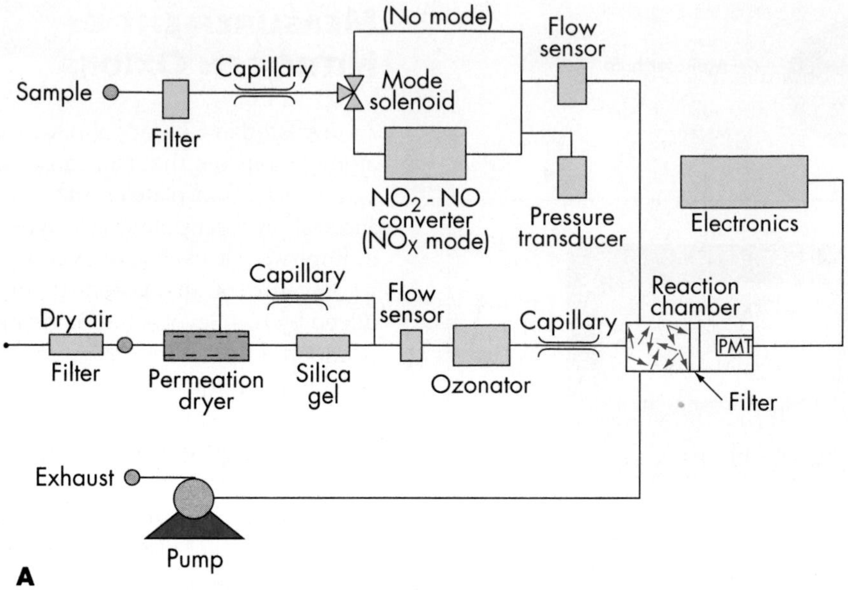

A

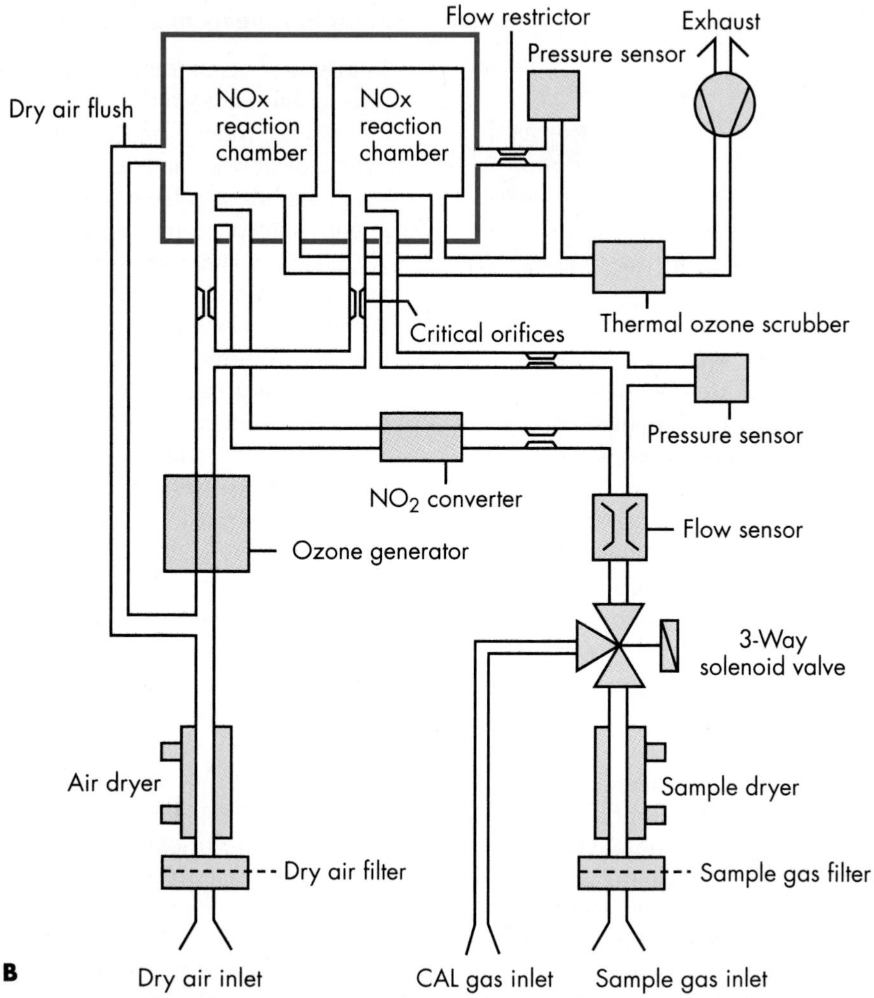

B

Figure 7-23 Schematic illustrating two types of chemiluminescence nitrogen oxide monitors. **A,** A single reaction chamber chemiluminescence device; **B,** A dual reaction chamber chemiluminescence device. (From Body S, et al: Nitric oxide: delivery, measurement, and clinical application, J Cardiothoracic Vasc Anesth 9(6):748, 1995, with permission.)

Variations in the composition of the sample gas can result from **quenching** of excited states of nitrogen dioxide, false identification of contaminant gases, such as NO_2, and alterations in the viscosity of the sample gas by background gases. Quenching occurs when NO_2^* is converted to ground state NO_2 by inadvertent collisions of the former gases with other background gases like oxygen, carbon dioxide, and water.[25] NH_2 and N_2O are two gases that can be falsely identified as NO_2. Increases in the viscosity of the sample gas (such as can occur with high percentages of oxygen) decrease the gas flow into the reaction chamber, thus reducing the number of NO molecules entering the chamber. Inaccuracies caused by photomultiplier tube interference are generally associated with photon emissions from contaminating gases in the sample reaction chamber and with thermal fluctuations.

Electrochemical Monitoring

This technique is based on a principle similar to that used with polarographic (Clark) electrodes. That is, gases diffusing across a semipermeable membrane react with an electrolyte solution, generating a current flow between two polarized electrodes as electrons are liberated or consumed.[25]

Figure 7-24 shows an example of an electrochemical NO analyzer. It consists of three electrodes (a sensing electrode, a counter electrode, and a reference electrode) immersed in an electrolyte solution that contains a highly conductive concentrated acid or alkali solution. The electrodes are separated from the gas sample to be analyzed by a semipermeable membrane. NO and NO_2 from the unknown gas sample diffuse across a semipermeable membrane and react with the electrolyte solution near the sensing electrode, generating electrons in the following oxidation reaction:

$$NO + 2H_2O \rightarrow HNO_3 + 3H^+ + 3e^-.$$

The electrons generated are consumed at the counter electrode through the reduction of oxygen, or:

$$O_2 + 4H^+ + 4e^- \rightarrow 2H_2O.$$

Balancing the equations at both electrodes yields the following equation,

$$4NO + 2H_2O + 3O_2 \rightarrow 4HNO_3.$$

NO_2 can be measured by electrochemical analysis using a similar principle. In this series of reactions, NO_2 is reduced to NO at the sensing electrode, and H_2O is oxidized at the counter electrode, or:

$$NO_2 + 2H^+ + 2e^- \rightarrow NO + H_2O$$
$$2H_2O \rightarrow 4H^+ + 4e^- + O_2.$$

The accuracy of NO/NO_2 electrochemical monitors can be altered by increases in ambient pressure (as occur with positive-pressure ventilation) and also by the presence of background gases, such as CO_2, CO, and NH_2, that have lower oxidation potentials than the sensor potential. The accuracy of these electrochemical monitors is also limited in the clinical setting for NO concentrations less than 0.1 ppm.[28]

Box 7-6 lists the Food and Drug Administration (FDA) standards for NO and NO_2 monitoring devices. Table 7-5 shows a comparison of chemiluminescence and electrochemical nitrogen oxide analyzers.

CAPNOGRAPHY (CAPNOMETRY)

Capnography, or capnometry, is the continuous measurement of carbon dioxide concentrations at the airway opening during respiration. The term *capnography* is used to describe the technique in which carbon dioxide concentration is displayed as a graphic waveform called a **capnogram;** capnometry is the technique in which carbon dioxide concentration is displayed as a numeric reading.[29] In both cases, the carbon dioxide concentration can be displayed in millimeters of mercury, representing the partial pressure or a percentage of carbon dioxide.[29]

Several methods are used to measure carbon dioxide, including infrared (IR) spectroscopy, mass spectroscopy, and Raman spectroscopy. Infrared and Raman spectrometers are portable devices used by individual patients. Mass spectrometers are shared devices that can sample gases from 10 to 12 patients. Infrared spectroscopy is currently the method of choice in critical-care settings, and mass spectroscopy is most often used in surgical suites. The use of Raman spectroscopy for capnography is limited.

Infrared Spectroscopy

Infrared spectroscopy is based on the principle that molecules containing more than one element absorb infrared light in a characteristic manner.[30] Normally, carbon dioxide maximally absorbs infrared radiation at 4.26 μm. The carbon dioxide concentration of a gas sample can be estimated because the amount of carbon dioxide in a gas sample is directly related to the amount of infrared light absorbed.[31]

As Figure 7-25 shows, the peak carbon dioxide absorption is very close to the absorption peaks for water and nitrous oxide. Thus if water or nitrous oxide are present, the carbon dioxide readings during infrared monitoring can be erroneous. The effects of water vapor can be eliminated by passing the gas sample through an absorbent (i.e., drying the sample) before it is analyzed. Nitrous oxide artifacts can be removed with filters or by using correction factors.[32]

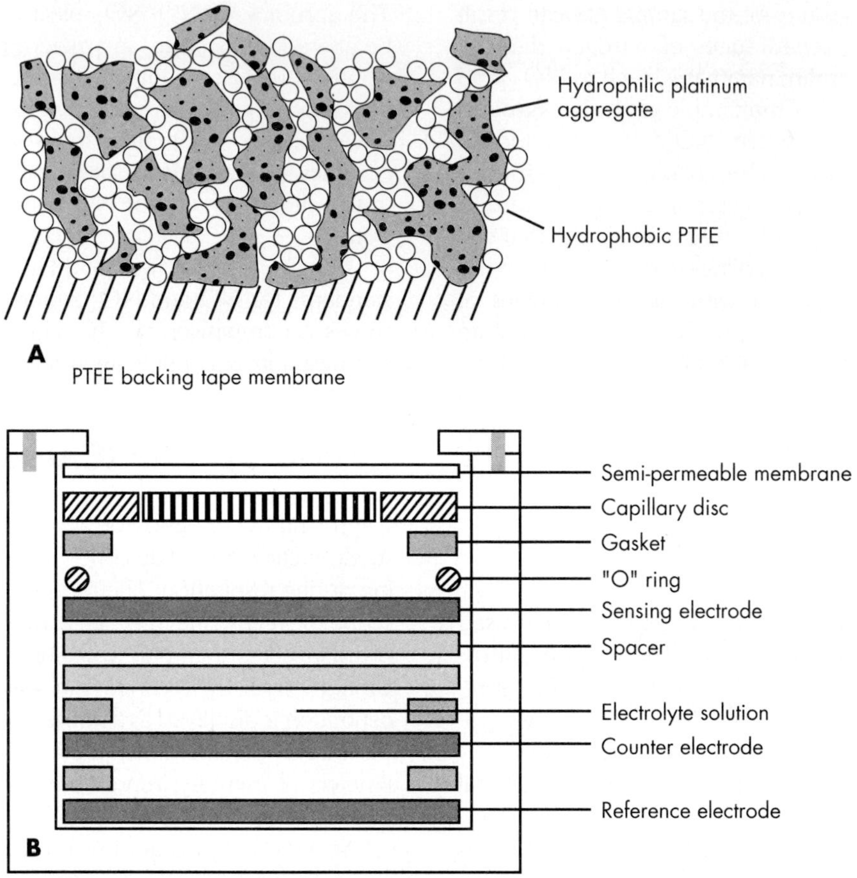

Figure 7-24 Schematic of an electrochemical nitrogen oxide monitor. (From Body S, et al: Nitric oxide: delivery, measurement, and clinical application, J Cardiothoracic Vasc Anesth 9(6):748, 1995, with permission.)

Figure 7-26 shows two types of infrared **capnographs:** *A* is a single-beam, negative filter device, and *B* is a double-beam, positive filter capnograph. With the single-beam device, the sample gas is directed to a sample chamber that lies between the infrared radiation source and a detection chamber. A chopper blade with two transparent cells (one containing carbon dioxide and the other containing nitrogen) is positioned between the sample chamber and the detector. Gas passing through the sample must pass through the circulating chopper cells before reaching the detection chamber. As the blade turns, two signals are generated, the ratio of which is detected and used to calculate the carbon dioxide concentration.

In the double-beam type of analyzer, gas is drawn into a sample chamber that contains a cuvette made of sodium chloride and sodium bromide.[30] Infrared radiation is beamed through the cuvette containing the sample of gas to be analyzed and through a reference chamber containing gas free of carbon dioxide. The carbon dioxide in the sample chamber absorbs some of the radiation, therefore decreasing the amount of radiation reaching the detector. The difference between the radiation transmitted through the sample cell and the radiation transmitted through the reference causes a diaphragm within the detector chamber to move. This diaphragm movement is converted into an electrical signal that is amplified and displayed in millimeters of mercury, representing the partial pressure or percentage of carbon dioxide.[33]

Clinicians generally classify infrared analyzers by the method used to sample gases at the airway. Figure 7-27 shows a **sidestream** and a **mainstream** device. With the sidestream devices, the gas to be analyzed is aspirated from the airway at a flow rate of approximately 500 mL/min through a narrow-bore polyethylene tube and transferred to the sample chamber, which is located in a separate console. With mainstream devices, analysis is performed at the airway, and gas passes into the sampling chamber that is attached directly to the endotracheal tube (ET).

Although sidestream devices are quite reliable, they show a slight delay between sampling and reporting times because of the time required to transport the sample from the airway to the sample chamber. Consequently, these devices may not be appropriate for patients breathing at high rates (e.g., neonates). The plastic tube that transports sample gas from the airway to the analyzer is prone to plugging by water and secretions, and therefore can lead to erroneous readings. Contamination with ambient air from leaks in the sample line is also a concern.

BOX 7-6

Proposed FDA Standards for Nitric Oxide and Nitrogen Dioxide Monitoring Devices

Monitoring Range

1 ppm NO lower limit. No upper limit specified.
1 to 5 ppm NO_2.

Accuracy*

≤20 ppm NO; ±20% of NO concentration, or 0.5 ppm—whichever is greater.
>20 ppm NO; ±10% of NO concentration.
NO_2; ±20% of NO_2 concentration.

Response Time

10% to 90% of full signal response time <30 seconds

Alarms

Audible and visual alarms: for NO, an upper level alarm able to be set from 2 ppm NO to maximum signal; for NO_2, an upper level alarm able to be set from 2 ppm NO_2 to maximum signal.

Other Considerations

Electrical safety (IEC601-1)
Electromagnetic compatibility and immunity (IEC601-1-2)
Environmental protection (temperature, humidity, and spill resistance)
Environmental pollution
Software safety (IEC601-1-4)

From Body SC and Hartigan PM: Manufacture and measurement of nitrogen oxides. In Hess D and Hurford WE, editors: Inhaled Nitric Oxide I, Respir Care Clin N Amer 3(3):414, 1997.
*The stated accuracy must be present in the following background gases: 0 and 5 ppm NO_2 (for NO monitoring); 0, 10, and 40 ppm NO (for NO_2 monitoring); 21%, 60%, and 95% oxygen and 0%, 50%, and 100% relative humidity. If the monitoring device is placed within the ventilator circuit and subject to lung inflation pressures, the accuracy must be maintained over a pressure range of −15 to +100 cm H_2O.

TABLE 7-5

Comparison of chemiluminescence and electrochemical monitoring devices

Factor	Electrochemical	Chemiluminescence
Cost	$2500–$5800	$11,000–23,000
Ease of use	+++	+
Ease of servicing	+++	+
Ease of setup	+++	+
Accuracy	+	+++
Response time	10–30 seconds	0.15–20 seconds
Measurement range	++	+++
Size	+++	+
O_2% correction required	No	Yes
Ozone production	No	Yes

Modified from Body S et al: Nitric oxide: delivery, measurement, and clinical application. J Cardiothoracic Vasc Anesth 9(6):748, 1995.

Box 7-7 illustrates a common problem that occurs with **sidestream capnographs.**

Mainstream devices do not show a delay between sampling and reporting times because the analyzer is attached directly to the ET. However, these devices add dead space to the airway, which must be quantified to prevent erroneous readings of the partial pressure of carbon dioxide. The additional weight placed on the artificial airway by this type of analyzer increases the possibility of dislodgment or complete extubation. It should also be recognized that because this type of analyzer is directly attached to the airway, it is subject to damage from mishandling (i.e., dropping the device on the floor).

Mass Spectroscopy

Mass spectroscopy is based on the principle that a gas molecules can be identified by their mass:charge ratio when they are passed through a magnetic field. Figure 7-28 is a schematic that shows this principle. The gas to be analyzed

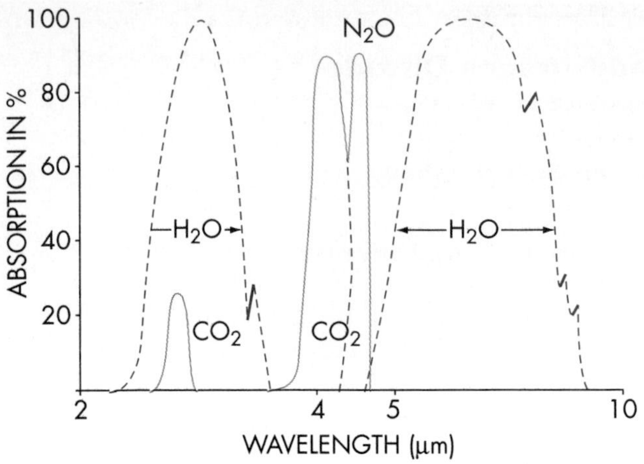

Figure 7-25 Infrared absorption spectra for carbon dioxide, nitrous oxide, and water. (From Hess D: Capnometry and capnography: technical aspects, physiologic aspects, and clinical applications, Respir Care 35:557, 1990.)

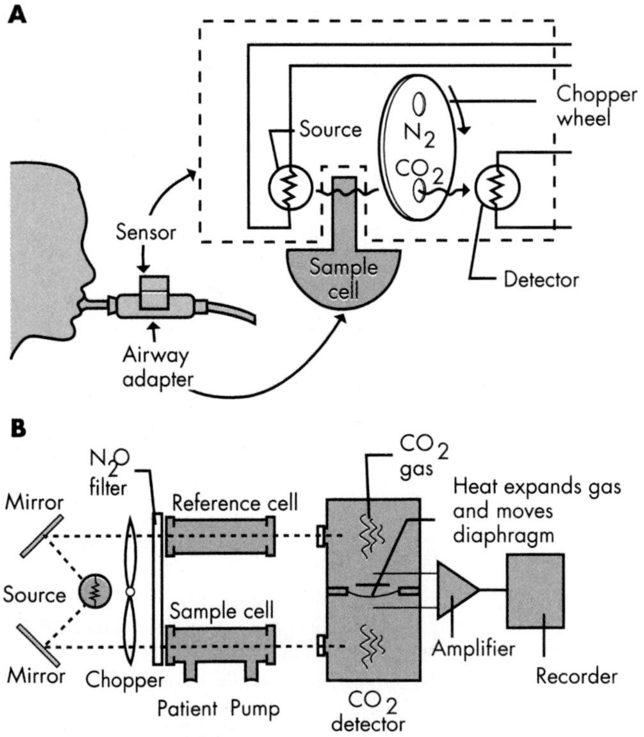

Figure 7-26 **A,** Single-beam nondispersive infrared capnograph; **B,** Double-beam, nondispersive infrared capnograph. (Redrawn from Gravenstein JS, Paulus DA, and Hayes TJ: Capnography in clinical practice, Boston, 1989, Butterworths.)

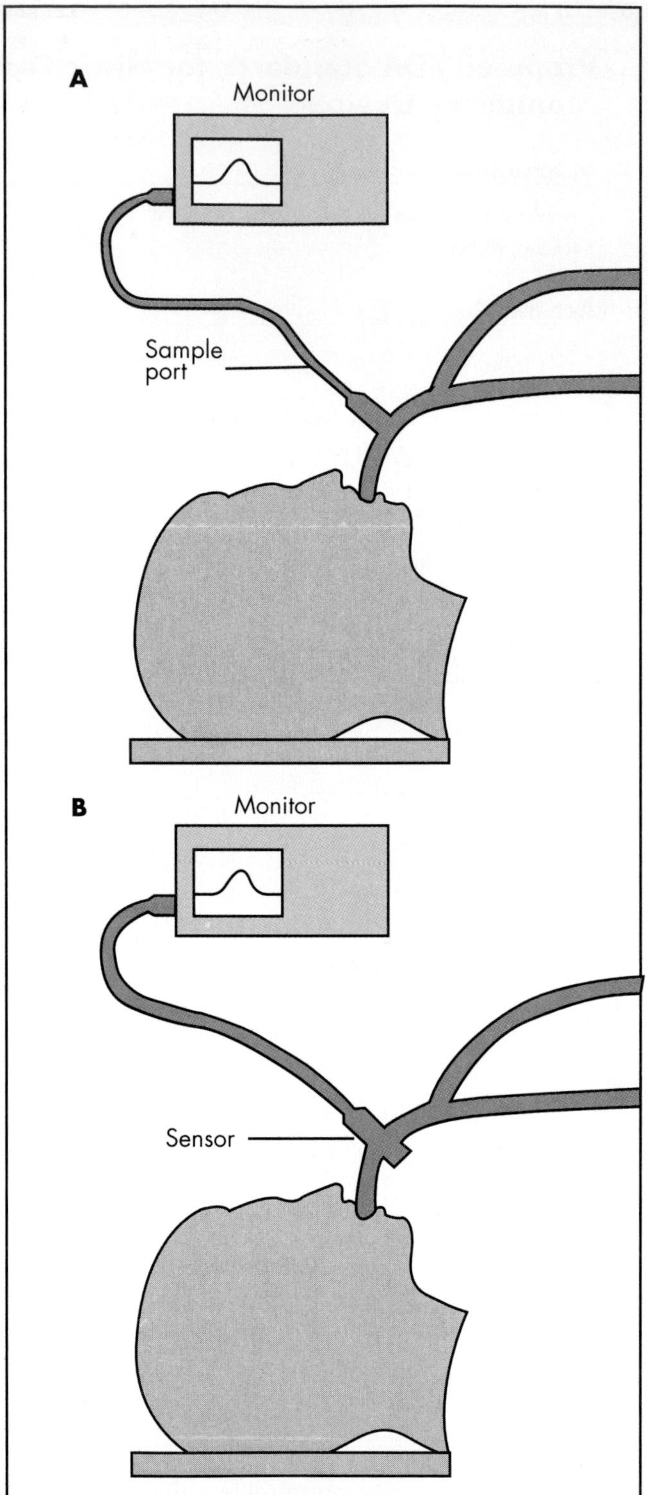

Figure 7-27 Capnographs can be classified by sampling technique. **A,** Sidestream capnograph: exhaled gas is extracted through small-bore tubing and transported to a console containing the infrared sensor; **B,** Mainstream capnograph: exhaled gas is measured at the airway.

is aspirated into a chamber and ionized by a stream of electrons emitted from a filament. The ionized gas molecules are accelerated and deflected by a magnetic field onto a collector plate. The amount of deflection depends on their mass:charge ratio. The gas molecules are then separated according to their mass:charge ratio, and as they reach the collector plate, they generate a signal that is picked up by a detector. The strength of the signal, which depends on the number of particles detected, can then be amplified and displayed.[33]

Although mass spectrometers are expensive, they can be used for several patients (i.e., multiplexing in the surgical suite) and can be used to measure gases other than carbon dioxide, including oxygen, nitrogen, and nitrous oxide. This added capacity does have drawbacks, however, because carbon dioxide and nitrous oxide have the same molecular weight. Therefore separation of the basis of weight alone can lead to erroneous readings. This problem is overcome by ionizing N_2O to N_2O^+ and CO_2 to C^+.[31,33]

BOX 7-7

Decision Making & Problem Solving

A patient is being monitored with a sidestream capnograph. Although no problems were noted during the initial period of monitoring, the capnograph now shows an irregular waveform because the percentage of carbon dioxide does not rise above 1%. What could cause this?

See Appendix A for the answer.

Raman Spectroscopy

This type of spectroscopy relies on the **Raman effect,** which occurs when light interacts with gas molecules to cause rotational or vibrational energy changes in the gas molecules. The light that is emitted from a gas molecule as it relaxes to its original state results in a shift in the wavelength that is characteristic of the molecule being analyzed. Monochromatic radiation that is passed through a gas mixture is therefore changed to a spectrum that depends on the structure of the individual molecules present in the gas mixture.[33]

Although Raman spectroscopy has been available for awhile, its use in clinical medicine is still somewhat limited.

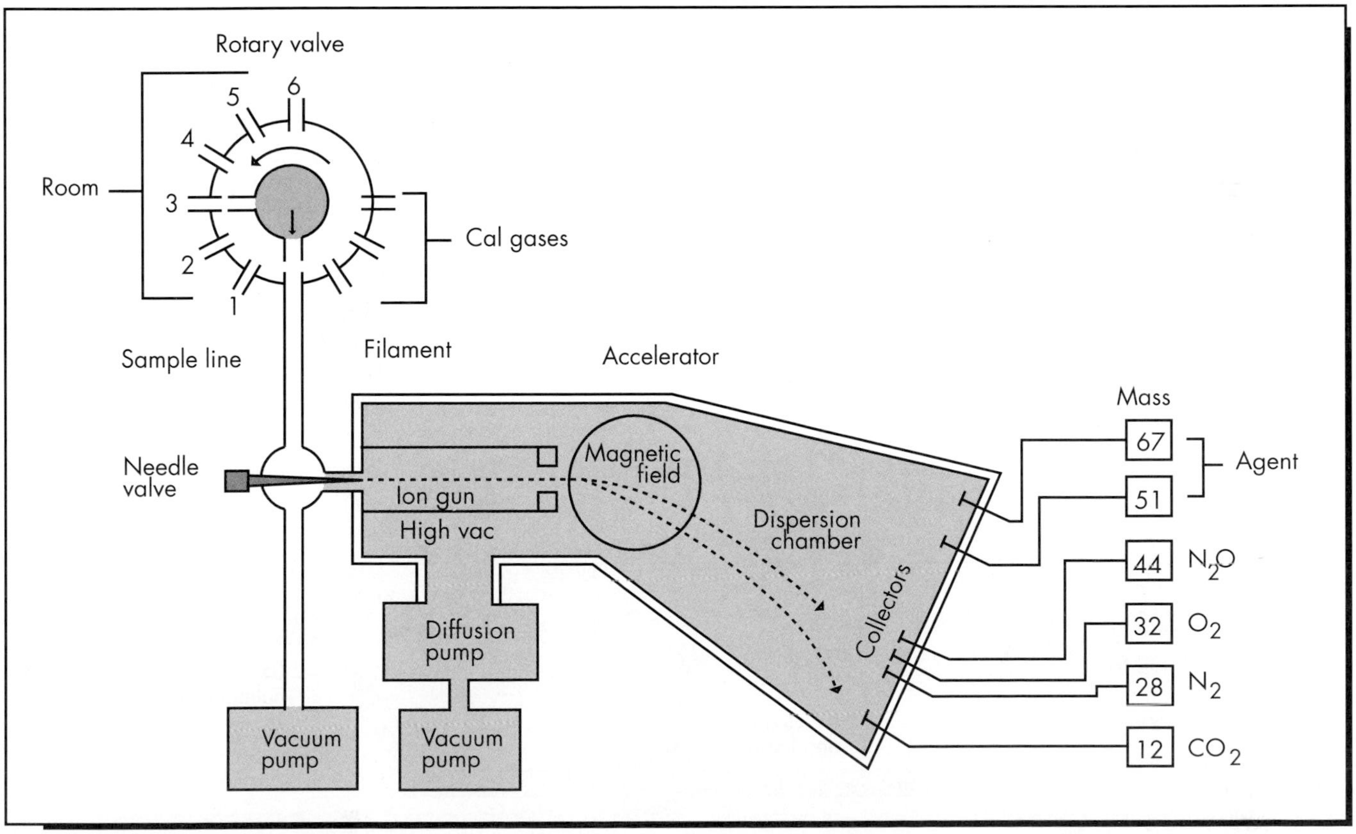

Figure 7-28 Schematic of a mass spectrometer. (Redrawn from Gravenstein JS, Paulus DA, and Hayes TJ: Capnography in clinical practice, Boston, 1989, Butterworths.)

Because the accuracy of these devices has been shown to be similar to mass spectroscopy, the future use of this technology remains promising.

Physiologic Basis of Capnography

Under normal circumstances, inspired air contains virtually no carbon dioxide (actually it contains about 0.3%). Expired air, on the other hand, contains about 4% to 6% carbon dioxide. Figure 7-29 is an idealized capnogram of a resting individual who is quietly breathing room air. This waveform, which is divided into four phases, reflects the elimination of carbon dioxide from the lungs during respiration. During Phase 1, gas is exhaled from the large conducting airways, which contain essentially no carbon dioxide. In Phase 2, some alveolar gas containing carbon dioxide mixes with gas from the smaller conducting airways, and the carbon dioxide concentration rises. During Phase 3, the carbon dioxide concentration curve remains relatively constant, as primarily alveolar gas is exhaled (alveolar plateau).* On inspiration (Phase 4), the concentration falls to 0.

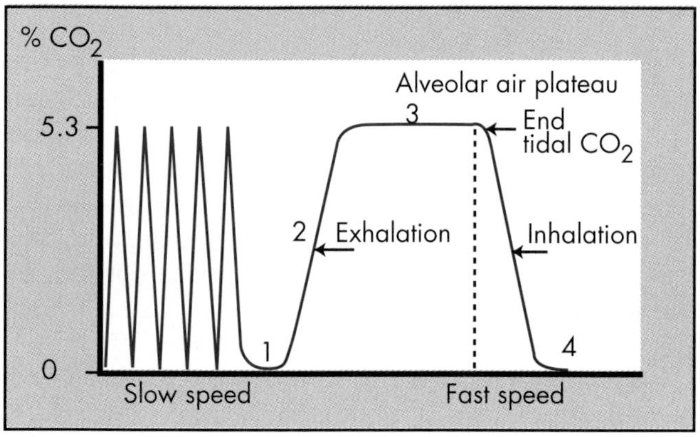

Figure 7-29 A normal capnogram. *1,* exhaled gas from conducting airways; *2,* a mixture of conducting airways and alveolar air; *3,* alveolar plateau; *4,* inspired air (0.3% CO_2).

The amount of carbon dioxide in exhaled air depends on a balance between carbon dioxide production and elimination. Production is primarily determined by the metabolic rate, but elimination is dependent upon alveolar ventilation, which is ultimately influenced by the ventilation/perfusion ($\dot{V}/\dot{Q}$) ratio of the lungs.

The relationship between $\dot{V}/\dot{Q}$ and gas exchange (i.e., the partial pressure of alveolar carbon dioxide [P_ACO_2]) can be expressed with $\dot{V}/\dot{Q}$ relationships. Figure 7-30 shows three $\dot{V}/\dot{Q}$ relationships that can potentially affect the level of partial pressure of arterial carbon dioxide ($PaCO_2$). In *A,* ventilation and perfusion are equally matched. $PaCO_2$ and P_ACO_2 are nearly equal. Note that

*The concentration of carbon dioxide at the end of the alveolar phase (just before inspiration begins) is called the end-tidal PCO_2, or $PetCO_2$.

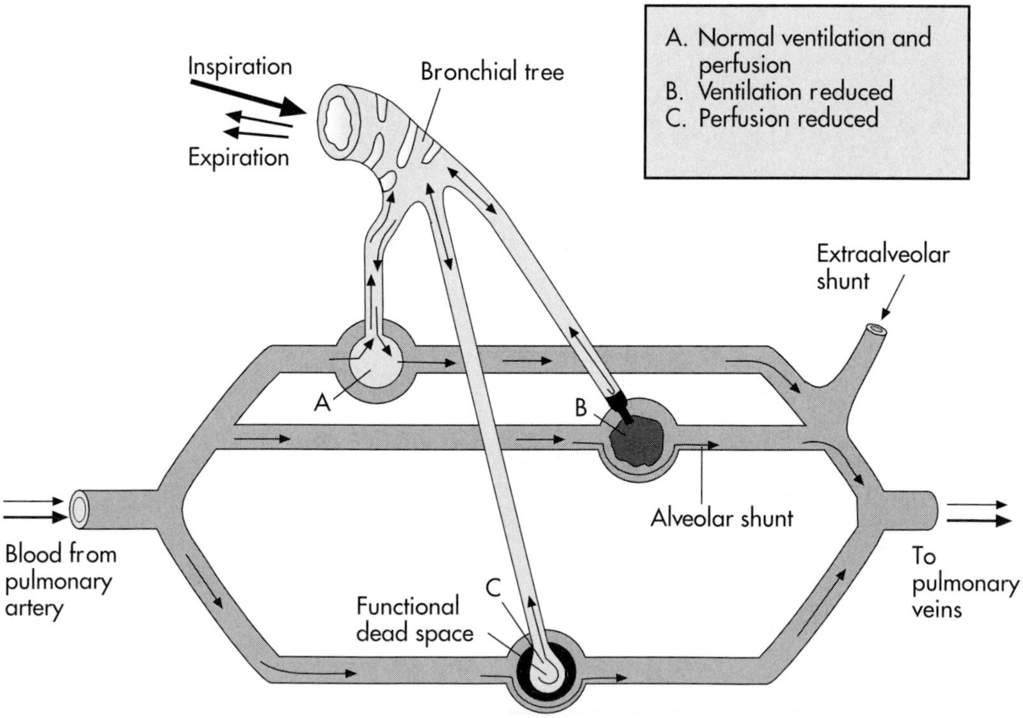

Figure 7-30 Ventilation/perfusion relationships: A, normal; B, Low V/Q; C, High V/Q. (In Pilbeam SP: Mechanical Ventilation: Physiological and Clinical Applications, ed 3, St Louis, 1998, Mosby. Modified from Despopoulos A, Silbernagl S: Color atlas of physiology, ed 4, New York, 1991, Thieme Medical Publishers.)

BOX 7-8

Clinical Practice Guidelines

Capnography/Capnometry during Mechanical Ventilation

Indications

Based on current evidence, capnography is useful for:

1. Monitoring the severity of pulmonary disease and evaluating the response to therapy, especially therapy intended to improve V_D/V_T and $\dot{V}/\dot{Q}$ relationships. It may also provide valuable information about therapy for improving coronary blood flow.
2. Determining that tracheal rather than esophageal intubation has taken place.
3. Monitoring the integrity of the mechanical ventilatory circuit and artificial airway.
4. Evaluating the efficiency of mechanical ventilatory support.
5. Monitoring the adequacy of pulmonary and coronary blood flow.
6. Monitoring carbon dioxide production.

Contraindications

There are no absolute contraindications to capnography in mechanical ventilated adult patients.

Monitoring

During capnography, the following should be recorded:

1. Ventilatory variables, including tidal volume, respiratory rate, positive end-expiratory pressure, inspiratory:expiratory ratio, peak airway pressure, and respiratory gas concentrations.
2. Hemodynamic variables, including systemic and pulmonary pressures, cardiac output, shunt, and $\dot{V}/\dot{Q}$ imbalances.

For a copy of the complete text, see Respiratory Care 40(12):1321, 1995.

although the partial pressure of end-tidal carbon dioxide ($PetCO_2$) should equal $PaCO_2$, it is actually about 4 to 6 mm Hg lower than the $PaCO_2$. In *B*, ventilation decreases relative to perfusion (low $\dot{V}/\dot{Q}$ or shunt). The P_ACO_2 eventually equilibrates with the partial pressure of carbon dioxide in mixed venous blood ($P_{\bar{v}}CO_2$). Clinical situations when this type of $\dot{V}/\dot{Q}$ relationship can exist throughout the lung, leading to higher than normal $PetCO_2$s include respiratory center depression, muscular paralysis, and COPD. In *C*, ventilation is higher than perfusion (high $\dot{V}/\dot{Q}$, or dead space ventilation). Physiologic dead space ventilation increases, and the P_ACO_2 approaches inspired air (0 torr). Decreased $PetCO_2$s are found with this type of $\dot{V}/\dot{Q}$ relationship in patients with pulmonary embolism, excessive PEEP (mechanical or intrinsic), and any disorder with pulmonary hypoperfusion.

Clinical Applications of Capnography

Capnography can be used for both spontaneously breathing and mechanically ventilated patients. Because it has been primarily used with mechanically ventilated patients, the AARC has prepared a guideline for using capnography to monitor such patients.[29] Box 7-8 summarizes the key points of this guideline. A discussion of how capnography can be used in the management of mechanically ventilated patients follows.

Capnograph Contours. Capnography can be used to detect increases in dead space ventilation, hyper- and hypoventilation, apnea or periodic breathing, inadequate neuromuscular blockade in pharmacologically paralyzed patients, and the presence of carbon dioxide rebreathing. It can also be used to effectively monitor gas exchange during cardiopulmonary resuscitation (CPR). Figure 7-31 shows various capnogram contours that are characteristic of several common situations.

In cases when physiologic dead space increases, as in COPD, Phase 3 becomes indistinguishable (see Figure 7-31, *A*). Hyperventilation is characterized by a reduction in $PaCO_2$ and therefore in $PetCO_2$ (*B*). Conversely, hypoventilation is associated with elevated $PaCO_2$s and $PetCO_2$s (*B*). *C* is a capnogram from a patient demonstrating Cheyne-Stokes breathing. During bradypnea, Phase 3 typically shows cardiac oscillations that result from the transferal of the beating heart motion to the conducting airways (*D*). Rebreathing exhaled gas is recognized because the capnogram does not return to baseline (*E*). *F* is a capnogram demonstrating the characteristic Phase 3 "curare cleft" that can occur when a patient is receiving insufficient neuromuscular blockade.[31,33]

Capnography can be used to detect cessation of pulmonary blood flow, as occurs with pulmonary embolism or during cardiac arrest.[29,31,33] Indeed, a number of investigators have advocated use of capnography as an adjunct to CPR. Laboratory studies suggest that capnography can be used as an indication of the progress and success of CPR, and demonstrated that $PetCO_2$ increases as $\dot{V}/\dot{Q}$ is restored to normal.[30,31]

Capnography can also be used during CPR to detect accidental esophageal intubation.[29,33] Gastric PCO_2 is generally equal to room air. Thus failure to detect the characteristic changes in carbon dioxide concentration during ventilation might indicate esophageal intubation. Although, low perfusion of the lungs is also associated with low $PetCO_2$ and should not be confused with esophageal

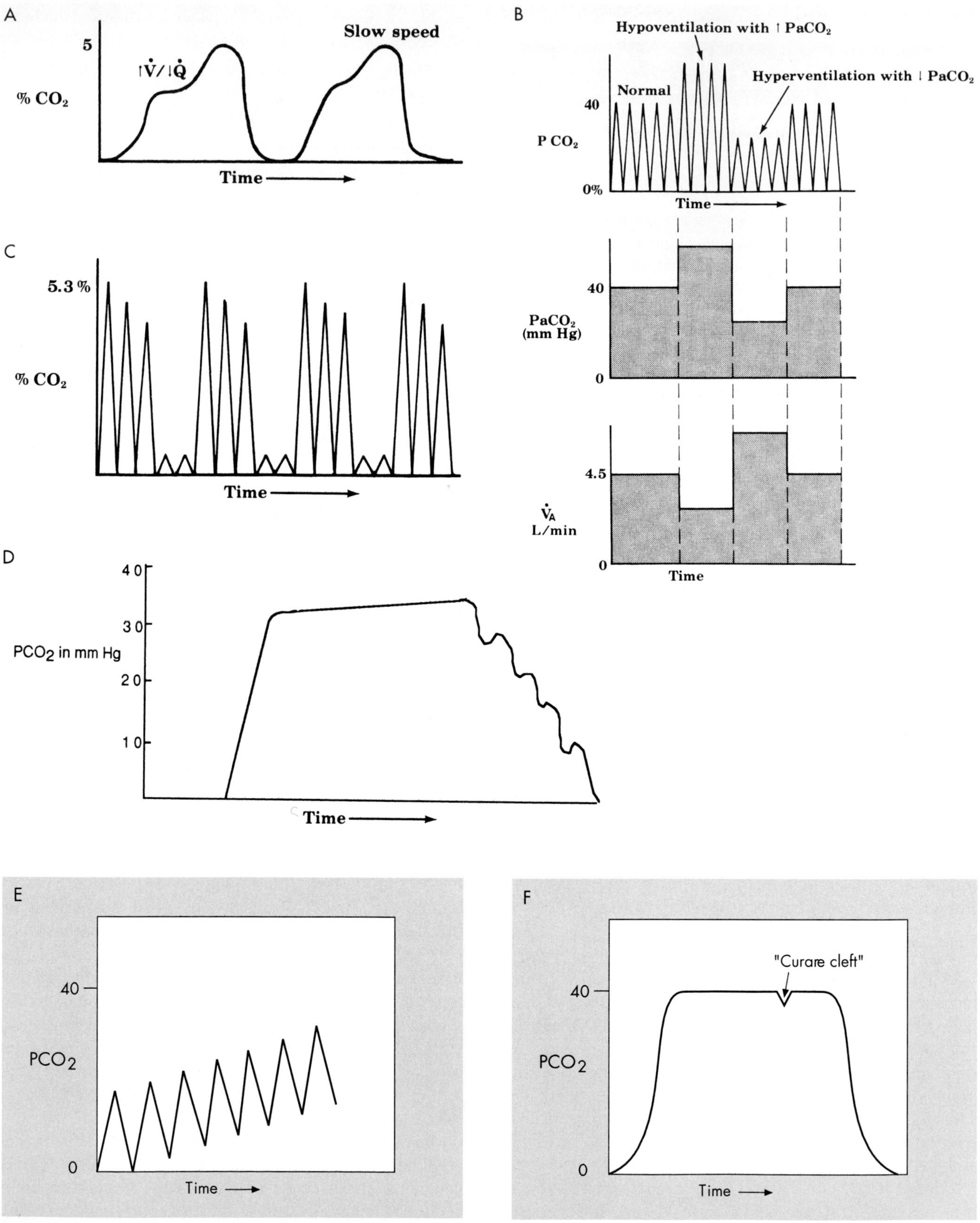

Figure 7-31 Capnogram contours associated with various breathing patterns: *A,* COPD; *B,* hyperventilation and hypoventilation; *C,* Cheyne-Strokes breathing; *D,* cardiac oscillations; *E,* rebreathing exhaled gases; *F,* curare cleft. (From Pilbeam SP: Mechanical ventilation, ed 3, St Louis, 1998, Mosby.)

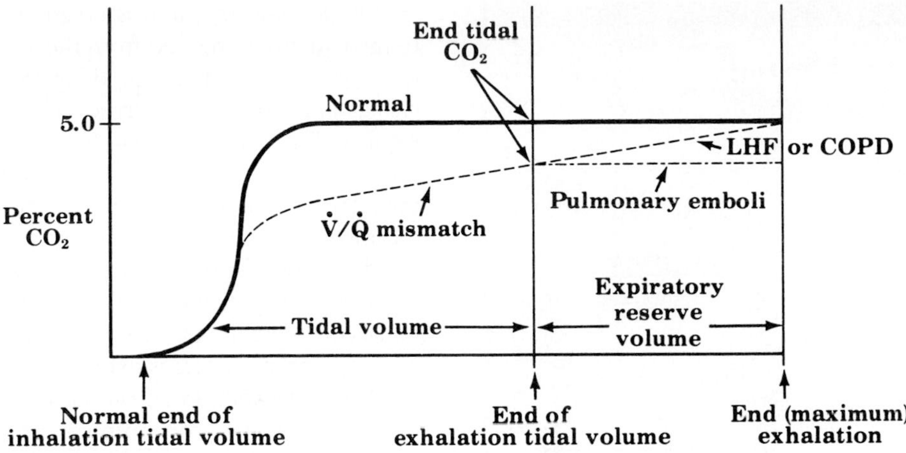

Figure 7-32 Capnogram illustrating exhaled carbon dioxide at the end of a quiet expiration and following a maximum expiration. The difference between these two values can be used to assess $\dot{V}/\dot{Q}$ relationships. A patient with COPD will typically show an end-tidal carbon dioxide less than that measured after a maximum expiration. For patients suspected to have pulmonary embolus, the end-tidal and maximum expiratory carbon dioxide measurements are nearly equal. (From Pilbeam SP: Mechanical ventilation, ed 3, St Louis, 1998, Mosby.)

intubation. Also, gastric PCO_2 may be elevated after mouth-to-mouth breathing or ingestion of a carbonated beverage.

Arterial-to-Maximum End-Expiratory PCO_2 Difference. As was previously mentioned, arterial-to-end-tidal partial pressure of carbon dioxide (a-et PCO_2) for tidal breathing should be negligible (essentially zero). It becomes elevated in patients with COPD, left heart failure, and pulmonary embolism due to an increase in their physiologic dead space.[29-31,33]

Another technique that can be used to further evaluate the severity of the disease is to compare the arterial PCO_2 measurements with the maximum expired PCO_2 measurements (the arterial to maximum expiratory PCO_2 gradient).[34,35] With this technique, the expired PCO_2 recorded at the end of a maximum exhalation to residual volume is compared to the $PaCO_2$. Normally, the difference between these two values is minimal. Interestingly, patients with COPD and left heart failure do not show an arterial-to-maximum expiration PCO_2 difference, whereas patients with pulmonary embolism do show an increased gradient. These differences are shown in Figure 7-32.

Indirect Calorimetry and Metabolic Monitoring

Most clinicians rely on equations derived by Harris and Benedict[36] in 1919 to estimate patient energy requirements. Although these formulae can be quite useful for normal subjects and non-critically ill patients, they may be limited for some critically ill patients. Kinney and associates[37] derived correction factors to compensate for the increased energy demands in critically ill patients (e.g., burns, bone fractures), but these factors are limited in their ability to account for situations where multiple conditions may exist simultaneously in a patient (e.g., sepsis, adult respiratory distress syndrome [ARDS]).

Recent advances in microprocessor technology have made it relatively easy for respiratory care practitioners to accurately measure energy needs and substrate utilization patterns in hospitalized patients. The technique used to accomplish this task is called **indirect calorimetry.**

Indirect Calorimetry

Indirect calorimetry is based on the theory that all of a person's energy is derived from the oxidation of carbohydrates, fats, and proteins, and that the ratio of carbon dioxide produced to oxygen consumed (i.e., the respiratory quotient, or $\dot{V}CO_2/\dot{V}O_2$) is characteristic of the fuel being burned.[38] **Energy expenditure** (EE) is calculated from $\dot{V}O_2$ and $\dot{V}CO_2$ measurements using the Weir equation, and substrate utilization patterns can be determined using equations like those derived by Burszein et al and Consolazio.[39-41] Box 7-9 summarizes these equations.

Indirect calorimeters are generally classified by their method of determining $\dot{V}O_2$. Thus two methods are usually described: the closed-circuit and the open-circuit methods. With the closed-circuit method, the patient breathes into and out of a container prefilled with oxygen. Oxygen consumption is determined by measuring the oxygen volume used by the patient. With the open-circuit method,

BOX 7-9

Formulae Used During Indirect Calorimetry

Energy Expenditure

Weir Equation[39]

$$EE = [3.941(\dot{V}O_2) + 1.106(\dot{V}CO_2)]1.44 - [2.17(UN)]$$

Modified Weir Equations

$$EE = [3.9(\dot{V}O_2) + 1.1(\dot{V}CO_2)] \times 1.44$$

Substrate Utilization[40]

Carbohydrates

$$dS = 4.115(\dot{V}CO_2) - 2.909(\dot{V}O_2) - 2.539(UN)$$

Fats

$$dF = 1.689\ (\dot{V}O_2 - \dot{V}CO_2) - 1.943(UN)$$

Proteins

$$dP = 6.25(UN)$$

dS, dF, and dP represent grams of carbohydrate, fat, and protein, respectively, for a fasting individual.

$\dot{V}O_2$ is determined by measuring the volume of inspired and expired gases, as well as the fractional concentrations of oxygen in the each. The $\dot{V}O_2$ is then determined by calculating the difference between the amount of oxygen in inspired gas ($\dot{V}_I \times FiO_2$) and the amount of oxygen in expired gas ($\dot{V}_E \times F_EO_2$).

Closed-Circuit Calorimeters

With closed-circuit devices, oxygen consumption can be determined by measuring either the oxygen volume removed from the device or by measuring the oxygen volume that must added to the system to maintain the original oxygen volume.

Figure 7-33 illustrates a closed-circuit system in which $\dot{V}O_2$ is determined by measuring the amount of oxygen removed from a reservoir over time. The system consists of a breathing circuit connected to a spirometer that is prefilled with oxygen. The patient's exhaled gases are directed to a mixing chamber, then through a carbon dioxide absorber, and back to the spirometer. Carbon dioxide production ($\dot{V}CO_2$) can be measured by incorporating the carbon dioxide analyzer positioned between the mixing chamber and the carbon dioxide absorber. **Closed-circuit calorimeters** can be used for both spontaneously breathing and mechanically ventilated patients.

Oxygen consumption is determined by measuring the oxygen volume removed from the spirometer. The volume of oxygen removed can be determined by measuring the change in the end-expiratory level. (Oxygen consumption is expressed in milliliters/ minute.) The fractional concentration of mixed expired carbon dioxide (F_ECO_2) is determined by aspirating a sample of the mixed expired gas (from the mixing chamber) into the carbon dioxide analyzer located between the mixing chamber and the spirometer. Carbon dioxide production is calculated by multiplying the fractional concentration of mixed expired carbon dioxide by the minute ventilation, and is expressed in milliliters/minute.

Another variation of the closed-circuit technique for estimating oxygen consumption involves measuring the oxygen volume that must be replenished while the patient removes oxygen from the reservoir. This system consists of a breathing circuit, a bellows containing oxygen, a carbon dioxide absorber, and an ultrasonic transducer to monitor the bellows position. As the patient breathes into and out of the bellows, oxygen that is used by the patient is replaced on demand by an external oxygen supply. The amount of oxygen that must be added back to the system is a measure of the oxygen consumption. These systems can be used for spontaneously breathing and mechanically ventilated patients.

Open-Circuit Calorimeters

Open-circuit calorimeters use mixing chambers, dilution techniques, and breath-by-breath measurements to determine oxygen consumption. With mixing chambers, expired gases are directed into a collecting chamber containing baffles to ensure adequate mixing of gases. A vacuum attached to the chamber aspirates a sample of the mixed-expired gas and directs it into the oxygen and carbon dioxide analyzers. Once analyzed, the gases are returned to the mixing chamber, and the entire volume of the mixing chamber is routed through a volume- or flow-sensing device.

Dilution systems also use a mixing chamber, but they use a bias flow of room air to dilute the gas sample and move it through the system. The amounts of oxygen and carbon dioxide exhaled are calculated by multiplying the fractional concentrations of oxygen and carbon dioxide by the total flow through the system, which is usually about 40 L/min.

Breath-by-breath devices measure the volume and fractional concentrations of oxygen and carbon dioxide in each breath. The amount of oxygen and carbon dioxide in inspired and mixed expired gases are actually determined by averaging the volumes and concentrations of several breaths. The number of breaths to be averaged can be preselected by the technologist or preset by the manufacturer.

Figure 7-34 is a schematic of an open-circuit, indirect calorimeter. A flow- or volume-sensing device is used to measure the inspired and expired gas volumes; a polaro-

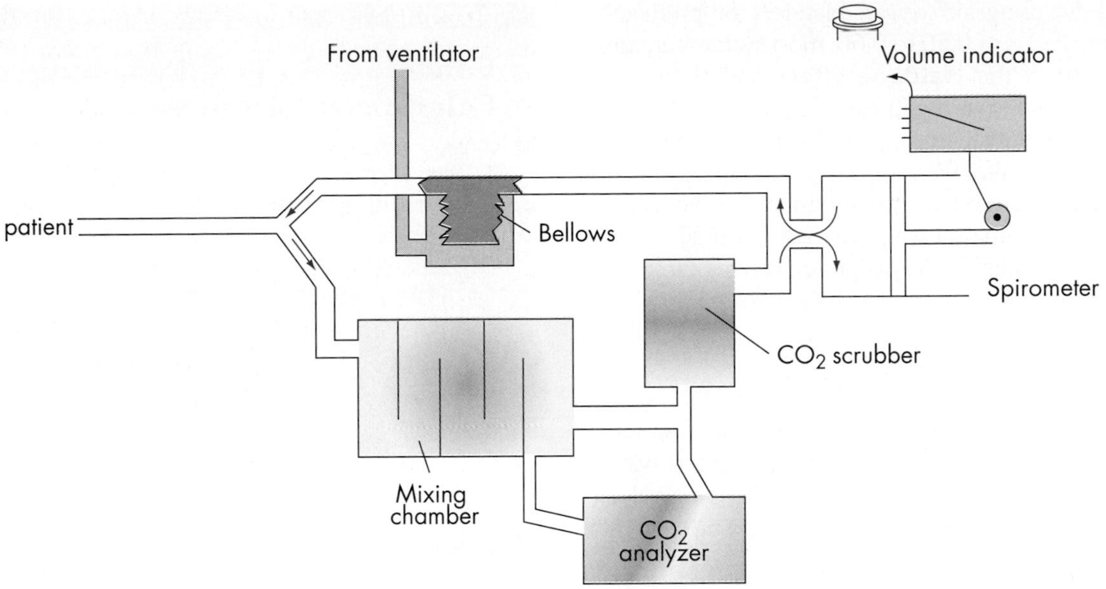

Figure 7-33 Closed-circuit indirect calorimeters. Oxygen consumption is estimated by measuring the amount of oxygen used from a reservoir. (From Branson RD: The measurement of energy expenditure: instrumentation, practical considerations, and clinical applications, Respir Care 35:640, 1990.)

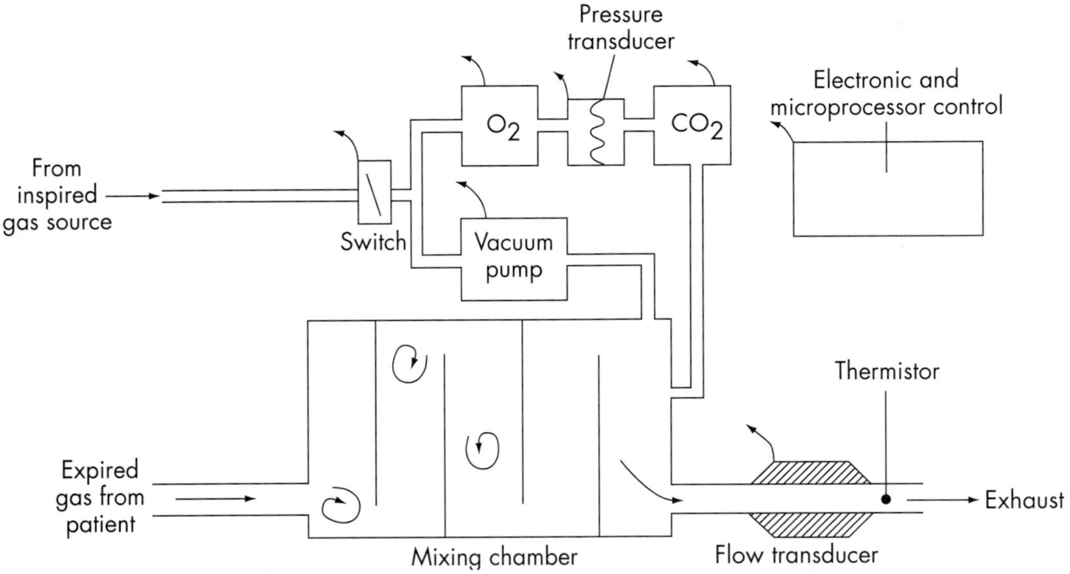

Figure 7-34 Open circuit indirect calorimeter. Oxygen consumption and carbon dioxide production are estimated by multiplying the minute ventilation by the fractional concentration of oxygen and carbon dioxide during inspiration and expiration. (From Branson RD: The measurement of energy expenditure: instrumentation, practical considerations, and clinical applications, Respir Care 35:640, 1990.)

graphic analyzer is used to measure the fractional concentrations of oxygen; and a nondispersive infrared analyzer is used to measure the fractional concentration of carbon dioxide. Because changes in ambient temperature and pressure can affect gas concentrations, a sensor for measuring the ambient temperature and barometric pressure of the gases being analyzed is also incorporated into the system design.

Although open-circuit devices can be used for both spontaneously breathing and mechanically ventilated patients, special problems can arise when these systems are used with mechanically ventilated patients. Some of these problems include fluctuations in FiO_2, separation of the patient's inspired and expired gases from the continuous gas flow from the ventilator, and handling of water vapor.[42] Problems with fluctuations in FiO_2 can be alleviated to some extent by using air/oxygen blenders or premixed gases.* Beyond FiO_2s of 0.50 to 0.60, most systems are unreliable because of the **Haldane effect** and should be viewed skeptically. Inspired and expired gases can be separated using isolation valves supplied by the manufacturer of the metabolic monitor. Water vapor is always a problem when performing continuous measurements on ventilator patients, but is accentuated when cascade humidifiers are used to supply humidity to the patient. Replacing these humidifiers with artificial noses may help to minimize the problem.

Practical Applications of Indirect Calorimetry

Spontaneously breathing patients who are breathing room air can be connected to the system by breathing through a mouthpiece or mask attached to a nonrebreathing valve. Specially designed canopies and hoods can also be used for spontaneously breathing patients who are not receiving ventilatory support.

Patients with ETs or tracheostomy tubes (TTs) can be connected to the system if the nonrebreathing valve is placed directly onto the airway opening and expired gases are routed into the system. It is important to inflate the cuffs of ETs and TTs when measuring inspired and exhaled gases, because failure to do so will result in loss of expired air around the tube and erroneous measurements of $\dot{V}O_2$ and $\dot{V}CO_2$. For patients receiving a continuous flow of gas during ventilatory support, such as occurs when a bias flow is present, an isolation valve must be used to ensure that only the patient's exhaled gases are delivered to the system.

As was already stated, oxygen consumption and carbon dioxide production are calculated by comparing the fractional concentrations of oxygen and carbon dioxide of inspired and expired air. When the patient is breathing room air, however, it is reasonable to assume that the fractional concentration of inspired oxygen is 20.9%, and the fractional concentration of inspired carbon dioxide is 0.3%. For patients receiving enriched oxygen mixtures, the fractional concentration of inspired oxygen must be measured by the system. Fluctuations in F_IO_2 can be caused by air leaks in the patient-ventilator/metabolic monitor system and also by varying gas volumes and pressure demands, as occur during intermittent mandatory ventilation (IMV). Unstable air-oxygen blending systems within the ventilator circuit may also contribute to unstable F_IO_2s. Additionally, clinical studies have demonstrated that currently available systems cannot provide accurate and reproducible $\dot{V}O_2$ measurements for patients breathing F_IO_2s greater than 0.5. Box 7-10 contains a summary of conditions that should be observed when making indirect calorimetry measurements.

*The latter solution is expensive considering the amount of gas that would be used during the measurement.

BOX 7-10

Conditions for Obtaining Indirect Calorimetry Measurements

1. The patient should be at rest and in a supine position for at least 30 minutes before the measurement is made.
2. Room temperature should be from 20° to 25° C.
3. The patient should remain relaxed during the measurement (i.e., no voluntary physical activity).
4. Measurements should be recorded for 15 to 30 minutes, or until there is less than a 5% variation in $\dot{V}O_2$ and $\dot{V}CO_2$.

Metabolic Monitoring

The main advantage of using indirect calorimetry instead of prediction equations like those of Harris and Benedict is that indirect calorimetry can provide actual measurements of patient caloric needs. When combined with measurements of nitrogen excretion, indirect calorimetry can also provide information about substrate utilization, thus giving the clinician valuable insight into the types of substrates that are being used by the patient to generate energy.

Energy Expenditure

Energy expenditure is typically expressed in kilocalories per day (kcal/day) or relative to an individual's body surface area (kcal/hr/m^2). A normal, healthy adult uses from 1500 to 3000 kcal/day, or about 30 to 40 kcal/hr/m^2.[42]

Many factors can influence the metabolic rate, including the type and rate of food ingested, the time of day of the measurement, the patient activity level, and if the patient is recovering from infection, surgery, or trauma.

Prolonged starvation is associated with a decreased metabolic rate. Feeding raises metabolic rate through a mechanism called specific dynamic action. It is thought that specific dynamic action is related to the digestion and absorption of food.[42] Energy expenditure shows diurnal variation (i.e., it is usually higher in the morning than in the evening), which may be related to the variations in hormone levels that naturally occur daily.[42] It is well recognized that changes in activity can alter metabolic rate. Figure 7-35 shows how changes in physical activity can affect energy expenditure in a hospitalized patient. Note that sleep is associated with a reduction in metabolic rate, and even the slightest exertion is associated an increase in metabolic rate. Fever, as can occur with bacterial and viral infection, can also have a profound effect on metabolic rate. For example, an increase in body temperature of 1°F will cause a 10% increase in metabolic rate. Burns, long bone fractures, and surgery can increase the metabolic rate by as much as 200%.[37]

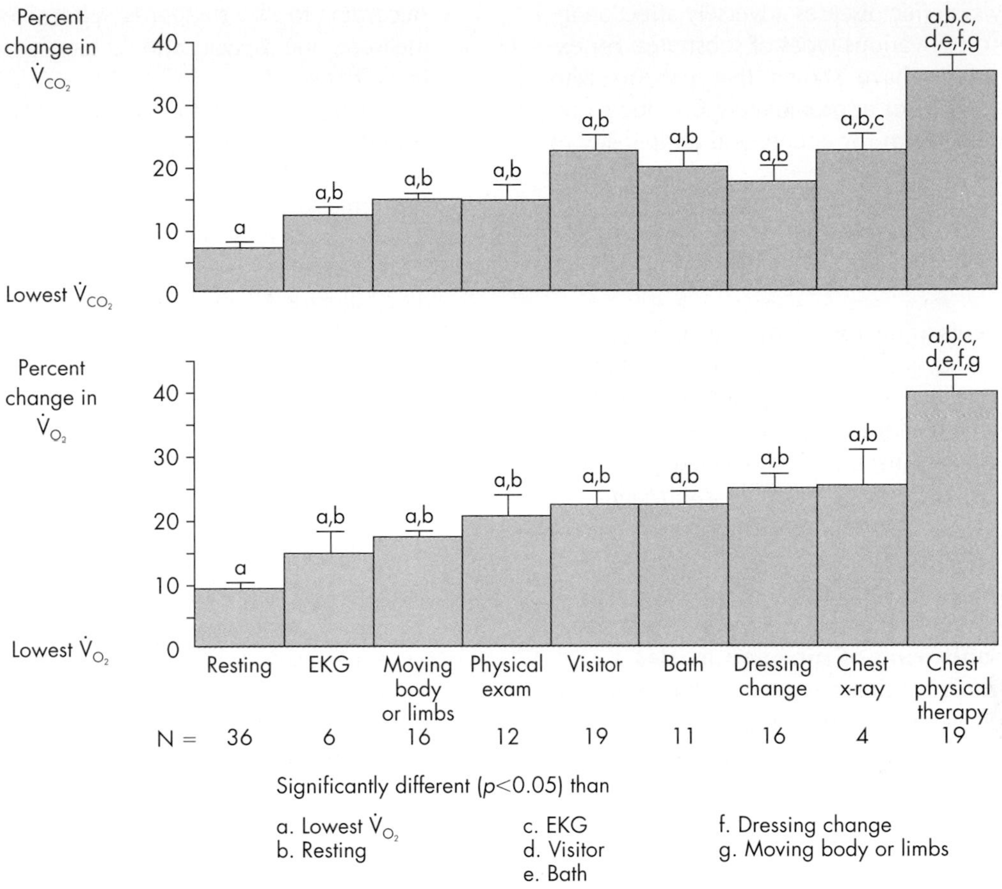

Figure 7-35 Variations in oxygen consumption and carbon dioxide production (expressed as percent change) associated with diagnostic and therapeutic interactions in an ICU patient. (From Weismann C, Kemper MC, and Damask M: The effects of routine interactions on metabolic rate, Chest 86(6):815, 1984.)

Substrate Utilization Patterns

The substrate utilization pattern is the proportion of carbohydrates, fats, and proteins that is contributing to the total energy metabolism. As was already stated, the percentage of the total energy that a substrate contributes can be determined using the respiratory quotient (RQ). Remember that the RQ is the ratio of $\dot{V}CO_2$ to $\dot{V}O_2$. The RQs for various foods are shown in Table 7-6. When pure fat is burned, the RQ is 0.7. The RQ for pure carbohydrate is 1.0, and the RQ for protein is approximately 0.8. RQs greater than 1.0 are associated with lipogenesis (fat synthesis) and hyperventilation. RQs less than 0.7 are associated with ketosis.

Healthy adults consuming a typical American diet derive 45% to 50% of their calories from carbohydrates, 35% to 40% from lipids, and 10% to 15% from proteins. The resultant RQ ranges from 0.80 to 0.85. Under normal conditions, proteins normally contribute only minor amounts to energy metabolism. Note that the percentage of protein used represents the normal turnover rate for replenishing structural and functional proteins in the body. Proteins may contribute significantly to EE, however, in cases of starvation. For this reason, a nonprotein RQ is usually reported to indicate the contribution to RQ made by carbohydrates and lipids.

TABLE 7-6

Variations in respiratory quotient

Substrate	RQ
Carbohydrates oxidation	1.0
Fats oxidation	0.7
Protein oxidation	0.8
Lipogenesis	>1.0

Substrate utilization is determined by the types of substrates ingested and the ability of an individual to use various types of foods. For example, eating a large amount of glucose raises the RQ to about 1.0, suggesting that carbohydrates are providing most of the energy expenditure. Prolonged starvation lowers the RQ to about 0.7, indicating that the individual is relying almost completely on fats for energy. Many systemic diseases adversely affect an individual's ability to use various types of substrates. For example, several studies have shown that patients with severe sepsis have RQs of approximately 0.7 due to reliance on lipid metabolism for energy and an inability to use carbohydrates.

Summary

Recent developments in microprocessor technology have significantly improved our ability to monitor the physiologic functions of patients with cardiopulmonary dysfunctions. Devices and techniques designed to assess respiratory system mechanics, inspired and exhaled gases, and metabolic function can provide valuable information for the clinician. Oxygen analyzers, capnographs, and indirect calorimeters are examples of devices that are routinely used by respiratory care practitioners in both the general and critical care settings. Chemiluminescence and **electrochemical monitoring of nitrogen oxides** are relatively newer techniques that are becoming common in the care of critically ill patients. Proper use of these devices requires an understanding of the operational theory of each, as well as how and when these devices can be used most effectively.

Review Questions

See Appendix A for answers.

1. Which of the following spirometers are classified as flow-sensing devices?
   I. Wright respirometers
   II. Hot wire anemometers
   III. Dry-rolling seal spirometers
   IV. Stead-Wells spirometers
      a. I and II only
      b. II and III only
      c. II and IV only
      d. I, II, and III only
2. Which of the following can influence the accuracy of spirometer measurements?
   I. The linearity and frequency response of the device
   II. The device's sensitivity to environmental condition
   III. Frequency of calibration
   IV. The presence of an obstructive or restrictive pulmonary disease
      a. I and II only
      b. II and III only
      c. I, II, and III only
      d. I, II, III, and IV
3. According to ATS standards, spirometers used to measure vital capacity should have an accuracy range (in BTPS) of:
   a. 5 liters ±10% of the reading, or 50 mL—whichever is greater
   b. 6 liters ±5% of the reading, or 50 mL—whichever is greater
   c. 7 liters ±3% of the reading, or 50 mL—whichever is greater
   d. 12 liters ±3% of the reading, or 50 mL—whichever is greater
4. The end of the nitrogen washout test is achieved when the:
   a. patient becomes fatigued
   b. exhaled nitrogen concentration is $<1.5\%$
   c. nitrogen percentage remains stable for 2 minutes
   d. exhaled volume equals the FRC
5. Which of the following can cause erroneous measurements with impedance pneumography?
   I. sinus tachycardia
   II. upper airway obstruction
   III. central apnea
   IV. tachypnea
      a. I only
      b. II only
      c. II and III only
      d. I, II, and III only
6. Which of the following lung volumes cannot be measured by simple spirometry?
   I. VC
   II. RV
   III. TLC
   IV. IC
      a. I and II only
      b. II and III only
      c. III and IV only
      d. I, III, and IV only
7. Maximum inspiratory pressures are normally:
   a. -20 to -40 cm H_2O
   b. -50 to -80 cm H_2O
   c. -60 to -100 cm H_2O
   d. -150 to -200 cm H_2O
8. The Beckman D2 oxygen analyzer is an example of a:
   a. paramagnetic oxygen analyzer
   b. polarographic oxygen analyzer
   c. galvanic oxygen analyzer
   d. electric (thermal conductivity) oxygen analyzer
9. Lack of a definitive Phase 3 on a capnogram is most often associated with:
   a. insufficient neuromuscular blockade
   b. cardiac oscillations

c. $\dot{V}/\dot{Q}$ imbalances, such as occur with patients with emphysema or chronic bronchitis
d. rebreathing exhaled gases

10. How many kilocalories of energy per day should a typical healthy adult ingest to maintain energy balance?
a. 500 to 1000
b. 900 to 1200
c. 1200 to 1800
d. 1500 to 3000

11. You notice that the FRC measured on a patient with COPD with the nitrogen washout technique is different than that measured with body plethysmography. In fact, the volume measured with the body box is ap proximately 500 mL greater than the FRC measured with nitrogen washout. Why might this difference exist?

12. Which of the following analyzers can be used to measure nitric oxide?
I. chemiluminescence analyzer
II. polarographic analyzer
III. electrochemical analyzer
IV. capnography
a. I only
b. II only
c. I and III only
d. I, II, and III only

13. A patient receiving mechanical ventilatory support via an ET is being monitored for oxygen consumption. Which of the following could lead to an erroneous measurement?
I. The patient appears agitated.
II. The measurement is performed immediately after the patient received a physical therapy treatment.
III. The FIO_2 is 0.8.
IV. The patient's ET cuff is inflated to seal the airway.
a. I and II only
b. II and III only
c. I, II, and III only
d. I, II, and III, and IV

14. The only source of nutrition administered to a patient is D5W (i.e., 5% dextrose in water). What would you expect to find when measuring RQ?
a. 0.7 to 0.75
b. 0.8 to 0.85
c. 0.9 to 0.95
d. 1.0

15. Which of the following patient conditions would you expect to be hypermetabolic (elevated $\dot{V}O_2$)?
a. starvation
b. fever
c. sedation
d. hypothermia

References

1. Wasserman K, et al: Principles of exercise testing and interpretation, Philadelphia, 1994, Lea & Febiger.
2. East TD: What makes noninvasive monitoring tick?: a review of basic engineering principles, Respir Care 35:500, 1990.
3. Snow M: Instrumentation. In Clausen JL, editor: Pulmonary function testing: guidelines and controversies, New York, 1882, Academic Press.
4. Fleisch A: Der pneumotachograph. Ein apparacat zur beischwindig-kertregstrier der ateniluft, Arch Ges Physiol 209:713, 1925.
5. Sullivan WJ, Peters GM, and Enright PL: Pneumotachography: theory and clinical application, Respir Care 29:736, 1984.
6. Kacmarek RM, Hess D, and Stoller JK: Monitoring in respiratory care, St Louis, 1993, Mosby.
7. American Thoracic Society: Snowbird workshop on standardization of spirometry, Am Rev Respir Dis 119:831, 1979.
8. American Thoracic Society: Standardization of spirometry, 1987 update, Am Rev Respir Dis 136:1285, 1987.
9. American Thoracic Society: Lung function testing: selection of reference values and interpretation, Am Rev Respir Dis 144:1202, 1991.
10. American Thoracic Society: Standardization of spirometry, 1994 update, Am Rev Respir Dis 152:1107, 1995.
11. American Association for Respiratory Care: Clinical practice guideline: spirometry, 1996 update, Respir Care 41:629, 1996.
12. American Association for Respiratory Care: Clinical practice guideline: assessing response to bronchodilator therapy at point of care, Respir Care 40:1300, 1995.
13. American Association for Respiratory Care: Clinical practice guideline: body plethysmography, Respir Care 39:1184, 1994.
14. Miller WF, Scacci R, and Gast LR: Laboratory evaluation of pulmonary function, Philadelphia, 1986, J.B. Lippincott.
15. American Association for Respiratory Care: Clinical practice guideline: static lung volumes, Respir Care 39:830, 1994.
16. Branson RD and Campbell RS: Impedance pneumography, apnea monitoring, and respiratory inductive plethysmography. In Kacmarek RM, Hess D, and Stoller JK, editors: Monitoring in respiratory care, St Louis, 1993, Mosby.
17. Southhall DP, et al: Undetected episodes of prolonged apnea and severe bradycardia in preterm infants, Pediatrics 72:541, 1983.
18. Wayburton D, Stork AR, and Taeusch HW: Apnea monitoring in infants with upper airway obstruction, Pediatrics 60:742, 1967.
19. Konno K and Mead J: Measurement of the separate changes of rib cage and abdomen during breathing, J Appl Physiol 22:407, 1967.
20. Krieger BP: Ventilatory pattern monitoring: instrumentation and application, Respir Care 35:697, 1990.
21. Marini JJ: Lung mechanics determination at the bedside: instrumentation and clinical application, Respir Care 35:669, 1990.
22. Osborne JJ and Wilson RM: Monitoring the mechanical properties of the lung. In Spence AA, editor: Respiratory monitoring in the intensive care, New York, 1980, Churchill-Livingstone.

23. Pauling L, Wood RE, and Sturdivant JH: Oxygen meter, J Am Chem Soc 68:795, 1946.
24. Bageant RA: Oxygen analyzers, Respir Care 21:410, 1976.
25. Etches PC, et al: Clinical monitoring of inhaled nitric oxide: comparison of chemiluminescence and electrochemical sensors, Biomed Instrum Technol 29:134, 1995.
26. Miller CC: Chemiluminescence analysis and nitrogen dioxide measurement, Lancet 34(3):300, 1994.
27. Body S, et al: Nitric oxide: Delivery, measurement, and clinical application, J Cardiothoracic Vasc Anesth 9:748, 1995.
28. Purtz E, Hess D, and Kacmarek R: Evaluation of electrochemical nitric oxide and nitrogen dioxide analyzers suitable for use during mechanical ventilation, J Clin Monit 13:25, 1997.
29. American Association for Respiratory Care: Clinical practice guideline: capnography, Respir Care 40:1321, 1995.
30. Stock MC: Capnography for adults, Critical Care Clinics 11:219, 1995.
31. Hess D: Capnometry and capnography: technical aspects, physiologic aspects, and clinical applications, Respir Care 35:557, 1990.
32. Kennel EM, Andrews RW, and Wollman H: Correction factors for nitrous oxide in the infrared analysis of carbon dioxide, Anesthesiology 39:441, 1973.
33. Gravenstein JS, Paulus DA, and Hayes TJ: Capnography in clinical practice, Boston, 1989, Butterworths.
34. Pilbeam SP: Mechanical ventilation, ed 3, St Louis, 1997, Mosby.
35. Davis PD, Parbrook GD, and Kenny GNC: Basic physics and measurement in anesthesia, 4 ed, Oxford, 1995, Butterworth-Heinemann.
36. Harris JA and Benedict F: Standard basal metabolism constants for physiologists and clinicians: a biometric study of basal metabolism in man, Philadelphia, 1919, J.B. Lippincott.
37. Kinney JM: The application of indirect calorimetry in clinical studies: assessment of energy metabolism in health and disease. In Kinney JM, editor: Report of the first Ross conference on medical research, Columbus, Ohio, 1980, Ross Laboratories.
38. Ferrannini E: The theoretical basis of indirect calorimetry: a review, Metabolism 37:287, 1987.
39. Weir JB: New method for calculating metabolic rate with special reference to protein metabolism, J Physiology 109:1, 1949.
40. Burszein P, et al: Utilization of protein, carbohydrate, and fat in fasting and postabsorptive subjects, Am J Clin Nutr 33:998, 1980.
41. Consolazio CJ, Johnson RE, and Pecora LJ: Physiological measurements of metabolic function in man, New York, 1963, McGraw-Hill.
42. Branson RD, Lacey J, and Berry S: Indirect calorimetry and nutritional monitoring. In Levine RL and Fromm RE, editors: Critical care conitoring, St Louis, 1995, Mosby.

Internet Resources

1. American Association for Respiratory Care:
   http://www.aarc.org
2. Critical Care Medicine:
   http://www.pitt.edu/~crippen/index.html
3. American Association of Cardiovascular and Pulmonary Rehabilitation:
   http://128.220.112.180/aacvpr/aacvpr.html
4. Canadian Journal of Respiratory Therapy:
   http://sam.serix.com/rrt/journal.htm
5. Virtual Hospital:
   http://indy.radiology.uiowa.edu/VirtualHospital.html
6. Gasnet, Global Anesthesiology Server Network:
   http://gasnet.med.yale.edu
7. Cyberspace Hospital:
   http://ch.nus.sg
8. SimBioSys Physiology Laboratory and Clinics:
   http://www.laketech.com
9. Medline Search Engine:
   http://www.healthgate.com/HealthGate/MEDLINE/search.shtml
10. National Library of Medicine:
    http://www.nlm.nih.gov

CHAPTER 8

CHAPTER OUTLINE

Blood Gas Analysis

J. M. Cairo

CHAPTER LEARNING OBJECTIVES

Upon completion of this chapter, the reader should be able to:

1. Describe how to perform and evaluate the modified Allen test.
2. Identify various sites used to obtain samples for blood gas analysis.
3. Label the components of a modern, in vitro blood gas analyzer.
4. Compare the operational principles of the pH, partial pressure of carbon dioxide (PCO_2), and partial pressure of oxygen (PO_2) electrodes.
5. Apply values for PO_2 at which 50% saturation of hemoglobin occurs (P_{50}), bicarbonate, buffer base, and base excess in the interpretation of ABGs.
6. Explain the operational principle of a standard Cardiac output (CO)-Oximeter.
7. Name the components of a quality assurance program for blood gas analysis.
8. Compare the effect of hyper- and hypothermia on ABGs.
9. Describe physiological and technical factors that can affect pulse oximeter readings.
10. Identify various factors that can influence transcutaneous PO_2 and PCO_2 measurements.
11. State criteria for identifying four types of acid-base disorders.

KEY TERMS

Absorbance Sensors
Acutal Bicarbonate
Allen Test
Amperometric
Base Excess/Deficit
Buffer Base
Capillary Blood Gas (CBG)
Central Processing Unit (CPU)
Clark Electrode
Clinical Laboratory Improvement Amendments of 1988 (CLIA-88)
Electrochemical Sensors
Electrodes
Fetal Hemoglobin (HbF)
Fluorescent Sensors
Fractional Hemoglobin Saturation
Functional Hemoglobin Saturation
Glucose Oxidase
Half-Cells
Henderson-Hasselbalch Equation
Hyperbilirubinemia
In Vitro
In Vivo
Invasive
Levy-Jennings Charts
Light-Emitting Diodes (LEDs)
Microcuvette
Nernst Equation
Noninvasive
One-Point Calibration
Optical Plethysmography
Optical Shunting
Oxygen Content (O_2ct)
$PaCO_2$
PaO_2
pH
Photoplethysmography
Potentiometric
Quality Assurance (QA)
Quality Control (QC)
Sanz Electrode
Servo-Controlled
Siggaard-Andersen Alignment Nomogram
Standard Bicarbonate
Sulfhemoglobin (HbS)
Superior Palpebral Conjunctiva
Temperature Correction
Three-Point Calibration
Total Hemoglobin (THb)
Two-Point Calibration

Measurements of arterial blood gases (ABGs) and pH are used extensively in the diagnosis and treatment of patients with acute and chronic illnesses. This is most evident in the management of critically ill patients, for whom ABG analysis can provide valuable information, such as acid-base status, ventilatory function, and oxygenation status.

Blood gas techniques are generally classified as either **invasive** or **noninvasive.** Invasive blood gas analysis, which involves the direct exposure of a sample of blood to a series of **electrochemical sensors** or **electrodes,** is considered the gold standard for measuring the pH, PCO_2, and PO_2 of arterial blood. Until recently, invasive blood gas analysis could only provide intermittent, **in vitro** measurements of a patient's blood gas and acid-base status; but the development of **fiberoptic** catheters has extended the possibilities of **in vivo** blood gas monitoring by allowing for real-time determinations of **pHa, $PaCO_2$,** and **PaO_2.**

Noninvasive techniques, which include pulse oximetry and transcutaneous monitoring, do not require blood samples and can be performed by sensors placed on the surface of the body. Both pulse oximetry and transcutaneous monitoring can provide continuous estimates of blood gases with minimal risk to the patient, so they are indispensable tools for managing patients with unstable ventilatory and oxygenation status. Appropriate use of noninvasive monitoring can significantly reduce the need for more expensive invasive blood gas analysis.

In this chapter, the various devices and techniques commonly used to determine ABGs and pH will be described. Some basic principles to ensure an understanding of how blood gas measurements can be used to assess a patient's acid-base and respiratory status will be presented. You should remember, however, that ABGs must be interpreted relative to other clinical indices, including laboratory tests (e.g., hematology and electrolytes), chest radiographs, patient history, and physical examination findings. Interpretation of blood gases without consideration of other clinical findings can lead to serious mistakes and, ultimately, patient harm.

INVASIVE BLOOD GAS ANALYSIS

Invasive blood gas analysis can be performed in a variety of settings, including hospitals, clinics, physician offices, and extended care facilities. The primary indications for invasive blood gas analysis are to quantify a patient's response to a diagnostic or therapeutic intervention and to monitor the severity and progression of a documented disease process.[1]

The American Association for Respiratory Care (AARC) has published a series of Clinical Practice Guidelines for ABG analysis to help ensure that these tests are performed in a safe and standardized manner.[1-3] Besides providing information on the equipment required to obtain blood samples, the guidelines also list the indications, contraindications, hazards, and complications of ABG analysis. Box 8-1 summarizes the Clinical Practice Guideline on sampling for ABG analysis. The AARC has also presented a Clinical Practice Guideline that relates to in vitro pH, blood gas analysis, and hemoximetry.[2]

Health care professionals performing blood gas analysis should understand patient assessment techniques, as well as the relationship of patient history, physical findings, and various cardiopulmonary dysfunctions. Therefore individuals involved in the performance of blood gas analysis should be formally trained in respiratory care, cardiovascular technology, clinical laboratory sciences, nursing, medicine, or osteopathy.[1,2] Periodic reevaluation of these individuals should focus on all aspects of blood gas analysis, including the proper technique for obtaining blood samples, postsampling care of the puncture site, and safe handling of blood, needles, and syringes.[1,2]

Collection Devices and Sampling Techniques

Specimens for ABG analysis can be drawn from a peripheral artery via a percutaneous needle puncture or from an indwelling intravascular cannula. Mixed venous blood samples can be obtained with a flow-directed (Swan-Ganz) intracardiac catheter. For percutaneous sampling, blood is most often drawn from the radial, brachial, or femoral arteries, or the dorsalis pedis artery of the foot.[3-5] Capillary blood samples from an earlobe or a side of the heel may be substituted when arterial blood cannot be obtained. As will be discussed later, **capillary blood gas (CBG)** values may vary considerably from ABG values.

In the case of percutaneous puncture of the radial artery, a modified **Allen test** should always be performed before obtaining the sample (Figure 8-1).[4,5] For the Allen test, patients clench their fist to force blood from their hand. While the fist is formed, pressure is applied to the radial and ulnar arteries. The patient is then instructed to release the fist, and the hand should appear blanched. When pressure on the ulnar artery is released, blood should return to the hand, causing the palm to blush and indicating that the ulnar artery is patent. If the palm does not blush, the ulnar artery is either absent or partially or totally occluded. Another sampling site, such as the brachial artery, should be chosen if the modified Allen test is negative. Note that a similar test can be performed when obtaining blood from the dorsal artery of the foot. The artery is occluded by applying pressure directly over it, and then pressure is applied to the nail of the big toe, causing it to blanch. When pressure on the big toe is released, color will return to the toe if there is sufficient collateral circulation from the posterior tibial and lateral plantar arteries.[6]

Once it has been determined that sufficient collateral circulation is present, the site should be prepared for puncture by being cleaned with 70% isopropyl alcohol or another suitable antiseptic solution.[7] In some cases, it may be necessary

BOX 8-1

Clinical Practice Guidelines

Sampling for ABG Analysis

Indications

1. Evaluation of a patient's acid-base, ventilation, or oxygenation status.
2. Quantification of a patient's response to therapeutic interventions and/or diagnostic evaluation.
3. Monitoring of the severity and progression of a documented disease process.

Contraindications

1. Negative results of a modified Allen test.
2. ABGs should not be performed through a lesion or distal to a surgical shunt, or if there is evidence of infection or peripheral vascular disease in the selected limb. If any of these conditions exists, another site should be selected.
3. Femoral punctures should not be performed outside of the hospital.
4. A coagulopathy or medium-to-high-dose anticoagulation therapy. (Streptokinase and tissue plasminogen activator may be a relative contraindication.)
5. An improperly functioning blood gas analyzer.
6. An analyzer that has not had its functional status validated by analysis of commercially prepared quality control products or tonometered whole blood.
7. A specimen containing visible air bubbles.
8. A specimen that has been kept at room temperature >5 minutes before analysis or has not been properlystored on ice-water slush for analysis in ≤ 2 hours, or has been stored on ice-water slush for >2 hours.

Hazards/Complications

1. Hematoma
2. Arteriospasm
3. Air or clotted-blood emboli
4. Anaphylaxis from local anesthetic
5. Hemorrhage
6. Trauma to the vessel
7. Arterial occlusion
8. Vasovagal response
9. Pain
10. Infection of the specimen handler from blood-borne pathogens
11. Inappropriate patient medical treatment based on erroneous ABG results

Limitations

1. Artery may be inaccessible.
2. Pulse may not be palpable.
3. Pain from the puncture may cause hyperventilation, which may be reflected in the ABG result.
4. Exercise ABGs should be drawn at peak exercise level or within 15 seconds or less from the termination of exercise.
5. Specimens from mechanically ventilated patients with minimal pathological pulmonary conditions can be drawn within 10 minutes of making changes in FiO_2; for spontaneously-breathing patients, 20 to 30 minutes should elapse after making FiO_2 changes before drawing a specimen for ABG analysis.
6. Specimens held at room temperature should be analyzed within 15 minutes of drawing; samples stored in an ice-water bath should be analyzed within an hour.

Validation

1. Sample must be drawn anaerobically, and all air bubbles must be immediately removed. Samples should be chilled and analyzed within 15 minutes.
2. Results should include documentation of the date and times of the test, along with the patient's body temperature, position, activity level, sample site, Allen test results, FiO_2, and mode of ventilatory support.
3. Appropriate sample size depends on the amount of anticoagulant used, the requirements of specific analyzers, and the need for other assays.

Assessment of Need

1. History and physical examination findings
2. Other abnormal diagnostic tests (e.g., pulse oximetry, chest radiograph)
3. Initiation, administration, discontinuation, or change in therapeutic modality
4. Projected surgical intervention for patients at risk
5. Projected enrollment in a pulmonary rehabilitation program

Infection Control

1. Universal precautions (standard precautions) published by the CDC should be taken.
2. Aseptic techniques should be employed whenever blood is sampled.
3. The site should be cleaned before a single puncture.
4. Blood specimens, contaminated needles, and syringes must be disposed into appropriate containers.

For a copy of the complete text, see AARC Clinical practice guideline: sampling for arterial blood gas analysis, Respir Care 37:913, 1992 and AARC Clinical practice guideline: in vitro pH and blood gas analysis and hemoximetry, Respir Care 38:501, 1993.

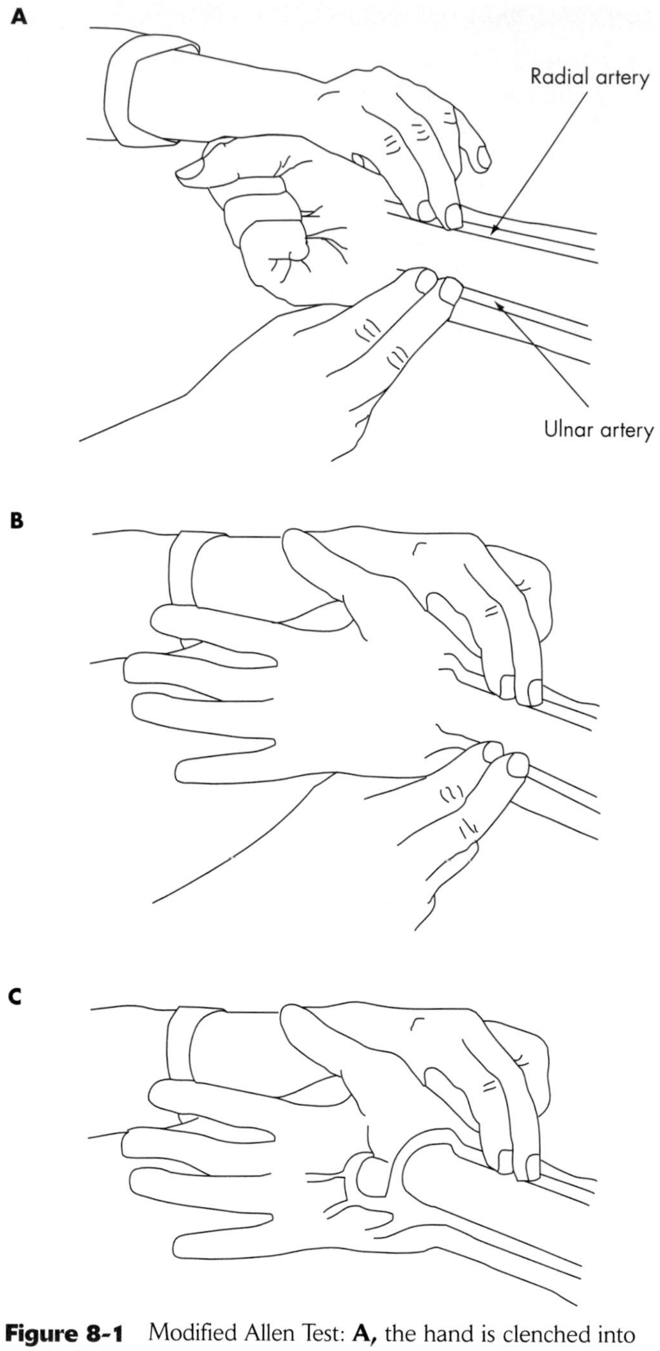

Figure 8-1 Modified Allen Test: **A,** the hand is clenched into a tight fist and pressure is applied to the radial and ulnar arteries; **B,** the hand is opened (but not fully extended), and the palm and fingers are blanched; **C,** pressure on the ulnar artery is removed, which should result in flushing of the entire hand. (From Shapiro BA, Peruzzi WT, and Templin R: Clinical application of blood gases, St Louis, 1994, Mosby.)

to anesthetize the puncture site by injecting a local anesthetic such as 1% lidocaine HCl.[1,4,5] Proper administration of the anesthetic can alleviate some of the pain associated with the procedure and reduce some patient anxiety.

Samples to be analyzed should be obtained with a small-gauge needle (23 to 25 gauge) attached to a glass or plastic syringe of low diffusibility containing an anticoagulant (sodium or lithium heparin, 1000 units/mL) (Figure 8-2).[1,2] For infants, 25- to 26-gauge scalp vein needles can be used to collect arterial samples. The blood should be drawn anaerobically to prevent contamination by room air. Room air that is inadvertently drawn into the syringe should be removed before analysis because contamination with room air can lead to erroneous results and ultimately compromise patient care. Box 8-2 gives an example of this type of problem in the clinical setting.

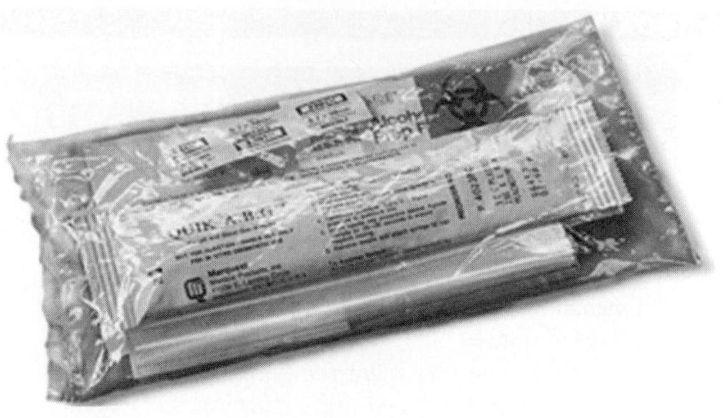

Figure 8-2 A commercially available blood gas kit. (Courtesy Marquest Medical Products, Vital Signs, Newark, NJ.)

After blood is withdrawn and the needle removed, direct pressure should be applied to the puncture site to prevent formation of a hematoma. For adult patients with indwelling cannulas, 1 to 2 mL of blood should be removed and discarded before blood is removed for analysis. For infants, the discarded volume is typically only about 0.2 to 0.5 mL.* After removing the blood sample to be analyzed, the cannula should be flushed with several milliliters of normal saline to prevent blood coagulation within the cannula and avoid loss of a functioning indwelling line.

As mentioned earlier, CBG samples obtained from an earlobe or the side of the heel may be substituted for arterial blood samples in certain situations.[8] CBGs are most often used in pediatrics, especially in the neonatal intensive care unit, to avoid multiple arterial sticks.[9-11] The site should be warmed before the sample is obtained in order to increase perfusion to the area (i.e., "arterializing"). "Arterialized" capillary samples actually contain a combination of arterial and venous blood and may therefore not be equivalent to an arterial blood sample.[11,12] The correlation between capillary and arterial pH and PCO_2 measurements is better than the correlation of capillary and arterial PO_2 measurements. Consequently, CBGs are used more often to discern acid-base status rather than to assess a patient's oxygenation status. Table 8-1 contains accepted normal ABG and CBG values, and Box 8-3 shows how CBGs can be used in clinical decision making.

Personnel responsible for performing blood gas analysis should understand that they are dealing with a poten-

*Remember that the volume of blood removed and discarded should be minimal; this is particularly important in neonates.

BOX 8-2

Decision Making & Problem Solving

How would a large air bubble affect the PCO_2 and PO_2 of an arterial blood sample taken from a normal person breathing room air?

See Appendix A for the answer.

BOX 8-3

Decision Making & Problem Solving

A CBG sample is obtained from a 2-day old infant in apparent respiratory distress. The results indicate respiratory alkalosis (high pH, low PCO_2) and apparent hypoxemia (low PO_2). How would you interpret these findings?

See Appendix A for the answer.

TABLE 8-1

Normal blood values*

pH	7.40 ± 0.05
$PaCO_2$	40 ± 5 mm Hg
PaO_2	80-100 mm Hg
HCO_3^-	24 ± 2 mEq/L
Base excess	± 2 mEq/L
O_2Hb	95%-100%
COHb	<1.5%
MetHb	<1.5%
THb	12-18 gm/dL
NA^+	140 ± 5 mWq/L
K^+	4 ± 0.5 mEq/L
CL−	101 ± 4 mEq/L
Ca^{++}	5 ± 0.5 mEq/L
Glucose	70-105 mg/dL
P_{50}	27 ± 2 mm Hg

*Values are expressed for a healthy adult..

tial **biohazard** and take appropriate precautions when performing these tests.[13,14] Such precautions include wearing gloves, protective eyewear (goggles), and other barriers deemed necessary for preventing exposure. Needles used for blood sampling should be recapped with the one-hand, "scoop" technique, or they can be removed after being inserted into a cork or similar device to shield the sharp end. Unused blood samples, needles, and other "sharps" should be discarded in appropriately marked containers. (See Chapter 13 for a full discussion of infection control principles in respiratory care.)

Specimens should be transported to the blood gas laboratory and analyzed as soon as possible after drawing because blood cells remain metabolically active in vitro, so a prolonged time delay (>5 minutes) between obtaining and analyzing a specimen can lead to erroneous results (i.e, a reduction in PO_2 and a rise in PCO_2). This problem is particularly evident for patients with high leukocyte counts.[4,5] Chilling the specimen to <5° C by placing the syringe in ice water can reduce the metabolic rate of the white blood cells, thus minimizing this problematic effect.

MODERN IN VITRO BLOOD GAS ANALYZERS

Modern in vitro blood gas analyzers (Figure 8-3) contain three electrodes for determining the pH, PCO_2, PO_2 of a blood sample. They also contain a **central processing unit (CPU)** for data management and outputs for displaying measured and derived variables. Many of these systems may also contain sensors for providing hemoglobin, oxyhemoglobin, carboxyhemoglobin, and methemoglobin measurements, along with serum electrolyte and blood glucose measurements. Table 8-2 lists the normal values for derived variables that are commonly recorded during blood gas analysis. Unlike early blood gas analyzers, which were cumbersome to operate and required large quantities of blood to make accurate measurements, modern analyzers are fully automated, self-calibrating devices that can analyze blood samples as small as 50 to 100 μL.

pH and Hydrogen Ion Concentration

S.P.L. Sorenson introduced the term ***pH*** as a shorthand way to express the hydrogen ion activity of solutions.[15,16] It is defined as the negative logarithm (base 10) of the hydrogen ion concentration, or

$$pH = -\log_{10}[H^+].$$

For example, a hydrogen ion concentration of 0.0000007 mol/L, or 1×10^{-7} mol/L, can be expressed as a pH of 7.0. Although there has been an increased scientific effort to express hydrogen ion concentrations in Système International (SI) units (i.e., nanomoles per liter [nmol/L]), the concept of pH is still recognized as a convenient and useful way of discussing a patient's clinical acid-base status.[16,17] Table 8-3 shows the relationship between hydrogen ion concentration and pH. Note that pH decreases as hydrogen ion concentration increases and increases as hydrogen ion concentration decreases. Despite the fact that hydrogen ion activity is not exactly equal to hydrogen ion concentration, these two terms are interchangable for practical purposes in clinical situations.

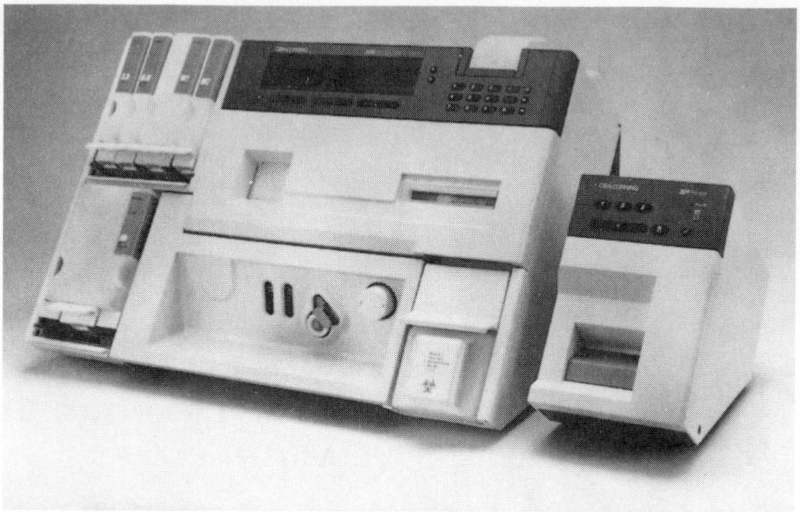

Figure 8-3 A modern in vitro blood gas analyzer. (Courtesy Corning Instruments, Chiron Diagnostics, Norwood, Mass.)

TABLE 8-2

Normal values for derived blood gases

Parameter	Symbol	Normal values	
Oxyhemoglobin	O_2Hb	≥95%	
Carboxyhemoglobin	COHb	<1.5%	
Methemoglobin	MetHb	<1.5%	
Deoxygenated hemoglobin	HHb	<2.0%	
Sulfhemoglobin	SulfHb	<1.0%	
Total hemoglobin	THb	Males:	15.8 ± 2.3 gm/dL
		Females:	14.0 ± 2.0 gm/dL
Partial pressure of oxygen at 50% Saturation	P_{50}	27.0 ± 2.0 mm Hg	

TABLE 8-3

Hydrogen ion–pH relationships

pH	$[H^+]$*	pH	$[H^+]$*
7.80	16	7.20	63
7.70	20	7.10	80
7.60	26	7.00	100
7.50	32	6.90	125
7.40	40	6.80	160
7.30	50		

*Reported in nanomols per liter.

In general chemistry textbooks, the pH scale is described as ranging from 1 to 14, with a pH of 7.0 representing universal neutrality. (Neutrality is defined as the pH of pure water, which contains 1×10^{-7} mol/L of hydrogen ions and 1×10^{-7} mol/L of hydroxyl ions.) A solution with a pH less than 7.0 is acidic, and a solution with a pH higher than 7.0 is alkaline. Although the pH of arterial blood can vary from 6.90 to 7.80, it normally ranges (±2 SD) from 7.35 to 7.45, with a mean pH of 7.40. For interpretative purposes, a blood pH less than 7.4 is considered acidic, and a blood pH higher than 7.4 is alkaline.

pH Electrode

The standard pH electrode, which is sometimes called the **Sanz electrode,** is composed of two **half-cells** that are connected by a potassium chloride (KCl) bridge (Figure 8-4).[18] One of the cells, which is the measurement half-cell, has a special glass membrane permeable to hydrogen ions (H^+); the measuring electrode is made of silver-silver chloride (Ag/AgCl) and immersed in a phosphate buffer solution with a pH of 6.840. The second cell, which is called the reference half-cell, is composed of mercury-mercurous chloride (Hg/HgO_2) (calomel) and is immersed in a solution of saturated KCl.

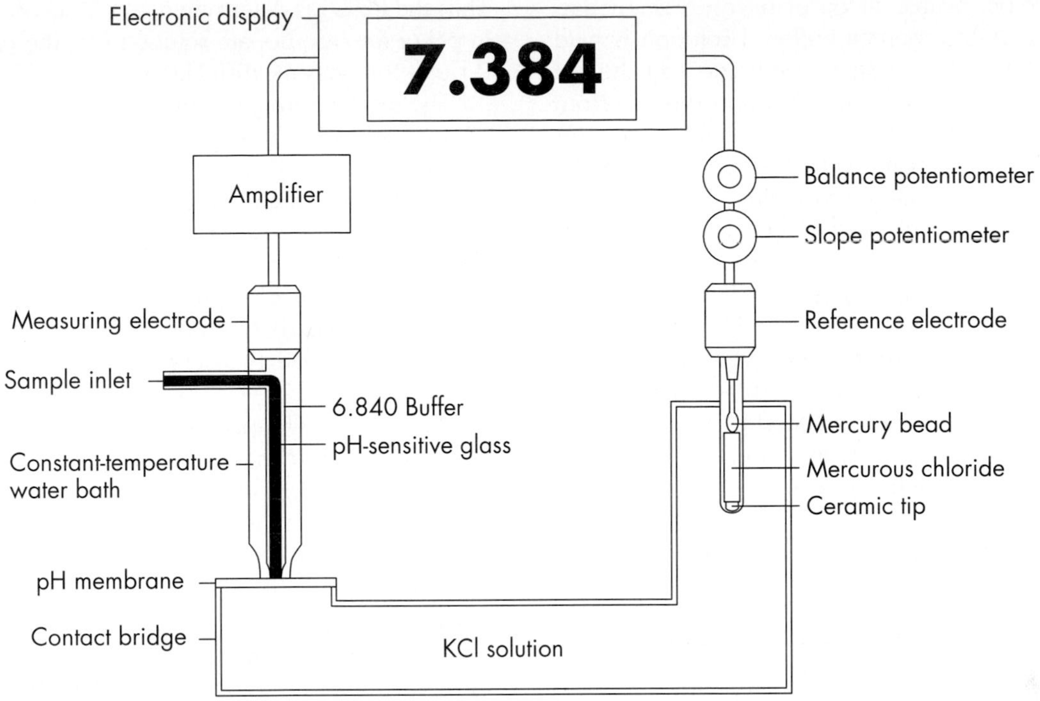

Figure 8-4 A schematic of the pH electrode. (From Shapiro, et al: Clinical application of blood gases, ed 4, St Louis, 1989, Mosby.)

According to the **Nernst equation,** the electrical potential generated as H^+ ions pass through the glass membrane (EH^+) is a logarithmic function of the ratio of hydrogen ion concentration across the membrane, or

$$EH^+ = (RT/F) \times \ln [(H^+{}_o)/(H^+{}_i)],$$

where R is the gas constant, F is Faraday's constant, T is the absolute temperature in Kelvin, $H^+{}_o$ is the hydrogen ion concentration outside the membrane, and $H^+{}_i$ is the hydrogen ion concentration inside the membrane. If you consider that at body temperature (37° C, or 310 K) the quantity (RT/F) is 61.5 mV, then the equation becomes,

$$EH^+ = 0.0615 \times \log_{10} [H^+], \text{ or}$$
$$EH^+ = 0.0615 \times \text{pH}.$$

Thus a voltage of 61.5 mV will be developed for every pH unit difference between the sample and the measuring electrode, which is constant (6.840). Consider the following example. A voltage difference of 30.75 mV is measured when a sample is analyzed. This voltage difference equals 0.500 pH units (30.750 ÷ 61.500 = 0.500). The resultant pH can be calculated as 6.840 + 0.500 = 7.34.

It should be apparent that these devices are quite sensitive, and therefore are adversely affected by changes in the permeability of the glass membrane as can occur when the electrode is damaged or coated with protein. As will be discussed later in this chapter, maintaining an effective **quality assurance** program can prevent these types of problems.

Partial Pressures of Carbon Dioxide (PCO_2) and Oxygen (PO_2)

In Chapter 1, it was stated that the partial pressure that a gas exerts in a gas mixture is calculated by multiplying the fractional concentration of the gas by the total pressure of the gas mixture. For example, if oxygen makes up about 21% of the atmosphere, and the barometric pressure is 760 mm Hg, then the partial pressure of oxygen in room air is approximately 159 mm Hg (0.21 × 760 mm Hg).

The **partial pressure of carbon dioxide in arterial blood ($PaCO_2$),** which is primarily regulated by the respiratory system, can vary from 10 to 100 mm Hg. Subjects breathing room air at sea level typically have a $PaCO_2$ in the range of 35 to 45 mm Hg (the mean is 40 mm Hg; the range represents ±2 SD). The **partial pressure of oxygen in arterial blood (PaO_2)** can range from 30 mm Hg to 600 mm Hg, depending on the fractional concentration of inspired oxygen. For healthy people breathing room air at sea level, the PaO_2 is usually from 80 to 100 mm Hg.

PCO_2 Electrode. The PCO_2 electrode was first described by Stowe in 1957, but later refined by Severinghaus and associates,[18] so the standard PCO_2 electrode is commonly called the **Stowe-Severinghaus electrode** (Figure 8-5). It is basically a pH electrode covered with a carbon dioxide-permeable Teflon or silicon elastic (Silastic) membrane. A bicarbonate buffered solution is held between the Teflon (or Silastic) membrane and the pH glass electrode by a nylon spacer. Carbon dioxide from the blood diffuses across the semipermeable Teflon (or Silastic) membrane and reacts with the water to form carbonic acid, which dissociates into hydrogen ions and bicarbonate. The reaction can be written as:

$$CO_2 + H_2O \rightarrow H_2CO_3 \rightarrow H^+ + HCO_3^-$$

H^+ ions from the bicarbonate buffered solution then diffuse across the glass electrode, and the pH of the solution is measured as described earlier. The pH is related to the PCO_2 by using the following modification of the **Henderson-Hasselbalch equation,**

$$pH = pK + \log(HCO_3^- \div PCO_2)$$

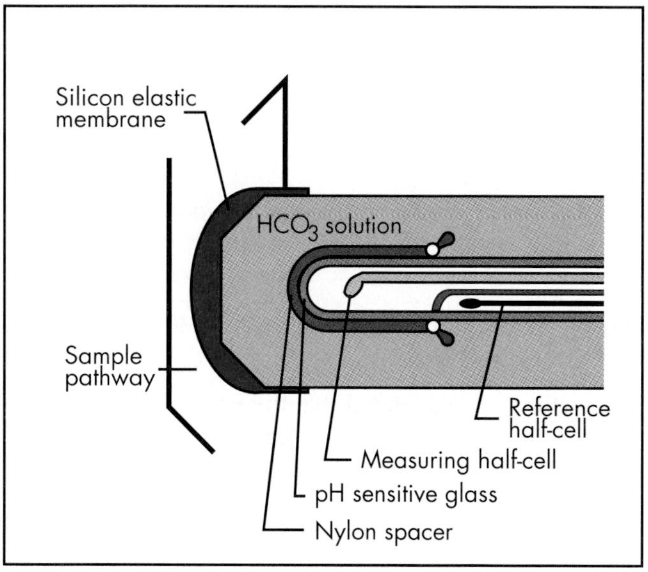

Figure 8-5 A Stowe-Severinghaus PCO_2 electrode. (Redrawn from Shapiro BA, Peruzzi WT, and Templin R: Clinical application of blood gases, ed 5, St Louis, 1994, Mosby.)

Thus the PCO_2 is determined as a function of the change in pH of the bicarbonate solution (i.e., the pH changes by 0.1 unit for every 10 mm Hg increase in PCO_2).

The most common problems encountered with PCO_2 electrodes involve interference with the diffusion of CO_2 across the Teflon (Silastic) membrane and the H^+ ions across the glass membrane (e.g., worn or cracked electrodes, protein deposits, etc.). If the bicarbonate solution dehydrates between the Teflon (Silastic) membrane and the pH glass electrode, erroneous data can result. As with the pH electrode, these problems can be minimized by using an effective quality assurance program.

PO_2 Electrode. The partial pressure of oxygen in blood is most commonly measured using the **Clark electrode.**[18] As Figure 8-6 shows, the Clark electrode consists of a negatively charged platinum electrode (cathode) and a positively charged Ag/AgCl reference electrode (anode) immersed in a phosphate/potassium chloride buffer, the pH of which can range from 7.0 to 10, depending on the manufacturer. The cathode and anode are connected together by a KCl bridge. An external voltage is applied to the platinum electrode, creating a small potential difference of about −0.5 to −0.6 mV between it and the anode.* The active surface of the electrode is separated from the blood to be analyzed by a polyethylene or polypropylene membrane that is permeable to oxygen.

Figure 8-7 illustrates the principle of PO_2 measurement. Oxygen from the blood sample diffuses across the semipermeable plastic membrane into the KCl solution and reacts with the platinum cathode, altering the conductivity of the electrolyte solution. Specifically, the platinum cathode donates electrons, which reduce oxygen to produce hydroxyl ions,

$$O_2 + 2H_2O + 4e^- \rightarrow 4OH^-$$

*Because an external polarizing voltage is applied to create this potential difference, the Clark electrode is called a polarographic electrode.

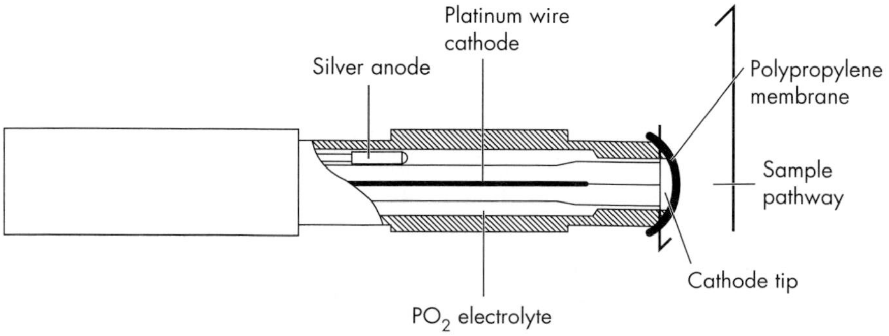

Figure 8-6 A Clark PO_2 electrode. (Redrawn from Shapiro BA, Peruzzi WT, and Templin R: Clinical application of blood gases, ed 5, St Louis, 1994, Mosby.)

The electrons donated by the cathode are derived from oxidation of Ag at the anode,

$$4Ag \rightarrow 4Ag^{+} + 4e^{-}$$
$$Ag^{+} + Cl^{-} \rightarrow AgCl$$

The volume of oxygen reduced at the cathode is directly proportional to the number of electrons used in the reaction. Therefore the amount of oxygen diffusing across the membrane into the electrolyte solution can be determined by measuring the current change that occurs between the anode and the cathode when the electrode is exposed to a blood sample containing oxygen. Because PO_2 is determined by measuring current changes that occur as oxygen is reduced, this technique is an example of an **amperometric** measurement; determinations of pH and PCO_2 as described above are examples of **potentiometric** measurements (i.e., they are based on voltage changes).

The electrical output of the Clark electrode, and thus its sensitivity for measuring PO_2, can be altered by several factors, including protein buildup, cracked electrodes, and loss of electrolyte. When analyzing blood samples, the consumption of oxygen by the electrode leads to an underestimation of the partial pressure of oxygen in a blood sample by 2% to 6%. This phenomenon, which has been called the **blood gas factor,** is due to the slow rate of oxygen diffusion in fluids (i.e., oxygen consumed by the electrode is not replaced by oxygen from the blood).[19] The magnitude of the blood gas factor depends on the diameter of the cathode and the thickness of the membrane between the sample and the cathode. Exposure of the PO_2 electrode to nitrous oxide and halothane (gaseous anesthetic agents) may also alter its electronic output by increasing the production of peroxide ions.[17]

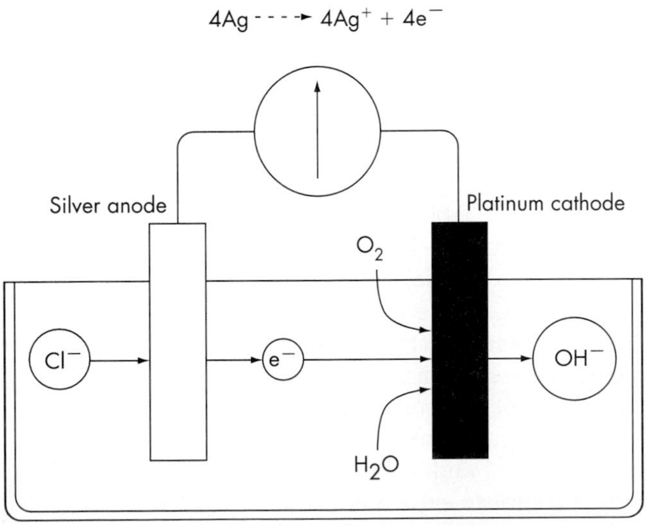

Figure 8-7 Principles of PO_2 measurements; see text for discussion. (From Shapiro BA, Peruzzi WT, and Templin R: Clinical application of blood gases, ed 5, St Louis, 1994, Mosby.)

Derived Variables

Several variables can be calculated from the measurements of pH, $PaCO_2$, and PaO_2. Oxygen saturation of hemoglobin, P_{50}, bicarbonate, **buffer base,** and **base excess/deficit** are examples of derived variables. Although most modern blood gas analyzers have computer software that automatically calculates these variables, they can also be determined using formulae or nomograms that incorporate accepted constants. Note, however, that these derived variables are calculated and not measured. As such, they may be inaccurate when compared with actual measurements because they may not necessarily account for all confounding factors. For example, calculations of oxygen saturation of hemoglobin do not account for the presence of **dyshemoglobins,** such as carboxyhemoglobin and methemoglobin.

Oxygen Saturation of Hemoglobin (SO_2)

The percentage of available hemoglobin that is saturated with oxygen can be calculated by using an equation empirically derived from the oxyhemoglobin saturation curve. These calculations do not account for all of the variables (e.g., the actual $PaCO_2$ or the presence of dyshemoglobins) that can affect this value, and therefore can lead to erroneous conclusions about the level of oxyhemoglobin saturation. Direct measurement of oxyhemoglobin saturation will be discussed along with oximetry later in this chapter. Directly measured values are more reliable and should be used instead of a derived oxygen saturation value when making decisions about a patient's oxygenation status. Notice that although both calculated and measured SO_2 are identical in many cases, this is not always true.

P_{50} Determinations

$\mathbf{P_{50}}$ is a convenient way of describing hemoglobin affinity for oxygen because it identifies the PO_2 in mm Hg when hemoglobin is 50% saturated with oxygen. It is determined by equilibrating a blood sample with various oxygen concentrations at 37° C, which can be accomplished with a tonometer connected to a series of certified gas mixtures.* As Figure 8-8 illustrates, alterations in hemoglobin affinity for oxygen are associated with shifting of the oxyhemoglobin dissociation curve. It is well established that the affinity of hemoglobin A (HbA, or normal adult hemoglobin) for oxygen, and thus the P_{50}, can be altered by changes in the pH, PCO_2, temperature, and 2,3 diphosphoglycerate concentration of arterial blood. The presence of **fetal hemoglobin (HbF)** and carboxyhemoglobin (COHb) can also alter the oxyhemoglobin curve. P_{50} determinations are not

*The P_{50} measurements are standardized for a pH of 7.40, $PaCO_2$ of 40 mm Hg, and a temperature of 37° C.[18,19]

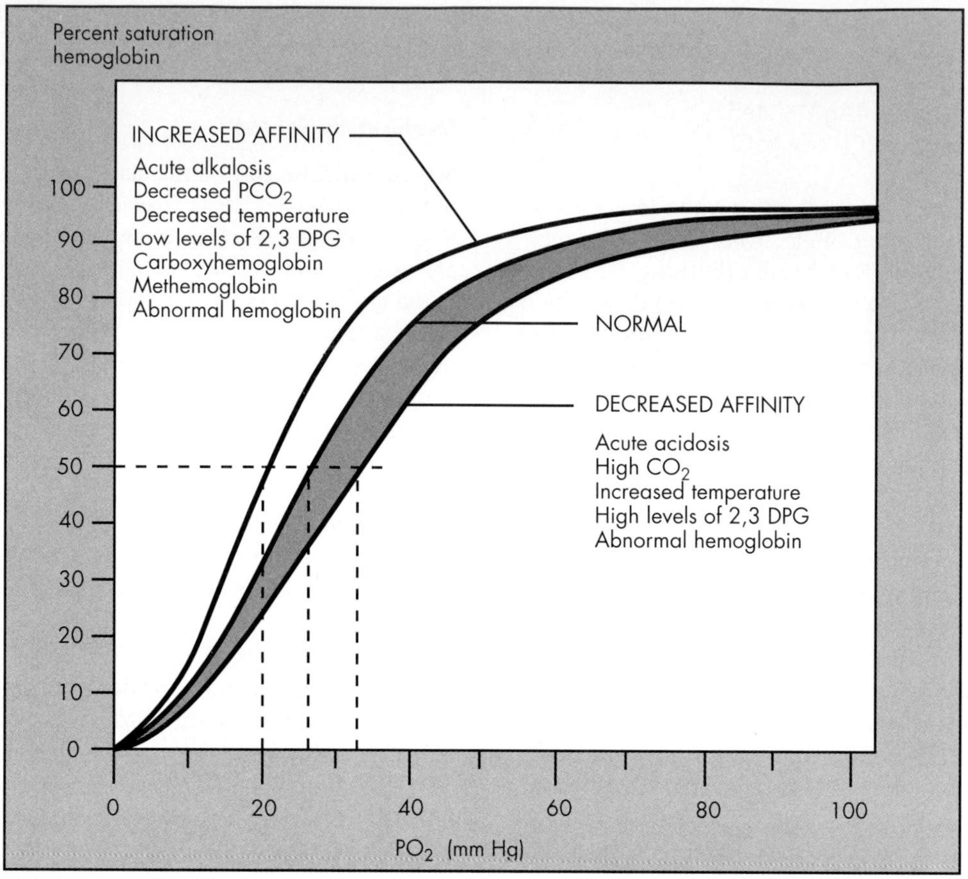

Figure 8-8 Effects of changes in pH, PCO_2, and 2,3 DPG on the oxyhemoglobin dissociation curve. (Redrawn from Lane EE and Walker JF: Clinical arterial blood gas analysis, St. Louis, Mosby, 1987.)

routinely performed, but they can be helpful in diagnosing and managing hypoxemia associated with various types of **hemoglobinopathies.**

Bicarbonate, Buffer Base, and Base Excess

The **actual bicarbonate** is the concentration of HCO_3^- in the plasma of anaerobically drawn blood.[16] It is derived from measurements of pH and $PaCO_2$ using the Henderson-Hasselbalch equation. (Note that the **standard bicarbonate** is also derived from the Henderson-Hasselbalch equation, but it represents the bicarbonate concentration in a fully oxygenated plasma sample measured at a temperature of 37° C and a $PaCO_2$ of 40 mm Hg.) Plasma bicarbonate levels are normally from 22 to 26 mmol/L. The HCO_3^- becomes elevated in metabolic alkalosis and chronic respiratory acidosis and reduced in metabolic acidosis and chronic respiratory alkalosis.

The buffer base represents the sum of all the anion buffers in blood, including bicarbonate, hemoglobin, inorganic phosphate, and negatively charged proteins.[18] The buffer base usually ranges from 44 to 48 mmol/L. The base excess/deficit is the number of millimoles of strong acid required to titrate a blood sample to a pH of 7.4 at a PCO_2 of 40 mm Hg. Theoretically, the buffer base and the base excess are not affected by changes in respiratory function, so they can be used to identify non-respiratory disturbances in acid-base status. Figure 8-9 is a **Siggaard-Andersen alignment nomogram** for calculating actual and standard bicarbonate, buffer base, and base excess concentrations.

Whole Blood Analysis: Electrolytes and Glucose

Many blood gas analyzers incorporate sensors for measuring electrolytes (e.g., Na^+, K^+, Cl^-, Ca^{++}) and metabolites (e.g., glucose). Table 8-4 contains the normal values for plasma electrolytes. The sensors used for electrolyte measurements are ion-selective electrodes, but those used to measure glucose are coated with an enzyme called **glucose oxidase.** Electrolytes are determined by potentiometric measurements, but metabolites are determined by amperometric measurements.

The typical electrolyte sensor is composed of a measuring half-cell and an external reference half-cell, which form a complete electrochemical cell. The measuring half-cell is made of a silver/silver chloride wire that is surrounded by an electrolyte-specific solution. For example, the electrolyte solution used in the sodium and chloride sensors contains a fixed concentration of sodium and chloride; the potassium sensor electrolyte contains a fixed con-

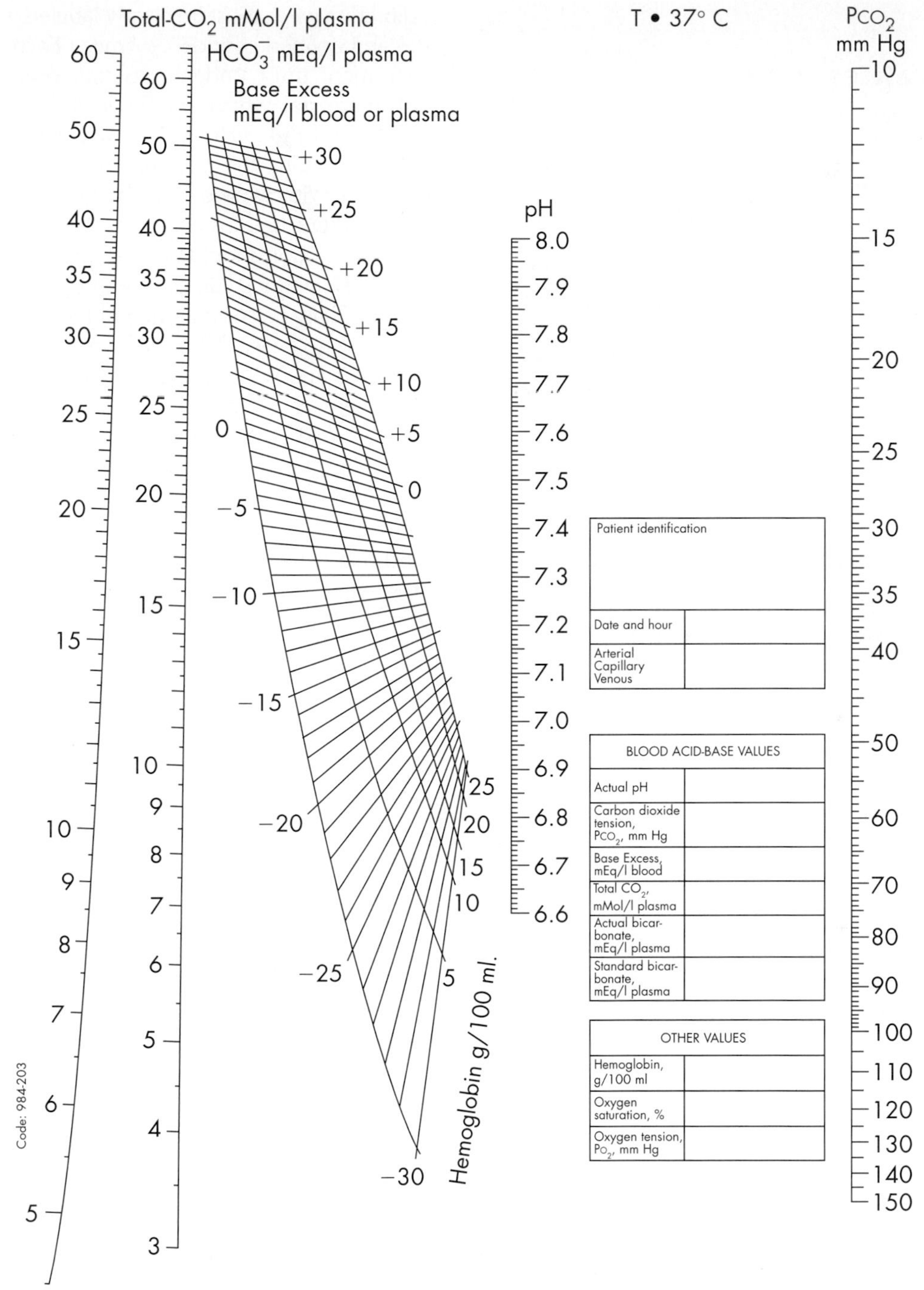

Figure 8-9 Siggaard-Anderson alignment nomogram: a line is drawn between pH and PCO_2, and actual bicarbonate is read directly at the intersection of this line. BE_b is hemoglobin dependent and can be read at the intersection of the constructed line and the patient's Hb value. Standard bicarbonate can be determined by constructing another line through the BE-Hb point and the PCO of 40 mm Hg, and by reading the HCO_3^- scale. Buffer base can be computed from the equation $BB = 41.7 + (0.42 \times Hb) + BE$. BE_{ECF} is calculated similarly to the BE_b, but the BE_{ECF} is read off at the intersection of the constructed line and one-third of the patient's Hb value. (Modified from Siggaard-Andersen O and Radiometer A/S: Arterial blood gas analizers. In Burton G, Hodgkin JE, and Ward JJ: Respiratory care: a guide to clinical practice, ed 4, Philadelphia, 1997, Lippincott.)

centration of potassium; and the calcium electrolyte contains a fixed concentration of calcium. The electrolyte solution is separated from the sample solution by an ion-selective membrane, and as the sample comes in contact with the membrane, a transmembrane potential develops across the membrane due to the exchange of ions across it. The potential developed across the membrane is compared with the constant potential of the external reference sensor, and the magnitude of the potential difference is proportional to the ion activity of the sample.

TABLE 8-4

Normal values for plasma electrolytes

Parameter	Symbol	Normal values
Sodium	Na^+	136-145 mEq/L
Potassium	K^+	3.5-5.0 mEq/L
Total Calcium	Ca^{++}	9.9-11.0 mEq/L
Magnesium	Mg^{++}	1.5-2.5 mEq/L
Chloride	$C1^-$	98-106 mEq/L
Glucose*	—	100 ± 20 mg/dL

*Although glucose is not classified as an electrolyte, it is included in this table for reference because many blood gas analyzers can now provide determinations of serum glucose concentrations.

A glucose type of sensor consists of four electrodes:

1. The measuring electrode, which is made of platinum and glucose oxidase, is enclosed in a binder.
2. A second reference electrode, which is composed of silver/silver chloride.
3. A "counter" electrode, which is composed of platinum, ensures that a constant polarizing voltage is applied to the sensor.
4. A second "counter" electrode, which does not contain the enzyme glucose oxidase, is used to quantify interfering substances in the sample.

As the sample contacts the measuring electrode, glucose oxidase on the surface of the electrode converts the glucose in the sample to hydrogen peroxide and gluconic acid. The polarizing voltage applied to the electrode causes the hydrogen peroxide to oxidize, resulting in the loss of electrons. The loss of electrons causes current flow to be directly proportional to the glucose concentration of the sample.

Quality Assurance of Blood Gas Analyzers

The Joint Commission on Accreditation of Healthcare Organizations (JCAHO), the Health Care Financing Administration (HCFA), and The College of American Pathologists (CAP) have published standards that clinical blood gas laboratories must follow to ensure the accuracy and reliability of blood gas measurements. These standards, which are based on recommendations from the **Clinical Laboratory Improvement Amendments of 1988 (CLIA-88),** require routine calibrations of instruments, as well as programs for assessing **quality control (QC)** and **quality assurance (QA).**[20,21]

Calibration standards for most blood gas analyzers are buffers for pH electrodes and specially prepared gases for the PCO_2 and PO_2 electrodes.[22] (Note that buffers and calibration gases must be clearly labeled with reference values and defined confidence limits.) Each day of use, every instrument must undergo routine **one-** and **two-point calibrations,** which should include high and low pH, PCO_2, and PO_2 values. The **one-point calibration** involves adjusting the electronic output to a single, known standard. With two-point calibrations, the electrode's electronic output is adjusted to two known standards. A one-point calibration should be performed before an unknown sample is analyzed, unless the analyzer is programmed to automatically perform a one-point calibration at regular intervals (e.g., every 20 to 30 minutes). **Two-point calibrations** are usually performed at least 3 times daily, usually every 8 hours. In many cases, analyzers can be programmed to perform a two-point calibration at predetermined intervals. A **three-point calibration** should be performed every 6 months, or whenever an electrode is replaced. Three-point calibrations involve adding a third standard that is intermediate to the other standards to ensure linearity of the electrode response.

The National Institute of Standards and Technology (NIST) and the International Federation of Clinical Chemistry (IFCC) have established standards for the calibration of blood gas electrodes. A nearly normal pH buffer (pH ~ 7.384) is used for one-point calibrations; a second, lower pH buffer (pH ~ 6.840) is analyzed in the two-point calibration to ensure that the electronic output of the electrode is linear over a wide range of pHs. The PCO_2 electrode is calibrated with two gas concentrations: a 5% CO_2 mixture for establishing the lower end of CO_2s encountered, and a 10% CO_2 mixture for the high end of the range. The 5% mixture is used for one-point calibrations, but both mixtures are used in the two-point calibration to establish a linear slope for the electrode's electronic output. The PO_2 electrode is also calibrated with two gas mixtures: usually a gas mixture with 0% O_2 and another with 12% or 20% O_2.[18] The accuracy of oxygen electrodes may vary by as much as 20% for high PO_2s because of the lack of linearity between electronic output and oxygen tensions above 150 mm Hg. It has been suggested that the latter problem can be minimized by using additional calibration gases with higher concentrations of oxygen (i.e., >20% O_2).

Quality control may be defined as a system that includes analyzing control samples (with known pH, PCO_2, and PO_2), assessing the measurements against defined limits, identifying problems, and specifying corrective actions. Internal quality control can be accomplished by periodically analyzing commercial products with known pH, PCO_2, and PO_2 values. Quality control materials include human or bovine whole blood samples that have been tonometered to exact gas tensions or commercially prepared aqueous buffers and perfluorocarbon emulsions that have been equilibrated with a series of known PCO_2 and PO_2 values by the manufacturer. Although **tonometry** remains the gold standard method for quality control of

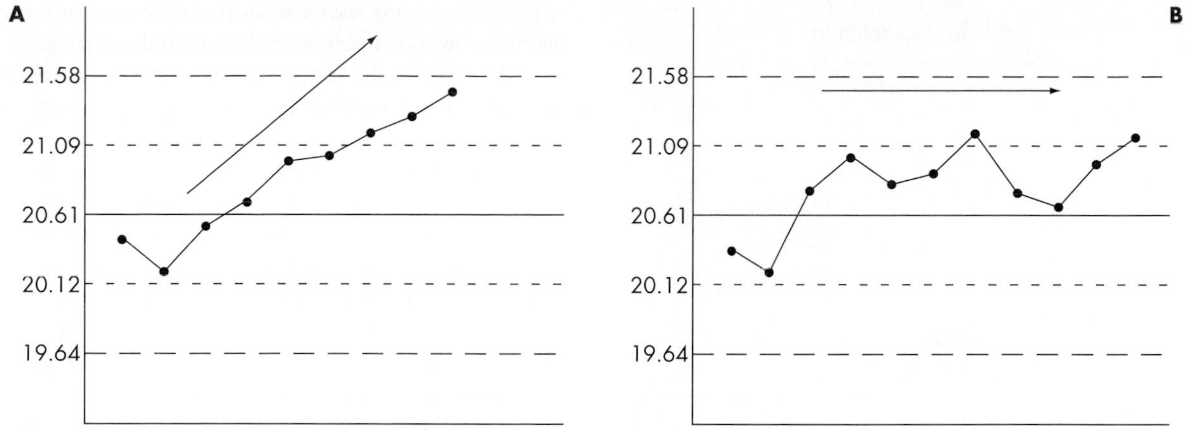

Figure 8-10 Levy-Jennings charts demonstrating two types of trend (**A**) and shift (**B**).

PCO_2 and PO_2 electrodes, most laboratories use commercially prepared quality control systems for biosafety and convenience. It should be mentioned, however, that commercially prepared controls provide information on the instrument's precision—not the accuracy of the data. (Remember that *precision* refers to the reproducibility of repeat measurements, and *accuracy* relates to how close the measurement is to the correct value.) Additionally, commercial controls are susceptible to variations in room storage temperature and do not reflect temperature and protein errors in blood gas analyzers.[18]

Regardless of the type of quality control material used to assess an instrument's performance, results should be recorded in a manner that allows the operator to detect changes in the operation of the blood gas analyzer. The most common method of recording quality control data involves the use of **Levy-Jennings charts** (Figure 8-10). These charts allow the operator to detect trends and shifts in electrode performance, thus helping to avoid problems associated with reporting inaccurate data due to analyzer malfunction. For example, a trend **(A)** is typically associated with protein buildup on an electrode membrane or an electrode nearing the end of its life expectancy. A shift **(B)** can be due to a tear in the electrode membrane or loss of the electrolyte that bathes the electrode.

Quality assurance involves testing the proficiency of both personnel and equipment, providing a dynamic process of identification, evaluation, and resolution of problems that affect blood gas measurements.[22] CAP and the American Thoracic Society (ATS) currently offer two proficiency testing programs that provide a means of assessing blind samples (periodically) and the technical competence of laboratory personnel, and a means of reporting the variability of individual blood gas analyzers.

Proficiency testing materials usually include a series of unknown samples with **target values** that have been established by previously identified reference laboratories. At regular intervals throughout the year (usually three times per year), all participating laboratories analyze unknown samples (typically three to five samples are used) and forward their results to the sponsoring organization collating the results from all laboratories. The criteria for acceptable results are defined, and the laboratory personnel are notified of their laboratory's performance. (Generally, an acceptable pH is within ± 0.04 of the target value; PCO_2 values must be ± 3 mm Hg or $\pm 8\%$ of the target value, whichever is greater; and PO_2 values must be within ± 3 standard deviations.)[18,19] An unsatisfactory performance, which is a failure to achieve any of the target values at a single event, necessitates that remedial action is taken and documented. Unsuccessful performance, which is a failure to achieve the target values for an analyte in two consecutive events or in two out of three consecutive events, can result in sanctions placed on the laboratory.[18-20] These sanctions can lose revenue for the laboratory because of suspension of Medicare and Medicaid reimbursement. The laboratory can only be reinstated by additional staff training, increased quality control procedures, and reapplication with evidence that the problems have been corrected.

Temperature Correction of Blood Gases

With most modern blood gas analyzers, the blood sample is heated and maintained at a constant temperature of 37° C during analysis. The term ***temperature correction*** refers to the application of mathematical formulae to adjust blood gas tensions to more accurately reflect the patient's core temperature (i.e., the temperature in the artery from which the blood sample was obtained). There is considerable debate as to whether it is necessary or even desirable to make these temperature corrections. Those favoring temperature corrections for blood gas analysis point out that corrected results are a true reflection of the oxygenation and acid-base status of an individual. According to Mohler and associates,[23] the PaO_2 changes approximately 7% for each degree Celsius; the $PaCO_2$ changes about 4% per degree Celsius; and the pH changes by 0.0146 per degree Celsius. Proponents of reporting blood gases at 37° C believe that pH and

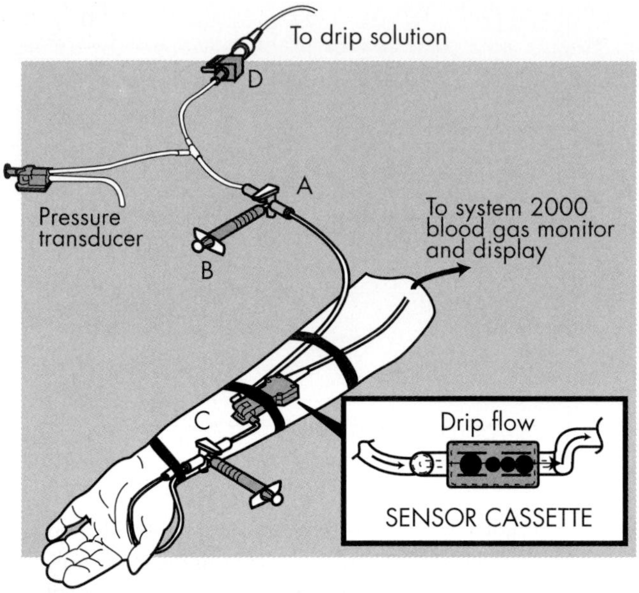

Figure 8-11 A fiberoptic blood-gas monitor. (Redrawn from Shapiro BA, et al: Clinical performance of a blood gas monitor: a prospective, multicenter trial, Crit Care Med 21:487, 1993. Used by permission.)

$PaCO_2$ values standardized to a body temperature of 37° C reliably reflect the in vivo acid-base status of the patient and that correction of pH and $PaCO_2$ do not affect the calculated HCO_3^-.[18] Furthermore, most acid-base nomograms are calculated for 37° C, and considerable errors occur if temperature-corrected blood gas data are used with these nomograms. Although all commercial blood gas analyzers contain solid-state circuitry that can easily perform temperature corrections, most laboratories still report blood gases at 37° C due to the lack of consensus on the topic.

In Vivo Blood Gas Monitors

As already mentioned, recent advances in fiberoptics technology have made it possible to obtain continuous, in-vivo ABG and pH measurements. A typical in vivo blood gas monitor contains one or more optical sensors that are imbedded in a gas or ion-permeable polymer matrix. The sensors are connected to a central processing unit via a fiberoptic cable. The fiberoptic sensor is inserted into the intravascular space through an indwelling 20-gauge cannula. Light of a specific wavelength and intensity from the central processing unit is transmitted along the fiber to a **microcuvette** containing a fluorescent dye. The incident light striking the microcuvette is modified in proportion to the PO_2, PCO_2, or pH levels of the blood, which is in contact with the microcuvette. The modified light is then transmitted back to the monitor, through either the same optical path or a second fiber parallel to the fiber carrying the incident light.[24] Figure 8-11 shows an alternative extra-arterial blood gas monitor. In this case, the blood gas sensor is located in series with the arterial catheter.

Optical blood gas sensors are generally categorized by how they modify the initial optical signal; they are classified as either **absorbance** or **fluorescent sensors.**[18] For **absorbance sensors,** when light of a known wavelength and intensity is transmitted down the fiber and through the microcuvette, a fraction of the incident light is absorbed, and the remaining light is transmitted. The concentration of the **analyte** can be determined by measuring the intensity of the light striking the photodetector because the amount of light transmitted is proportional to the concentration of the analyte in question (i.e., the pH, PCO_2, or PO_2).

Fluorescent sensors use dyes that fluoresce when they are struck by light in the ultraviolet or nearly ultraviolet visible range. Light from the monitor is transmitted to the microcuvette containing the dye. The dye absorbs the light energy of the optical excitation signal and emits a fluorescent signal that is returned to the monitor along the fiberoptic cable. The concentration of the analyte in question can be measured by determining the ratio of fluorescent light emitted to the original excitation light signal. The pH, PCO_2, or PO_2 of arterial blood can be determined by using sensing fibers containing dye systems that are analyte-specific (i.e., most commercially available systems contain three analyte-specific sensing fibers).

Fluorescent sensors currently in use can measure pH values from 6.8 to 7.8, PCO_2 values from 10 to 100 mmHg, and PO_2 values from 20 to 600 mm Hg. When compared with in vitro blood gas analysis, intraarterial blood gas monitoring systems are comparable for pH, however, the correlation may not be as good for PCO_2 and PO_2 measurements.[24]

Calibration of Intraarterial Blood Gas Monitors

Intraarterial blood gas monitoring systems must be calibrated before being inserted into a patient by immersing the sensor in a buffer containing known pH, PCO_2, and PO_2 values. In vivo calibrations are complicated and subject to error because adjustment must be made using single-point measurements from laboratory (in vitro) ABG analysis.

In many cases, temperature corrections may be required because the sensor may be in a peripheral artery where the measured temperature may not equal the patient's core temperature. Temperature corrections are usually accomplished by combining a temperature measuring thermocouple with the analyte-specific sensor. By measuring the sensor's temperature, the pH or blood gas value may then be displayed as measured, or corrected to 37° C (or some other user-entered patient temperature).

Point-of-Care (POC) Testing

These are lightweight, portable devices (total weight is approximately 1 lb) that allow in vitro ABG and pH measurements in the emergency room, intensive care unit (ICU), physician's office, or in a transport vehicle.[25] Figure 8-12

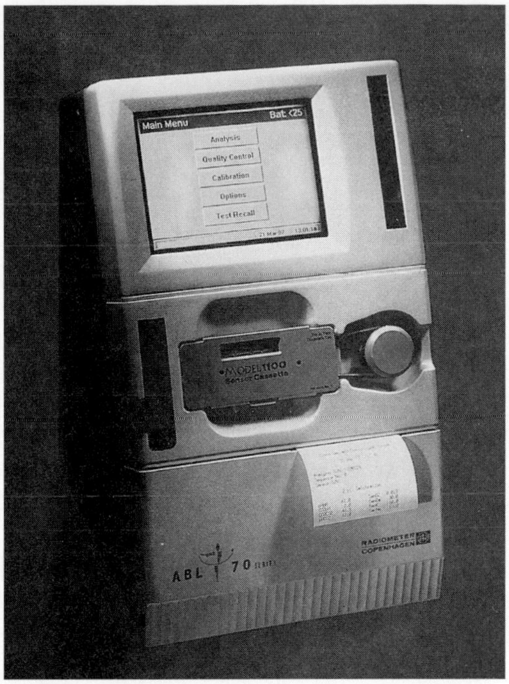

Figure 8-12 A point of care blood gas analyzer. (Courtesy Radiometer America, Cleveland.)

shows a typical POC blood gas analyzer. POC devices are usually battery-powered but can be powered by a standard AC electrical outlet. The system uses solid-state sensors, which rely on either fluorescence technology or thin-film electrodes that have been fabricated onto silicon chips. The microelectrodes are incorporated into a single-use disposable cartridge that also contains calibration reagents, a sampling stylus, and a waste container. In addition to the standard blood gas cartridges, several cartridge configurations are also available for the analysis of electrolytes (e.g., sodium, potassium, and chloride), blood urea nitrogen (BUN), glucose, and hematocrit. Results are shown on a liquid crystal display.

Measurements can be made on blood samples less than a milliliter in volume in 60 to 120 seconds. Manufacturers of POC devices state that these devices are accurate over a wide range of pH, $PaCO_2$, and PaO_2 values. For example, iSTAT states that their device has a range of 6.8 to 8.0 for pH, 10 to 100 torr for $PaCO_2$, and 5 torr to 800 torr for PaO_2. Although the use of these devices is limited, there is much potential for this technology, especially as a replacement for "stat" laboratory services. Table 8-5 compares four commercial POC blood gas analyzers currently available.[25]

CO-OXIMETRY

An **oximeter** is a device that can measure the **oxyhemoglobin** saturation of arterial, venous, mixed venous, or intracardiac blood. Two types of oximeters are routinely used in respiratory care: **CO-oximeters** and **pulse oximeters.** A CO-oximeter can provide simultaneous in vitro measurements of various hemoglobin gases, including oxyhemoglobin (HbO_2), **carboxyhemobin (HbCO), methemoglobin (HbMet), Sulfhemoglobin (HbS),** and **fetal hemoglobin** using whole blood samples. Pulse oximeters are noninvasive devices that can only provide measurements of arterial oxyhemoglobin saturation. Pulse oximeters will be discussed in detail in the section on noninvasive assessment of ABGs.

Oximeters operate on the principle of **spectrophotometry,** which is based on the relative transmission and/or absorption of portions of the light spectrum.[26] The various forms of hemoglobin mentioned earlier can be identified because each form has its own absorption spectrum. (Figure 8-13 illustrates the light spectra for each hemoglobin.) The concentration of a certain hemoglobin type can be determined using the **Lambert-Beer law,** which states that the transmission of a specific wavelength of light through a solution is a logarithmic function of the concentration of the absorbing species in the solution.[18,27]

Figure 8-13 illustrates the principle of operation of a typical CO-oximeter. A blood sample is heated to 37° C and hemolyzed (either chemically or by high frequency vibrations), creating a translucent solution. The solution is placed in a cuvette, which is positioned between a light source and a condenser and two **photodetectors.** A series of monochromatic light beams are simultaneously directed through the cuvette containing the sample of blood and through a blank solution (containing no hemoglobin).[18] The condenser lense system focuses the light passing through the sample cuvette onto a photodetector, which generates an electric current that is proportional to the intensity of the transmitted light and inversely proportional to the amount of light absorbed by the sample. The light passing through the blank solution is simultaneously focused onto a reference photodetector, which generates an electric current proportional to the light transmitted through the blank solution. The absorbance of the blank solution is then subtracted from the absorbances of the blood sample, and the resultant values are used to calculate the concentration of each type of hemoglobin in the blood sample. The normal concentrations of the various hemoglobin types are shown in Table 8-1.

Although blood can contain six different types of hemoglobin, most commercially available CO-oximeters provide measurements of only four types: oxyhemoglobin (HbO_2), deoxyhemoglobin (Hb), methemoglobin (HbMet), and carboxyhemoglobin (HbCO). Sulfhemoglobin and fetal hemoglobin are not usually determined by CO-oximetry, although Radiometer has introduced a CO-oximetry procedure to determine fetal hemoglobin. Although these results are different from reference methods such as radioimmunoassay and chromatographic procedures, CO-oximeter analysis of fetal hemoglobin has been clinically

TABLE 8-5

Comparison of four point-of-care blood gas analyzers

Analyzer	StatPal II	Gem 6	Gem Stat	Gem Premier
Measured values	pH PCO_2 PO_2	pH PCO_2 PO_2 Hct Ca^{++} K^+	pH PCO_2 PO_2 Hct Ca^{++} K^+ Na^+	pH PCO_2 PO_2 Hct Ca^{++} K^+ Na^+
Calculated values	6	5	4	4
Sample volume	0.2 mL	2 mL	0.5 mL	0.2 mL
Analysis time	60 sec	130 sec	109 sec	92 sec
Samples/module	25	50 in 72 hr	50 in 72 hr	150 or 300 in 7 d
Interface	—	RS 232	RS 232	RS 232
Data management	—	hard copy of module in use	hard copy of module in use	hard copy or floppy disk storage of module in use
Price $	5000	21,500 auto sampler adapter: 3,500	25,000	35,000
Module $	75 cal syr: 75/25	335	350	150 300 600 900 bg only: 525 750 lytes only: 450 600

PCO_2, Partial pressure of carbon dioxide; *PO_2*, partial pressure of oxygen; *Hct*, hematocrit; *Ca*, calcium; *K*, potassium; *cal syr*, calibrant syringe; *bg*, blood gases; *lytes*, electrolytes.

StatPal II (PPG Industries, Inc.), Gem 6, Gem Stat, and Gem Premier (Mallinckrodt Sensor Systems).

From Levine RL and Fromm Jr. RE: Critical care monitoring: from pre-hospital to the ICU, St Louis, 1995, Mosby.

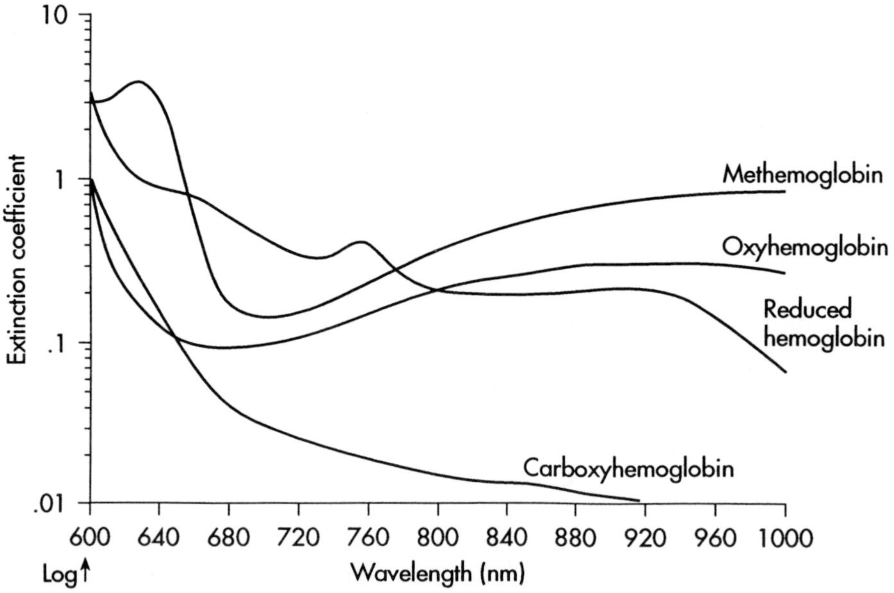

Figure 8-13 Absorption spectra for various species of hemoglobin. (From Pilbeam S: Mechanical ventilation: physiological and clinical applications, ed 3, St Louis, 1998, Mosby.)

BOX 8-4

Decision Making & Problem Solving

Assessment of a patient admitted to the emergency department after exposure to an enclosed fire included evaluation of SpO_2 and ABGs. Results were obtained while the patient was breathing room air: SpO_2 = 98%, pH = 7.38, $PaCO_2$ = 35 mm Hg, PaO_2 = 95 mm Hg, and SaO_2 = 97%. What is your interpretation of these findings?

See Appendix A for the answer.

acceptable. Other reported values may include **total hemoglobin (THb)** and **oxygen content (O_2ct).**

A number of factors can interfere with CO-oximetry measurements. Incompletely hemolyzed red blood cells or lipids or air bubbles in the sample can scatter some of the incident light, thus producing erroneous measurements.[28,29] The presence of bilirubin (>20 mg/dL of whole blood), as well as intravenous dyes (particularly methylene blue and indocyanine green) can also alter measurements because they absorb near-infrared and infrared light. Absorbance of light by these substances lowers the actual oxyhemoglobin measured. The presence of fetal hemoglobin can also lead to false HbCO readings. Oxygenated fetal hemoglobin produces a 4% to 7% false carboxyhemoglobin level; reduced fetal hemoglobin yields a 0.2% to 1.5% false carboxyhemoglobin level.[18]

Calibration of CO-Oximeters

CO-oximeters should be routinely calibrated with solutions supplied by the manufacturer. These solutions are typically dye-based propylene glycol solutions that only allow for the calibration of total hemoglobin. Determination of the various forms of hemoglobin is accomplished by relating the relative absorbances recorded at the wavelengths tested. That is, the percentage of a particular hemoglobin type reported is derived from absorbance ratios at predetermined wavelengths.

NONINVASIVE ASSESSMENT OF ABGS

Noninvasive blood gas monitoring has become a standard practice in respiratory care and anesthesiology. The importance of these devices in the management of patients with cardiopulmonary dysfunctions cannot be overstated. In just 30 years, pulse oximeters and transcutaneous pH, PCO_2, and PO_2 monitors have gone from expensive, bulky units to compact, affordable devices that can provide both continuous and intermittent pH, PCO_2, and PO_2 measurements that are reliable and accurate.

Pulse Oximetry

Pulse oximetry provides continuous, noninvasive measurements of arterial oxygen saturation and pulse rate via a sensor placed over a digit, an earlobe, or the bridge of the nose that measures the absorption of selected wavelengths of light beamed through the tissue. Advances in microprocessor technology, coupled with improvements in the quality of **light-emitting diodes (LED)** and photoelectric sensors have greatly improved the accuracy and reliability of these devices. Pulse oximetry is now considered by most clinicians as an indispensable tool for monitoring the oxygenation status of patients at risk of hypoxemia.

Theory of Operation

Pulse oximetry is based on the principles of spectrophotometry and **photoplethysmography.**[30-32] Like CO-oximeters, pulse oximeters use spectrophotometry to determine the amount of hemoglobin (and deoxyhemoglobin) in a blood sample. Oxyhemoglobin and deoxygenated hemoglobin are differentiated by shining two wavelengths of light (660 and 940 nm) through the sampling site. As Figure 8-13 shows, at a wavelength of 660 nm (red light), deoxygenated hemoglobin absorbs more light than oxyhemoglobin. Conversely, oxyhemoglobin absorbs more light at 940 nm (infrared light [IR]) than deoxygenated hemoglobin.

Photoplethysmography, or **optical plethysmography,** estimates heart rate by measuring cyclic changes in light transmission through the sampling site during each cardiac cycle. That is, as the blood volume in the finger, toe, or ear lobe increases during ventricular systole, light absorption increases and transmitted light decreases. Conversely, as blood volume decreases during diastole, absorbency decreases and transmitted light increases. The pulsatile and non-pulsatile components of a typical pulse oximetry signal are shown in Figure 8-14.

The percentage of oxyhemoglobin in a sample can be determined by first calculating the ratio of absorbencies for pulsatile and non-pulsatile flow at the two specified wavelengths, or

$$\text{Red/Infrared} = \frac{\text{Pulsatile}_{660\text{ nm}} / \text{Non-pulsatile}_{660\text{ nm}}}{\text{Pulsatile}_{940\text{ nm}} / \text{Non-pulsatile}_{940\text{ nm}}}$$

This ratio is then applied to an algorithm that relates the ratios of these two absorbencies to oxyhemoglobin saturation.[32]

As mentioned earlier, four types of hemoglobin can be measured by oximetry: reduced or deoxygenated hemoglobin (HHb), oxyhemoglobin (O_2Hb), carboxyhemoglobin (COHb), and methemoglobin (MetHb). Two terms that are often used when describing oxyhemoglobin saturation determinations are **fractional** and **functional** saturations. **Fractional hemoglobin saturation** is calculated by

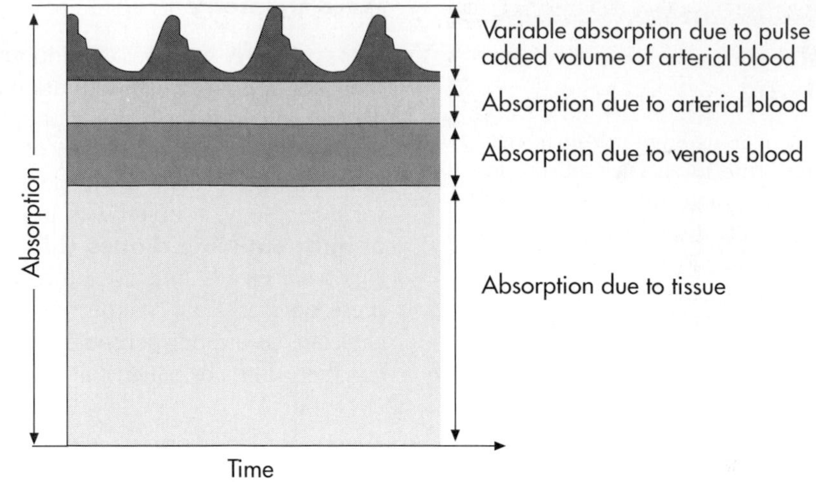

Figure 8-14 Pulsatile and nonpulsatile components of a typical pulse oximetry signal. (From McGough EK and Boysen PG: Benefits and limits of pulse oximetry in the ICU, J Crit Ill 4(2):23, 1989.)

dividing the amount of oxyhemoglobin by the amount of all four types of hemoglobin present, or

$$\text{Fractional } O_2Hb = O_2Hb \div [HHb + O_2Hb + COHb + MetHb]$$

Functional hemoglobin saturation is calculated by dividing the oxyhemoglobin concentration by the concentration of hemoglobin capable of carrying oxygen. It may be written as,

$$\text{Functional } O_2Hb = O_2Hb \div [HHb + O_2Hb]$$

Although laboratory CO-oximeters measure all four types of hemoglobin by using a series of wavelengths of light to identify each species, pulse oximeters use only two wavelengths to quantify the amount of O_2Hb and HHb present. Thus laboratory CO-oximeters can report fractional oxyhemoglobin saturation, and pulse oximeters can estimate functional oxyhemoglobin saturation.

Physiological and Technical Considerations

It is important to recognize that both physiological and technical factors can influence the accuracy of pulse oximetry measurements. A brief discussion of how each factor can affect pulse oximeter accuracy follows.[33]

Low Perfusion States. The accuracy of a pulse oximeter reading depends on the identification of an arterial pulse, therefore many conditions can interfere with proper pulse oximeter function. Hypovolemia, peripheral vasoconstriction from drugs or hypothermia, and heart-lung bypass (i.e., extracorporeal membrane oxygenation [ECMO]) are associated with a diminished pulsatile signal resulting in either an intermittent or absent SpO_2 reading.[30] Some oximeters compensate for the weak signal associated with low perfusion states by increasing the signal output. The problem with this approach is that augmenting the signal also causes an increase in the signal-to-noise ratio, which can result in high levels of background noise that can contribute to erroneous results. A simpler approach is to reposition the oximeter sensor in an area of higher perfusion. For example, placement of the oximeter probe on the ear instead of the finger may alleviate some of the problems associated with reductions in peripheral perfusion.

Dysfunctional Hemoglobins. It is well established that high levels of dysfunctional hemoglobins (i.e., carboxyhemoglobin [COHb] and methemoglobin [MetHb]) can adversely affect oxyhemoglobin measurements by pulse oximeter.[30] High carboxyhemoglobin (COHb) levels can alter SpO_2 measurements because O_2Hb and COHb have similar absorption coefficients for red light (660 nm), but COHb is relatively transparent to infrared light (940 nm). Accordingly, significant levels of HbCO, as occur in carbon monoxide poisoning, lead to an overestimation of SpO_2.[30] (See Box 8-4 for a decision making problem involving pulse oximetry.)

Methemoglobinemia, a complication associated with administering certain types of drugs (e.g., nitrites, benzocaine [a local anesthetic], and dapsone [an antibiotic used to treat malaria and Pneumocystis carinii]), can lead to erroneous SpO_2 values because MetHb absorbs both red and infrared light.[30] Methemoglobinemia is also associated with nitrate poisoning. If enough MetHb is present to dominate all pulsatile absorption, the pulse oximeter will measure a red to infrared ratio of 1:1, corresponding to a SpO_2 of about 85%. Consequently, the pulse oximeter reading will over- or underestimate the true oxyhemoglobin saturation.[30]

Dyes. Intravascular dyes can adversely affect SpO_2 values by absorbing a portion of the incident light emitted by the pulse oximeter diodes. Injection of methylene blue and indigo carmine during cardiac catheterization causes a false drop in SpO_2; indocyanine green has been shown to have little effect on pulse oximeter readings.[33]

Dark nail polishes (particularly blue and black nail polish) can severely affect SpO_2 readings. It has been suggested that nail polish may affect pulse oximetry values by causing the shunting of light around the finger periphery.[34,35] In **optical shunting,** transmitted light never comes in contact with the vascular bed, so SpO_2 values can be erroneously high or low, depending on whether this light is pulsatile. This problem can be alleviated to a large extent by placing the device over the lateral aspects of the digit instead of over the nail. Theoretically, skin pigmentation should not effect pulse oximeter readings; but in practice, SpO_2 readings are inconsistent for patients with dark pigmentation possibly because of optical shunting.[36] **Hyperbilirubinemia,** which is a yellow discoloration of the skin associated with hepatic dysfunction, does not seem to affect pulse oximetry readings.[18]

Ambient Light. Fluorescent lights and other external light sources (e.g., heat lamps, fiberoptic light sources, and surgical lamps) have been shown to adversely affect heart rate and SpO_2 readings.[37] Most commercially available pulse oximeters attempt to compensate for this interference by continually cycling the transmitted red and infrared light on and off at a rate of about 480 cycles per second. In this process, the pulse oximeter cycles in three modes:

1. Red light on, IR off.
2. IR on, red light off.
3. Red light and IR off.

By using this sequence, ambient light interference can be determined when both red and IR light sources are off. Subtracting any light measured during Phase 3 from that measured during Phases 1 and 2 provides a means of minimizing ambient light interference.

Calibration of Pulse Oximeters

Pulse oximeters are calibrated by manufacturers with data obtained from studies of healthy humans. Specifically, pulse oximeter oxyhemoglobin saturations (SpO_2) are compared with invasive hemoximetry oxygen saturations (SaO_2) measured simultaneously while each subject breathes several gas mixtures of different F_IO_2s. Therefore the accuracy and reliability of a pulse oximeter is ultimately dependent on the initial calibration algorithm that is programmed into the device by the manufacturer. Generally, pulse oximeters are accurate for oxygen saturations higher than 80%. Pulse oximeter saturations lower than 80% are questionable and should be confirmed with ABG analysis and hemoximetry.

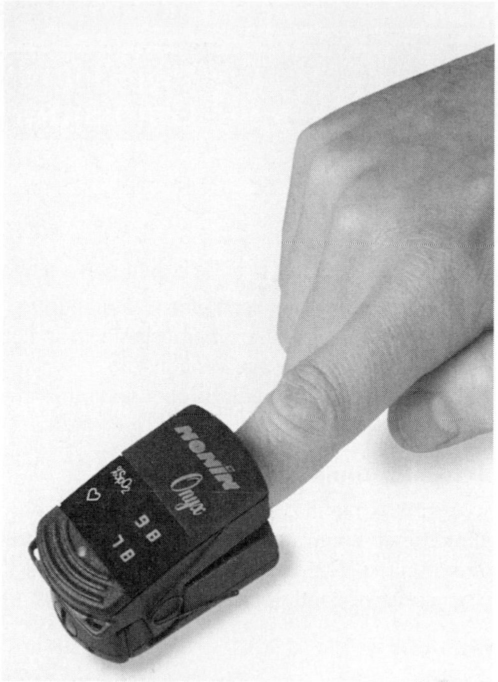

Figure 8-15 A hand-held pulse oximeter. (Courtesy Nonin Medical, Inc., Plymouth, Minn.)

Clinical Applications of Pulse Oximetry

Pulse oximetry probes are available in neonatal, pediatric, and adult sizes. Advances in light-emitting electrode (LED) and solid-state technology have led to the miniaturization of pulse oximeters and the manufacture of hand-held devices (Figure 8-15). The response time of a pulse oximeter (i.e., how long it takes for a change in central [left heart PO_2] to be detected by the pulse oximeter) depends on the location of the probe. Probes placed on fingers show a delay of 12 seconds or more than when the probe is placed on the ear lobe. Probes placed on the toe show an even greater lag time for detecting PO_2 changes.

Pulse oximetry is well recognized as an early warning system for detecting hypoxemia of patients with unstable oxygenation status. It can provide a continuous display of oxygen saturation, which can be used to monitor the oxygenation status of patients during surgery, mechanical ventilation, or bronchoscopy. It can also provide intermittent measurements of SpO_2, which can be useful, for example, in the management of home-care patients.

Although pulse oximetry can be quite effective when adjusting oxygen therapy in hospitalized patients, its use in prescribing oxygen therapy for home-care patients is questionable. Therefore caution should be exercised when using pulse oximeter readings to prescribe oxygen therapy. Carlin and associates[38] demonstrated that using only pulse oximetry measurements could disqualify a significant number of patients applying for reimbursement for oxygen therapy. The Health Care Financing Administration (HCFA) guidelines for

BOX 8-5

Clinical Practice Guidelines

Pulse Oximetry

Indications

Based on current evidence, pulse oximetry is useful for:

1. Monitoring arterial oxyhemoglobin saturation.
2. Quantifying the arterial oxyhemoglobin saturation response to therapeutic intervention.
3. Monitoring arterial oxyhemoglobin saturation during bronchoscopy.

Contraindications

Pulse oximetry may not be appropriate in situations where ongoing measurements of pH, $PaCO_2$, and total hemoglobin are required. The presence of abnormal hemoglobins may be a relative contraindication.

Limitations

A number of factors, agents, and situations may affect readings, limit precision, and performance of pulse oximetry, including:

1. Motion artifacts.
2. Abnormal hemoglobins (especially COHb and MetHb).
3. Intravascular dyes.
4. Exposure of the measuring sensor to ambient light sources.
5. Low perfusion states.
6. Skin pigmentation.
7. Nail polish.
8. Low oxyhemoglobin saturations (i.e., below 83%).

Monitoring

The following information should be recorded during pulse oximetry:

1. Probe type, and measurement site, date and time of measurement, and patient position and activity level
2. FiO_2 and mode of supplemental oxygen delivery
3. ABG measurements and CO-oximetry results that may have been made simultaneously
4. Clinical appearance of the patient (e.g., cyanotic, skin temperature)
5. Agreement between pulse oximeter heart rate and heart rate determined by palpation or ECG recordings

For a copy of the complete text, see AARC Clinical practice guideline: pulse oximetry Respir Care 36:1406, 1991.

qualifying for oxygen therapy require that the patient demonstrate a PaO_2 of ≤55 torr or a saturation of ≤85% saturation.[39] Because any of the physiological or technical problems discussed above can significantly affect pulse oximetry measurements, it is wise to use invasive ABG analysis to establish the need for oxygen therapy for chronically ill patients.

Box 8-5 summarizes the AARC Clinical Practice Guideline for pulse oximetry, which provides valuable information to ensure that SpO_2 values are valid.

Transcutaneous Monitoring

Transcutaneous monitoring provides another method of indirect ABG assessment. Unlike pulse oximetry, which relies on spectrophotometric analysis, transcutaneous monitoring uses modified blood gas electrodes to measure the oxygen and carbon dioxide tension at the skin surface.[41-43] The conjunctival PO_2 electrode, which is a modification of the standard transcutaneous PO_2 electrode, measures the PO_2 of the palpebral conjunctiva surrounding the eyeball.

Transcutaneous PO_2

Figure 8-16*A* is a schematic of a **transcutaneous PO_2 ($PtcO_2$)** electrode, which consists of a **servo-controlled** heated (Clark) polarographic electrode connected to a CPU.[41,43] The electrode is covered with a Teflon membrane, and the entire electrode assembly attaches to the skin surface with a double-sided adhesive ring. The electrode is heated to 42° to 45° C to produce capillary vasodilation below the surface of the electrode. Heating improves gas diffusion across the skin because it increases local blood flow at the site of the electrode, as well as alters the structure of the stratum corneum. The stratum corneum has been described as a mixture of fibrinous tissue within a lipid and protein matrix. It has been suggested that heating the skin to temperatures greater than 41° C melts the lipid layer, thus enhancing gas diffusion through the skin.[40]

The ratio of transcutaneous PO_2 to PaO_2 measured by hemoximetry (i.e., the $PtcO_2/PaO_2$ index) has been shown to be good for neonatal use, but it is often unreliable for critically ill adults.[44,45] Decreases in peripheral perfusion caused by reductions in cardiac output or increases in peripheral (cutaneous) resistance can significantly affect the accuracy of $PtcO_2$ measurements.[45,46] Current data indicate that when the cardiac index is >2.2 L/min/m^2, the $PtcO_2/PaO_2$ index is 0.5, but when the cardiac index is <1.5 L/min/m^2, it is only 0.1.[47] Thus hypoperfusion of the skin caused by pathologic states (e.g., septic shock, hemorrhage, or heart failure) or by increased vascular resistance (e.g., hypothermia or pharmacological intervention) can lead to erroneous data. Because $PtcO_2$ is influenced by blood flow to the tissues as well as by oxygen utilization by the tissues, changes in $PtcO_2$ may be an early indicator of

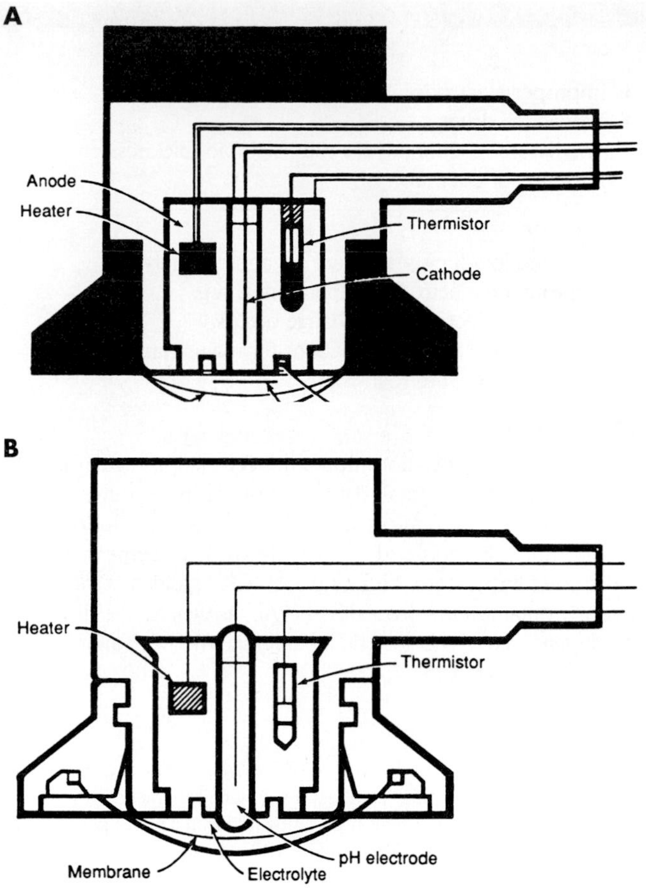

Figure 8-16 Transcutaneous electrodes: **A,** $PtcO_2$; **B,** $PtcCO_2$. (From Deshpande VM, Pilbeam SP, and Dixon RJ: A comprehensive review in respiratory care, 1988, Appleton & Lange, Stamford, Conn.)

vascular compromise or shock. In fact, many $PtcO_2$ monitors display the power supplied to the electrode heater as a way of identifying perfusion problems at the site.

Transcutaneous PCO_2

The standard transcutaneous carbon dioxide ($PtcCO_2$) electrode is a modified Stowe-Severinghaus blood gas electrode composed of pH-sensitive glass with a Ag/AgCl electrode (see Figure 8-16, *B*). As with the $PtcO_2$ electrode, the $PtcCO_2$ electrode is heated to 42° to 45° C. The $PtcCO_2$ values are slightly higher than the $PaCO_2$ value primarily because of the higher metabolic rate at the site of the electrode caused by heating the skin. Most commercial instruments incorporate correction factors into their system's software to remove the discrepancy between $PtcCO_2$ and $PaCO_2$.

Technical Considerations for Transcutaneous Monitoring

Box 8-6 contains guidelines for transcutaneous monitoring of neonatal and pediatric patients that relate to care, placement, and calibration of the electrodes. Several points deserve special attention:

1. Transcutaneous signals are adversely affected by dirt and hair, so before an electrode is placed on the patient's skin, the site should be cleansed with an alcohol swab. In cases when hair may be present, the site should be shaved to ensure good contact between the electrode and the skin. When attaching the electrode to the patient, placing a drop of electrolyte gel or deionized water on the electrode surface enhances gas diffusion between the skin and the electrode.
2. Transcutaneous PO_2 monitors are calibrated with 2-point calibration in which room air ($PO_2 \sim 150$ torr) is the high PO_2 of the calibration and an electronic zeroing of the system is the low PO_2 of the calibration. The $PtcCO_2$ electrodes are also calibrated with a 2-point calibration procedure. In this latter calibration, a 5% CO_2 calibration gas and a 10% CO_2 calibration gas are used for low and high calibration points respectively. Electrodes should be calibrated before their initial use on a patient. Manufacturers typically suggest that an electrode should be calibrated each time it is repositioned.
3. Transcutaneous electrodes are bathed with a small volume of electrolyte solution that can easily evaporate because heat is applied to the electrode. Loss of electrolyte either through evaporation or leakage from a torn membrane can adversely affect electrode operation. The electrolyte and the sensor's membrane should be checked regularly and changed weekly or whenever a signal drift during calibration is noticed. Because silver can deposit on the cathode, the electrode should be periodically cleaned per manufacturer recommendations.
4. When transcutaneous PO_2 and PCO_2 readings are reported, the date and time of the measurement, the patient's activity level and body position, the site of electrode placement, and the electrode temperature should be noted. The inspired oxygen concentration and the type of equipment used to deliver supplemental oxygen should always be included. The clinical appearance of the patient, including assessment of peripheral perfusion (i.e., pallor, skin temperature), is important data to note. When invasive ABG measurements are available, they are recorded for comparison with $PtcO_2$ and $PtcCO_2$ readings.[46]

Burns are probably the most common problem that clinicians encounter during transcutaneous monitoring because the site of measurement must be heated to 42° to 45° C. Repositioning the sensor every 4 to 6 hours can minimize this problem. For transcutaneous monitoring of neonates, the sensor should be repositioned more often.

Conjunctival PO_2

This technique uses a miniaturized polarographic electrode embedded in a plastic eyepiece. As shown in Figure 8-17, the eyepiece is placed in the **superior palpebral**

BOX 8-6

Clinical Practice Guidelines

Transcutaneous Blood Gas Monitoring for Neonatal and Pediatric Patients

Indications

1. Monitoring the adequacy of arterial oxygenation and/or ventilation.
2. Quantifying a patient's response to diagnostic and therapeutic interventions.

Contraindications

Transcutaneous monitoring may be a relative contraindication in patients with poor skin integrity or adhesive allergy.

Hazards/Complications

1. False-negative or false-positive results may lead to inappropriate treatment of patients.
2. Tissue injury at the measuring site (e.g., blisters, burns, skin tears).

Limitations

The following factors may increase the discrepancy between arterial and transcutaneous values:

1. Hyperoxemia ($PaO_2 > 100$ mm Hg)
2. Hypoperfused state (e.g., shock)
3. Improper electrode placement
4. Vasoactive drugs
5. The nature of the patient's skin (skinfold thickness or presence of edema)

Validation

1. High and low limit alarms are set appropriately.
2. Appropriate electrode temperature is set.
3. Systematic electrode site change occurs.
4. Manufacturer recommendations for maintenance, operation, and safety are followed.

Monitoring

The following information should be recorded at regular intervals (e.g., 1 to 4 hours): date and time of measurement, patient position, respiratory rate, activity level, FiO_2, mode of ventilatory support and settings, electrode placement site, electrode temperature, time of placement, results of simultaneously obtained in vitro ABG analysis, as well as the clinical appearance of the patient, including perfusion, pallor, and skin temperature.

For a copy of the complete text, see AARC Clinical practice guideline: transcutaneous blood gas monitoring for neonatal and pediatric patients, Respir Care 39(12):1176, 1994.

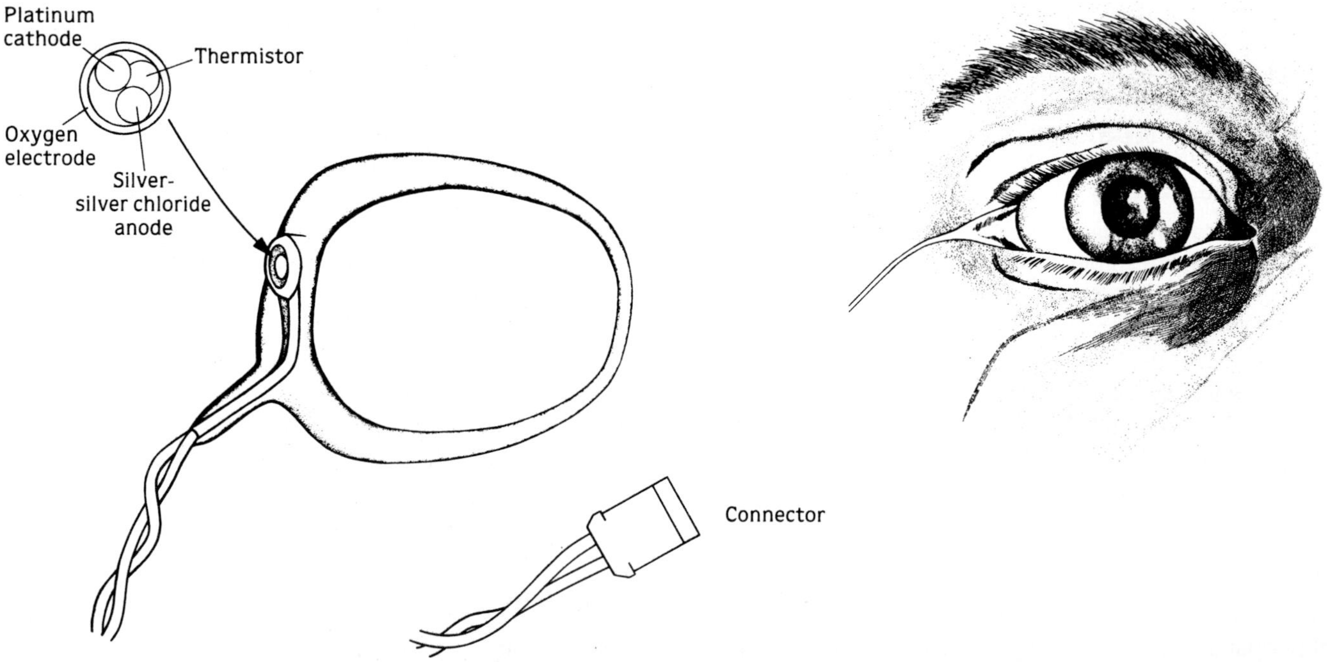

Figure 8-17 A conjunctival eyepiece for measuring PO_2. (Courtesy Orange Medical Instruments, Costa Mesa, Calif. In Wilkins RL, Krider SJ, and Sheldon RL: Clinical assessment in respiratory care, ed 3, St Louis, 1995, Mosby.)

conjunctiva. The conjunctiva receives its O_2 supply from a branch of the ipsilateral carotid artery. Gases can readily diffuse across the conjunctiva to contact the electrode, so it is not necessary to heat the site of measurement as with transcutaneous PO_2 and PCO_2 devices. Because of this increased sensitivity, these devices can detect hypoxemia and decreased perfusion sooner than transcutaneous monitoring. Conjunctival PO_2 rings can be left in place for up to 30 days, as long as the eyes are lubricated and taped shut.

INTERPRETATION OF BLOOD GAS RESULTS

As stated previously, ABGs can provide valuable information about a patient's acid-base, ventilatory, and oxygenation status. Blood gas analysis is also an integral part of more sophisticated procedures, such as cardiopulmonary and hemodynamic monitoring. It is beyond the scope of this book to fully discuss the interpretive value of blood gas measurements. We will therefore only provide a framework for ABG interpretation, but the titles of several texts and monographs on blood gas analysis are listed at the end of the chapter.

Acid-Base Status

Acid-base disorders can be categorized as either acidosis or alkalosis. Acidosis is associated with an increase in the plasma hydrogen ion concentration and a fall in the pH. Alkalosis is associated with a decrease in plasma hydrogen ion concentration and a rise in pH. The Henderson-Hasselbalch equation can be used to describe how changes in HCO_3^- and $PaCO_2$ can be used to determine if a metabolic, respiratory, or a combined acid-base disorder is present. Consider the following equations:

$$pH = pKa + \log (HCO_3^-) \div (PaCO_2 \times 0.03),$$

or

$$pH \sim (HCO_3^-) \div (PaCO_2)$$

Acute decreases in HCO_3^- and increases in $PaCO_2$ are associated with decreases in pH and metabolic and respiratory acidosis, respectively. Conversely, acute increases in HCO_3^- and decreases in $PaCO_2$ are associated with increases in pH and metabolic and respiratory alkalosis, respectively. If only one of the parameters changes and the other stays within normal limits, then the problem can be classified as an acute or uncompensated acid-base disorder. For example, a reduced pH with an increase in $PaCO_2$ and a normal HCO_3^- is indicative of an acute or uncompensated respiratory acidosis. If the reduced pH is associated with a decreased HCO_3^- and a normal $PaCO_2$, then an acute or uncompensated metabolic acidosis is suggested.

Figure 8-18 provides an algorithm that can be used to interpret ABG measurements by determining if evidence of compensation for the acid-base disorder exists. First, look at the pH and determine if an acidosis or alkalosis is present. To determine the primary disorder, look at the

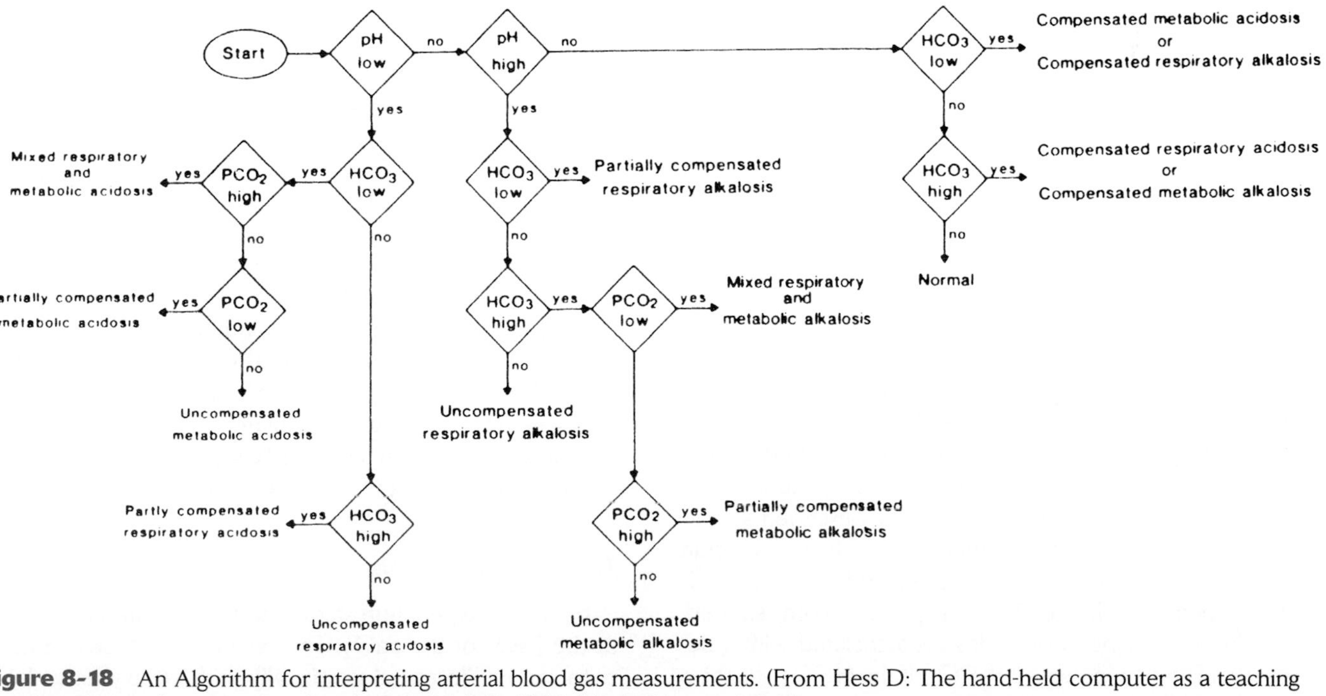

Figure 8-18 An Algorithm for interpreting arterial blood gas measurements. (From Hess D: The hand-held computer as a teaching tool for acid-base interpretation, Respir Care 29:375, 1984. Used with permission.)

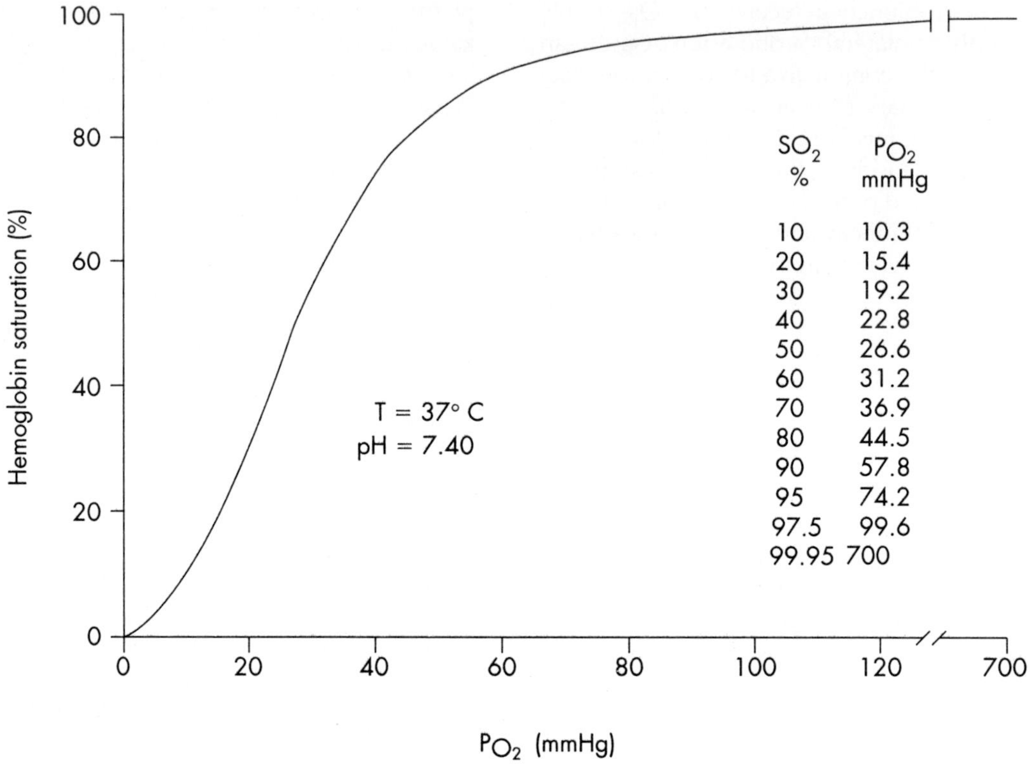

Figure 8-19 Oxyhemoglobin dissociation curve. (From Lane EE and Walker JF: Clinical arterial blood gas analysis, St Louis, 1987, Mosby.)

$PaCO_2$ to decide if a respiratory problem could have caused the altered pH. Next, look at the HCO_3^- to determine if a metabolic disorder is responsible for the altered pH. Once the origin of the acid-base disorder has been established, it can be determined if compensation has occurred by seeing if the other variable has also changed. Consider the following situation. If a patient's pH is below 7.40, then the original problem could be caused by an increase in $PaCO_2$ (i.e., respiratory acidosis) or a decrease in HCO_3^- (i.e., metabolic acidosis). The compensation for a respiratory acidosis would be a rise in the HCO_3^-, whereas the compensation for a metabolic acidosis would be a reduction in $PaCO_2$. The converse of this situation would follow the same line of logic. If the patient's pH is greater than 7.40, then the original problem could be caused by a reduction in $PaCO_2$ (i.e., respiratory alkalosis) or an increase in HCO_3^- (i.e., metabolic alkalosis). The compensation for a respiratory alkalosis is to retain HCO_3^- while the compensation for a metabolic alkalosis is CO_2 retention.

The level of compensation is usually described as partially compensated or fully compensated. If the pH is within the range of normal limits, then the acid-base disorder is fully compensated. If not, then it is partially compensated. For example, a respiratory acidosis is associated with a decreased pH and an increased $PaCO_2$. If the HCO_3^- has also increased, then there is evidence of metabolic compensation. If the pH is between 7.35 and 7.40, then this is interpreted as a fully compensated respiratory acidosis.

Ventilatory Status

A patient's ventilatory status can be assessed by looking at the $PaCO_2$. An increase in $PaCO_2$ is associated with hypoventilation and a respiratory acidosis. Conversely, a decrease in $PaCO_2$ is associated with hyperventilation and a respiratory alkalosis. As a general rule, a $PaCO_2$ greater than 50 mm Hg is classified as ventilatory failure and is often used as a criterion for initiating mechanical ventilatory support. Note that changes in $PaCO_2$ must be interpreted relative to the patient's clinical condition. For example, patients with COPD often demonstrate chronic ventilatory failure (e.g., $PaCO_2$ higher than 50 mm Hg with pH within normal limits). Thus acute ventilatory failure is only said to exist in COPD patients if the $PaCO_2$ increases well above 50 mm Hg and the pH is below 7.30.

Oxygenation Status

A patient's oxygenation status can be evaluated by looking at the PaO_2 or the SaO_2. The relationship between these then can be illustrated graphically with an oxyhemoglobin dissociation curve, like the one shown in Figure 8-19. Note

TABLE 8-6

Criteria for classifying hypoxemia using PaO_2/SaO_2 measurements

Hypoxemia	PaO_2
Conditions: room air is inspired; the patient is <60 yr	
Mild*	<80 mm Hg
Moderate*	<60 mm Hg
Severe*	<40 mm Hg
Conditions: supplemental oxygen is inspired; the patient is <60 yr	
Uncorrected	Less than room air acceptable limit
Corrected	Within the room air acceptable limit; <100 mm Hg
Excessively corrected	>100 mm Hg; less than the minimal level predicted in Table 3-4

Adapted from Shapiro BA, et al: Clinical application of blood gases, ed 4, Chicago, 1989, Mosby.

*Subtract 1 mm Hg of oxygen to limits of mild and moderate hypoxemia for each year over 60. A PaO_2 <40 mm Hg indicates severe hypoxemia in any patient at any age.

BOX 8-7

Examples of Disease States Associated with Various Types of Acid-Base Disorders

Metabolic Acidosis

Diabetes mellitus
Diarrhea
Methanol ingestion
Renal dysfunction
Salicylate intoxication

Metabolic Alkalosis

Administration of excessive amounts of bicarbonate
Diuretic therapy
Ingestion of excessive amounts of antacids
Nasogastric suctioning
Vomiting

Respiratory Acidosis

Acute airway obstruction
Ingestion of excessive amounts of sedative, opiates, and other respiratory depressants
Neuromuscular disorders
Pneumothorax
Restrictive pulmonary disease

Respiratory Alkalosis

Anxiety
Encephalitis
Excessive mechanical ventilatory support
Progesterone

that a PaO_2 of 45 mm Hg is associated with an SaO_2 of approximately 80%; a PaO_2 of about 60 mm Hg corresponds to an SaO_2 of 90%; and a PaO_2 of 75 mm Hg is equivalent to an SaO_2 of 95%. For interpretative purposes, a PaO_2 from 60 to 80 mm Hg is classified as mild hypoxemia; a PaO_2 from 40 to 60 mm Hg is classified as moderate hypoxemia; and a PaO_2 less than 40 mm Hg is classified as severe hypoxemia. Table 8-6 provides PaO_2 and SaO_2 ranges for evaluating a patient's oxygenation status.

Box 8-7 lists examples of conditions and disease states associated with various acid-base disorders. As mentioned earlier, blood gas measurements are only meaningful when they are interpreted relative to other clinical findings. Interpretation of ABGs without other supporting clinical data can be misleading and lead to potentially harmful decisions in patient management.

Summary

Blood gas analysis is an integral part of managing patients with cardiopulmonary dysfunctions. Modern in vitro blood gas analyzers are fully automated systems that only require small amounts of blood for analysis and can provide intermittent measurements of pH, $PaCO_2$, and PaO_2, which give valuable information about a patient's acid-base, ventilatory, and oxygenation status. Many blood gas analyzers also allow for determinations of plasma electrolytes and metabolites, such as sodium, potassium, calcium, and glucose. Noninvasive devices, including pulse oximetry and transcutaneous monitoring, provide an alternative to the standard in vitro blood gas analysis and allow for continuous blood gas surveillance. Two relatively new devices, the in vivo intraarterial catheter and the point-of-care blood gas analyzer, hold considerable promise for providing accurate and reliable blood gas analysis at the bedside.

The importance of blood gas analysis cannot be overstated. It is important to recognize that blood gas measurements should be interpreted relative to other clinical indices, including history and physical examination, chest radiographs, and other clinical laboratory tests.

Review Questions

See Appendix A for answers.

1. Which of the following are current safety guidelines for the protection of the therapist drawing an ABG sample?
   I. gloves
   II. gown
   III. protective eyewear (goggles)
   IV. shoe covers
   a. I and III only
   b. II and III only
   c. II and IV only
   d. I, II, and III only

2. A positive Allen test indicates the presence of:
   a. an occluded radial artery
   b. a patent ulnar artery
   c. inadequate arterial oxygenation to the hand
   d. inadequate collateral circulation to the hand

3. The site most often used for sampling arterial blood in adults is which of the following arteries?
   a. brachial
   b. dorsal foot
   c. radial
   d. femoral

4. Interpret the following ABG findings:

pH = 7.50; $PaCO_2$ = 30 mm Hg; PaO_2 = 60 mm Hg; HCO_3 = 24 mEq/L.
   a. acute metabolic alkalosis with mild hypoxemia
   b. chronic metabolic acidosis with moderate hypoxemia
   c. acute respiratory alkalosis with mild hypoxemia
   d. chronic respiratory alkalosis with moderate hypoxemia

5. Which of the following conditions is associated with an acute respiratory acidosis?
   a. barbiturate intoxication
   b. excessive ingestion of antacids
   c. emphysema
   d. anxiety

6. A patient is admitted to the emergency department of the hospital after a motor vehicle accident. In your initial assessment of the patient, you find that he is pale and his pulse is weak. You are unable to obtain a steady pulse oximeter reading. Which of the following is the most probable cause of the erratic pulse oximetry readings?
   I. poor perfusion state
   II. increased levels of carboxyhemoglobin
   III. low PaO_2
   IV. anemia
   a. I only
   b. I and II only
   c. I, II, and III only
   d. I, II, III, and IV

7. Which of the following can alter pulse oximeter readings?
   I. low perfusion states, such as hypovolemic shock
   II. dark blue nail polish
   III. methemoglobinemia
   IV. hyperbilirubinemia
   a. I and III only
   b. II and III only
   c. II and IV only
   d. I, II, and III only

8. A patient's P_{50} is 37 mm Hg. Which of the following conditions could be responsible?
   I. hypercarbia
   II. decreased plasma levels of 2,3 diphosphoglycerate
   III. acute acidosis
   IV. carbon monoxide poisoning
   a. I and III only
   b. II and III only
   c. II and IV only
   d. I, II, and IV only

9. To function effectively, the reference pH electrode must be bathed in which of the following solutions?
   a. 1% sodium bicarbonate
   b. saturated potassium chloride
   c. 5% hydrochloric acid
   d. 0.9% sodium chloride

10. While assessing the Levy-Jennings graphs for PCO_2 values, you notice that results for the last five QA tests have increased progressively. Which of the following is the most likely cause of this finding?
    a. a leak in the electrode membrane
    b. protein build-up on the electrode
    c. a damaged wire
    d. this is a normal membrane function

11. Which of the following is NOT an anion buffer?
    a. hemoglobin
    b. inorganic phosphate
    c. bicarbonate
    d. organic calcium

12. Based on CLIA standards, laboratory instruments used in the hospital for blood sample testing should have three-point calibrations performed at least:
    a. daily
    b. weekly
    c. monthly
    d. every 6 months

13. Compare the processes of quality control and quality assurance.

14. Arterial blood was obtained from a patient after open-heart surgery. The patient's temperature is 35° C, and the measured PaO_2 is 80 mm Hg before temperature correction. The patient's actual PaO_2 is approximately:
    a. 70 mm Hg
    b. 80 mm Hg
    c. 90 mm Hg
    d. it cannot be determined from the information provided

15. What are the consequences of maintaining the temperature of the transcutaneous PO_2 probe at 48° C?
    a. thermal injury
    b. low $PtcO_2$ readings
    c. fire hazard
    d. malignant hyperthermia

16. Which of the following tests is indicated for determining the presence of carbon monoxide poisoning?
    a. pulse oximetry
    b. ABGs
    c. CO-oximetry
    d. transcutaneous $PtcO_2$

References

1. American Association of Respiratory Care: Clinical practice guideline: sampling for arterial blood gas analysis, Respir Care 37:913, 1992.
2. American Association of Respiratory Care: Clinical practice guideline: in vitro pH and blood gas analysis and hemoximetry, Respir Care 38:505, 1993.
3. Browning JA, Kaiser DL, and Durbin CG: The effect of guidelines on the appropriate use of arterial blood gas analysis in the intensive care unit, Respir Care 34:269, 1989.
4. Bruck E, et al: Percutaneous collection of arterial blood for laboratory analysis, National Committee for Clinical Laboratory Standards 1985, H11A, 5(3):39.
5. National Committee for Clinical Laboratory Standards: Procedures for the collection of diagnostic blood specimens by skin puncture, ed 3, Villanova, Penn. 1992, The Committee.
6. Koch G and Wendel H: Comparison of pH, carbon dioxide tension, standard bicarbonate and oxygen tension in capillary blood and in arterial blood during the neonatal period, Acta Paediatr Scand 56:10, 1967.
7. Burritt MF and Fallon KD: Blood gas preanalytical considerations: specimen collection, calibration, and controls, National Committee for Clinical Laboratory Standards 1989, C27-T 9(11):685.
8. Ehrmeyer S and Laessig RH: Measurement of the proficiency of pH and blood gas analyses by interlaboratory proficiency testing, J Med Tech 2:33, 1985.
9. Koch G and Wendel H: Comparison of pH, carbon dioxide tension, standard bicarbonate and oxygen tension in capillary blood and in arterial blood during the neonatal period, Acta Paediatr Scand 56:10, 1967.
10. Duc GV and Cumarasamy N: Digital arteriolar oxygen tension as a guide to oxygen therapy of the newborn, Biol Neonate 24:134, 1974.
11. McLain BI, Evans J, and Dear PFR: Comparison of capillary and arterial blood gas measurements in neonates, Arch Dis Child 63:743, 1988.
12. Desai SD, et al: A comparison between arterial and arterialized capillary blood in infants, S Afr Med J 41:13, 1967.
13. Centers for Disease Control: Update: universal precautions for prevention of transmission of human immunodeficiency virus, hepatitis B virus, and other blood-borne pathogens in health care settings, MMWR 37:377, 1988.
14. Department of Labor, Occupational Safety and Health Administration: Occupational exposure to bloodborne pathogens, 29 CFRR Part 1910.1030, Federal Register, December 6, 1991.
15. Moran RF, et al: Oxygen content, hemoglobin oxygen, "saturation," and related quantities in blood: terminology, measurement, and reporting, National Committee for Clinical Laboratory Standards 1990, C25-P 10:1.
16. Davenport HW: The ABC of acid-base chemistry, ed 3, Chicago, 1975, University of Chicago Press.
17. Brensilver JM and Goldberger E: A primer of water, and acid-base syndromes, ed 8, Philadelphia, 1996, FA Davis.
18. Shapiro BA, et al: Clinical application of blood gases, ed 4, Chicago, 1989, YearBook Medical Publishers Inc.
19. National Committee for Clinical Laboratory Standards: Clinical laboratory technical procedure manual, ed 2, Publication GP2-A2, Illinois, 1992, Villanova.
20. Clinical Laboratory Improvement Amendments of 1988: Final rule, subpart H, Federal Register, February 1992.
21. Clinical Laboratory Improvement Amendments of 1988: Final rule, subpart H, Federal Register, February 1992.
22. Hansen JE, et al: Assessing precision and accuracy in blood gas proficiency testing, Am Rev Respir Dis 141:1190, 1990.
23. Mohler JG, et al: Blood gases. In Clausen JL, editor: Pulmonary function testing: guidelines and controversies, New York, 1982, Academic Press.
24. Barker SJ and Hyatt J: Continuous measurement of intraarterial pH, $PaCO_2$, and PaO_2 in the operating room, Anesthesia Analg 73: 43, 1991.
25. MacIntyre NR, et al: Accuracy and precision of a point-of-care blood gas analyzer incorporating optode, Respir Care 41(9):800, 1996.
26. Brown LJ: A new instrument for the simultaneous measurement of total hemoglobin, % oxyhemoglobin, % carboxyhemoglobin, % methemoglobin, and oxygen content in whole blood, IEEE Trans Biomedical Engineering 27:132, 1980.
27. Falholt W: Blood oxygen saturation determinations by spectrophotometry, Scan J Clin Lab Invest 15:67, 1963.
28. Severinghaus JW and Astrup PB: History of blood gas analysis, VI oximetry, J Clin Monitoring 2:270, 1986.
29. Nillson NJ: Oximetry, Physiol Rev, 40:1, 1960.
30. Tremper KK and Barker SJ: Pulse oximetry, Anesthesiology 70:98, 1989.
31. Yang K, Brown SD, and Gutierrez G: Noninvasive assessment of blood gases. In Levine RL and Fromm RE, editors: Critical care monitoring, from pre-hospital to ICU, St Louis, 1995, Mosby.

32. Pilbeam S: Mechanical ventilation, ed 3, St Louis, 1998, Mosby.
33. Scheller MS, Unger RJ, and Kelner MJ: Effects of intravenously administered dyes on pulse oximetry readings, Anesthesiology 65:550, 1986.
34. Cote CJ, et al.: The effect of nail polish on pulse oximetry, Anesth Analg 67:685, 1988.
35. Rubin AS: Nail polish color can affect pulse oximeter saturation, Anesthesiology 68:825, 1988.
36. Emery JR: Skin pigmentation as an influence on the accuracy of pulse oximetry, J Perinatology 7:329, 1987.
37. Amar D, et al: Fluorescent light interferes with pulse oximetry, J Clin Monit 5:135, 1989.
38. Carlin BW, Claussen JL, and Ries AL: The use of cutaneous oximetry in the prescription of long-term oxygen therapy, Chest 94:239, 1988.
39. Kacmarek RM, Hess D, and Stoller JK: Monitoring in respiratory care, St Louis, 1993, Mosby.
40. Baecjert P, et al: Is pulse oximetry reliable in detecting hypoxemia in the neonate, Adv Exp Med Biol 220:165, 1987.
41. Lubbers DW: Theory and development of transcutaneous oxygen pressure measurement, Int Anesthesiol Clin 25:31, 1987.
42. Severinghaus JS and Bradley FA: Electrodes for blood PO_2 and PCO_2 determination, J Appl Physiol 13:515, 1958.
43. Severinghaus JS, Stafford M, and Bradley FA: Transcutaneous PO_2 electrode design, calibration, and temperature gradient problems, Acta Anesthesiology Scan (suppl) 68:118, 1978.
44. Reed RL, et al: Correlation of hemodynamic variables with transcutaneous PO_2 measurements in critically ill patients, J Trauma 25:1045, 1985.
45. Lubbers DW: Theoretical basis of transcutaneous blood gas measurements, Crit Care Med 9:721, 1981.
46. American Association of Respiratory Care: Clinical practice guideline: transcutaneous blood gas monitoring for neonatal and pediatric patients: Respir Care 39(12):1176, 1994.
47. Wahr JA and Tremper KK: Non-invasive oxygen monitoring techniques, Crit Care Clin 11(1):199, 1995.

Internet Resources

1. AARC Clinical Practice Guidelines:
http://www.aarc.org
2. CPT codes—Blackwell Science International Publishers:
http://www.healthgate.com/healthgate/free/dph/static/dph.0015.shtml
3. Acid-Base Balance (Alan W. Grogono, MD):
http://www.tmc.tulane.edu/anes/acidbase/practical.html
4. Carbon monoxide headquarters (David G. Penney, Ph.D.):
http://www.phymac.med.wayne.edu/facultyprofile/penney/COHQ/col.htm
5. Anesthesia for Elephants:
http://www.csen.com/anesthesia/elephants.htm
6. NIH Clinical Center Nursing Department—procedure for obtaining blood samples from pediatric patient with arterial lines:
http://cc.nih.gov/nursing/obspparl.html
7. Joint Commission on Accreditation of Healthcare Organizations:
http://www.jcaho.org
8. American College of Physicians—Annals of Internal Medicine:
http://www.acponline.org/journals/annals/annaltoc.htm
9. New England Journal of Medicine:
http://www.nejm.org
10. The Virtual Hospital:
http://www.vh.org
11. American Lung Association:
http://www.lungusa.org/index2.html
12. Medical Vendors with Internet Addresses:
http://www.med.utah.edu/usrc/national.htm
13. Respiratory Care Textbooks:
http://www.mosby.com

CHAPTER 9

CHAPTER OUTLINE

Introduction to Ventilators

Susan P. Pilbeam

CHAPTER OUTLINE (cont'd)

CHAPTER LEARNING OBJECTIVES

Upon completion of this chapter, the reader will be able to:

1. List the two primary power sources used in mechanical ventilators.
2. Compare and contrast negative- and positive-pressure ventilation.
3. Give an example of an intelligent or closed-loop ventilator system.
4. Define volume and pressure ventilation and provide three additional names for each.
5. Name three volume-displacement designs and three flow-control valves.
6. Compare the location of expiratory valves on current ICU ventilators with that on older model ventilators.
7. Draw the flow and pressure curves produced by linear drive and rotary drive pistons.
8. Explain the two fundamental principles of fluidics.
9. Identify the output port on a fluidic device.
10. Describe the four phases of a breath and the terms *trigger* and *cycle*.
11. Graph the flow/time, volume/time, and pressure/time curves for time-triggered, volume- or pressure-limited, time-cycled breaths.
12. Define the modes of ventilation by their triggering, limiting (controlling), and cycling mechanisms.
13. Evaluate patient information and determine which expiratory maneuver is appropriate: NEEP, CPAP, PEEP, expiratory pause, or expiratory retard.
14. Analyze findings from pressure, flow, and volume scalars and flow/volume and pressure/volume loops in terms of mode of ventilation and common problems that occur during ventilation.
15. Compare the servo-control modes of ventilation by intended function.
16. Explain the five common methods of delivering high-frequency ventilation.
17. List the common causes of high- and low-pressure alarms.
18. Determine from a clinical situation whether a problem with a ventilated patient is in the ventilator system or the patient.
19. From a diagram, identify the expiratory threshold resistor shown.
20. Diagram a demand flow and a continuous flow IMV system.
21. Assess the cause of a problem situation using either an IMV system or a freestanding CPAP system.

KEY TERMS

Adaptive Support Ventilation (ASV)
Airway Pressure-Release Ventilation (APRV)
AND/NAND Gate
Assist
Assist/Control Mode
Assisted Breaths
Autoflow
Auto-PEEP
Back-Pressure Switch
Baseline Pressure
Beam Deflection
Bi-level Positive Airway Pressure (BiPAP, Bi-level Pressure-Assist, Bi-Level Pressure-Support)
Bistable
Blowers
Chest Cuirass
Closed-Loop System
Coanda Effect
Combined-Powered Ventilators
Combined Pressure Devices
Compressors
Continuous-Flow IMV and CPAP Systems
Continuous Positive Airway Pressure (CPAP)
Control Mode
Control Panel
Control Variables
Control Ventilation
Cycle Variable
Demand Flow IMV and CPAP Systems
Differential Output
Direct Drive Pistons
Drive Mechanisms
Dual Modes of Ventilation
Electrically Powered
Expiratory Hold (End-Expiratory Pause)
Expiratory Positive Airway Pressure (EPAP)
Expiratory Retard
External Circuit
Flip-Flop Valves
Flow-Control Valves
Flow Resistors
Flow Triggering
Fluidics
Fluid Logic
Gas Streaming
High-Frequency Flow Interruption (HFFI)
High-Frequency Jet Ventilation (HFJV)
High-Frequency Oscillatory Ventilation (HFOV)
High-Frequency Percussive Ventilation (HFPV)
High-Frequency Positive-Pressure Ventilation (HFPPV)
High-Frequency Ventilation (HFV)
Inspiratory Pause
Inspiratory Positive Airway Pressure (IPAP)
Inspiratory Hold
Intensive Care Unit (ICU)
Intermittent Mandatory Ventilation (IMV)
Internal Circuit
Iron Lung
Linear Drive Piston
Loop
Mandatory Breath
Mandatory Minute Ventilation (MMV)
Microprocessor Controlled
Monostable
Negative End-Expiratory Pressure (NEEP)
Negative Pressure Ventilators
Open-Loop System
OR/NOR Gate
Patient Circuit
Patient Triggering
Peak Inspiratory Pressure (PIP)
Pendelluft
Phase Variables
Plateau Pressure (Pplateau)
Pneumatic
Pneumatic Circuit
Pneumatically Powered
Pressure Triggering
Positive End-Expiratory Pressure (PEEP)
Positive-Pressure Ventilators
Power Source
Power Transmission Systems
Pressure-Controlled Ventilation (PCV)
Pressure-Controlled, Inverse Ratio Ventilation (PCIRV)
Pressure-Regulated Volume Control (PRVC)
Pressure-Support Ventilation (PSV)
Pressure Triggering
Pressure Ventilation (PV) (Pressure-Limited Ventilation, Pressure-Controlled Ventilation, Pressure-Targeted Ventilation)
Proportional Amplifier
Proportional Assist Ventilation (PAV)
Rotary Drive Pistons
Rotary Compressors
Scalars
Schmitt Trigger
Separation Bubble
Sinusoidal
Splitter Configuration
Spontaneous Breaths
Spring-Loaded Bellows
Static Compliance
Synchronized Intermittent Mandatory Ventilation (SIMV)
Taylor Dispersion
Threshold Resistors
Total Cycle Time (TCT)
Trigger Sensitivity
Trigger Variable
User Interface
Variable Pressure Control
Variable Pressure Support
Ventilator Circuit
Volume-Controlled Inverse Ratio Ventilation (VCIRV)
Volume-Displacement Devices
Volume Support
Volume Ventilation
Work of Breathing (WOB)
Wye Connector

Part I: Physical Characteristics of Ventilators

There are a wide variety of mechanical ventilators available for managing patients of different ages in different settings. Although there is a large number of available units, all ventilators share certain physical properties, as well as important functional characteristics that describe breath delivery. These concepts are reviewed in this chapter.

Another important aspect of mechanical ventilation is the use of specific ventilator modes. This chapter's discussion of these modes includes not only those most commonly used but also servo-controlled and high-frequency ventilation methods. Managing the patient-ventilator system is less difficult with an understanding of ventilator alarms, an ability to identify problems using ventilator graphics, and a knowledge of some of the fundamentals of troubleshooting. Finally, an explanation of expiratory valves and spontaneous breathing systems completes this chapter.

Physical Characteristics of Mechanical Ventilators

Historical Perspective of Ventilator Classification

When compared with other types of medical practices, the use of ventilators in patient management is relatively young. In the United States, the earliest ventilators appeared in the 1950s and '60s and were originally classified by a system used by Mushin and associates,[1] the purpose of which was to try to describe ventilator function. The technology behind mechanical ventilation has since expanded so rapidly that the original system needed modification, so in the late 1980s and early 1990s Chatburn and Branson[2-4] established a newer classification system. Although a welcome change, this system was difficult for some practitioners to adopt.[5]

Historically, classification systems tried to describe the physical function of the ventilator, but current systems do two things. They describe certain characteristics of the ventilator and provide a description of the breath or breathing pattern that is delivered to the patient.[5] An introduction to current methods of ventilator classification follows.

Current Ventilator Classification

A ventilator is basically a "black box." It is connected to a **power source** and provides a breath or inspiratory flow to a patient. The operator sets certain controls on the **control panel,** or **user interface,** that determine the pattern of gas flow to the patient. Box 9-1 summarizes the basic physical and performance characteristics of ventilators.

BOX 9-1

Physical Characteristics of Ventilators[6]

Ventilator power source or input power (electric or gas source)
- electrically powered ventilators
- pneumatically powered ventilators
- combined power ventilators

Positive- or negative-pressure ventilators

Control systems and circuits
- open- and closed-loop systems to control ventilator function
- control panel (user interface)
- pneumatic circuit

Power transmission and conversion system
- volume-displacement, pneumatic designs
- flow-control valves

(From Pilbeam SP: Mechanical ventilation: physiological and clinical applications, St Louis, 1998, Mosby.)

POWER SOURCE

Power sources, which provide the energy to perform the work required to ventilate a patient, fall into three categories: **pneumatically powered, electrically powered,** or **combined-powered ventilators.**

Pneumatically Powered Ventilators

Pneumatically powered ventilators connect to high pressure gas sources, relying on them to ventilate the patient. In general, pneumatically powered ventilators operate using two 50 psi gas sources (oxygen and air) and have built-in reducing valves so that the operating pressure is lower than the source pressure. There are two basic types of pneumatic ventilators: **pneumatic** and fluidic. Pneumatic ventilators may incorporate things such as Venturi or air entrainers, needle valves, flexible diaphragms, and spring-loaded valves to perform their function. For example, Venturis, flexible diaphragms, and spring-loaded valves may be used to control an expiratory valve (see the section on resistive expiratory valves in Part IV of this chapter). A needle valve may control the rate of gas flow during inspiration. On the other hand, fluidic ventilators use fluidic components that are based on special pneumatic principles. The section on fluidics later in this chapter provides a more detailed description of fluidic function.

Electrically Powered Ventilators

Electrically powered ventilators most often use standard electrical outlets to power the internal components. They may also contain internal DC (direct-current) batteries, which can provide electrical power during patient transport or if there is a power failure. Some ventilators can also be connected to external DC batteries. Electrically powered ventilators may use the electricity to power internal motors for running air compressors, pistons, electrical solenoids, transducers, and microprocessors, all of which either provide gas flow to the patient or help control gas flow to the patient.

Combined Power Ventilators: Pneumatically-Powered and Electronically or Microprocessor-Controlled

One of the most common types of ventilators used in the **ICU (intensive care unit)** today is pneumatically powered and **microprocessor-controlled.** Two 50 psi gas sources provide the pressure (force) to deliver inspiratory gas flow. This gas flow is often the same air that goes into the patient during inspiration. Control of the inspiratory flow waveform is governed by a microprocessor. For example, the waveform or pattern of gas flow may be constant, producing a constant flow waveform, or it may be rapid at the beginning of inspiration and gradually taper down, producing a descending ramp waveform (see the section on inspiratory waveform and ventilator graphics later in this chapter). It is the programming of the microprocessor and its interaction with electrically operated flow valves or mechanical devices that control this function. These ventilators require both electric and pneumatic power sources.

BOX 9-2

Types and Examples of Pressure Ventilators

Negative-Pressure Ventilators
iron lung
chest cuirass

Positive-Pressure Ventilators
most ventilators in use today are this type

Positive/Negative Ventilators
high-frequency oscillators

PRESSURE DELIVERY

To provide the **work of breathing (WOB)** for the patient, a ventilator can increase lung volume during inspiration either by creating negative- or positive-pressure gradients, which represent the type of force that the unit applies to the body to produce ventilation (see Box 9-2).

Positive-Pressure Ventilators

There must be a pressure gradient for flow to occur. During normal spontaneous breathing, inspiration occurs due to contraction of the inspiratory muscles. During inspiration, the diaphragm contracts and descends and the external intercostal muscles contract. The action of these muscles, especially the diaphragm, results in an increase in the intrathoracic volume. A subambient intrapleural, then intraalveolar, pressure results, producing a pressure gradient from the mouth, which is at ambient pressure, to the alveoli, which are at less than ambient pressure. Air flows into the lungs. Expiration then occurs as passive relaxation of the respiratory muscles reduces the intrathoracic volume. Intraalveolar pressure become slightly positive (above ambient), and air flows out of the lungs.[6]

During positive-pressure ventilation, a pressure above ambient is created at the mouth while intraalveolar pressure is ambient. As a result, air flows into the lungs, expanding them and the chest wall (see Figure 9-1). **Positive-pressure ventilators** are by far the most common method of ventilation used today.

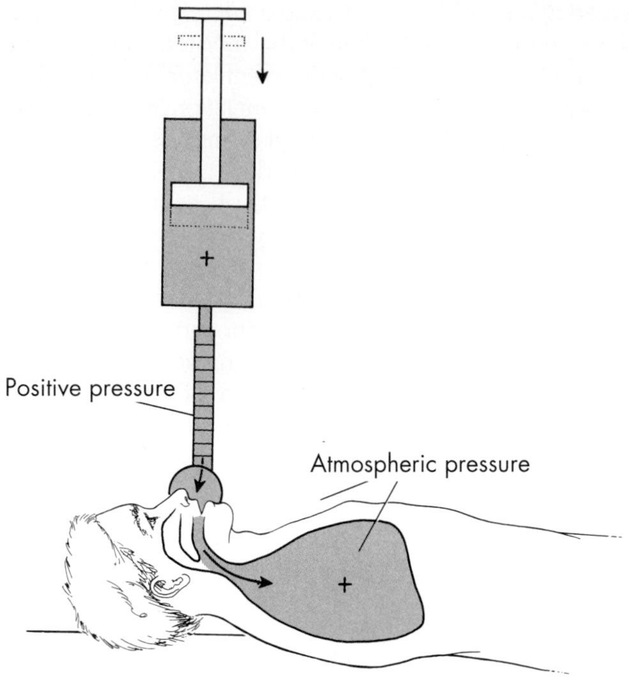

Figure 9-1 Application of positive pressure at the airway provides a pressure gradient; therefore gas flows into the lungs.

Negative-Pressure Ventilators

Negative-pressure ventilators generally enclose the thoracic area and create a negative pressure around the chest wall (Figure 9-2). This negative pressure is transmitted across the chest wall, resulting in reduced intrapleural and intraalveolar pressure. The pressure at the mouth is at atmospheric pressure, creating a pressure gradient between

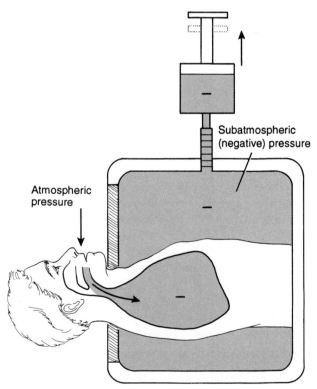

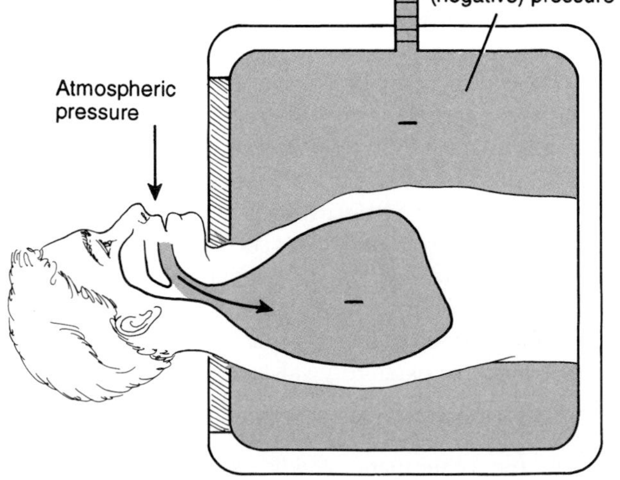

Figure 9-2 By applying subatmospheric pressure around the chest wall, a pressure drop in the alveoli and gas flow into the lungs can be produced.

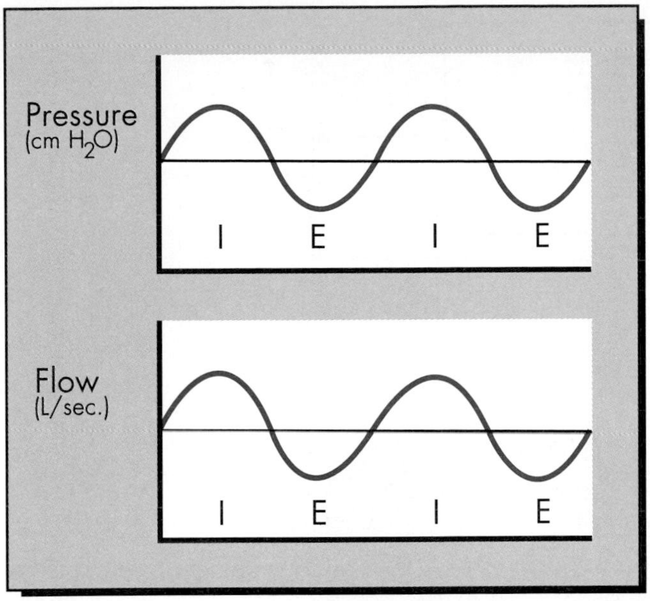

Figure 9-3 The sinusoidal waveform produced by an oscillator. *I* is inspiration, and *E* is expiration.

the mouth and alveoli similar to the normal spontaneous pressure gradient. Air flows into the lungs. During exhalation, the negative pressure around the chest is returned to ambient, the alveolar pressure becomes slightly positive, and air flows out of the lungs. Examples of these types of units are the **iron lung** and the **chest cuirass.**

Combined-Pressure Devices

The most common example of a **combined-pressure device** is a high-frequency oscillator. This is a form of **high-frequency ventilation (HFV)** that produces oscillating gas pressure waveforms at the upper airway. The waveform is a **sinusoidal** pattern with positive- and negative-pressure oscillations produced at the upper airway by an oscillating device (Figure 9-3). The section in this chapter on high-frequency ventilation explains oscillator function.

CONTROL SYSTEMS AND CIRCUITS

A combination of mechanical, pneumatic, and/or electronic devices within the ventilator represent the control or decision-making functions of the unit. They govern ventilator operation and can either be an **open-loop** or a **closed-loop system.**

Open- And Closed-Loop Systems

The terms open and closed loop describe the level of computer control within a ventilator. Units that are unintelligent are called open-loop systems. When the operator sets a control, such as tidal volume (V_T), the unit delivers the set amount of volume. In reality, this volume might leak into the room and never reach the patient. Unfortunately, an open-loop system cannot monitor the difference between the volume actually delivered and the set volume and respond to this difference (Figure 9-4 **A**).[2]

Closed-loop systems are intelligent systems. For example, the manufacturer programs a responsive system into the computer that can deliver a set parameter (e.g., V_T). This system measures the volume provided and exhaled, makes a comparison, and adjusts volume delivery based on this comparison. Figure 9-4 **B** shows an example of an algorithm for a closed-loop system.[2]

Control Panel

The control panel or user interface is located on the top, outside surface of most ventilators and contains the controls for the operator to set desired parameters such as respiratory rate (f), tidal volume (V_T), pressure (Pset), and inspiratory time (T_I).

Pneumatic Circuit

The **pneumatic circuit** consists of a series of tubing that directs gas flow both within the ventilator (the **internal circuit**) and from the ventilator to the patient (the external or **patient circuit**).

Internal Circuit

The internal circuit takes gas generated by the power source, passes it through various mechanical and/or pneumatic mechanisms, and finally directs it to the **external circuit.** Internal circuits are either single or double circuits (see Box 9-3). Figures 9-5 and 9-6 show examples of each type of circuit.

External Circuit

The external circuit conducts the gas from the ventilator to the patient and from the patient through an expiratory valve to the room. The external circuit is commonly called the **ventilator circuit,** or the patient circuit. Basic components of the patient circuit are listed in Box 9-4. Figure 9-7 **A** shows an example of a ventilator circuit with an externally mounted expiratory valve, and **B** shows a ventilator circuit with an internally mounted exhalation valve.

POWER TRANSMISSION SYSTEM

The power sources, gas and/or electricity, provide the energy to power mechanical devices, which ultimately generates a pressure gradient. The pressure gradient, negative or positive, provides all or part of the patient's work of breathing. We call these internally powered mechanical devices

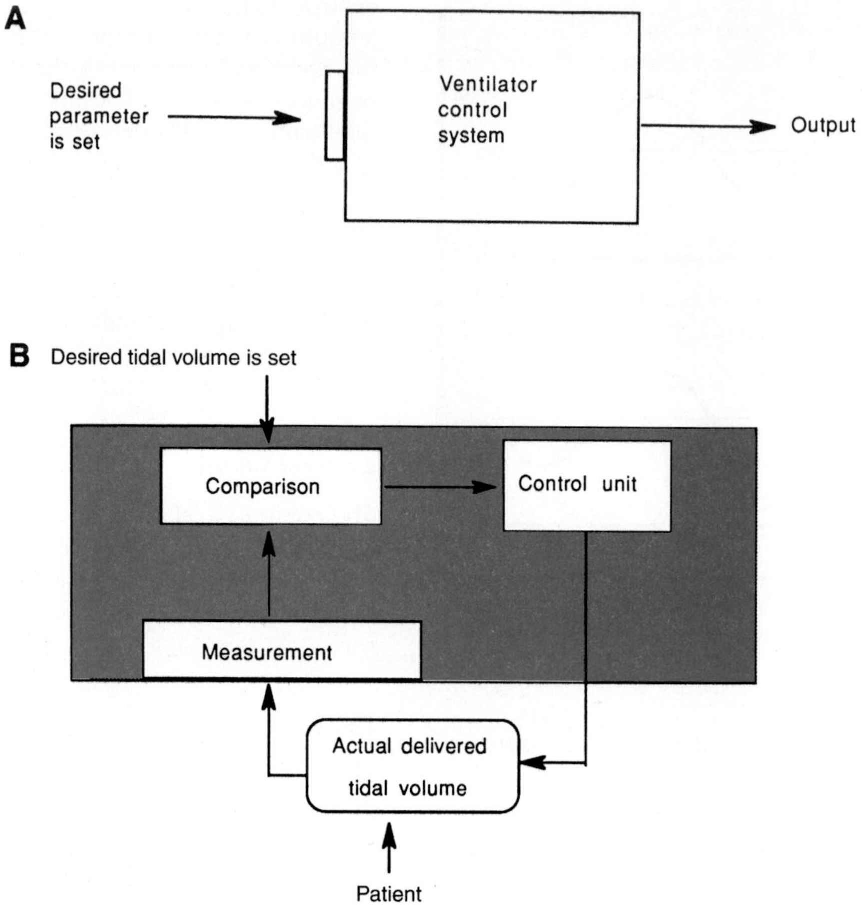

Figure 9-4 **A,** open-loop system; **B,** closed-loop system using tidal volume as the measured parameter. (From Pilbeam SP: Mechanical ventilation: physiological and clinical applications, ed 3, St Louis, 1998, Mosby.)

BOX 9-3

Types of Internal Circuits

- A single circuit is one in which the gas supply that powers the ventilator is the same gas that goes to the patient.
- A double circuit has a source gas that powers the unit by compressing a bag or bellows containing the gas that will go to the patient.

the **power transmission systems,** but they are sometimes called the **drive mechanisms.**

From an engineering point of view, there are two basic categories that describe the power transmission system in most conventional ventilators: those controlling volume delivery, and those controlling flow delivery.[7-11] For electrically powered ventilators that control volume delivery, these systems might be **compressors** or **blowers,** and **volume-displacement devices.** For pneumatically powered systems, the power transmission unit may consist of Venturi entrainers, flexible diaphragms, or specially designed pneumatic or fluidic elements. For pneumatically powered, microprocessor-controlled units the power transmission devices might be **flow-control valves.** The following section reviews examples of power transmission systems.

Compressors or Blowers

Compressors can be driven by pistons, rotating blades (vanes), moving diaphragms or bellows. Large, piston-type, water-cooled compressors are used by hospitals to supply high-pressure air for wall air outlets. Small portable compressors are used for powering small-volume nebulizers and similar devices. The most common type of compressor used for ventilators are **rotary compressors.** The rotor acts as a fan, drawing air from the room, compressing it, and directing it through the ventilator's internal circuit. Add-on compressors (those not built into the unit) can provide a 50-psi gas source to power the ventilator when a wall outlet is not available. Box 9-5 and Figure 9-6 provide a historical perspective on ventilators that used compressors as power sources.

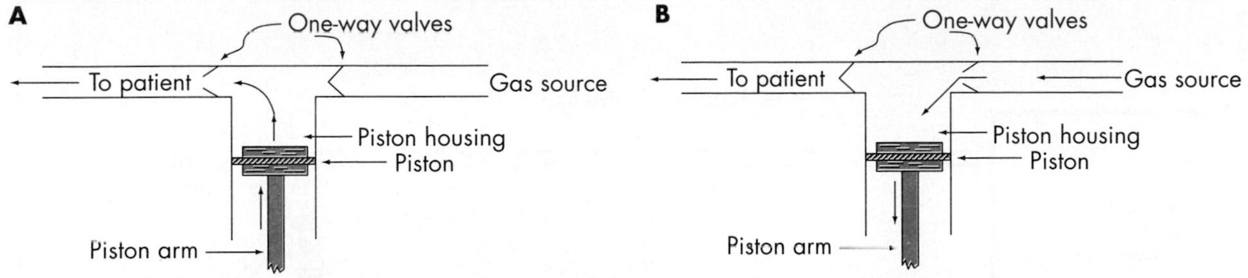

Figure 9-5 A ventilator using a single-circuit design. Gases drawn into the device's power source, which is a piston in this case, are sent directly into the patient circuit. (From Pilbeam SP, Mechanical ventilation: physiological and clinical applications, ed 3, St Louis, 1998, Mosby.)

BOX 9-4

Basic Elements of a Patient Circuit

1. A main inspiratory line that connects the ventilator output to the patient's airway adapter or connector.
2. An adapter that fits this tube to the patient's airway; it is also called a patient adapter or "wye" connector because of its shape.
3. An expiratory line that carries expired gas from the patient to the expiratory valve.
4. An expiratory valve that conducts the patient's exhaled gas from the expiratory line to the room.

(From Pilbeam SP: Mechanical ventilation: physiological and clinical applications, St Louis, 1998, Mosby.)

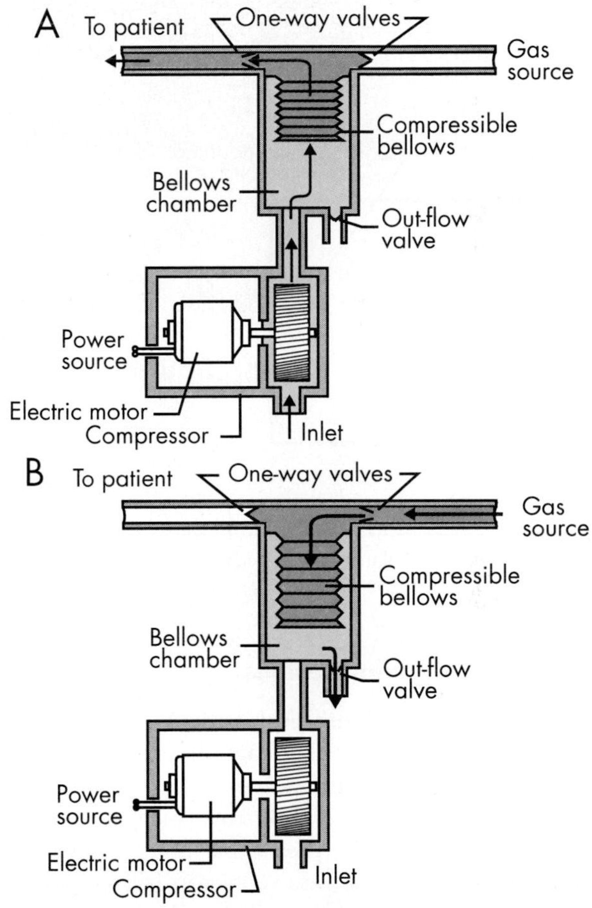

Figure 9-6 A ventilator is using a double-circuit design. The compressor produces a high-pressure gas source, which is directed to a chamber that holds a collapsible bellows. The bellows contains the desired gas mixture that will go to the patient. The pressure from the compressor forces the bellows upward, resulting in a positive-pressure breath (A). After the inspiratory breath is delivered, the compressor no longer directs pressure to the chamber and exhalation occurs. The bellows drops to its original position and fills with the desired delivery gas in preparation of the next breath (B). (From Pilbeam SP: Mechanical ventilation: physiological and clinical applications, ed 3, St Louis, 1998, Mosby.)

BOX 9-5

Historical Note

Use of the Rotary Compressor

Some of the older ventilators developed in the 1950s and '60s were never connected to wall air sources because at that time wall outlets for air were scarce. An internal compressor was sometimes used within the ventilator as the power source itself. For example, the rotating vane compressor in the MA-1 provided the driving pressure to power the drive mechanism. In this case, an electric motor powered a blower that held a series of blades, similar to a fan. The rotary blower caused gas to flow to a cannister containing a bellows, which forced air into the cannister. The bellows emptied, sending the gas inside it to the patient (see Figure 9-6).

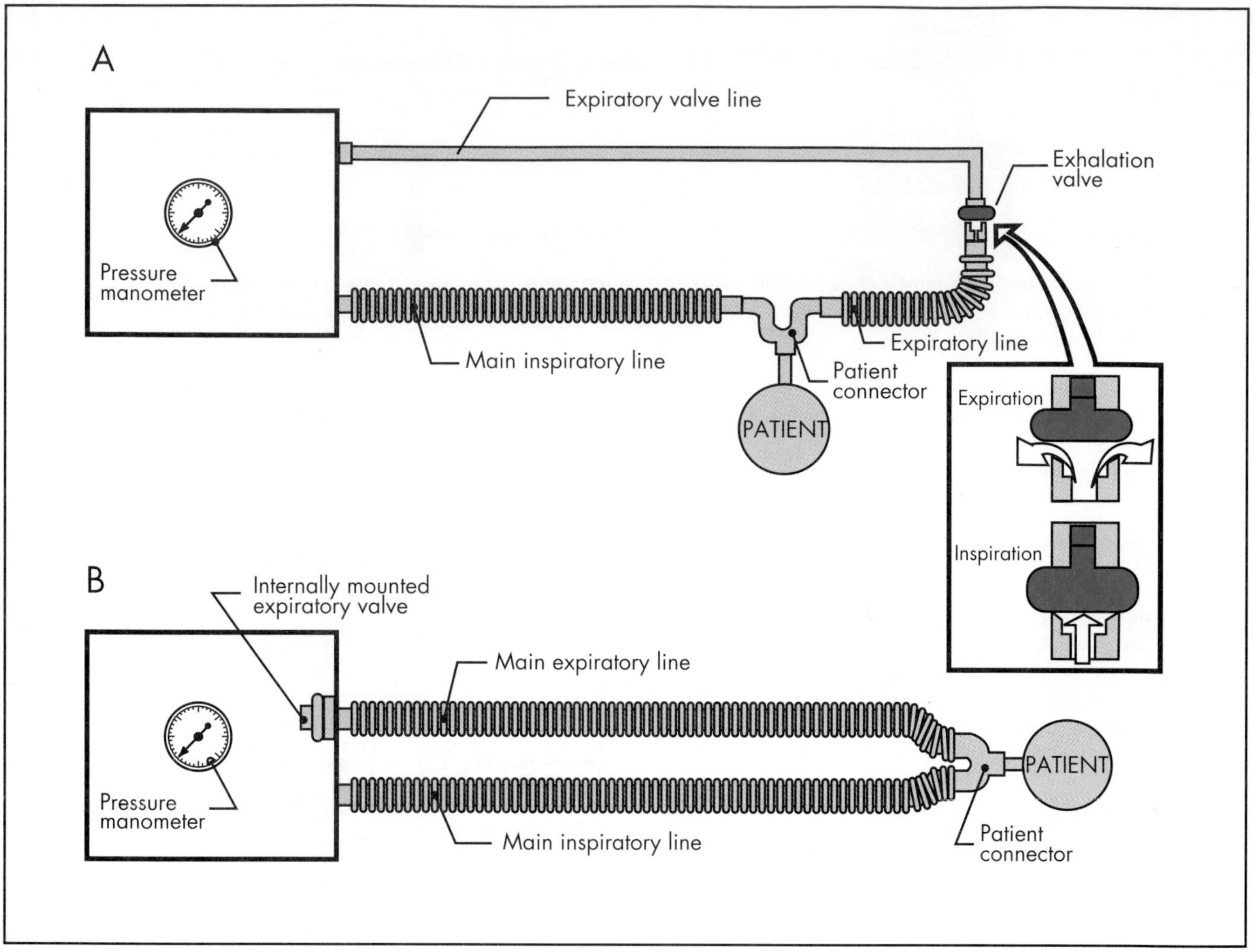

Figure 9-7 **A,** a ventilator circuit with an externally mounted expiratory valve; **B,** a ventilator circuit with an internally mounted exhalation valve.

Volume-Displacement Designs

Some ventilators use volume-displacement devices, including pistons, bellows, concertina bags, or similar "bag-in-a-chamber" mechanisms, to deliver a positive-pressure breath.[9] Many of the older ventilators, such as the MA-I and the Emerson Post-Op, used a bag-in-a-chamber or a piston design. Some home-care ventilators still use pistons, and one of the newer ICU ventilators, Cardiopulmonary Corporation's Venturi, uses a bag-in-a-chamber circuit.

Pistons

There are two commonly used piston designs: the direct drive and the indirect drive. In a direct, or **linear drive piston,** special gearing connects an electrical motor to a piston rod or arm (Figure 9-8 **A**). The rod moves the piston forward linearly inside the cylinder housing at a constant rate. This produces a constant or rectangular waveform of gas flow to the patient, an ascending ramp volume waveform, and a relatively linear ascending ramp pressure waveform (Figure 9-9). Ventilators that use linear drive pistons are usually single-circuit units. Some high-frequency ventilators use **direct drive pistons.** The recently incorporated use of the rolling-seal or low-resistance materials have helped eliminate the friction of the early piston/cylinder designs. For example, the Nellcor Puritan Bennett 740 uses a very low-resistance piston that provides all the gas flow to patient and does not require an external high-pressure gas source to function (electrically powered).[9]

Rotary or nonlinear drive pistons are sometimes called eccentric drive pistons (see Figure 9-8 **B**). Gas flow is slowest at the beginning and end of inspiration and the fastest at mid-inspiration, producing a sine-wavelike flow pattern. Figure 9-10 shows a complete forward cycle of such a unit. The piston is connected to the outer edge of the drive wheel. The piston's forward motion is short at the beginning of inspiration (A1 to B1), rapid at mid-inspiration (B1 to C1), and slow again at the end of inspiration (C1 to D1). This change in speed produces the sine-wavelike flow

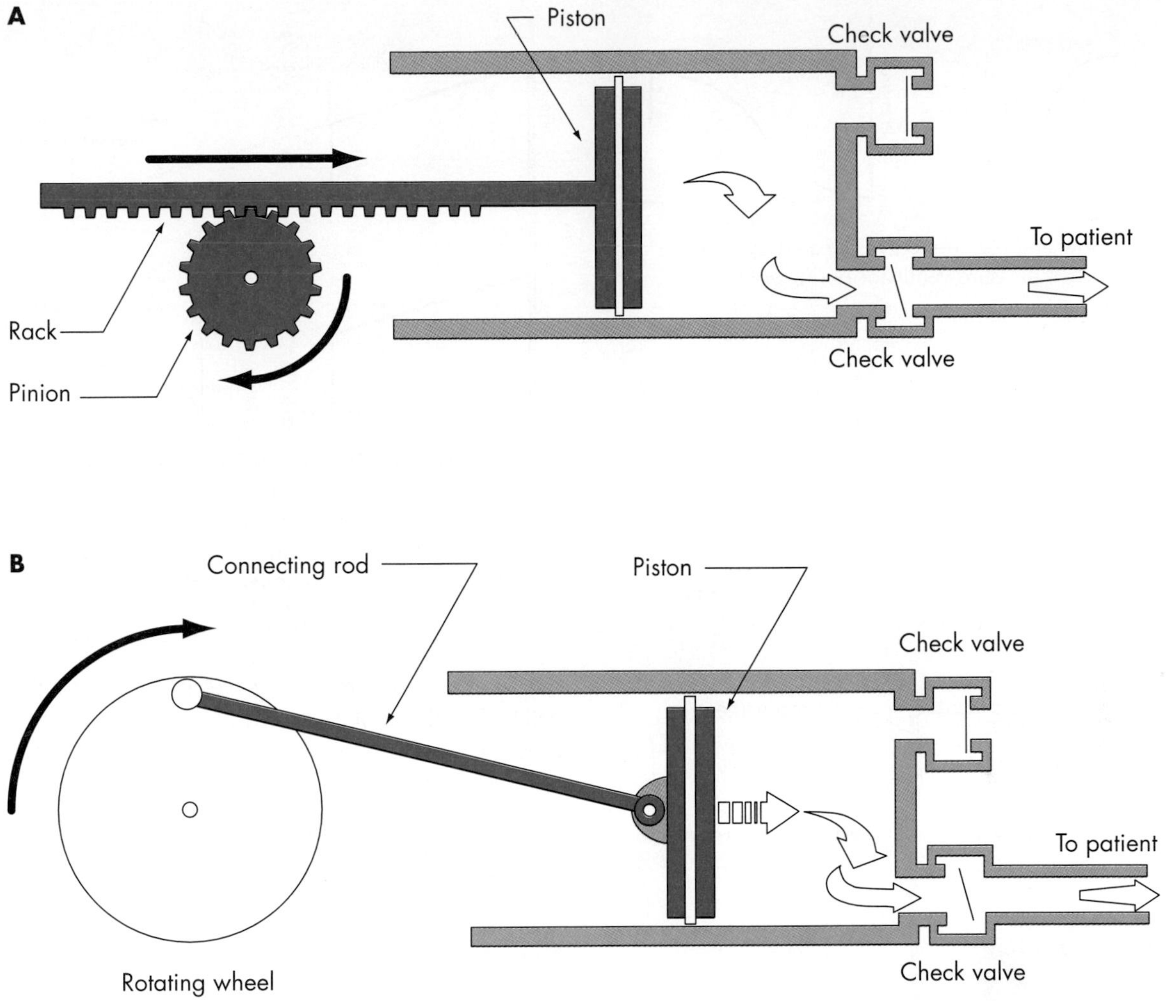

Figure 9-8 **A,** linear, and **B,** rotary, piston-driven mechanisms for ventilators. (Redrawn from Dupuis Y: Ventilators, ed 2, St Louis, 1992, Mosby.)

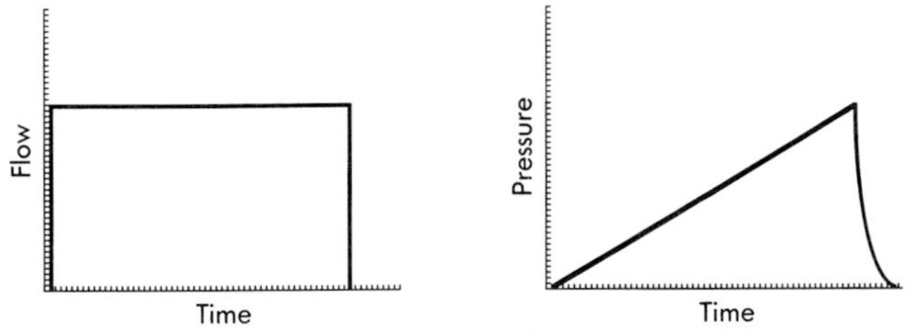

Figure 9-9 The flow/time and pressure/time curves for a linear drive piston.

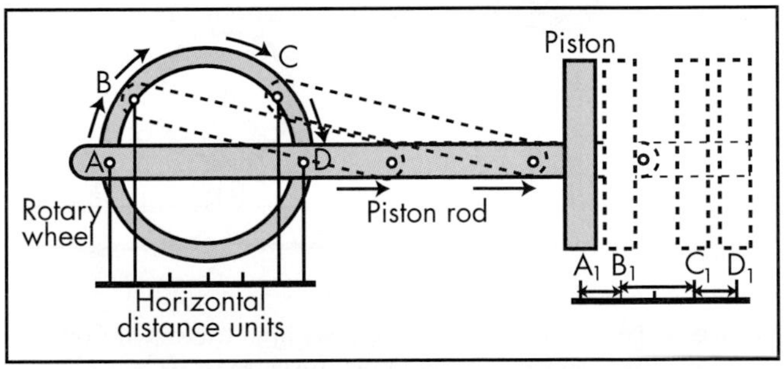

Figure 9-10 A diagram of the rotary-driven piston's movement. The times between points *A* and *B*, *B* and *C*, and *C* and *D* are equal.

curve (Figure 9-11). Note that the **rotary drive piston** produces half of the sinusoidal wave during the inspiratory phase, but it is commonly referred to as a sine wave or sinewavelike pattern.

Bag in a Chamber

Piston-driven ventilators can be double- as well as single-circuit ventilators. A double-circuit, piston-driven ventilator is shown in Figure 9-12. A piston drives air into a chamber, which compresses a bag containing the gas for the patient. Although not a common design for most ICU ventilators, the recently introduced Venturi ventilator uses this concept in its patient circuit.

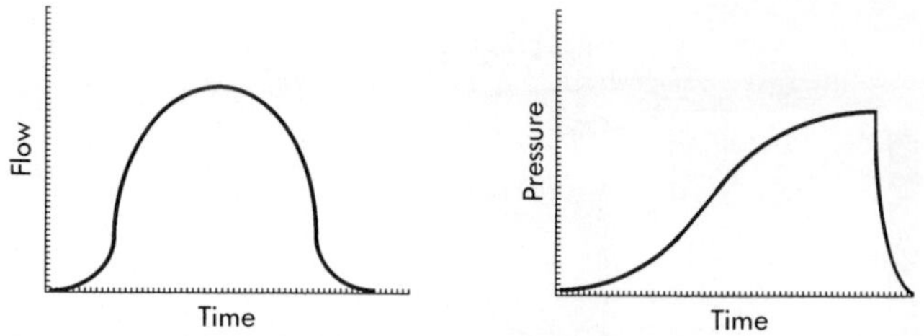

Figure 9-11 Flow and pressure curves created by a rotary-driven piston, positive-pressure ventilator during volume delivery.

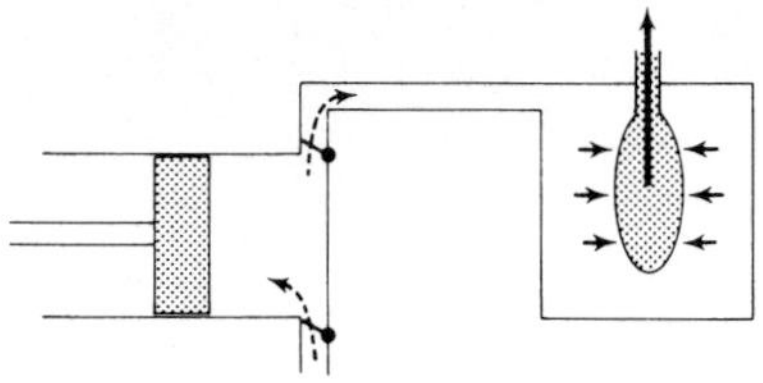

Figure 9-12 A simple diagram of a piston-driven, double-circuit system (i.e., bag-in-a-chamber).

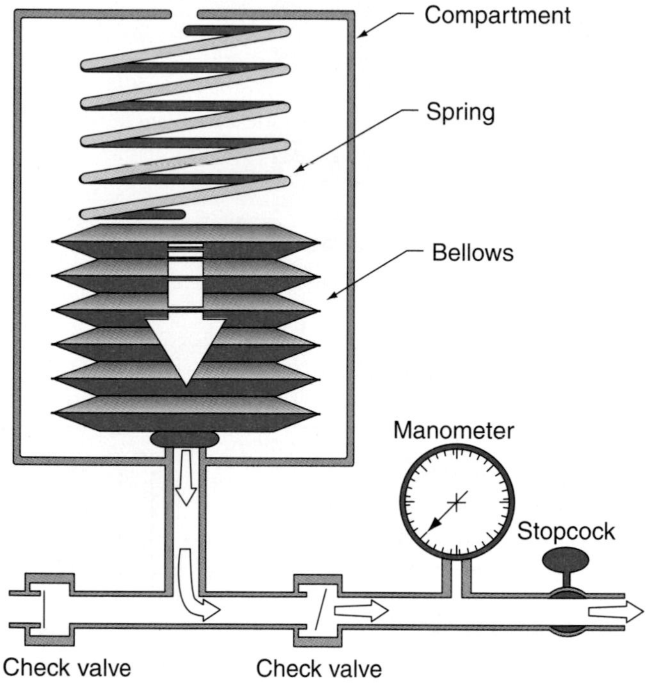

Figure 9-13 A spring-loaded bellows unit. (Redrawn from Dupuis Y: Ventilators, ed 2, St Louis, 1992, Mosby.)

Spring-Loaded Bellows

Another volume design unit uses a **spring-loaded bellows** to act as the force behind the breath (Figure 9-13). A mixture of oxygen and air at the desired FiO_2 flows into a bellows, which has a spring that applies a force to the unit (Pressure = force/area). The operator can tighten the spring to increase the force and pressure delivered to the patient. The Servo 900C ventilator uses this type of power transmission system and can be adjusted up to 120 cm H_2O.

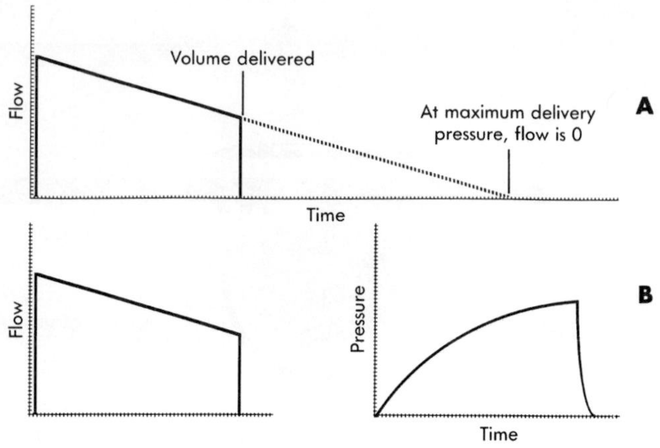

Figure 9-14 **A,** The primary flow curve from a spring-loaded bellows with a low working pressure and a high system resistance (i.e., high patient airway resistance and low lung compliance). **B,** Flow/time and pressure/time curves for this system when the breath is time-cycled.

The flow and pressure curves produced by this system will be like those of a linear drive piston when the working pressure is high and the system resistance (patient lung condition and patient circuit) is low (SEE Figure 9-9). When the working pressure is low, especially when the system resistance is high, the flow curve descends during inspiration (Figure 9-14).

Flow-Control Valves

Most of the current ICU ventilators use valves that precisely control flow to the patient. In general, high-pressure sources of air and oxygen are mixed and delivered at the desired FiO_2 to accumulator chambers. From these chambers, gas is sent through a valve that controls the inspiratory gas flow to the patient. These valves can be moved in small precise increments and varying rates because their activity is governed by a microprocessor. Flow-control valve function is so rapid that these valves have almost exclusively replaced the volume-delivery "bag-in-a-chamber" drive mechanisms in ICU ventilator operation. Some ventilators still use pistons, and operating room anesthetic machines use bag-in-a-chamber designs to help separate the breathing gas and help avoid any contamination. Three common flow-controlling valves are worth further discussion: proportional solenoids, stepper motors with valves, and digital valves with on/off configurations.

Proportional Solenoid Valves

Proportional solenoid valves control flow by using an on/off switch (Figure 9-15). A common example of this valve contains a gate or plunger, a valve seat, an electromagnet, a diaphragm, a spring, two electrical contacts, and an adjustable electrical current. The current flows through a coil and creates a magnetic field (e.g., an electromagnet.)

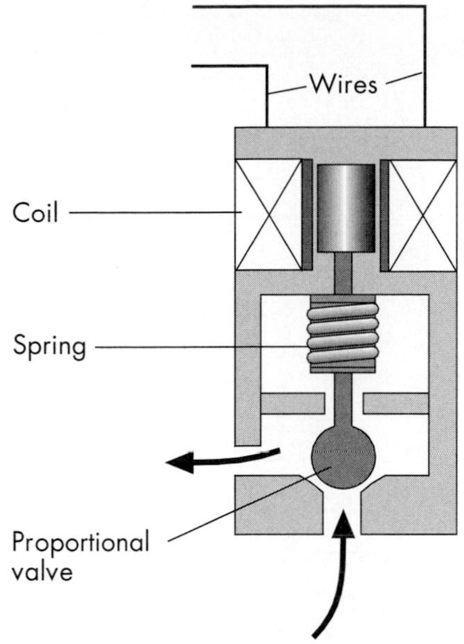

Figure 9-15 A proportional solenoid valve. (Redrawn from Sanborn WG: Respir Care 38:72, 1993)

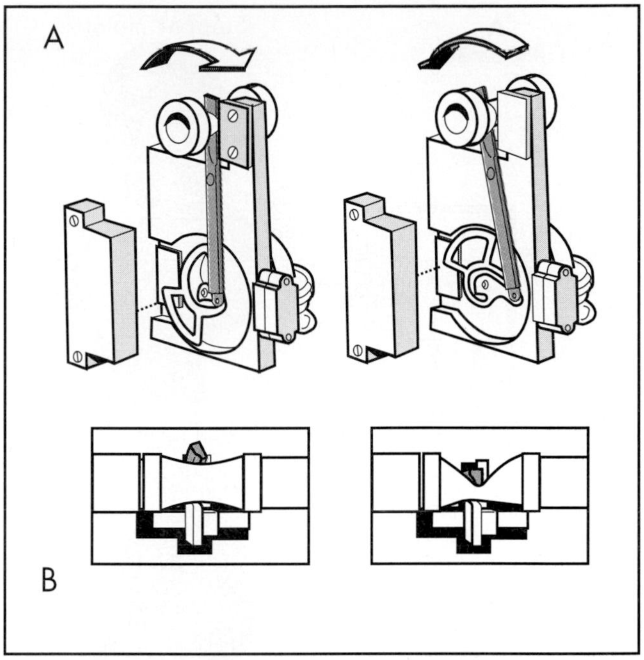

Figure 9-16 A stepper motor with a scissor valve in the Siemens Servo 900C ventilator. **A,** A cam on the motor controls the moving arm. On the left, the valve is shown in the closed position, and on the right, it is completely open. (Courtesy of Siemens Life Support Systems, Schaumburg, Ill.) **B,** The closing and opening of the internal circuit by the scissor valve.

The strength of the magnetic field produced depends on the amount of current used. The magnetic field results in movement of the gate or plunger and causes the plunger to assume a specific position. The design of a proportional solenoid varies by manufacturer.

Besides using an electrical current, which is often microprocessor-controlled or controlled by an electric timer, solenoids can also be controlled by manual operation and by pressure. Manual operation closes a switch, which sends a current to the electromagnet and alters the valve position. Air pressure changes often caused by an actively breathing patient can cause a diaphragm to descend, closing an electric contact and altering valve position. Examples of ventilators with proportional solenoid valves are the Nellcor Puritan Bennett 7200, the Hamilton VEOLAR and GALILEO, the Dräger Evita, and the Siemens Servo 300.

Stepper Motor with Valve

Stepper motors can move in very rapid, discreet steps to open or close a valve. Electricity is used to power the motor that controls the movement of a lever arm on a hinged clamp that is similar to a scissors valve. Stepper motors are considered digital valves as opposed to analog valves, which do not move in discreet steps. An example of a stepper motor occurs in the Siemens Servo 900C ventilator. Flow metering is accomplished by a stepper-motor–driven scissors valve that pinches a silicon tube, thus controlling gas flow to the patient (Figure 9-16).

Figure 9-17 shows a microprocessor-controlled stepper motor, which consists of a cam connected to a stepper motor and a spring-loaded plunger attached to a wheel. The tension of the spring pushes the wheel against the perimeter of the cam. During exhalation, the plunger occludes the gas outlet and stops flow to the patient. During inspiration, the motor turns the cam, and the spring tension relaxes, although contact is still maintained. Because of this action, the plunger moves to the right (Figure 9-17 **B**), and gas flows to the patient. There is an optical sensor and a shutter, which sends information to the microprocessor about the position of the cam, and thus the plunger. Through microprocessor control, the motor can rotate the cam in many specific steps and at different speeds, allowing the microprocessor to deliver gas flow in the pattern and amount the operator selects.[12]

Although several ventilators incorporate stepper motors as flow-control valves, there are several different motor and cam designs for controlling valve or poppet position in each. For example, in the Infrasonics Adult Star Ventilator, there is a flow-metering orifice directly coupled to a stepper motor. In the Bear 1000 and the Bird 8400 ventilators, stepper-motor–driven cam devices actuate flow-control valves. Figure 9-18 shows one example of an externally actuated proportional valve, but there are several different motor and cam designs for controlling valve or poppet position.

Digital Valve On/Off Configuration

With a digital valve on/off configuration, several valves operate simultaneously, assuming either an open or closed position (Figure 9-19). A given valve produces a specific flow by opening or closing a certain size orifice. Depending

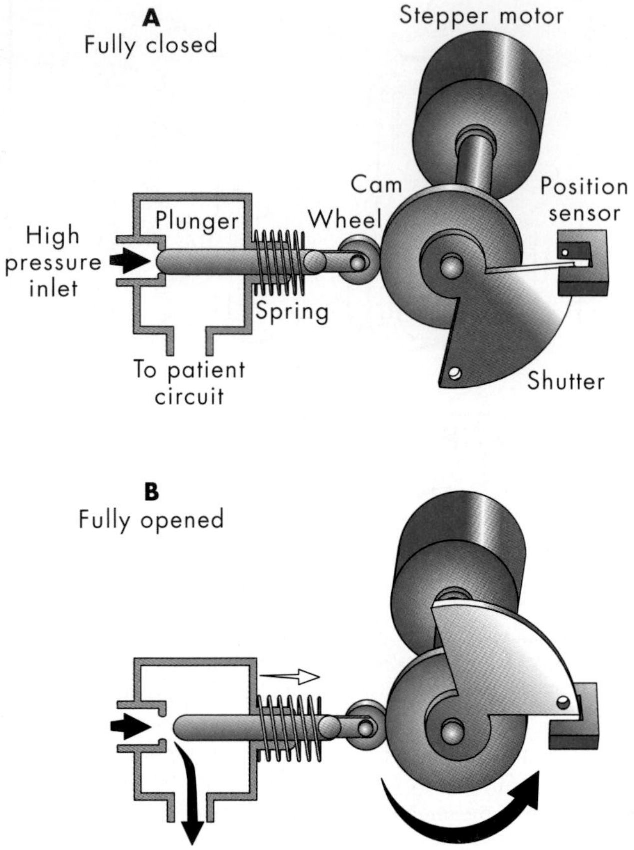

Figure 9-17 A schematic of a microprocessor-operated flow valve. (See text for description). (Redrawn from Dupuis Y: Ventilators, ed 2, St Louis, 1992, Mosby.)

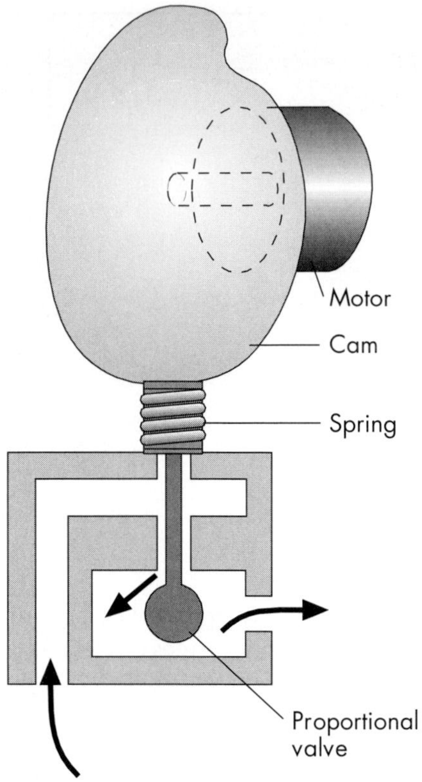

Figure 9-18 This is an example of an externally actuated proportional valve. (Redrawn from Sanborn WG: Respir Care 38:72, 1993.)

on which valves are open, the amount of flow can be varied. The Infrasonics Infant Star ventilator uses this type of valve configuration.

Fluidic Elements in Power Transmission Design

Units using **fluidics** or **fluid logic** to deliver gas flow to the patient do not require moving parts or electrical circuits to function. Control is provided solely through fluid dynamics. Fluidic units use air and/or oxygen as the operating medium and employ all of the same basic functional controls as electrically operated ventilators.[12-14] The Sechrist IV-100B and the Monaghan 225 are examples of fluidic ventilators.

Fluidic devices use two basic physical principles: wall attachment and **beam deflection.** The principle of wall attachment is commonly called the **Coanda effect** (Box 9-6 and Figure 9-20), a phenomenon that occurs when an air stream (jet stream) is forced through an opening. The jet exits the opening, creating a localized drop in pressure adjacent to itself. Ambient air is drawn toward the jet stream on all sides as a result of the localized low pressure associated with the rapid movement of the jet through the air

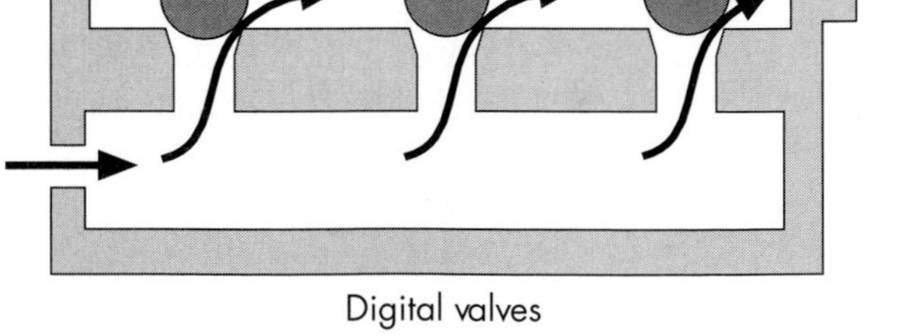

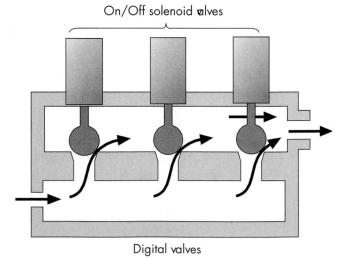

Figure 9-19 An on/off digital-valve design for flow control. Each valve controls a critical orifice and thus a specified flow. The number of discreet flow steps (from zero upward) becomes 2^n, where n is the number of valves. (Redrawn from Sanborn WG: Respir Care 38:72, 1993.)

BOX 9-6

Historical Note

The Coanda Effect

In 1932, Dr. Henri Coanda, a Romanian aeronautical engineer, first described the "wall attachment" phenomenon. Consequently, this effect now carries his name.[14]

BOX 9-7

The Coanda Effect

As gas travels faster over a pocket of turbulent air, the increased forward molecular velocity of the gas causes a decreased lateral pressure by the pocket as adjacent molecules are sheared away by the jet stream. The surrounding gas molecules (i.e., those not in the stream) then possess a higher pressure, thus holding the stream against the wall (see Figure 9-20 **B**).

(Figure 9-20 **A**). When a wall is added to one side of the jet stream, as seen in **B,** the entrained gas can only enter from the opposite side. However, a **separation bubble** (a low-pressure vortex) develops between the wall and the jet stream. The bubble attracts or bends the jet stream toward the wall. The pocket of turbulence forms an air foil, similar to that seen with an airplane wing (Box 9-7).[12-14] When the gas entrained into the bubble from the jet stream equals the amount of air moving from the vortex flow of the bubble back to the jet stream, the attachment is stable.

The second important phenomenon of fluid logic is beam deflection. When a beam or jet of gas is moving through a fluid device, the direction of the beam can be changed by hitting the beam with another jet of gas. The second gas jet usually comes from the side, at a right angle to the main jet stream. Beam deflection is best understood by studying some of the fluidic elements (components) of ventilator function (Box 9-8). The nomenclature used in fluidics has its origin in digital electronics, which is why many of the terms seem unusual in relation to those for medical terminology.

A **flip-flop valve** is a basic element of fluidic devices and uses the principles of wall attachment (Coanda effect) and beam deflection. As shown in Figure 9-21 **A,** when a pressurized gas source enters at P_S, wall attachment occurs. In this example, the gas has entered at C_2, resulting in wall attachment toward the left. The separation bubble occurs on the left, which results in the gas stream exiting at outlet 2 (O_2). The gas flow continues to exit at outlet 2 unless a single, controlled pulse of gas is directed at the main jet

BOX 9-8

Some Common Examples of Fluidic Elements Used in the Design of Fluidically Operated Ventilators

1. Flip-flop component
2. OR/NOR gate
3. AND/NAND gate
4. Back-pressure switch
5. Proportional amplifier
6. Schmitt trigger

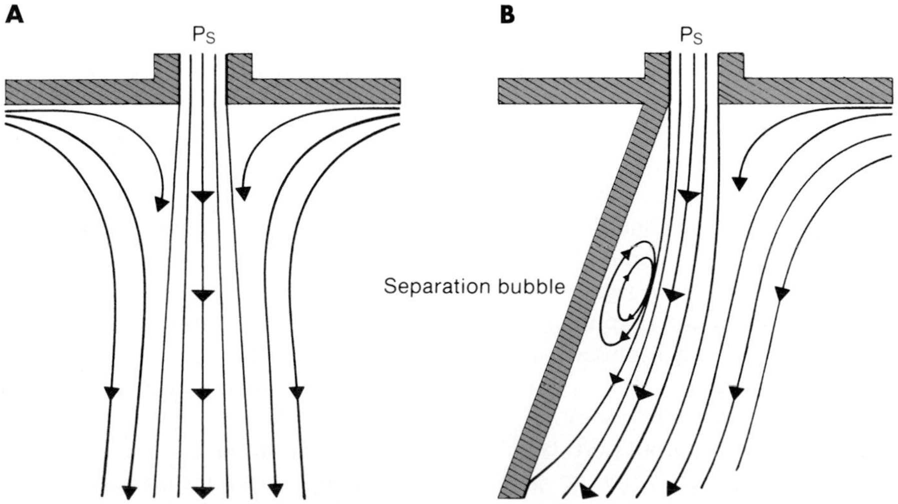

Figure 9-20 The Coanda effect, or the wall attachment phenomenon: **A,** turbulent jet flow causes a local drop in lateral pressure and draws air inward; **B,** a wall placed adjacent to the jet stream creates a low-pressure vortex or separation bubble. The gas stream tends to bend toward that wall. (From Dupuis Y: Ventilators, ed 2, St Louis, 1992, Mosby.)

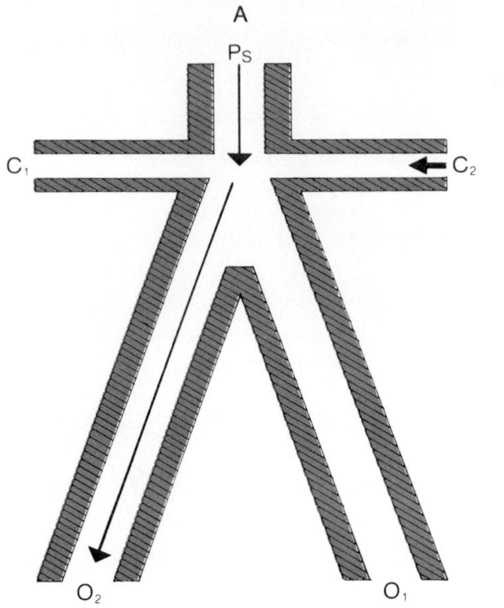

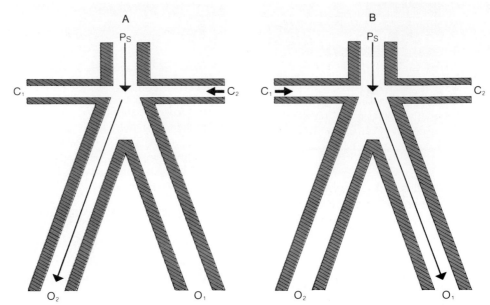

Figure 9-21 A diagramatic representation of a flip-flop valve. (See text for explanation.) (From Dupuis Y: Ventilators, ed 2, St Louis, 1992, Mosby.)

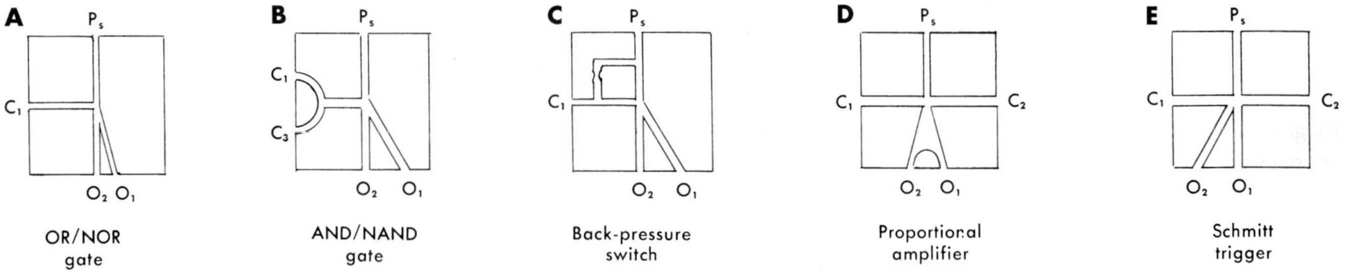

Figure 9-22 Symbols for some common fluidic elements, as established by the National Fluid Power Association.[14] **A,** OR/NOR; **B,** AND/NAND; **C,** Back-Pressure switch; **D,** Proportional amplifier; and **E,** Schmitt trigger.

stream. On the right side of **B,** the controlled pulse of gas enters at C_1 and redirects the main gas flow to exit at outlet 1 (O_1). The flip-flop valve is a **bistable** device, which means that it is capable of two stable output states and has no preference for either wall.

The **OR/NOR gate** is a **monostable** device, which means that it can direct to only one outlet unless acted upon (Figure 9-22 **A**). The OR/NOR gate only has one input and two possible outputs. Without a control signal from C_1, output is normally at O_2. Input of a control beat at C_1 causes beam deflection to output O_1 (see Figure 9-21 **A**). When the control signal is removed, the output returns to O_2. Note that OR/NOR gates generally have several input choices, any one of which can be used.

The **AND/NAND gate** is another monostable device with two control ports and two output ports (see Figure 9-22 **B**). The primary outlet is O_2 when no control signal is present. Simultaneous input signals from C_1 and C_2 change the outlet to O_1.

The **back-pressure switch** (see Figure 9-22 **C**) allows most gas to outlet at O_2, and some gas from P_S to escape out C_1, the control port, because of the construction of the control port and the restriction built into this loop. When C_1 is occluded, pressure is redirected, which causes beam deflection and an outlet switch (from O_2 to O_1).

A **proportional amplifier** has two opposing control ports, C_1 and C_2 (see Figure 9-22 **D**), and two outlets, O_2 and O_1. It also has a different **splitter configuration** than the AND/NAND and OR/NOR gates (Box 9-9), and because of this difference, wall attachment does not occur and gas from P_S leaves from both outlets. When the input at C_1 equals that at C_2, the output from O_2 and O_1 is equal, and the **differential output** is zero. (Differential output is the difference between the output of O_1 and O_2.) When C_1 is greater than C_2, O_1 has the higher output, and vice versa (Box 9-10).

The **Schmitt trigger** is actually an integrated circuit made up of several proportional devices (3 proportional amplifiers and 2 flip-flop valves) connected in a series. Figure 9-22 **E** shows the fluidic symbol for the Schmitt Trigger. In the absence of control signals from ports C_1 and C_2, the outlet is O_1. Beam deflection occurs with a control signal

BOX 9-9

Definition of a Splitter

The splitter is the intersecting point that the main input gas hits as it descends into the device. When gas hits the splitter in the proportional amplifier, the gas is directed down both the right and left legs of the unit to outlets O_2 and O_1, respectively (see Figure 9-22 **D,** proportional amplifier).

BOX 9-10

Decision Making & Problem Solving

Compare the slitter configuration of the OR/NOR device to that in the proportional amplifier. How does the design of each affect the function of the element?

See Appendix A for the answer.

from C_2. When the control signal is removed, output automatically returns to O_1. Because of this, the Schmitt trigger is classified as a monostable device. The utility of Schmitt triggers lies in their ability to sense very small pressure changes between C_1 and C_2 to cause outputs at O_1 and O_2. They are often used in pressure-cycled fluidic ventilators.

Because of the variety of functions that can be performed by fluidic elements, it becomes apparent this technology can be used in many ventilation devices.

BASIC COMPONENTS OF BREATH DELIVERY

For a ventilator to accomplish breath delivery, it must be able to provide the four basic phases of a breath and assume all or part of the work of breathing. The four phases, which are controlled by **phase variables,** are listed in Box 9-11.[8] The following sections discuss these concepts in more detail.

Model Description of Shared Work of Breathing

Two forces are available to perform work of breathing: the patient's muscles and the ventilator. The ventilator must also be adjustable so the operator can balance the work between these two components. This balance is best described by the equation of motion (Box 9-12) and is shown in Figure 9-23. For a single breath, the compliance and resistance of the respiratory system do not change significantly, but the volume, pressure, flow and time can vary and are regulated by the ventilator.[2,15]

BOX 9-11

The Four Phases of a Breath During Mechanical Ventilation

1. End of expiration and beginning of inspiration
2. Delivery of inspiration
3. End of inspiration and beginning of expiration
4. Expiratory phase

Phase variables are controlled by the ventilator and are responsible for each of the four parts of a breath.

The Phase Variables

Triggering: begins inspiratory gas flow
Cycling: ends inspiratory gas flow
Limiting: places a maximum value on a control variable (pressure, volume, flow, and/or time) during delivery of a breath

BOX 9-12

Equation of Motion

Muscle Pressure + Ventilator Pressure = Elastic Recoil Pressure + Flow Resistance Pressure, or
$Pmus + P_{TR} = V/C + (Raw \times flow)$

Pmus is the pressure generated by the muscles of ventilation (i.e., muscle pressure). If these muscles are not active, this is equal to zero.
P_{TR} is the transrespiratory pressure (Pawo − Pbs [i.e., the airway opening pressure minus the body surface pressure]) and basically is the pressure read on the ventilator gauge during inspiration with intermittent positive-pressure ventilation (ventilator pressure).
V is volume delivered.
C is respiratory system compliance.
V/C is elastic recoil pressure.
Raw is respiratory system resistance.
Flow is the gas flow during inspiration (i.e., Raw × flow, flow resistance).
Because P_{TA} = Raw × flow, and alveolar pressure (P_A) = V/C, the following substitutions can be made in the equation above:

$$P_{mus} + P_{TR} = P_A + P_{TA}$$

(From Pilbeam SP: Mechanical ventilation: physiological and clinical applications, St Louis, ed 3, 1998, Mosby.)

Type of Breath Delivery

As mentioned, work of breathing can be provided by the ventilator and the patient, so there is more than one possible type of breath delivery. If the ventilator does all the work of breathing (i.e., starts the breath, controls inspiratory gas delivery, and ends inspiration), this is called a **mandatory breath. Assisted breaths,** on the other hand, are

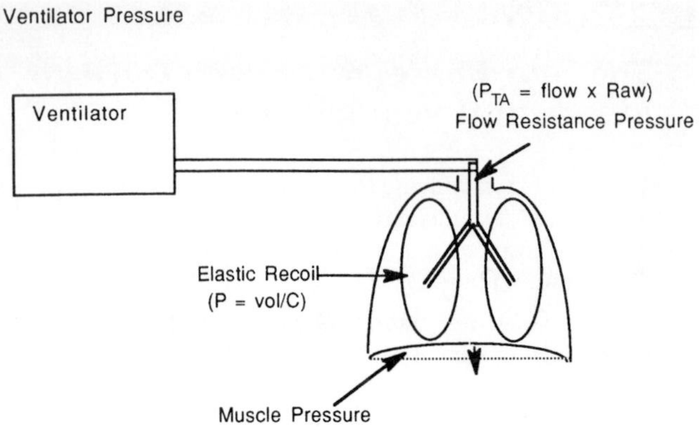

Figure 9-23 Equation of motion model. (From Pilbeam SP: Mechanical ventilation: physiological and clinical applications, ed 3, St Louis, 1998, Mosby.)

BOX 9-13

Other Names for Volume and Pressure Ventilation

Volume Ventilation

Volume-limited ventilation
Volume-controlled ventilation
Volume-targeted ventilation

Pressure Ventilation

Pressure-limited ventilation
Pressure-controlled ventilation
Pressure-targeted ventilation

those in which inspiration is begun by the patient, but the ventilator controls the inspiratory phase and ends inspiration. **Spontaneous breaths** are those in which the patient controls all phases of inspiration.

Another important aspect of breath delivery is whether the operator wishes to control the volume or the pressure delivered to the patient. **Volume ventilation (VV)** involves setting a desired tidal volume, and **pressure ventilation (PV)** refers to setting a desired pressure. Box 9-13 lists alternative names for each; it can be very confusing with so many names meaning basically the same thing.

Phases of a Breath

When the term *breath* is used, it is usually used for inspiration, but a breath really consists of a total respiratory cycle; that is, the time required for both inspiration (T_I) and expiration (T_E) and the events that occur during that time. This time frame is also called the **total cycle time (TCT).** A ventilator must be capable of separating a breath into the following four parts (see Box 9-11):

1. The **trigger variable** begins inspiration.
2. Breath delivery (inspiration) is accomplished when the ventilator establishes the control variables (pressure, flow, volume, and time).
3. The **cycle variable** ends the inspiratory phase and begins exhalation.
4. Pressures can be controlled during exhalation, thus the ventilator can be involved in the expiratory phase.

Beginning of Inspiration: the Triggering Variable

The trigger variable begins the inspiratory phase. Ventilators can be either time-, pressure-, flow-, or volume-triggered. For example, when the variable is time, the ventilator controls the beginning of inspiration, starting the breath after a specific measured time (time triggering). When pressure, flow, or volume begin the breath, the patient controls the beginning of inspiration. This is called **patient triggering.**

The triggering variable must not be confused with the cycling variable. Triggering begins inspiration; cycling, which is discussed later, ends inspiration. The purpose for mentioning this difference is that the term *cycle* used to mean the variable that began the breath, although some journal articles and technical manuals still occasionally use this terminology.

Time Triggering

With time triggering, the ventilator controls the beginning of inspiration based on the rate or the inspiratory time set on the control panel by the operator. When a patient's breathing is being time triggered, this is sometimes called **control ventilation.** The breath is mandatory.

Patient Triggering

Ventilators can be adjusted to sense patient inspiratory effort. The control set by the operator is commonly called the sensitivity setting, or **trigger sensitivity.** Pressure and flow are the most common variables used for patient triggering. **Pressure triggering** occurs when the ventilator senses a drop in pressure below baseline in the circuit. Pressure triggering is usually set from -0.5 to -2.0 cm H_2O (i.e., the pressure must drop by this amount below baseline to begin inspiration). **Baseline pressure** is the pressure maintained at the airway during exhalation and the pressure from which inspiration begins. (See the discussion of the expiratory phase later in this section.)

Pressure is commonly measured in three different locations on ventilators because pressure transducers or sensors can be placed at three common locations:

BOX 9-14

Decision Making & Problem Solving

A patient has a baseline pressure of +10 cm H_2O during mechanical ventilation. The trigger sensitivity is set at −1 cm H_2O. At what pressure will the ventilator sense a patient effort and start inspiration?

See Appendix A for the answer.

BOX 9-15

Decision Making & Problem Solving

The operator decides to use flow triggering for a patient and sets the base flow at 6 L/min and the trigger flow at 2 L/min. The base flow measurement must drop to what value before the ventilator will begin the inspiratory phase?

See Appendix A for the answer.

1. within the internal ventilator circuit near the point where the main gas flow leaves the unit,
2. where expired gas enters the unit, or
3. at the proximal airway (near the **wye connector**).

In the latter case, there is small-bore plastic tubing that runs from the front of the ventilator to the patient's wye connector (Box 9-14). (See Chapter 7 for further information on pressure monitoring devices.)

Flow triggering occurs when a drop in flow is detected. The operator commonly sets a base flow, which is present during the expiratory phase. This is set from approximately 5 to 10 L/min. A flow trigger is also set and can range from about 1 to 5 L/min, although this value varies with the type of ventilator being used and the patient's size (baby vs. adult) and inspiratory effort. Most manufacturers recommend a value with their units.

The ventilator measures the baseline flow during exhalation. When the flow drops by the amount set on the flow trigger, inspiration begins (Box 9-15). Figure 9-24 shows a flow-triggering device. Flow is most often measured near the expiration valve.

Other methods of triggering include the following:

1. Manual triggering in which the operator activates the "manual breath" control and delivers a mandatory breath based on the set variables.
2. Triggering from chest wall movement as is available in the Infrasonics Star Sync module on the Infant Star ventilator (see Chapter 11).
3. Volume triggering that occurs after a specific volume has been exhaled by the patient. This is currently used in infant ventilation (see Chapter 11).

THE INSPIRATORY PHASE

One of the most important ventilator functions is delivery of inspiratory gas flow. The first positive-pressure volume ventilators were often classified by how strong the force was behind inspiratory delivery and by the evaluation of the pressure, flow, and volume curves produced during inspiration (Box 9-16). Many current ICU ventilators, such as the Servo 300, the Bear 1000, and the T-Bird, can actually alter their function so that different inspiratory gas flow can be selected by the operator. A ventilator can now be instructed to produce specific waveform patterns for

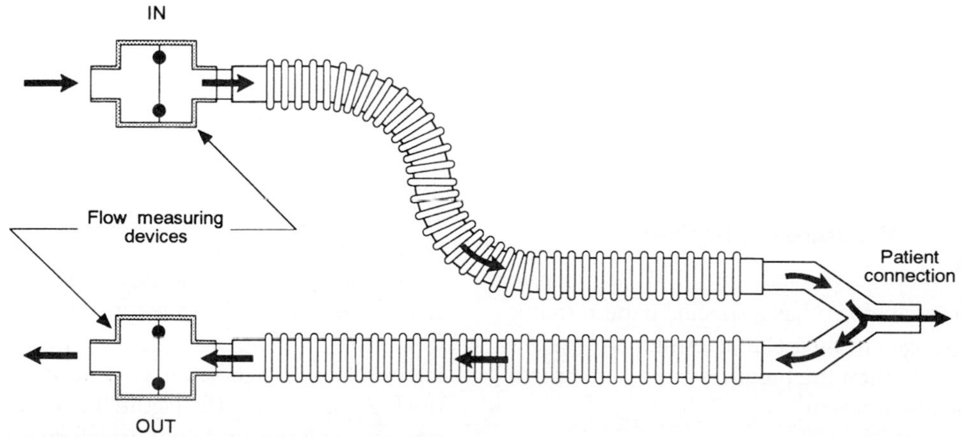

Figure 9-24 A schematic representation of flow triggering, which occurs when the patient makes an inspiratory effort and drops the flow through the patient circuit to the trigger level. (From Dupuis Y: Ventilators, ed 2, St Louis, 1992, Mosby.)

BOX 9-16

Historical Note

Classification[1,7]

Classification Was Previously Based on the Power Source

For example, the IMV Emerson ventilator was described as a high-pressure drive ventilator. A powerful electric motor was used to drive its rotary piston. Regardless of changes in patient lung characteristics, the ventilator could deliver the set volume, although pressure would increase as the work load increased.

Classification Was Also Based on the Flow Waveform Produced

For example, the IMV Emerson was also referred to as a nonconstant-flow generator because the flow produced was not constant (in this case, it was sine-wavelike) and produced the same sine pattern breath after breath, regardless of changes in patient lung characteristics.

pressure, volume, flow, or time. The two most commonly controlled variables during inspiration are volume and pressure, as mentioned previously. The type of breath being delivered is defined or identified by the waveforms produced for pressure, volume, flow, and time.

A Volume Breath (Volume-Controlled, Volume-Limited)

When the volume waveform is maintained in a specific pattern, the delivered breath is a volume breath. The volume stays the same, but the pressure waveform varies with changes in the patient lung characteristics. Ventilators capable of measuring flow and time during inspiration can use them to calculate volume.

Note that any ventilator with a set volume waveform has a set flow waveform (flow = volume/time). So a volume breath is one in which flow is also controlled (i.e., a flow-controlled breath) (Box 9-17).*

A Pressure Breath (Pressure-Controlled, Pressure-Limited)

When the pressure waveform has a specific pattern that is not affected by changes in lung characteristics, but where volume and flow vary, then the breath is a pressure breath or a pressure controlled breath.

*In this text, the terms *volume-limited* or *volume-controlled* also mean flow-limited or flow-controlled.

BOX 9-17

A Flow-Controlled Breath

Any breath that has a set flow waveform that does not change from one breath to the next—regardless of changes in lung characteristics—is a flow-controlled breath. If flow is controlled, the volume is also controlled. Thus the breath is also a volume-controlled breath.

A Time-Controlled Breath

When a ventilator delivers a breath that is time controlled, pressure, volume and flow may vary with changes in lung characteristics. Time is constant. An example of timed breaths are those produced during **high-frequency jet ventilation** and high-frequency oscillation. Time-controlled ventilation is less commonly used than pressure or volume ventilation. Compare time controlled ventilation to time-triggered, pressure-limited, time-cycled breaths (see the section on limiting factors during inspiration).

Inspiratory Waveform and Ventilator Graphics

The operator of a ventilator can select any of the following:

1. The type of pressure delivery (positive- vs. negative-pressure ventilation).
2. The type of control variable (pressure-, volume-, flow-, or time-controlled).
3. The type of triggering (time or patient), which helps determine if the breath is mandatory, assisted, or spontaneous.
4. The type of flow or pressure waveform.

The two most common flow waveforms used for volume ventilation are the constant (rectangular) and the descending ramp (decelerating ramp) waveforms. The two most commonly occurring pressure waveforms are the constant and the ascending exponential.

Monitoring and evaluating graphic waveforms produced during ventilation has become a popular way to determine how patients are being ventilated and whether or not problems are occurring during ventilation. Although more detailed descriptions of waveform use are available elsewhere,[6] a summary of the more common waveforms produced during ventilation is provided here.

Pressure, volume, and flow graphed over time are also called **scalars** (i.e., pressure/time, volume/time, and flow/time).[16] There are six basic waveforms produced during ventilation for pressure, volume, and flow over time (Figure 9-25 and Box 9-18). Figure 9-26 shows examples of the pressure, volume, and flow waveforms produced with several methods of pressure and volume ventilation. Another type of graphic is called a **loop,** which is a display of two variables plotted on the x (horizontal) and y (vertical) axes.

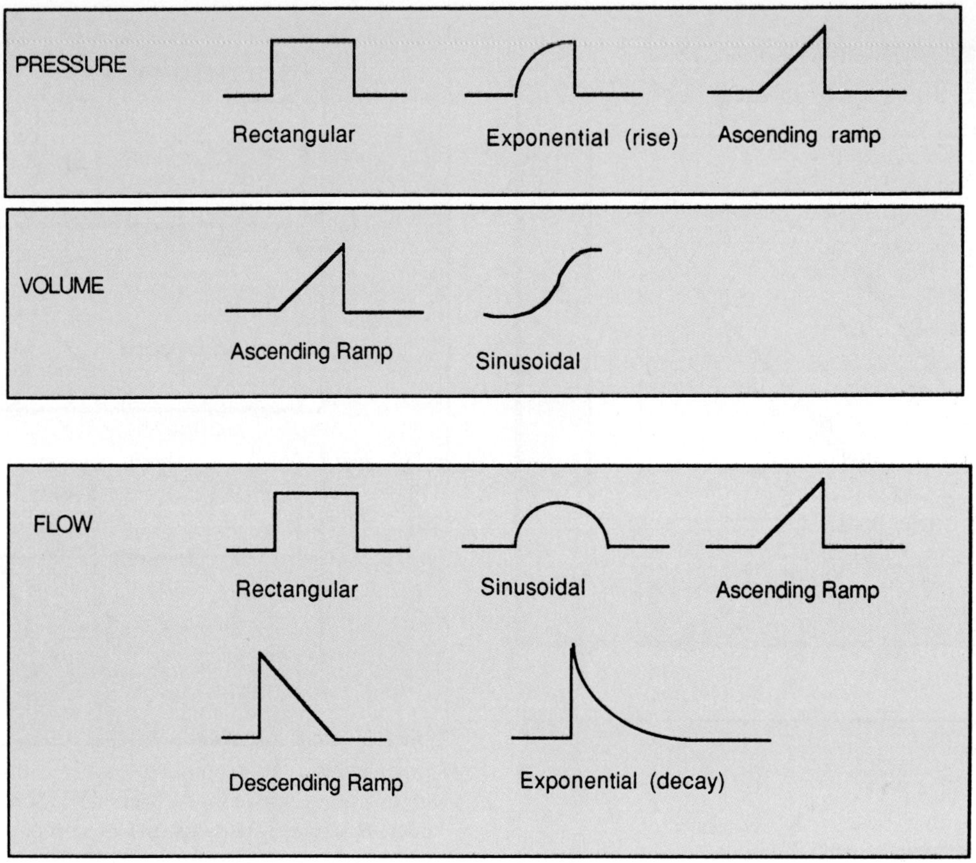

Figure 9-25 Examples of curves for pressure, volume, and flow. Pressure curves are usually constant, rising exponential, or ascending ramps. Volume curves are usually ascending ramp or sinusoidal (sine-wavelike). Flow curves are commonly rectangular (constant), sine, ramp (ascending or descending), and decaying exponential. (From Pilbeam SP: Mechanical ventilation: physiological and clinical applications, ed 3, St Louis, 1998, Mosby.)

BOX 9-18

Six Basic Curves or Waveforms

Rectangular
Often called the square wave

Descending ramp
Also referred to as a decelerating ramp

Ascending ramp
Also called an accelerating ramp

Sinusoidal
Often called the sine wave; only a half or part of this wave is present

Exponential (rising)
Exponential (decaying)

(From Pilbeam SP: Mechanical ventilation: physiological and clinical applications, ed 3, St Louis, 1998, Mosby.)

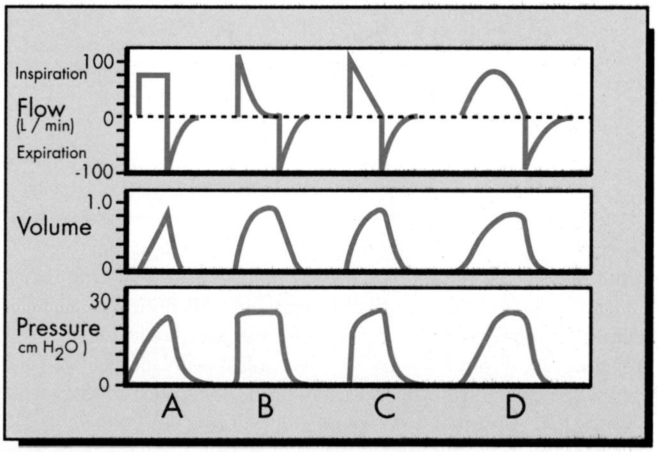

Figure 9-26 Characteristic waveforms for pressure, volume, and flow in the following forms of ventilation: **A,** a volume breath with constant flow; **B,** a pressure breath (pressure-controlled) with a constant pressure delivery, a long T_I time (flow returns to zero), and time-cycling; **C,** a volume breath with a descending ramp flow pattern; and **D,** a volume breath using a sinelike flow pattern.

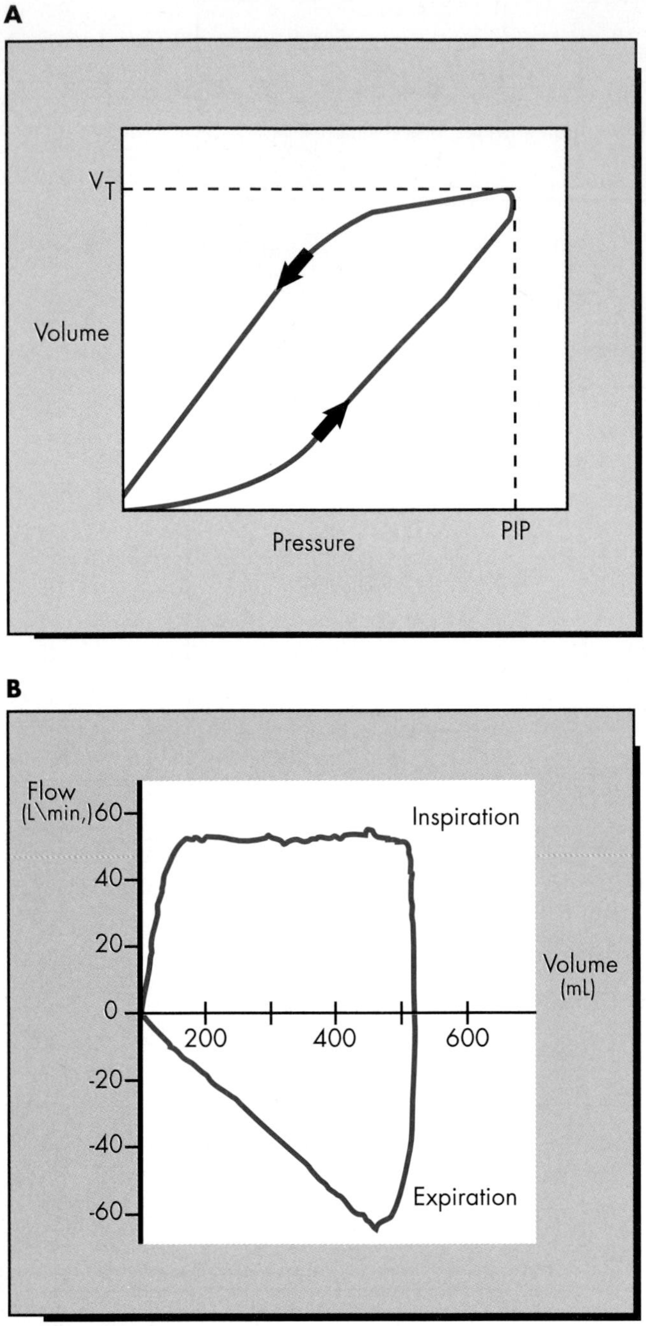

Figure 9-27 **A,** A typical pressure/volume curve for a positive-pressure breath. The highest points for tidal volume (V_T, vertical axis) and peak inspiratory pressure (*PIP,* horizontal axis) represent the dynamic compliance for the pressure/volume relationship. (From Pilbeam SP: Mechanical ventilation: physiological and clinical applications, ed 3, St Louis, 1998, Mosby.) **B,** A normal flow/volume loop during volume ventilation. The inspiratory curve is on the top here; the expiratory curve is on the bottom. Note the linear change in expiratory flow from peak to end-expiration. Note also that end-expiratory flow is zero.

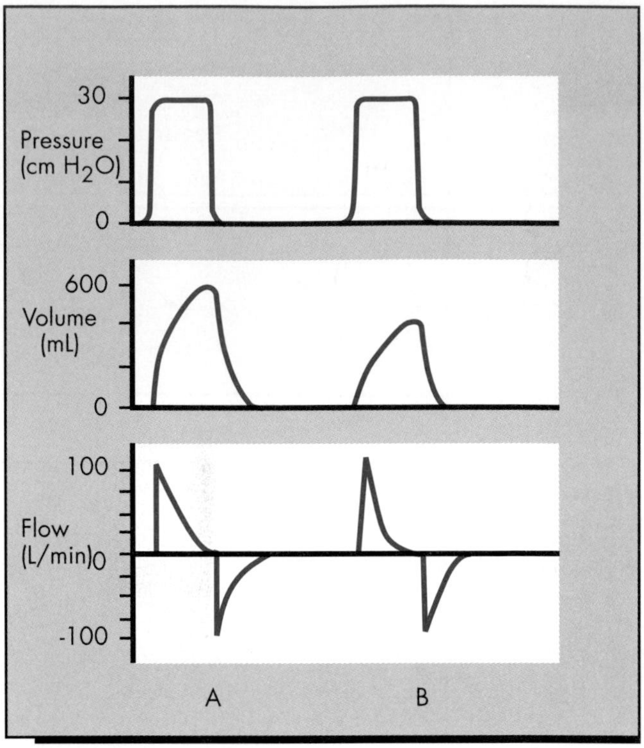

Figure 9-28 An example of patient's lungs getting worse with pressure ventilation: **A,** normal pressure, volume, and flow curves; **B,** curves with reduced lung compliance, showing reduced volume delivery.

Pressure/volume (Figure 9-27 **A**) and flow/volume loops (**B**) are the two most frequently used.

Remember that during pressure ventilation the delivered set pressure pattern stays the same, regardless of changes in the patient's lung condition, but volume and flow delivery vary (Figure 9-28). During volume ventilation, the selected volume and flow wave patterns stay the same, but the pressure varies (Figure 9-29).

Limiting Factors During Inspiration

As reviewed, the ventilator controls one of the four **control variables** during inspiration and can also limit the remaining variables. A limiting variable has a maximum value that cannot be exceeded during inspiration; reaching its limit does not end inspiratory flow. For example, in a piston-driven ventilator, the volume is limited to the gas volume within the piston housing. It cannot exceed that volume; however, delivering the volume does not necessarily end the breath. The forward movement of the piston rod may control the time of inspiratory delivery (time-cycling), and this is considered volume-limited and time-cycled. The two events may occur simultaneously, but whichever actually ends the breath specifies the cycling mechanism.

A ventilator is considered flow-limited if the flow reaches a maximum value before the end of inspiration but does not exceed that value. For example, if the forward

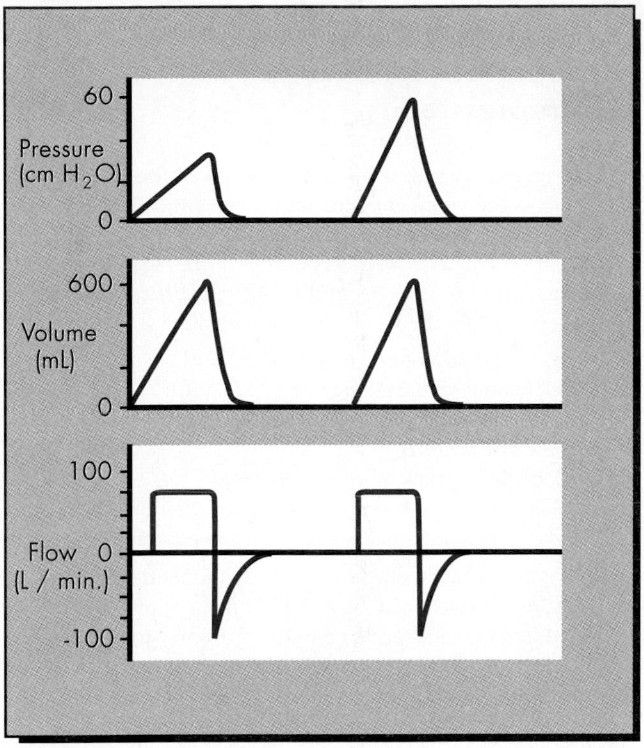

Figure 9-29 An example of patient's lung getting worse with volume ventilation: **A,** normal pressure, volume, and flow curves; **B,** curves with reduced lung compliance, showing increased pressure delivery. Volume stays constant.

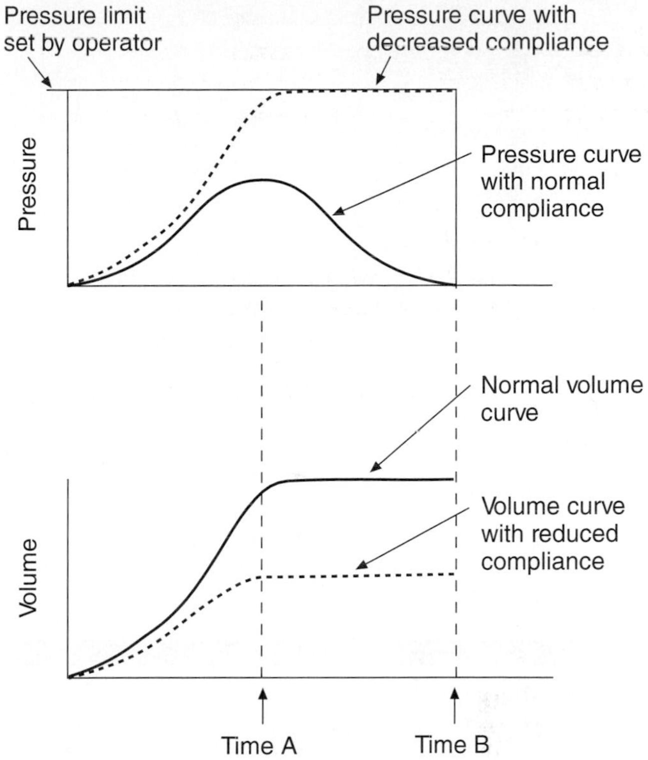

Figure 9-30 This is an example of a sine wave pressure curve. The pressure and volume lines for normal compliance show pressure peaking at time *A,* and the normal volume delivered by time *A.* Inspiration ends at time *B.* With a reduced compliance, the pressure rises higher during inspiration (volume ventilation). Excess pressure is vented so that the pressure reaches the set limit and stays constant. No more flow enters the patient's lungs. Volume delivery has reached its maximum at time *A* when the pressure starts venting. Again, inspiration is time-cycled at *B.* (From Pilbeam SP: Mechanical ventilation: physiological and clinical applications, ed 3, St Louis, 1998, Mosby.)

motion of a linear drive piston is constant, then the flow is constant and limited to the rate of forward motion and the volume within the piston housing (flow = volume/time).

Pressure limiting sets a maximum value for pressure, which is not exceeded during inspiration. Once the pressure is reached, inspiration may continue, but no more pressure (and thus no more volume) is delivered to the patient (Figure 9-30). Excess pressure is vented through a pressure-release mechanism. Many infant ventilators have pressure-limited capabilities.

Maximum Safety Pressure

All ventilators come with some type of feature that allows inspiratory pressure to reach—but not exceed—a maximum value during inspiration. This pressure is usually set by the operator at 10 cm H_2O above the peak pressure reached during inspiration. This particular control on the control panel can have a variety of names (Box 9-19); the purpose of this feature is to prevent excessive pressure from damaging lung tissue. In most adult ventilators, reaching this pressure ends inspiratory gas flow; thus the ventilator pressure cycles out of inspiration. Unfortunately, the labeling used on the control panel of most ventilators includes the term *pressure limit,* which leads to a lot of confusion because this feature usually cycles the ventilator out of inspiration and does not just limit the pressure.

BOX 9-19

Common Names for Maximum Safety Pressure Control

Pressure limit
Upper pressure limit
Normal pressure limit
High pressure limit
Peak/Maximum pressure

TERMINATION OF THE INSPIRATORY PHASE: CYCLING MECHANISM

The phase variable measured and used to end inspiration is called the cycle variable. A breath can be volume-cycled, pressure-cycled, time-cycled, or flow-cycled (Boxes 9-20 and 9-21). It is worth mentioning that even though the ventilator

BOX 9-20

Cycling Variables

Volume-Cycled

The ventilator ends inspiration after a predetermined volume has been reached.

Pressure-Cycled

The ventilator ends inspiration after a predetermined pressure has been reached.

Time-Cycled

The ventilator ends inspiration after a predetermined time has been reached.

Flow-Cycled

The ventilator ends inspiration after a predetermined flow has been reached.

BOX 9-21

Decision Making & Problem Solving

During volume ventilation in current ICU ventilators, the operator sets a volume, flow, and respiratory rate. The ventilators do not measure volume. They calculate and set the inspiratory time needed to achieve the set volume based on the set variables (volume, flow, and time [rate]). This technically makes them time-cycled.

However, clinicians commonly consider them volume-cycled because they do achieve volume delivery by the time inspiratory flow ends, but technically do not "measure" the volume using a volume-measuring device like a bellows or bag.

Defend the argument that these ventilators are volume- instead of time-cycled.

See Appendix A for a discussion.

may measure a specific volume output during volume-cycled ventilation, the amount delivered to the patient may be less than the measured value. This can be due to leaks in the system or compression of some of the volume in the patient circuit (tubing compressibility [Box 9-22]).

The Expiratory Phase

Normally, when inspiratory flow ceases during ventilation, the expiratory valve opens and allows expiratory flow to begin. The expiratory phase is the time between inspiratory phases. Expiratory flow can be delayed by keeping the expiratory valve closed, thus preventing gas flow from the circuit. This maneuver is referred to as an **inspiratory pause,** or inflation hold, and extends inspiratory time.

BOX 9-22

Tubing Compliance or Compressibility

During positive-pressure ventilation, part of the volume that exits the ventilator expands the patient circuit due to the compliance of the circuit and does not reach the patient's lungs. This is based on Boyle's law. To calculate tubing compliance, perform the following procedure before connecting the ventilator to a patient:

1. Set ventilator volume to 100 or 200 mL.
2. Select a low flow setting (e.g., 40 L/min).
3. Set the upper pressure limit to the maximum and the PEEP to zero.
4. Occlude the patient wye connector.
5. Manually cycle the ventilator, record the measured peak pressure, and measure the exhaled volume.

Tubing compliance equals measured volume divided by measured pressure ($C_T = V \div PIP$). Most adult ventilator patient circuits have a compliance from 1 to 3 mL/cm H_2O. In other words, for every centimeter of pressure generated during ventilation of a patient, 1 to 3 mL is lost to tubing compliance. Example, if PIP = 10 cm H_2O, and $C_T = 2$ mL/cm H_2O, what is the volume lost to the circuit? 10 cm $H_2O \times 2$ mL/cm H_2O = 20 mL. If the V_T leaving the ventilator is 500 mL, only 480 mL will reach the patient.

Inspiratory Pause (Plateau or Inflation Hold)

Inflation hold actually extends inspiratory time (T_I) and is not a part of the expiratory phase. Inspiratory pause can occur in either pressure or volume ventilation. In volume ventilation, it is commonly used to obtain a reading of **plateau pressure ($P_{plateau}$)** for estimating alveolar pressure and calculating **static compliance** ($C_S = V/P_{plateau} - EEP$) (Box 9-23 and Figure 9-31). It can also be used to extend inspiratory time and increase mean airway pressure for mandatory breaths. There is a control for this function on the operating panel with which you can select a time period from fractions of a second up to about 2 seconds.

During pressure ventilation, an **inspiratory hold** can also be observed when T_I is sufficient to allow the selected pressure delivery to equilibrate with the patient's lungs. In this situation, inflation hold is not actually selected as a parameter on the control panel. Flow is seen to read zero during this time, before expiratory flow is allow to begin (see Figure 9-26 *B*). This same phenomenon can be observed with pediatric ventilators when a pressure-relief valve is used. In this situation, the pressure-relief valve opens during the inspiratory phase and allows the pressure to main-

BOX 9-23

Peak, Plateau, and Transairway Pressure

As volume is delivered, pressure rises to a peak (peak inspiratory pressure [PIP]) at the end of inspiration. PIP represents the pressure needed to overcome both airflow resistance and elastic compliance.

When an inspiratory pause is selected, the volume is held in the lungs at the end of inspiration, and the pressure reading drops to a plateau. The plateau or static reading indicates the pressure needed to overcome the static (lung) compliance alone. $C_S = Vol \div (P_{plateau} - PEEP)$.

The difference (PIP − Pplateau) is the transairway pressure (P_{TA}) and represents pressure associated with airflow resistance and is used to calculate airway resistance: $Raw = P_{TA} \div flow$.

BOX 9-24

PEEP and CPAP

PEEP is the term most commonly used when mandatory ventilator breaths are being delivered with a positive baseline pressure.

CPAP is the term most commonly used to describe the positive baseline pressure continuously applied to the airway of a spontaneously breathing patient. Patients doing well on CPAP alone do not require mandatory breaths from a ventilator.

tained at a constant level within the circuit until the breath time-cycles into expiration (pressure-limited, time-cycled ventilation)(see Figure 9-30).

Baseline Pressure

Baseline pressure is the pressure level at which inspiration begins and ends. It is a variable controlled by the ventilator during the expiratory phase. Baseline pressures above zero are commonly called **PEEP (positive end-expiratory pressure)** or **CPAP (continuous positive airway pressure)** (Box 9-24 and see Figure 9-31).

Expiratory Retard

Expiratory retard is a technique that offers resistance to expiratory gas flow by incorporating a variable orifice in the expiratory outflow tract (Figure 9-32). Its purpose is to maintain pressure in the circuit and thus the airway during expiration to help prevent flaccid airways from collapsing in patients with chronic obstructive pulmonary disorders. This maneuver is thought to mimic pursed-lip breathing, which is prevented with an endotracheal or tracheostomy tube,[17] and it may increase mean intrathoracic pressure, potentially increase expiratory time (especially during spontaneous breathing), and alter inspiratory to expiratory (I:E) ratios. An expiratory retard control, although present on older ventilators, is rarely seen in newer ventilator designs.

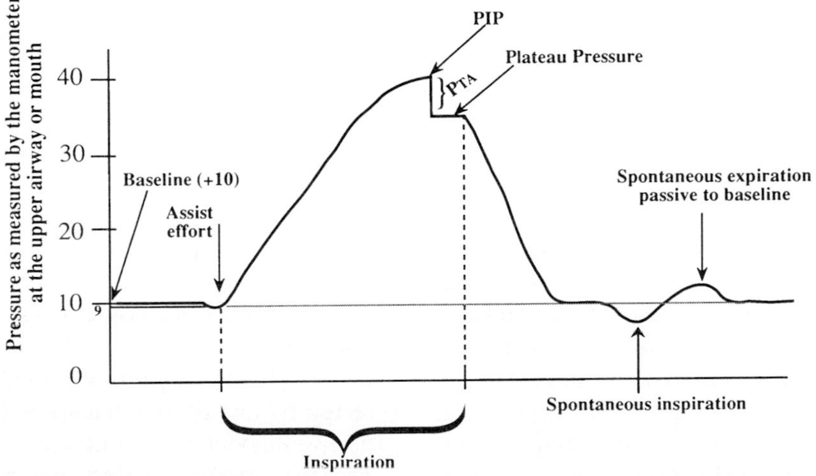

Figure 9-31 An example of a volume breath with an inspiratory hold giving a pause before expiratory flow begins, allowing plateau (alveolar) pressure to be estimated. To be performed accurately, the patient cannot be making spontaneous breathing efforts. Also shown is baseline pressure, which is at a PEEP of 10 cm H_2O, transairway pressure (P_{TA} = PIP − Pplateau), and pressure changes during a spontaneous breath. (From Pilbeam SP: Mechanical ventilation: physiological and clinical applications, ed 3, St Louis, 1998, Mosby.)

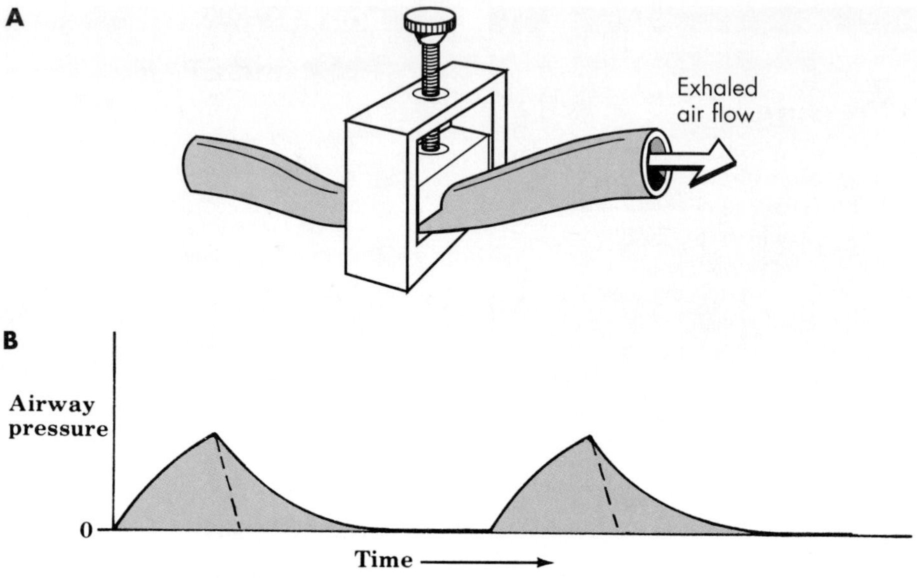

Figure 9-32 **A,** a screw clamp showing a flow resistor; **B,** a pressure/time curve for a normal breath with normal exhalation (*dashed line*) and with expiratory retard (*solid line*). (From Pilbeam SP: Mechanical ventilation: physiological and clinical applications, ed 3, St Louis, 1998, Mosby.)

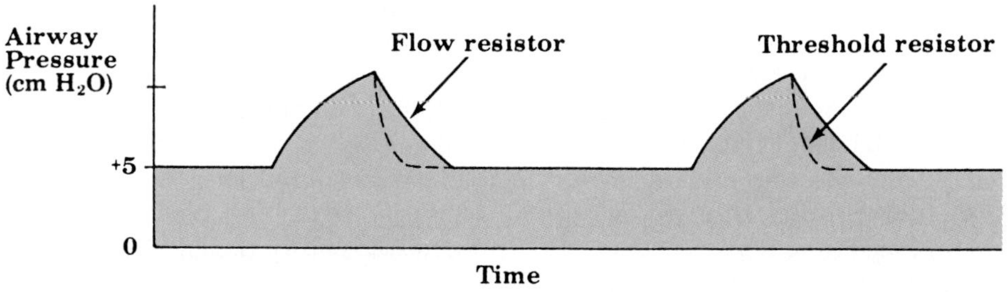

Figure 9-33 This airway pressure curve shows a mandatory breath plus PEEP with two different expiratory flow curves. The solid line illustrates pressure with a flow resistor. Pressure can vary with flow. The dashed line represents a threshold resistor. Flow leaves the lungs rapidly until the set baseline is reached. (From Pilbeam SP: Mechanical ventilation: physiological and clinical applications, ed 3, St Louis, 1998, Mosby.)

Positive End-Expiratory Pressure (PEEP)

PEEP occurs because a resistance is applied during exhalation, which limits lung emptying and increases functional residual capacity (FRC) to increase mean airway pressure and improve oxygenation. Increased pressure is accomplished by using a resistance device, which can be either a flow or threshold resistor.

Flow resistors direct expiratory flow through an orifice or resistor, such as a screw clamp, and act as expiratory retard devices (see Figure 9-32). The higher the rate of gas flow, the higher the pressure generated. If the expiratory period is extended, the baseline pressure can return to zero. One example of the use of flow resistors is in a positive expiratory pressure (PEP) mask used for combating atelectasis and aiding secretion removal (see Chapter 6). It is used less commonly in ventilator circuits because the rapid flow from a patient's cough can cause pressure to be very high.

Threshold resistors allow expiratory flow to continue unimpeded until the pressure in the circuit equals the threshold value set. A true threshold resistor is unaffected by rate of flow (Figure 9-33). Most newer generation ventilators have PEEP capabilities built into their design and operate through the expiratory valves that are generally located internally. Older generation ventilators such as the MA-1 and the IMV Emerson had PEEP valves located near or built into the expiratory valve, which was located outside the ventilator in the patient circuit. Part IV of this chapter contains a section on expiratory valves and devices.

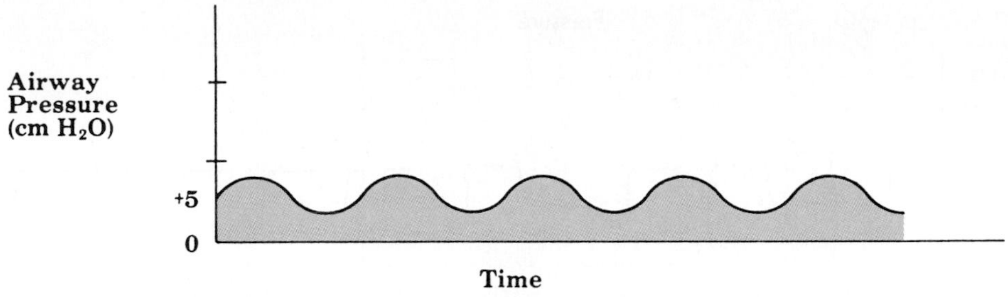

Figure 9-34 Curve of pressure and time for CPAP. (From Pilbeam SP: Mechanical ventilation: physiological and clinical applications, ed 3, St Louis, 1998, Mosby.)

Continuous Positive Airway Pressure (CPAP)

CPAP (constant or continuous positive airway pressure) refers to a technique in which a patient breaths spontaneously at an elevated baseline pressure (Figure 9-34). As with PEEP the increased pressure is accomplished with the use of some type of expiratory resistance device. CPAP can be performed through a mechanical ventilator or with a free-standing spontaneous breathing system (see section in this chapter on spontaneous breathing circuits).

Like PEEP, CPAP can be used to increase functional residual capacity (FRC) to increase mean airway pressure (MAP) and improve oxygenation. It is also used for the treatment of sleep apnea (see Chapter 14).

Continuous Gas Flow During Exhalation

Ventilators that provide flow-triggering have a continuous flow of gas passing through the circuit throughout expiration, providing immediate flow to a patient at the beginning of the inspiratory effort.

Subambient Pressure, or Negative End-Expiratory Pressure (NEEP)

Historically, negative pressure during expiration was called **negative end-expiratory pressure (NEEP).** One of the designs for NEEP used a Venturi at the upper airway to actively draw air from the airway (Figures 9-35 and 9-36).

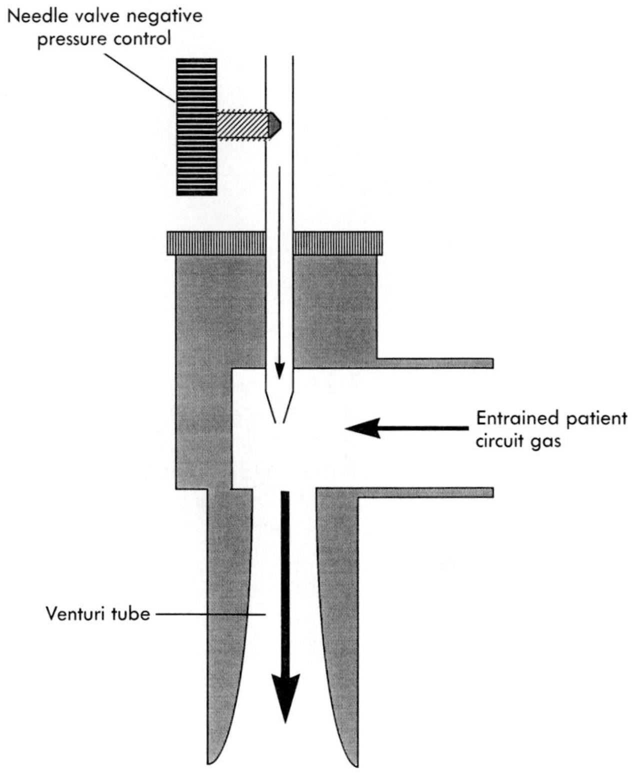

Figure 9-35 Example of a NEEP mechanism.

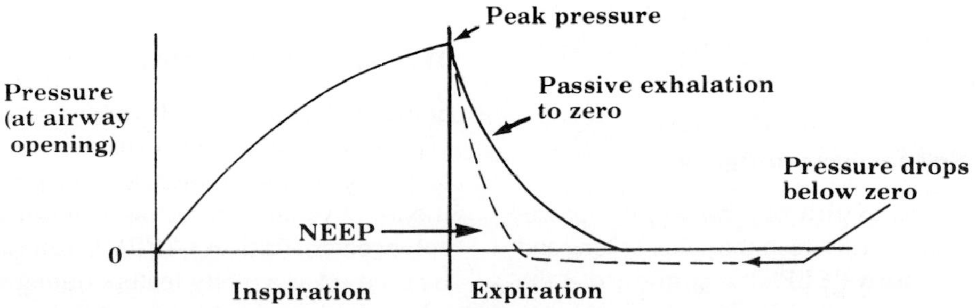

Figure 9-36 Pressure/time curve for a mandatory breath, showing normal passive exhalation to zero baseline (*solid line*) and exhalation using NEEP (*dashed line*). (From Pilbeam SP: Mechanical ventilation: physiological and clinical applications, ed 3, St Louis, 1998, Mosby.)

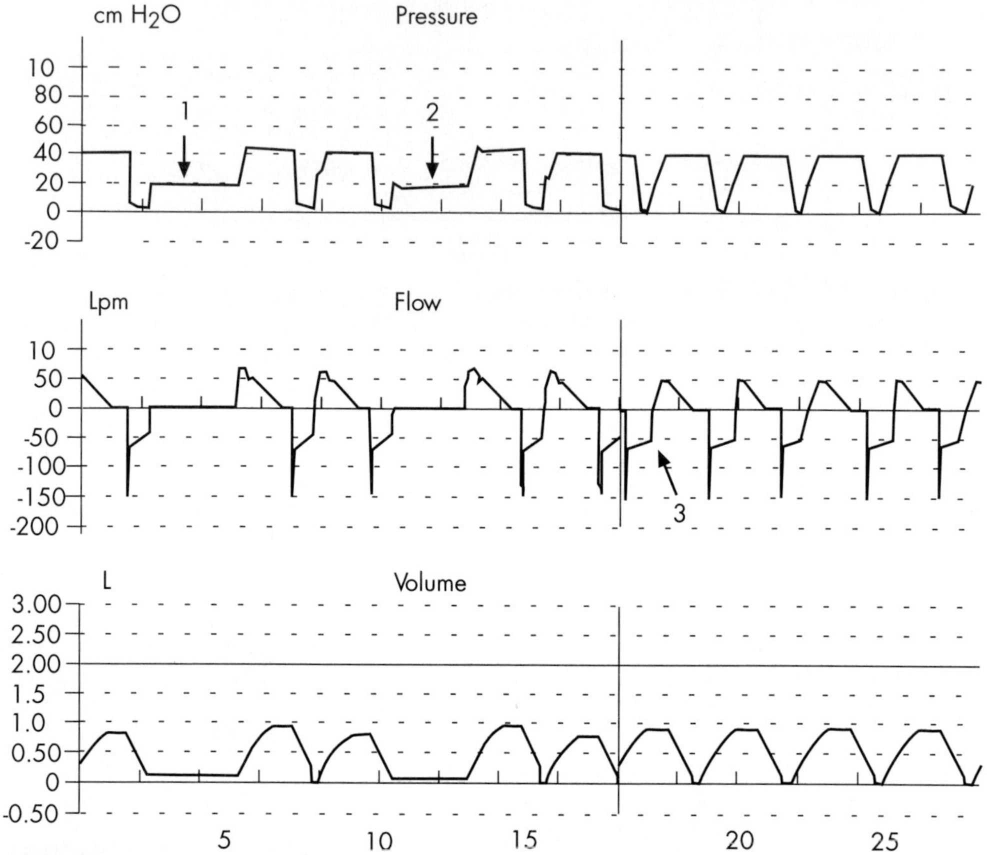

Figure 9-37 Pressure, flow, and volume curves showing the use of end-expiratory pause, allowing the estimation of auto-PEEP (*1* and *2*). Without using a pause, the presence of auto-PEEP can be detected from the flow curve. Flow does not return to zero before the next mandatory breath (*3*). (Redrawn from Nilsestuen JO and Hargett K: Managing the patient-ventilator system using graphic analysis: an overview and introduction to Graphics Corner, Respir Care, 41:1105, 1996.)

This older technique was intended to counterbalance the increase in mean intrathoracic pressures caused by positive-pressure ventilation and permit more rapid respiratory rates in infants.

Current use of negative pressure during expiration occurs during high-frequency oscillation (see Figure 9-3). The ventilator actually creates a wave of negative pressure, drawing air out of the airway.

Expiratory Hold: End Expiratory Pause

Expiratory hold or **end-expiratory pause,** is a procedure performed to estimate pressure in the patient's lung and circuit from trapped air (**auto-PEEP**). It is performed at the end of exhalation, following a mandatory breath. Some ventilators come equipped with a control for this purpose. Activating the control closes both the inspiratory and expiratory valves at the end of expiration and delays delivery of the next mandatory breath, allowing time for equilibration of pressures in the system and for the operator to obtain a reading of end-expiratory pressure (Figure 9-37). The valves reopen when the control is released or after a set time frame.

Time-Limited Exhalation

Some ventilators allow the operator to set expiratory time (T_E). In these situations, exhalation is time-limited. An example of its use is discussed in this chapter under the modes of ventilation section reviewing **airway-pressure release ventilation (APRV).** Time limiting of exhalation is also used as a safety feature during ventilation of infants when rapid respiratory rates dictate a very short total cycle time (TCT). Breath stacking can occur and become a hazard (see Chapter 11).

Part II: Modes of Ventilation

BASIC MODES OF VENTILATION

Modes of ventilation are terms used to describe the pattern of breath delivery to a patient. The use of the terms associated with ventilator modes tells users what type of breath is being delivered and how breaths are triggered, controlled, and cycled. Most ventilator control panels have a mode-selection switch. Unfortunately, naming of modes varies by manufacturers, which leads to confusion.

For a discussion of the purpose of different ventilator modes and how they are set, the reader is referred elsewhere.[6,11] The following discussion will focus on definitions of the modes and technical aspects of their function.

Controlled Mechanical Ventilation, or the Control Mode

The **control mode** is the delivery of a preset volume (volume-targeted) or pressure (pressure-targeted) breath at set timed intervals (time-triggered breaths). Breaths are time- or volume-cycled and pressure- or volume-limited, and each breath is mandatory. Control ventilation is generally used when patients have no inspiratory effort, such as patients with drug overdoses, neurological or neuromuscular disorders, or seizure activity, that require sedation and/or paralysis. Box 9-25 provides a historic note about the control mode. Figure 9-38 shows the pressure, flow, and volume scalars for controlled ventilation, **A,** volume, and **B,** pressure ventilation.

Note that control ventilation should never be deliberately selected on the operating panel. That is, the ventilator should never be insensitive to the patient's inspiratory effort. Generally, if a practitioner wants to control breathing, the patient is sedated and paralyzed. Control of breathing can be provided by any mode of ventilation except spontaneous mode settings (i.e., CPAP and pressure support). Newer ventilators do not have pure "control mode" options (i.e., a knob that says "control mode.")

Note also that when practitioners in the clinical setting hear the term *control mode* or ***assist/control mode*** (which is described in the following section), they assume that volume ventilation is being used. This has come about through the historical development of this mode. On the other hand, the phrase ***pressure-controlled ventilation*** **(PCV)** is assumed to mean controlled ventilation that is pressure targeted (pressure-limited). Likewise, in the clinical setting when "control or assist/control" is heard, it is commonly understood to mean the assist/control mode with volume targeted breaths.

The misuse of modes described above, however, is beginning to change, as is described in the following section.

BOX 9-25

Historical Note

The Control Mode

Early volume ventilators had no sensitivity control to monitor and respond to patient efforts at inspiration. If patients tried to breathe on their own, they simply ended up "fighting the ventilator." Sensitivity controls were soon added to allow patient triggering. When this control was first added, clinicians would sometimes turn the sensitivity off so that patients could be controlled. When patients did make efforts at inspiration under these conditions, their "fighting the ventilator" was sometimes treated by sedation and/or paralysis.

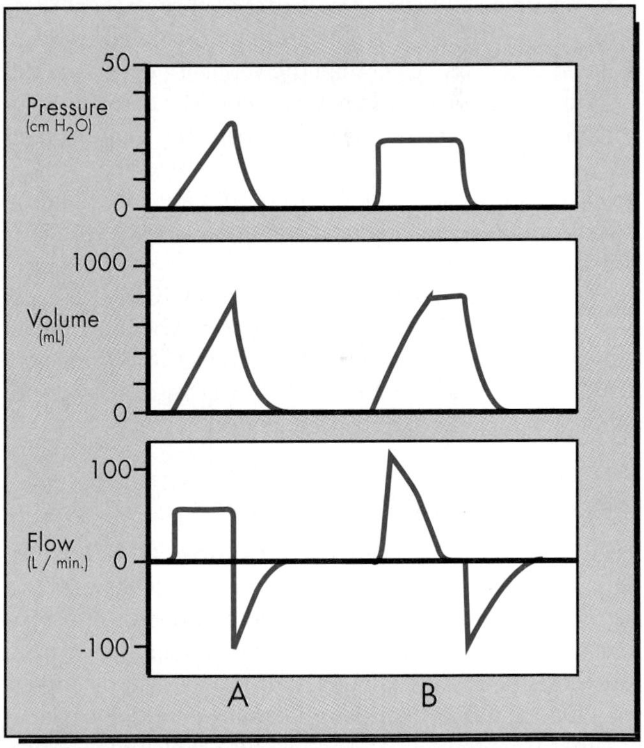

Figure 9-38 Pressure, volume, and flow scalars for volume ventilation with constant flow (**A**) and pressure ventilation (**B**) in the control mode.

Assist, Assist/Control Ventilation

Sensing mechanisms are designed to detect a drop of pressure or flow (and sometimes volume) in the circuit when a patient makes an inspiratory effort (patient triggering). When all breaths are patient-triggered, this is referred to as the **assist** mode. When a backup rate is set and some

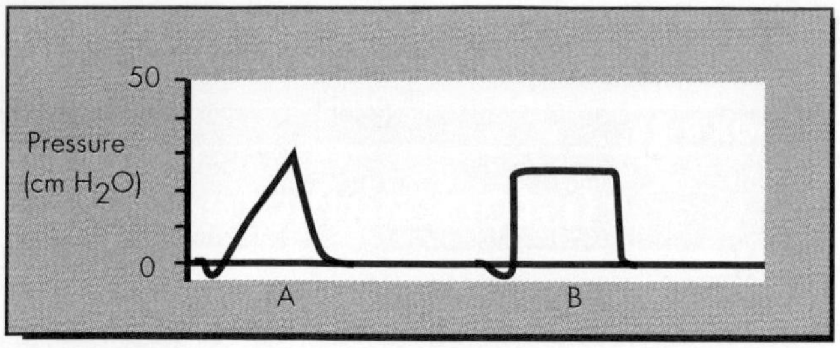

Figure 9-39 Pressure/time curves for volume (**A**) and pressure (**B**) ventilation in the assist/control mode. Note the deflection of the pressure below baseline prior to breath delivery.

breaths are time- as well as patient-triggered, this mode is referred to as the assist/control mode. Operators set a backup rate when using assist/control to ensure patient safety.

The pressure/time waveform reflects the downward deflection of a patient-assisted breath when breaths are patient-triggered (Figure 9-39). Breath intervals may be irregular, but each breath will deliver the set volume or pressure, regardless of how it was triggered. If the patient's rate drops below the set rate (i.e., if the time between patient-initiated breaths is longer than the ventilator cycle time [60 seconds/set rate]), timed breaths occur. Mandatory breaths continue at the set rate until the patient's rate increases again or patient effort occurs before the timed ventilator interval. Control and assist/control modes are commonly labeled continuous mandatory ventilation (CMV) on newer generation ventilators.

In summary, assist and assist/control (CMV) are patient- (pressure or flow) or time-triggered, volume- or pressure-targeted, and volume- or time-cycled. In volume ventilation, breaths are volume- or flow-limited. In pressure ventilation, breaths are pressure-limited.

Intermittent Mandatory Ventilation

Intermittent mandatory ventilation (IMV) is designed to deliver volume- or pressure-targeted breaths at a set minimum frequency (time-triggered). Between mandatory breaths, the patient can breathe spontaneously from the ventilator circuit without getting the set volume or pressure. During this spontaneous breathing period, the patient breathes from the set baseline pressure, which may be ambient pressure or a positive baseline pressure (PEEP/CPAP). Spontaneous breaths can also be aided by the use of pressure support (see the section on pressure support later in this chapter). Because patients have an opportunity to spontaneously breathe, they must assume part of the work of breathing. For this reason, IMV and SIMV (which is described later) are used for weaning patients from ventilatory support.

Figure 9-40 illustrates the pressure/time graph for IMV with volume or pressure ventilation. During IMV with volume ventilation (IMV vol.), mandatory breaths are time-triggered, volume-targeted, and volume-cycled. During IMV with pressure ventilation (IMV press.), mandatory breaths are time-triggered, pressure-targeted, and time-cycled.

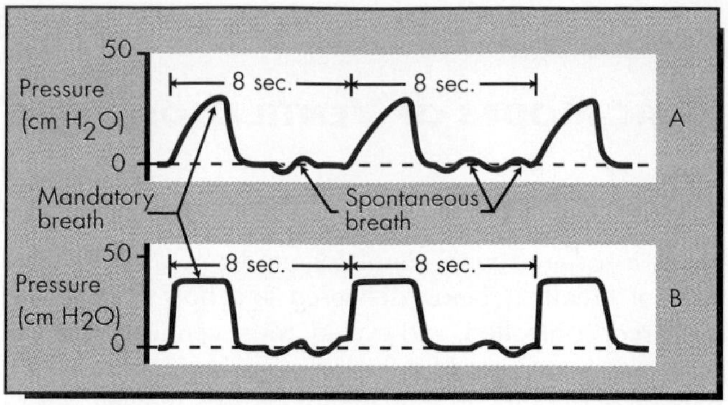

Figure 9-40 Pressure/time curves for volume (**A**) and pressure ventilation (**B**) with IMV.

Historically, IMV circuits had to be added to the patient circuit to provide for IMV ventilation. Newer ventilators have this system built-in and provide SIMV rather than IMV (which is described later in this chapter), but IMV circuits are still added to home-care ventilators. For this reason, Part III of this chapter contains a section on the structure of an add-on IMV system.

When IMV or SIMV are used for weaning, the mandatory breath rate can be progressively decreased, allowing for more spontaneous breaths from the patient.

Synchronized Intermittent Mandatory Ventilation (SIMV)

Synchronized intermittent mandatory ventilation (SIMV) delivers a set volume or pressure breath to the patient in response to the patient's effort. Similar to IMV, with SIMV the operator sets a minimum respiratory rate. These breaths can be volume- or pressure-targeted. Between these assisted breaths, the patient can breathe spontaneously and will not receive the set volume or pressure.

During the spontaneous period, the patient breathes from the baseline pressure, which may be ambient or positive (PEEP/CPAP). Spontaneous breaths can also be aided by the use of pressure support (see the section later in this chapter on pressure support). The main difference between IMV and SIMV is that SIMV tries to synchronize delivery of the mandatory breath with patient effort (patient triggering). When it is time for a mandatory breath, the unit waits briefly for a patient effort. If the patient triggers the breath, then the ventilator automatically delivers the mandatory breath.

The use of the terms *mandatory* and *assist* in relation to IMV/SIMV should be noted. Recall that a mandatory breath is completely machine-controlled, and an assisted breath is patient-triggered with the ventilator determining how inspiration is delivered and when it ends (cycles). If a

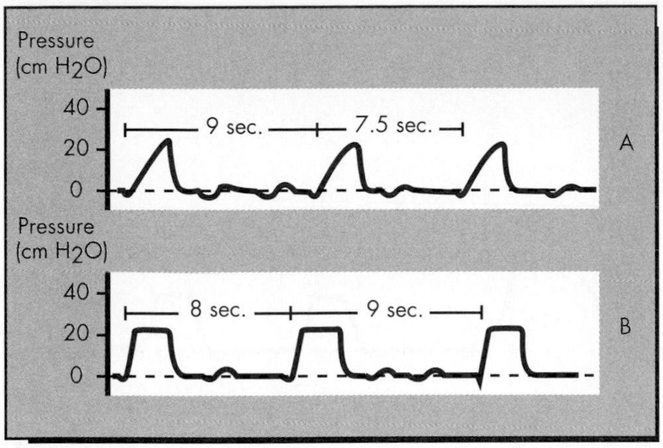

Figure 9-41 Pressure/time curves for volume (**A**) and pressure (**B**) breaths with SIMV.

patient fails to trigger a breath during SIMV, the machine will time-trigger the breath, which makes it a "mandatory" breath. If the patient triggers the breath, it is technically an "assisted" breath. However, when referring to the IMV/SIMV mode, it is easier to call breaths that are volume- or pressure-targeted "mandatory" breaths, regardless of how they are triggered. This will become clearer as the function of SIMV, PCV, and PSV are reviewed.

In SIMV, as in IMV, the operator sets a minimum respiratory rate and a desired volume (volume-targeted, SIMV-vol.) or pressure (pressure-targeted, SIMV-press). Between mandatory breaths, the patient breathes spontaneously.

If the pressure waveform has a downward deflection before the delivery of a mandatory breath, the breath is patient triggered (Figure 9-41). If there is no downward deflection of the pressure waveform prior to a mandatory breath, the breath is time triggered.

Current ICU ventilators have controls on the front panel labeled SIMV that can actually deliver IMV or SIMV (IMV/SIMV). Sometimes there are labels on the control panel such as "SIMV(vol.)" and "SIMV(press.)" to distinguish between volume- and pressure-targeted SIMV.

In summary, SIMV has both mandatory and spontaneous breaths. Mandatory breaths are patient- or time-triggered, pressure- or volume-targeted, and time- or volume-cycled. Spontaneous breaths are from the set baseline and can be assisted with pressure support.

Pressure-Controlled Ventilation (PCV)

Pressure-controlled ventilation (PCV) is the common name applied to pressure-targeted (pressure-limited) ventilation in the assist/control mode. The operator sets a target pressure. Sensitivity is also set to allow for patient triggering. A rate and an inspiratory time are set to establish the total cycle time. The rate guarantees a minimum respiratory rate.

When the breath is triggered, the ventilator produces a very rapid inspiratory flow to achieve the set pressure. When the pressure is reached as the lungs fill, the flow decreases (descending ramp). The breath ends when the inspiratory time has passed. Volume delivery varies with the set inspiratory time and the patient's lung characteristics—whether or not the patient is actively inspiring. For example, when the patient's lungs are stiff, less volume is delivered for the same amount of pressure. As the lungs improve, less pressure is required to deliver the same volume. If the patient actively inspires, the ventilator will increase flow delivery to maintain the set pressure, which can increase volume delivery. If inspiratory time is too short, the ventilator won't have sufficient time to deliver all the pressure to the lungs, and the volume may be lower than desired.

In its early development, PCV was used with inverse I:E ratios and was termed **pressure-controlled inverse ratio ventilation (PCIRV).** Inverse ratios were used to increase the mean airway pressure, in the hope of improving oxygenation of the patient.

Operator-Selected Controls for Volume- and Pressure-Targeted Breaths in Assist/Control and IMV/SIMV

For volume-targeted breaths in assist/control and IMV/SIMV, the operator normally selects from two options:

1. In volume-cycled (or flow/time*) ventilators, volume, flow, and rate are set.
2. In time cycled ventilators, volume, rate and inspiratory time are set.

For pressure-targeted breaths in assist/control and IMV/SIMV modes, the operator normally selects the following:

1. pressure
2. respiratory rate
3. inspiratory time

Pressure-Support Ventilation (PSV)

Pressure-support ventilation is a spontaneous mode of ventilation that allows the operator to select a pressure to help support the patient's work of breathing. It is patient-triggered, pressure-limited, and flow-cycled.[18] PSV can also be used to support the work of breathing for spontaneous breaths during IMV/SIMV ventilation. Figure 9-42 shows the waveforms for SIMV + PSV for both volume- and pressure-targeted mandatory breaths.

As with pressure-controlled ventilation, when a breath is triggered during pressure-support ventilation, the ventilator delivers a high flow of gas to the patient. As the lungs fill, the flow and the pressure gradient between the machine and the patient decrease (descending ramp). The flow curve never falls all the way to zero during inspiration

*Flow and time are measured, and the ventilator cycles when it estimates that set volume has been delivered.

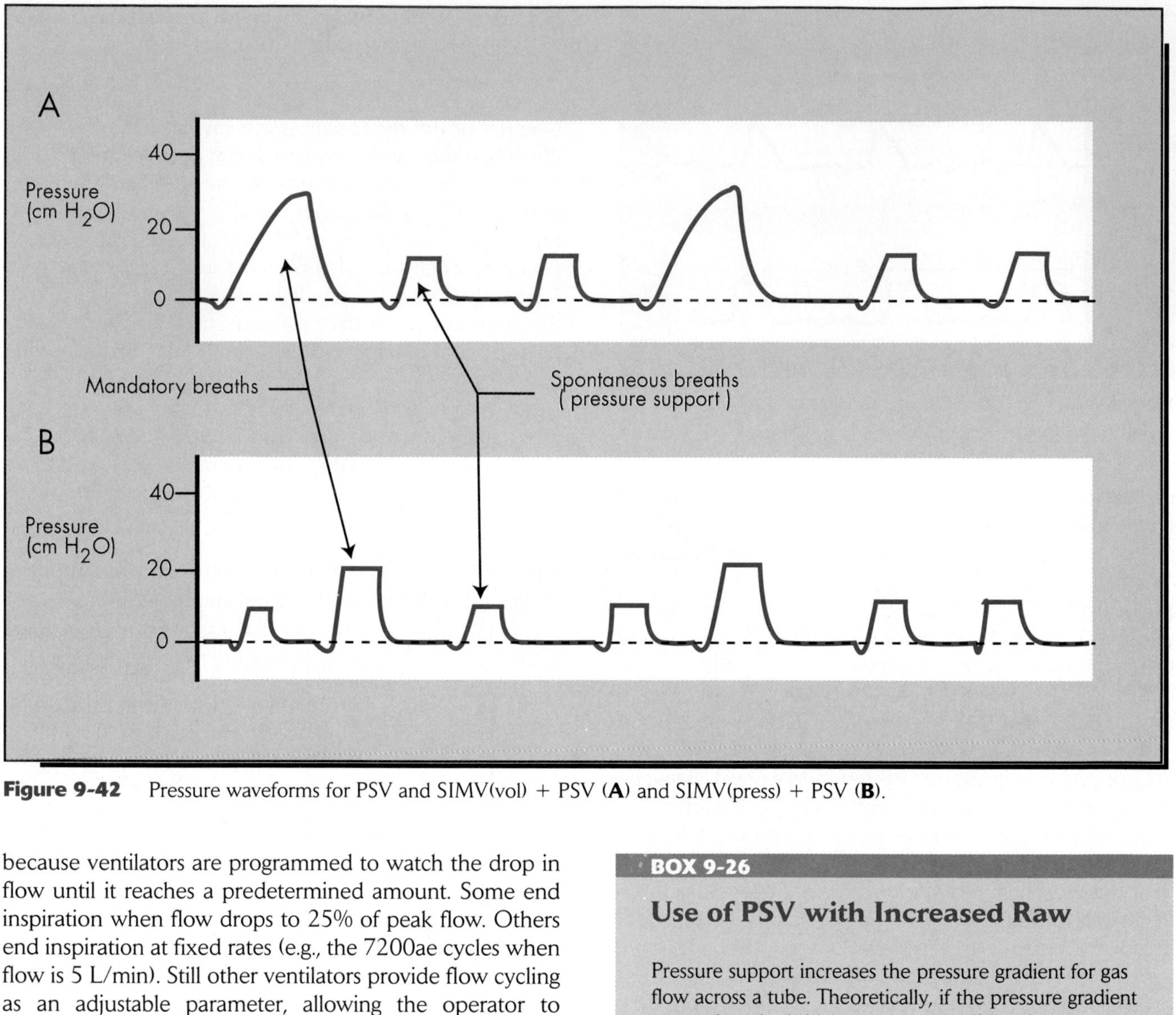

Figure 9-42 Pressure waveforms for PSV and SIMV(vol) + PSV (**A**) and SIMV(press) + PSV (**B**).

because ventilators are programmed to watch the drop in flow until it reaches a predetermined amount. Some end inspiration when flow drops to 25% of peak flow. Others end inspiration at fixed rates (e.g., the 7200ae cycles when flow is 5 L/min). Still other ventilators provide flow cycling as an adjustable parameter, allowing the operator to change the cycle level (% flow) based on the type of patient being ventilated.

If the flow does not decrease (e.g., there is a leak in the system), inspiration will be either time-cycled (1 to 5 seconds) or pressure-cycled (set pressure + 2 to 3 cm H_2O), which are safety back-up systems available with any ventilator providing PSV.

The volume delivery in PSV is determined by the set pressure, the patient's lung characteristics (resistance and compliance), and the patient's inspiratory effort.

There are two common uses for PSV. The first is to reduce the patient's work of breathing when resistance to breathing is increased due to the artificial airway or the ventilatory circuit. The work of breathing imposed by small endotracheal tubes can be a major contributor to fatigue. A review of Poiseuille's law illustrates the basic theory of pressure support when airway resistance (Raw) is increased (see Chapter 1). Decreasing the diameter of the airway significantly increases the resistance to gas flow, which can be a contributing factor to the difficulty of weaning some patients (Box 9-26).

BOX 9-26

Use of PSV with Increased Raw

Pressure support increases the pressure gradient for gas flow across a tube. Theoretically, if the pressure gradient across the tube is high enough, the effect of the increased resistance due to the tube is negated.

In a situation of increased work of breathing associated with the artificial airway or the ventilator system, the initial pressure-support level can be estimated from the transairway pressure (P_{TA}, which is the difference between peak and plateau pressure). P_{TA} reflects the resistance caused by the ventilator system, endotracheal tube, and patient airways.[6] (Note that resistance = (P_{TA})/flow, but only P_{TA} must be calculated because the operator actually sets a pressure with PSV.) The P_{TA} value is a safe starting point for PS but must be readjusted once it is activated so it accommodates the patient's needs. Resistance is influenced by flow rate and flow pattern.

BOX 9-27

Candidates for Pressure-Support Ventilation

Patients with an artificial airway in place and
- airways smaller than optimal size.
- spontaneous respiratory rates >20 breaths/min (adults).
- minute ventilation >10 L/min.

Patients being supported with IMV/SIMV or CPAP (with spontaneous breaths) and:
- a history of COPD.
- evidence of ventilatory muscle weakness requiring ventilatory support.

BOX 9-28

Decision Making & Problem Solving

If the algorithm that controls the ventilator's function is what determines the cycling time in PSV, then how would you argue that this is classified as a spontaneous breath? Isn't the ventilator determining cycling time and not the patient?

See Appendix A for the answer.

A second use for PSV is as a mode of ventilation for patients with intact respiratory centers who are spontaneously breathing. PSV can be adjusted so that much of the work of breathing is provided by the ventilator with a simple increase of the set pressure level. This can be accomplished by measuring volume delivery while adjusting pressure. A desired V_T is based on the patient's ideal body weight (IBW) and lung condition. For example, 8 to 12 mL/kg may be appropriate for a normal patient, but tidal volume needs vary with different lung conditions.[6] Box 9-27 lists patients who might benefit from PSV; Box 9-28 provides an exercise in PSV.

Bi-level Positive Airway Pressure, or Bi-level Pressure-Assist (BiPAP)

Bi-level positive airway pressure is similar to CPAP in that it can provide positive pressure during inspiration and expiration. With CPAP, the pressure tends to stay at a fairly constant baseline with a slightly negative pressure as the patient breathes in and a slightly positive pressure as the patient breathes out (see Figure 9-34). With bi-level positive airway pressure, **inspiratory positive airway pressure (IPAP)** is usually at a higher pressure than **expiratory positive airway pressure (EPAP)** (Figure 9-43).

This form of patient ventilatory assistance is called by several names including bi-level positive airway pressure, **bi-level pressure-assist,** bi-level PEEP, bi-level CPAP, bi-level positive pressure, and **bi-level pressure-support.** One of the original units manufactured is the Respironics BiPAP S/T unit. The term **BiPAP,** although a brand name for this unit, became the popular term used to describe this method of ventilation. BiPAP is most commonly used to treat obstructive sleep apnea using a nasal or face mask. Units that provide BiPAP generate a high gas flow through a microprocessor-controlled valve. There are operator controls for both IPAP and EPAP. Inspiration is normally patient-triggered, but it can be time-triggered when a rate control is provided. BiPAP units can be flow- or time-cycled.

Hospitals also use these units for noninvasive positive-pressure ventilation (NIPPV) for patients who do not necessarily require intubation.

Most BiPAP units also provide leak compensation. The normal interface between the unit and the patient is a mask, and because masks commonly have leaks around them, these units can measure flow to the patient and flow from the patient. If there is a discrepancy between these flows (i.e., a leak), the unit can determine the amount of leak and increase its output to compensate. It can continue its normal triggering and cycling, even with a small leak.

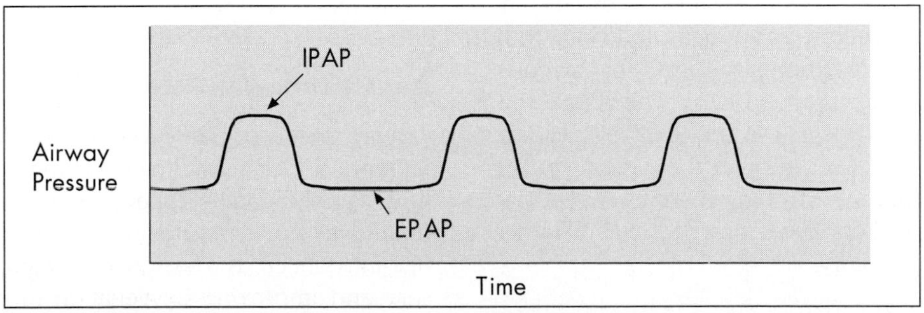

Figure 9-43 Bi-level positive airway pressure (BiPAP) showing inspiratory positive airway pressure (IPAP) and expiratory positive airway pressure (EPAP). (From Pilbeam SP: Mechanical ventilation: physiological and clinical applications, ed 3, St Louis, 1998, Mosby.)

BOX 9-29

Interrelation of Tidal Volume, Flow Rate, Inspiratory Time, Expiratory Time, Total Cycle Time, and Respiratory Rate

Total cycle time equals inspiratory time plus expiratory time.

$$TCT = T_I + T_E$$

Respiratory rate (f) equals 1 min (60 sec) divided by total cycle time.

$$f = \frac{1\text{ min}}{TCT} = \frac{60\text{ seconds}}{TCT\text{ (seconds)}} = \text{breaths/min}$$

Calculate TCT from f.

$$TCT = \frac{60\text{ sec}}{f}$$

Inspiratory to expiratory ratio equals inspiratory time divided by expiratory time.
Calculate I/E ratio from TCT and T_I.

$$TCT = T_I + T_E$$
$$TCT - T_I = T_E$$

Calculate T_E from f and T_I.

$$f = \frac{60\text{ sec}}{TCT}\text{ and } TCT = T_I + T_E$$
$$T_E = TCT - T_I$$

Reducing the I:E ratio to its simplest form, divide the numerator and denominator by T_I.

$$I/E = (T_I/T_I)/(T_E/T_I)$$

Inverse ratio ventilation equals the division of both the numerator and the denominator by the expiratory time.

$$I{:}E = (T_I/T_E)/(T_E/T_E)$$

Calculate T_I, T_E, and TCT from I:E and f.

$$TCT = T_I + T_E \text{ and } f = 60\text{ sec}/TCT$$
$$f = 60\text{ sec}/(T_I + T_E)$$
$$T_I + T_E = 60\text{ sec}/f$$

Calculate T_I from V_T and flow rate ($\dot{V}$).

$$T_I = V_T/\dot{V}$$

Calculate V_T from T_I and $\dot{V}$.

$$V_T = \dot{V} \times T_I$$

Calculate $\dot{V}$ from V_T and T_I.

$$\dot{V} = V_T/T_I$$

(From Pilbeam SP: Mechanical Ventilation, 3rd ed, St Louis, 1998, Mosby.)

INVERSE RATIO VENTILATION

In the early 1970s, Reynolds reported success using mechanical ventilation in infants when the inspiratory phase lasted longer than the expiratory phase and a pressure hold was used.[19,20] Since then, much more extensive use of inverse ratios has occurred both in infants and adults. The primary purpose of this technique is for treatment of acute respiratory distress syndrome (ARDS). By extending inspiratory time, mean airway pressure is increased and oxygenation can be improved. Sometimes air-trapping (auto-PEEP) occurs, which increases the functional residual capacity of the lung. The occurrence of auto-PEEP in this instance is not always a drawback and can, in fact, keep alveoli open that would otherwise collapse on exhalation. Auto-PEEP should be monitored and measured along with the PEEP levels selected by the operator so that alveolar pressures do not exceed 35 cm H_2O. Levels above this value are known to be damaging to the lungs of a variety of experimental animals. Even though the clinical studies on humans are limited, it is strongly recommended that pulmonary pressures be kept lower than 35 cm H_2O rather than risk potential lung injury.[6]

PCIRV and VCIRV

Inverse ratio ventilation can be done using either pressure ventilation **(pressure-controlled inverse ratio ventilation [PCIRV])** or volume ventilation **(volume-controlled inverse ratio ventilation [VCIRV]).** When inspiration is time-cycled, it is not difficult to extend inspiratory time and shorten expiratory time, provided that the ventilator in use allows for this procedure. ICU ventilators are normally time-cycled when pressure-controlled ventilation is used. With volume ventilation, however, not all units have controls for inspiratory time. To extend the inspiratory time, the operator can reduce flow rates, use a descending ramp waveform (extends T_I in non-time–cycled volume ventilation), and/or use an inspiratory pause. Box 9-29 provides a list of equations describing the relationship of inspiratory time, expiratory time, I:E ratio, flow, respiratory rate, and volume. For a more detailed explanation of these, the reader is referred elsewhere.[6,11]

Airway Pressure-Release Ventilation

Airway pressure-release ventilation (APRV) provides two levels of CPAP and allows for spontaneous breathing at both. Patients can be apneic, and this mode still works. It is time-triggered, pressure-limited, and time-cycled. It was first introduced as a way of controlling mean airway pressure and improving oxygenation in patients with severe lung injuries, and often employs inverse I:E ratios.[21] Patients are given an elevated baseline pressure that approximates their optimum CPAP level. The baseline pressure is periodically released to a lower level (usually above zero)

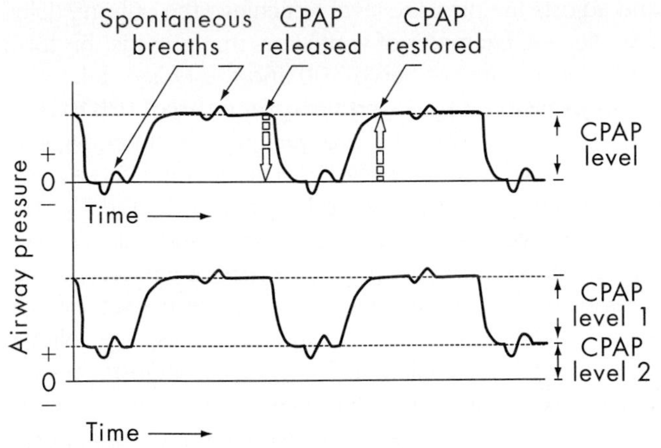

Figure 9-44 Pressure/time curve for airway pressure release ventilation. (Redrawn from Dupuis Y: Ventilators, ed 2, St Louis, 1992, Mosby.)

for a very brief period (about 1 to 1.5 sec).[22] The high CPAP level increases mean airway pressure and helps improve oxygenation. The periodic timed intervals that briefly drop pressures to a lower CPAP level reduce the patient's functional residual capacity and allow for ventilation (i.e., exhalation of carbon dioxide). As soon as this expiratory period is complete, pressures return to the higher CPAP level (Figure 9-44).

At the present time, APRV is available on the Dräger Evita and the Dräger E4 ventilators, but other current and newly developed ICU ventilators will undoubtedly be reprogrammed to make this mode available if further clinical research supports its benefits, and clinicians become more familiar with its operation.

SERVO-CONTROLLED MODES OF VENTILATION

Intelligent, closed-loop ventilator systems have been available for several decades. The advent of faster computer systems, more sophisticated programming and higher levels of technology in monitoring have provided for a variety of intelligent systems. There are now several forms of closed-loop or servo-controlled modes. One such system that has been available since the 1970s is **mandatory minute ventilation (MMV),** which guarantees delivery of a minimum minute ventilation ($\dot{V}_E$) setting and has been used as a method of weaning as well as a method of backing-up ventilation (see the following section on MMV).

Other forms of servo-controlled ventilation sprang from a solution to a problem that clinicians had with pressure-controlled ventilation (PCV). When lung characteristics change during PCV, the volume delivery changes and can affect overall $\dot{V}_E$, acid-base status, and oxygenation. Two closed-loop modes of ventilation were developed and became available in the 1990s to overcome this problem.

BOX 9-30

Servo-Controlled Modes of Ventilation

1. Mandatory minute ventilation, as in the Bear 1000, the Hamilton Veolar, the Ohmeda Advent, and several others.
2. Pressure-targeted ventilation with volume guaranteed every breath: as in pressure augmentation (Paug) in the Bear 1000 ventilator and volume-assured pressure support (VAPS) in the Bird T-Bird and the Bird 8400STi.
3. Pressure-targeted ventilation with volume guaranteed over several breaths as in pressure-regulated volume control (PRVC) and volume support (VS) in the Servo 300, and Autoflow in the Dräger E4.
4. Proportional Assist Ventilation (PAV) as a prototype in development (possibly available in the Drager E-4 upgrade and with other ventilators when upgrades are available).
5. Adaptive Support Ventilation (ASV) in the Hamilton Galileo.

These modes guaranteed volume delivery using pressure target ventilation. One such method guarantees the volume for each breath delivered, and the other guarantees the volume over a several breaths. Thus the benefits of pressure ventilation (i.e., limiting maximum pressure and allowing a more compatible flow pattern) can still be incorporated while volume is guaranteed. Both methods have also been referred to as **dual modes of ventilation.**[23] These and other more recently developed modes are described in the following section (Box 9-30).

Mandatory Minute Ventilation (MMV)

Mandatory (or minimum) minute ventilation is a closed-loop form of volume or **pressure-targeted ventilation** used in patients who can perform part of the work of breathing and are progressing toward weaning from ventilation. MMV guarantees a minimum $\dot{V}_E$, even though the patient's spontaneous ventilation may change. The minimum $\dot{V}_E$ set by the operator in MMV is usually less than the patient's projected spontaneous $\dot{V}_E$. When the measured $\dot{V}_E$ falls below the minimum level, the ventilator increases either pressure or rate to return the ventilator to the minimum $\dot{V}_E$. The Hamilton Veolar is an example of a unit that increases pressure using pressure-support breaths for MMV. The Bear 1000 is an example of a unit using rate to adjust MMV during volume ventilation. The operator must set high rate and low tidal volume alarms in most units to indicate when the patient's rate rises too high and tidal volume falls too low (Box 9-31), which indicates an increased work of breathing—even if the patient could maintain the desired $\dot{V}_E$ (Table 9-1).

BOX 9-31

Decision Making & Problem Solving

A patient on MMV has a set minute ventilation of 4 L/min and a measured $\dot{V}_E$ of 6 L/min (spontaneous $V_T = 0.6$; spontaneous rate = 10 breaths/ min). Over several hours, the patient's tidal volume drops to 0.3 L, and the rate increases to 25 breaths/min. Will the ventilator increase its ventilation delivery to reduce the patient's work of breathing?

See Appendix A for the answer.

TABLE 9-1

Constant minute ventilation with changing alveolar ventilation

Tidal volume (mL)	Dead space (mL)	Respiratory rate (breaths/min)	Alveolar ventilation (L/min)	Minute ventilation (L/min)
800	150	10	6.50	8.0
667	150	12	6.20	8.0
533	150	15	5.75	8.0
400	150	20	5.00	8.0
250	150	32	3.20	8.0

If a patient has a constant dead space of 150 mL, minute ventilation can stay constant while alveolar ventilation decreases, rate increases, and tidal volume falls.

(From Pilbeam SP: Mechanical ventilation, ed 3, St Louis, 1998, Mosby.)

Pressure-Targeted Ventilation with Volume Guaranteed for Every Breath

Pressure augmentation (Paug; Bear 1000 ventilator) and volume-assured pressure-support (VAPS; T-Bird and Bird 8400st) are examples of dual modes that provide **pressure-limited ventilation** with volume guaranteed every breath. In Paug and VAPS, the patient initiates a breath (patient-triggering), and pressure climbs to the set level. During inspiration, the ventilator monitors V_T delivery. If volume is delivered before flow drops to its set value (value on flow control), then inspiration flow-cycles. If volume is not delivered by the time flow drops to its set value, then flow continues at the amount set until the set V_T is delivered and inspiration becomes volume-cycled (based on measured flow and time elapsed). Figure 9-45 provides examples of these types of breaths.

Pressure-Targeted Ventilation with Volume Guaranteed over Several Breaths

Another dual control mode of ventilation uses patient-triggered (or time-triggered), pressure-limited ventilation and adjusts the pressure level to achieve the volume delivery selected. Examples of ventilators that provide this form of ventilation are the Servo 300 and the Dräger E4.

In **pressure-regulated volume control (PRVC)** on the Servo 300, breaths are patient- or time-triggered, pressure-limited and time-cycled. The operator sets a maximum safety pressure, a desired V_T and a desired $\dot{V}_E$. The ventilator gives a test breath at 5 cm H_2O and calculates system compliance. Then it gives a few more test breaths and determines the pressure needed to deliver the set volume. As it ventilates the patient, it monitors pressure, volume, rate, and minute ventilation. The ventilator adjusts pressure delivery to accomplish volume delivery in increments of 1 to 3 cm H_2O at a time—up to the maximum (upper pressure limit minus 5 cm H_2O) and as low as the set baseline (PEEP level). If the volume cannot be delivered within these parameters, the ventilator alarms alert the clinician.

If the patient's respiratory rate declines, there is a set back-up rate. The **autoflow** mode on the Dräger E4 and the **variable-pressure control** mode on Cardiopulmonary Corporation's Venturi ventilator are similar to PRVC on the Servo 300.

Volume support (VS; Servo 300) is similar to PRVC, except that there is no back-up rate, so it is a purely assist mode. VS is patient-triggered, pressure-limited, and flow-cycled, which basically makes it a form of PSV except that volume delivery is guaranteed over a time-frame of several breaths. As with PRVC, pressure increases and decreases within the same limits described to maintain V_T. If the patient's respiratory rate drops and the set $\dot{V}_E$ is not being maintained, the Servo 300 increases V_T delivery (up to 150%) in an attempt to achieve the set $\dot{V}_E$. If the patient becomes apneic, the ventilator automatically switches to PRVC, delivers whatever respiratory rate is set, and sounds an alarm to alert the practitioner. The **variable pressure support** mode available on Cardiopulmonary Corporation's Venturi ventilator is similar to VS on the Servo 300.

Proportional Assist Ventilation

Proportional assist ventilation (PAV) is a method of assisting spontaneous ventilation in which the practitioner adjusts the amount of work it wants the ventilator to perform. It is an approach to ventilatory support in which pressure, flow, and volume delivery at the airway increase in proportion to the patient's inspiratory effort. PAV augments the underlying breathing pattern of a patient who has problems with work of breathing associated with worsening lung characteristics (increasing airway resistance [Raw] or decreasing compliance [C]). The more the patient breathes in, the more pressure the machine provides. PAV allows patients to comfortably reach whatever ventilatory pattern suits their system.[24-26] PAV operation is based on the equation of motion previously described (see Box 9-12). The

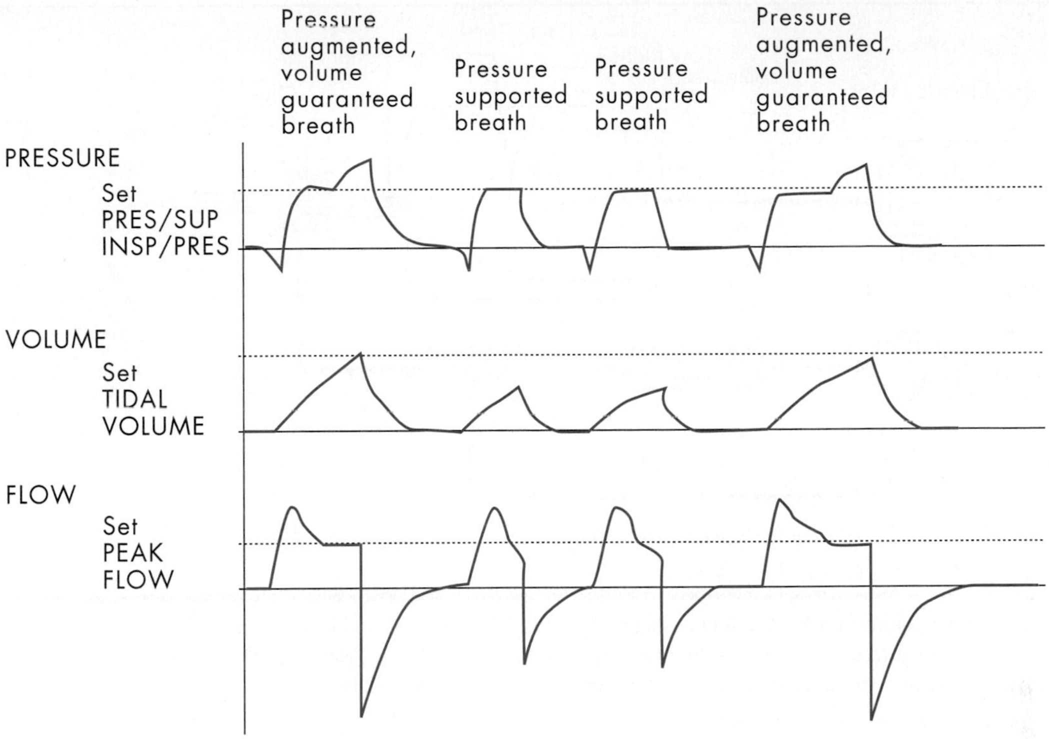

Figure 9-45 Examples of breath delivery in Paug with SIMV plus PSV. Note that the flow curve for a mandatory breath rises rapidly, descends to the set value, and remains constant at the set value until the volume is delivered. For PSV breaths, flow is a descending-ramplike curve and ends when it is about 30% of peak. (Courtesy Bear Medical Corp., Riverside, Calif.)

amount of pressure generated by the patient's own respiratory muscles is used as an index of inspiration effort:

$$Pmus = (V \times e) + (flow \times R) - Paw,$$

where *Pmus* is pressure generated by the respiratory muscles, *V* is volume, *e* is elastance (1/compliance), *R* is resistance, and *Paw* is airway pressure. Pmus can be calculated when e and R are known. The signal obtained from these can be used as a reference for the amount of pressure the ventilator needs to produce.[24]

Figure 9-46 shows an example of a device for delivering proportional assist ventilation. A rolling-seal piston is filled with air intended for a patient. It is connected to the patient by way of the artificial airway. The piston operates on a very low resistance arm connected to an electrically powered motor. When the patient breathes in, air moves from the piston toward the patient, and the piston moves forward to assist the patient's inspiration. The air movement is sensed by a flow-measuring device, which creates flow and volume signals that are sent to a microprocessor. The processor then signals the piston in a positive feedback manner. The greater the patient effort, the greater the piston force. The electric motor supplies current to the piston in proportion to the flow and volume signals. These signals are added, and the total signal determines the amount of current going to the motor. There is also a gain control that determines how much force (pressure) will be exerted based on where the gain is set. The gain set for the flow determines how much pressure is generated for each unit of flow (cm H_2O/L/sec [i.e., resistance units]). The gain set on the volume signal establishes how much pressure will result for each unit of the volume signal (cm H_2O/L [i.e., elastance units]).[25]

For a better understanding of the concept behind this technique, consider the following example. Suppose a patient is connected by endotracheal tube to a sealed rigid box. When the patient spontaneously breathes in, the pressure inside the box decreases in proportion to the volume the patient inspires. This represents an increased workload. If the box is replaced with a ventilator that provides instantaneous pressure delivery as soon as the patient breathes in, and does so in proportion to the amount inspired, then the ventilator basically "unloads" the amount of work. This represents "volume" proportional assist. Figure 9-47 compares a patient on CPAP to a patient on volume proportional assist ventilation.[27,28]

Here is another example. A patient is connected by endotracheal tube to a narrow tube. When the patient inspires, pressure in the tube drops. In flow-proportional assist ventilation (flow-PAV) the ventilator increases pressure during inspiration in proportion to the rate of inspiratory flow

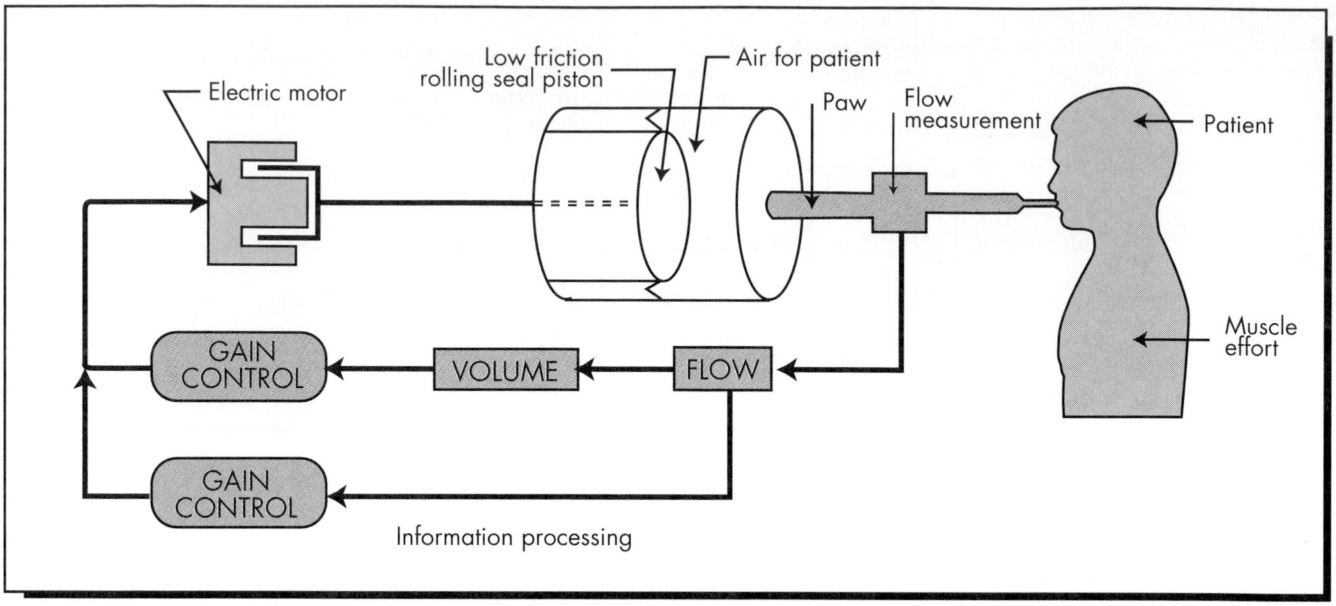

Figure 9-46 A simple diagram of a PAV-delivery system. A piston is coupled to an electric motor that generates force in proportion to the supplied current. The current is determined by the measured rate of volume delivery and gas flow to the patient. The gain controls are set by the operator and determine what proportion of patient effort will be assisted.

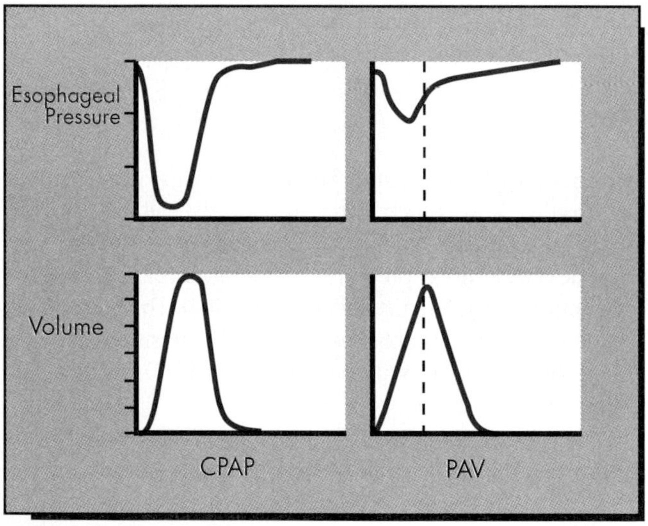

Figure 9-47 Volume and esophageal pressure curves for a CPAP breath and a volume proportional assist. (Redrawn from Schulze A, et al:, Am J Respir Crit Care Med 153:671, 1996.)

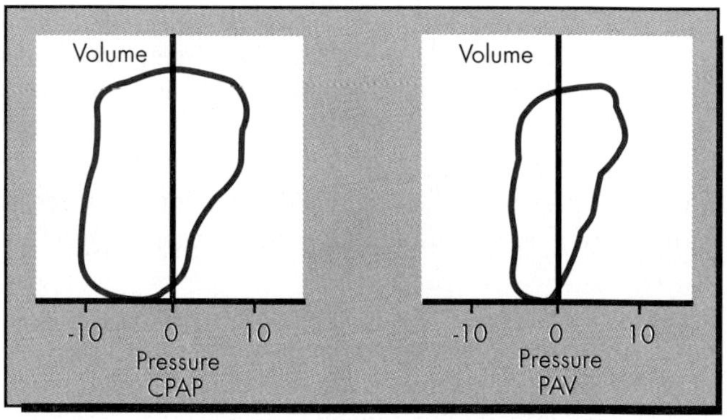

Figure 9-48 Pressure/volume loop changes comparing CPAP with PAV. PAV reduces work of breathing. (Redrawn from Schulze A, et al: Am J Respir Crit Care Med 153:671, 1996.)

generated by the patient. This has the affect of unloading the work (Figure 9-48).[27,28]

When volume- and flow-proportional assist ventilation are used together, they respond to both the elastic (1/C) and resistance (R) components of breathing and help to unload work of breathing in proportion to patient effort. The greater the volume and flow demand of the patient, the higher the force (pressure) provided by the ventilator.

For PAV the operator sets the following:

1. Baseline pressure
2. Gain for volume (elastance component)
3. Gain for flow (resistance component)

For example, if gain is set at 50% of the patient's elastance and 50% of the resistance, the ventilator will provide half the work performed by the patient required to overcome the forces of elastance and resistance (Box 9-32). If the patient makes no effort, the ventilator does no work. Thus PAV is better suited for patients with abnormalities in resistance and compliance and less so for those with neuromuscular weakness with an inability to generate a strong inspiratory effort.

BOX 9-32

Determining Proportional Assist

Paw = (f1 × volume) + (f2 × flow),
where *f1* is the ventilator-supported elastic load, or the amount of volume assist; and *f2* is the ventilator-supported resistive load, or the amount of flow assist.

An example of a ventilator with PAV is the Stephan Medizintechnik's Stephanie Infant Ventilator. This mode may soon be available on ventilators in the United States.

Adaptive Support Ventilation in the Hamilton Galileo

Adaptive support ventilation (ASV) is a closed-loop mode of ventilation in which the ventilator determines dynamic compliance ($C_D = V_T/PIP - PEEP$) and expiratory time constant (exhaled V_T/peak expiratory flow rate) for the patient and establishes a respiratory rate and V_T delivery based on monitored and set parameters. Its purpose is to target respiratory rate and V_T to establish the least amount of work possible for the patient based on lung characteristics.[29] The clinician sets the following parameters:

1. Patient's ideal body weight (IBW) and percentage of $\dot{V}_E$ that the operator wants the ventilator to supply
2. Maximum pressure limit and baseline pressure (PEEP)
3. Pressure or flow trigger
4. Rise time (pressure ramp)

When the patient is apneic, breaths are time-triggered, pressure-targeted, and time-cycled. Both respiratory rate and V_T are calculated to establish the optimum $\dot{V}_E$ based on the patient's IBW and lung mechanics. The maximum pressure limit determines the upper limit of pressure delivery.

When the patient can perform some spontaneous breaths, patient-triggered breaths are supported at a calculated pressure using PSV (minimum P = PEEP + 5 cm H_2O). The difference between the actual number of spontaneous breaths and the calculated number established by the ventilator equals the number of mandatory breaths delivered.

In spontaneously breathing patients with an adequate spontaneous rate, the ventilator adjusts pressure delivery to keep patients in the optimal calculated range for rate and V_T. The parameter range for respiratory variables in ASV are presented in Table 9-2. Chapter 10 provides a more in-depth discussion of ASV and the Hamilton Galileo ventilator.

TABLE 9-2

Parameter range for respiratory variables in adaptive-support ventilation in the Hamilton Galileo

Parameter	Range
Respiratory rate range	5 to 60 breaths/min
Tidal volume range	4.4 to 22.0 mL/kg
Inspiratory time	0.5 sec (or expiratory time constant [RCe]) to 2 × RCe or 3 seconds

HIGH-FREQUENCY VENTILATION[30]

High-frequency ventilation (HFV) is a technique of ventilation rather than a mode. It uses respiratory rates higher than normal and tidal volumes lower than normal. The Food and Drug Administration (FDA) defines high-frequency ventilation as any form of mechanical ventilation in which respiratory rates are >150 breaths/min; there are five basic types:

1. **High-frequency positive-pressure ventilation (HFPPV)**
2. High-frequency jet ventilation (HFJV)
3. **High-frequency oscillatory ventilation (HFOV)**
4. **High-frequency flow interruption (HFFI)**
5. **High-frequency percussive ventilation (HFPV)**

For particularly high rates, frequencies are usually given in Hertz (Hz) or cycles per second, with 1 Hz equalling 60 cycles (breaths)/min.

High-Frequency Positive-Pressure Ventilation (HFPPV)

HFPPV uses a conventional volume- or pressure-limited ventilator with a low compliance patient circuit. With HFPPV, the airway is intermittently pressurized with gas with no air entrainment. Respiratory rates are about 60 to 110 breaths/min. Breath rates are sometimes given in Hertz (1 Hz = 1 cycle/sec). In this case 60 to 100 breaths/min would be 1 to 1.8 Hz. HFPPV was developed by Sjöstrand and associates in the late 1960s to minimize the cardiovascular side effects of positive-pressure ventilation.[31] Animal studies also showed its effectiveness in eliminating intracranial pressure variations normally associated with breathing, thus providing a better surgical field for microneurosurgical procedures.

Early prototypes used an H-valve assembly in which the circuit was connected to an insufflation catheter attached

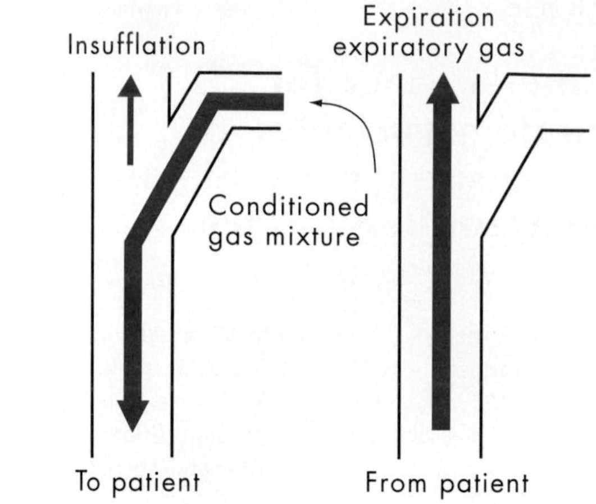

Figure 9-49 This pneumatic valve assembly used with HFPPV introduces a gas mixture during inspiration. Because of the Coanda effect, the gas stream hugs the channel. No air entrainment occurs, and only a small amount of gas leaks from the expiratory limb. (From Pilbeam SP: Mechanical ventilation: physiological and clinical applications, ed 1, St Louis, 1986, Mosby.)

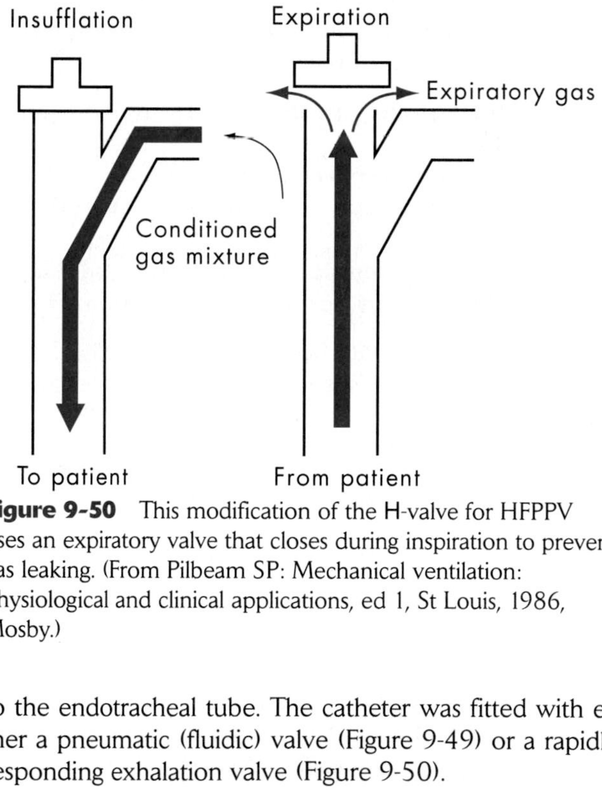

Figure 9-50 This modification of the H-valve for HFPPV uses an expiratory valve that closes during inspiration to prevent gas leaking. (From Pilbeam SP: Mechanical ventilation: physiological and clinical applications, ed 1, St Louis, 1986, Mosby.)

to the endotracheal tube. The catheter was fitted with either a pneumatic (fluidic) valve (Figure 9-49) or a rapidly responding exhalation valve (Figure 9-50).

Two possible problems could occur with the use of HFPPV: the short inspiratory times and high rates can prevent adequate V_T delivery; and breath stacking can occur with these rates and with only passive exhalation occurring.[32] That is, when respiratory rates are this rapid, sometimes the air has enough time to enter the lungs but not enough to leave. Breaths begin to "stack up" in the lungs, resulting in trapped air, which creates pressure called auto-PEEP. With other modes of HFV now becoming more popular and the use of other techniques for the management of acute lung injury (e.g., permissive hypercapnea), HFPPV is not often used in the clinical setting.

BOX 9-33

Historical Note

Early Uses of HFJV

1. To provide surgical fields undisturbed by ventilatory movement.
2. For use with bronchoscopy and laryngoscopy to provide better surgical field access while maintaining ventilation.
3. To reduce cardiovascular side effects associated with IPPV.
4. To reduce the risk of barotrauma.
5. To maintain ventilation when large air leaks are present (e.g., bronchopleural fistula)

(From Pilbeam SP: Mechanical ventilation: physiological and clinical applications, ed 1, St Louis, 1986, Mosby.)

High-Frequency Jet Ventilation (HFJV)

In 1977 Klain and Smith developed a method of HFJV ventilation that used a percutaneous transtracheal catheter. The catheter was connected to an air source that provided a jet injection of air controlled by a fluidic logic ventilator. Rates up to 600 breaths/min (10 Hz) were employed. Later this technique used a catheter that allowed for air entrainment.[33]

This technique offers rates of about 100 to 600 breaths/min (1.7 to 10 Hz) with V_T smaller than dead space. Box 9-33 lists some of the earlier uses of HFJV. In general, HFJV operates by passing gas from a high pressure source through a variable regulator that reduces the pressure to the desired working level. The gas then passes through a device, usually a solenoid or a fluidic valve, that governs the amount and duration of flow. The gas jet is then delivered through a specially made triple-lumen endotracheal tube (Figure 9-51, *A*), which is similar to conventional endotracheal tubes except that two additional small lines are added. One is for delivering jet ventilation and the other is for monitoring distal airway pressures. The jet stream exits the tube at about one third of the tube's length from the distal end. The pressure tube is located at the distal tip of the tube. If a jet tube is not used, a special jet adapter can be attached to the endotracheal tube (Figure 9-51, *B*). Another technique to use when a special jet tube is not in place is to use a small catheter inserted either through a conventional endotracheal or tra-

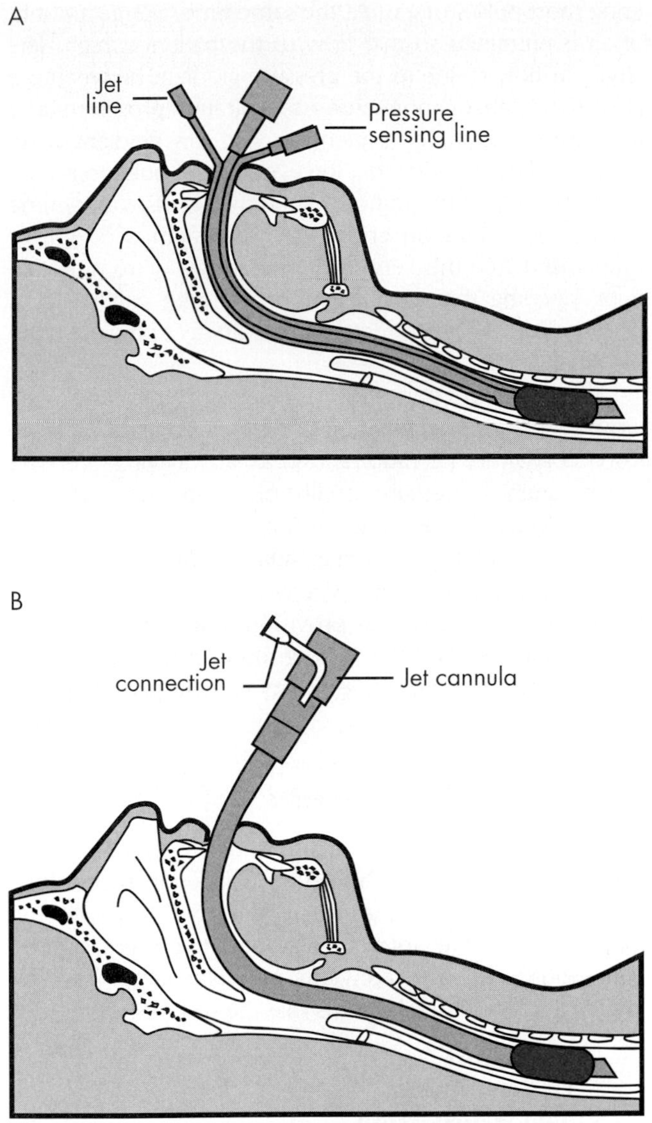

Figure 9-51 A diagram of a high frequency tube (*A*) and a jet connection with a jet cannula (*B*).

cheostomy tube. Studies have shown that the best position for the jet is close to the proximal end of the trachea near the vocal cords.[34]

The operational principle of HFJV involves the delivery of short breaths or pulsations (20 to 34 msec) under pressure through a small lumen at high rates (4 to 11 Hz).[34] The tidal volume of the breath depends on the following four basic factors:

1. Length of the pulsation
2. Amplitude or driving pressure of the jet
3. Jet orifice size
4. Patient lung characteristics

Under certain conditions, gas can be entrained around the jet through the physical process of jet mixing. It results from the viscous shearing of the jet gas layer with stagnant gas in the airway. This gas is dragged downstream in an entrainment-like effect. The volume of entrained gas can alter V_T delivery depending on patient lung characteristics.[30] Examples of jet ventilators include the Bunnell's Life Pulse and Intrasonics's Adult Star 1010.

High-Frequency Oscillatory Ventilation (HFOV)

High-frequency oscillatory ventilation (HFOV) uses some type of reciprocating pump to generate an approximation of a sine wave (see Figures 9-3 and 11-37). Examples of devices that provide this function are reciprocating pumps (usually pistons), diaphragms, and loudspeakers. Although not true oscillators, high frequency flow interrupters (HFFI) (see the following section) can be used in ventilators to provide a similar effect. These ventilators are called "pseudo-oscillators."

With HFOV, pressure is positive in the airway during the inspiratory phase (forward stroke) and negative during the expiratory phase (return stroke). Thus both inspiration and expiration are active, and there is bulk flow rather than jet pulsations. HFOV uses frequencies in the range of 1 to 50 Hz (60 to 3000 cycles/min), and V_T is less the dead space. Some ventilators have a fixed I:E ratio, and others allow the I:E ratio to be adjusted.

HFOV is one of the most widely used forms of HFV in infants and pediatric patients. One example of an oscillator is the Sensormedics Corporation's 3100A (see Chapter 11). The 3100A uses a diaphragm-shaped piston that is driven magnetically, much like a stereo speaker (see Figure 11-37). The mean airway pressure control sets the tension on the diaphragm. Gas is oscillated back and forth by the action of the diaphragm. The amplitude of the wave set by the power control determines the forward and backward excursion of the piston, which helps determine V_T. In the 3100A, rigid plastic circuits provide the bias flow of warmed and humidified air that is delivered to the patient.

High-Frequency Flow Interruption (HFFI)

High-frequency flow interruption is similar to HFJV, but differs in its technical design. In HFFI a control mechanism interrupts a high-pressure gas source. One common mechanism is a rotating ball with a flow port in the center. Another example is a rotating bar (Figure 9-52). Frequencies with HFFI are as high as 15 Hz. As in HFJV, the high pressure bursts of gas can entrain static gas supplied by the addition of a bias flow circuit, which enhances volume delivery. An example of this device was invented by Emerson, whose HFFI uses a spinning ball and consists of a conduit that conducts a gas flow. Inside the conduit is a ball with a flow port in its center. The ball is moved back and forth in the conduit by an electric motor at rates up to 200 cycles/min. As it moves, it interrupts the outflow of gas

(Figure 9-53).[30] An example of a HFFI (a pseudo-oscillator) is Infrasonics's Infant Star ventilator (see Chapter 11).

High-Frequency Percussive Ventilation (HFPV)

Dr. Forrest M. Bird, a pioneer in ventilatory devices, designed a high-frequency percussive ventilation device in which he incorporated the beneficial characteristics of both a conventional positive-pressure ventilator and a jet ventilator. It operates in such a way that high-frequency breaths are superimposed onto conventional breaths and can be compared with time-cycled, pressure-limited ventilation when high-frequency pulsations (up to 100 to 225 cycles/min, or 1.7 to 5 Hz) are injected throughout the inspiratory phase (Figure 9-54). The resulting unit is called a high-frequency percussive ventilator.

A ventilator that incorporates this principle is the Bird VDR-4, which operates using a sliding Venturi (Figure 9-55). At the mouth of the Venturi is a jet orifice. Around the jet is a continuous bias flow of warm, humidified air. During inspiration, a diaphragm connected to the Venturi fills with gas. This action slides the Venturi forward, toward the patient's airway, simultaneously blocking the expiratory port. During this time, the jet is activated and begins delivering short pulses of gas. At the same time, a large amount of air is entrained so that flow to the patient is high. The large gas flow is due to the pressure gradient between the jet and the patient connector. As inspiration progresses and pressure builds in the patient airway, this gradient is reduced, so flow is reduced. However, the jet pulsations continue throughout inspiration. When the set inspiratory time is reached, inspiration ends. The diaphragm is no longer pressurized, and the Venturi slides back away from the patient, opening the expiratory port. During exhalation, a counterflow of gas is directed at the airway to maintain the set PEEP level.[30]

Ventilation is controlled by respiratory rate and peak airway pressure. Oxygenation is determined by PEEP level, inspiratory time, I:E ratio, and peak airway pressure. The high-frequency pressure oscillations also affect gas exchange, which makes clinical monitoring of these variables an important part of frequency adjustments.

Clinical benefits of HFPV may include facilitation of secretion removal, as well as provision of a mode of continuous ventilation. HFPV has been used prophylactically in patients with thermal airway injury to help prevent pneumonia and atelectasis.[30]

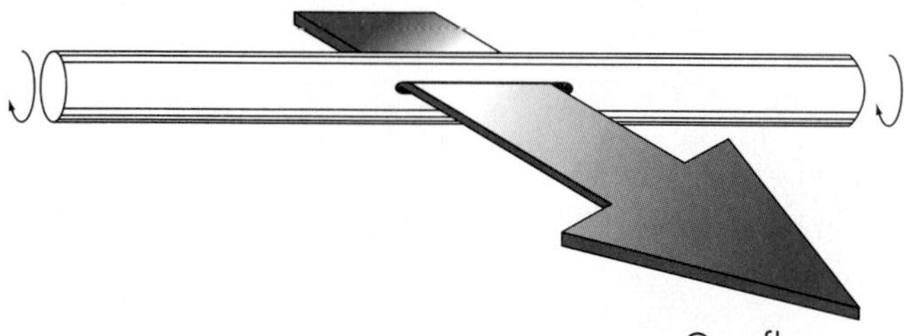

Figure 9-52 A flow interruptor. Flow is interrupted at high frequencies as a rotating metal bar allows it during some portions of the breath and blocks it at others. (From Pilbeam SP: Mechanical ventilation: physiological and clinical applications, ed 1, St Louis, 1986, Mosby.)

Mechanisms of Action of HFV

The mechanisms of action of the various forms of HFV are not clearly understood; however, ventilation successfully occurs even when V_T is less than dead space (V_D). Alveoli located close to the airways are thought to be ventilated by convection, just as in conventional ventilation.* The following additional mechanisms may be responsible:

1. **Pendelluft**
2. **Gas streaming**
3. **Taylor dispersion**
4. Molecular diffusion

*Convection is the movement of air molecules associated with the pressures of ventilation.

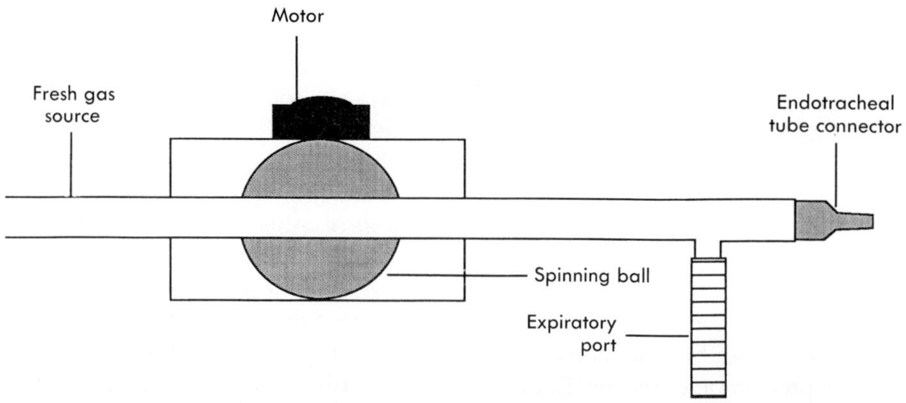

Figure 9-53 An example of a high-frequency oscillatory device, the spinning ball.

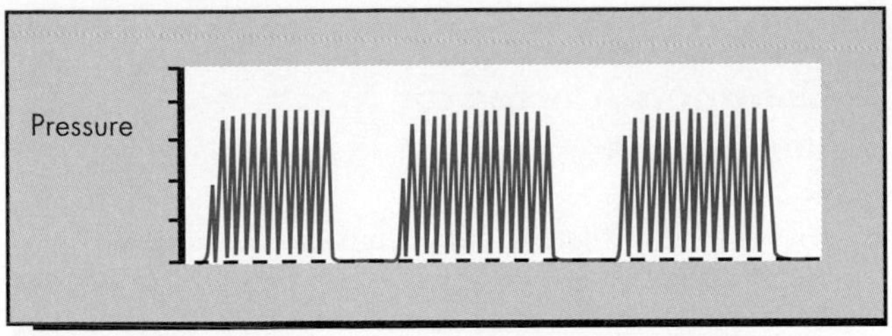

Figure 9-54 An example of a pressure/time waveform created during HFPV.

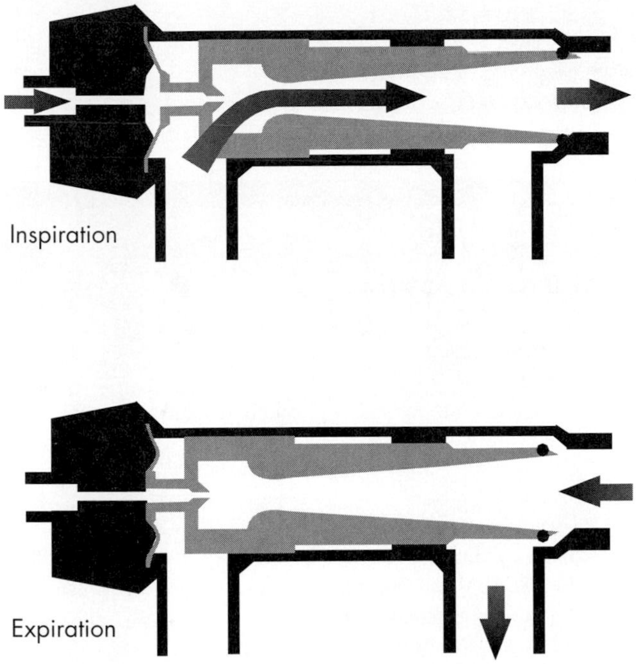

Figure 9-55 Design of the sliding venturi for a high-frequency percussive generator used to provide HFPV (see text for explanation). (From Pilbeam SP: Mechanical ventilation: physiological and clinical applications, ed 3, St Louis, 1998, Mosby.)

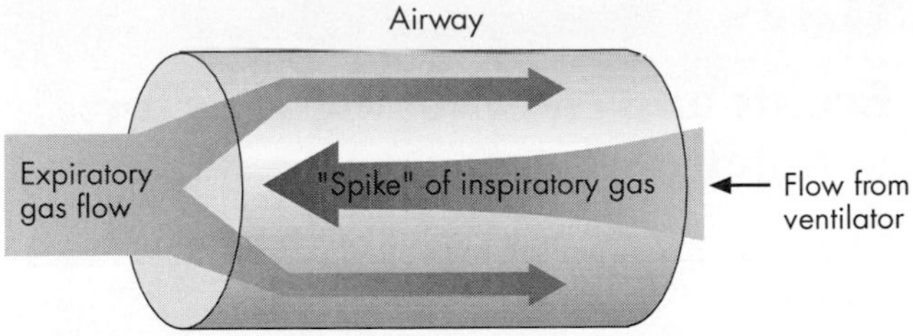

Figure 9-56 Effects of streaming in HFJV: forward movement of the gas in the center produced by pulsations from the jet cause gas along the airway walls to be pushed backward. (From Pilbeam SP: Mechanical ventilation: physiological and clinical applications, ed 3, St Louis, 1998, Mosby.)

Pendelluft is the movement of gases from one area of the lungs to another due to differences in the compliance and resistance of various lung regions. This movement occurs through normal anatomic channels (e.g., alveolar ducts, the pores of Kohn, and the canals of Lambert). When lung tissue is oscillated, as occurs with HFV, this phenomenon may be enhanced.

Streaming or asymmetric velocity profiles occur when gas flows in both directions at once through a conductive airway. Inspired gas is thought to move down the center of the airway in a parabolic fashion, while exhaled gas tends to move near the walls and out (Figure 9-56).

Taylor dispersion is thought to occur in HFOV. It is the enhanced mixing of gases associated with the turbulent flow of high velocity gases moving through small airways and their bifurcations. The erratic pattern of eddies and streams created is thought to enhance gas mixing and diffusion.

Simple molecular diffusion also occurs, at least at the terminal air spaces and is another mechanism which adds to gas mixing.

Because HFV is used infrequently in many institutions, and because it has not been proven to show improved outcomes in comparison with conventional ventilation, HFV has not been a dominant technique of ventilatory support of patients. It has, however, gained popularity in some hospitals, especially in the management of infants and children. How important its position will be is still uncertain and depends on not only further clinical research but also increased popularity with a larger group of clinicians.

Part III: Troubleshooting During Mechanical Ventilation

VENTILATOR ALARMS

A variety of alarms are available with all mechanical ventilators that can be audible, visible, provide written messages on a display screen, or do a combination of these. Some can be inactivated by the operator, but others cannot. Alarms that are critical to unit function, such as loss of power (electric or pneumatic) or detection of an internal operational error (technical error), cannot be silenced and require immediate attention. The American Association for Respiratory Care (AARC) has suggested a classification system for the levels of priorities of alarms (Table 9-3). Box 9-34 lists the most common types of alarms available. Appendix A-1 (at the end of this chapter) provides algorithms to help solve common alarm situations.

TABLE 9-3

Events and monitoring sites for ventilator alarms

Event	Possible monitoring site
Level 1	
Power failure (including when battery in use)	Electrical control system*
Absence of gas delivery (apnea)	Circuit pressure,* circuit flows, timing monitor, CO_2 analysis
Loss of gas source	Pneumatic control system*
Excessive gas delivery	Circuit pressures,* circuit flows, timing monitor
Exhalation valve failure	Circuit pressures, circuit flows, timing monitor
Timing failure	Circuit pressures, circuit flows, timing monitor
Level 2	
Battery power loss (not in use)	Electrical control system*
Circuit leak*	Circuit pressures,* circuit flows
Blender failure	FiO_2 sensor
Circuit partially occluded	Circuit pressures, circuit flows
Heater/humidifier failure	Temperature probe in circuit
Loss of/or excessive PEEP	Circuit pressures
Autocycling	Circuit pressures, circuit flows
Other electrical or preventive subsystem out of limits without immediate overt gas delivery effects	Electrical and pneumatic systems monitor
Level 3	
Change in central nervous system drive	Circuit pressures, circuit flows, timing monitor
Change in impedances	Circuit pressures, circuit flows, timing monitor
Intrinsic PEEP (auto) > 5 cm H_2O	Circuit pressures, circuit flows

*Alarms currently defined in the ISO and ASTM standards.

From AARC consensus statement on the essentials of mechanical ventilation, Respir Care 37:1007, 1992; with permission.

BOX 9-34

Common Alarms for Mechanical Ventilators

1. Loss of power (electric or pneumatic)
2. Apnea
3. Pressure alarms: low and high circuit pressure, low and high baseline pressures (PEEP/CPAP), and failure of pressure to return to baseline
4. High and low expired V_T or $\dot{V}_E$
5. Low and high respiratory rate
6. Inappropriate T_I or T_E
7. Inspired temperature alarm
8. High and low FiO_2 alarms

BOX 9-35

Common Causes of Low-Pressure Alarm Situations

Patient disconnect
Circuit leaks
- Mainline connections to humidifiers, filters, and/or water traps
- In-line metered dose inhalers
- In-line nebulizers
- Proximal pressure monitors
- Flow monitoring lines
- Exhaled gas monitoring devices
- In-line closed suction catheters
- Temperature monitors
- Exhalations valve leaks: cracked or leaking valves, unseated valves, and/or improperly connected valves

Airway leaks
- Use of minimum leak technique
- Inadequate cuff inflation
- Leak in pilot balloon
- Rupture of tube cuff

Chest tube leaks

(From Pilbeam SP: Mechanical ventilation. In Burton GG, Hodgkin JE, and Ward JJ, editors: Respiratory care: a guide to clinical practice, ed 4, Philadelphia, 1997, Lippincott.)

Identifying and Solving Alarm Situations

Alarms may inform the operator of a potential problem, but the problem still must be solved. Most of the time this is easy because the alarm provides a light or message telling the operator what problem has occurred or is currently present. For example, when a ventilator reaches its high pressure limit, it normally provides an audible high-pressure alarm, which only sounds once to signal the event. Most ventilators have a small light that remains lit until a manual reset button is activated by the operator. In this way, the ventilator keeps a visual record of the alarm event that the operator can observe even after the alarm has ceased.

Some of the common causes of low- and high-pressure alarms are provided in Boxes 9-35 and 9-36 respectively.

BOX 9-36

Common Causes of High-Pressure Alarm Situations

Common causes
- Patient coughing
- Secretions or mucus in the airway
- Patient biting tube (oral intubation)

Airway problems
- Kinking of tube inside the mouth or in the back of the throat
- Impinging of the tube on the carina
- Change in the tube position
- Cuff herniated over the end of the tube

Patient-related conditions
- Reduced compliance (e.g., pneumothorax or pleural effusion)
- Increased airway resistance (e.g., secretions, mucosal edema, or bronchospasm)
- Patient "fighting the ventilator" (e.g., dyssynchrony with ventilator settings)

Ventilator circuit
- Accumulation of water in the patient circuit
- Kinking in the circuit
- Ventilator's inspiratory or expiratory valves malfunctioning

(From Pilbeam SP: Mechanical ventilation. In Burton GG, Hodgkin JE, and Ward JJ, editors: Respiratory care: a guide to clinical practice, ed 4, Philadelphia, 1997, Lippincott.)

Whenever an alarm is activated, the clinician's primary responsibility is to be sure that the patient is being adequately ventilated. Sometimes the solution is immediately obvious. For example, a patient may be disconnected from the ventilator at the wye connector. If this is easily seen, it is easily solved by reconnecting the patient. Other times the problem is less obvious. When the problem is not apparent, the most immediate and important solution is to disconnect the patient from the ventilator and perform manual ventilation with a resuscitation bag. If the patient improves, the problem resides with the ventilator. Examples of mechanical problems include leaks, expiratory valve failures, power source failures, inappropriately assembled circuits, I:E ratio problems, and incompatible settings. If the patient does not improve, the problem is with the patient. Patient problems can include airway obstructions, pneumothorax, pulmonary thromboembolism, cardiac problems, and air trapping.

Troubleshooting Problems Using Ventilator Graphics

Clinicians can rely on ventilator alarms, changes in patients' signs and symptoms, and changes in ventilator data to help solve problems and alarm situations. In the last few years, ventilator graphic display screens have become more widely available and are another tool for evaluating and determining problems. Although it is beyond the scope of this text to cover all the possible graphic changes that can help determine problems, the most common methods of identifying these problems will be reviewed.[6] For some additional introductory information on the basics of ventilator graphics, check "www.saminc.com," a web site course on graphics designed by Yvon Dupuis, MS, RRT of the Respiratory Care Program at Fanshaw College in London, Ontario, Canada.

Increased Airway Resistance

Figure 9-57 shows the difference between PIP and $P_{plateau}$ increases (increased P_{TA}) as one method of identifying an increase in Raw. In addition, prolonged expiratory flows in a flow/time curve (Figure 9-58 **A**), reduced flows in flow/volume loops (**B**), and an increase in the hysteresis of a pressure/volume loop (**C**) can all help establish the presence of increased airway resistance.

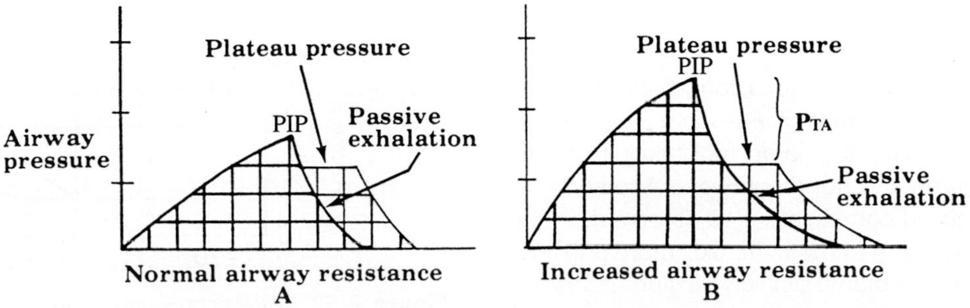

Figure 9-57 **A,** Normal pressure difference between peak and plateau pressure when airway resistance is normal during volume ventilation. When airway resistance is increased, the difference between peak and plateau pressure is increased (i.e., more pressure is lost to the airways [P_{TA}]). **B,** Note that peak inspiratory pressure is also increased. (From Pilbeam SP: Mechanical ventilation: physiological and clinical applications, ed 3, St Louis, 1998, Mosby.)

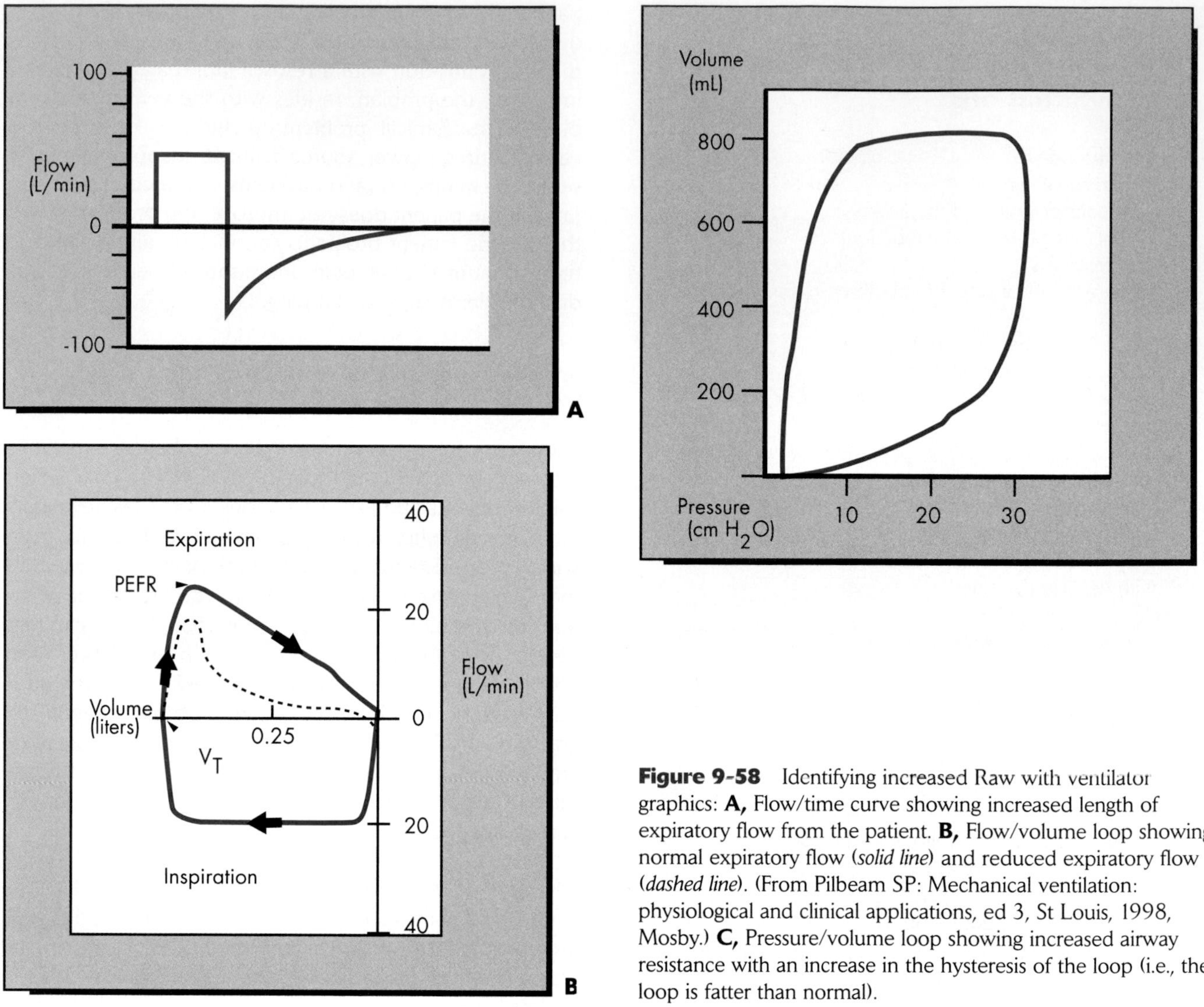

Figure 9-58 Identifying increased Raw with ventilator graphics: **A,** Flow/time curve showing increased length of expiratory flow from the patient. **B,** Flow/volume loop showing normal expiratory flow (*solid line*) and reduced expiratory flow (*dashed line*). (From Pilbeam SP: Mechanical ventilation: physiological and clinical applications, ed 3, St Louis, 1998, Mosby.) **C,** Pressure/volume loop showing increased airway resistance with an increase in the hysteresis of the loop (i.e., the loop is fatter than normal).

Decreased Compliance

When both PIP and $P_{plateau}$ increase proportionally during volume ventilation, lung compliance is decreased. In this example, P_{TA} will remain the same, indicating that the problem is in the lungs and not the airways. Another way of identifying a reduced compliance is to observe the shift of a pressure/volume loop to the right, (i.e., more pressure is required for a similar volume delivery) (Figure 9-59).

Auto-PEEP

Air-trapping or auto-PEEP can be identified when the expiratory flow curve does not return to zero before the next breath triggers into inspiration. This can be seen in the

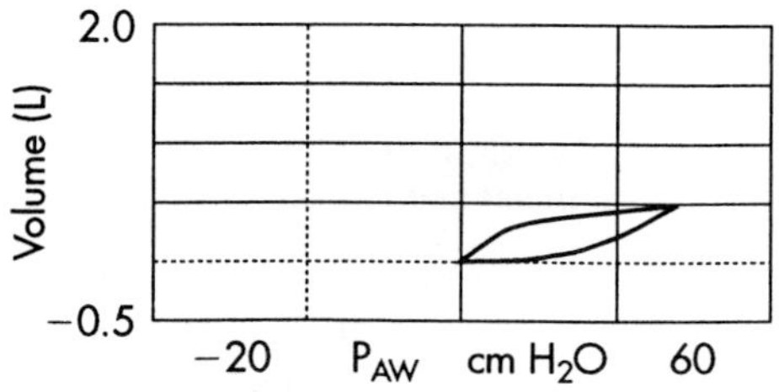

Figure 9-59 Airway pressure/volume loop recorded on a patient with reduced lung compliance. Note the decrease in area (i.e., the loop is thinner), representing nonelastic inspiratory and expiratory work. The curve is "shifted" (i.e., leans) to the right. (Redrawn from Kacmarek RM, Hess D, and Stoller JK: Monitoring in respiratory care, St Louis, 1993, Mosby.)

flow/time and the flow/volume loops (see Figure 9-37 and Figure 9-60).

Inadequate Flow

When a fixed flow is delivered during volume ventilation, sometimes the amount of flow is inadequate for the patient. This is seen as a concave pressure/time curve (Figure 9-61).

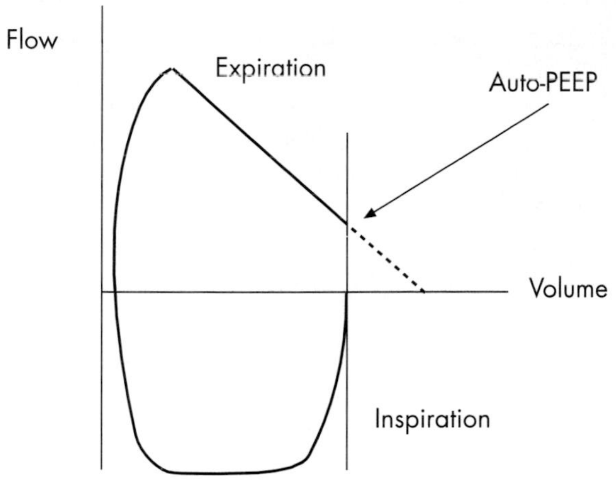

Figure 9-60 A flow/volume loop showing the presence of auto-PEEP. Flow does not return to zero during exhalation.

Inadequate Sensitivity Setting

If the patient appears to be struggling for a breath and inspiratory pressures are deflecting below baseline, then the ventilator is not sensitive enough to patient effort (Figure 9-62). Sometimes sensitivity is set appropriately, but the patient still cannot trigger a breath. This can occur if auto-PEEP is present, making it more difficult for the patient to drop upper airway pressures low enough to trigger inspiration.

Active Exhalation or Out of Calibration

When a volume/time curve shows expiratory volume going below baseline, two possible problems are suggested. The patient is air trapping and is forcibly exhaling, or the expiratory flow transducer is out of calibration and is recording expiratory flow below the baseline (Figure 9-63).

Overinflation

When a pressure/volume loop shows a sharp, beak-shaped spike to the right (i.e., pressure increases without much or any volume change during volume ventilation), then the patient's lungs are overinflated (overdistended) (Figure 9-64).

Leaks

Leaks in the circuit can be quickly identified when the expiratory volume curve does not return to baseline or zero.

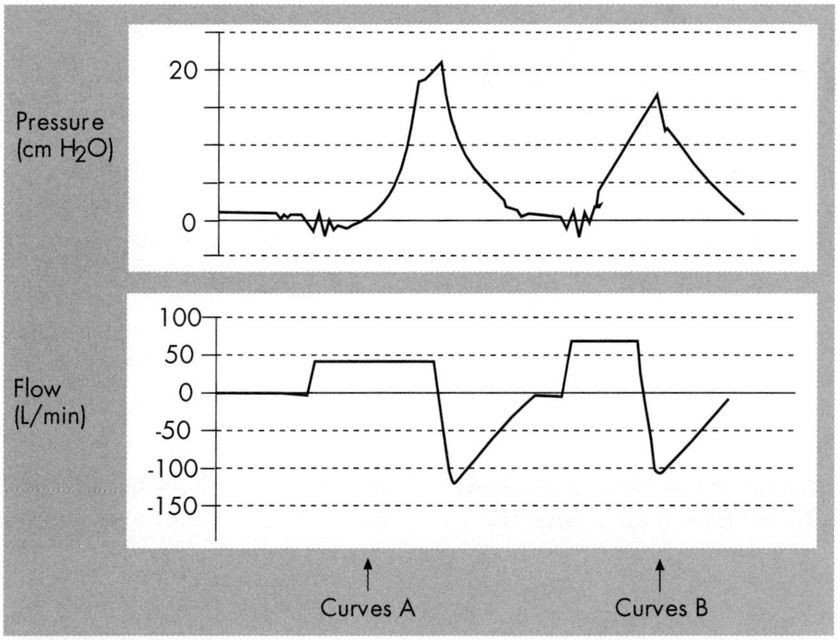

Figure 9-61 These are examples of volume breaths with constant flow delivery. **A,** The flow, which is set at 50 L/min, is too low for patient demand. Note the concave appearance of the pressure curve. **B,** In this curve, flow has been increased to 75 L/min, and pressure rise is normal. The erratic pattern of pressure just before the mandatory breath suggests that sensitivity may not be set appropriately. (From Pilbeam SP: Mechanical ventilation: physiological and clinical applications, ed 3, St Louis, 1998, Mosby.)

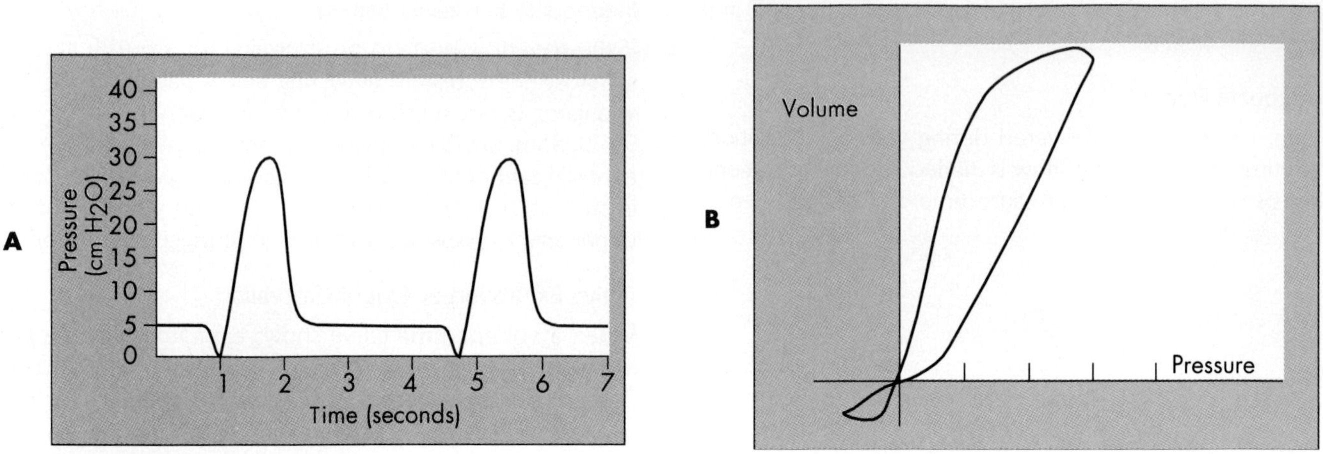

Figure 9-62 Inadequate sensitivity: **A,** pressure drops well below baseline before a breath delivery. In this case, baseline is 5 cm H_2O of PEEP. **B,** a pressure/volume loop showing a deflection to the left on inspiration much higher than normal. (From Pilbeam SP: Mechanical ventilation: physiological and clinical applications, ed 3, St Louis, 1998, Mosby.)

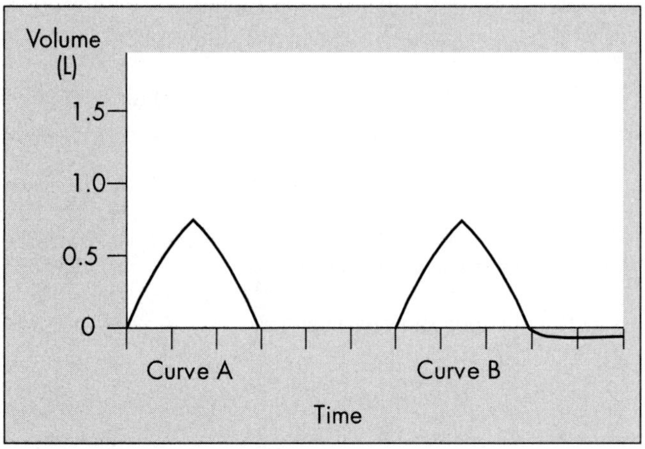

Figure 9-63 Curve A is a normal volume/time curve. Curve B shows the expiratory portion of the volume below the zero baseline (see text for explanation). (From Pilbeam SP: Mechanical ventilation: physiological and clinical applications, ed 3, St Louis, 1998, Mosby.)

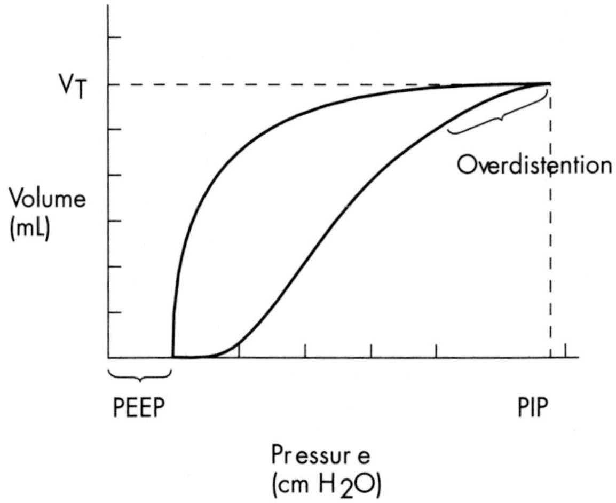

Figure 9-64 A pressure/volume loop in a patient with acute overdistention of the lung during positive-pressure ventilation. Notice the duck-billed appearance of the top, righthand portion of the curve (overdistention). (From Pilbeam SP: Mechanical ventilation: physiological and clinical applications, ed 3, St Louis, 1998, Mosby.)

This is true for volume/time curves (Figure 9-65 **A**), volume/pressure loops (**B**), and flow/volume loops (**C**).

Ringing or Oscillation in the Circuit

The initial flow of gas in PSV may be the maximum flow for the ventilator. If this flow is too rapid, it can cause a spike in the pressure curve. When it is extremely high, "ringing" occurs. For example, if the working pressure is set too high on the Servo 900, this has been shown to cause "ringing" or oscillations in pressure delivery, which can create patient discomfort, end a breath prematurely, and reduce volume delivery (Figure 9-66).[35] Oscillations can also occur when there is water in the circuit.

Solving Problems During Alarm Situations

Box 9-37 and Appendix 9-1 provide some solutions to problems encountered during ventilation by identifying alarm situations, establishing the cause of the alarm, and finding some potential solutions. For more in-depth coverage of ventilator graphics and management of patient-ventilator problems, readers are referred elsewhere.[6,16,36-39]

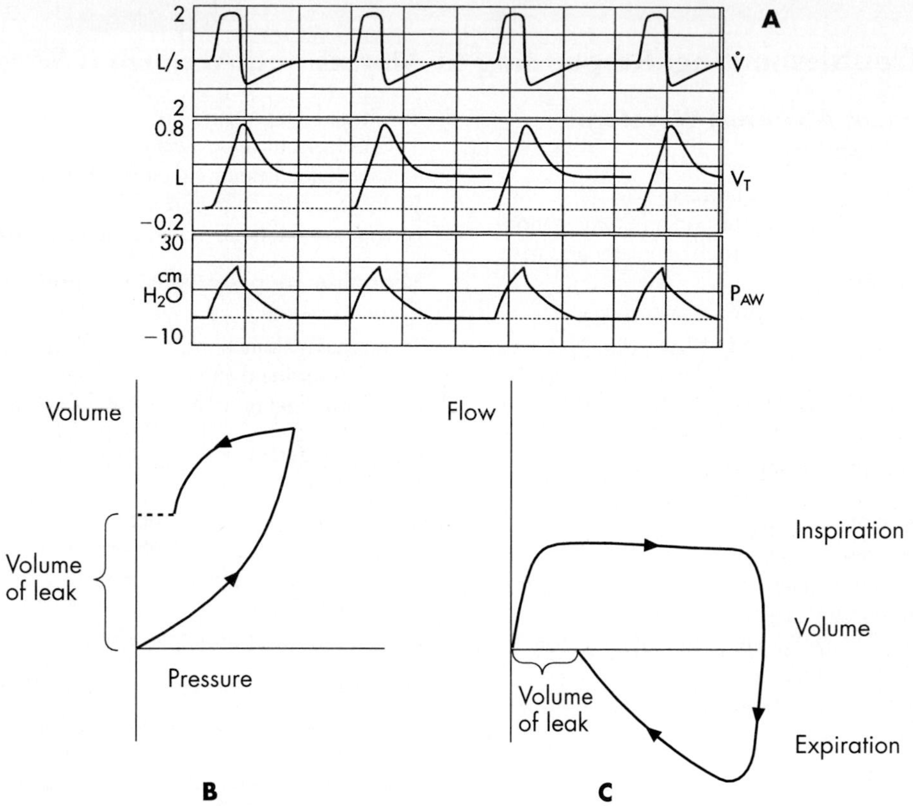

Figure 9-65 **A,** Airway pressure (*Paw*), tidal volume (V_T), and flow (V̇) curves during volume ventilation. Note that the exhaled volume curve does not return to zero. The ventilator's computer returns the curve to the baseline at the beginning of the next breath. By measuring the difference between inspired and expired volume, the leak can be quantified. (Redrawn from Kacmarek RM, Hess D, and Stoller JK: Monitoring in respiratory care, St Louis, 1993, Mosby.) **B,** A pressure/volume loop showing an air leak. **C,** A flow/volume loop showing an air leak. (From Pilbeam SP: Mechanical ventilation: physiological and clinical applications, ed 3, St Louis, 1998, Mosby.)

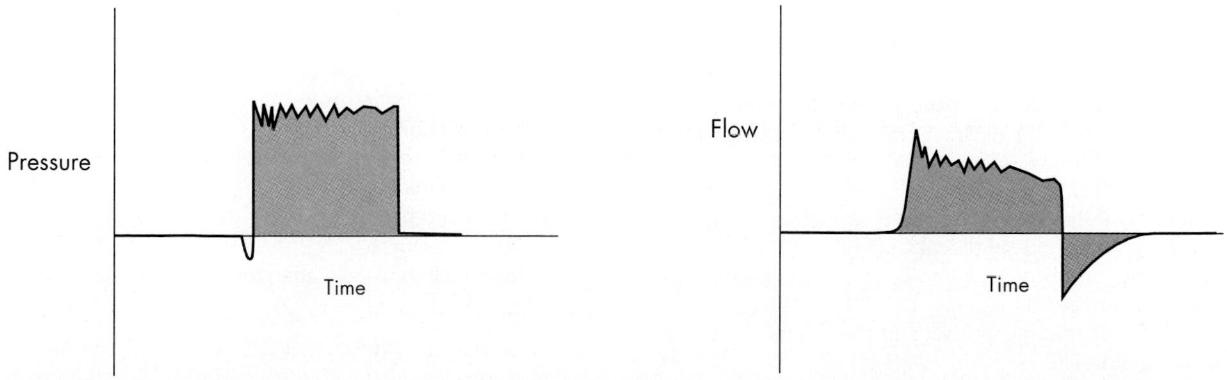

Figure 9-66 Ringing or oscillation in the circuit, occurring when working pressure is high, which results in high flow. (From Pilbeam SP: Mechanical ventilation: physiological and clinical applications, ed 3, St Louis, 1998, Mosby.)

BOX 9-37

Ventilator Troubleshooting: Responding to Alarms and Abnormal Waveforms

Alarm Situation, or Abnormal Waveform Present, in All Situations

1. Look at the patient to evaluate distress.
2. Assess patient to be sure of ventilation and oxygenation.
3. If necessary, disconnect patient from ventilator and manually ventilate, increasing FiO_2.
4. Check that alarm parameters are set appropriately.
5. Once the cause of problem has been determined, resolve the cause.
6. If the problem cannot be resolved, change the ventilator.

Common Alarm Situations

Low-Pressure Alarm

1. Check for patient disconnection.
2. Check for leaks in the patient circuit, related to the artificial airway, and through chest tubes.
3. Check the proximal Paw line to be sure that it is connected and not obstructed.
4. This alarm may be accompanied by a low $\dot{V}_E$ or low V_T alarm.

High-Pressure Alarm

1. If patient is coughing, be sure that secretions have not built up in the airway and that patient is not biting the tube.
2. Check for kinking of the endotracheal tube, displacement of the tube balloon, and position of the tube.
3. Check to see if the patient's Raw has increased or if C_L has decreased.
4. Be sure that the main inspiratory or expiratory lines are not kinked or obstructed.
5. Check that patient is breathing synchronously with ventilator.
6. Determine if auto-PEEP has developed.
7. Be sure the expiratory valve is functioning properly.

Low PEEP/CPAP Alarms

1. Check the low PEEP alarm setting to be sure it is below the PEEP level.
2. See if the patient is actively inspiring below baseline.
3. Determine if a leak is present.
4. Check to be sure that the patient is not disconnected.
5. Assess the proximal Paw line to be sure it is not occluded.

Apnea Alarm

1. Determine if the patient is apneic.
2. Check for the presence of leaks.
3. Check the sensitivity setting to be sure the ventilator can detect patient effort.
4. Check the alarm-time interval and the volume setting, when appropriate.

Low Source-Gas Pressure or Power Input Alarm

1. Check 50 psi gas source (e.g., wall connection or air compressor).
2. Check high-pressure hose connections to the ventilator.
3. Check electrical power supply, and reconnect if necessary.
4. Check line fuse or circuit breaker.
5. Try using the reset button.
6. If alarms continue, replace the ventilator.

Ventilator Inoperative Alarm and/or Technical Error Message

1. Internal malfunction present; try turning ventilator off and restarting it.
2. If alarm continues, replace the ventilator.

Operator Settings Are Incompatible with Machine Parameters

1. Error message usually indicates that a parameter must be reset (e.g., flow is not high enough to deliver V_T within an acceptable T_I to keep I:E ratio below 1:1 [based on f, V_T, and flow]).
2. Readjust the appropriate controls.

I:E Ratio Indicator and Alarm Activated

1. Usually indicates an I:E ratio of greater than 1:1.
2. If inverse I:E ratio is a goal, disable the I:E ratio limit.
3. If normal I:E ratios are a goal, check alarm causes:
   - Has increased Raw or decreased C_L resulted in a lower flow? Treat the cause.
   - Is the flow setting too low for the desired V_T delivery? Increase flow or change flow waveform.

Other Possible Alarms

1. High PEEP/CPAP alarms
   - Similar to causes of high-pressure alarms.
   - In flow-cycled modes, check for system leaks.
2. Low V_T, low $\dot{V}_E$, and/or low f alarms
   - Similar to situations that cause low-pressure alarms.
   - The patient's spontaneous ventilation has decreased for some reason.
   - The alarms may be set inappropriately.
   - Flow sensor disconnection or malfunction.
3. High V_T, high $\dot{V}_E$, and/or high f alarms
   - Check machine sensitivity for auto-triggering.
   - Check for possible cause of increased patient $\dot{V}_E$.
   - Be sure alarms are set appropriately.
   - If external nebulizer is in use, reset the alarm setting until the treatment is finished.
   - Check flow sensors for miscalibration, contamination, or malfunction.
4. Low FiO_2 and high FiO_2 alarms
   - Check gas source.
   - Check built-in oxygen analyzer for proper functioning.

(From Pilbeam SP: Mechanical ventilation: physiological and clinical applications, ed 3 St Louis, 1998, Mosby.)

Part IV: Ancillary Equipment Used During Patient Ventilation

RESISTIVE EXPIRATORY VALVES TO ALLOW FOR PASSIVE EXHALATION OF PEEP/CPAP

Expiratory valves in a ventilator normally close during inspiration, directing gas flow into the patient's lungs, and open on exhalation, allowing the patient to exhale through the valve. When PEEP is selected, it is the threshold-resistive characteristics of the expiratory valve that provide PEEP. PEEP valves can also be used in the freestanding PEEP/CPAP systems described later in this chapter. Optimally designed expiratory valves allow unrestricted flow from the patient circuit. Newer ventilator systems try to accommodate this function because older valves often increased resistance to gas flow when expiratory flow was high or the patient coughed into the circuit.[40]

In newer ventilators, the PEEP valve is often located inside the ventilator housing. Older ventilators, such as the Bear 3 and the MA-1, have expiratory valves both external to the ventilator and integrated into the patient circuit (see Figure 9-7 **A**).

The two major categories of threshold expiratory resistor valves are gravity-dependent and non-gravity–dependent.[17,41] Gravity-dependent resistors include underwater columns (Figure 9-67), water-weighted diaphragms (Figure 9-68), and weighted balls (Figure 9-69). Non-gravity–dependent devices include spring-loaded valves (Figure 9-70), balloon or diaphragm type of expiratory valves (Figure 9-71), opposing gas flow systems (Figure 9-72), and magnetic and electromagnetic PEEP valves (Figures 9-73 and 9-74).[42]

The following three devices (underwater column, water-weighted diaphragm, and weighted ball) are added here as a historical note because they are seldom—if ever—used at this time.

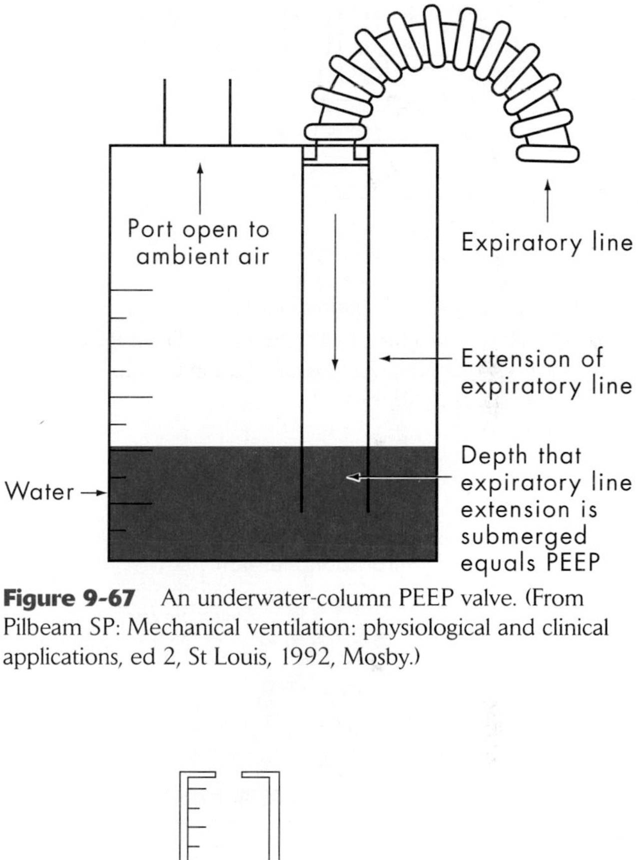

Figure 9-67 An underwater-column PEEP valve. (From Pilbeam SP: Mechanical ventilation: physiological and clinical applications, ed 2, St Louis, 1992, Mosby.)

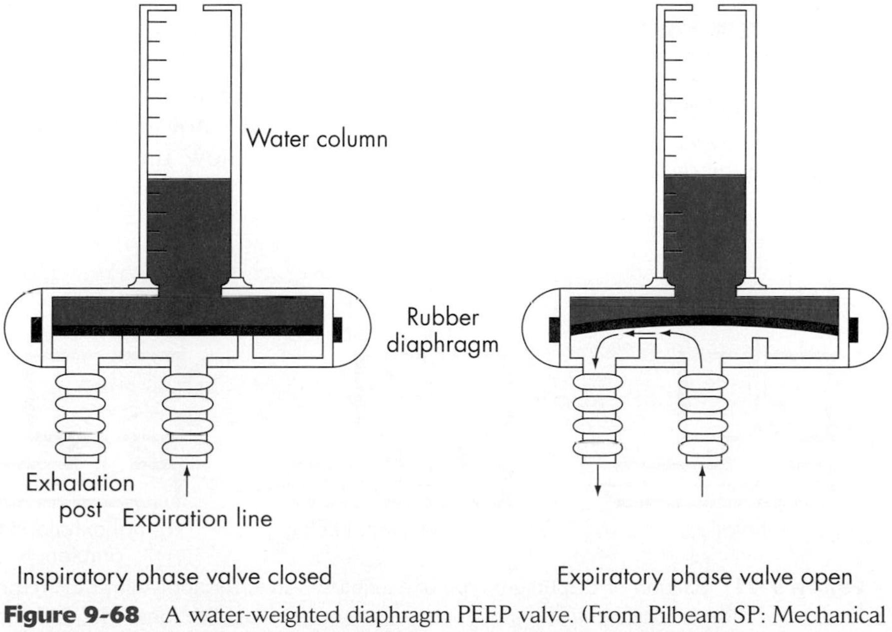

Figure 9-68 A water-weighted diaphragm PEEP valve. (From Pilbeam SP: Mechanical ventilation: physiological and clinical applications, ed 2, St Louis, 1992, Mosby.)

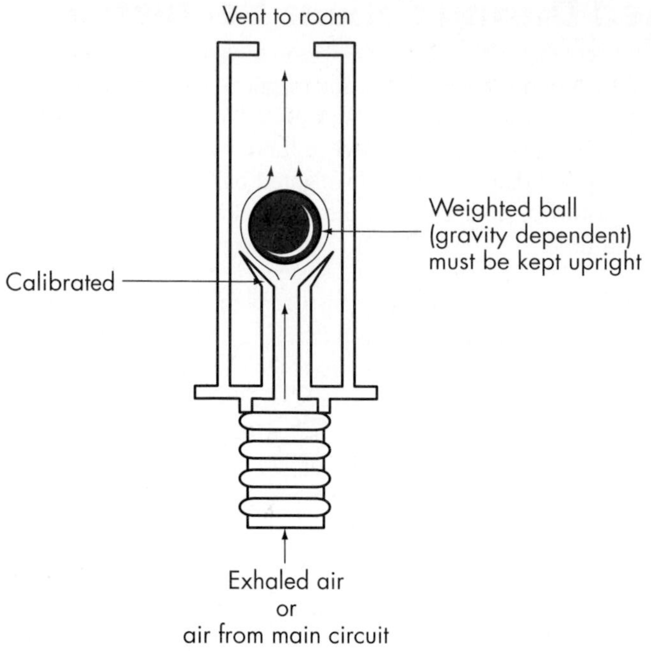

Figure 9-69 A weighted-ball PEEP valve. (From Pilbeam SP: Mechanical ventilation: physiological and clinical applications, ed 2, St Louis, 1992, Mosby.)

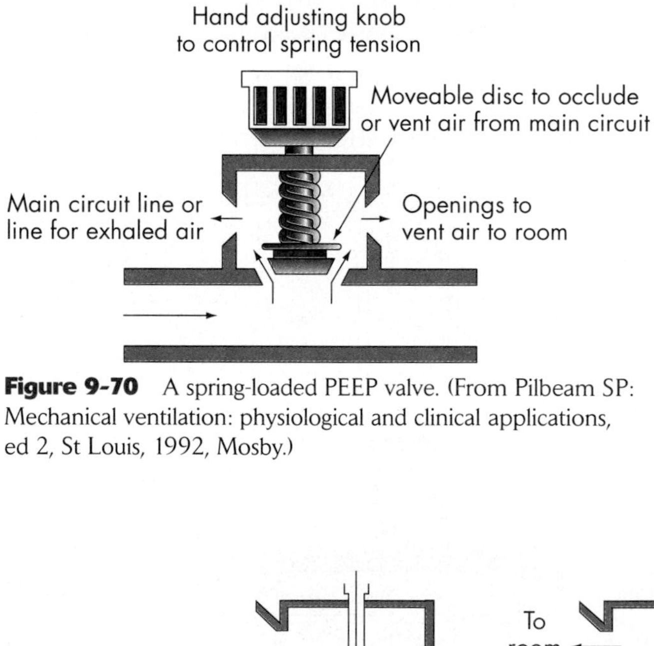

Figure 9-70 A spring-loaded PEEP valve. (From Pilbeam SP: Mechanical ventilation: physiological and clinical applications, ed 2, St Louis, 1992, Mosby.)

BOX 9-38

Water-Weighted Diaphragm for PEEP Administration

In this device, the calibrations on the column for centimeters of water pressure are not the actual centimeter distance because of the relationship between the surface areas on the water side of the diaphragm and on the diaphragm's seat.

Underwater Columns

Figure 9-67 shows a simple device for adding PEEP to ventilator tubing circuits. The expiratory flow from the patient's tubing circuit is directed underwater through a column or tower. The amount of pressure exerted is directly related to the height of the water in the submerged tube. The cross-sectional area of the tube must be equal to or greater than the cross-sectional area of the main expiratory line of the patient circuit. Coughing or forced exhalation can increase PEEP levels transiently, but the valve functions primarily as a threshold resistor.

Water-Weighted Diaphragm

The J.H. Emerson Co. produces a water-column PEEP device that uses the weight of the water to push on the expiratory diaphragm (Figure 9-68). During active expiration the pressure in the patient circuit is greater than that exerted by the water and the diaphragm is pushed up, opening the outflow port. When the pressure in the tubing circuit equals the pressure exerted by the water, the diaphragm closes, keeping pressure within the circuit and the patient's airway. The weight of the water above the diaphragm and the surface area of the diaphragm determine the PEEP level (Box 9-38). This is a true threshold resistor that is not significantly affected by changes in expiratory gas flow until flows exceed approximately 200 L/min.[12]

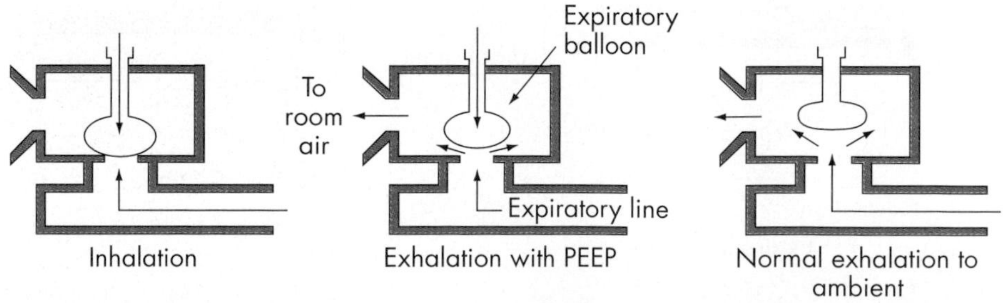

Figure 9-71 Balloon or diaphragm type of expiratory valves for applying PEEP. (From Pilbeam SP: Mechanical ventilation: physiological and clinical applications, ed 2, St Louis, 1992, Mosby.)

The Weighted Ball

Figure 9-58 illustrated a weighted-ball threshold resistor. A device containing a weighted valve is connected vertically to the main expiratory line of a patient circuit. The pressure generated varies directly with the weight of the ball. The diameter of the expiratory line and the opening connected to this valve must be equal to or greater than the valve connector to prevent flow resistance, which would affect the PEEP level. An example of this is the Boehringer valve.

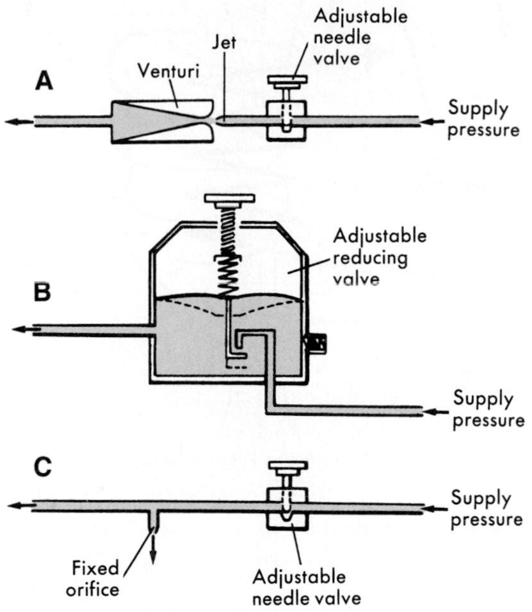

Figure 9-72 Three methods for pressurizing the expiratory line to provide PEEP with balloon or diaphragm expiratory valve devices: **A,** Using a Venturi device to control pressure in the balloon. Opening the needle valve increases pressure. **B,** Using a reducing valve to provide pressure to the balloon. Tightening the spring increases the pressure. **C,** Using a fixed orifice and an adjustable needle valve. As the needle valve is opened, more gas flows from the supply pressure, increasing pressure against the leak of the fixed orifice. This increased pressure is applied to the expiratory line for the balloon and increases PEEP.

Spring-Loaded Valves

A spring-loaded valve may also be used to create PEEP (see Figure 9-70). Changing the spring tension adjusts the amount of pressure needed to move the valve off its seat and allow expiration to occur. Once the circuit pressure equals the force applied on the valve by the spring, the valve closes. Some of these devices may have flow-resistor characteristics when expiratory flows are high. Examples include Vital Signs (multiple springs against a disc) and Ambu (single spring and disc).

Balloon or Diaphragm Type of Expiratory Valves

These devices commonly incorporate the balloon or diaphragm that is a part of the patient-circuit expiratory valve assembly (see Figure 9-71). During inspiration, the expiratory valve line pressurizes the balloon (or diaphragm) and closes the expiratory orifice. During normal expiration, pressure in the line is released and the patient's expiratory gas flow occurs unimpeded. When PEEP is selected, a proportional pressure is held within the expiratory tubing, partially inflating the balloon, which provides resistance to expiratory gas flow. When expiratory flow varies, PEEP also varies (flow resistance). Thus these valves have both flow- and threshold-resistor properties. Figure 9-72 illustrates three methods of pressurizing the expiratory line.

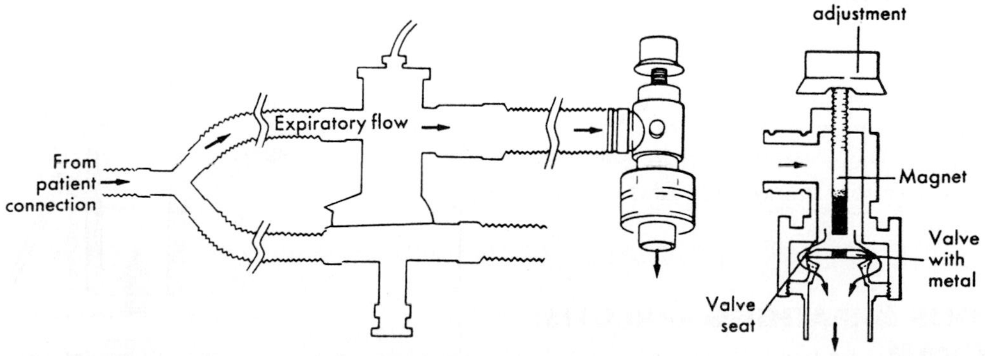

Figure 9-73 A magnetic PEEP valve. **A,** The valve is connected to a typical ventilator circuit with the expiratory valve mounted in-line. Arrows show the direction of expiratory flow. **B,** Detail of the magnetic valve. The threaded adjustment moves the magnet closer to or farther from the metal valve, which increases or decreases, respectively, the magnetic attraction. The greater the attraction, the greater the pressure needed to lift the valve from its seat.

Opposing Gas Flow Systems

The output pressure from a Venturi can be used to oppose gas flow to a one-way valve. Figure 9-72 **A** shows a system in which a Venturi applies pressure against a one-way valve (expiratory diaphragm). The valve normally opens, allowing a patient's expiratory gas to flow out. Gas flow from the Venturi creates a pressure that opposes opening of the valve resulting in PEEP in the patient circuit. When pressure on the patient circuit side of the valve is greater than Venturi pressure, gases flow through the one-way valve and out the open ports near the Venturi jet. When pressure on the patient circuit side is less, the valve closes. Examples of this include the Bourns BP 200, the Bear Cub, the Ohmeda CPU-1, and the Nellcor Puritan Bennett 7200a.

Magnetic PEEP Valves

Some PEEP valves use magnetic forces to oppose gas pressure (see Figure 9-73). A metallic valve is held on its seat by magnetic attraction supplied by an adjustable magnet. The threaded adjustment moves the magnet closer or farther from the metal valve, causing an increase or decrease, respectively, in magnetic attraction. The greater the attraction, the greater the pressure needed to push the valve off its seat and allow gas flow from the circuit. If the cross-sectional area of the device is small or restricted, it can act as a flow resistor. Instrumentation Industries designs a magnetic PEEP valve.

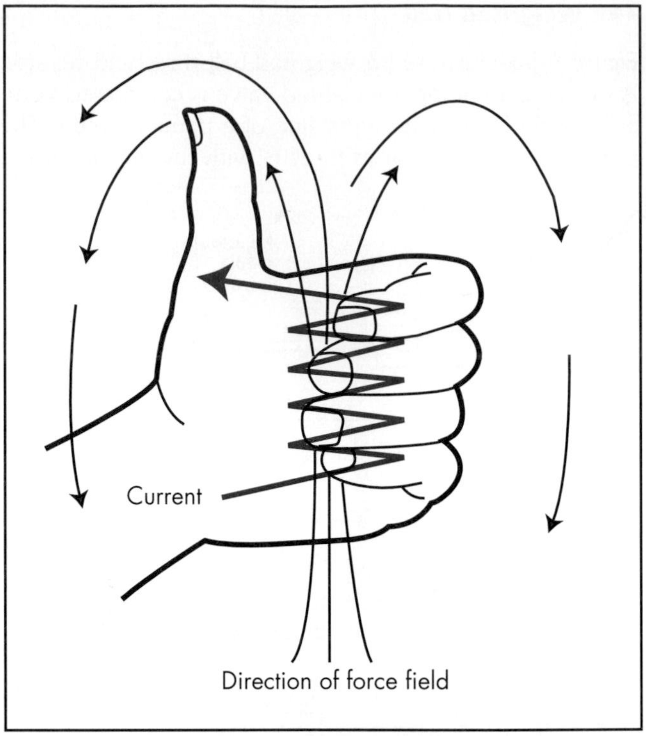

Figure 9-74 A solenoid uses a coil of wire. An electrical current is passed through the coil, generating a magnetic field. The direction of the magnetic field is indicated by the arrows. If you hold your hand with your thumb pointed up and your fingers slightly curved, the curve of your fingers are the direction of the electric current through the coil, and your thumb is the direction of the magnetic field.

Electromagnetic Valves

Electromagnetic valves often use solenoids in their construction (see Figure 9-74). Figure 9-75 shows the electromagnetically activated piston used in the Hamilton Veolar and Amadeus, which uses a solenoid in its construction. The amount of electric current to a solenoid is regulated by a rheostat. The solenoid creates a downward force through an actuating shaft. The actuating shaft pushes against a diaphragm that opposes expiratory gas flow. The stronger the current, the stronger the downward force and the higher the PEEP level.

Low–resistance threshold resistors are the expiratory valve of choice when ventilating patients or using free-standing CPAP systems. These valves can help reduce expiratory resistance (expiratory work) and reduce the potential for barotrauma.

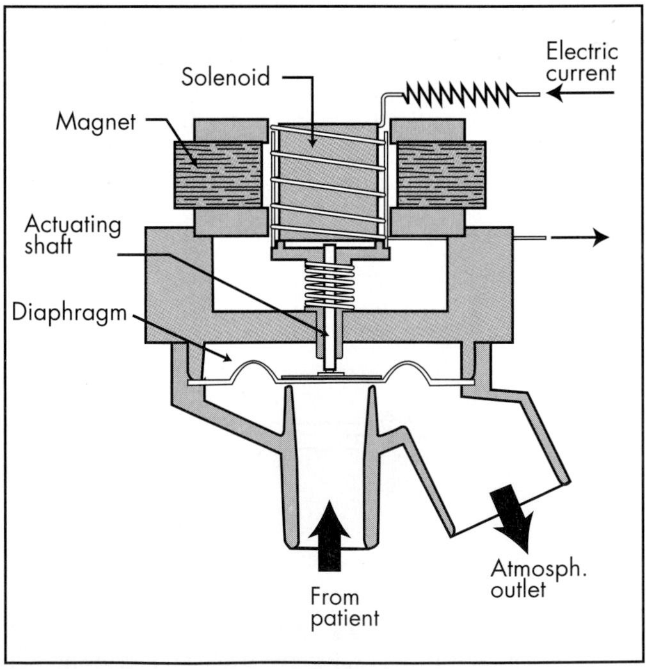

Figure 9-75 The electromagnetic threshold resistor of the Hamilton Veolar. (*SA* is surface area; *P* is pressure.) (Redrawn from Hamilton Medical Corp., Reno, Nev.)

SPONTANEOUS BREATHING CIRCUITS: IMV AND CPAP

The techniques of IMV and CPAP were defined earlier in this chapter. Both of these techniques allow for spontaneous breathing. Current generation ventilators can pro-

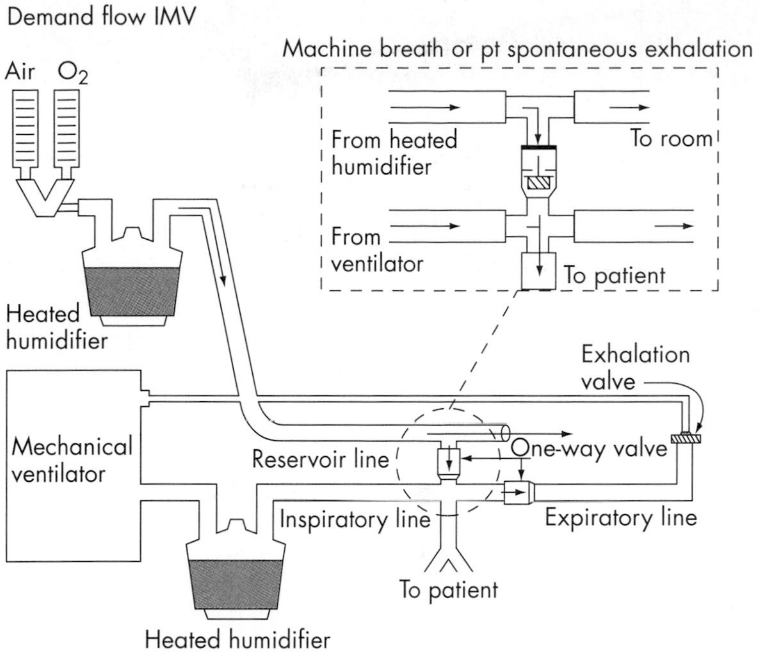

Figure 9-76 Demand flow IMV. (From Pilbeam SP: Mechanical ventilation: physiological and clinical applications, ed 2, St Louis, 1992, Mosby.)

vide for both of these techniques, unlike older models. Clinicians using ventilators such as the MA-1 must add an IMV circuit to the ventilator. Add-on IMV circuits are also used with some home ventilators (see Chapter 12).

It is possible to construct freestanding CPAP systems for use in spontaneously breathing patients who are not adequately oxygenated.[6] This way, ventilators can be spared for patients who cannot support their own ventilation.

Because of the continued need in special situations for both of these systems, the following section reviews their design.

Setting up a Ventilator with IMV

There are two basic types of designs for an IMV system: demand flow and continuous flow. Demand-flow systems, also called parallel flow or open-circuit IMV, were the earliest type of design. **Demand-flow IMV** requires the patient to open a one-way valve that needs an effort of -0.5 to -2 cm H_2O. In the demand-flow system pictured (Figure 9-76), a one-way valve is positioned near the patient's wye connector. When the ventilator provides a mandatory breath, the expiratory valve closes and the pressure from the breath closes the one-way valve, connecting the demand system with the patient circuit, so air goes to the patient. During spontaneous inspiration between mandatory breaths, the patient opens the one-way valve and receives gas from a separate heated, humidified source that is usually two flowmeters (air and oxygen) or a blender. Sometimes a one-way valve is placed in the main expiratory line to reduce the chance of the patient rebreathing exhaled air. Figure 9-76 is a schematic of a volume ventilator with a demand-flow IMV circuit added. The enlarged portion of the demand IMV circuit shows the connection between the two circuits. During spontaneous breathing, the one-way valve near the patient opens and warm, humidified air from a separate source goes to the patient. There is an additional piece of tubing at the end of the spontaneous circuit that vents to the room and also acts as a reservoir when inspiratory flow demand is high.

The problem with the original demand-flow design was that it was close to the patient's airway and tended to add weight or pull on the artificial airway. In addition, the patient was required to perform the work of opening the valve. When PEEP was in use, the patient had to reduce patient-circuit pressure to below ambient to receive airflow from the IMV circuit, which was at atmospheric pressure, while the patient-circuit pressure was at the set PEEP level (Figure 9-77).

Continuous-flow or closed-circuit IMV systems are slightly different. For example, the design takes advantage of the heated humidifier used with the ventilator so that a separate heated humidification system does not have to be added. Also, it incorporates a reservoir, along with a continuous flow of gas, so that the one-way valve going toward the patient circuit is kept open by the continuous flow and does not have to be opened by the patient. Figure 9-78 shows an example of a **continuous-flow IMV system.** A blended gas source (i.e., air and oxygen flowmeters or a blender) provides gas flow to a reservoir bag. The gas reservoir is attached to the ventilator circuit by a one-way

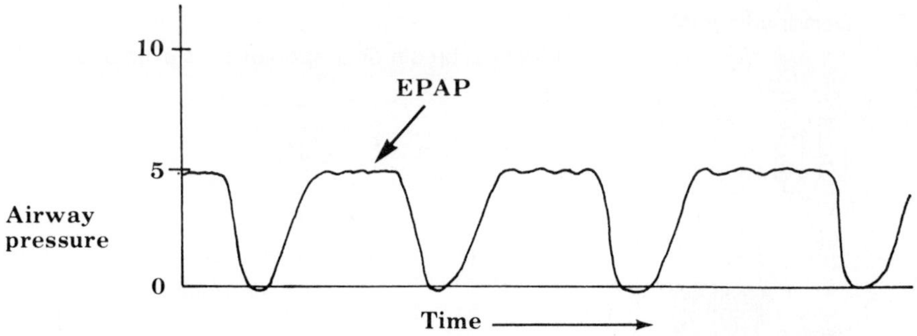

Figure 9-77 Spontaneous breathing with a demand-flow IMV system with PEEP in use. During inspiration, the pressure drops to slightly below ambient, which is required to open the one-way valve. IPAP is at or below zero, and EPAP is at the set-PEEP level. (From Pilbeam SP: Mechanical ventilation: physiological and clinical applications, ed 3, St Louis, 1998, Mosby.)

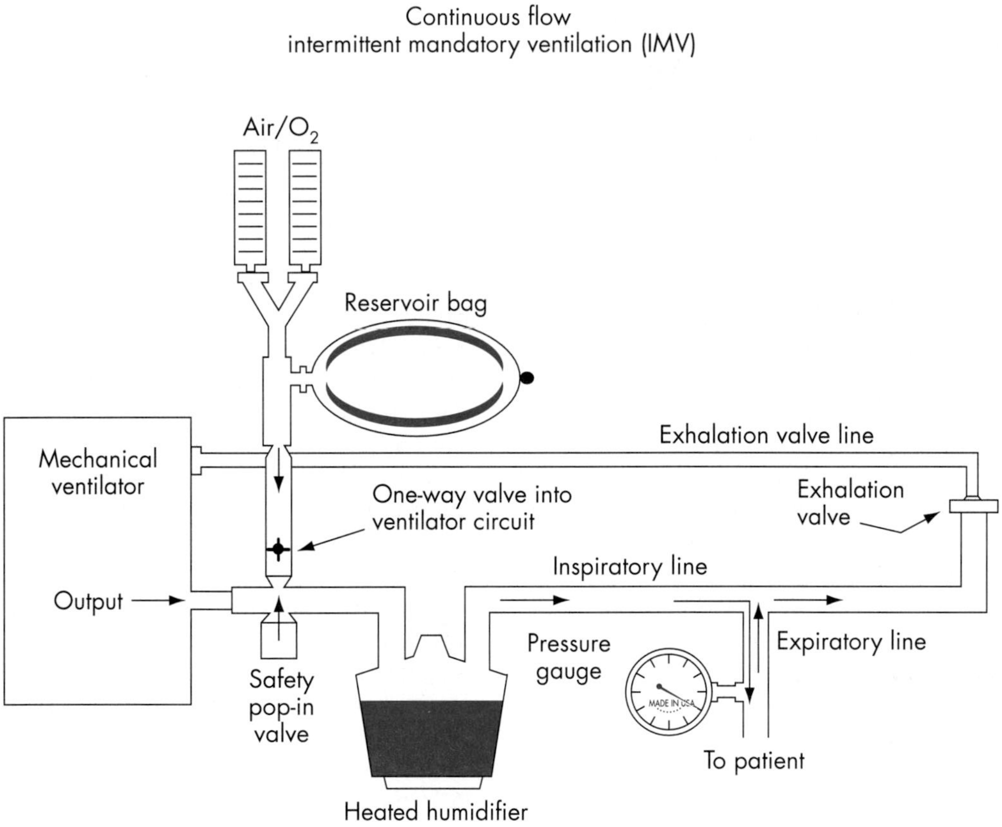

Figure 9-78 A continuous-flow IMV system added to a volume ventilator. (See text for explanation.) (From Pilbeam SP: Mechanical ventilation: physiological and clinical applications, ed 2, St Louis, 1992, Mosby.)

valve on the proximal side of the humidifier (the side closest to the main outlet of the ventilator). The function of this valve is to remain open during the spontaneous breathing period, so that the patients can receive a continuous flow of gas past their airways. During a mandatory breath, the pressure of the breath delivery closes the one-way valve so that the mandatory breath is delivered to the patient and not the reservoir. It is wise to add a safety pop-in valve, as shown in Figure 9-78. If gas flow from the outside source is accidentally shut off, patients can open the one-way valve and receive ambient air.

Figure 9-79 shows another example of a continuous-flow IMV assembly. Blended gas fills the reservoir and flows through the one-way valve into the patient circuit.

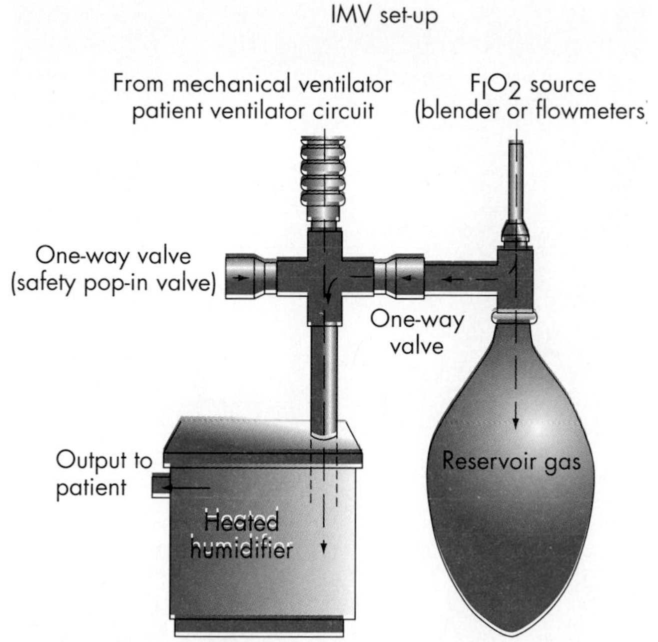

Figure 9-79 A schematic of a continuous-flow IMV circuit. (From Pilbeam SP: Mechanical ventilation: physiological and clinical applications, ed 2, St Louis, 1992, Mosby.)

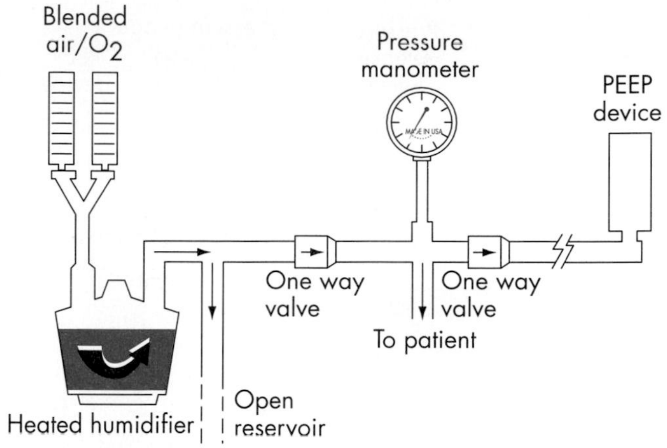

Figure 9-80 A freestanding demand-flow sPEEP (CPAP) circuit (open system). (From Pilbeam SP: Mechanical ventilation: physiological and clinical applications, ed 2, St Louis, 1992, Mosby.)

Because of their shape, add-on systems are sometimes called H-valve assemblies. If it is desirable to use PEEP, the reservoir can be pressurized to keep its pressure at or near the set PEEP level.

There are some disadvantages to the continuous-flow system. First, because of the continuous flow, there is often an inadvertent level of PEEP at the patient's airway. Second, because flow is constantly coming out the expiratory valve during the spontaneous period, an inspiratory plateau cannot be used to measure plateau pressure. Closing the expiratory valve for any reason with this type of assembly results in continuous flow of gas into the circuit and the patient's lungs, increasing system pressure. Third, it is not possible to measure V_T at the exhalation valve because of the constant gas flow, so it must be measured at the endotracheal tube. By placing a respirometer directly between the endotracheal tube and the ventilator wye connector, an accurate measurement of exhaled V_T can be obtained.

When this system is in use, the ventilator sensitivity is either turned off (as long as a safety pop-in valve allowing access to room air is added) or reduced so that it does not normally respond to patient effort. The pressure limit must be set at about 10 cm H_2O above peak inspiratory pressure for a mandatory breath. This is very important because a mandatory breath may occur just after a spontaneous inspiration, which could result in a very high volume delivery. When adjustments are made to the FiO_2 control on the ventilator front panel, the FiO_2 must also be changed at the source providing flow to the IMV system.

Freestanding CPAP Systems

Similar to add-on IMV systems, freestanding CPAP systems can be either demand- or continuous-flow devices. Unlike the IMV systems, they are not attached to ventilators but operate on their own. Figure 9-80 shows an example of a **demand-flow CPAP** (spontaneous PEEP [sPEEP]) system. It is called *sPEEP* in this situation because pressure is only positive during exhalation—not during inhalation. The patient must open a one-way valve to receive gas flow from a warmed, humidified, blended gas (air/oxygen) source. The patient must drop circuit pressures from the set CPAP level to ambient in order to open the valve and receive flow. This is similar to the demand-flow IMV system with PEEP added (see Figure 9-77). There are demand valves available that can balance the pressure on both sides of the demand flow one-way valve so that very little drop in pressure occurs during inspiration.

In a **continuous-flow CPAP system,** blended gas passes into a reservoir that can be pressurized to equal the desired positive pressure. The blended gas can come from air and oxygen flowmeters, from a blender, or from a CPAP generator. The gas is then warmed and humidified. A threshold resistor is attached to the expiratory end of the system (Figure 9-81), and a manometer is used to monitor circuit pressure. There is a safety pressure-release valve added, the threshold resistance of which equals the desired CPAP level plus 5 cm H_2O. For example, if the CPAP is 10 cm H_2O, the safety pressure release is 15 cm H_2O. If the normal threshold resistor jams, preventing gas flow from the system, the valve can act as a pop-off valve. Adding a safety pop-in valve is also important in case the source gas is accidentally turned off so that there is a source of ambient air for the patient. Some institutions add a one-way valve in the main expiratory lines to keep gas flowing in one direction, which can be important in patients with

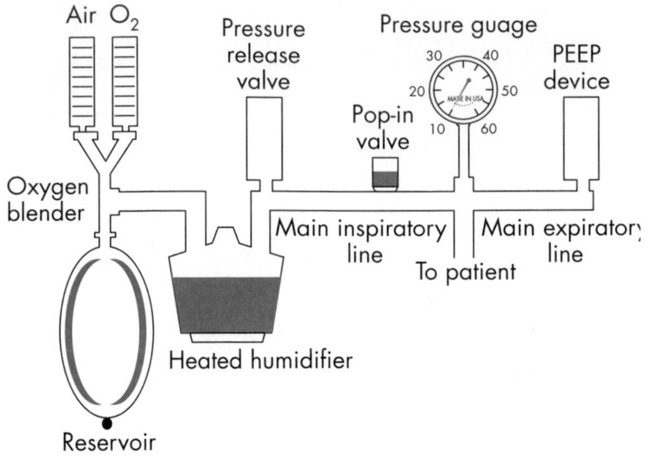

Figure 9-81 A freestanding, continuous-flow CPAP system. (From Pilbeam SP: Mechanical ventilation: physiological and clinical applications, ed 2, St Louis, 1992, Mosby.)

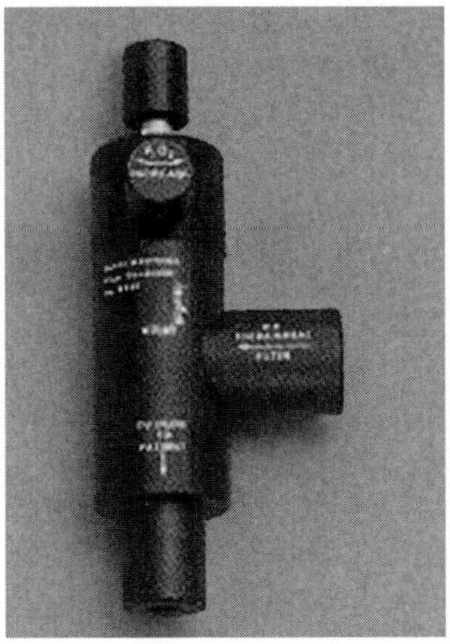

Figure 9-82 A diagram of the Downs CPAP generator. (Courtesy Vital Signs Corp., Totowa, NJ.)

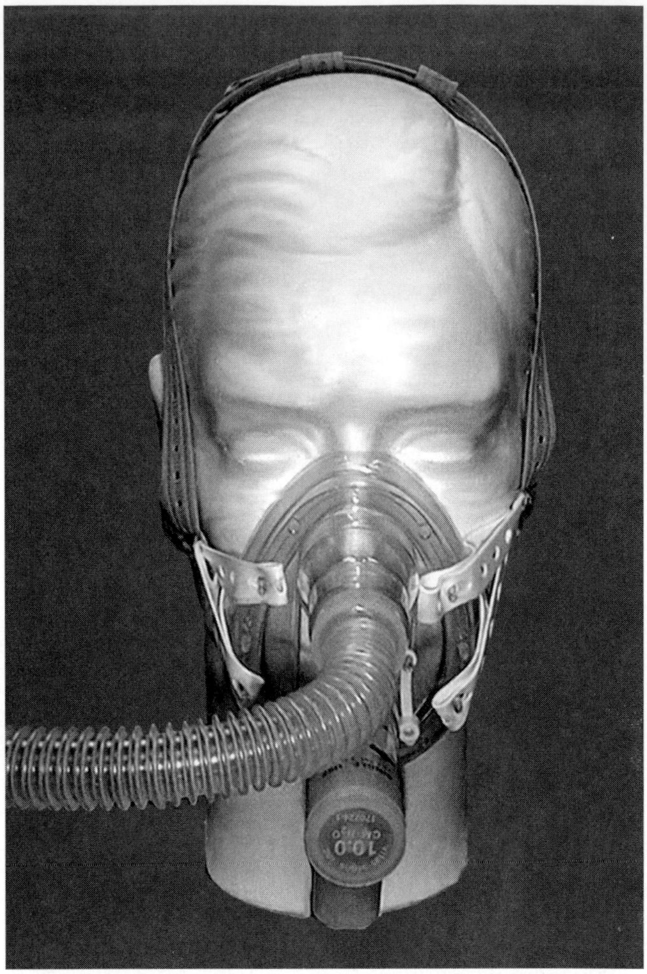

Figure 9-83 A photo of a patient with a CPAP mask connected to the Downs CPAP generator. (Courtesy Vital Signs Corp., Totowa, NJ.)

high flow demands who may begin to rebreathe some of their own exhaled air.

As mentioned, one possible gas source for a freestanding CPAP system is a CPAP generator. Figure 9-82 shows an example of a Downs CPAP generator that is connected to a high-pressure gas source and then connected by large-bore tubing to a CPAP mask. The mask has a CPAP valve attached to its face. Most valves are spring-loaded with fixed pressures (e.g., 5 cm H_2O, 7.5 cm H_2O, etc.), but others can be adjusted by tightening the spring (Figure 9-83).

A variety of problems can occur with a freestanding CPAP system, so it is important that the operator is sure that the safety systems (i.e., pop-off and pop-in valves) are in

BOX 9-39

Decision Making & Problem Solving

Problem 1

A patient on a freestanding, continuous-flow CPAP system set at 10 cm H_2O appears to be in distress (e.g., supraclavicular retractions, accessory muscle use, pale and diaphoretic). The operator notices that the manometer drops to -1 cm H_2O during inspiration and rises to +10 cm H_2O during expiration. What do you think is the problem?

Problem 2

The low oxygen saturation alarm is sounding on a patient connected to a freestanding, continuous-flow CPAP system. The operator notices that the manometer fluctuates around the zero point during both inspiration and expiration. What is the problem?

See Appendix A for the answers.

place. The following are some examples of problems that can occur: (1) inadequate flow to the patient; (2) leaks in the system; (3) loss of source gas flow; and (4) jamming or obstruction of the expiratory threshold resistor (Box 9-39).

Summary

There are many important aspects of mechanical ventilation that must be understood before a practitioner begins managing a patient-ventilator system. Most common aspects of mechanical ventilation related to the physical characteristics and technical operation of ventilators have been reviewed here, with a main focus on physical function and terms and explanations of fundamental concepts related to mechanical ventilation. Chapters 10, 11, and 12 review the use and operation of a variety of mechanical ventilators.

Review Questions

(See Appendix A for answers.)

1. Name the two common power sources for mechanical ventilators.
2. A ventilator measures a drop in tidal volume during pressure ventilation and automatically increases the pressure to return the volume to its original value. What type of system is this?
3. During operation of a ventilator, the respiratory care practitioner sets the tidal volume, respiratory rate, and flow, which are appropriate parameters for:
   a. pressure (-limited) ventilation
   b. volume (-limited) ventilation
4. Give three additional names for pressure ventilation.
5. Which of the following represent flow-control valves:
   I. rotary drive piston
   II. proportional solenoid
   III. bag-in-a-chamber
   IV. stepper motor with valve
      a. I only
      b. II only
      c. II and IV only
      d. I, III, and IV only
6. When a jet stream passes through an opening and there is a wall adjacent to its left side, the jet will deflect away from the wall because of the formation of a separation bubble—true or false?
7. Classify and describe controlled volume ventilation with a constant flow waveform.
8. What is the trigger mechanism in assisted ventilation?
9. During volume ventilation, the volume/time curve shows that inspired volume is greater than expired volume. The expired volume curve does not return to zero during exhalation. What is the most likely problem?
10. Graphic findings on a patient indicate an increase in the difference between the peak pressure and the plateau pressure and a prolonged expiratory flow on a flow/time curve. What do you think is the problem?
11. An apneic patient is severely hypoxemic. The physician wishes to use an elevated baseline pressure. Which would you recommend: PEEP or CPAP?
12. The flow/time curve for a paralyzed and sedated patient on PCIRV reveals that a mandatory breath occurs before flow returns to zero at the end of exhalation. Which of the following maneuvers would you preform?
    a. inflation hold
    b. cuff pressure measurement
    c. maximum inspiratory pressure measurement
    d. end-expiratory pause
13. A physician wants to use a pressure-limited mode of ventilation that guarantees volume delivery of every breath. Which of the following would you recommend?
    a. pressure-regulated volume control
    b. pressure augmentation
    c. proportional-assist ventilation
    d. airway pressure-release ventilation
14. What HFV techniques provides an active inspiratory and expiratory phase?
15. Which of the following is NOT a cause of high-pressure alarm?
    a. patient coughing
    b. increased airway resistance
    c. a ruptured endotracheal tube cuff
    d. water in the patient circuit
16. Which of the following is an example of a PEEP valve (expiratory resistor) that primarily has threshold resistor quality and is gravity-dependent?
    a. balloon type of expiratory valve
    b. underwater column
    c. spring-loaded diaphragm
    d. restrictive orifice
17. A patient is on a continuous-flow IMV system. The respiratory care practitioner notices that during spontaneous inspiration the reservoir bag completely collapses and fills slowly during expiration. To solve this problem the practitioner might:
    a. check the function of the one-way valve between the reservoir bag and the ventilator circuit
    b. increase the flow to the reservoir
    c. increase the sensitivity setting on the ventilator
    d. check the expiratory valve line connection

Internet Resources

1. Virtual Hospital:
   http://vh.radiology.uiowa.edu
2. American Association for Respiratory Care:
   http://www.aarc.org
3. National Board for Respiratory Care:
   http://www.nbrc.org
4. Critical Care Medicine:
   http://ccm-l.med.edu
5. Nellcor Puritan Bennett:
   http://www.nellcorpb.com
6. Respiratory Care source pages:
   http://www.sourcepages.com
7. The RT Corner for Students:
   http://www.rtcorner.com
8. Sechrist Industries:
   http://www.sechristind.com
9. Siemens Medical:
   http://www.sms.siemens.com
10. Medscape:
    http://www.medscape.com
11. Respironics:
    http://www.respironics.com
12. Internet Based Learning (ventilator graphics):
    http://www.saminc.com

References

1. Mushin WW, et al: Automatic ventilation of the lungs, Philadelphia, 1980, FA Davis.
2. Chatburn RL: Classification of mechanical ventilation, Dallas, 1988, American Association for Respiratory Care.
3. Chatburn RL: A new system for understanding mechanical ventilators, Respir Care 36:1123, 1991.
4. Branson RD, Hess DR, and Chatburn RL: Respiratory care equipment, Philadelphia, 1995, JB Lippincott.
5. Blanch PB and Desautels DA: Chatburn's ventilator classification scheme–a poor substitute for the classic approach, Respir Care 39:762, 1994.
6. Pilbeam SP: Mechanical ventilation: physiological and clinical applications, ed 3, St Louis, 1998, Mosby.
7. McPherson SP: Respiratory care equipment, ed 5, St Louis, 1996, Mosby.
8. Mushin WW, et al: Automatic ventilation of the lungs, Philadelphia, 1980, FA Davis.
9. Sanborn WG: Microprocessor-based mechanical ventilation, Respir Care 38(1):72-109,1993.
10. Desautels D: Ventilator classification: a new look at an old subject, Current Rev Respir Ther, (lesson 11) 1: 81-88, 1979.
11. Scanlan CL, Spearman CB, and Sheldon RL: Egan's fundamentals of respiratory therapy, ed 6, St Louis, 1995, Mosby.
12. Dupuis Y: Ventilators: theory and clinical application, ed 2, St Louis, 1992, Mosby.
13. Spearman CB and Sanders HG Jr: Physical principles and functional designs of ventilators. In Kirby RR and Desautels DA, editors: Mechanical ventilation. New York, 1985, Churchill Livingston.
14. Smith RK: Respiratory care applications for fluidics, Respir Ther 3:19, 1973.
15. Chatburn RL: Dynamic respiratory mechanics, Respir Care 31:703, 1986.
16. Nilsestuen JO and Hargett K: Managing the patient-ventilator system using graphic analysis: an overview and introduction to Graphics Corner, Respir Care 41:1105, 1996.
17. Kacmarek RM, et al: Technical aspects of positive end-expiratory pressure (PEEP) (I,II, and III), Respir Care 27:1478, 1490, 1505, 1982.
18. Campbell RS and Branson RD: Ventilatory support for the '90s: pressure support ventilation, Respir Care 38:526, 1993.
19. Reynolds EOR: Effect of alterations in mechanical ventilator settings on pulmonary gas exchange in hyaline membrane disease, Arch Dis Child 46:152, 1971.
20. Reynolds EOR and Taghipadeh A: Improved prognosis of infants mechanically ventilated for hyaline membrane disease, Arch Dis Child 49:405, 1974.
21. Stock MC and Downs JB: Airway pressure release ventilation: a new approach to ventilatory support during acute lung injury, Respir Care 32:517, 1987.
22. Martin LD and Wetzel RC: Optimal release time during airway pressure release ventilation in neonatal sheep, Crit Care Med 22:486,1994.
23. Branson RD and MacIntyre NR: Dual-control modes of mechanical ventilation, Respir Care 41:294, 1996.
24. Younes M: Proportional assist ventilation. In Tobin MJ, editor: Principles and practice of mechanical ventilation, New York, 1994, McGraw-Hill.
25. Younes M: Proportional assist ventilation: a new approach to ventilatory support, part I: theory, Am Rev Respir Dis 145:114, 1992.
26. Younes M, et al: Proportional assist ventilation: results of an initial clinical trial, Am Rev Respir Dis 145:121,1992.
27. Schulze A and Schaller P: Proportional assist ventilation: a new strategy for infant ventilation? Neonatal Respir Dis 6:1, 1996.
28. Schulze A, et al: Effects of ventilator resistance and compliance on phrenic nerve activity in spontaneously breathing cats, Am J Respir Crit Care Med 153:671-676, 1996.
29. Otis AB, Fenn WO, and Rahn H: Mechanics of breathing in man, J Appli Physiol 2:592, 1950.
30. Watson K: Ventilatory support in newborn and pediatric patients. In Pilbeam SP: Mechanical ventilation: physiological and clinical applications, ed 3, St Louis, 1998, Mosby.
31. Sjöstrand U: High-frequency positive pressure ventilation (HFPPV): a review, Crit Care Med 8:345, 1980.
32. Boros SJ, et al: Using conventional infant ventilators at unconventional rates, Pediatrics 74:487, 1984.
33. Klain M and Smith RB: High-frequency percutaneous transtracheal jet ventilation, Crit Care Med 5:280, 1977.
34. Calkins JM: High-frequency jet ventilation: experimental evaluation. In Carlon CG and Howlan WS, editors: High-frequency ventilation in intensive care and during surgery, New York, 1985, Marcel Dekker.

35. Cohen IL, Bilen Z, and Krishnamurthy S: The effects of ventilator working pressure during pressure support ventilation, Chest 103:588, 1993.
36. Pilbeam SP: Mechanical ventilation. In Burton GG, Hodgkin JE, and Ward JJ: Respiratory care: a guide to clinical practice, Philadelphia, 1997, Lippincott.
37. Kacmarek RM, Hess D, and Stoller JK: Monitoring in respiratory care, St Louis, 1993, Mosby.
38. Meliones JN, Cheifetz IM, and Wilson BG: Use of airway graphic analysis to optimize mechanical ventilation strategies, L1312, Palm Springs, Calif., 1995, Bird Products Corporation.
39. Wilson BG, Cheifetz IM, and Meliones JN: Optimizing mechanical ventilation in infants and children with the use of airway graphics, L1326 Rev B, Palm Springs, Calif., 1995, Bird Products Corporation.
40. Banner MJ: Expiratory positive pressure valves and work of breathing, Respir Care 32:431, 1987.
41. Woods R, et al: An inexpensive continuous positive end-expiratory pressure (PEEP) adaptor for positive pressure respirators, Chest 61:376, 1972.
42. Spearman CB: Positive end-expiratory pressure: terminology and technical aspects of PEEP devices and systems, Respir Care 33:434, 1988.

APPENDIX 9-1

Algorithms for Alarm Situations

In any alarm situation, it is imperative that patients be assessed to determine if they are in urgent distress. If so, they should be disconnected from the ventilator and manually ventilated with 100% oxygen. If the patient improves, the problem is most likely in the ventilator system. If the patient does not improve, the problem is with the patient or the artificial airway. The following algorithms review common alarm situations when the problem is with the ventilator or the artificial airways. Patient problems, such as pneumothorax and pulmonary embolism, are beyond the scope of this text.

Because some alarms often occur at about the same time, the situations are grouped together and include the following:

1. Increased V_T, $\dot{V}_E$, or rate alarms (Figure A9-1)
2. Low pressure, low PEEP/CPAP, low $\dot{V}_E$, low V_T, and/or low rate alarms (Figure A9-2)
3. High pressure or high PEEP/CPAP alarms (Figure A9-3)

Additional alarms to be reviewed are as follows:

1. Inverse I:E ratio indication (Figure A9-4)
2. Apnea alarm (Figure A9-5)
3. Loss of power alarm (Figure A9-6)

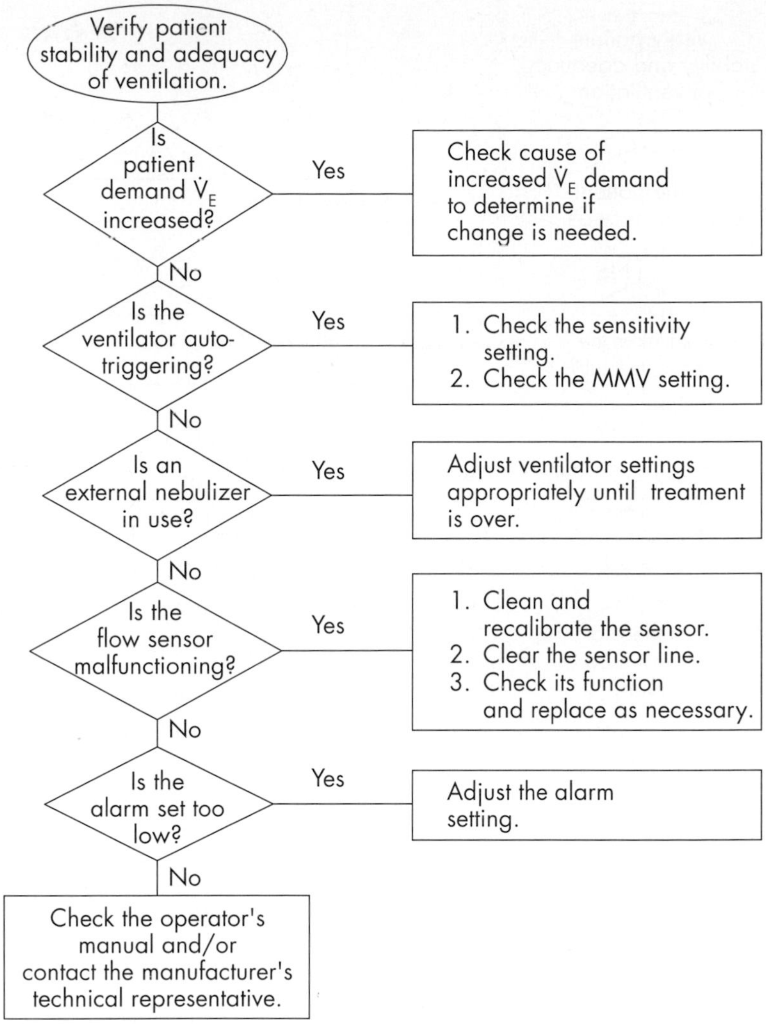

Figure A9-1 Increased V_T, $\dot{V}_E$, or rate alarm.

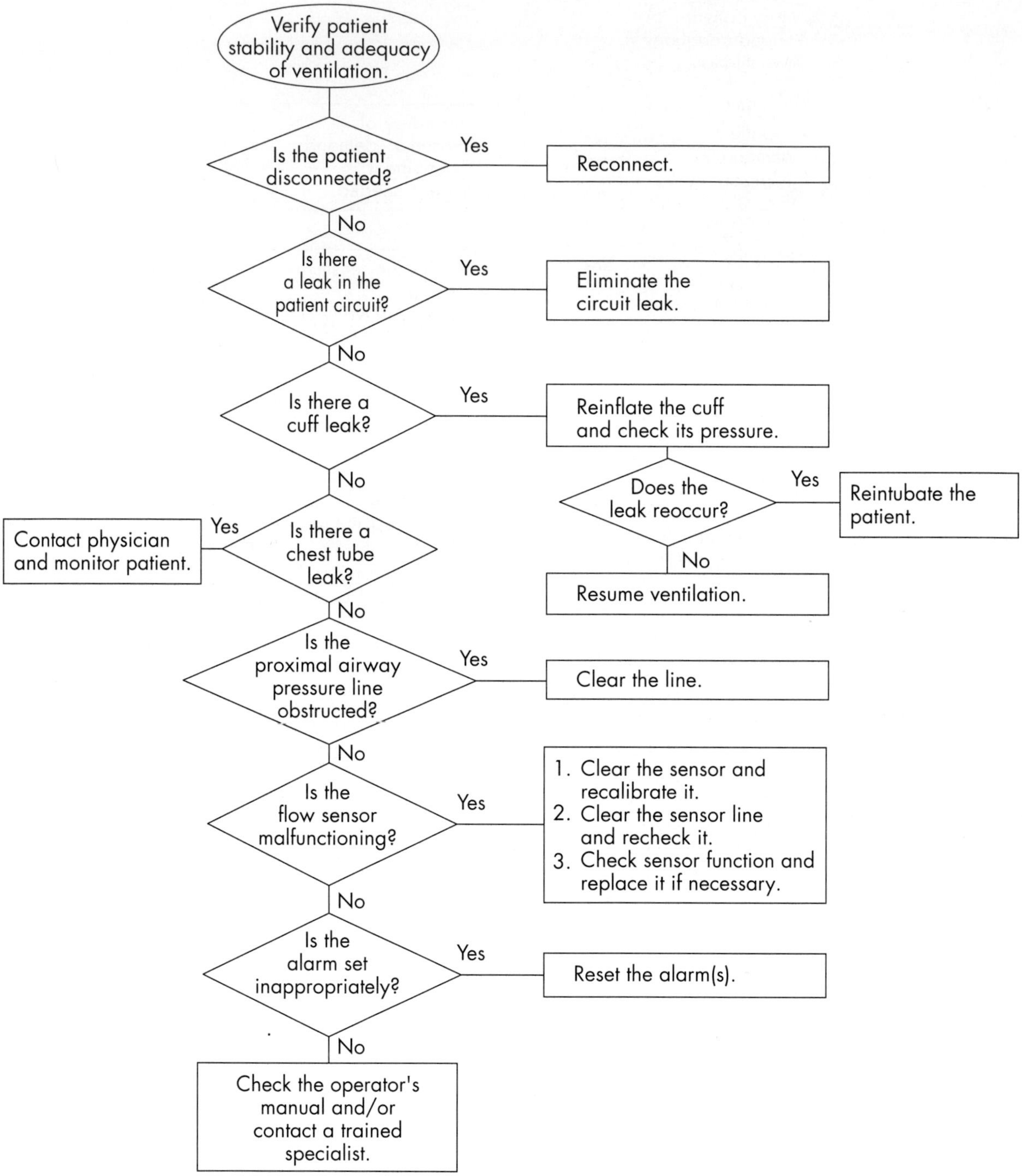

Figure A9-2 Low pressure, low PEEP/CPAP, low $\dot{V}_E$, low V_T, and/or low rate alarms.

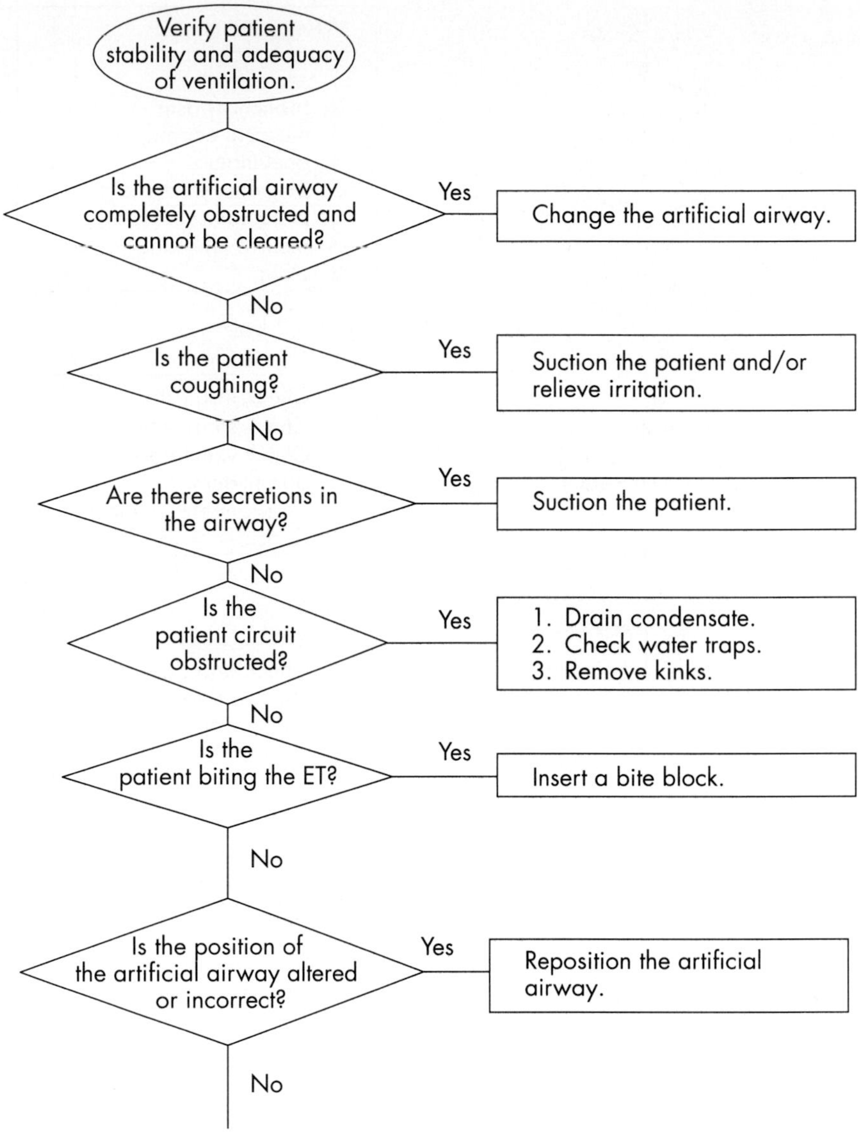

Figure A9-3 High-pressure or high-PEEP alarms.

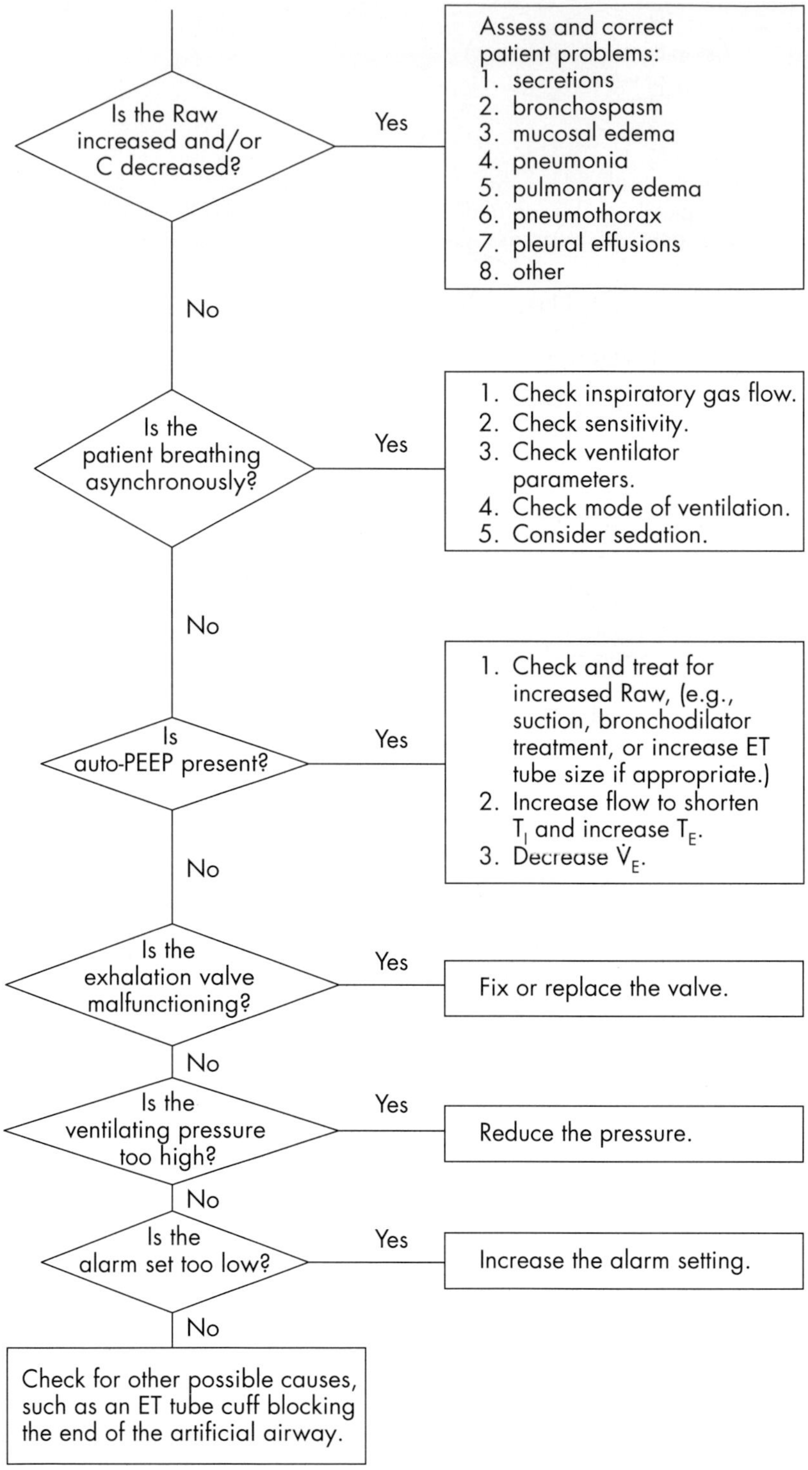

Figure A9-3, cont'd.

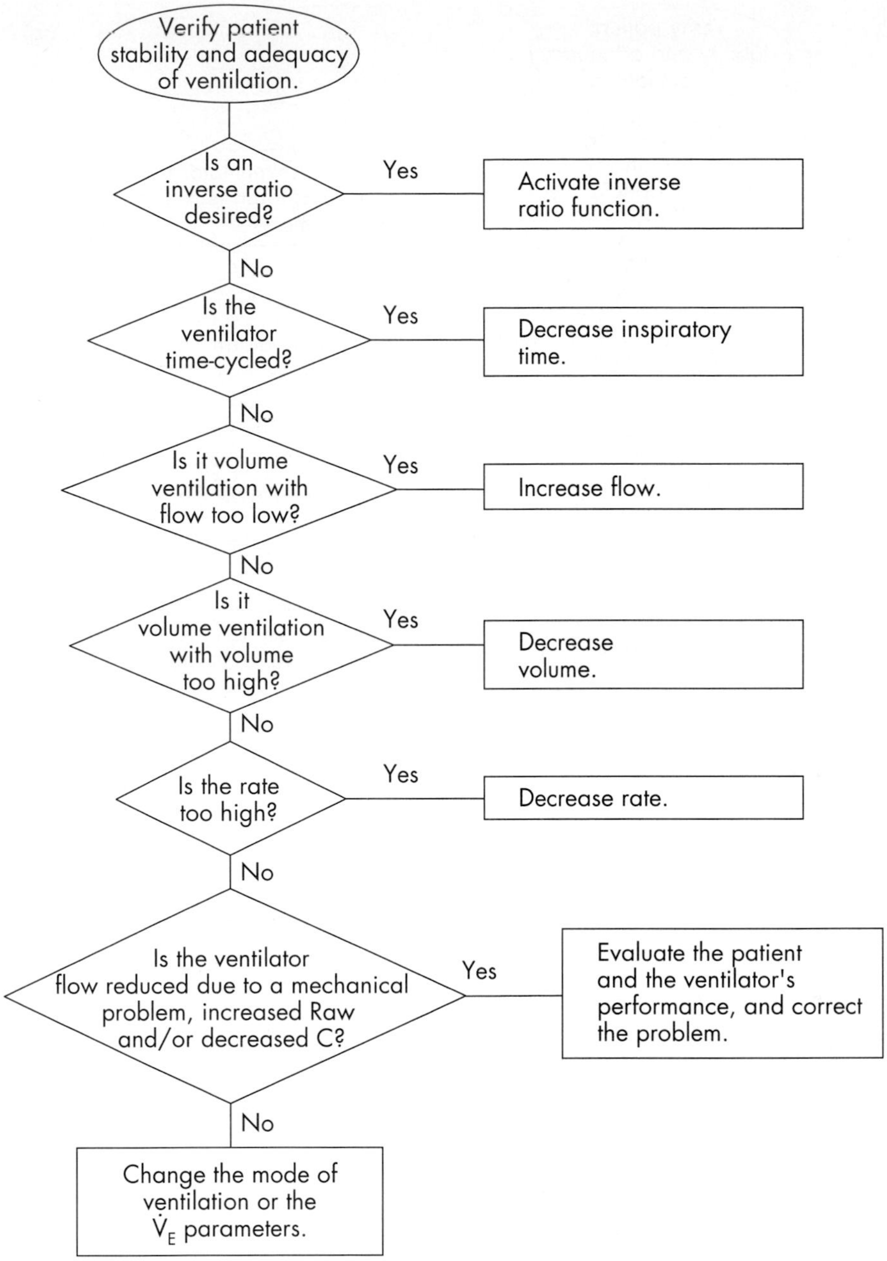

Figure A9-4 Inverse I: E ratio indicator activated.

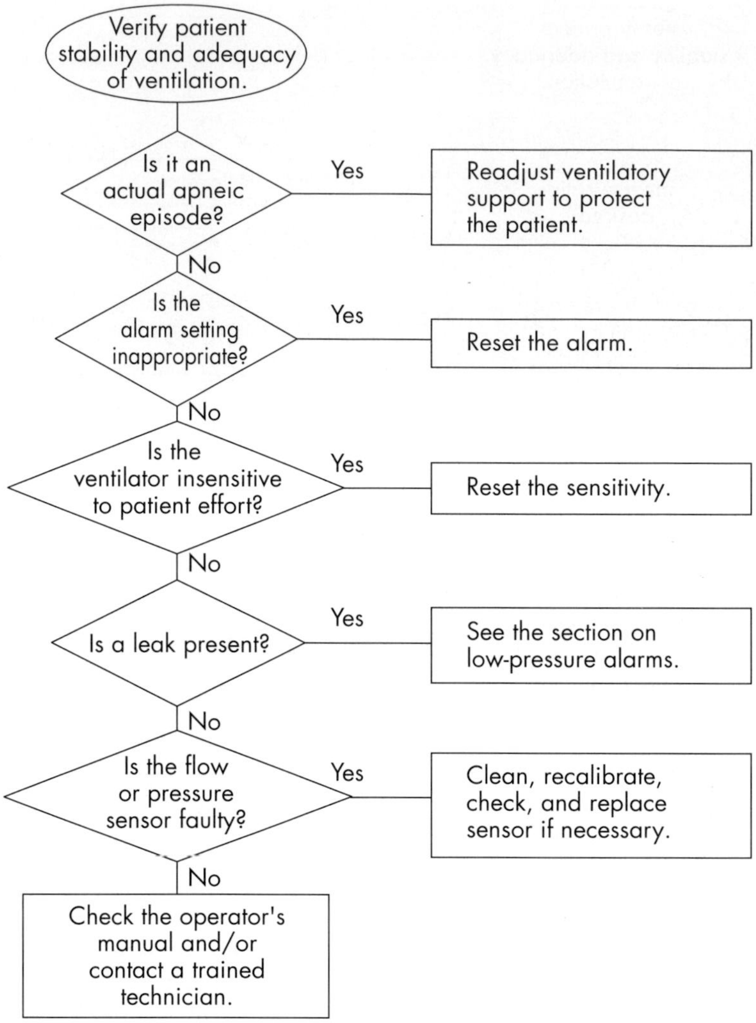

Figure A9-5 Apnea alarm.

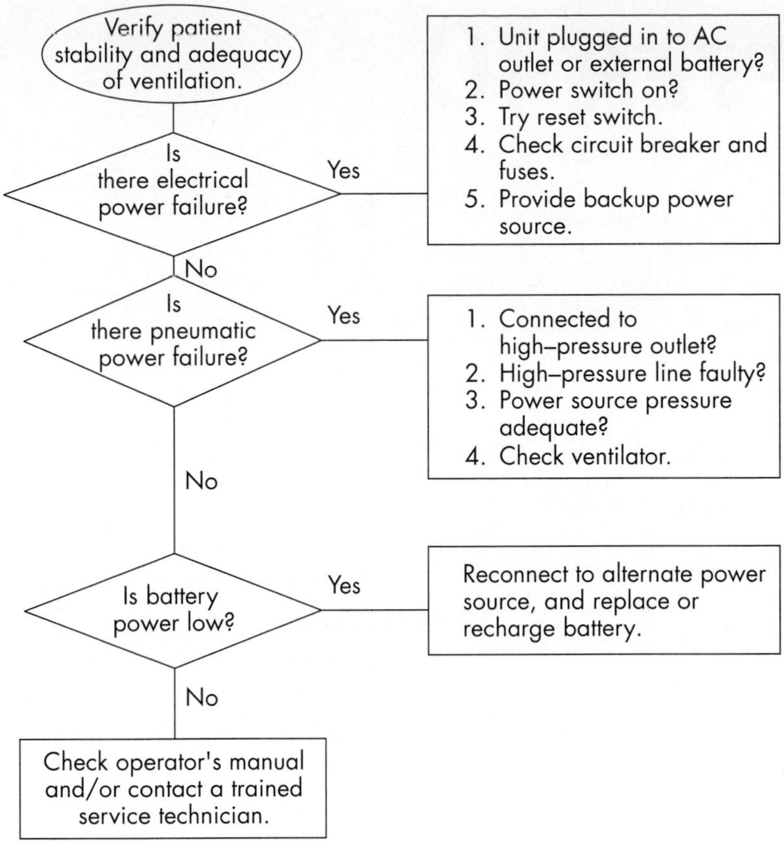

Figure A9-6 Loss of power alarm.

CHAPTER 10

CHAPTER OUTLINE

Mechanical Ventilators: General-Use Devices

KEY TERMS

100% Oxygen Suction
Accumulator
Airway Pressure-Release Ventilation (APRV)
Alarms
Alarm Silence
Alternating Current (AC)
Analog Pressure Manometer
Antisuffocation Valve
Apnea Ventilation
Apneic Period
Assist/Control (A/C)
Autoflow
Base Flow
Baseline Pressure
Bias Alert
Bias Flow
Continuous Mandatory Ventilation (CMV)
Control Panel
Continuous Positive Airway Pressure (CPAP)
Cyber Knob
Cyber Pad
Default
Diffuser
Direct Current (DC)
Display Window
Drag Turbine
Electrically Powered
Electromagnetic Frequency Interference (EFI)
Electronic Logic
Expiratory Hold
Expiratory Pause
Expiratory Time (T_E)
External Battery
Flow Trigger
Flow Waveforms
Graphics
Hardware
High Pressure Servo Valves
Inspiratory Hold
Inspiratory Pause
Inspiratory Time (T_I)
Internal Battery
Internal Demand Valve
Internal Mechanisms
Intrinsic Positive End-Expiratory Pressure (PEEP)
Inverse Ratio Ventilation (IRV)
Light-Emitting Diodes (LEDs)
Mandatory Breaths
Mandatory Minute Volume Ventilation (MMV)
Manual Trigger
Maximum Pressure Limit (Pmax)
Message Window
Microprocessor
Monitor
Nebulizer Control
Occlusion Pressure ($P_{0.1}$)
Optical Encoder
Over Pressure-Relief Valve
Oxygen Analyzer
Oxygen Sensor
Pneumatically Powered
Pneumotachograph
Positive End-Expiratory Pressure (PEEP)
Power Indicators
Pressure Augmentation (Paug)
Pressure-Control Ventilation (PCV)
Pressure Slope
Pressure Support
Pressure-Support Ventilation (PSV)
Pressure-Targeted Ventilation
Pressure Trigger
Proximal Pressure Line
Radio Frequency Interference (RFI)
Sensitivity
Service Verification Test (SVT)
Slope
Sloping
Software
SmartTrigger
Smart Window
Subambient Overpressure-Relief Valve (SOPR)
Subambient Pressure Valve
Subambient Relief Valve
Synchronized Intermittent Mandatory Ventilation (SIMV)
Total Cycle Time (TCT)
Turbine
User Verification Test (UVT)
Ventilator Inoperative Alarm (VENT. INOP.)
Volume-Assured Pressure Support (VAPS)
Volume-Targeted Ventilation

The incorporation of **microprocessors** into mechanical ventilators in the 1980s forever changed their design. Ventilators with microprocessing features can process and store information. Manufacturers can change or add functions by simply adding new programming instructions, a circuit board, or maybe even a new face to the device.

Buyouts are another phenomenon that has affected the character of ventilator purchases and use. For example, Bear Medical Corporation was bought out by Allied Health Corporation, which was then purchased by Thermo Electron Corporation, which now owns Bird Ventilator Products, as well. The original Bird company was owned by Dr. Forrest Bird, who sold it to the 3M Corporation. Likewise, Nellcor purchased the Puritan-Bennett Corporation as well as Infrasonics. In turn, Nellcor Puritan Bennett was bought out. And so goes the buyout phenomenon, affecting the competition and the availability of ventilators.

Both the economic situation and technological advances have resulted in a rapidly changing environment for mechanical ventilators. It is important for consumers to keep these factors in mind and to be aware that units used or purchased should have the appropriate manufacturer support.

COMMON FEATURES OF VENTILATORS

Fierce competition among manufacturers has created an advantageous situation for consumers. Because ventilators can be reprogrammed (and technology now allows this process), whenever a manufacturer comes out with a new feature, its usually not long until other manufacturers offer a similar feature. For example, the Puritan-Bennett 7200 ventilator was one of the first—if not the first—to offer a back-up mode of ventilation. Back-up ventilation has preprogrammed parameters, such as tidal volume (V_T), rate, FiO_2, and flow, which become active if the ventilator detects the presence of apnea. Most ventilators now used in acute care have this feature.

Distinguishing Different Models

Because programmable features can be added, clinical facilities can purchase a unit and then add new features as they are developed. This add-on concept has resulted in much confusion about the names and numbers given to various machines. For example, you initially purchase a unit called the Magnolia 500; but after developing several new alarm or monitoring capabilities, the manufacturer now calls it the Magnolia 500a or maybe the Magnolia 500 version 2.0. Keeping track of what features have been added is truly an art for both the purchaser and the sales representative, putting an important responsibility on clinicians to learn about updates and understand how they affect a product's function.

Common Internal Mechanisms

The **internal mechanisms** of many microprocessor-controlled machines have several similarities. For example, they usually require high-pressure air and oxygen gas sources for pneumatic power, as well as electricity to power the internal computer and various electronically operated components. Once gas enters, it is filtered, temperature and pressure are measured, pressure is regulated, and both gases are mixed. The mixture is sometimes fed into a holding tank that acts as a reservoir for gas under pressure. Then the gas is routed to a microprocessor-controlled flow valve. Although these valves vary by manufacturer, they all provide rapid response and a variety of gas delivery methods. For example, they can give a constant flow and preset volume, or they can give a constant pressure while volume delivery varies. They can change the shape of the inspiratory flow waveform during volume ventilation and respond rapidly to a patient's spontaneous demand for gas flow.

Patient Monitoring

Sophisticated new technology enables flow and pressure delivery to be monitored rapidly and accurately and allows a variety of **monitors** and **alarms** to be used. Pressure and flow are often measured internally, near the main ventilator outlet and return line (i.e., expiratory valve area), but some ventilators monitor flow and/or pressure at the patient's upper airway. Although types of monitors vary, their function is usually the same. For example, ventilators incorporate flow-measuring devices, which may be variable-orifice **pneumotachographs** or heated thermistor beads, depending on manufacturer preference. Chapter 7 reviews the function of several of these devices.

Ventilators usually have digital displays of the following: V_T, rate (spontaneous and total), peak inspiratory pressure (PIP), plateau pressure ($P_{plateau}$), PEEP/CPAP, peak flow, oxygen percentage, and inspiratory:expiratory (I:E) ratio. Many also offer a graphic display screen as an add-on feature.

Parameters and Displays

Most ventilators now have **light-emitting diodes (LEDs)** on their **control panels** to show the operator the mode and parameters currently active. These control panels usually include a **display window** that can provide the operator with a written message.

The range of available volume, pressure, and flow, also tends to be very similar in current ventilators. For example, tidal volume range for units used for pediatric and adult patients tends to be from 50 to 2000 mL, although the range may be lower than 50 mL for units that can volume ventilate infants. The typical range of inspiratory pressure limits is from 0 to 120 cm H_2O; PEEP/CPAP values are usually from 0 to 50 cm H_2O; and pressure-support pressure levels generally range from 0 to 100 cm H_2O. Most units provide three **flow waveforms** in volume ventilation: constant, descending ramp, and sine waveforms.

Nearly every ventilator for use in acute care provides the following ventilatory modes: **assist/control (A/C)** and SIMV (either volume- or pressure-targeted), and spontaneous, which includes PEEP/CPAP and **pressure support.**

Alarms

Common alarms include high/low pressure, high/low oxygen percentage, high/low minute volume, high rate, and low PEEP/CPAP. Ventilators also include alarm-silencing buttons that usually silence audible alarms for 1 to 2 minutes. Sometimes the type of alarm that is active is shown in a display window. In their memory, microprocessors can save which alarms have occurred and can report these back to the operator in some form. Some illuminate the LEDs next to the violated alarms to indicate which alarms are being or have been set off. Some units scroll through the chronological order of the alarm events as the operator reads the display screen. Some units do both.

Low gas supply and **ventilator inoperative alarms** (i.e., internal error detected by the microprocessor) are available and cannot be silenced on every unit.

Understanding Individual Ventilators

Once clinicians have mastered the use of a newer, more sophisticated ventilator, it is usually not difficult for them to understand another brand. Manufacturers have tried to make their equipment user-friendly and provide a wide variety of materials and services to explain their operation: training videotapes, instruction and operation manuals, trained technicians and representatives, CD-ROM interactive programs, and product specialists via telephone or Internet. And, as always, users are encouraged to read the directions.

Presentation of Specific Ventilators

It is assumed that readers have a basic understanding of the physical properties of ventilators as outlined in Chapter 9. The machines are presented in such a way as to help prepare readers to use them in a clinical setting, so the discussions do not focus too much detail on internal function or classification.

The Bear 3 Ventilator

OUTLINE

Power Source

Internal Mechanisms

Controls and Alarms
- Main Control Panel
- Top Monitoring Panel

Modes of Operation
- SIMV
- Pressure Support
- Special Features

Troubleshooting

LEARNING OBJECTIVES

Upon completion of this section, the reader should be able to:

1. Describe the major components of the internal mechanisms on the Bear 3 as well as explain their primary functions.
2. Identify and discuss the function of each control on the front panel.
3. Assess an alarm situation based on the LEDs and alarms activated and state a possible cause.
4. Explain each mode of ventilation on the Bear 3, including the trigger and cycling mechanisms and the target variable (pressure or volume).
5. Troubleshoot a malfunction caused by inappropriate positioning of the expiratory flow sensor.

In 1988, the Bear 3 ventilator[1-3] was introduced by Bear Medical Systems, Inc., a subsidiary of Thermo Electron Corporation. It is the third model of a type of Bear ventilator. Because the Bear 1, Bear 2, and Bear 3 are similar and because the Bear 3 is currently the most common of these used in the United States, only the Bear 3 is described here.

Power Source

The Bear 3 ventilator (Figure 10-1) is currently produced by Bear Medical Systems, Inc. It is **electrically powered** by a 120-volt **alternating current (AC)** and **pneumatically powered** by external air and oxygen sources. It has

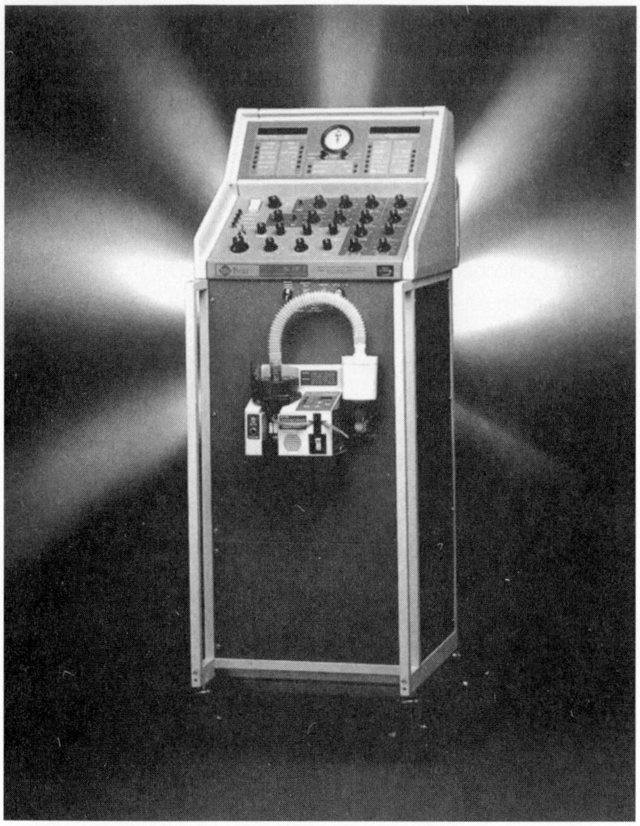

Figure 10-1 Photograph of the Bear 3 ventilator. (Courtesy Bear Medical Systems, Inc, Riverside, Calif.)

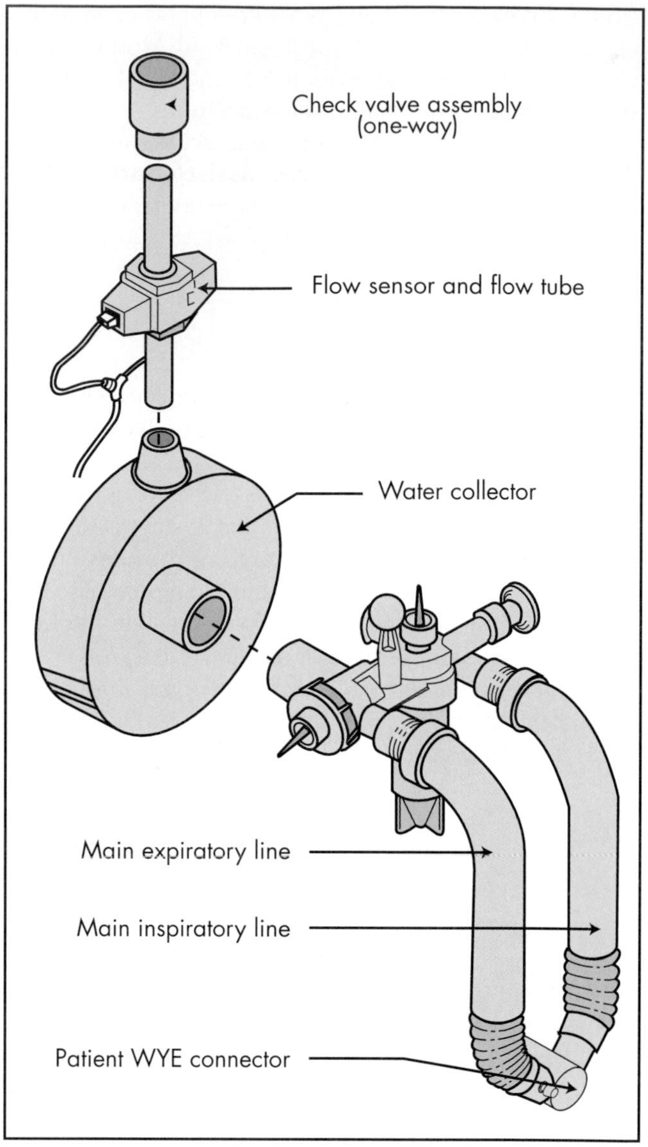

Figure 10-2 Ultrasonic flow transducer, flow tube, and patient circuit. (Courtesy Bear Medical Systems, Inc, Riverside, Calif.)

an internal, belt-driven, rotary air compressor that provides a high-pressure air source if an external source is not available or the external air pressure drops below 25 psig.

The Bear 3 is designed to ventilate pediatric and adult patients and is most commonly used in the acute care setting. The patient circuit has standard features, which in this case include an externally mounted exhalation valve. After leaving the exhalation valve, expired gases are directed through a large-bore corrugated tube to an external flow sensor (Figure 10-2), which is an important part of the patient alarm and monitoring system and is described later in this section in the discussion of special features. In addition, airway pressures are monitored at the proximal airway via a small-bore clear plastic tube that connects at the patient wye connector.

Internal Mechanisms

Compressed air and/or oxygen (30 to 100 psig sources) are the driving force of the ventilator (see Figure 10-3, *1* and *2*). If a malfunction reduces one of the external gas sources, a crossover solenoid (*3*) is activated, and the ventilator continues to operate from the remaining gas source. If external air pressure fails, a switchover valve (*4*) activates the internal compressor.

The two gas pressures are reduced to about 10 to 11 psi after entering the ventilator. They are then blended in the internal oxygen-mixing system, from which they pass through the waveform control system and the main solenoid (on/off switch, [*5*]). The pressure is then further reduced to about 1.8 to 3 psi as the gas passes the peak- and/or taper-flow control system (*6*).

Some of the gas bypasses the main solenoid (*7*) and provides gas for spontaneous breathing in the SIMV mode and in CPAP. This flow comes from the **internal demand valve** (*8*). A patient-sensing pressure line controls gas flow from the demand valve. During spontaneous breaths in SIMV and CPAP, the valve opens when pressure drops to 1 cm H_2O below **baseline pressure** to provide flow to the patient. Blended gases enter the

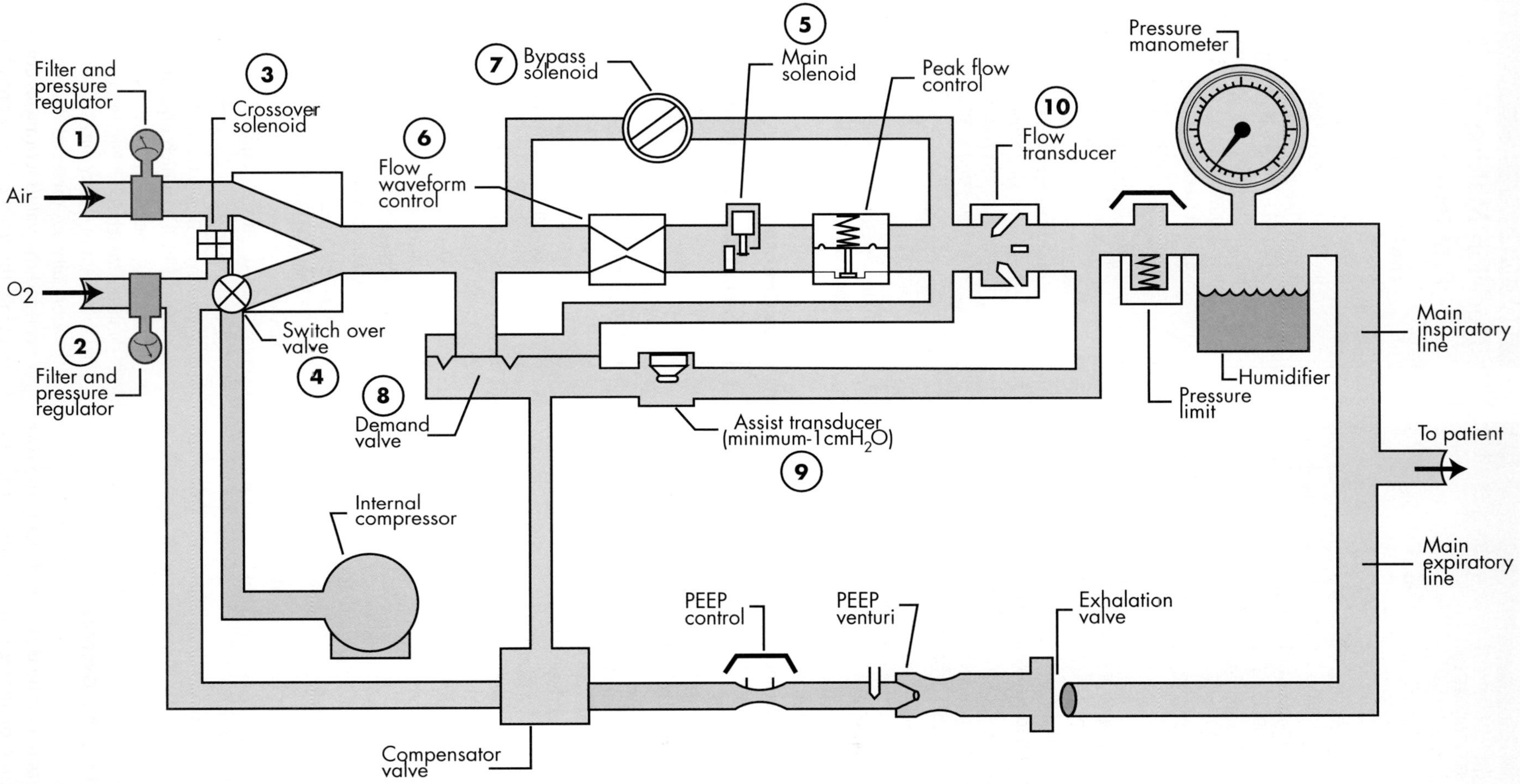

Figure 10-3 Diagram of the internal operating system.

BOX 10-1

The Assist Transducer

Under certain circumstances, a patient can draw a significant volume of gas from the demand valve without triggering a mandatory breath. This can occur when the patient's inspiratory effort creates a very slow change in flow; that is, a change that is not rapid enough to cause sudden cooling of the thermistor bead (assist transducer). Without an adequate temperature change, the electrical output from the transducer is not strong enough to result in a mandatory breath delivery.

ventilator circuit at a rate proportional to patient effort at flows from 0 to 100 L/min. The flow stops when pressure rises above the threshold.

The **internal demand valve** is also involved with patient-triggered breaths in SIMV and A/C for volume-targeted breaths. When the patient effort decreases pressure 1 cm H_2O below baseline, gases from the pneumatic demand valve begin to flow. These gases pass the assist transducer (9), which is a heated thermistor bead (see Figure 10-3). If the transducer detects a large enough change in flow from a patient effort, a signal is sent to the main solenoid, triggering a preset V_T or a sigh volume breath. The operator determines the amount of flow change required by adjusting the ASSIST SENSITIVITY control on the front panel. The assist transducer is actually more sensitive to the suddenness of a flow change than it is to actual flow or pressure change (Box 10-1).

Volume delivery is determined by a vortex-shedding sensor, which is also called the flow transducer (*10*), that measures gas flow during inhalation. The volume setting on the control panel sets a reference signal for the **electronic logic.** When the signal from the vortex sensor matches the setting on the control panel, inspiration ends.

During spontaneous inspiration in SIMV and CPAP, the assist transducer senses flow coming from the demand valve and relays this information to the following sites:

1. The rate display and counting circuit
2. The spontaneous indicator light
3. The exhaled volume display and counting circuit
4. The apnea timing circuit

Because of these various functions, it is important that ventilator **sensitivity** is properly adjusted—even during spontaneous breathing (Box 10-2).

A **subambient pressure valve** allows the patient to breathe room air if the ventilator malfunctions.

CONTROLS AND ALARMS

The front (operator) panel of the Bear 3 is divided into two main sections: the top monitoring panel (Figure 10-4) and the main operating panel (Figure 10-5). The operating panel controls will be reviewed first.

BOX 10-2

Decision Making & Problem Solving

The Importance of Setting Sensitivity on the Bear-3

If the ASSIST SENSITIVITY CONTROL knob is set in the least sensitive position during CPAP with the Bear 3, the detection of spontaneous rate and volume can be affected. When spontaneous breaths go undetected, the display shows zero (0) breaths and zero (0) volume, or the last counted volume that was detected. Eventually, the apnea alarm sounds.

Problem

Suppose that a patient is set on SIMV at a rate of 6 breaths/min on the Bear 3; the ASSIST SENSITIVITY is at the less-sensitive setting. Would the patient still be able to breathe from the demand valve? Would the ventilator recognize spontaneous breaths and correctly report rate and volume?

See Appendix A for the answers.

Main Control Panel

The control panel is visually divided into several sections. There is a section on the top row for rate and volume, a section on the right for alarms, a section on the second row for sighs, and a section on the left side and the lower left side for a variety of controls. To simplify a review of these controls, they will be described row by row.

The top row of controls on the operating panel of the Bear 3 are as follows (left-to-right; Figure 10-5):

1. Main ON/OFF switch.
2. MODE CONTROL switch (control, assist/control, SIMV, and CPAP).
3. SINGLE BREATH switch, which is a **manual trigger** that delivers the set V_T and has a 340 msec delay after cessation of expiratory gas flow to prevent breath stacking.
4. NORMAL TIDAL VOLUME control (ranges from 0.10 to 2.0 L).
5. NORMAL RATE control (ranges from 0.5 to 60 breaths/min).
6. NORMAL PRESSURE LIMIT control (ranges from 0 to 120 cm H_2O), which ends inspiratory gas delivery and activates the PRESS.LIMIT ALERT alarm when the set value is reached.
7. LOW INSPIRATORY PRESSURE ALARM, which activates when airway pressure during inspiration has not exceeded the value set on this control or has not dropped below the level on this control during exhalation.

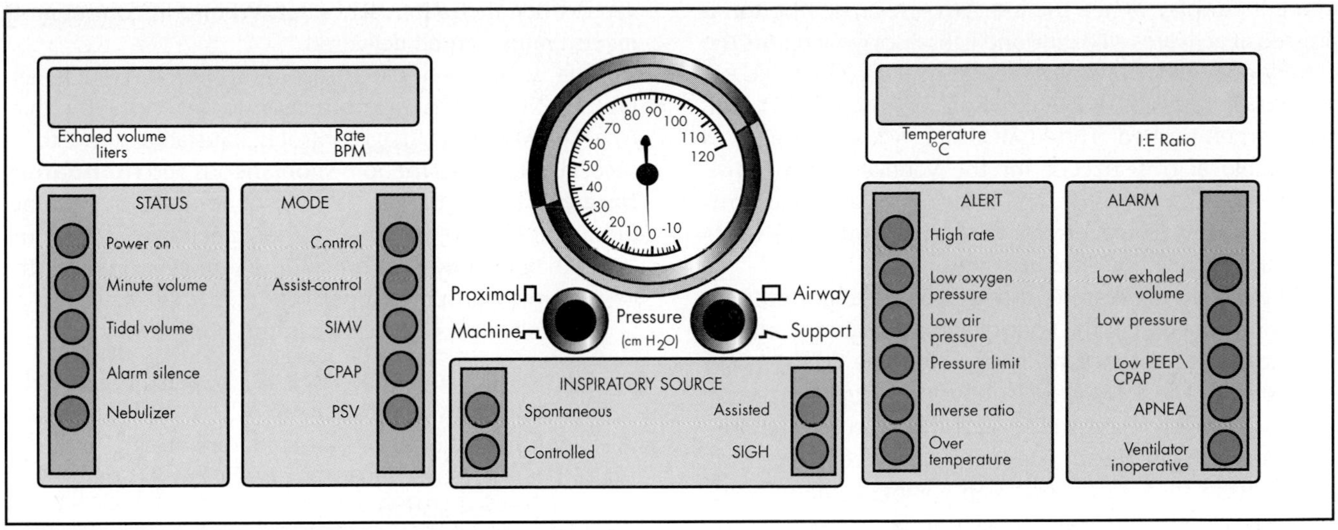

Figure 10-4 Monitor and alarm display panel of the Bear-3.

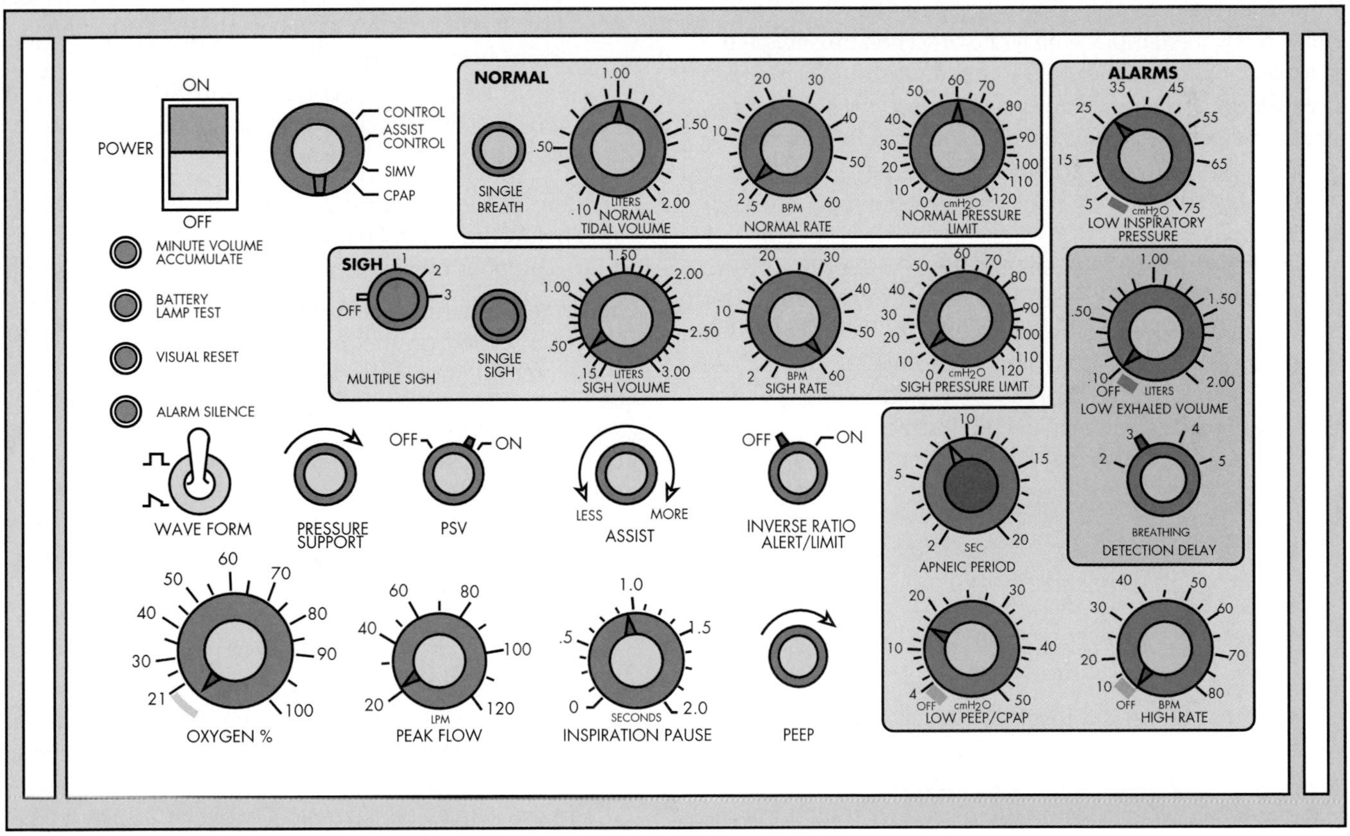

Figure 10-5 Control panel of the Bear-3.

The second horizontal row of controls comprises several features. At the far left, there are four manual buttons, as follows:

1. MINUTE VOLUME ACCUMULATOR
2. BATTERY/LAMP TEST
3. VISUAL RESET
4. **ALARM SILENCE** button

When the MINUTE VOLUME ACCUMULATOR button is pushed, it activates the volume monitor to accumulate tidal volumes measured for 1 minute. During this minute, the minute volume indicator blinks. Accumulated $\dot{V}_E$ is displayed during the second minute, and the $\dot{V}_E$ indicator remains lit. The displayed digital value automatically returns to the normal V_T after the 2 minutes have passed. Pressing the button a second time immediately returns the monitor to the V_T display. When the BATTERY/LAMP TEST button is pressed, it activates all digital and light displays and tests the battery-powered, power-loss sensing circuit. A VISUAL RESET button resets all activated visual alarms and alert indicators when pushed. The ALARM SILENCE button silences all audible alarms—except for the ventilator inoperative alarm—for 60 seconds or until it is pressed a second time. There is a light on the display panel that illuminates when the alarm silence button is activated.

The sigh controls are to the right of these four buttons. Sighs only function in the control and assist/control modes. The MULTIPLE SIGH switch allows up to three sighs to occur sequentially. The SINGLE SIGH button manually triggers a single-sigh breath in any mode once the patient's expiratory flow from the last breath has stopped. The SIGH VOLUME control (0.15 to 3.0 L) allows sigh volume to be selected. The SIGH RATE control permits sighs to occur from 2 to 60 times per hour and determines the interval between sigh breaths. The **total cycle time (TCT)** during a sigh is based on the normal rate setting, which is doubled when a sigh is delivered. For example, with a rate of 12 breaths/min on the normal rate control, the TCT is 5 seconds. When a sigh breath occurs, the ventilator waits 10 seconds after the sigh breath before delivering another mandatory breath. The SIGH PRESSURE LIMIT control allows a pressure range of 0 to 120 cm H_2O. Reaching this limit during a sigh ends inspiration.

The LOW EXHALED VOLUME ALARM control (0.10 to 2.0 L, or off) is on the far right of the second row. This alarm activates the audiovisual LOW EXH. VOL. alarm that occurs when the exhaled volume does not exceed the setting for the number of consecutive breaths selected on the DETECTION DELAY switch located just below it.

The third row contains the following controls:

1. WAVEFORM SELECTION
2. PRESSURE-SUPPORT LEVEL and ON/OFF switch
3. ASSIST SENSITIVITY control
4. INVERSE RATIO ALERT/LIMIT
5. **APNEIC PERIOD** control
6. DETECTION DELAY control

The first control is a toggle switch allowing WAVEFORM SELECTION for either a constant flow or a descending ramp waveform. When CONSTANT is selected, the flow to the patient equals what is set on the peak flow control (on the 4th row). When DESCENDING RAMP is selected, flow drops to 50% of the set peak flow during inspiration. The next control sets the PRESSURE-SUPPORT LEVEL, and to the right of it is the ON/OFF switch for **pressure-support ventilation (PSV).** This mode will be reviewed under the section of modes of ventilation. Next is the ASSIST (SENSITIVITY) control, which adjusts the trigger sensitivity to the patient from "less" to "more" sensitive. The INVERSE RATIO ALERT/LIMIT control is next. When it is on, the set I:E ratio cannot become inverse, so the inverse I:E ratio alert is activated when the ratio reaches 1:1. When this control is off, inverse ratios can be delivered.

The APNEIC PERIOD control and the DETECTION DELAY switch are in the alarm section at the end of the third row. The APNEIC PERIOD control is adjustable from 2 to 20 seconds and works for both spontaneous and **mandatory breaths.** The DETECTION DELAY control sets the number of breaths (2 to 5) that must occur sequentially at a volume lower than the low exhaled volume setting in order for the low-volume alarm to activate.

The following controls are in the bottom row:

1. OXYGEN CONTROL knob (21% to 100% [± 3%])
2. PEAK FLOW control (10 to 120 L/min), which determines the flow of a mandatory breath
3. **INSPIRATORY PAUSE** control (0 to 2.0 sec), which delays exhalation
4. PEEP control (0 and 40 cm H_2O), which sets the end-expiratory pressure
5. LOW PEEP/CPAP ALARM (off, or up to 40 cm H_2O), which activates when the baseline pressure drops below the set value
6. HIGH RATE ALARM control (0 to 80 breaths/min), which activates when respiratory rate exceeds the set value

There is another control on the Bear 3, which is located below the control panel on the front face of the ventilator. This control is an ON/OFF switch on the right side next to the three small-bore, metal nipple connectors (i.e., proximal pressure, expiratory valve, and nebulizer connectors). The switch turns an electronic connector for the expiratory flow sensor on the internal nebulizer pump, allowing medications to be intermittently administered during mandatory breaths. The operating pressure for the nebulizer is 14 psig at 11 L/min. The nebulizer system will not function if the PEAK FLOW control is set at 30 L/min or less. V_T and FiO_2 delivery are not affected by operation of the nebulizer pump.

Top Monitoring Panel

Figure 10-4 shows the top monitoring display panel of the Bear 3. This panel is visually divided into three sections: left, central, and right.

The top left section contains a digital display of EXHALED VOLUME (in liters) and BREATHS/MINUTE. When it is displaying TIDAL VOLUME, the V_T light is illuminated in the left column below. When it is displaying MINUTE VENTILATION (in liters/minute) the MINUTE VOLUME light in the column below will flash to indicate that the volume is being accumulated and will be lit constantly when the accumulated volume for 1 minute is displayed.

The digital display of rate (in breaths/min) gives the average for the past 20 seconds and continually updates the breath rate every second. This display includes all detected breaths; that is, the sensitivity must be set so that a reasonable patient effort is sensed and counted as a breath.

The boxed section to the left of the display panel contains two columns of parameters, one labeled *STATUS* and the other *MODE*. The STATUS section gives information about the current operating status of the ventilator, including the following:

1. POWER ON indicator, which illuminates when the ventilator is plugged into an operating AC outlet and the power switch is on
2. MINUTE VOLUME indicator (described previously)
3. TIDAL VOLUME indicator (described previously)
4. ALARM SILENCE indicator, which illuminates when the alarm silence button is pressed
5. NEBULIZER ON indicator, which illuminates when the nebulizer is on during a mandatory delivered breath

The mode section includes light indicators for CONTROL, A/C, SIMV, CPAP, and PSV, which illuminate when the designated mode is selected.

The central portion of the monitor display panel has an airway pressure manometer that is calibrated between -10 and 120 cm H_2O and displays a pressure reading depending on the position of the two buttons below it. It reads proximal airway pressure (through the wye connector line), machine pressure (detected upstream of the main flow bacteria filter), or support pressure (read internally from the output of the PSV regulator). The central portion of the display panel also has inspiratory source lights that illuminate depending on how inspiration was delivered: SPONTANEOUS breath, CONTROLLED (mandatory) breath, ASSISTED breath (patient-triggered, volume-targeted breath), or SIGH breath.

The right portion of the display panel contains a digital display of temperature and I:E ratio (breath-by-breath). The digital temperature reading represents the temperature measured by an external sensing probe generally placed at the proximal airway. An audiovisual alarm occurs if the temperature exceeds 41° C (106° F) or the probe is disconnected from the ventilator during use. The I:E ratio display functions in the control and A/C modes. When it flashes, an I:E ratio $\leq$ 1:9.9 exists.

The boxed-in section to the right of the display panel below the digital display contains a list of alert and alarm indicators.

The following indicators are under the alert section:

1. HIGH RATE: lights when the total breath rate (spontaneous and mandatory) exceeds the setting on the high rate alarm; ranges from off to 80 breaths/min
2. LOW OXYGEN PRESSURE: lights when the pressure at the oxygen inlet line is less than 27.5 $\pm$ 2.5 psi and the O_2% control is set at >21%
3. LOW AIR PRESSURE: lights when the pressure at the air inlet line is <27.5 $\pm$ 2.5 psi, or the compressor pressure is <9.5 psi
4. PRESSURE LIMIT: activates when the pressure limit setting has been reached; inspiratory gas flow ends, and an audible alarm sounds; delivered volume will likely be less than the set volume
5. INVERSE I:E RATIO: lights when $T_I > T_E$; if the I:E control is on and the ventilator is in the control mode, the 1:1 ratio limit will end inspiration and provide an audible and visible alarm indicating that a 1:1 I:E ratio has been reached
6. OVER-TEMPERATURE: activates when setting is exceeded.

Any of the alarms under the alarm section give both a visual indicator and an audible alarm. The following are in the alarms section:

1. LOW EXHALED VOLUME: has an off position; when on, is adjustable from 0.10 to 2.0 L. Activates when the exhaled volume has not exceeded the low exhaled volume alarm setting for the number of consecutive breaths indicated on the detection delay control. If the expiratory flow sensor is disconnected, the alarm activates on the next breath (see the discussion of the exhaled volume sensor).
2. LOW INSPIRATORY PRESSURE: adjustable from 3 to 75 cm H_2O. Activates when the inspiratory pressure of a mandatory breath stays below the set value on the LOW INSPIRATORY PRESSURE control on the operating panel, or during exhalation when the pressure does not drop below the level set on the low inspiratory pressure alarm setting.
3. LOW PEEP-CPAP(audiovisual alarm): activates when the PEEP/CPAP measured baseline pressure is less than the set value on the operating panel for the LOW PEEP-CPAP control (adjustable from off to 40 cm H_2O). Is also activated if flow through the transducer exceeds 25 L/min for 7 to 9 seconds, which occurs when large leaks are present when A/C, SIMV, or CPAP is set, or when the patient is disconnected while receiving PEEP in any of these modes. The alarm can be silenced for 60-second intervals by the ALARM SILENCE/BYPASS button.
4. APNEA: activates when 0 to 20 seconds elapse, depending on the apneic period control setting. Time is measured from the beginning of the last breath (either spontaneous or mandatory). The sensitivity (ASSIST knob) must be set appropriately.
5. VENT. INOPERATIVE: activates when there is a total gas failure, the AC power fails, or certain electronic failures occur. Activation of this alarm shuts down the electrical functions. Pneumatic systems can still operate unless the alarm was due to loss of gas supplies.

MODES OF OPERATION

The mode selection switch allows the operator to select volume ventilation with control, A/C, or SIMV. (These modes are described in Chapter 9.) Spontaneous ventilation is

BOX 10-3

Decision Making & Problem Solving

A patient is being ventilated at an SIMV rate of 4 breaths/min. The patient initiates a volume-targeted breath, but then becomes apneic. When will the next mandatory volume-targeted breath be delivered, and will an apnea alarm be activated?

(See Appendix A for the answers.)

available in the CPAP setting. PEEP/CPAP can give an elevated baseline pressure in any of the available modes.

In the control mode, the Bear 3 is time-triggered based on the rate setting, volume-targeted based on the set volume, and volume-cycled (i.e., inspiration ends when the ventilator determines the volume has been delivered based on flow and T_I). Inspiration can be extended with the INSPIRATORY PAUSE control (time-cycled). A/C is similar to control, except that inspiration can be patient- or time-triggered.

SIMV

With the SIMV mode, the ventilator provides a set breath rate for volume-targeted breaths based on the set normal rate, which is patient- or time-triggered and usually volume-cycled. Between these volume-targeted breaths, patients may breathe spontaneously at baseline pressure from the demand valve without triggering a mandatory breath. Spontaneous breaths are patient-triggered and pressure-limited. PSV can also be added to the spontaneous breaths, in which case they become flow- instead of pressure-cycled.

The ventilator uses a signal period or synchronous period equal to 60 seconds/rate to monitor mandatory breath delivery. If the patient fails to take a breath that triggers a volume-targeted breath, the machine delivers a breath at the beginning of the next period (Box 10-3).

Pressure Support

Pressure-support ventilation has been added and can be adjusted up to 66 cm H_2O and is activated by the assist signal. Inspiration is terminated when patient circuit flow drops to 25% of the initial peak flow.

As mentioned previously, the two pressure-support controls are located on the left side of the control panel, below the multiple sigh control. The ON/OFF switch activates the pressure-support mode when either SIMV or CPAP are selected.

The monitor panel includes an indicator light under the mode section for pressure-support ventilation. When the indicator is lit and SIMV or CPAP has been selected, PSV is on. If the PSV control is on and control or A/C has been selected, the PSV light will flash, but no PSV breaths will be delivered. When pushed, the button below and to the right of the pressure manometer in the display panel measures pressure support.

When the rate setting dictates that it is time for a mandatory breath in the SIMV mode, the next assist signal initiates a volume-targeted breath. When PSV has also been selected, all subsequent assist signals trigger a PSV breath.

Special Features

In order to monitor volume and rate and display them on the Bear 3 display panel, the ventilator uses a vortex-shedding ultrasonic flow transducer to measure gas flow. (Chapter 7 explains this type of flow device.) To allow for continuous monitoring, the expiratory flow sensor (ultrasonic flow transducer) is heated to avoid excess water condensation from accumulation of exhaled gases on the transducer head. This sensor is commonly mounted in a vertical position for the same reason. The ultrasonic transducer collar can be unsnapped from the flow tube, which simply conducts exhaled gas from the exhalation valve into ambient air.

TROUBLESHOOTING

The operating manual also provides a table for troubleshooting the ventilator that lists symptoms, possible causes, and solutions.

Review Questions

(See Appendix A for answers.)

1. Which of the following devices is the drive mechanism for the Bear 3?
   a. volume-displacement bellows
   b. electrically operated solenoid
   c. spring-loaded bellows
   d. linear drive piston
2. The on/off switch for the Bear 3 is located on the:
   a. front control panel
   b. back of the ventilator
   c. side of the ventilator
   d. electrical cord to the AC outlet

3. The flow-measuring sensor at the exhalation valve of the Bear 3 determines volume delivery by measuring:
   a. vortices using ultrasonic detection
   b. volume-displacement of a bellows
   c. resistance changes of an electrical current
   d. current requirements to heat a bead
4. During ventilation of a patient with the Bear 3, PIP rises to 18 cm H_2O, and pressure drops to the set PEEP of 7 cm H_2O during exhalation. The high inspiratory pressure is set at 25 cm H_2O, and the low inspiratory pressure at 5 cm H_2O. Which of the following will occur?
   a. The ventilator will operate normally
   b. A peak inspiratory pressure alarm will sound
   c. A low inspiratory pressure alarm will sound
   d. A low PEEP alarm will sound
5. A patient is on a CPAP setting of 10 cm H_2O. A small leak develops in the circuit. This will result in which of the following:
   a. an apnea alarm will activate
   b. the flow through the patient circuit will increase
   c. the ventilator will switch to a back-up mode of ventilation
   d. the ventilator will operate normally
6. Although a patient is making an inspiratory effort and his chest wall is moving, the Bear 3 does not trigger a volume-targeted breath in the SIMV mode. This may be a result of which of the following?
   I. inappropriate sensitivity setting
   II. inspiratory flow too weak to activate the assist transducer
   III. too high a baseline pressure
   IV. an inadequate PEEP/CPAP level
   a. III only
   b. I and II only
   c. II and IV only
   d. I and III only
7. The electrical cord on the Bear 3 suddenly becomes disconnected while the ventilator is in use on a patient. Which of the following is true?
   a. the patient will be unable to obtain air
   b. the ventilator high-pressure alarm will sound
   c. the patient will be able to receive room air through the subambient pressure valve
   d. back-up ventilation will begin
8. The LOW EXHALED VOLUME control is set at 0.15 L, and the DETECTION DELAY control is set at 4 breaths/min. A patient exhales three consecutive breaths at 0.1 L, and then one breath at 0.3 L. The low exhaled volume alarm will activate in this situation—true or false?
9. The normal V_T control determines volume-targeted breath delivery in all modes—true or false?
10. Pressure-support ventilation on the Bear 3 is normally patient-triggered, pressure-targeted, and flow-cycled—true or false?
11. A respiratory therapist notes that the exhaled V_Ts on the display panel vary from about 0.1 L to 0.5 L while the set V_T is 0.8 L. She also finds the expiratory flow sensor mounted in a horizontal position. What is a possible cause of the difference between the set and measured V_T readings?

References

1. Dupuis YG: Ventilators: theory and clinical application, ed 2, St Louis, 1992, Mosby.
2. McPherson SP: Respiratory care equipment, ed 5, St Louis, 1995, Mosby.
3. Burton GG, Hodgkin JE, and Ward JJ: Respiratory care: a guide to clinical practice, ed 4, Philadelphia, 1997, Lippincott.

Bear 1000 Ventilator

OUTLINE

Power Source

Internal Mechanisms

Controls and Alarms
- Control Panel
- Monitors and Alarms
- Alarms

Modes of Operation
- Changing Ventilator Modes
- Special Features

Graphics

Troubleshooting

LEARNING OBJECTIVES

Upon completion of this section, the reader should be able to:

1. Describe the major components of the internal mechanisms of the Bear 1000.
2. Identify the controls and discuss the function of each.
3. Explain how the controls are set.
4. Discuss how the alarms are set.
5. Assess what alarm-activated LEDs and alarm messages indicate, and state possible causes.
6. Compare each of the modes of ventilation on the Bear 1000, including the trigger and cycle mechanisms and the target variable (pressure or volume).
7. Evaluate a graph or a description of a graphic display that shows pressure **sloping** or **pressure augmentation (Paug)** to determine if the ventilator is set appropriately.
8. Explain the function of the COMPLIANCE COMP. control.
9. Identify a resource that can help determine the causes of a functional problem of the Bear 1000.

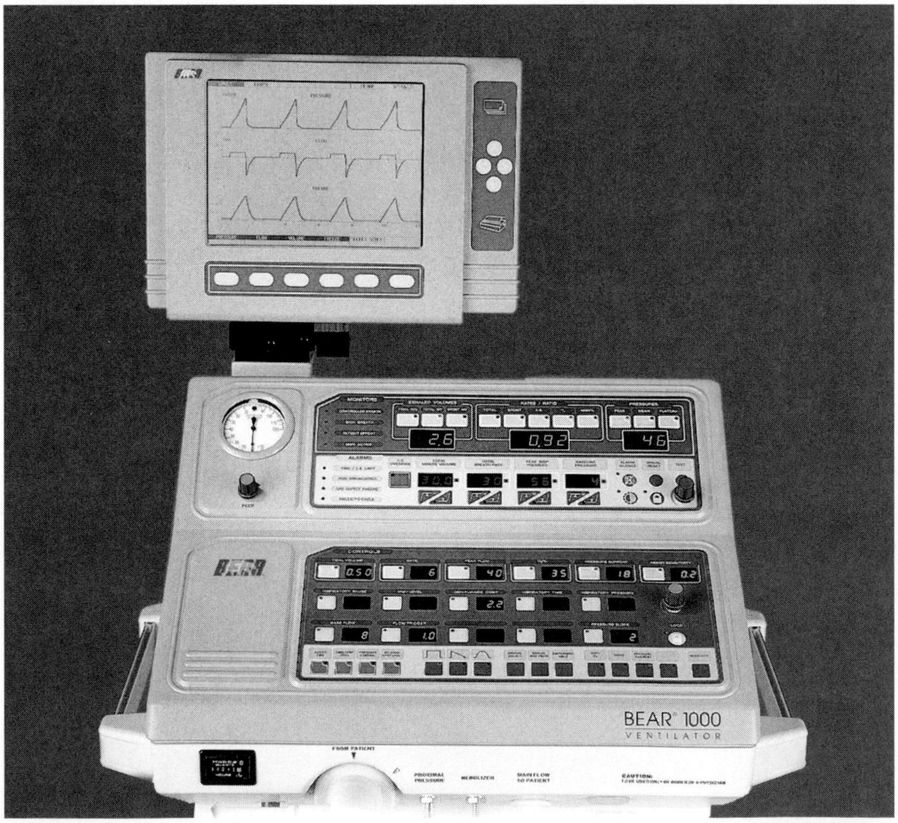

Figure 10-6 The Bear 1000 ventilator. (Courtesy Bear Ventilator Products, Riverside, Calif.)

BOX 10-4

Bear 1000 Exhalation Flow Sensor

Remember from Chapter 7 that a hot wire anemometer measures gas flow as the rate of heat loss from the hot wire. Therefore the greater the flow, the greater the current needed to maintain a high constant temperature.

The Bear 1000 ventilator[1,2] is manufactured by Bear Medical Systems, Inc., which is a subsidiary of Thermo Electron Corporation (Figure 10-6). It can be programmed to provide ventilation for children and adults. Updates to the Bear 1000 have resulted in changes in the operating panel, the most recent version of which is reviewed in this section because it includes both the previous controls and some newer ones.

POWER SOURCE

The Bear 1000 is pneumatically powered and microprocessor-controlled. It is normally connected to external high-pressure sources of air and oxygen (30 to 80 psig), but an air compressor can be added to the unit so that the ventilator can operate from a high-pressure air source without external gas connections but cannot provide increased FIO_2s. The power switch for the unit is on the back of the ventilator.

The patient circuit has a **proximal pressure line** to monitor airway pressure at the wye connector. The exhalation valve is mounted internally. Gas from the patient exits through the exhalation diaphragm and the external flow sensor, which is a hot wire anemometer (Box 10-4).

INTERNAL MECHANISMS

Compressed oxygen and air enter the Bear 1000 through filters and check valves to regulators that reduce the pressures to an internal driving pressure of 18.0 psig. Gas flow passes to a blender and is then directed to an **accumulator** that holds 3.5 L of gas under driving pressure. The accumulator acts both as a mixing chamber to blend gases and as a source of high peak outflow (≥200 L/min). Gas exits the accumulator and passes to a flow-control valve that is positioned by a stepper motor, so that rapid changes in flow are possible (see Chapter 9). The flow delivery logic of the microprocessor uses information from the monitors and the control panel to determine outflow from the valve. There are six pressure transducers that provide information to the microprocessor: (1) a proximal pressure transducer, (2) a differential pressure transducer, (3) a flow valve pressure transducer, (4) a machine pressure transducer, (5) air, and (6) oxygen source pressure transducers.

Both control panel settings and patient flow demand determine the output from the flow-control valve. The flow-control valve allows for delivery of flows from 10 to 150 L/min for volume breaths and in excess of 200 L/min for pressure breaths or on patient demand. From the flow-control valve, gas travels through the **subambient overpressure-relief valve (SOPR)** and out of the ventilator through the outlet check valve (Figure 10-7).

CONTROLS AND ALARMS

The operating panel of the Bear 1000 is separated into two sections (Figure 10-8 and 10-9). The lower section contains the control functions, and the upper section contains the alarms and monitors. Both panels contain a key that must be unlocked before any settings can be changed. Once unlocked, both panels also contain a CONTROL knob that adjusts the numerical value of any parameter selected. To select a parameter, the operator must simply press the touch pad for the parameter, and an LED illuminates and flashes to show that it has been selected.

Control Panel

The most recent control panel is organized into four rows of controls (see Figure 10-9). With the exception of the CONTROL knob, each control variable (e.g., volume and rate) has a touch pad, a small LED to show when it is active, and a digital window to give the operator its selected value. A control can only be selected and changed if the LED for the variable is illuminated, and only those controls available in the current mode of ventilation illuminate. For example, to change V_T during volume ventilation, the touch pad next to the parameter is pushed, and then the CONTROL knob at the far right on the second row of controls is turned until the desired value for V_T appears. The change in the parameter's actual value occurs immediately.

The top row of controls on the control panel includes (from left to right) TIDAL VOLUME (0.1 to 2.0 L), RATE (0, or 0.5 to 120 breaths/min), FLOW (10 to 150 L/min), O_2% (21% to 100%), PRESSURE SUPPORT (0 to 80 cm H_2O), and ASSIST SENSITIVITY (0.2 to 5.0 cm H_2O). Units programmed for lower volumes can provide lower tidal volumes (30 to 99 mL) and flows (5 to 150 L/min). To obtain these lower variables, the operator must press and hold the touch pad for V_T or flow while turning the control knob. When a "P" is displayed in the adjacent digital window, the lower volume range has been obtained. When a pediatric circuit is used, it is recommended that the **PRESSURE SLOPE** control (on the third row) be turned to 0 or P0. This control can be readjusted using the ventilator's graphic display once the patient is attached (see the discussion of pressure sloping).

The second row of controls includes INSPIRATORY PAUSE (0.0 to 2.0 seconds), MMV LEVEL (0 to 50 L/min), COMPLIANCE COMPENSATION (0.0 to 7.5 mL/cm H_2O),

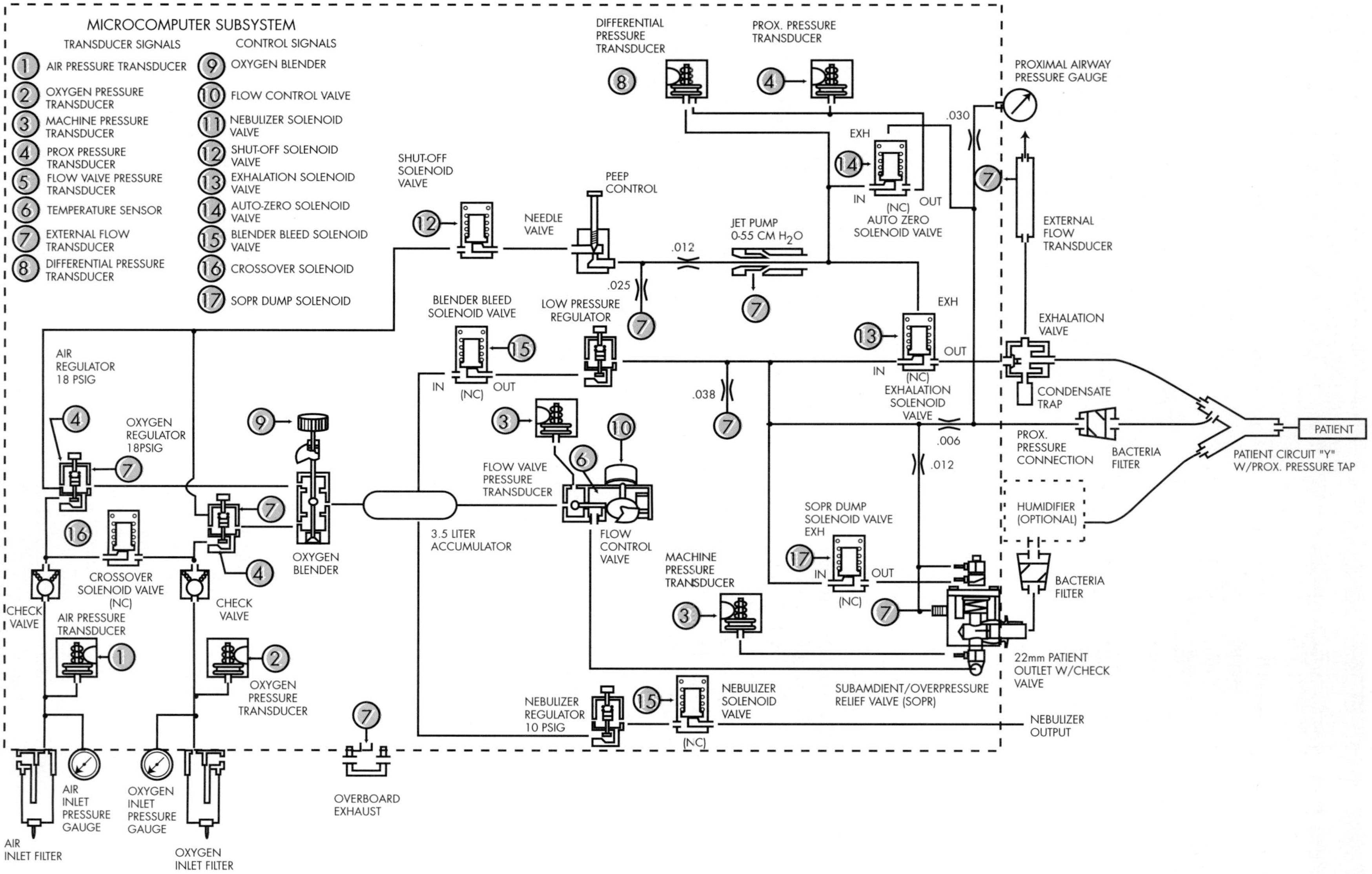

Figure 10-7 The internal circuit of the Bear 1000. (Courtesy Bear Ventilator Products, Riverside, Calif.)

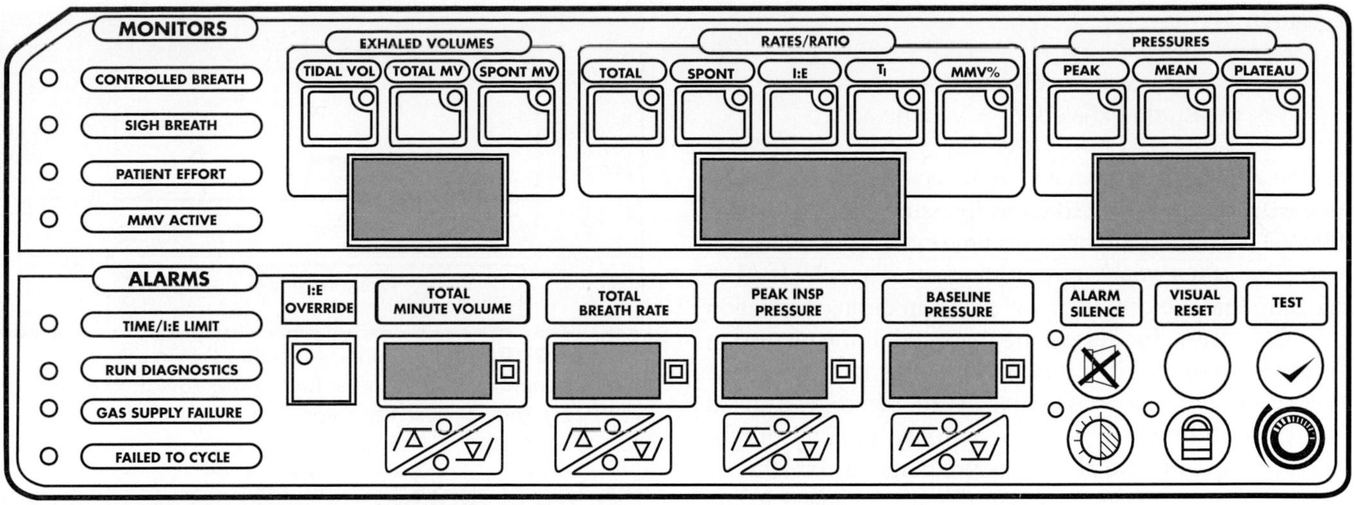

Figure 10-8 Monitor and alarm panel of the Bear 1000.

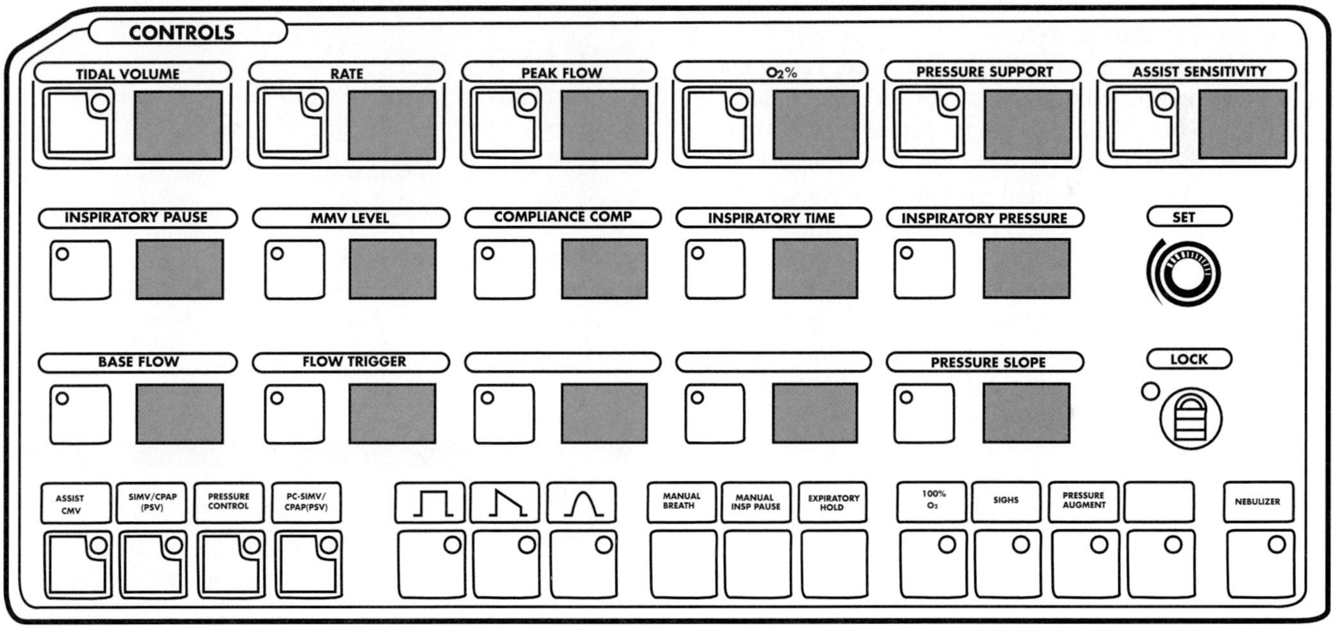

Figure 10-9 Control panel.

INSPIRATORY TIME (0.1 to 5.0 sec), INSPIRATORY PRESSURE (0 to 80 cm H_2O), and the control knob. With inspiratory pause, both the inspiratory and expiratory valves close and hold the delivered breath in the patient and the patient circuit after inspiration. Inspiratory pause is commonly used to measure plateau pressure for the calculation of static compliance. The MMV control sets the minimum $\dot{V}_E$ that the operator wants the ventilator to provide for the patient (see the discussion on modes later in this chapter). The COMPLIANCE COMP. control compensates for the volume lost due to tubing compressibility (tubing compliance). The operator enters the numerical value of tubing compliance for the patient circuit being used. The ventilator adds volume to the set V_T (Equation 1) to establish volume output (Equation 2), so the desired V_T is delivered to the patient. The monitor display of V_T (monitor and alarm panel) shows the measured exhaled V_T minus the additional volume (Equation 3).

Equation 1:

$$\text{volume added} = (\text{compliance comp. setting}) \times (\text{PIP}^* - \text{PEEP})$$

Equation 2:

$$\text{volume output from ventilator} = \text{volume added (for tubing compliance)} + \text{set } V_T$$

*PIP is the peak pressure from the previous breath.

Equation 3:

$$\text{volume displayed} = \text{measured exhaled } V_T - \text{volume added}$$

When the INSPIRATORY TIME control is used with **pressure-control ventilation** (pressure control and PC-SIMV/CPAP[PS]), the breath is time-cycled out of inspiration. The INSPIRATORY PRESSURE control sets the level of pressure that the ventilator will maintain during inspiration for PCV. (These modes will be reviewed in the discussion of modes later in this section.) In the original panel of the Bear 1000, the INSPIRATORY PRESSURE control was called "PRES SUP/INSP PRES," and controlled the pressure for pressure-support breaths, pressure-targeted breaths in PCV, and pressure augmentation. It was changed in the updated version so that SIMV could provide mandatory PCV and spontaneous PSV with different pressure levels for each. The control knob allows the operator to adjust the value of a selected parameter.

The third row of controls includes the **BASE FLOW** control (0, or 2 to 20 L/min), **FLOW TRIGGER** control (from 1 to 10 L/min), two blank controls for future updates, PRESSURE SLOPE control (from -9 to +9 for adult settings and P-9 to P+9 for pediatric settings), and the lock control. Base flow is the flow added to the circuit during exhalation in order to provide flow triggering. Flow trigger is the amount the flow must drop from the base flow value to trigger a patient-flow–triggered breath (see Chapter 9). The FLOW TRIGGER control can only be set if base flow is active. (Note that the unit can be set so that pressure and flow transducers for triggering a breath are active. The ventilator selects the signal that is most sensitive to patient effort and has the fastest response. The manufacturer calls this the "**SmartTrigger**" option.)

PRESSURE SLOPE provides control over the speed at which the inspiratory pressure level is achieved and can be monitored by observing the amount the pressure curve tapers at the beginning of a pressure breath (pressure control, pressure support, pressure augmentation). Significant tapering reduces pressure delivery at the beginning of the breath (negative values). Positive values for pressure slope provide rapid delivery of pressure at the beginning of the breath (Figure 10-10). The LOCK function locks and unlocks the control panel. When controls are locked, they cannot be changed.

The fourth row of controls are listed in Box 10-5. The mode controls are explained in the discussion of modes later in this section. The original version of the Bear 1000 did not provide a mode for SIMV with pressure-targeted breaths, but the newer version does. This control is called "PC-SIMV/CPAP(PSV)." The FLOW WAVEFORM controls only operate during volume-targeted breaths. The constant flow waveform delivers flow at the peak flow setting. The descending ramp rapidly rises to the peak flow setting, then descends linearly until flow decreases to about 50% of peak. The sine flow progressively rises to peak flow and gradually falls to zero in a sinusoidal pattern (Box 10-6).

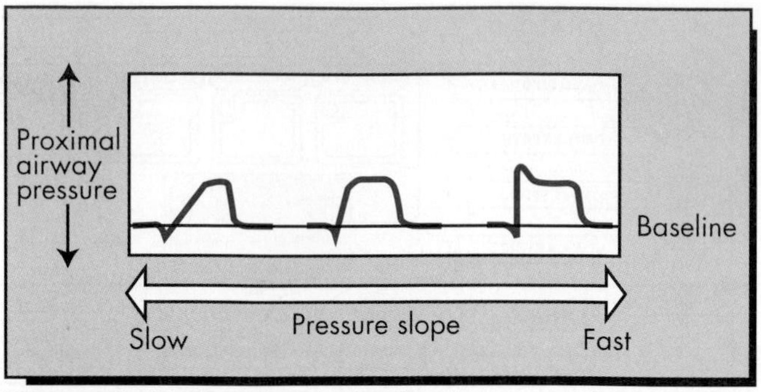

Figure 10-10 Pressure sloping function shown during pressure-support breaths on the Bear 1000; slow (P-9) to fast (+9). (Courtesy of Bear Ventilator Products, Riverside, Calif.)

BOX 10-5

The Fourth Row of Controls on the Bear 1000 Operating Panel

Mode Controls

Assist CMV, SIMV/CPAP (PSV), Pressure Control, PC-SIMV/CPAP (PSV)

Flow Waveform Controls

Constant (rectangular), descending ramp, sinelike wave

Miscellaneous Controls

Manual breath, manual inspiratory pause, expiratory hold, 100% O_2, sighs, pressure augment, blank control (for future option), nebulizer

BOX 10-6

Decision Making & Problem Solving

During volume ventilation with the Bear 1000, the length of inspiration depends on the flow, volume, and rate. For example, the following parameters are set:

- Peak flow = 60 L/min (1 L/second)
- Flow waveform = constant
- Volume = 500 mL
- Rate = 12 breaths/min (TCT = 5 seconds)

Calculate the inspiratory time (T_I). What happens to T_I when the flow curve is changed to a descending ramp?

When activated during expiration, the MANUAL BREATH control delivers one mandatory breath in any mode based on the set values. (Note that the unit will not allow this to be delivered during inspiratory flow of another breath.) MANUAL INSPIRATORY PAUSE triggers a pause at the end of inspiration of the next volume breath and operates for as long as it is depressed—up to a maximum of 2 seconds. It can be used to obtain a plateau pressure reading.

EXPIRATORY HOLD delays breath delivery when pressed during the end of exhalation. It closes the expiratory and inspiratory valves at the moment the next mandatory breath would have been delivered and stops breath delivery for as long as it is pressed (maximum time is 9 seconds). It is used for measuring auto-PEEP.

100% O_2 delivers 100% oxygen through the patient circuit until it is pressed a second time or 3 minutes have passed, whichever comes first.

Selecting the SIGH control provides a sigh breath every 100th breath. The conditions of delivery vary with the mode. Sigh is not available with pressure control in either A/C or SIMV modes. With CPAP, only volume breaths are counted until the 100 breath, so sigh delivery is infrequent. The volume delivery is 150% of the set V_T. The pressure limit for sigh is 150% of the set pressure limit. When it is time for delivery, the sigh breath replaces the next volume breath. With A/C, total cycle time (TCT) is doubled. With SIMV, TCT does not change.

PRESSURE AUGMENTATION is another control in this row; it is reviewed in the discussion of modes of ventilation later in this section.

When **NEBULIZER** control is selected, a 10 psig gas source is available to the nebulizer port, which can be connected to a small-volume nebulizer for delivery of medication. Approximately 6 L/min of flow comes from this port. The ventilator automatically subtracts 6 L/min from the flow that would be delivered during inspiration so that V_T delivery does not change significantly. In addition, the nebulizer only operates when the flow from the main inspiratory line is exceeds 20 L/min—regardless of the mode, pressure slope, or waveform selected. The nebulizer port operates for 30 minutes unless the control is turned off first.

The only control not part of the control panel is the PEEP control, which is a knob below the analog manometer. The PEEP control has no numerical values next to it, so adjustment is determined by the PEEP value indicated on the analog manometer. PEEP ranges from 0 to 50 cm H_2O and is available with all modes. If a leak occurs in the patient circuit when baseline is above zero, the ventilator increases flow through the circuit to try to maintain the selected PEEP level.

The **analog pressure manometer** reads from -10 to 120 cm H_2O and provides monitoring in all modes. It is a back-up method of verifying digitally displayed pressure values (peak, mean, and plateau pressure).

Monitors and Alarms

The top panel of the Bear 1000 contains the alarms and monitors. The first row of this section contains monitored information, and the second row contains alarm information. On the left of the panel is a list of four possible breath functions: CONTROLLED BREATH, SIGH BREATH, PATIENT EFFORT, and MMV ACTIVE. An LED adjacent to each of these illuminates to indicate the type of breath that has just been initiated. For example, the CONTROLLED-BREATH LED lights if a set volume or pressure breath is either patient- or time-triggered. It also lights for a sigh breath or a manually triggered breath. The SIGH BREATH LED lights during the inspiratory phase of a sigh breath. The PATIENT EFFORT LED indicates that patient effort was equal to or greater than the set assist sensitivity or flow trigger. The MMV ACTIVE LED indicates that the ventilator is giving back-up breaths to maintain a minimum level of ventilation (see MMV in the section under modes) and remains lit as long as the MMV backup is active.

The next section of the monitor panel is the exhaled volume section. There is one digital readout window and three potential volume readings: V_T, total $\dot{V}_E$, and spontaneous $\dot{V}_E$. The operator selects the desired displayed volume by pressing the touch pad below the volume. Volumes are measured by the flow sensor near the main expiratory line. The expiratory flow sensor reads flow and converts it to volume readings at STPD (standard temperature [77° F, or 25° C], ambient pressure, dry gas). The microprocessor subtracts the volume attributed to humidity from the exhaled volumes to help correct readings.

V_T represents the most recent breath of any type. $\dot{V}_E$, total or spontaneous, is the average of the most recent breaths. Any changes represent the actual exhaled volumes accumulated over a 1 minute. The V_Ts range from 0.00 to 9.99 L and the $\dot{V}_E$s (total and spontaneous) range from 0 to 99.9 L.

The next panel displays either respiratory rate (total or spontaneous), I:E ratio, or % MMV. Likewise, there is one digital display window, so the operator selects which parameter is to be displayed. Rate is an average of the most recent breaths and reflects a 60-second accumulated value. Available readings are from 0 to 155 breaths/min. The total represents all breaths, and the spontaneous rate only represents patient spontaneous breaths for CPAP or pressure-support breaths.

The I:E ratio ranges from 1:0.1 to 1:99.9 and can be calculated with the following ratio: $1{:}(T_E/T_I)$. The reading is based on the last breath and updates at the beginning of the next inspiration. It does not measure spontaneous or pressure-support breaths (Box 10-7).

T_I displays the inspiratory time for the previous breath. Similar to the I:E ratio, it does not work for spontaneous or pressure-supported breaths. Its values range from 0 to 9.99 seconds.

The MMV % monitor (0% to 100%) displays the average percentage of time in the last 30 minutes that the MMV backup rate has been used instead of the normal breath rate control.

The pressure monitors include peak, mean, and plateau. As with the other monitors, the operator must select which of the three is to be displayed. Peak pressure (0 to 140 cm H_2O) shows PIP for the most recent breath, but does not read spontaneous peak pressure. Mean (0 to 140 cm H_2O) shows the average mean pressure at the wye connector for the last breath. Plateau (0 to 140 cm H_2O) requires that an inspiratory pause of at least 0.1 seconds be

BOX 10-7

Calculating I:E Ratios on the Bear 1000

A patient on A/C volume ventilation on the Bear 1000 has the following settings: V_T = 1.0 L; rate = 10/min; flow = constant; peak flow = 60 L/min. Calculate the I:E ratio.

$$TCT = 60/10 \text{ breaths/min} = 6 \text{ seconds}$$
$$T_I = V_T/\text{flow}$$

Change flow to liters/second.

$$60 \text{ L/min} = 1 \text{ L/sec}$$
$$T_I = V_T/\text{flow} = 1 \text{ L}/(1 \text{ L/sec}) = 1 \text{ second}$$
$$T_E = TCT - T_I = 6 \text{ seconds} - 1 \text{ second} = 5 \text{ seconds}$$
$$I{:}E = 1{:}5$$

(If you had trouble with this calculation, refer to Chapter 9.)

BOX 10-8

Measuring Plateau Pressure

Plateau pressure measurement is an attempt to estimate the pressure in the patient's lungs at the end of inspiration; but it really measures pressure in both the lungs and the patient circuit.

When plateau pressure is measured, a patient cannot be actively breathing. If the patient tries to breathe in or out against the closed valves, which is only natural, the plateau reading will be inaccurate.

provided. This can be done using the INSPIRATORY PAUSE control on the second row of controls or the MANUAL INSPIRATORY PAUSE on the fourth row of controls. It displays the plateau pressure of the previous breath. If no measurable plateau was present on the previous breath, it reads zero (Box 10-8).

Alarms

The alarms being monitored appear in the second row on the monitor and alarm panel. The left column of alarms are built-in alarms. The TIME/I:E LIMIT alarm is set off under two circumstances: when T_I is ≥5 sec + inspiratory pause time and T_I exceeds T_E, and when the I:E ratio exceeds 1:1 for mandatory breaths. For example, if an attempt is made to alter the ratio to 2:1, the alarm will sound. If these limits are exceeded, the ventilator ends inspiration. The first alarm circumstance cannot be disabled. To disable the second alarm condition, the operator must select the I:E OVERRIDE key, which is to the right of the time/I:E limit alarm. When the LED for the I:E OVERRIDE key is on, then the ventilator will allow inverse ratios up to 4:1.

The RUN DIAGNOSTICS indicator tells the operator that the microprocessor has detected a system or electronic problem during the self test or normal operation. A troubleshooting code can be viewed in the total minute volume digital display by pressing the TEST key. The GAS SUPPLY FAILURE alarm activates if either source gas pressure falls below 27.5 psig. The ventilator will continue to operate from the remaining gas source, but this can alter FiO_2 delivery. The FAILED TO CYCLE alarm activates if the ventilator does not cycle due to an external or internal condition. The error code appears in the total minute volume digital display window. An internal safety valve opens, allowing the patient to breathe room air. These four built-in alarms are both visual (flashing light) and audible. If any of these LEDs are lit but not flashing, this indicates that the alarm condition occurred but was corrected. Pressing the VISUAL RESET near the right side of this row of alarms turns the light off.

There are also four sets of adjustable alarms in the second row. The alarm sequence from left to right is: TOTAL MINUTE VOLUME, TOTAL BREATH RATE, PEAK INSPIRATORY PRESSURE, and BASELINE PRESSURE. They can all be adjusted in the same way. For each alarm panel, there is one digital display window used for both the high and low settings of a particular alarm. To the right of the digital window is an LED that lights when the alarm is violated. There are two touch pads below the digital window: the left one has an upward-pointing triangle and sets the upper limit; the right one has a downward-pointing triangle and sets the lower limit. To adjust either, the alarm panel must be unlocked with the LOCK control. Either the upper or lower limit touch pad should be touched for the desired alarm parameter. For example, if the upper alarm key for total minute volume is touched, its current numerical value appears in the digital display window. At the same time, the touch pad light that was touched begins to flash and will do so for 15 seconds or as long as the control knob continues to be turned. While it is flashing, the touch pad light can be adjusted by turning the ALARM CONTROL knob on the far right side of the alarm panel. It is important to note that the alarm level changes as soon as the knob is turned, even while the alarm indicator is flashing. While the first selected alarm parameter is still flashing, the operator can select another alarm to adjust by repeating the same process. Even though the indicators may be flashing, only one parameter can be adjusted at a time.

When the alarm parameters set by the operator have been exceeded, the small light to the right of the digital display (the alarm trigger indicator for that control) flashes and an audible alarm sounds. Once the alarm condition is corrected, the alarm trigger indicator stays lit until the VISUAL RESET pad is pressed.

The HIGH and LOW $\dot{V}_E$ alarms range from 0 to 80 and 0 to 50 L, respectively. HIGH and LOW V_T RATE alarms range from 0 to 155 and 1 to 99 breaths/min, respectively.

BOX 10-9

Situations Affecting Baseline Pressure

PEEP is set at 8 cm H_2O, and the high and low PEEP alarms are set at 13 and 3 cm H_2O, respectively. If a leak occurs and pressure during expiration falls to zero, the low baseline pressure alarm activates. If the patient actively exhales or coughs during expiration and prevents pressure from falling to at least 8 cm H_2O, the high baseline pressure alarm will sound.

HIGH and LOW PIP alarms are slightly more involved. The high PIP range is from 0 to 120 cm H_2O, and reaching this alarm ends inspiration. For a sigh breath, the PIP is 150% of the set high PIP limit, or 120 cm H_2O, whichever occurs first. When a high PIP alarm occurs, the pressure in the proximal line must drop to within 5 cm H_2O of the PEEP level (baseline). If there is a kink in the main expiratory line, the line pressure may not be able to drop, and the delivery of the next breath is delayed until pressure in the proximal line decreases. The range for the low PIP alarm is from 3 to 99 cm H_2O and cannot be set below 3 cm H_2O. It is not active for spontaneous breaths and is also inactive in PSV and PCV under the following condition:

$$[\text{PEEP} + (\text{Pres Sup/Insp Pres})] \leq 3 \text{ cm } H_2O$$

If the abbreviation *Pro* occurs in the PIP alarm display window, the machine pressure is greater than the sum of the high PIP alarm setting + 10 cm H_2O. This alarm is most commonly caused by a disconnection of the proximal pressure line from the machine or the patient circuit, but large leaks can also be to blame.

HIGH AND LOW BASELINE PRESSURE alarms (0 to 55 cm H_2O and 0 to 50 cm H_2O, respectively) occur when monitored pressure limits are violated. Box 10-9 gives some examples of when these events can occur.

Five touch pads and the control knob are to the right of the alarms in this row. The top three touch pads are as follows:

1. ALARM SILENCE: silences audible alarms for 60 seconds or until pressed again; cannot silence the FAILED TO CYCLE alarm
2. VISUAL RESET: resets visual alarms after alarm conditions are corrected
3. TEST: has three functions: (1) activates the visual and audible indicators for 4 seconds during normal operation in order to check function; (2) displaces any troubleshooting codes that might have occurred in the total minute ventilation digital window; (3) if pressed before the ventilator is turned on and held while the power is turned on, it causes the ventilator to enter Operator Diagnostics, and the operating manual should be consulted

The bottom two touch keys are the DIMMER key and the LOCK key. The DIMMER key adjusts the brightness of the LEDs on the control panel, and the LOCK key locks the alarm control panel so values cannot be accidentally changed. The LED near this key is lit when the panel is locked. Changes to alarm controls cannot be made until this key is pressed to unlock it.

MODES OF OPERATION

The mode controls on the Bear 1000 include the following: ASSIST CMV, SIMV/CPAP(PSV), PRESSURE CONTROL, PC-IMV/CPAP(PSV), and PRESSURE AUGMENT. Each of these will be reviewed, and they are all changed in the same way.

Changing Ventilator Modes

The first four mode keys are on the lower left row of the control panel. The last, PRESSURE AUGMENTATION, is the farthest right control in this row. Mode keys have three conditions: OFF, SETUP, and ON. When changing an operating mode on the Bear 1000, the following procedure is used. The operator first presses the mode key for the new mode desired: OFF to SETUP. This causes the LED by that mode's touch pad to flash while the original mode key LED stays lit. The control panel illuminates the controls available for the new mode. Then the operator adjusts each control variable for the new mode to the desired setting, along with all desired alarm settings. Once everything is set, the operator presses the new mode touch pad a second time: SETUP to ON. It stays illuminated and the old mode switches to OFF.

Assist CMV

Assist CMV is **volume-targeted ventilation** that can be time- or patient- (pressure- or flow-) triggered. All of the controls are available except MMV, inspiratory time, pressure support, or inspiratory pressure.

SIMV/CPAP (PSV)

SIMV/CPAP (PSV) is volume-targeted SIMV. The operator can provide a positive baseline (PEEP/CPAP) in this mode by using the PEEP control. Pressure support is also available for spontaneous breaths. Volume breaths can be patient-triggered or, if that fails, time-triggered. Volume breaths are based on the V_T, rate, peak flow, and flow waveform selected. Spontaneous breaths occur from the set baseline pressure. In addition, pressure-support ventilation (PSV) can be provided for spontaneous breaths based on the set

BOX 10-10

Reviewing Definitions of Breath Types

Mandatory breath delivery is completely determined by the ventilator (i.e., triggering, delivery of inspiration, and cycling are ventilator-controlled). Breaths are commonly volume- or pressure-targeted.

An assisted breath is patient-triggered. The delivery of inspiration and the ending of inspiration (cycling) is determined by the ventilator.

With spontaneous breaths, the patient controls all phases of the breath.

pressure-support level. The set pressure is added to the PEEP level. For example, if the PEEP is 5 cm H_2O, and the PSV is set at 15 cm H_2O, PIP during a PSV breath will be 20 cm H_2O. The PSV breaths are patient-triggered, pressure-limited, and flow-cycled at about 30% of the initial peak flow reached at the beginning of the breath.

When this mode control is active and the RATE is turned to zero, the ventilator can provide either CPAP alone or PSV. Baseline can also be positive with PSV alone.

Pressure Control

Pressure control is **pressure-targeted ventilation** in which each breath is time- or patient- (flow- or pressure-) triggered, and the ventilator provides the set pressure on the inspiratory pressure control for each breath. Pressure-delivered equals the inspiratory pressure plus PEEP. In addition to inspiratory pressure, the operator sets the RATE, T_I, ASSIST SENSITIVITY and/or BASE FLOW and FLOW TRIGGER, and PRESSURE SLOPING. Most other controls, including the waveforms, sigh, and pressure augment, are not available. It is very important to set the upper pressure limit in this mode because pressure can go above the set inspiratory pressure level. For example, if the patient coughs, the pressure may exceed the set value.

PC-SIMV/CPAP(PSV)

PC-SIMV/CPAP(PSV) is ventilation in which mandatory or assisted breaths are pressure-targeted and time-cycled. Remember the definitions of *mandatory* and *assisted* (Box 10-10; see Chapter 9). Baseline can be positive. Spontaneous breaths can occur with pressure support or simply from the set baseline. As in pressure control, the operator sets the RATE, INSPIRATORY PRESSURE, TRIGGERING MECHANISMS, and T_I. PEEP and PRESSURE SUPPORT can also be set. Both the inspiratory pressure setting and the pressure support setting are added to the PEEP level. If the inspiratory pressure is 20 cm H_2O, the pressure support is 10 cm H_2O, and the baseline 10 cm H_2O, PIP for mandatory or assisted breaths will be 30 cm H_2O, and all spontaneous breaths will be at 20 cm H_2O.

If rate is turned to zero, the ventilator allows the patient to spontaneously breathe at the set baseline (zero or PEEP/CPAP). If the sensitivity is appropriately set, the ventilator can monitor spontaneous breaths, which occurs when the patient's inspiratory effort meets or exceeds the set trigger value. These spontaneous breaths can also be pressure-supported.

Pressure slope can also be used in this mode and can affect the rate of flow during pressure-targeted mandatory or assisted breaths, pressure-support breaths, or spontaneous breaths.

Pressure Augment

Pressure augment, or pressure augmentation (PAug), is a servo-control (closed-loop) mode of ventilation that guarantees volume delivery on a breath-by-breath basis. Because it is a fairly unusual form of ventilation, more time is spent reviewing its function.

PAug provides the benefits of pressure-targeted ventilation, such as high initial gas flows, a descending-ramp type of flow pattern, and a limited pressure, with the added benefit that it can guarantee volume delivery. Key criteria for using pressure augmentation are that a patient must be able to initiate breaths and must have a consistent respiratory rate and a reasonable inspiratory effort.

PAug is currently designed to work in any patient-triggered, volume breath. For this reason, it only works in assist CMV and SIMV/CPAP(PSV). It is selected by pressing the PRESSURE AUGMENT control so that it is illuminated. The operator also selects a V_T, a rate, an inspiratory pressure level above baseline, a peak flow, and a sensitivity setting. It is also important to set an appropriate pressure limit of about 10 cm H_2O of the inspiratory pressure plus PEEP. Regarding flow pattern, it is currently recommended that a constant flow pattern be selected to help keep T_I shorter.

PAug operates in the following manner. When the patient triggers a breath, the ventilator provides a high inspiratory gas flow in order to achieve the set pressure level. As it delivers this flow, it monitors flow and volume delivery. From this point, one of two possible scenarios unfolds. If patient inspiratory flow demand and the set pressure are high, the ventilator will see that the minimum volume is delivered quickly and it does not need to take any action. Inspiration ends when the flow drops to 30% of measured peak flow. If the patient demand is modest, however, the ventilator may find that the volume has not been delivered by the time the measured flow has dropped to a value equal to the flow set on the peak flow control. In this case, it will not allow the flow to drop further, but will maintain flow at the set peak flow and continue to provide this flow until it determines that the minimum volume has been delivered, at which point the breath ends.

Figure 10-11 illustrates some of the potential outcomes of PAug. Waveform *A* is an example of a typical pressure-

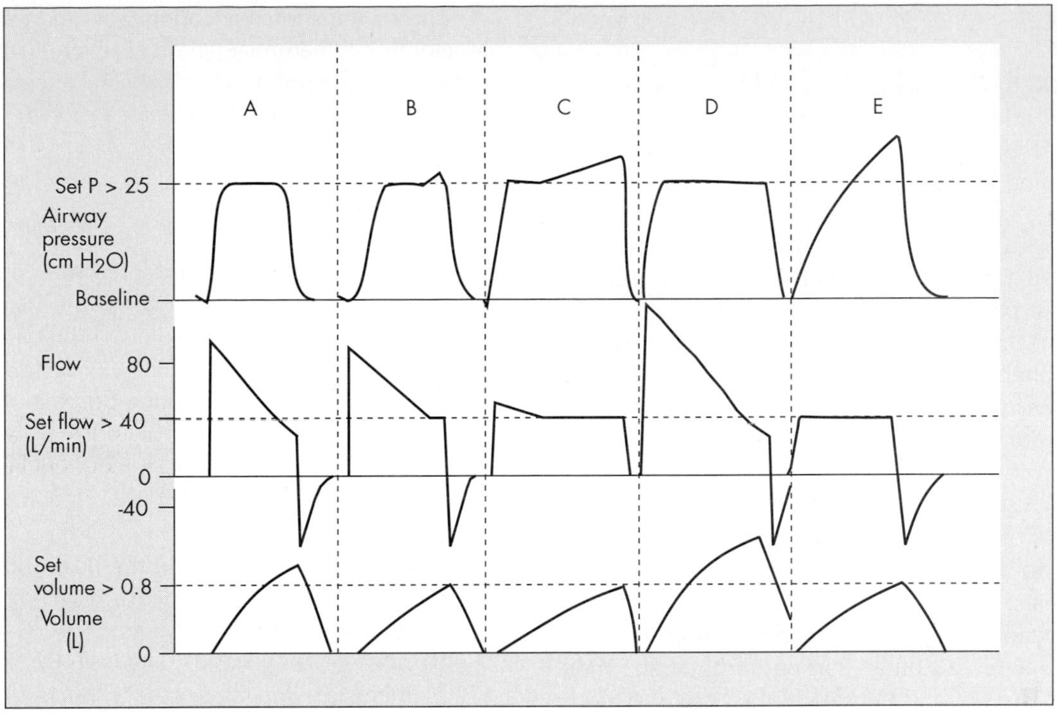

Figure 10-11 Various waveforms achievable with pressure augmentation. (From Pilbeam SP: Mechanical ventilation: physiological and clinical applications, ed 3, St Louis, 1998, Mosby.)

support breath instead of a pressure-augmented breath, so that readers can make some comparisons with pressure augmentation. In *A*, the breath is patient-triggered, pressure-limited (25 cm H_2O), and flow-cycled at approximately 30% of the peak flow reached (100 L/min), and the patient achieved a V_T of about 1.0 L. In Waveform *B*, the patient has a moderate inspiratory demand, and flow rises to reach and maintain the pressure (25 cm H_2O).

Flow drops to the set value of 40 L/min and the ventilator determines that the set volume of 0.8 L has not been reached. It maintains the flow at 40 L/min. Because more flow is going into the patient's lungs, the pressure rises above the set value. When the ventilator determines that the volume was delivered, the breath ends. This is a classic pattern of a pressure-augmented breath. In Waveform *C*, it appears that the set pressure of 25 cm H_2O is not adequate to quickly meet the volume setting for this particular patient. When the flow drops to the set value (40 L/min), it is maintained until the 0.8 L volume is delivered. Notice how long inspiration is compared with Waveforms *A* and *B*. To more appropriately provide pressure augmentation, the inspiratory pressure needs to be increased. The flow may need to be increased as well. In Waveform *D*, the patient has a high inspiratory demand, flow rises rapidly to reach and maintain the set pressure, inspiratory pressure is set high, and minimum volume is surpassed. Volume delivery is high. In this situation, inspiration ends when the flow drops to about 30% of peak flow. PAug can provide whatever volume and flow the patient desires and still remain within a safe pressure limit. In Waveform *E*, no patient effort is detected. The ventilator delivers a typical volume breath at a constant flow setting. Pressure rises to a peak, which depends on the volume delivered and the patient's lung characteristics.

When PAug is used in assist CMV, every breath is potentially augmented. With SIMV, only the assisted breaths are augmented. It is strongly recommended that practitioners use the graphic waveforms for pressure, volume, and flow against time when adjusting PAug for a patient.

Because of its ability to perform pressure augmentation, the ventilator can also augment flow and volume. If patient inspiratory demand drops the measured airway pressure below the baseline pressure, the ventilator automatically increases flow to maintain baseline. This augments flow to the patient and also increases volume delivery above the set value if the patient demands it. For example, in the CPAP mode or with SIMV + CPAP, if baseline pressure during spontaneous breathing drops below the set value due to patient demand, the ventilator increases flow to the patient to maintain the baseline and augment the patient's needs.

Special Features

The most significant special features of the Bear 1000 are pressure augmentation, pressure slope, and SmartTrigger. Undoubtedly, the manufacturer will be able to develop newer available modes in the near future.

Graphics

The Bear 1000 has a **graphics** monitor and program that can easily be added to the ventilator unit. The graphics panel has a viewing screen (see Figure 10-6), below which are six operating keys. To the right of the screen are two icons and four operating keys that look like arrowheads. The POWER switch for the screen is on the back panel of the unit, and the screen is activated by touching the icon (that looks like pages of paper) on the upper right corner of the panel to the right of the screen. The icon at the bottom of the panel looks like a printer and allows the information on the screen to be printed when connected to a printer. The four directional arrows have two main functions: they can change the lighting on the screen; and when they are being used for functions, they can change the amplitude scale of the graphs. For example, if a pressure graph goes from 0 to 10 cm H_2O, the arrows can be used to change the range to 0 to 100 cm H_2O.

The instruction manual provides information about setting time and date and other start-up information. There are menus at the top and bottom of the basic waveform pages of the screen. The top menu provides access to waves, loops, set-up, and time and has several blank positions for future updates. The bottom menu provides information about what parameter is on the screen (e.g., flow or volume) and allows it to be selected and changed. The bottom menu also can freeze a screen, mark a particular graph for reference, and scale the x-axis of the graph.

Between one and three graphs can be placed on the screen. For example, the operator may want to view pressure, volume, and flow per unit time. These parameters can be selected by highlighting the desired parameter with the adjacent touch pads just below the screen and can be removed by simply unhighlighting the parameters. Loops or graphs can be provided by highlighting the options appearing at the top menu on the screen. The graphic display also has a mechanics page, which offers flow/volume and pressure/volume loops as well as compliance, resistance, and work of breathing calculations.

Troubleshooting

The variety of alarms and monitors and the availability of graphic monitoring make everyday troubleshooting fairly simple. In addition, the operating manual contains a troubleshooting section with a table of symptoms, possible causes, and corrective actions.

Radio frequency interference (RFI)/electromagnetic frequency interference (EFI) can affect the operation of the Bear 1000, just as it can with any medical device that uses a microprocessor. Walkie-talkies and cellular phones should not be used near these types of medical devices.

The manufacturer is continually updating the various programs and features that are available with the unit. It is important to be sure to check which system is in operation when troubleshooting a ventilator problem.

Review Questions

(See Appendix A for answers.)

1. The flow-control valve of the Bear 1000 is positioned by which type of device so that rapid changes in flow are possible?
   a. an electronic flow transducer
   b. a linear drive, microprocessor-controlled piston
   c. a proportional rotary microswitch
   d. a stepper motor
2. To adjust the V_T setting on the Bear 1000, which of the following should be performed?
   a. turn the TIDAL VOLUME knob to the desired value
   b. press TIDAL VOLUME, key in the value on the numeric key pad, and press ENTER
   c. press the VOLUME touch pad and rotate the control knob (at the far right on the second row of controls) until the desired value for V_T appears
   d. reduce the $\dot{V}_E$ setting, then change the rate until the desired V_T appears in the **message window**
3. To set the high total $\dot{V}_E$ alarm on the Bear 1000, which of the following must be performed?
   I. unlock the alarm panel
   II. touch the left upward pointing triangle below the total $\dot{V}_E$ digital window
   III. turn the ALARM CONTROL knob until the desired value is displayed
   IV. press the activated touch pad to the right of the alarm
   a. III only
   b. I and II only
   c. II and IV only
   d. I, II, and III only
4. An alarm sounds, and the respiratory therapist notes that the GAS SUPPLY FAILURE LED is illuminated. This indicates which of the following?
   a. one or more of the gas sources is <35 psi
   b. if one gas supply is still available, the ventilator will continue to operate
   c. measured F_{IO_2} has dropped below the set value
   d. inspiratory pressure in the patient circuit is below the set value
5. The Bear 1000 requires both an air and an oxygen gas source and an electrical power source—true or false?
6. Both volume- and pressure-targeted mandatory breaths are available with the SIMV mode—true or false?

7. A nurse is trying to readjust the V_T on the Bear 1000 ventilator. Although the V_T reading is 0.5 L and the LED next to the V_T control is illuminated, turning the control has no effect. What could be the problem?
8. A physician is attempting to change the V_T setting during ventilation of a patient, but the digital display on the V_T control is blank and turning the control knob gets no response. What could be the problem?
9. The graphic display of pressure and time for a pressure-support breath shows the following:
   - a slight dip in the curve below baseline at the beginning of inspiration
   - a sharp rise in pressure to a peak, which falls to a plateau value during inspiration
   - a smooth drop in pressure to baseline at the end of inspiration

   Does this description fit an appropriate PSV breath delivery?
10. The COMPLIANCE COMP. control indicates a value of 3 cm H_2O. The set V_T is 0.7 L; the PIP is 25 cm H_2O. The digital exhaled volume fluctuates from 0.68 to 0.71 L. If a respirometer is placed in the main inspiratory side coming out of the ventilator and going to the patient, what would the volume read?
11. A patient is on pressure augmentation. The pressure/time graph shows a rapid rise to the set value, which is maintained constantly during inspiration. Flow rapidly rises to a peak, which progressively descends to 30% of peak flow and ends. Set volume is 0.5 L, but delivered volume is 0.75 L. Is the patient actively breathing? How do you know?

References

1. Bear 1000 ventilator instruction manual, Publication No. 50-10613-00, Riverside, Calif, 1995, Bear Medical Products, Inc.
2. Pilbeam SP: Mechanical ventilation: physiological and clinical applications, ed 3, St Louis, 1998, Mosby.

Bird 8400STi Ventilator

OUTLINE

Power Source
Internal Mechanism
Controls and Alarms
- Controls
- Monitors and Alarms

Modes of Operation
- Assist/Control
- SIMV
- Spontaneous Mode
- Volume-Assured Pressure Support (VAPS)

Graphic Display Screens
Special Features
Troubleshooting

LEARNING OBJECTIVES

Upon completion of this section, the reader should be able to:
1. Describe the internal mechanism.
2. Explain the location and function of the controls on the front panel.
3. From a description, establish which alarm is active and state a possible cause for the alarm.
4. Recommend a solution to an alarm situation.
5. Compare the pressure-targeted breath setting to the volume-targeted breath setting.
6. Determine what parameter is cycling the breaths in VAPS based on the description of a pressure/time graph.

The Bird 8400STi ventilator[1-4] is a second-generation unit derived from the Bird 6400, which has largely replaced that unit. It is manufactured by Bird Medical Technologies, Inc., which is a subsidiary of Thermo Electron Corp. (Figure 10-12 *A* and *B*) and is designed for use with pediatric and adult patients.

The patient circuit has the usual main inspiratory and expiratory limb and an expiratory valve that is mounted within the unit.

POWER SOURCE

The Bird 8400STi is pneumatically powered and microprocessor-controlled. It requires a blender so that a blend of gases may enter the back panel and usually uses a Bird 3800 Microblender, which has two 50 psig (ranging from 30 to 70 psig) gas sources: air and oxygen. The blended and pressurized gas is used for pneumatic operation. A

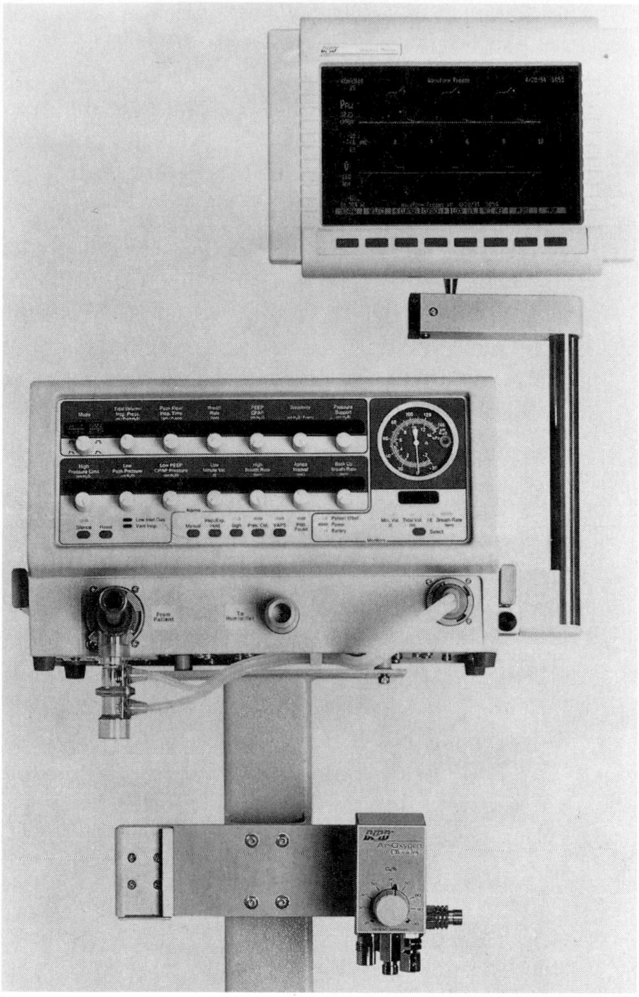

A

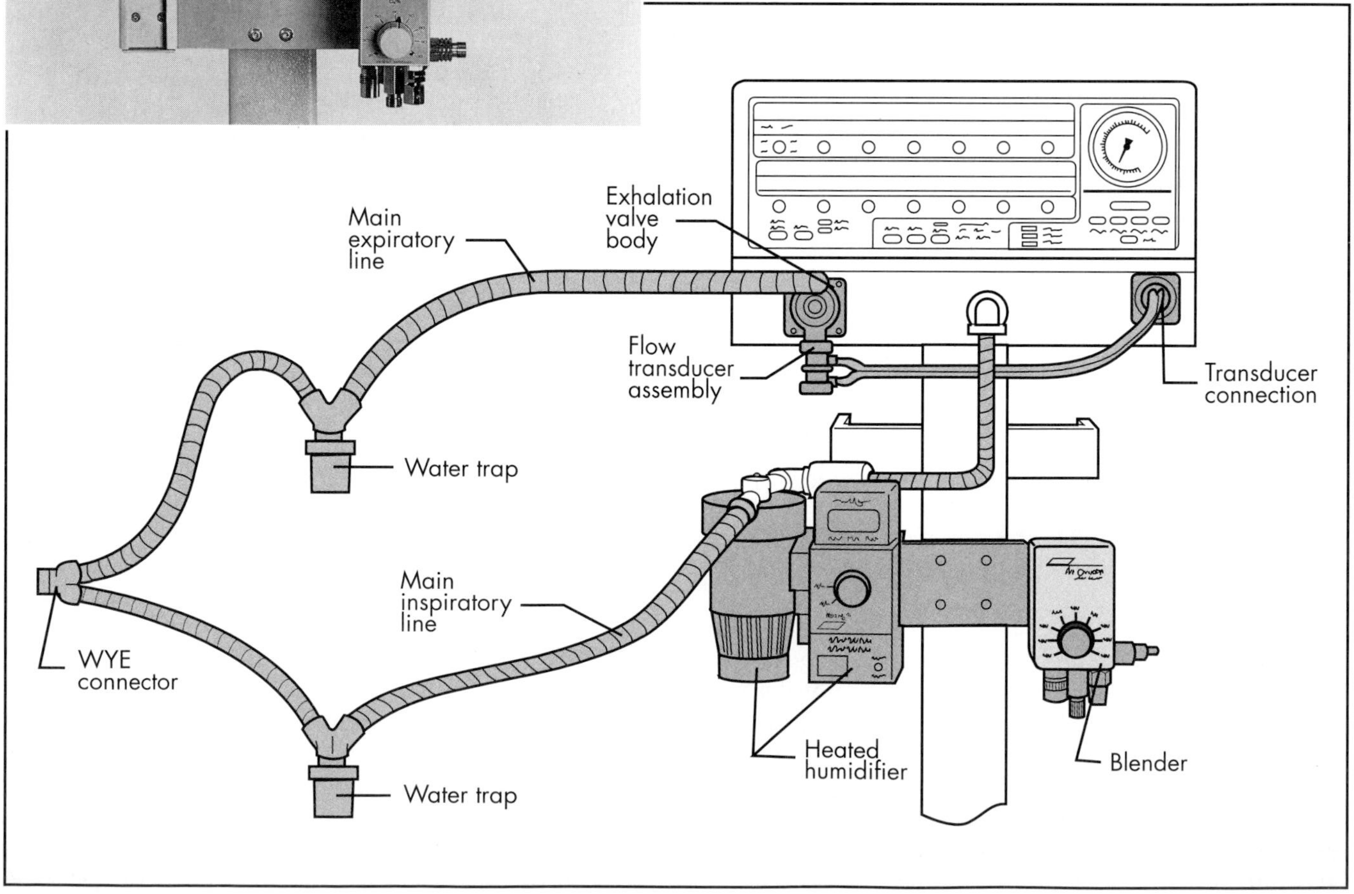

B

Figure 10-12 **A,** photo of the Bird 8400 STi ventilator; **B,** the Bird 8400 STi with a patient circuit attached. (Courtesy Bird Corp., Palm Springs, Calif.)

standard 120-volt AC outlet powers the microprocessor and the electrically operated components.

INTERNAL MECHANISM

Only the basic internal circuit of the Bird 8400STi ventilator is described here. The blended gases enter the unit where they are filtered and flow into a high-pressure, 1.1 liter reservoir (Figure 10-13). This large, pressurized reservoir allows for an augmented gas flow of up to 120 L/min to the patient. Gas passes from the reservoir to a pressure regulator, where the pressure is adjusted to 20 psi. From the regulator, gas passes to the pulsation dampener, a rigid chamber that dampens pressure pulses that may originate from the reservoir, thus minimizing pressure fluctuations.

Gas flow is then directed to the servo-control valve, which is an electromechanical stepper valve that works in the following way. Signals from the microprocessor cause an electric motor to rotate a shaft. These rotations occur in a series of precise steps, each of which opens or closes a poppet type of orifice inside the servo-control valve (see Chapter 9). The information about valve position, orifice size, and the relative flow output from the valve is programmed into the microprocessor, allowing it to precisely deliver the flow, flow pattern, volume, and/or pressure designated by the operator. The operator determines these by selecting the appropriate parameters and modes on the control panel. Flow from the inspiratory flow valve is then directed to the patient.

There is a flow transducer assembly used to monitor flow from the expiratory valve (see Figure 10-13). It operates on the principle of a variable-orifice transducer (see Chapter 7). The two small-bore connecting hoses from this unit send pressure information to an internal differential pressure transducer. This information is monitored and interpreted by the microprocessor and used to display information such as $\dot{V}_E$, V_T, respiratory rate, and I:E ratio.

CONTROLS AND ALARMS

The front panel of the Bird 8400STi has two rows of control knobs and a bottom row of touch pad controls (Figure 10-14). Display windows are above the knob controls, and the values displayed there are set, not measured, values.

Controls

The top row of controls has a MODE and WAVEFORM SELECTION switch on the far left (see Figure 10-14), which allows either A/C or SIMV to be selected. These modes can be either volume- or pressure-targeted. (Note that pressure-targeted ventilation is an option available on the 8400STi ventilator, but is not a standard function.) In volume ventilation, the operator can choose either the constant flow or the descending ramp flow waveform. The next control knob determines either the target volume or pressure, but it normally regulates volume (ranges from 50 to 2000 mL). Pressure-targeted or pressure-controlled ventilation (PCV) requires the use of the touch pad on the bottom row marked PRESS. CTRL. Pressing this pad activates the pressure-control mode. The desired pressure can then be selected with the TIDAL VOLUME/INSP.PRESS. control. The letter *P*, followed by the amount of inspiratory pressure chosen by the operator (ranges from 5 to 100 cm H_2O) is displayed in the window above the knob. How to set up pressure control will be reviewed in the discussion of modes of ventilation in this section.

The next knob on the top row controls either PEAK FLOW (volume ventilation) or INSPIRATORY TIME (PCV). When PCV is used, the numerical value is proceeded by the letter *P*. For example, if the digital value is 50, the flow is 50 L/min (10 to 120 L/min). If it reads "P 0.5," the inspiratory time in PCV is 0.5 seconds (0.1 to 9.8 sec).

The third knob on top regulates the respiratory rate (0 to 80 breaths/min), which determines the minimum mandatory rate in the A/C or SIMV mode. This is followed by the PEEP/CPAP control (0 to 30 cm H_2O) and the SENSITIVITY knob. The unit can be pressure- or flow-triggered. **Pressure triggering** ranges from -1 to -20 cm H_2O, or can be turned off. Flow triggering uses a base flow of 10 L/min and a flow trigger range of 1 to 10 L/min (see Chapter 9). When flow triggering is used, the letter *F* precedes the numerical value for the liters/minute trigger sensitivity. For example, if the number *2* appears in the window above the knob, the machine is pressure triggering at -2 cm H_2O. If "F 2" is in the window, the unit is flow triggering at 2 L/min. The last knob in this row controls pressure-support settings (1 to 50 cm H_2O, or is off). The pressure set by this control is above the set baseline or PEEP level. Pressure support is normally flow cycled at 25% of measured peak flow, but it will time cycle if inspiratory flow time exceeds 3 seconds. The second row of alarm controls is dicussed in the section on monitors and alarms.

The final row of touch pads and indicators (the right portion after the alarm section) contains some additional controls. The first is the MANUAL touch pad, which provides a manual breath at the set mandatory settings. The INSP/EXP HOLD control can provide either an **inspiratory hold** for measuring plateau pressure for a mandatory volume breath or an expiratory hold for measuring auto-PEEP when pressed. To obtain an inspiratory hold, the pad must be pressed, so the display window below the pressure manometer reads "I HLD." Pressing and holding the SELECT key displays the inspiratory hold pressure. The pad must be pressed three times after this maneuver to return the display to its normal reading. To obtain an expiratory hold, the insp/exp hold pad must be pressed twice until "E HLD" is displayed in the monitor window. Next, the SELECT key must be pressed and held to display the

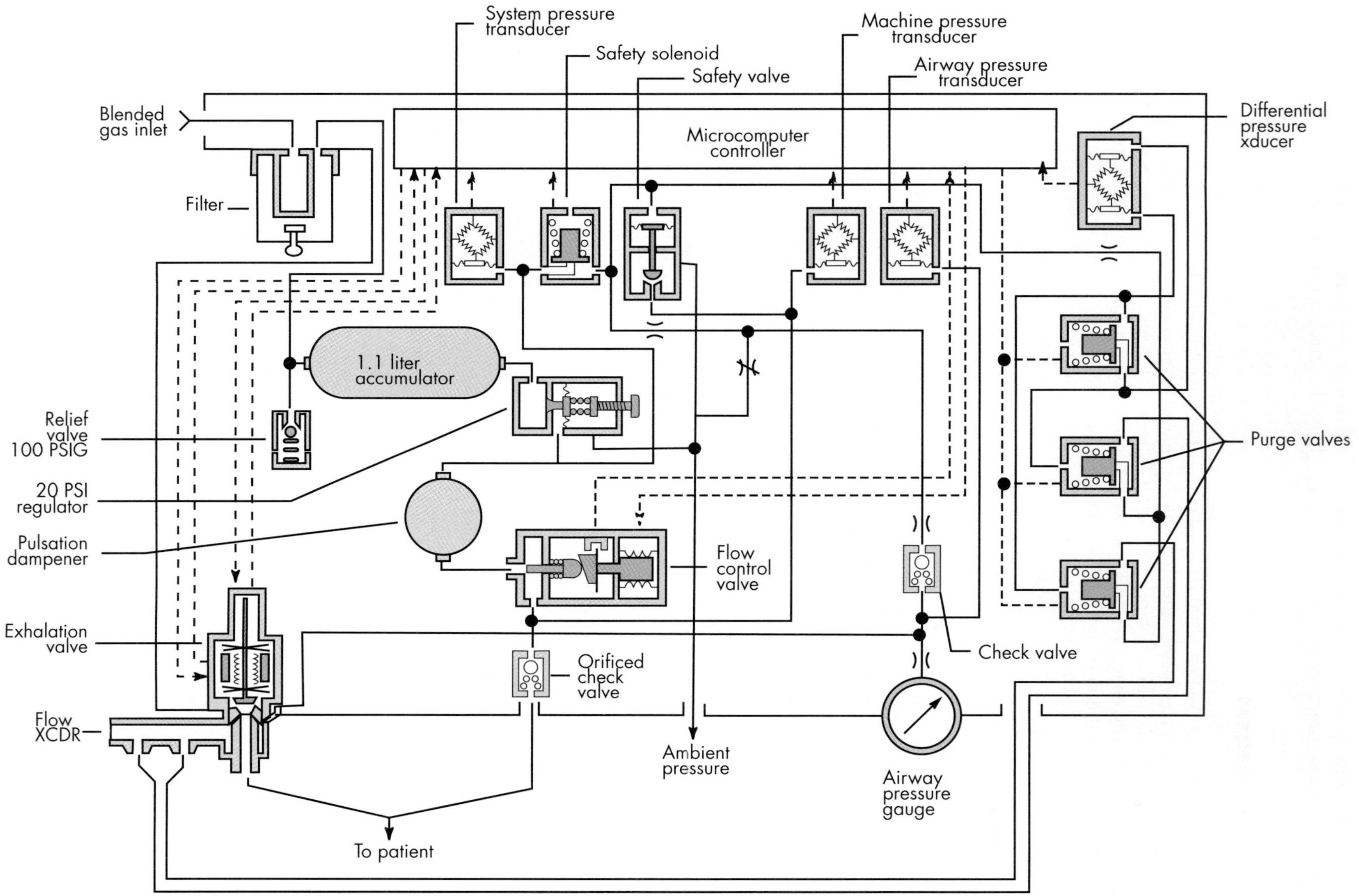

Figure 10-13 Pneumatic Diagram for the Bird 8400STi (see text for further discussion).

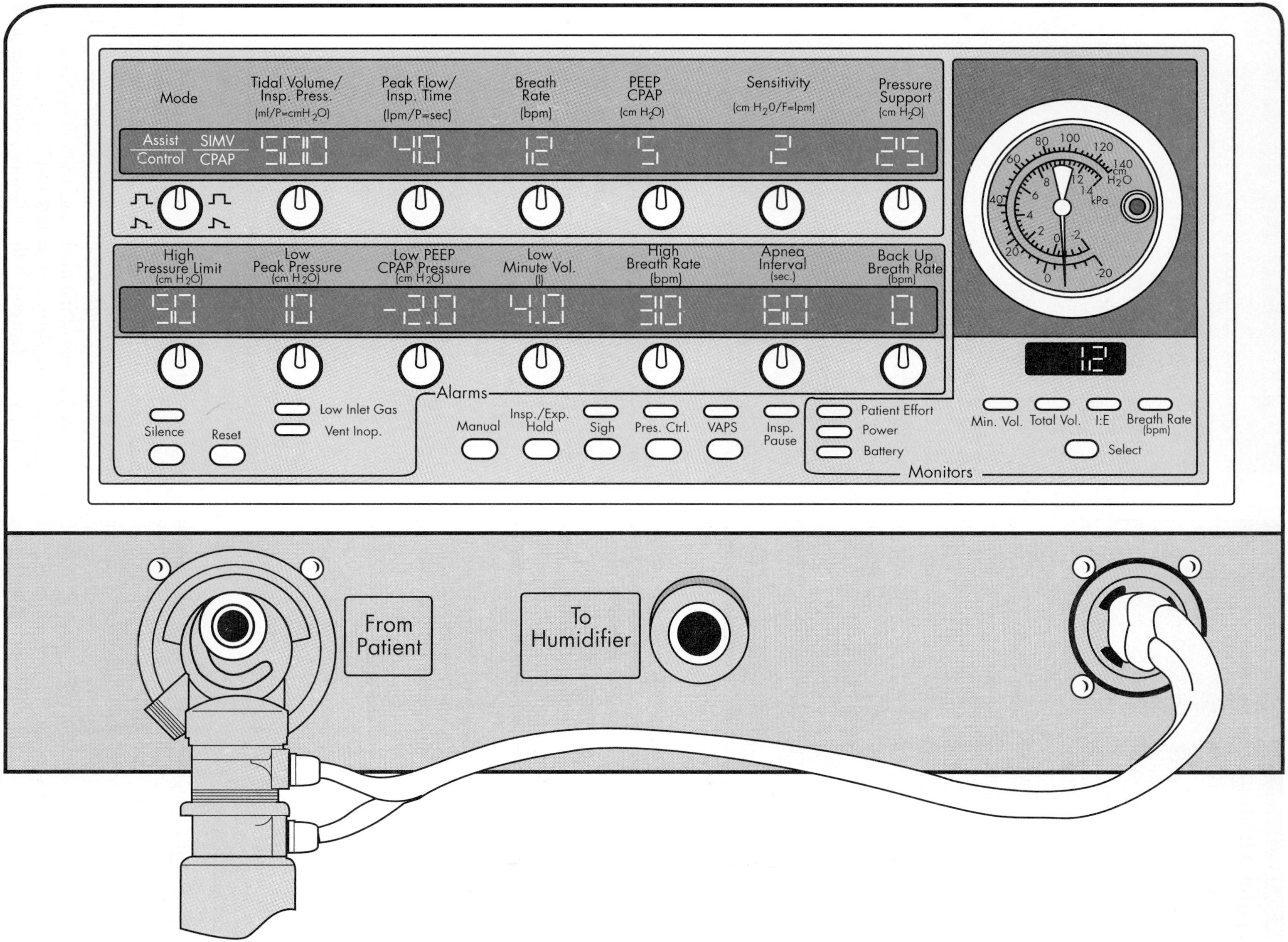

Figure 10-14 The control panel of the Bird 8400STi ventilator.

BOX 10-11

Decision Making & Problem Solving

A respiratory therapist suspects that a ventilated patient has air trapping. How can she determine the end-expiratory pressure on the Bird 8400 STi?

See Appendix A for the answer.

expiratory pressure (auto-PEEP). After this maneuver, the pad must be pressed twice to return the display to its normal reading. The maximum length for either inspiratory or expiratory hold is 6 seconds. (See Box 10-11 for an exercise in performing this function.)

Activation of the SIGH control provides a sigh breath every 100 breaths. The sigh breath is a mandatory breath equal to 150% of the set V_T (75 to 3000 mL). The upper pressure limit increases to 150% of the set value for this breath (maximum is 140 cm H_2O). The sigh function is available in all modes.

The PRES. CTRL. touch pad is used to set pressure control. The VAPS control is used to set **volume-assured pressure support (VAPS)** ventilation (see the discussion of modes of ventilation in this section).

At the end of the row of touch pads is an LED marked INSP. PAUSE. Inspiratory pause (0.1 to 3.0 seconds) can be selected for volume-targeted mandatory breaths in A/C or SIMV modes. To activate an inspiratory pause, the INSP./EXP HOLD key must be pressed three times until "IP 0.0" appears in the monitor window. Then the SELECT key must be pressed as many times as necessary to obtain the desired value for pause time. Each time the pad is pressed, pause time increases by 0.1 seconds. Once the desired value is obtained, the INSP./EXP HOLD touch pad must be pressed one more time. The INSP. PAUSE LED stays lit, and the display window returns to its original reading. To cancel inspiratory pause, the HOLD pad must be pressed four times until "IP X.X" appears in the display window. Pressing the RESET key returns the pause time to "IP 0.0." Pressing the INSP./EXP HOLD pad once more turns off the INSP. PAUSE LED.

Monitors and Alarms

To the right of the bottom row of controls is a section marked "Monitors." The first three monitors are LEDs for PATIENT EFFORT, POWER, and BATTERY. The PATIENT EFFORT LED is lit whenever the ventilator detects a patient inspiratory effort sufficient to trigger a breath (spontaneous or mandatory). The POWER LED lights when the unit is turned on and connected to an AC power source. The BATTERY LED is illuminated when an **external battery** is used. An external 12-volt (ranges from 11.8 to 16 volts) direct-current battery can be connected to the unit, but the back panel switch must be changed to the ALT PWR source setting for the battery to become the source of power.

On the bottom right section of the control panel, there is a touch pad marked SELECT. Pressing this pad allows several parameters (listed in Box 10-12) to be displayed in the monitor window below the pressure manometer. The last front panel monitor is the pressure manometer, which displays airway pressure (ranges from -20 to 140 cm H_2O).

Alarms on the Bird 8400STi are both audio and visual. The second row of the front panel controls contains most of the available alarm settings. Box 10-13 lists the adjustable alarms, which function in the following fashion. Reaching the high-pressure limit ends inspiration, so if the ventilator

BOX 10-12

Parameters Shown in the Display Window Using the Select Touch Pad on the Bird 8400STi

Minute Volume (liters/minute)

Calculated from the last eight breaths (average volume per minute) and the rate for spontaneous and mandatory breaths, as follows:

$$\dot{V}_E = \text{Total breath rate} \times \{[\text{Sum of last 8 } V_T \text{ (mL)}] \div 8\} \times (1\text{ L}/1000\text{ mL})$$

Tidal Volume (milliliters)

Breath-by-breath

I:E Ratio

Calculated for mandatory breaths only; updated breath-by-breath; range of 1:1.0 to 1:99, or 1:0 to 99:1

Breath Rate (breaths/minute)

Based on an average of the last eight breaths (spontaneous or mandatory), calculated as follows:

$$\text{Breath rate} = 8 \text{ breaths} \div \text{sum of the last 8 breath periods (minutes)}$$

BOX 10-13

Adjustable Alarm Controls for the Bird 8400 STi

High-pressure limit (1 to 140 cm H_2O)
Low peak pressure (2 to 140 cm H_2O, or off)
Low PEEP/CPAP pressure (-20 to +30 cm H_2O)
Low minute volume (0 to 99.9 L/min)
High breath rate (3 to 150 breaths/min)
Apnea interval (10 to 60 seconds)
Back-up breath rate (0 to 80 breaths/min)

BOX 10-14

Low PEEP/CPAP Alarm in the Bird 8400STi

The low PEEP/CPAP alarm can be valuable in detecting the return of the inspiratory effort in patients who have been apneic. This alarm can be set below baseline. For example, if the alarm is set at -2 cm H_2O on a patient who is being heavily sedated, the clinician can be alerted to a change in the level of ventilatory effort. When the patient's inspiratory effort is sufficient to drop baseline pressure to -2 cm H_2O for just half a second, the low PEEP/CPAP alarm sounds. The clinician can then identify the circumstances and take appropriate actions.

detects circuit pressures above the upper pressure limit for more than 0.3 seconds and/or above the baseline pressure + 3 cm H_2O for more than 3 seconds, an internal safety valve opens that reduces the pressure. Once pressure returns to baseline + 3 cm H_2O, the ventilator attempts another mandatory breath. If the problem isn't resolved, such as with a kinked expiratory line, the process repeats itself. Once the problem is resolved, the ventilator resumes normal operation.

The LOW PEAK PRESSURE alarm is activated if the airway pressure does not exceed the set value during inspiration. The LOW PEEP/CPAP alarm is activated if the airway pressure drops below the set value at any time during a complete respiratory cycle (inspiration plus expiration) for more than 0.5 seconds (Box 10-14). The LOW MINUTE VOLUME alarm is activated whenever the minute ventilation drops below the value set on the alarm. The volume is measured by the flow transducer connected to the exhalation valve body outlet. (This applies to all types of breaths.) The HIGH RATE ALARM is activated when the patient's total respiratory rate exceeds the set value on the alarm.

The apnea interval determines the amount of time that must pass before an apneic condition is detected, based on all breaths—spontaneous and mandatory. When apnea is present, the ventilator will switch to apnea back-up ventilation. The APNEA BACK-UP VENTILATION BREATH RATE is the final control knob in this row and can be set to zero or some value greater than the breath rate control. (Note that if the back-up ventilation breath rate is lower than the primary breath rate, the display value will be limited to the primary breath rate and will flash.) During back-up ventilation, the ventilator switches back to the A/C mode. The back-up breath rate becomes dominant, and the regular rate control is no longer functional. The settings for V_T (or inspiratory pressure), peak flow (or inspiratory time), PEEP/CPAP, and sensitivity remain active. Normal ventilation resumes if one of two conditions occur: two consecutive spontaneous breaths occur and at least 50% of the set

BOX 10-15

Decision Making & Problem Solving

A respiratory therapist is using a Bird 8400 STi to ventilate a patient. Suddenly a beep is heard, and the window above the apnea interval displays "AP" alternating with "20" seconds. The respiratory rate control is set at 6 breaths/min, and the mode was set on SIMV. However, the ventilator has switched to apnea back-up ventilation. The therapist presses the alarm reset button, but the ventilator remains in apnea back-up ventilation.

What mode will the ventilator switch to if apnea is detected? What will be the rate and V_T delivery? How can the ventilator be switched back to normal operation?

See Appendix A for the answers.

V_T is exhaled with each (but in the pressure ventilation mode, two consecutive spontaneous breaths will reset the unit), or the operator presses the RESET button and activates the control setting for breath rate (Box 10-15).

The next row contains several alarm indicators as well as several controls. The alarm indicators are on the left side of the panel. The first is the ALARM SILENCE control, which silences most audible alarms for 1 minute when touched. A loss of electrical power alarm, a ventilator inoperative alarm, a low inlet gas alarm, or a circuit alarm, however, cannot be silenced by a simple touch of this control (see Box 10-16 for information on the circuit alarm). During a loss of electrical power, the alarm can be silenced by pressing this button for 3 to 5 seconds.

The low inlet gas pressure (LOW INLET GAS) alarm can be caused by insufficient gas supply pressure, a clogged inlet filter, malfunction of the internal regulator, and/or malfunction of the system pressure transducer. It cannot be silenced.

The ventilator inoperative alarm (VENT INOP.) will activate with one of the following three conditions:

1. Loss of electrical power
2. Detection of an internal system problem
3. Prolonged detection (>1 sec) of excessively high (>24 psig) or low (<16 psig) pressure at the blended gas inlet in an older ventilator version

(Note that current unit production has changed this function because low inlet gas no longer produces a VENT INOP. condition.) If a VENT. INOP alarm situation occurs, a safety valve opens to provide the spontaneously breathing patient access to room air.

Although these alarm controls are easily seen on the control panel, there are two additional, nonprogrammable alarms (see Box 10-16). The cause of these alarms can be determined by viewing the monitor window on the right

BOX 10-16

Nonadjustable Alarms Shown in the Display Window of the Bird 8400STi

"CIRC": Possible Circuit or Pressure Transducer Fault

How measured: compares measurements of the airway pressure transducer with those of the machine pressure transducer (both located internally).

Activates during inspiration if machine pressure is 29 cm H_2O greater than or 9 cm H_2O less than the airway pressure for >100 msec.

Activates during expiration if machine pressure is 29 cm H_2O greater than or 9 cm H_2O less than the airway pressure for >1.0 sec.

Results in opening of the expiratory valve and ending inspiratory flow. PEEP/CPAP is maintained. If prolonged (>12 seconds), the safety and expiratory valves open to allow spontaneous breathing of room air.

Common causes:

- Blocking of the airway pressure sensing port
- Occlusion or kinking of either the main inspiratory or the main expiratory line
- Transducer failure

"MODE/WAVEFORM" Discrepancy Display

A square appears in the display window, the corners of which flash sequentially. This indicates that the mode selection switch is not properly positioned and the ventilator is in operation. The 8400STi stays in the previous mode and settings. If this situation occurs when the ventilator is first turned on, the ventilator provides SIMV with a descending-flow waveform.

side of the front panel, between the pressure manometer and the row of LEDs.

MODES OF OPERATION

The Bird 8400STi provides the usual modes of ventilation with volume- or pressure-targeting. In addition, it also has a servo-controlled, pressure-targeted mode that guarantees volume delivery, which is called volume-assured pressure support (VAPS).

Assist/Control

This mode is patient- (pressure or flow) or time-triggered. Each breath can be either volume- or pressure-targeted. When volume-targeted, inspiration ends when the unit determines that the volume has been delivered (volume-cycled, based on flow and time calculations). When pressure-targeted, it is time cycled out of inspiration based on the set T_I.

Because pressure-targeted breaths for either A/C or SIMV are set slightly differently than on most ventilators, the setting of pressure-controlled (targeted) breaths is reviewed here. After selecting the desired mode, the operator presses the PRESSURE-CONTROL touch pad, and the LED above the touch pad flashes. The current settings are still operational, and a "P" flashes in the V_T control window. The operator selects the desired pressure delivery in this location by using the TIDAL VOLUME/INSP. PRESS control knob, and a flashing "P" appears in the PEAK FLOW/INSP. TIME window. The operator selects the desired T_I with this control. When these controls have been set and all other controls are at their desired settings, the operator presses the PRESSURE-CONTROL touch pad again to activate pressure-targeted mandatory breaths in the selected mode. The "P" stays continuously lit in the INSP. PRESS. and INSP. TIME display windows, and the PRES. CTRL. LED is also continuously illuminated.

When switching from pressure-controlled breaths back to volume ventilation, the inspiratory pressure must first be reduced to 5 cm H_2O to ensure that the V_T is not set too high and can be readjusted upward. Pressing the PRESSURE-CONTROL pad turns off pressure ventilation (so the LED is no longer lit).

SIMV

The function of the SIMV mode of ventilation on the Bird 8400STi is similar to the SIMV mode on most ventilators. Mandatory breaths are patient- or time-triggered, but when they are volume-targeted, inspiration ends when the unit determines that the volume has been delivered. When mandatory breaths are pressure-targeted, they are time-cycled out of inspiration. Spontaneous breaths can occur at baseline pressure or with pressure support.

Spontaneous Mode

To provide spontaneous ventilation, the BREATH RATE control is set at zero, and the patient breathes spontaneously from the desired baseline pressure, allowing for CPAP. Spontaneous breaths can also be pressure-supported. For example, the clinician may select 5 cm H_2O of CPAP and PSV of 10 cm H_2O. The baseline pressure will be 5 cm H_2O, and the inspiratory pressure will reach 15 cm H_2O during a pressure-supported spontaneous breath.

Volume Assured Pressure Support (VAPS)

Volume-assured pressure support (VAPS) is a pressure-targeted mode of ventilation that guarantees volume delivery in each breath. It is a servo-control (closed-loop) mode (see Chapter 9). VAPS is similar in its function to the PAug

BOX 10-17

Control Settings During VAPS

Mode: A/C, SIMV, or SIMV + PS
Flow Waveform: constant (rectangular)
Pressure Support: at a pressure sufficient to provide the patient's current V_T; estimate using plateau pressure
Tidal Volume: set a minimum value
Flow: should be set high and readjusted after starting
Breath Rate: set a minimum guaranteed value
Back-up Breath Rate: below set rate
PEEP: appropriate for the patient
Trigger Sensitivity below PEEP: appropriate for the patient
Alarm Limits: appropriate for the patient

For example, the mode selected is SIMV with a constant flow waveform and a flow of 60 L/min. The breath rate is set at 10 breaths/min. The back-up rate is set at 8 breaths/min. V_T is 0.5 L. Pressure support is 20 cm H_2O, which is 2 cm H_2O above the patient's plateau pressure during volume ventilation at the same volume. PEEP is 3 cm H_2O, and trigger sensitivity is set so that a breath patient triggers at 2 cm H_2O (-1 cm H_2O below baseline).

mode discussed previously with the Bear 1000. Box 10-17 lists the control settings used in this mode.

VAPS is intended for use with spontaneously breathing patients. It functions as follows: when a patient triggers a breath, the ventilator pressure targets the breath and delivers the set PS level. Flow is rapid at the beginning of inspiration and gradually tapers down in a descending ramp pattern. As flow is delivered, the microprocessor monitors flow and volume delivery, and two common patterns emerge. If the volume delivered is greater than or equal to the set minimum V_T, the ventilator ends the breath by flow cycling at the set flow value. If volume delivered is less than the set volume, and the flow drops to the set flow value, the set flow is maintained until the volume is delivered. Figure 10-15 shows examples of different types of respiratory patterns that can occur during this mode of ventilation.

GRAPHIC DISPLAY SCREENS

Figure 10-16 provides an overview of the basic controls on the Bird graphics monitor. The menu along the bottom provides a variety of functions. Waveforms of pressure, flow,

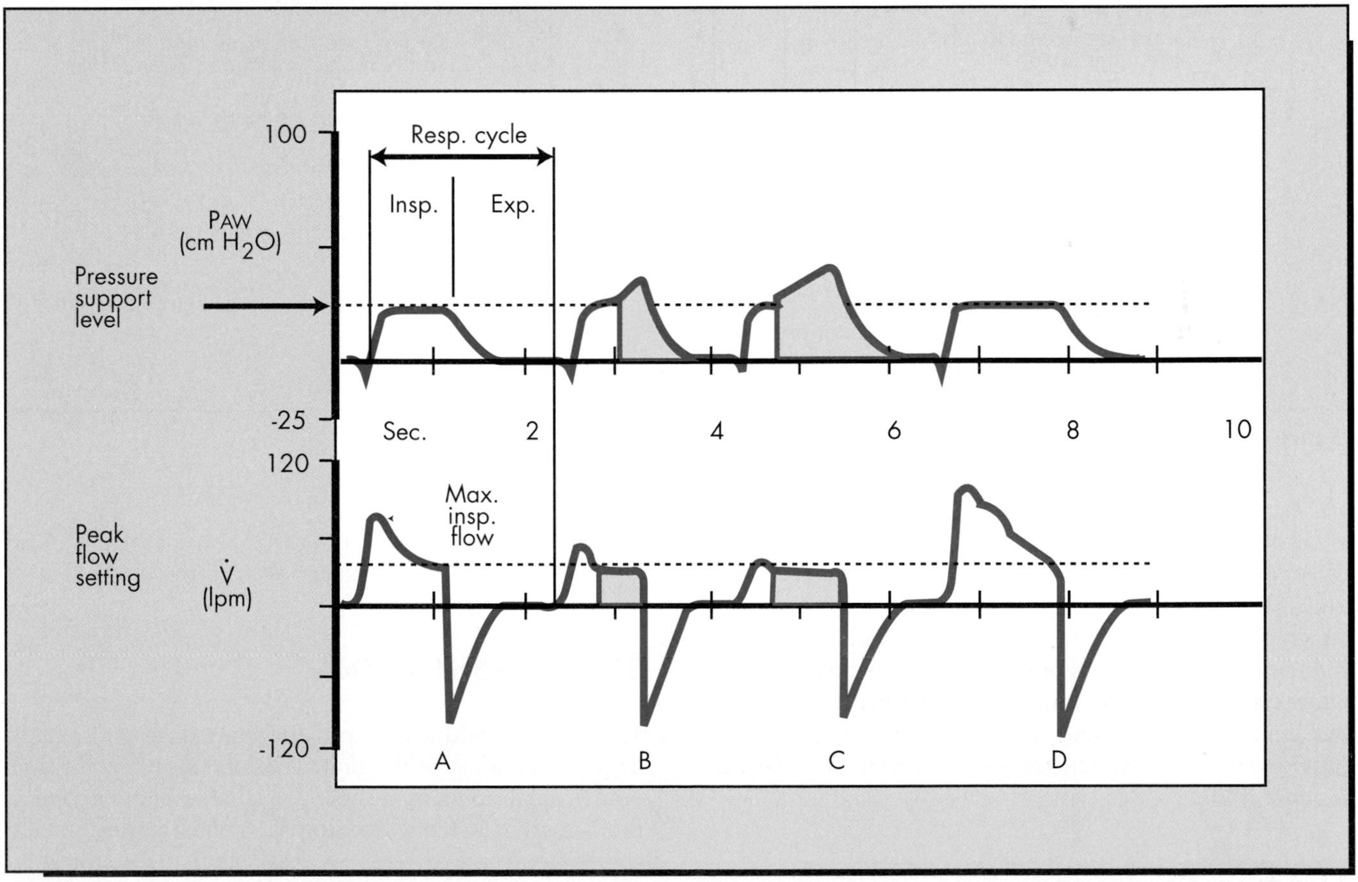

Figure 10-15 Examples of potential VAPS breath patterns: **A,** a pressure-generated breath with flow cycling at the set flow value. The V_T was $\geq$ set V_T. **B,** an example where flow has dropped to the set value, but V_T has not been delivered, so flow is sustained until V_T is delivered. Note the rise in pressure as flow is continued. **C,** a breath where the set pressure is inadequate for the patient's lung conditions and inspiration is prolonged. **D,** an example of a breath in a patient with a high inspiratory flow demand. The ventilator responds by delivering an increased flow and V_T (not shown). (Courtesy Bird Corp., Palm Springs, Calif.)

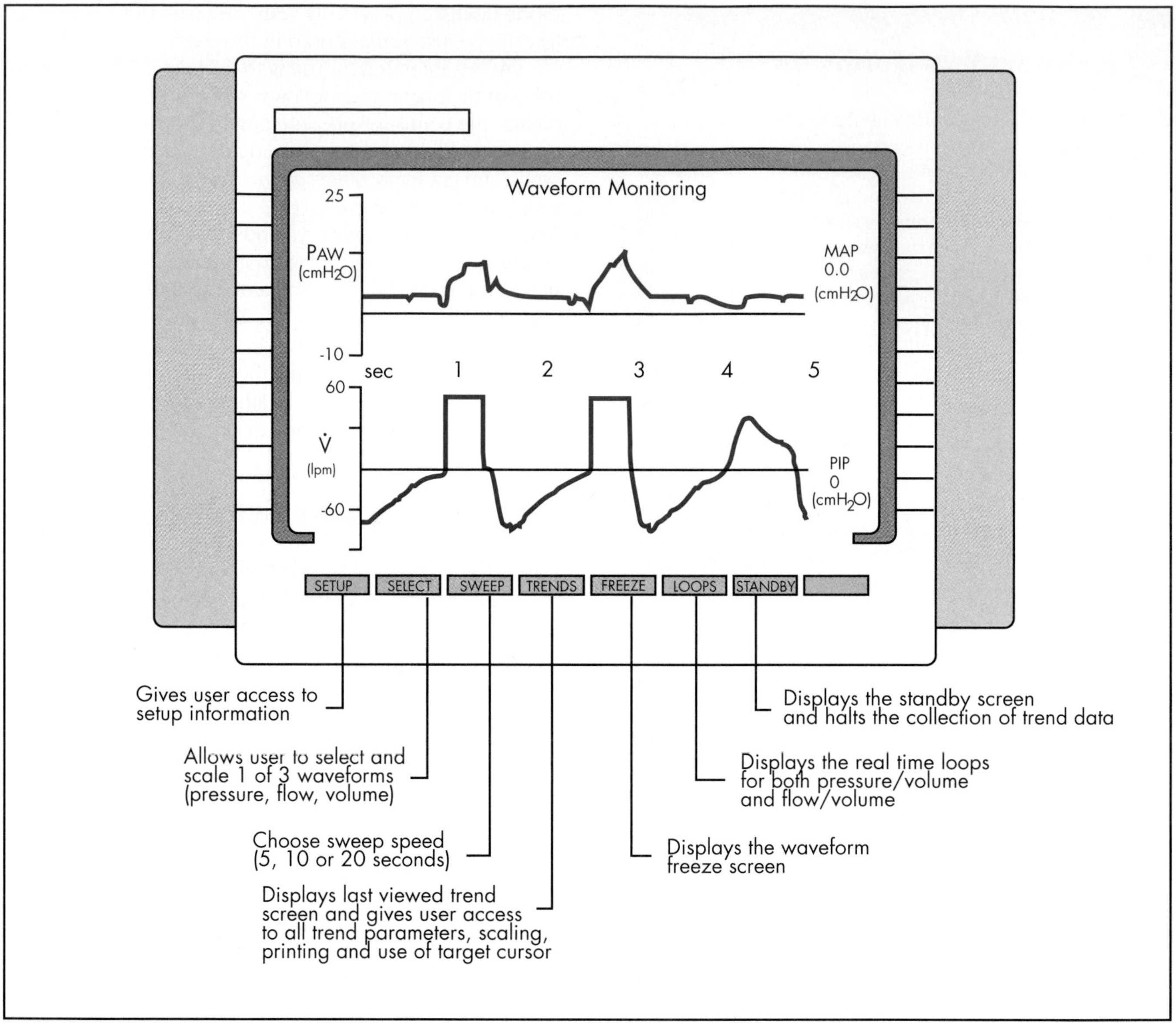

Figure 10-16 The Bird 8400STi waveform graphics monitor. (Courtesy Bird Corp., Palm Springs, Calif.)

and volume vs. time are available, in addition to a variety of loops including flow/volume and pressure/volume loops. The graphics package can also freeze screens, overlap graphs and loops, and indicate trending. Information on the screen can be printed out when a compatible printer is attached to the unit. Complete instructions for operating the graphics package and troubleshooting guidelines are provided by the manufacturer's Instruction and Service Manual (PIN L 1282).

Special Features

Perhaps the most significant features of the Bird 8400 are its new mode of ventilation (VAPS) and its graphic monitor. An air compressor (Bird 6500) is also available and can be used to provide pneumatic power to the unit.

Troubleshooting

The monitors and alarms provide immediate information about functioning of the unit. The manufacturer's instruction manual contains a table for troubleshooting clinical problems that includes symptoms, potential causes, and the corrective action to take. As with other microprocessor-controlled medical equipment, it should be kept away from RFI and EFI equipment. In addition, Chapter 9 of this text reviews common problems encountered during mechanical ventilation.

Review Questions

(See Appendix A for answers.)

1. The Bird 8400STi uses which of the following flow control valves?
   a. variable-orifice solenoid
   b. low resistance piston
   c. electromechanical stepper valve
   d. Venturi injector
2. The PRES. CTRL key is used to set the:
   a. high-pressure limit
   b. pressure-support level
   c. pressure-control mode
   d. low-pressure alarm
3. Pressure reaches 30 cm H_2O, ending inspiration and causing an audio and visual alarm. This alarm is most likely the:
   a. HIGH-PRESSURE LIMIT alarm
   b. LOW PEAK PRESSURE alarm
   c. HIGH PEEP/CPAP alarm
   d. VENT. INOP. alarm
4. A respiratory therapist is switching a patient from pressure-control ventilation to volume ventilation (A/C mode). Inspiratory pressure is set at 10 cm H_2O and PEEP is at 5 cm H_2O for a total PIP of 15 cm H_2O. Whenever the therapist presses the pressure-control pad to switch to volume ventilation, the unit will not do so. The most likely problem is:
   a. the mode must be SIMV
   b. the pressure-control setting must be reduced to 5 cm H_2O
   c. the ventilator cannot perform volume ventilation
   d. an alarm is active
5. "F 2" is shown in the sensitivity control display window. This indicates that the sensitivity is:
   a. set for flow trigger at 2 L/min below base flow
   b. set for pressure trigger at -2 cm H_2O, but is in fault (F)
   c. favorable (F) for the patient based on patient size
   d. set outside of available range
6. In which of the following conditions will the ventilator give a VENT INOP. alarm?
   I. loss of electrical power
   II. detection of an internal system problem
   III. improper installation of the expiratory valve
   IV. prolonged occurrence (>1 sec) of excessive high pressure (>24 psi)
   a. I only
   b. II and IV only
   c. I and III only
   d. I, II, and IV only
7. Following an interval of back-up ventilation, the 8400STi will resume normal ventilation when which of the following events occurs?
   I. two consecutive spontaneous breaths occur with a $V_T \geq$ the set V_T for each breath during volume ventilation
   II. two consecutive spontaneous breaths occur during pressure-targeted ventilation
   III. the operator presses the reset button and activates the control setting for breath rate
   IV. the ALARM SILENCE button is pressed
   a. IV only
   b. I and II only
   c. II and IV only
   d. I, II, and III only
8. On the Bird 8400STi, the control knob for V_T is also the control knob to set inspiratory pressure for pressure-targeted breaths—true or false?
9. All Bird 8400STi units can provide pressure-control ventilation—true or false?
10. The unit is operating in the VAPS mode and the pressure/time curve on the graphics display shows a slight dip in the curve just before inspiration begins, then a rapid rise in pressure during inspiration where it reaches and sustains a plateau. The pressure drops rapidly to baseline during exhalation. How would you describe the patient's breathing pattern? Is the breath volume- or flow-cycled.

References

1. Bird 8400STi Ventilator operation manual and options L1297, Palm Springs, Calif., 1994, Bird Products Corp.
2. Bird 8400STi Volume ventilator instruction manual L1141R2, Palm Springs, Calif., 1994, Bird Products Corp.
3. Bird graphics monitor instruction and service manual L1282, Palm Springs, Calif., 1995, Bird Products Corp.
4. Pilbeam S: Mechanical ventilation: physiological and clinical applications, ed 3, St Louis, 1998, Mosby.

Bird T-Bird

OUTLINE

LEARNING OBJECTIVES

Upon completion of this section, the reader should be able to:

1. Describe the power source, patient circuit, and internal mechanism of the T-Bird.
2. Explain how the control parameters and adjustable alarms are set.
3. Assess an alarm situation and name possible causes and solutions.
4. Compare VAPS on the T-Bird with PAug on the Bear 1000.
5. Recommend an information source for reviewing user verification tests.
6. Explain the operation of the special functions.

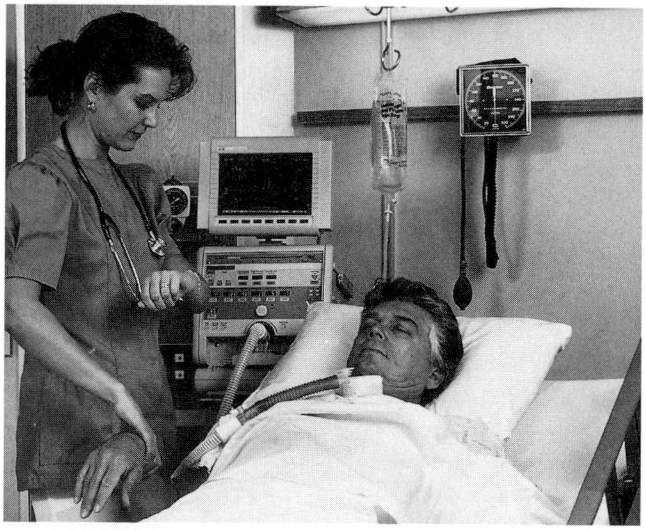

Figure 10-17 The Bird T-Bird AVS. (Courtesy Bird Products Corp., Palm Springs, Calif.)

The T-Bird AVS is manufactured by Bird Products Corp., which is a division of Thermo Electron Corp. (Figure 10-17). The AVS comes in three configurations, depending on what options have been added. The AVS III comes with PCV and VAPS modes and also has the following options added: expiratory hold, inspiratory time, and MIP/NIF measurements. The AVS I does not have these options. Of these features, the AVS II has expiratory hold and MIP/NIF measurements.

Power Source

Similar to many of the newer generation ventilators, the T-Bird is also a microprocessor-controlled unit. It requires an electrical source to power the microprocessor and the electrical components of the internal circuits. Unlike some of the newer units, however, the T-Bird, does not require a high-pressure gas source to function because it possesses an electrically powered internal **turbine.** Silencers help to suppress the noise generated by turbine intake. Oxygen can be provided to the patient by using either or both of the two available high pressure oxygen connectors (range from 40 to 65 psig). Using two oxygen sources rather than one allows the T-Bird to transfer sources without interruption.

The ON/STANDBY power switch, as well as the high-pressure oxygen connectors and the air inlet filter, is on the back panel of the ventilator. There is an **internal battery** (48 volts, **direct current [DC]**) that can provide a backup power source. In addition, there is an external battery, which is manually loaded on the lower right side of the unit and provides another power source.

The patient circuit has an expiratory valve mounted inside the front of the unit and the standard main inspiratory and expiratory lines that connect to the patient wye adapter.

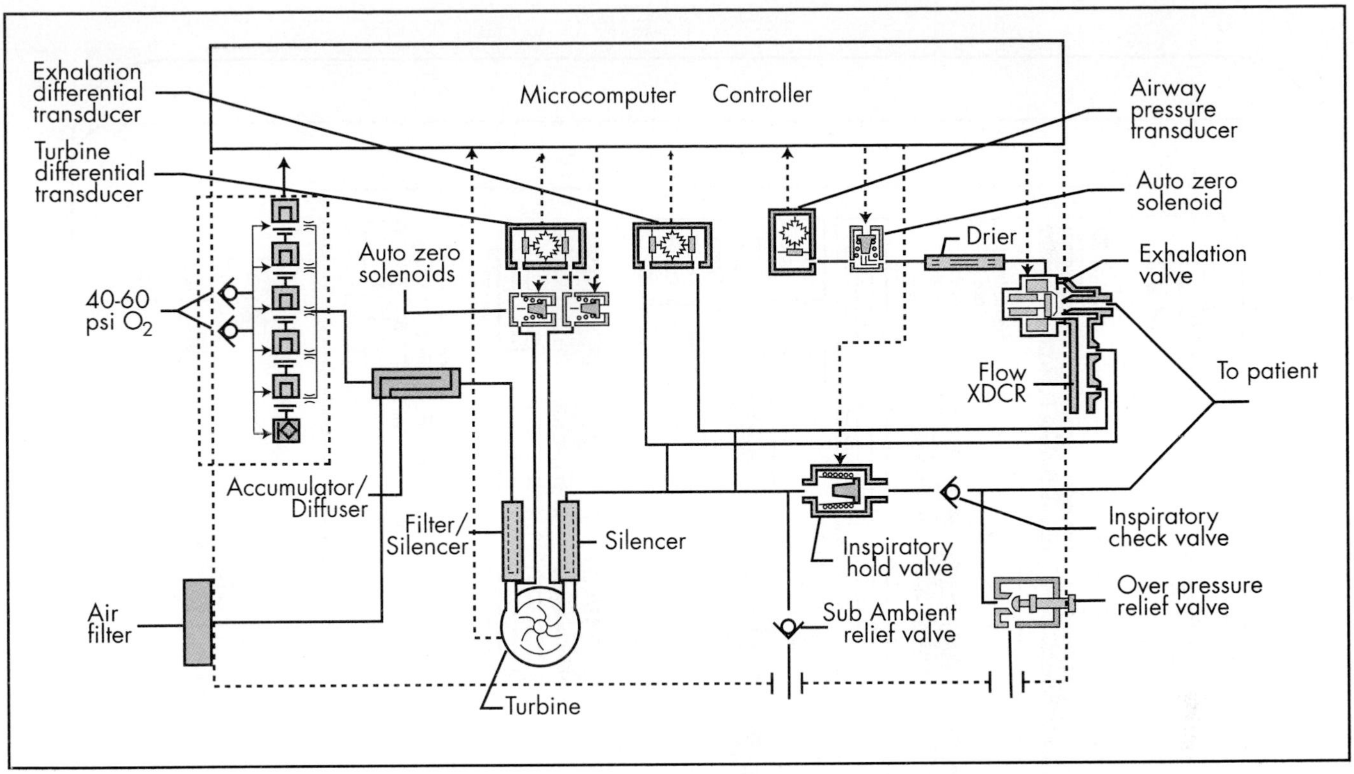

Figure 10-18 The internal circuit of the T-Bird AVS. (Courtesy Bird Products Corp., Palm Springs, Calif.)

INTERNAL MECHANISM

Ambient air enters the unit through the air filter, and oxygen enters through one or both of the oxygen connections. The T-Bird is equipped with an internal blender that uses a series of electronically operated, microprocessor-controlled solenoids (Figure 10-18). The microprocessor evaluates the oxygen setting on the control panel and selects and mixes the appropriate blend of gases from the air inlet and the solenoids receiving oxygen to provide the desired FiO_2 for the patient. Blended gases are sent to the accumulator/**diffuser** for initial mixing. The accumulator/diffuser also helps silence the noise caused by the built-in turbine (see Figure 10-18).

The gas is then directed to the turbine inlet (filter/ silencer). The microprocessor monitors the speed and output pressure from the turbine and uses this information to establish breath delivery to the patient. The flow-control device in this unit is called a **drag turbine.** Inlet and outlet pressures for the turbine are monitored by the turbine differential-pressure transducer. The microprocessor uses information about the pressure difference and the turbine speed (from the **optical encoder**) to control the precise flow delivered to the patient from the turbine. Volume delivery is the integration of flow for each unit of time (volume = flow × T_I).

An internal **subambient relief valve,** or **antisuffocation valve,** opens if the ventilator cannot provide an assisted breath to the patient. The patient can then inhale to open the valve and receive room air. This would occur, for example, during a ventilator inoperative condition (see the discussion of alarms in this section).

There are also internal transducers to measure expiratory and airway pressures. The expiratory flow transducer is a differential-pressure transducer (see Chapter 7).

CONTROLS AND ALARMS

The front panel of the T-Bird AVS provides a wide variety of controls, monitors, and alarms (Figure 10-19), some of which are touch pads that allow actions such as mode selection, mandatory breath delivery, or variable adjustment to be made.

When a touch pad is active, the LED on its surface is lit. Above the touch pads controlling different variables (e.g., pressure and volume) are display windows that provide digital values of the set parameters. These windows may be bright or dim. A control is dim when it is not available in the currently active mode. For example, V_T is not available during pressure-controlled ventilation, so the V_T digital value is dim. Fortunately, the previous setting remains visible so that if the mode is changed, that setting is still available. In addition, a dimmed control can be adjusted so that it is at the desired setting before a ventilator mode is changed.

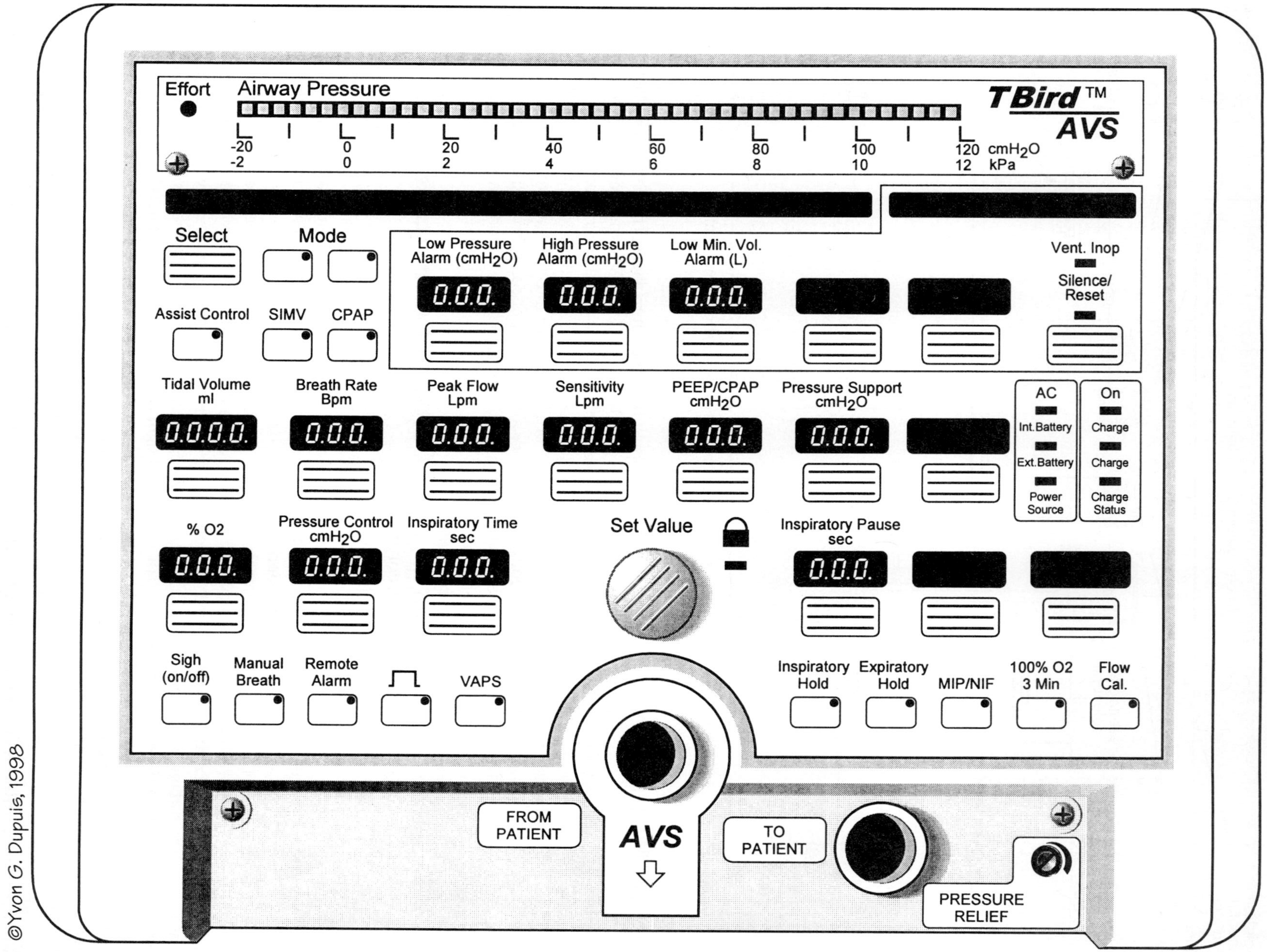

Figure 10-19 The front Panel of the T-Bird AVS. (Courtesy Yvon Dupuis)

BOX 10-18

Flashing Controls on the T-Bird

Flashing Occurs

When the following settings are used:

- $T_E < 250$ msec
- $T_I < 300$ msec
- High pressure alarm setting < 5 cm H_2O above set PEEP
- I:E > 4:1 (e.g., 5:1)
- Peak flow setting < bias flow setting
- Bias flow setting > peak flow

When a required control has not been set for the mode selected; for example, a low peak pressure alarm that has been turned off will flash until it is set.

When an alarm is active.

When the mode pad has been pressed once. It flashes for 15 seconds or until the mode is activated by pressing the pad a second time.

Sometimes the window for a control will be flashing to show that a parameter has been set incorrectly. Box 10-18 provides the usual reasons for these to be flashing.

In the center, there is a control knob for adjusting all control and alarm levels. This knob has three basic functions:

1. To set variable controls (V_T, breath rate, pressure, etc.)
2. To select special functions
3. To activate tests during **user verification testing (UVT)**

To set a parameter (control variable), the operator presses the touch pad for the parameter and turns the control knob to change the numerical value of the parameter.

To select special functions, the control knob is pressed and held down until "VENT SETUP" appears in the monitor window (i.e., the window below the pressure manometer). The control knob is then released (see the discussion of special functions later in this section).

The UVT permits the operator to review several ventilator functions, such as a lamp test, a filter test, a leak test, etc. The operator's manual for the T-Bird covers this information, so it is not included here. These tests may be run during the set-up and check-out procedure before patient use.

A lock control allows the operator to lock the front panel and prevent accidental or unauthorized adjustments. Pressing the control knob locks it, preventing adjustable parameters from being changed. A green LED next to a lock icon lights when the control knob is locked. Pressing the knob again unlocks it. The only controls that do not lock are MONITOR SELECT, MANUAL BREATH, and ALARM SILENCE/RESET.

There are also digital display windows above the alarm control touch pads that show their settings. Across the top of the front panel is a horizontally mounted pressure monitor. The main outlet to the patient is at the lower right corner of the front panel.

BOX 10-19

Setting the Over Pressure-Relief Valve

1. Attach the patient circuit to a test lung.
2. Set the high-pressure limit to the maximum (120 cm H_2O).
3. Set high V_T and peak flow in order to achieve ≥100 cm H_2O (monitored display value).
4. During breath delivery, monitor PIP.
5. Adjust the pressure-relief valve until the desired maximum pressure is seen on the manometer.
6. Remember the high-pressure limit must be reset appropriately for the patient and the over pressure-relief valve must be 5 to 15 cm H_2O above this.

Connections for the main inspiratory and expiratory flow lines are below the operating controls of the front panel. In the lowest right corner is an adjustable control for the **over pressure-relief valve,** with which the maximum pressure allowed by the system can be set. Reaching this pressure does not end inspiration, but vents excess pressure to the room. It is set from 5 to 15 cm H_2O above the high-pressure limit. Box 10-19 describes this procedure.

Controls

Looking at the front of the control panel, the upper left area is where the mode control touch pads are located (see Figure 10-19).

The first touch pad in this section is the MONITOR SELECT control, which is used to do three things:

1. Select monitored parameters
2. Select special functions
3. Run UVTs

It is also used to clear some alarms.

Table 10-1 lists the monitored parameters visible in the top display window during normal operation. Their appearance is controlled by the SPECIAL FUNCTIONS control (explained in the later discussion of special functions) or by the MONITOR SELECT button. The parameters are displayed in sets of two or three and are automatically scanned (autoscanning) when either of these functions are turned on (i.e., enabled). Using the monitor select control, the display can hold at a particular set of parameters or can be manually advanced through parameters.

To access SPECIAL FUNCTIONS, press and hold the main control knob for about 2 seconds until "VENT SETUP" appears in the monitor window. Then release the

TABLE 10-1

T-Bird monitored parameters

Parameter	Range
Total breath rate (f)	0 to 250 breaths/min
I:E ratio	99:1 to 1:99
$\dot{V}_E$	0 to 99.9 L/min
PIP	0 to 140 cm H_2O
Mean airway pressure (MAP)	0 to 99 cm H_2O
T_I	0.01 to 99.99 sec
PEEP	0 to 99 cm H_2O
Exhaled V_T (Vte)	0 to 4000 mL

TABLE 10-2

Special functions and parameters

Special function	Parameter available
Vent set-up	Autoscan on/off
	Bias flow setting
	Enables/disables control lock function
	Bird graphic monitor (BGM) on/off
	Select display language
	Display software version
	Total hours of operation
	Display turbine serial no.
	Altitude compensation
Alarm set-up	Apnea interval
	Remote alarm status
Transducer data	Readings from various transducers*
Transducer test group	Autozero flow transducer
	Autozero expiratory flow transducer
	Autozero turbine pressure transducer
Events code group	Displays previous 256 event codes*

*See operator's manual for codes.

control knob. Turning the control knob now allows display of the special functions that can be selected (Table 10-2; see the later section on special functions).

The UVT can be accessed in the same way in which special functions are accessed. The UVT and the **service verification test (SVT)** appear after event codes, but cannot be accessed while the ventilator is in operation. The UVT and SVT are described in the operator's manual, so they are not covered here.

The next controls in this row are the mode touch pads, which are activated by pressing them. Modes include A/C, SIMV, and CPAP. When the selected mode is pressed twice, the LED on the corner of the pad is illuminated, and the mode becomes active. Set-up and operation of the modes will be covered in the discussion of modes of ventilation later in this section.

BOX 10-20

Back-up Ventilation

When setting the controls for any mode of ventilation on the T-Bird, it is wise to set all settings. For example, even if you plan to use a pressure-targeting form of ventilation such as pressure control, you still need to set the V_T, f, peak flow, flow pattern, FIO_2, and pressure limit. This way, if the apneic back-up mode of ventilation becomes active, its parameters will be appropriately set.

Alarm settings are to the right of the mode touch pads (see the discussion of alarms in this section).

The row of controls in the central part of the panel are as follows: TIDAL VOLUME, BREATH RATE, PEAK FLOW, SENSITIVITY, PEEP/CPAP, and PRESSURE SUPPORT. There is a blank control at the end of this row to be used in future upgrades.

Tidal Volume

The V_T control (ranges from 50 to 2000 mL) sets the V_T for volume ventilation and sets the volume goal for VAPS. The V_T is delivered in the selected flow waveform with the maximum flow as the peak flow setting. Even when a pressure-targeted mode or CPAP is selected, this control must be set at the appropriate level for back-up ventilation in case the patient becomes apneic. The value is dimmed in pressure ventilation (Box 10-20).

Breath Rate

The BREATH RATE control (2 to 80 breaths/min) sets the number of mandatory breaths. It is available in A/C, SIMV, and apnea back-up modes and should always be set in case the patient becomes apneic.

Peak Flow

The PEAK FLOW control (10 to 140 L/min) sets the maximum inspiratory flow during volume ventilation and interacts with the FLOW WAVEFORM control. When a constant waveform is selected, the peak flow is sustained during inspiration. When a descending ramp is selected, the set peak flow occurs at the beginning of inspiration, and flow gradually tapers toward the end of inspiration.

With VAPS, the PEAK FLOW control sets the minimum flow generated, determines expiratory criteria, and establishes minimum flow for a guaranteed volume delivery (see the discussion of VAPS under the section on modes of ventilation).

Sensitivity

The SENSITIVITY control (1 to 8 L/min, or off) sets the threshold flow. When the base flow drops to this amount in any mode, a breath is triggered (Figure 10-20). When

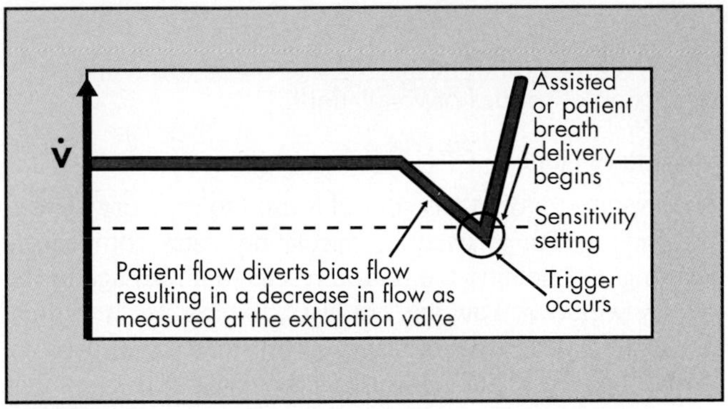

Figure 10-20 A graph showing the function of the flow trigger (sensitivity control). (Courtesy Bird Products Corp., Palm Springs, Calif.)

sensitivity is off, the unit can not be triggered by the patient, so it is recommended that the sensitivity never be turned off. (Note that the T-Bird does not use pressure triggering.)

PEEP/CPAP

The PEEP/CPAP control (0 to 30 cm H_2O) sets the baseline pressure and maintains the airway pressure between breaths in all modes of ventilation. The HIGH PRESSURE ALARM setting must be set at least 5 cm H_2O above the PEEP/CPAP setting.

Pressure Support

The PRESSURE SUPPORT control (1 to 60 cm H_2O, or off) sets the pressure level above PEEP for all pressure-support breaths. It is functional for spontaneous breaths in SIMV and CPAP modes.

Blank Control

Blank control is the last touch pad in this row and is for future upgrades.

Power Indicators

The section to the right of the row of controls described above contains battery and power source indicators.

The AC POWER SOURCE indicator activates when the unit is connected to a wall outlet (AC power). While the unit is connected, the optional external and internal battery are being charged. If power fails, the unit switches to the external battery source, if present. If no external battery is connected, it switches to the internal battery. An alarm occurs when the power source changes from AC to DC. To the right of this indicator is the ON indicator, which shows that the unit is turned on.

The internal battery has two light indicators, one to indicate battery use (INT. BAT.) and one to indicate battery charge status (CHARGE). Both lights change colors.

The INT. BAT. light comes on when it is in use. It is green when fully charged (about 7 to 24 minutes remain), yellow at medium charge (about 5 to 14 minutes remain), and red at low power (about 4 to 10 minutes remain). OFF indicates the unit is using either an AC wall outlet or the external battery for power. When the color changes (from green to yellow or yellow to red), an audible alarm is activated to alert the operator. The length of battery use depends on the amount of power being used by the unit.

The internal battery charge status indicators are as follows:

- green = 90% to 100% charged
- yellow = battery is being charged
- red = low battery, needs to be charged*

When the external battery indicator is lit (EXT. BAT.), the unit is operating on external battery power. The available time from a fully charged battery depends on the power demand of the unit, but ranges from about 1.0 to 3.5 hours. Colors provide the following information about battery status:

- green = sufficient power
- yellow = charge is getting low (about 20 min to 1.5 hours remain)
- off = not in use

When the battery is fully discharged, the ventilator switches to the internal battery and the EXT. BAT. alarm is activated.

The color of the external battery charge indicator (CHARGE) shows that the external battery is being charged and changes depending on the amount of charge present:

- green = 90% to 100% charged
- yellow = being charged (charge time about 7 to 11 hours)
- red = low battery, needs to be charged
- off = battery is not present or properly connected

Immediately below this row of controls are the following: % O_2, PRESSURE CONTROL, INSPIRATORY TIME, the control knob, INSPIRATORY PAUSE, and two blank parameter positions for use in future upgrades.

% O_2

The % O_2 control sets the delivered oxygen percentage from 21% to 100%.

Pressure Control

The PRESSURE CONTROL position (AVS III only; ranges from 1 to 100 cm H_2O, or off) sets inspiratory pressure above baseline for pressure-targeted breaths in A/C, SIMV, and VAPS.

Inspiratory Time

The INSPIRATORY TIME control (AVS III only; T_I in seconds, ranges from 0.3 to 10.0 seconds) sets the inspiratory time for pressure-control breaths. When selected, the new time begins with the next pressure-targeted mandatory breath.

*Charge time is about 6 to 7 hours.

Control Knob

The control knob is used to set each parameter as it is selected by the operator.

Indicator

The indicator shows whether or not the control knob has been locked or unlocked.

Inspiratory Pause

The INSPIRATORY PAUSE control (0.1 to 2.0 seconds, or off) sets an inspiratory pause time for volume-targeted breaths in A/C and SIMV. Inspiratory pause occurs on the next and on all subsequent volume breaths.

The bottom row of controls consists of a series of touch pads as follows (left-to-right): SIGH, MANUAL BREATH, REMOTE ALARM, FLOW WAVEFORM CONTROL, VAPS (AVS III), INSPIRATORY HOLD, EXPIRATORY HOLD (AVS II OR III), MIP/NIF (AVS II OR III), 100% O_2 3 min, and FLOW CAL.

Sigh

When the SIGH control (on/off) is activated, the ventilator delivers a sigh breath at the next mandatory breath and then at every 100th breath or 7th minute—whichever comes first. The sigh volume is 150% of the set V_T. Inspiratory time increases by 50% (to a maximum of 5.5 sec); and PIP increases by 50% (to a maximum of 120 cm H_2O). (Note that the over pressure-relief valve setting must be adjusted when sigh is selected.)

Manual Breath

Pressing the MANUAL BREATH touch pad delivers a mandatory breath based on set parameters. For example, during volume ventilation, the set V_T and the peak flow are delivered using the set flow waveform. During pressure ventilation, the set pressure and T_I are active. The manual breath touch pad can only be activated after inspiration and the minimum T_E (250 msec) have occurred.

Remote Alarm

The REMOTE ALARM control turns the optical remote alarm transmitter on and off. The transmitter is a special feature that must be added to the unit (see the operating manual). When purchased, this feature provides a remote receiver that can be placed at an appropriate location and activated in case an alarm is triggered.

Square Waveform

The SQUARE WAVEFORM (on/off) button is located adjacent to the REMOTE ALARM control and provides a constant (rectangular) or descending (decelerating) ramp flow waveform during volume ventilation. The LED lights when the square waveform is active. Pressing the button changes the waveform.

VAPS

The VAPS control turns the VAPS mode on and off (see the discussion of modes of ventilation).

Inspiratory Hold

The INSPIRATORY HOLD control is used to measure plateau pressure, which is used in calculating static compliance. Pressing and holding the button results in a message in the display window: "Paw xxx cm H_2O," where *xxx* is the real time value of airway pressure. At the end of inspiration, "Pplat xxx cm H_2O" appears, where *xxx* is the measured plateau pressure. The value is continually updated as it is displayed. Inspiratory pause ends when the button is released or 6 seconds has elapsed—whichever occurs first. After the maneuver, the window reads "Palvd xxx cm H_2O Cst xxx ml/cmH_2O," where *Palvd xxx* is the alveolar distending pressure, and *Cst xxx* is the static compliance. This maneuver fails if the INSPIRATORY HOLD button is released too soon or a stable plateau cannot be obtained, which can occur if the patient is actively breathing against the closed valves.

Expiratory Hold

The EXPIRATORY HOLD control (AVS II and AVS III) is used to measure auto-PEEP during A/C and SIMV ventilation. When the button is pressed, the display window shows "Paw nn Pex mm AUTOPEEP pp cm H_2O," where *nn* is a display of actual airway pressure, *mm* is the end-expiratory pressure, and *pp* is the measured auto-PEEP. First, the button is pressed. At the moment when the next mandatory breath would have been delivered, both the inspiratory and expiratory valves close. The value of *Pex* (total end expiratory pressure) is updated in the display window every 6 seconds or until the button is released. At the end of the maneuver, the auto-PEEP level is calculated by determining the difference between PEEP (regular baseline pressure) and Pex.

MIP/NIF

The MIP/NIF control (AVS II and AVS III) allows the operator to perform an MIP (i.e., an NIF maneuver). The MIP/NIF control is pushed and held to initiate and perform an MIP maneuver. At the end of expiratory flow, the ventilator closes the inspiratory and expiratory valves, measures pressures in the patient circuit, and displays values in the display window as "Pstart ____," "Paw ____," and "MIP ____ cm H_2O." The value for MIP is updated each time a new maximum negative pressure is detected until the button is released or 30 seconds have passed—whichever occurs first.

100% O_2 3 min

Pushing this pad (LED illuminated) provides 100% oxygen through the patient circuit for 3 minutes. Touching it a second time turns the control off before the 3 minute limit.

BOX 10-21

Inactivating T-Bird Alarms

1. Once an alarm condition no longer exists, the audible alarm usually is silenced.
2. The visual alarms and messages usually clear once the alarm condition is resolved, as well.
3. If the visual alarm remains on, press the ALARM SILENCE/RESET button.
4. Some alarm conditions, such as the "BATTERY ON" alarm, require that the ALARM SILENCE/RESET button is pressed twice for deactivation.

Flow Cal

The FLOW CAL control allows the operator to perform a manual flow calibration that measures the **bias flow** passing through the expiratory flow valve transducer. When the unit is first turned on, the display window gives the message "FLOW CAL." To clear the message, a flow calibration must be performed by pressing and holding down the FLOW CAL pad down during the expiratory phase of a breath. The message "FC nn.n," where *nn.n* is the bias flow (L/min), appears. When "FC nn.n OK" appears, the FLOW CAL touch pad can be released because calibration is complete. (Note that the unit will still operate with a "FLOW CAL" alert, but the accuracy of V_T and $\dot{V}_E$ measurements may be off.)

BOX 10-22

Nonadjustable Alarms/Alerts on the T-Bird

AC power lost alarm
Apnea alarm
Bias alert
Check apnea back-up settings alert
Check filter alert
Circuit fault alarm
Control settings limit alert
Controls locked alert
Default setting alarm
EEPROM failure alert
Fan fault alarm
Flow calibration required alert
Flow sensor alert
Hardware fault alarm
High oxygen inlet pressure alarm
Internal operations check alarm
Invalid calibration values alert
Low external battery alarm
Low internal battery alarm
Low oxygen inlet alarm
New sensor alert
Remote alarm transmission fault alarm
Transducer fault alarm
Ventilator inoperative alarm

Monitors

Across the top of the control panel is the airway pressure manometer (-20 to 120 cm H_2O), which contains a series of LEDs, each equal to 2 cm H_2O when lit. LEDs to the right of zero represent positive pressure and to the left of zero represent negative pressure. The amber LEDs indicate the current high- and low-pressure alarm settings.

Just to the left of the pressure manometer is the EFFORT LED, which (when lit) verifies that a patient's inspiratory effort has been detected once it reaches the sensitivity setting. Below the pressure manometer, there is a monitor window that displays ventilator parameters, messages, and other information.

Alarms

Most ventilator alarms are both audio and visual. In the top right section of the front panel is an alarm window. It displays messages for alarms and alerts (Box 10-21).

Nonadjustable Alarms

Nonadjustable alarms (Box 10-22) are briefly reviewed here. The adjustable alarm controls are located in the next row of controls and are discussed later.

Apnea Alarm. The message window reads "xx sec APNEA." This alert occurs immediately following the power-on self-test (POST) and gives the operator the amount of seconds set on the apnea interval setting.

AC Power Lost Alarm. The message window reads "BATTERY ON." This alarm occurs if the ventilator has been operating from a standard AC electrical power source, which has failed. The ventilator immediately switches to an external or internal battery power source.

Bias Alert. The message window reads "BIAS xx LPM." After the POST test, this informs the operator of the current bias flow setting.

Check Apnea Back-Up Settings Alert. The message window reads "CHECK BKUP," which reminds the operator to set the parameters needed for back-up ventilation. All parameters should be appropriate for the patient's size, age, and condition. This will ensure that the back-up ventilation parameters are also set. For example, in SIMV with pressure-targeted breaths inspiratory pressure above PEEP rate, T_I would be needed.

Internal Operations Check Alarm. The message window reads "CHECK EVENTS," which occurs when the ventilator detects an unusual condition during one of its ongoing self-tests. The ventilator runs the POST test to recheck itself and records the type of error that occurred into memory (EEPROM). If the unit detects an error that compromises safe operation, it gives a VENT. INOP. alarm.

Circuit Fault Alarm. The message window reads "CIRC FAULT." This alarm occurs if the patient circuit becomes kinked, occluded, or disconnected, but also occurs if the internal transducer that measures patient circuit pressure has a problem that is detected by the ventilator.

Default Setting Alarm. The message window reads "DEFAULTS." The ventilator has a number of **default** settings that are set at the factory, but the operator actually overrides these default values when a new value is set. For example, the default value for V_T is 500 mL, but setting a different V_T overrides this value. The new setting is stored into memory (EEPROM) and replaces the set value. In this way, the ventilator can be turned off and it keeps the new settings when it is turned back on. If an error occurs that prevents retrieving the new value from memory, the factory-set values are always available.

EEPROM Failure Alert. The message window reads "EEPROM FAULT." This alert is caused when a **hardware** failure occurs, preventing the unit from retrieving ventilator settings from memory (EEPROM). If this fault occurs, a Bird technician should be contacted.

Low External Battery Alarm. The message window reads "EXT BATTERY." This alarm occurs when the ventilator switches from external to internal battery power.

Fan Fault Alarm. The message window reads "FAN FAULT." When the speed of the cooling fan falls below its set acceptable low limit, this alarm is activated.

Check Filter Alert. The message window reads "FILTER." Every 500 hours, this alert will appear to remind the operator to check the air inlet filter because it may need cleaning or replacing.

Flow Calibration Required Alert. The message window reads "FLOW CAL" and occurs only when the unit is turned on. It requires that the operator perform a flow calibration.

Flow Sensor Alert. The message window reads "FLOW SENSOR." This alert occurs if the unit cannot detect that the expiratory valve body has been connected to the exhalation valve. The valve may need to be reseated or replaced.

High Oxygen Inlet Pressure Alarm. The message window reads "HIGH O_2." If the inlet pressure is >65 psi, and the oxygen percentage is set at >21%, the alarm will be activated.

BOX 10-23

Decision Making & Problem Solving

A respiratory therapist is changing a ventilator from pressure support of 18 cm H_2O to A/C using volume ventilation. The following parameters are set: Mode = A/C; V_T = 0.7 L; f = 20 breaths/min; sensitivity = 2 L/min; peak flow = 20 L/min using a constant flow waveform; inspiratory pause = 1.2 seconds; and O_2% = 35%. An alarm sounds, and the message window reads "LIMITED." What does the alert indicate, and what should the therapist do to correct the situation?

See Appendix A for the answers.

Hardware Fault Alarm. The message window reads "HW FAULT." If a self-test detects a ventilator hardware problem, this alarm is activated. It also occurs if the internal temperature of the unit is too high for normal operation.

Control Settings Limit Alert. The message window reads "LIMITED" and appears if an incompatible setting is made. Box 10-23 gives an example. (Note that T_I must be at least 300 ms, T_E no less than 250 msec, I:E $\leq$ 4:1 [e.g., 1:1], and the high-pressure limit must be $\geq$ the set PEEP level + 5 cm H_2O.)

Controls Locked Alert. The message window reads "LOCKED." This alert appears if you try to change a control when the front panel is locked.

Low Internal Battery Alarm. The message window reads "LOW BATTERY." If the ventilator is operating from the internal battery and the charge in the battery drops to the medium level, this alarm appears. The audible portion of this alarm is a chirping sound heard every 3 seconds, and the internal battery light indicator is yellow. If the alarm is continuous, the power level is low and the light indicator is red. The low power level alarm can be cleared by plugging the ventilator into an AC power source.

Low Oxygen Inlet Alarm. The message window reads "LOW O_2." If the oxygen inlet pressure is <35 psi, and the oxygen percentage is set at >21%, this message appears and an alarm activates.

New Sensor Alert. The message window reads "NEW SENSOR." The alert appears when a newly installed sensor is present in the exhalation valve body. A flow-sensor calibration is required when the valve body is replaced.

Invalid Calibration Values Alert. The message window reads "NO CAL DATA." During a POST, if the unit detects a problem with transducer calibration data that have been stored in memory (EEPROM), this alert will appear and cannot be cleared. Although the unit will still function, the accuracy of the volume and pressure measurements is reduced, so it is advisable to take the unit out of service and contact a Bird representative.

Remote Alarm Transmission Fault Alarm. The message window reads "REMOTE FAULT." This only occurs if a remote alarm transmitter has been installed, and the unit fails to transmit valid data to the remote receiver. The alarm remains active until the problem is corrected or the remote alarm button is turned off.

Transducer Fault Alarm. The message window reads "XDCR FAULT." This alarm occurs if the zero point of a transducer has drifted out of range. The unit will continue to operate, but volume and pressure measurements will be less accurate. Replacing the exhalation valve body and recalibrating the flow sensor usually clears the error.

Ventilator Inoperative Alarm. The message window reads "VENT INOP." The ventilator has detected an unsafe operating condition and ceases to operate if this alarm occurs. The patient is able to breathe room air through the circuit, but the unit must be removed and replaced.

Adjustable Alarms

The adjustable alarm controls can be set using the control knob and the appropriate touch pad and digital display window. The adjustable alarm controls include the following: LOW PRESSURE, HIGH PRESSURE, LOW MINUTE VOLUME, and HIGH RATE.

The LOW PRESSURE ALARM control (2 to 60 cm H_2O) sets the lowest pressure that must be achieved in the patient circuit during a breath. If the unit fails to produce at least the set pressure, a LOW PRESS alarm occurs.

The HIGH PRESSURE ALARM control (5 to 120 cm H_2O) sets the maximum amount of pressure in the patient circuit that the unit will allow, regardless of the type of breaths. Its lowest setting is 5 cm H_2O over the set PEEP. If a HIGH PRESS alarm is activated, inspiration ends (pressure-cycling). If circuit pressure does not drop to PEEP + 5 cm H_2O within 3 seconds, all flow from the unit stops. When pressure falls below PEEP + 5 cm H_2O, the alarm is automatically cleared, flow is restarted, and the next breath is delivered. During a sigh breath, the alarm is increased to 150% of the set high-pressure limit, but this value does not appear in the display above the alarm control.

The LOW MINUTE VOLUME ALARM control (ranges from 0.1 to 99.9 L) sets the minimum $\dot{V}_E$ level that must be exceeded to prevent an alarm. The expiratory flow transducer measures exhaled volume (average of last 8 breaths extrapolated to 1 minute) and compares measured values to the alarm settings. If exhaled $\dot{V}_E$ is below the set low $\dot{V}_E$ alarm setting, the LOW MINUTE VOLUME alarm is activated.

The HIGH BREATH RATE alarm (ranges from 3 to 150 breaths/min) counts both spontaneous and mandatory breaths before being activated and can be turned off. The display window gives the total respiratory rate (spontaneous + mandatory) actually measured. If this equals or exceeds the alarm setting, the alarm is activated.

At the far right of the alarm control panel is the ALARM SILENCE/RESET touch pad, which silences most audible alarms for 1 minute when pressed. Touching it again reactivates the controls. If a VENT. INOP. alarm occurs (indicator in same area), the manufacturer recommends that the unit be turned off before the ALARM SILENCE pad is touched. Of course, the patient should be disconnected from the machine and be manually ventilated. The VENT. INOP. indicator is activated whenever the ventilator detects a condition that could affect safe operation of the unit. The ventilator ceases to operate, opens the exhalation valve, and stops turbine flow so the patient can breathe spontaneously from room air. This requires that the operator immediately provide for patient ventilation and obtain another ventilator for the patient. The unit in question must be serviced by a certified Bird technician.

MODES OF OPERATION

The modes of ventilation include A/C, SIMV, CPAP, and VAPS. A/C and SIMV can provide volume- or pressure-targeted breaths. CPAP provides spontaneous ventilation at the desired baseline and can also provide PSV, which is available whenever spontaneous breaths are provided (e.g., SIMV or CPAP). VAPS is a pressure-targeted breath with volume guarantee.

To select a mode, the operator presses the desired mode button. The LED flashes for 15 seconds, notifying the operator that the unit is ready to switch modes. The mode becomes operational at the selected parameters once the mode pad is pressed a second time, while the LED is still flashing. If the pad is not pressed a second time, the operation is canceled and the ventilator stays in the current mode.

Assist/Control

The A/C mode provides a mandatory breath at the minimum set rate or whenever the patient triggers a breath. Volume ventilation is provided whenever PCV is off. When PCV is on, pressure control and inspiratory time are set by the operator, and any volume setting is ignored. The pressure delivered is in addition to any baseline (PEEP) set. (Note that PCV is available on the AVS III.)

SIMV

SIMV can provide volume ventilation for mandatory breaths (PCV off) or pressure ventilation for mandatory breaths (PCV on). PEEP can also be set, and all volumes or pressures are delivered from the baseline pressure. Spontaneous breaths can occur at baseline pressures only or can be provided with pressure support (PS set where desired).

Pressure Support

PSV can be provided during SIMV or CPAP for the patient's spontaneous breaths. The operator sets the desired pressure-support level above the PEEP (baseline) setting. Sensitivity must be set appropriately. All PSV breaths are patient-triggered. Inspiration is flow-cycled at 25% of the measured peak flow.

CPAP

CPAP is a purely spontaneous breathing mode setting. The patient can breathe from baseline pressure (CPAP level) and also receive pressure-support during inspiration if the pressure-support level is set above zero. During CPAP, certain parameters must be set on the control panel even though they are not operational. These parameters are the default settings if the ventilator switches to apnea back-up ventilation. In the display window, "CHECK BKUP" appears, telling the operator to verify that back-up rate, volume, flow, etc., have been set.

VAPS

The VAPS mode (AVS III only) is a servo-control mode of ventilation (see Chapter 9). The operator must select appropriate settings for the following based on the patient's size, age, and condition: V_T, peak flow, pressure control, PEEP/CPAP, sensitivity, pressure support (available with SIMV), inspiratory pause, and appropriate alarm settings. When VAPS is first turned on, the ventilator delivers a VAPS breath using whatever pressure-control level (plus baseline) is set. Two common events then result, as follows:

1. The ventilator ends inspiration if the V_T has been delivered by the time inspiratory flow decreases to the set value. That is, the ventilator flow cycles at the set peak flow value.
2. If V_T has not been delivered by the time flow has dropped to this value, the flow is maintained (constant waveform pattern) at the peak flow value until the V_T has been delivered. In this situation the unit volume cycles at the set V_T. Box 10-24 gives an example of delivery of a volume during VAPS (Figure 10-21).

Note that if a VAPS breath meets the minimum V_T criteria and inspiratory pause is set at some value above zero, the

BOX 10-24

Decision Making & Problem Solving

The following parameters are set on a patient being ventilated by the T-Bird: mode = assist/control/VAPS; V_T = 0.65 L; f = 10 breaths/min; sensitivity = 3 L/min; flow pattern = constant; peak flow = 60 L/min; pressure control = 20 cm H_2O; O_2% = 30%.

While monitoring the patient, the respiratory therapist notices a breath that appears as shown in Figure 10-21. Was this breath flow- or volume-cycled out of inspiration? How this be determined?

See Appendix A for the answers.

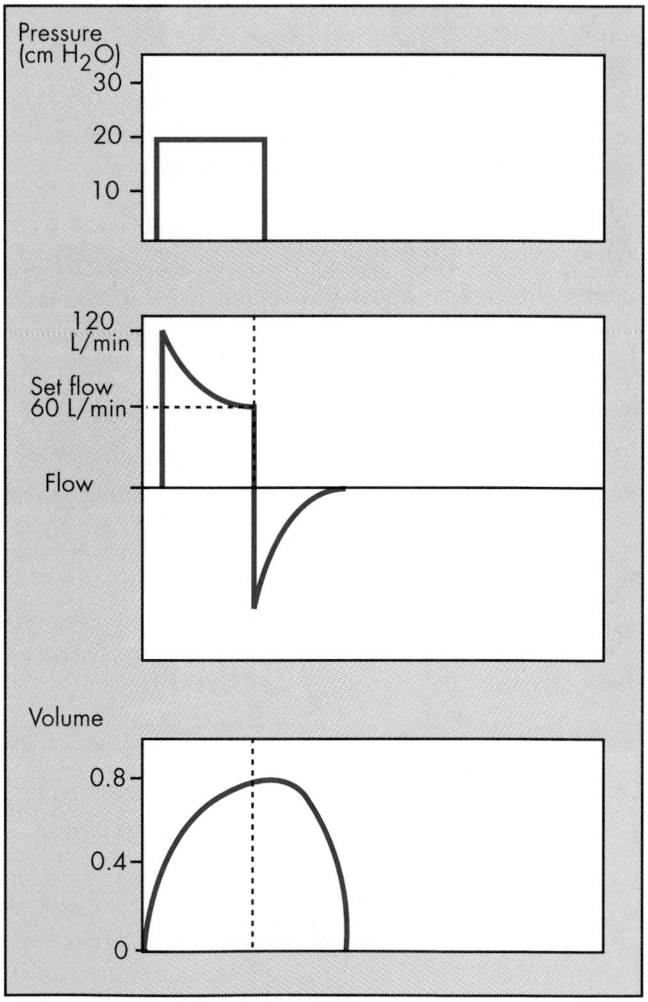

Figure 10-21 A graph of pressure, flow, and volume vs. time for a breath during VAPS on the T-Bird. The top curve shows constant pressure delivery at the set PC level. The baseline is 0 cm H_2O. The middle curve shows the flow rising rapidly at the beginning of inspiration and then descending to the set flow value, and at which point the breath ends. The V_T achieved is higher than the set value, so the patient must have been actively breathing.

inspiratory pause is active. However, if a VAPS breath does not meet the minimum V_T criteria and transitions to a volume-cycled breath, the ventilator will ignore inspiratory pause if it is set.[1]

GRAPHIC DISPLAY SCREENS

The graphics monitor for the T-Bird is the same as the one adapted to use with the Bird 8400STi, so readers are referred to that section for more details.

SPECIAL FEATURES

One of the advantages of the T-Bird is the availability of several unique features (see Table 10-2). For example, under the VENTILATOR SET-UP options, it allows the operator to adjust for altitudes ranging from -1000 to 10,000 feet. Because of this, the unit can compensate for lower gas pressures and improve the accuracy of volume and flow delivery at varying elevations. The VENTILATOR SET-UP options also contain the BIAS FLOW (10 to 20 L/min) control, which sets the level of continuous gas flow through the patient circuit.

The special functions alarm group allows for setting the apnea interval(ranges from 10 to 60 sec), which sets the time between breaths before the apnea alarm is activated. The ventilator then switches to apnea back-up and stays in this mode until the patient initiates two successive breaths or the operator hits the ALARM SILENCE/RESET button twice.

The two groups of special controls that are most likely to be frequently used are the ventilator set-up group and the alarm set-up group (Table 10-3). The reader is directed to the operating manual for full descriptions of all the special function groups and tests.

TABLE 10-3

Ventilator and alarm set-up special function

Ventilator set-up group

Function	Description
Altitude	Altitude setting (-1000 to 10,000 ft)
Autoscan	Turns automatic scanning of monitored parameters on/off
BGM (MCH) interface	Switches ventilator interface with graphics monitor to activate or deactivate lung mechanics
Bias flow	Sets the bias flow from 10 to 20 L/min
Control lock enable	Turns on/off control lock function
Display language selector	Selects the display language preferred by the operator
Hour meter	Shows the total number of hours the unit has been in operation
Software Versions	Displays the current software versions in use by the unit
Turbine	Shows the serial number of the internal turbine

Alarm set-up group

Function	Description
Apnea interval	Sets the apnea time interval from 10 to 60 seconds
Remote alarm status	Displays the remote alarm ID

TROUBLESHOOTING

The alarms and monitoring functions reviewed in this section provide the basic information needed to troubleshoot common problems. In addition, the operating manual contains a section on troubleshooting that describes potential problems, possible causes, and appropriate actions.

Review Questions

(See Appendix A for answers.)

1. The internal mechanism that establishes breath delivery to the patient on the T-Bird is called a(n):
   a. drag turbine
   b. air compressor
   c. rotary drive piston
   d. stepper motor

2. Flow waveforms available for volume ventilation on the T-Bird include which of the following?
   I. descending ramp
   II. ascending ramp
   III. constant
   IV. sine waveform
      a. I and III only
      b. II and IV only
      c. I, III, and IV only
      d. I, II, III, and IV

3. During patient transport, a respiratory therapist hears an alarm coming from the T-Bird ventilator. The external battery indicator is yellow, and the message window reads "EXT. BATTERY." Which action should be taken?
   a. the alarm should be silenced, and no other action
   b. the ventilator should be immediately plugged into a grounded AC electrical outlet

c. the ventilator should be manually switched from the external battery to the internal battery source
d. the patient should be disconnected from the ventilator, and manual ventilation begun

4. A respiratory therapist is trying to measure plateau pressure and have the T-Bird calculate a patient's static compliance, but after repeated attempts using the INSPIRATORY HOLD control, the therapist cannot get a plateau pressure reading to appear in the message window. Which of the following are possible causes of this problem?
   I. The patient is trying to breathe actively during the maneuver.
   II. The therapist is holding down the INSPIRATORY HOLD touch pad for too long.
   III. Inflation hold is not the correct control to use.
   IV. The internal computer is detecting a problem.
   a. I only
   b. I and III only
   c. II and IV only
   d. III and IV only

5. Which of the following is a reliable information source for reviewing the UVT for the T-Bird?
   a. operator's manual
   b. head nurse
   c. respiratory care clinical specialist
   d. pulmonologist

6. Which of the following modes are available on the T-Bird AVS III?
   I. SIMV
   II. PCV
   III. PSV
   IV. VAPS
   a. I only
   b. II and III only
   c. I, II, III only
   d. I, II, III, and IV

7. The T-Bird requires two high-pressure gas sources (air and oxygen) as part of its power source—true or false?

8. The exhalation valve is mounted within the unit and can be located in the lower central portion of the front—true or false?

9. Setting the value of a parameter requires the use of both the parameter's touch pad and the central control knob on the T-Bird—true or false?

10. Comparing pressure augment on the Bear 1000 with VAPS on the T-Bird, what is the difference in the cycling mechanism when the set V_T is met during inspiration without having to sustain flow?

Reference

T-Bird: the seamless solution, T-Bird AVS, ventilator series, operator's manual L1331, Palm Springs, Calif., 1997, Bird Products Corp.

Dräger Evita

OUTLINE

LEARNING OBJECTIVES

Upon completion of this section, the reader should be able to:

1. Describe and label the components of the front panel on the Dräger Evita.
2. Discuss the function of each control on the front panel.
3. Explain the CMV mode, including the associated features of pressure limiting and PCV.
4. Given appropriate ventilatory parameters, determine the spontaneous breathing window during SIMV ventilation.
5. Identify and correct an alarm situation.
6. Draw or describe a pressure/time graph for a patient breathing spontaneously during APRV.
7. Describe the method for setting APRV ventilation.
8. Explain the set-up and measurement of **intrinsic PEEP** and **occlusion pressure ($P_{0.1}$)** on the Dräger Evita.

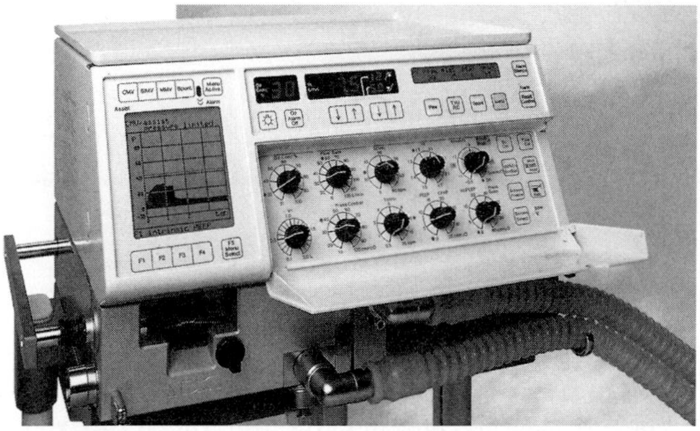

Figure 10-22 The Dräger Evita ventilator. (Courtesy Dräger Corp., Telford, Penn.)

The Dräger Evita ventilator was the first in a series of ventilators manufactured by Drägerwerk in Lubeck, Germany and represented in the United States by the Dräger Corporation (Figure 10-22). The Evita 2 was a modified version of the Evita (Evita 1), but was never marketed in the United States. A second version, the E-2 Dura, replaced the Evita 2 and is sold internationally. And, finally, the Evita 4, or E-4, is the newest edition to the series. (There was never an Evita 3.) All three of these units are presented here, starting with the Evita, which was designed primarily for adult use in the acute care setting.

POWER SOURCE

The Evita normally uses two high-pressure gas sources (40 to 87 psig) as its pneumatic power source, but it can also operate with a single-gas source, such as an air compressor with version 14.0 **software** or higher. Using a single-gas source, however, alters oxygen delivery capability. A standard AC 120-volt outlet is used to power the microprocessor and the electrical components. The on/off switch is located in the upper right corner of the unit's back panel.

INTERNAL MECHANISM

In the Evita, the gas source enters the unit through high-pressure gas connections on the back panel (Figure 10-23). The gas is filtered, and the pressure is reduced to a lower working pressure. The incoming flow is then directed to two electromagnetically operated **high-pressure servo valves.** Gases are blended to match the FiO_2 to be delivered, depending on the setting and assuming that oxygen and air are the source gases. Information from the settings on the front panel, the internal flow, the pressure transducers, and the position of the valves is sent to the microprocessor. The microprocessor uses this information to regulate the action of the servo valves and govern the amount and flow pattern of gas delivered to the patient.

A variety of multiple-pressure transducers monitor the internal gas flow, the output from the unit, and the return of expired gas from the patient through the expiratory valve.

CONTROLS AND ALARMS

The Evita's front panel (Figure 10-24) is divided into the following three main sections:

1. A lower control panel covered by a protective cover
2. An upper section for displaying parameters and alarm settings
3. A main monitoring screen on the left

Control Parameters

The lower control panel consists of two rows of knobs and a section of touch pads (*right side*). The top row comprises the following (see Figure 10-24):

1. O_2 % control (ranges from 21% to 100%).
2. INSPIRATORY FLOW (6 to 120 L/min) sets the peak flow for all time-cycled breaths. In volume-targeted breaths,

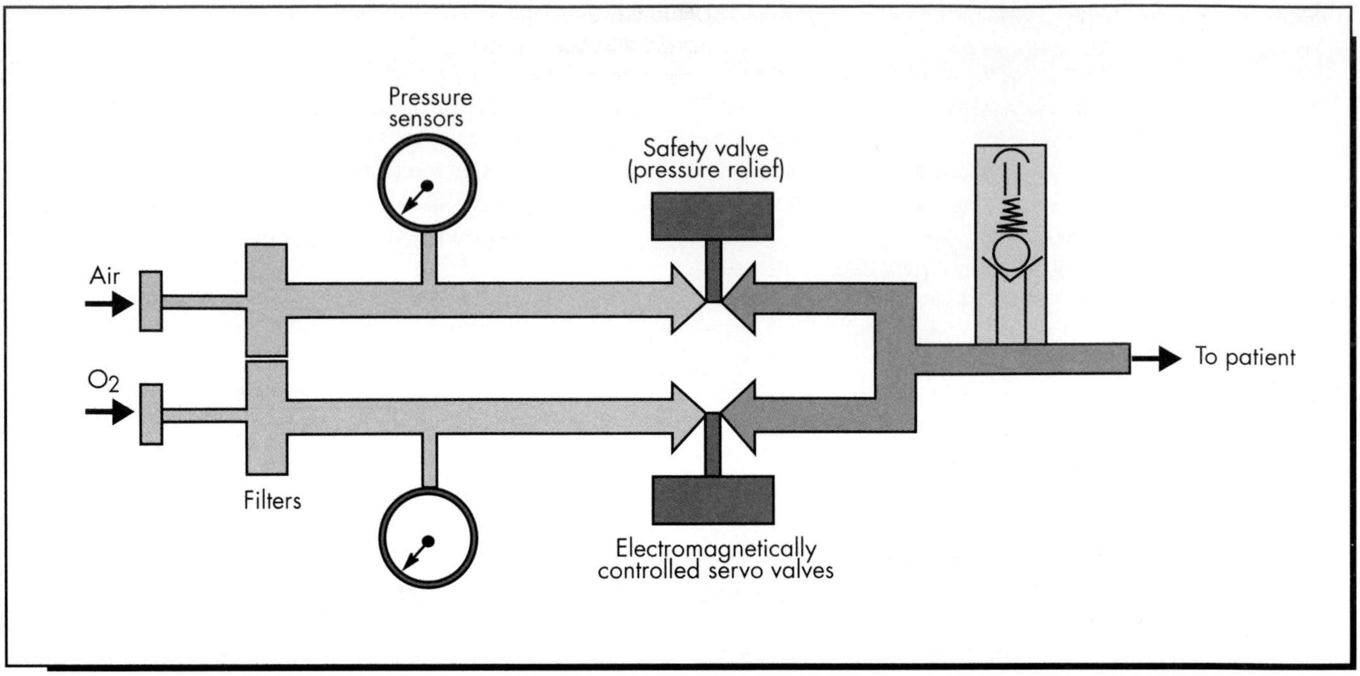

Figure 10-23 A simplified diagram of the internal mechanism of the Evita ventilator that shows the flow-control valves.

the flow waveform is constant. For pressure-control ventilation and pressure-limiting, it sets the maximum flow at the beginning of the breath. Flow then decreases in a ramplike fashion. (Note that for pressure-support breaths, flow is governed by the rise time or **SLOPE** control.)

3. CMV RATE control knob (5 to 60 breaths/min) sets the breath rate and the inspiratory time in SIMV and MMV.
4. I:E RATIO control (4:1 to 1:5).
5. Knob for SENSITIVITY in CMV and for SLOPE in pressure support.
   - For mandatory breaths in CMV, this knob controls the sensitivity (−0.5 to −5 cm H_2O). When the patient triggers a breath, the green ASSIST LED at the top left corner of the main monitoring screen lights. (Note that in SIMV and MMV, the pressure trigger is fixed at −0.7 cm H_2O, and in CPAP it is fixed at −0.2 cm H_2O.)
   - When pressure support is active, this knob controls the rate of rise or slope in the pressure and flow curves for PS breaths in the SIMV, MMV, and PSV modes (ranges from 0 to 2 seconds). The knob determines how fast the high-pressure servo valves open. The time selected is the time it takes pressure to rise to the set value after the beginning of inspiratory flow. (For a further explanation of rise time, see the discussion of the pressure-support mode in later section on modes of ventilation).

Pressure support is flow-triggered (ranges from 1 to 15 L/min) instead of pressure triggered. Box 10-25 shows how trigger sensitivity is set for pressure-support breaths.

The second row of controls includes the following:

1. TIDAL VOLUME (0.1 to 2.0 L) sets V_T delivery for volume-targeted breaths in CMV, SIMV, and MMV.
2. PRESS. CONTROL (ranges from 10 to 100 cm H_2O).
   - Sets the target pressure for mandatory breaths (pressure-controlled breaths) in CMV, SIMV, and MMV.
   - Sets the pressure limit for all breaths in all modes. The microprocessor uses the set pressure control value plus 10 cm H_2O to establish the maximum pressure that may be reached in the patient circuit. For this reason, this control must be set at all times
3. IMV RATE control, or "f(SIMV)," (0.5 to 20 breaths/min) sets the mandatory breath rate in the SIMV mode.
4. PEEP/CPAP (0 to 35 cm H_2O). To set the PEEP value, rotate the knob while observing the value for measured PEEP in the measured values window. (Note that to view the PEEP value, press the PAW touch pad below the measured values screen at the upper right of the top monitor panel [an LED appears] and rotate the PEEP/CPAP knob until the desired value appears in the measured values window.)
5. Rotary knob for INT.PEEP and PRESS. SUPP.
   - The INTERMITTENT PEEP knob is turned to the desired pressure level. The baseline pressure is increased by the value set on the INT. PEEP knob (0 to 35 cm H_2O for two consecutive breaths every 3 minutes) during CMV only (Figure 10-25). The function becomes active as soon as it is set, and the top of the main monitoring screen reads "int.PEEP active" when

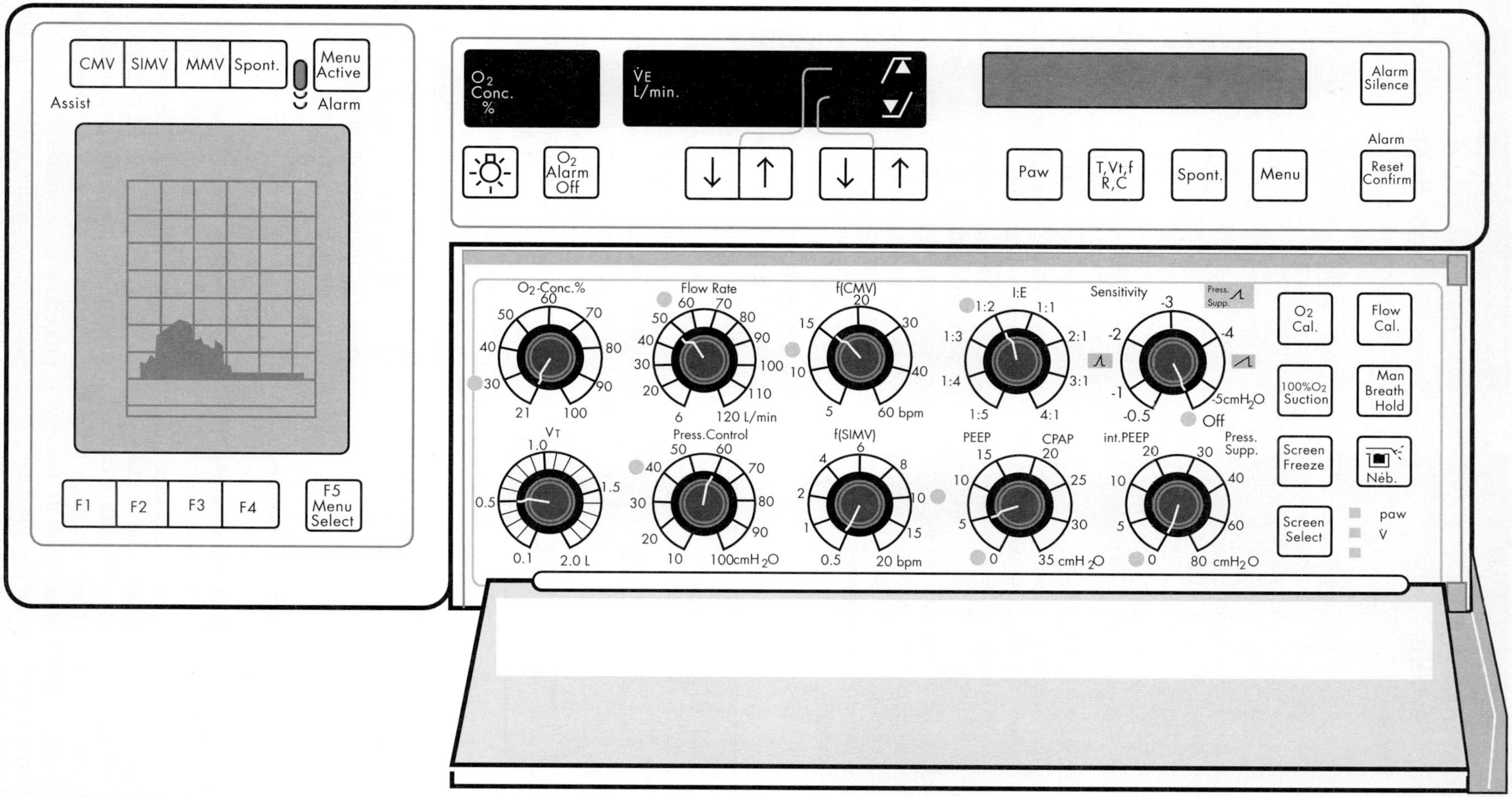

Figure 10-24 The front control panel of the Dräger Evita. (Redrawn from Dräger Corp., Telford, Penn.)

BOX 10-25

Adjusting Sensitivity for Pressure-Support Breaths on the Dräger Evita

Setting the flow triggering for PSV is performed by using the function touch pads or keys below the main monitor. They are selected in the following order:

1. Press menu select (F5)
2. From the displayed menu options appearing on the main monitor screen, use the F3 key to scroll through and select SET VALUE.
3. Activate the set value by using the F1 or F2 key. The set value appears on the screen against a dark background.
4. Confirm the set value using the F3 key. The value now appears dark against a light background.
5. To return the main monitor to its normal waveform display, press F5 or wait and the main screen will appear in 2 minutes.

Note that once the F5 key is activated and a menu appears, the menu provides enough information for you to proceed with the desired change. You do not need to memorize a list of steps or refer to the operator's manual to perform these exercises.

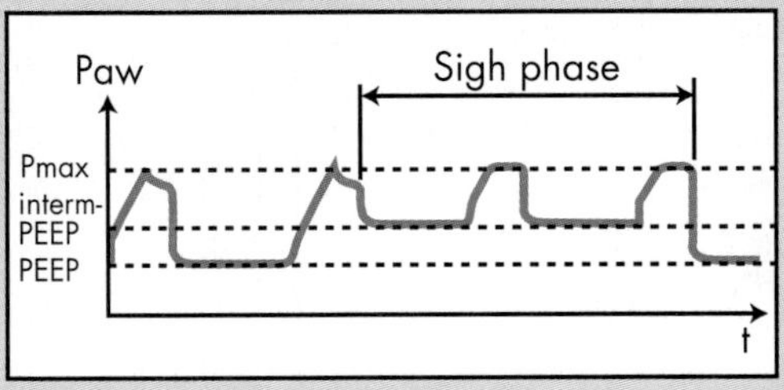

Figure 10-25 Intermittent PEEP for the delivery of sigh breaths. (Redrawn from Dräger Corp., Telford, Penn.)

it is selected. Setting this function is similar to setting sigh breaths on other ventilators.

- The pressure-support function of this control sets the PS level during SIMV, MMV, and PSV ventilation (3 to 80 cm H_2O). The value set on this control determines the maximum amount of pressure the ventilator will deliver with a pressure-support breath (Box 10-26). When the pressure-support function is active (SIMV, MMV, or SPONT. mode touch pad lit), the sigh (INTER PEEP) is not active. (Note that the green LEDs adjacent to and on either side of the knob appear to show which function is active.)

BOX 10-26

Setting the Pressure Level for Pressure Support on the Dräger Evita

If you want a pressure support of 15 cm H_2O, you must set the desired value above the baseline pressure (PEEP/CPAP). For example, if you want 15 cm H_2O of PS and the PEEP is set at 5 cm H_2O, set the PRESS. SUPPORT knob to 20 cm H_2O.

Each of these operating controls has a green LED indicator adjacent to it that illuminates when the knob needs adjustment or is operational. (Note that a flashing LED is warning of an extreme setting, such as an I:E ratio >1:1 or <1:3, and indicates that the knob is functional and the change has occurred, but is asking you to confirm that you do want this setting. Verify the setting by using the RESET/CONFIRM keypad. If multiple LEDs, such as V_T, flow, and I:E, are flashing, this is a warning that parameters are set incorrectly. For example, the V_T set may be too high to be achieved with the set flow and inspiratory time, so the settings must be readjusted. The ventilator will stay at the original setting prior to the change until the error is corrected.)

The touch pad controls on the right side of the panel serve the following functions:

1. Calibration of the built-in **oxygen sensor** (LED is yellow during calibration).
2. **100% O_2 SUCTION,** which provides 100% oxygen during suctioning. When pressed, the ventilator delivers 100% oxygen through the circuit for 3 minutes. The main screen reads "O_2 enrichment 180 s," and the time remaining is displayed. A pressure of 4 cm H_2O is applied if a PEEP of <4 cm H_2O is set to help the ventilator identify when the circuit is disconnected and reconnected. All other parameters are unchanged. After disconnection has been identified, the unit provides 100% oxygen for 2 minutes after suctioning. During these 2 minutes, the audible alarm is silenced so that it is not a nuisance, and a flow of 4 L/min is provided through the circuit. This low flow is intended to reduce humidifier splash. After the patient is reconnected, ventilation is resumed, and an additional 2 minutes of 100% oxygen are provided to the patient. The alarms are reactivated, and the Evita returns to its normal operating mode. The main display screen reads "final O_2 enrich. 120 s." Pressing the RESET/CONFIRM key at any time stops the oxygenation procedure, which cannot be restarted for 15 seconds. (Note that the oxygenation procedure is interrupted if the Evita does not detect a disconnection within the first 3 minute period.)
3. SCREEN FREEZE freezes the waveform on the main monitor screen.

BOX 10-27

Viewing the Inspiratory Flow Curve on the Dräger Evita

1. Press the SCREEN SELECT key (lower right panel) repeatedly until the LED for flow lights.
2. The waveform for flow/time appears on the left of the main monitoring screen.

4. SCREEN SELECT allows selection of pressure/time or flow/time waveforms to appear on the main monitor screen. For example, the flow/time curve can be viewed by following the procedure in Box 10-27.
5. FLOW CAL cleans and calibrates the sensor (LED is yellow during calibration).
6. MANUAL BREATH HOLD either delivers a mandatory breath or performs an inspiratory breath hold. (LED is yellow when this key is pressed; maximum time is 15 seconds.)
7. NEBULIZER CONTROL; the nebulizer operates for 10 minutes and is synchronized with the inspiratory flow phase of a breath and provides 1.5 L/min (air or oxygen). (LED is green when the nebulizer is operating.) It is recommended that the Dräger reusable nebulizer provided be used for this function to maintain FiO_2 and volume delivery as much as possible. Software upgrades (version 14.0) allow for flows of 6 to 9 L/min when other nebulizers are used. Cleaning and calibration of the flow sensor automatically occurs after the nebulizer function is used. (Note that the flow sensor is located on the expiratory end of the internal pneumatic circuit.)

Monitors and Alarms

At the top of the display panel are three small LED screens or windows to provide digital information. The left screen displays the O_2 % being measured by the **oxygen analyzer.** The next screen shows the measured expired $\dot{V}_E$ with the set upper and lower $\dot{V}_E$ alarm limits. The right screen is the MEASURED VALUES display, which provides a digital display of selected measured values based on using the touch pads below the window.

To select ALARM SETTINGS and MEASURED VALUES, the operator uses the touch pads adjacent to the LED windows. For example, below the O_2 % window is a key (touch pad) marked with a picture of a light bulb that is used to change the back lighting on the main viewing screen and the measured values screen. Next to it is the touch pad to turn the oxygen analyzer function on and off. When it is off, the yellow LED flashes. The displayed measured value may differ by ±4% of the value set on the control knob. If it differs by more than this, an alarm is activated to indicate that the oxygen sensor needs to be calibrated or replaced (see the operator's manual).[1]

BOX 10-28

Touch Pads on the Dräger Evita for Selecting Data Display

First Touch Pad (at Left) Provides the Following Values:
Peak pressure
Plateau pressure
PEEP
Mean airway pressure

Second Touch Pad Provides the Following Values:
Inspiratory gas temperature (T)
Exhaled tidal volume (V_{Te})
Frequency (f)
Resistance (R)
Compliance (C)

Third Touch Pad Provides the Following Data:
Spontaneously breathed exhaled $\dot{V}_E$
Spontaneously respiratory rate (f-spo)
Spontaneous respiration with positive airway pressure

Below the $\dot{V}_E$ window are four touch pads that contain arrows (up and down) for changing the upper alarm and lower alarm limits for $\dot{V}_E$.

There are four more touch pads below the measured values display screen. The first three allow the selection of the measured and calculated data listed in Box 10-28. When any of the three are activated, a green LED appears. When any of these pads are touched a second time, the dimensions (units) of the measurement are indicated. The fourth touch pad is the MENU SELECT button, which is used to adjust the contrast setting on the display and screen and to adjust the clock.

Main Monitoring Screen

The left side of the front panel contains a large LED screen, the main monitoring screen, which provides a constant display of the waveform pattern selected. At the top of this screen are the status and alarm displays. For example, the status display might indicate the mode of ventilation.

Above and below the monitoring screen are touch pads for selecting ventilator modes and specific functions. The top pads are used to select CMV, SIMV, MMV, and SPONTANEOUS modes of ventilation. (Note that when a mode is being set, these keys must be pressed and held until the LED lights.) In addition, there is a MENU ACTIVE key, which places the Evita in **apnea ventilation** or **airway pressure-release ventilation (APRV),** depending on which is selected from the menu. The touch pads below the screen give access to many additional menu functions. A few main functions are reviewed in the material here, but readers are

BOX 10-29

Alarm Messages for the Dräger Evita

Ventilation Alarms

MV low or high
Airway pressure low or high
Oxygen concentration low or high
Apnea
High rate
High temperature

Equipment Alarms

Compressed air low
Oxygen pressure low, or oxygen cal. inactive
Pressure measurement inoperative
Mixer inoperative
Malfunction fan
Fan defect
Flow measurement inoperative
Suction inactive
Expiratory valve inoperative
Failure to cycle
Oxygen measurement inoperative
Service needed
Pressure-relief opened
RS 232 inoperative (defect in digital interface)

advised to check the operator's manual for a complete review of the function keys.[1]

Alarm Conditions

When an alarm is activated, a red light flashes at the upper right corner of the main screen and an intermittent sound is emitted. An alarm message is displayed in the upper right corner of the main monitor screen. Box 10-29 lists the ventilation and equipment alarm messages that may occur. To silence the audible alarm for 2 minutes, the ALARM SILENCE key should be pressed. When the problem is corrected, the alarm stops. Pressing the ALARM RESET key removes the alarm message from the main screen.

Airway Pressure Alarms

The alarm thresholds for pressure and PEEP are automatically set by the ventilator. The upper pressure limit is 10 cm H_2O above the setting on the PRESS. CONTROL knob, and is always active regardless of the mode. When this upper pressure limit is reached in the circuit, inspiratory gas flow stops and the expiratory valve opens. If the level reaches 15 cm H_2O above the setting, a second valve opens to vent the pressure more quickly.

The lower pressure limit is 5 cm H_2O below the PEEP/CPAP setting and is active in CMV, SIMV, MMV, and spontaneous.

Front Connections

There are several connectors below the front control panel (see Figure 10-22). There are large-bore connectors for the main inspiratory and expiratory lines of the patient circuit and a small connector for the nebulizer line. The expiratory flow transducer housing is below the main monitoring screen. To the right of the main inspiratory line connection is a screw adjustment for the protective cover over the oxygen analyzer and the room air intake filter (not shown in the figure).

MODES OF VENTILATION

Modes of operation available on the Evita include CMV, SIMV, spontaneous (PSV and CPAP), MMV, apnea ventilation and APRV. Before using the ventilator with a patient, a series of tests are performed as a part of standard maintenance. The operator's manual describes all of the essential steps for testing the unit's readiness.[1]

CMV (Continuous Mandatory Ventilation)

The **CMV** mode is an A/C volume ventilation mode. The operator presses the CMV key until its LED remains continuously lit. The parameters that are set include V_T, FLOW, f (CMV), I:E, SENSITIVITY, PEEP, FiO2, PRESS. CONTROL, and desired alarm settings. Breaths are patient- or time-triggered, volume-targeted, and time-cycled. (Note that if the sensitivity is turned all the way clockwise, the Evita is placed in controlled ventilation, [i.e., time triggering] and an "assist" message disappears from the top left portion of the main screen.) T_I is based on the rate and the I:E control settings. For example, if the rate is set at 10 breaths/min and the I:E at 1:2, the inspiratory time will be as follows:

1. TCT = 60 seconds ÷ (10 breaths/min) = 6 seconds
2. I:E = 1:2, T_I = 2 seconds, and T_E = 4 seconds (see Chapter 9)
3. T_I = 2 seconds

All breaths deliver the set V_T. Flow to the patient is restricted to the flow setting value. The flow waveform is constant. If flow is high and V_T is delivered before T_I is achieved, the inspiratory valve closes (expiratory valve is already closed) and the breath is held. This can be identified by an inspiratory pause pressure in the pressure/time curve and the flow returning to zero on the flow/time curve. Using high flow rates provides a longer pause time but also produces a higher peak pressure (Figure 10-26). (Note that when setting up volume-targeted breaths in CMV or any

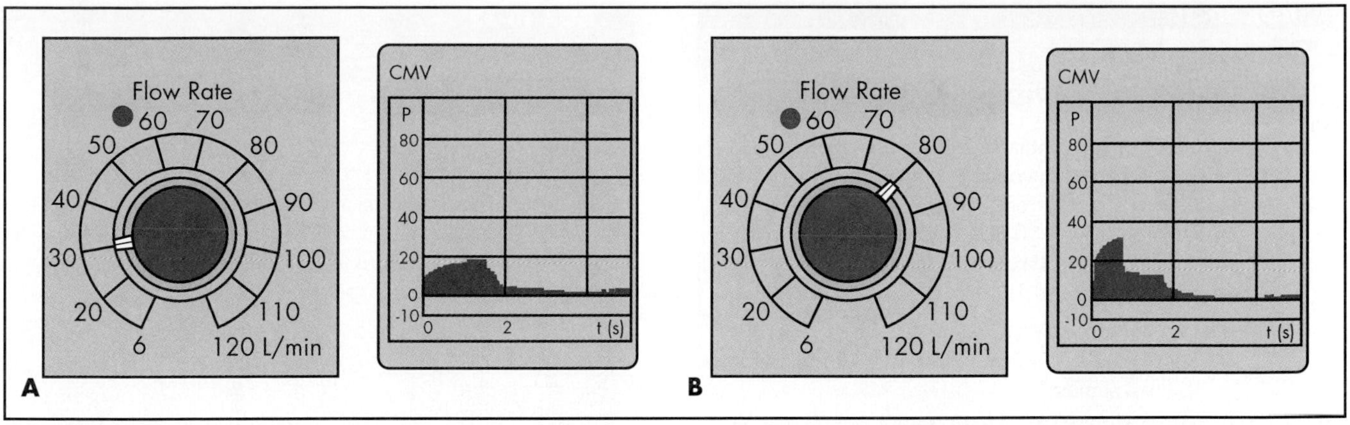

Figure 10-26 Comparison of high and low flow rates during CMV ventilation. Curve **A** shows a slow filling rate with a low peak pressure and a short pause. Curve **B** shows a rapid flow rate with a higher peak pressure and a longer pause time. (Redrawn from Dräger Corp., Telford, Penn.)

BOX 10-30

Ventilating Infants with the Dräger Evita

Tidal volume may be reduced to approximately 50 mL by using the Pmax setting and inspiratory flow settings to limit pressure during inspiration during CMV.

volume mode, the PRESSURE CONTROL knob must be set high enough to deliver a constant (square) flow waveform. If there is a descending flow waveform, pressure and flow delivery are being limited.)

Once the patient is connected, the MEASURED VALUES window can be accessed using the T, V_T, f, R, and C touch pads below the window. The values for each variable are then displayed in the window. Some adjustments can be made to accommodate pediatric patients (Box 10-30).

Pressure Limit Function

The high peak pressures that may occur with volume ventilation can be avoided by using a lower flow or by using the pressure limit function,which is controlled by the PRESS. CONTROL knob. (Note that the pressure limit function is also called "**Pmax**" and "pressure-limited ventilation (PLV)" by the manufacturer and is available on the E-4 and the Evita 2 Dura, as well.)

When pressure limit is selected, it changes the pressure and flow delivery pattern during volume ventilation in CMV, SIMV, and MMV modes. The unit can still provide the set V_T, but it limits the pressure delivered during the breath. This function operates in the following manner. When a breath begins, the pressure in the circuit rapidly reaches the maximum pressure set (knob labeled PRESS. CONTROL). The speed at which the pressure is reached depends on how high the peak flow is set. Flow rises rapidly to its set value and maintains this value until the set pressure is reached. When the pressure is reached, flow gradually descends to keep the pressure constant (Figure 10-27). Inspiration continues for the set T_I, but the amount of pressure in the circuit does not go above the set value. The V_T initially remains constant at the set value *as long as flow drops to zero before the end of inspiration* (i.e., an inspiratory hold). If flow does not drop to zero for the pressure being provided by the unit, the volume cannot be delivered.

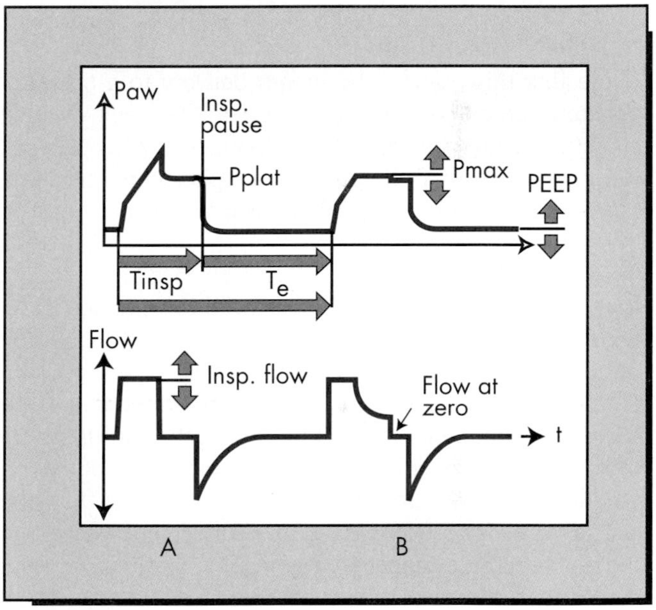

Figure 10-27 The pressure limit function operating during volume targeted mandatory breaths. The top curve is a pressure/time curve showing a typical volume delivered breath with a constant flow delivery (**A**) and a second breath delivery when pressure limit is selected (**B**). (Redrawn from Dräger Corp., Telford, Penn.)

BOX 10-31

Decision Making & Problem Solving

A patient being ventilated with the Dräger Evita is being switched from volume ventilation in the CMV mode to PCV. Current V_T is 0.65 L, rate is 10 breaths/min, flow is 50 L/min, Ppeak is 20 cm H_2O, and Pplateau is 16 cm H_2O. Answer the following questions:

1. How do you activate PCV?
2. Where would you set an initial pressure setting to deliver a similar V_T?
3. Where would you set the upper and lower $\dot{V}_E$ alarm values?
4. Once PCV is activated, how do you check the delivered V_T?

See Appendix A for the answers.

(Note that this changes the breath delivery to a pressure-targeted breath. As the condition of the patient's lung changes, the volume delivery also changes, so peak pressure must be at least 3 cm H_2O above the plateau to guarantee V_T. A plateau pressure will not appear if T_I is too short.)

Pressure Control and Inverse Ratio Ventilation

In the CMV or SIMV modes, the Evita can provide PCV, which is activated by rotating the PRESS. CONTROL knob until the desired (target) pressure ("Ppeak") appears in the MEASURED VALUES window. It is recommended that V_T be set at 2.0 L, and it is important to turn off the VOLUME NOT CONSTANT alarm in the function key pads, otherwise whenever a breath does not reach the set V_T (2.0 L), the alarm will be set off. Displays of pressure can be viewed on the digital monitoring screen by pressing the PAW key pad.

When a pressure value is set on the PRESS. CONTROL knob, pressure limit takes priority over volume delivery. For example, if the volume is set at 2 L and the pressure is set at 20 cm H_2O, the Evita will go to the set pressure (20 cm H_2O) as soon as inspiration begins. It will stay there for the allotted T_I (based on rate and I:E ratio) and time-cycle out of inspiration. V_T delivery depends on the patient's lung compliance and the set pressure value (Box 10-31).

Flow waveforms during PCV resemble those occurring when the pressure limit feature is used (i.e., a descending ramp waveforms). If flow reaches zero at the end of inspiration, the pressure generated by the ventilator is equivalent to the pressure in the lungs. Remember that changes in lung characteristics (resistance and compliance) will alter the volume delivered during pressure ventilation, so it is recommended that the HIGH and LOW $\dot{V}_E$ alarms be set carefully so that they will be activated when a significant change in compliance or resistance has occurred (see Box 10-31).

BOX 10-32

Setting Inverse Ratio Ventilation (IRV)

1. Select the flow/time curve on the main monitor to observe flow delivery while IRV is being adjusted. Avoid developing auto-PEEP during the procedure. The flow must return to zero before the next breath is delivered (see Chapter 9).
2. If PEEP is being used, it should be reduced for safety purposes. In other words, IRV increases mean Paw, as does PEEP, so you do not want the mean Paw too high to begin with.
3. Gradually increase the I:E ratio from 1:1 to 2:1, and so on while monitoring the patient.
4. The top of the main monitor screen reads "confirm I:E," and the green LED on the I:E knob flashes.
5. Confirm to the microprocessor that you want to go to IRV by pressing the RESET CONFIRM touch pad (at the top right of the front panel) until the change is confirmed; the LED stops flashing, and the message disappears.
6. Readjust the following control knobs: FLOW, PRESSURE LIMIT (PRESS. CONTROL), PEEP, and I:E as necessary.
7. Be sure that $\dot{V}_E$ alarm limits are set appropriately.

Inverse ratio ventilation (IRV) can be provided in either volume- or pressure-targeted ventilation by using the I:E RATIO control knob, but is only available in the CMV mode. In Box 10-32, the procedure for setting and confirming the desired IRV is reviewed.

SIMV (Synchronized Intermittent Mandatory Ventilation)

SIMV provides a minimum number of mandatory breaths and allows the patient to breathe spontaneously between these breaths (see Chapter 9). Mandatory breaths can be patient- or time-triggered, volume- or pressure-targeted and time-cycled. In the SIMV mode, as in CMV mode, the volume breaths can be changed to pressure-targeted breaths by using the PRESS. CONTROL knob. They can also be set as pressure-targeted breaths by using the procedure for setting PCV described in the previous section on the CMV mode.

The operator selects the mandatory rate using the f(SIMV) control knob, which determines the time between mandatory breaths. This value is always set lower than the f(CMV) knob. The f(CMV) rate and the I:E ratio are also set and establish the inspiratory time of a mandatory breath. For example, suppose the following are set: f(CMV) = 10 breaths/min, I:E = 1:2, and f(SIMV) = 5 breaths/min. The T_I will be 2 seconds (Box 10-33). The patient can receive the set volume or pres-

BOX 10-33

Calculations of T_I and SIMV Cycle Time in the Evita

Calculation:

60 seconds ÷ 10 breaths/min = 6 seconds cycle time
TCT/(sum of I:E) = T_I
6/3 = 2 seconds

The mandatory breath is delivered in 2 seconds. Expiratory time is 4 seconds. The time between mandatory breaths is 60 seconds ÷ 5 breaths/min, or 12 seconds.

sure in 2 seconds (T_I), have the next 10 seconds to exhale, and then breathe spontaneously. The V_T and flow controls determine what part of the T_I is spent delivering flow to the patient and what part provides a pause (Box 10-34).

All other adjustable parameters in SIMV are the same as those described in the previous section on CMV. Spontaneous breaths can be provided using pressure support. Pressure support breaths are patient-triggered, pressure-limited, and normally flow-cycled (see the following section on PSV).

When SIMV is first started, the patient has a 5-second window during which to make an inspiratory effort and trigger a mandatory breath. For example, suppose the following values are set:

- f(CMV) = 10 breaths/min
- f(SIMV) = 5 breaths/min
- T_I = 2 seconds, based on I:E and f(CMV)

The set SIMV time is 12 seconds (60 seconds ÷ 5 breaths/min). Following a mandatory breath, the patient has 10 seconds during which to exhale and breathe spontaneously (12 seconds − 2 seconds = 10 seconds of spontaneous breathing time).

Suppose that the patient does not make a spontaneous effort and the ventilator time triggers the first mandatory breath at the end of the 5-second window (Figure 10-28, *A*). The next mandatory breath will occur 12 seconds after the beginning of this breath if the patient remains apneic.

Suppose that a patient breathes the first time-triggered mandatory breath spontaneously (see Figure 10-28, *B*). The patient has 5 seconds to do so before the next 5-second window appears. During the window, an adequate inspiratory effort triggers the next mandatory breath. Figure 10-28 shows the following example:

1. Mandatory inspiration (T_I) = 2 seconds
2. Spontaneous breathing time = 12 seconds − 2 seconds = 10 seconds
3. Mandatory window = 5 seconds
4. Spontaneous time without breath-triggering window = 10 seconds − 5 seconds

BOX 10-34

Decision Making & Problem Solving

A respiratory therapist is ventilating a patient with the Dräger Evita in the SIMV mode. The ventilator parameters are as follows: V_T = 0.5 L; f (CMV) = 15 breaths/min; I:E = 1:3; f (SIMV) = 4 breaths/min; flow = 60 L/min; PRESS. CONTROL is set at zero. Answer the following questions:

1. What will the flow waveform pattern look like?
2. What is the T_I of a mandatory breath?
3. What part of T_I is spent in flow delivery and what part in inspiratory pause?
4. What is the time interval between mandatory breaths?

See Appendix A for the answers.

The patient breathes spontaneously for 5 seconds, and then the 5-second window begins. The next patient effort triggers a mandatory breath 1 second into the 5-second window. This is 4 seconds before the next mandatory breath (time-cycled) is due. If this early triggering continues, the actual mandatory breath rate will be higher than its set value. To compensate, the microprocessor calculates the difference between the actual breath delivery (see "patient trigger" in Figure 10-28, *B*) and the expected breath delivery (which is 4 seconds in this example). This amount of time is added to the next spontaneous window. The 4-second extension is added onto the spontaneous breathing time for the next mandatory breath delivery, preventing mandatory breaths from occurring too frequently and thus increasing the mandatory rate over the set SIMV rate.

In the Evita, the mandatory volume is also compensated in SIMV. Suppose that the patient spontaneously breathes in a large volume of air at the beginning of a mandatory breath. The ventilator takes this volume into account and reduces the inspiratory flow and time enough to keep the V_T constant at the set value, thus avoiding excessive volume delivery. The combination of adjustments to the SIMV rate and the V_T delivery helps to maintain a stable minimum $\dot{V}_E$.

Pressure Support Ventilation (PSV)

The Dräger Evita can provide PSV during SIMV, MMV, and spontaneous ventilation modes. To activate PSV in these modes, dial the desired PS level using the INT.PEEP/PRESS. SUPP knob. The main monitor will read "CPAP/press.supp." PS breaths are patient-triggered, pressure-targeted, and usually flow-cycled (25% of the peak measured flow). Patient triggering is based on the set flow-trigger value or when the inspired volume exceeds 25 mL (volume-triggering). The machine then provides the set pressure. Flow delivery is in a descending waveform pattern.

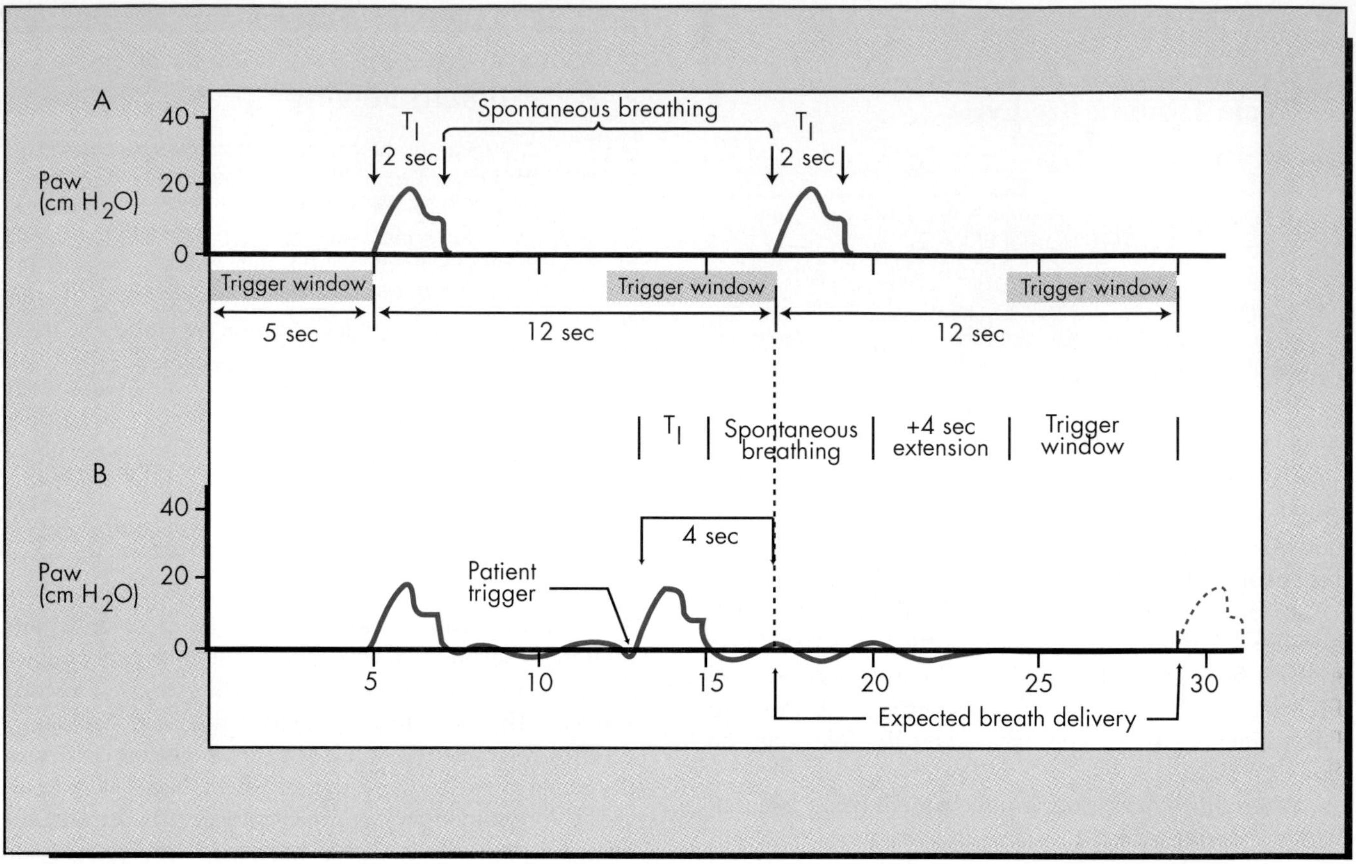

Figure 10-28 SIMV rate timing; see text for further explanation.

When PSV is active, the rate of rise in pressure and flow that occurs at the beginning of a PS breath can be adjusted using the SENSITIVITY/PRESS. SUPP control. When the left portion of the range is used, pressure and flow rise rapidly (ranging from 0 to 1 seconds). When the right portion of the range is used, pressure and flow rise slowly (about 1 to 2 seconds) (Figure 10-29).

If the patient actively exhales or fights the ventilator during the start of a PS breath, inspiratory flow ends. This happens when either the flow goes to zero at the beginning of a breath or the patient is actively exhaling during the early portion of inspiration. Inspiratory flow during PSV will also time-cycle at 4 seconds. Prolonged T_I occurs most commonly if a leak is present. In this situation, an alarm (audio and visual) is activated.

When switching from spontaneous ventilation modes (PSV or CPAP) to CMV, the INT.PEEP/PRESS. SUPP knob must be readjusted. Remember that in switching back to CMV, the SENSITIVITY/PRESS. SUPP control now controls trigger sensitivity—not the rate of pressure and flow delivery, which must also be readjusted.

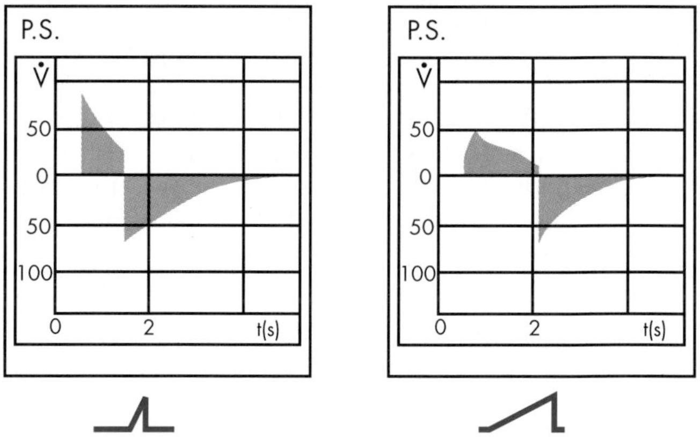

Figure 10-29 The sloping (adjustment of rise time) of the flow/time curve using the SENSITIVITY/PRESS. SUPP control with the Dräger Evita. Curve **A** shows a very rapid flow. Curve **B** shows a very slow flow. (Redrawn from Dräger Corp., Telford, Penn.)

Continuous Positive Airway Pressure (CPAP)

CPAP is available on the Evita by selecting the SPONTANEOUS MODE touch pad. Set the desired CPAP level (cm H_2O) with the PEEP/CPAP knob. Set PS if spontaneous breaths are to be aided with PSV. The set PS level is the peak pressure for the breath (see Box 10-26). Be sure to set upper and lower $\dot{V}_E$ alarm limits, and remember that when switching from a spontaneous mode back to CMV, the INT. PEEP and SENSITIVITY/PRESS. SUPP controls must be readjusted.

Mandatory Minute Volume Ventilation (MMV)

As described in Chapter 9, a patient can spontaneously breathe and contribute a portion or all of the overall $\dot{V}_E$ in the MMV mode. The difference between the spontaneous and the set $\dot{V}_E$ is provided by mandatory breaths at the set volume.

A desired minimum $\dot{V}_E$ is set using an appropriate rate and V_T to maintain the desired arterial blood gas values. A pressure-support level should also be selected to help the patient's spontaneous breathing efforts between any mandatory set V_T breaths. Pressure-support rise time can be used to slope the pressure/time curve during PSV. A HIGH RESPIRATORY RATE alarm is also set to monitor increased work of breathing.

The frequency of a mandatory breath is determined by the level of spontaneous breathing. If the patient is providing sufficient spontaneous $\dot{V}_E$, no mandatory breaths occur. However, if spontaneous $\dot{V}_E$ falls below what the ventilator anticipates to occur based on the set $\dot{V}_E$ ($V_T \times f$), mandatory breaths begin as soon as the balance between the set and the spontaneous $\dot{V}_E$ becomes negative. The software program for MMV ventilation is designed to allow for irregular patterns of spontaneous breathing with occasional short intervals of apnea. It permits these irregularities without allowing excessive time to pass with no spontaneous or mandatory breathing.

Apnea Ventilation

Apnea ventilation is an independent mode setup in the menu. It is not a backup for other modes and only supplies CPAP and PSV modes with backup. Apnea ventilation provides volume ventilation with a minimum breath rate if the patient becomes apneic. If the patient quits breathing for the length of time set on the APNEA ALARM control, the alarm is activated, the ventilator switches to CMV based on the control knob settings, and apnea ventilation begins.

Box 10-35 describes how to set apnea ventilation. If an apneic event occurs, the Evita will give an audio/visual alarm after 15 seconds. After the set apnea time has elapsed (15 to 60 seconds), ventilation with the CMV mode begins, using all rotary knobs that have green LEDs lit. The main screen shows a flashing "CMV" message, and the unit remains in apnea ventilation regardless of what the patient is doing. Pressing the RESET/CONFIRM key returns the ventilator to its previous function.

Airway Pressure-Release Ventilation (APRV)

APRV is a mode of ventilation that can be selected from the EXTENSIONS menu (F5). It provides two levels of CPAP (P_{high} and P_{low}) (Figure 10-30) and is intended for spontaneously breathing patients. Patients are able to breathe spontaneously at any time. P_{high} and P_{low} range from 0 to 35 cm H_2O. Changing from P_{high} to P_{low} or from P_{low} to P_{high} is sensitive to and synchronized with the patient's spontaneous respiratory efforts. Chapter 9 provides additional information about this mode.

To set APRV, select the APRV mode from the VENTILATOR MODES menu. The upper and lower pressure levels are set using the F1 and F2 function keys and are confirmed with the F3 key. The unit also times the length of both pressure levels. "T_{high}" is the length of time that high pressure is provided, and "T_{low}" is the length of time that low pressure is provided. APRV time levels range from 0.5 to 60 seconds. The duration of each is selected by first choosing F3 in the APRV menu. Then the settings are adjusted and confirmed using the F1, F2, and F3 keys. (The menu prompts you through the steps.) Return to the last menu (F5). To activate APRV, press F1 and press the MENU ACTIVE key until its green LED stays lit. (Note that to switch to another mode of ventilation, that mode key should be pressed and held until its LED remains lit. The menu from the mode that was previously active stays on the screen until it is changed with the function keys.)

BOX 10-35

Setting Apnea Ventilation on the Evita

1. Touch the F5 function key.
2. Select the APNEA VENT. menu using the F2 key.
3. Select apnea time using F2.
4. Set the desired apnea time using the F1 and F2 keys.
5. Confirm the new value by pressing the F3 key.
6. Return to the original screen using F5.
7. Press F1 to select APNEA VENTILATION.
8. Press the MENU ACTIVE button until its LED is lit continuously; the new apnea time is set and apnea ventilation is now active.
9. Press the F5 key twice to return to the normal waveform screen.

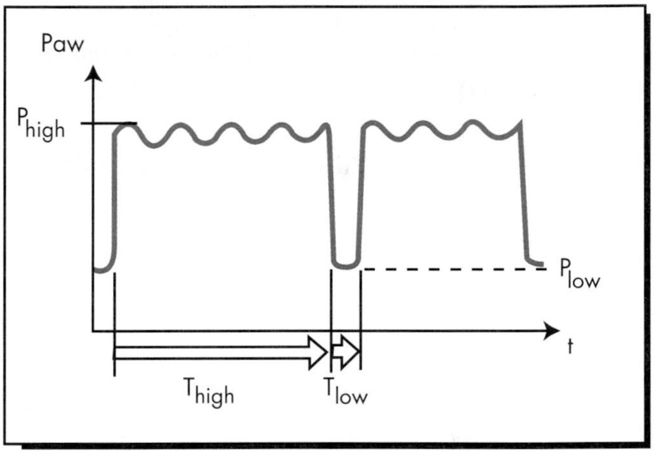

Figure 10-30 Airway pressure-release ventilation; see text for further explanation. (Redrawn from Dräger Corp., Telford, Penn.)

BOX 10-36

Performing an Intrinsic PEEP Maneuver with the Evita

1. Push the MENU SELECT (F5) key.
2. From the screen menu select F4, MEAS. MANEUVER.
3. With F1, select INTRINSIC PEEP.
4. Use F5 to select the waveform display (pressure/time curve).
5. The measurement is automatically performed when the F1 key is pressed; the measured values are displayed on the screen.
6. After measurement, return to the pressure/time curve display (F5). (This screen automatically returns in 2 minutes.)

BOX 10-37

Measurement of Occlusion Pressure in the Evita

1. Push the MENU SELECT (F5) key.
2. From the screen menu, select F4: MEAS. MANEUVER.
3. With F2, select OCCLUSION PRESSURE.
4. Use F5 to select the waveform display (pressure/time curve).
5. The measurement is automatically performed when the F1 key is pressed.
6. After the measurement is performed, return to the pressure/time curve display (F5). (This screen automatically returns in 2 minutes.)

Occlusion pressure can be set up in any mode, but can only be measured during the spontaneous mode.

SPECIAL FUNCTIONS

Additional features on the Dräger Evita are the measurement of intrinsic PEEP and occlusion pressure.

Intrinsic Positive End-Expiratory Pressure (PEEP)

An estimate of the amount of auto-PEEP present in the patient can be determined in addition to an estimate of the trapped volume (Vtrap) by using the intrinsic PEEP (PEEPi) function. These measurements can be performed only in the CMV mode and as long as no patient activity occurs during the measurement.

Box 10-36 describes the steps of performing this measurement. During the maneuver, the inspiratory and expiratory valves close, allowing for equilibration of pressure in the patient circuit during the expiratory phase. On the screen, values for PEEPint and trapped volume (Vtrap) are shown. The auto-PEEP level can be viewed at any time on the pressure/time curve display.

Occlusion Pressure

Measurement of occlusion pressure ($P_{0.1}$) is available as a special function in the Evita, but can only be done during spontaneous breathing. Occlusion pressure is used to evaluate a patient's neuromuscular drive. At the beginning of inspiration, the ventilator occludes the inspiratory and expiratory valves 0.1 second after the beginning of inspiratory flow. The pressure measured at that time is displayed. The normal values range from -3 to -4 cm H_2O. Values below -6 cm H_2O may indicate impending exhaustion and respiratory muscle fatigue.

This procedure can be automatically performed using the steps outlined in Box 10-37. The value for occlusion pressure is shown on the screen; this measurement can only be carried out in the spontaneous breathing mode. Preparation for measurement, however, can be accomplished in any mode.

VENTILATOR GRAPHIC WAVEFORMS

The graphics monitor of the Dräger Evita is part of the main computer screen during standard operation. It can provide pressure/time or flow/time waveforms.

TROUBLESHOOTING

The alarms and monitored information provided by the Evita are a great help in solving most problems that might occur. In addition, the operator's manual contains a troubleshooting section that lists ventilation and equipment alarm messages, common causes, and appropriate remedies.

Review Questions

(See Appendix A for answers.)

1. Which of the following variables are functional during CMV ventilation on the Dräger Evita?
   I. V_T
   II. PRESS. CONTROL (PRESS. LIMIT)
   III. f(SIMV) rate
   IV. pressure-support rise time
   a. I and II only
   b. II and IV only
   c. III and IV only
   d. I, II, and III only
2. What mode touch pad is pressed to activate the PCV mode with the Evita?

a. PCV
b. CMV
c. SPONT.
d. MMV

3. During PCV, the pressure set on the PRESS. CONTROL knob equilibrates with pressure in the lungs when which of the following conditions occurs?
   a. The patient actively inspires and increases flow delivery above the set flow value.
   b. The pressure limit is set below the current plateau pressure.
   c. The flow/time curve shows flow returning to zero before the end of inspiration.
   d. The flow is set at 60 L/min, and the I:E ratio is 1:3.
4. During PSV on the Evita, the LOW $\dot{V}_E$ alarm activates. The respiratory therapist notes that T_I is 4 seconds long on the pressure/time curve. The most likely cause of the problem is which of the following?
   a. patient's respiratory rate has dropped
   b. patient's lung compliance is reduced
   c. leak in the circuit
   d. trigger sensitivity is not sensitive to patient effort
5. Which of the following parameters can be used to assess a patient's neuromuscular drive?
   a. intrinsic PEEP
   b. plateau pressure
   c. occlusion pressure
   d. sensitivity setting
6. Which of the following procedures is used to begin the set-up of APRV ventilation in the Evita?
   a. press the APRV mode key until the LED remains lit
   b. set the pressure limit at $P_{plateau}$ + 3 cm H_2O during CMV ventilation
   c. activate the MMV mode touch pad and set the SIMV RATE knob to the desired rate
   d. select the F5 MENU SELECT function key and proceed with other function keys, depending on the menu provided
7. Which of the following statements is (are) true about the measurement of occlusion pressure with the Evita?
   I. The procedure is first begun by selecting F5 to obtain a menu screen.
   II. The procedure is automatically performed once all the steps in its selection have been completed.
   III. The INSPIRATORY and EXPIRATORY HOLD touch pads are pressed when the message "measure P 0.1" appears at the top of the main screen.
   IV. The ventilator performs this measurement 0.1 seconds after inspiratory flow has started.
   a. I only
   b. IV only
   c. II and III only
   d. I, II, and IV only
8. The majority of controls on the Evita are rotary knobs and touch pads—true or false?
9. A patient can breathe spontaneously at any time during APRV—true or false?
10. Describe APRV ventilation.

Reference

Dräger Evita: intensive care ventilator operator's manual, 90 28 225, Telford, Penn.,1993, Dräger, Inc.

Dräger E-4 (Evita-4)

CHAPTER OUTLINE

LEARNING OBJECTIVES

Upon completion of this section, the reader should be able to:

1. Describe the front panel on the Dräger E-4.
2. Discuss the function of each control on the E-4 front panel.
3. Compare the set-up of a ventilator mode on the E-4 with that on another microprocessor-controlled ICU ventilator.
4. Assess an alarm situation, describe its priority level, and suggest a possible cause and solution.
5. Identify a pressure/time graph for a patient breathing spontaneously during PCV ventilation.
6. Compare upper Paw alarm limit to the Pmax pressure limit.
7. Describe the method for setting PCV+ and APRV and compare it with the two modes of ventilation.
8. Discuss the similarities and differences between **AutoFlow** and PRVC on the Servo 300 (see Chapter 9).
9. List the features available when Neoflow is added as an upgrade to the Dräger E-4.
10. Explain the set-up and function of proportional pressure support.

The Dräger E-4[1] and the Evita 2 Dura were developed after the original Evita ventilator. The Dräger E-4 ventilator was originally manufactured by Drägerwerk in Lubeck, Germany. Production of the E-4 and the E-2 Dura is now at Dräger, Inc. in Telford, Penn. The E-4 and the E-2 Dura have many functional similarities. The E-4 is presented first here (Figure 10-31). Note that the manufacturer refers to the E-4 as the Dräger E-4 Pulmonary Work Station because it can monitor a variety of patient information.

The unit has a front panel that contains touch pads, a rotary (dial) knob, and a computer screen. The infrared touch screen uses light beam interruption technology, and there are images or icons on the computer screen. Some of these are shaped like knobs (soft knobs, or **cyber knobs**), and some are shaped like touch pads (soft pads, or **cyber pads**). All of these dials and knobs are used to control the unit and are discussed later in this section.

Below the front operating panel are the connections for the main inspiratory and expiratory lines, the expiratory valve, and the nipple connector for the nebulizer line. The expiratory flow sensor is on the left of the expiratory valve. On the far right side below the unit's main control knob (rotary knob) is a protective cover that hides the oxygen sensor and the ambient air filter.

Power Source

The E-4 normally uses two 50 psig gas sources (air and oxygen, ranging from about 40 to 87 psig). The unit will operate on a single gas source, but it will issue an alert when the other gas source runs low, altering oxygen-delivery capabilities. A standard AC 120-volt outlet is used to power the microprocessor and the electrical components. The on/off switch is located on the back panel of the unit.

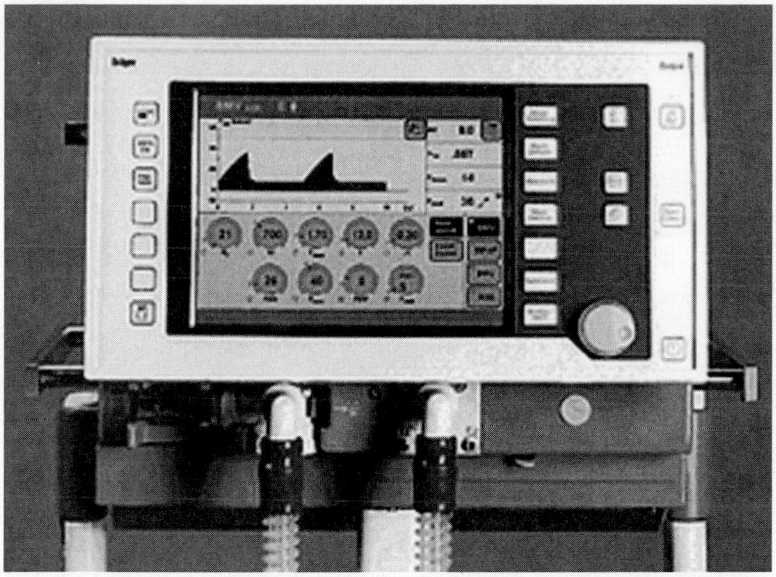

Figure 10-31 **A,** the Dräger E-4 ventilator (Courtesy of Dräger Corp., Telford, Penn.)

INTERNAL MECHANISM

The internal mechanism is similar to those of many of the recently released ICU ventilators. The gas sources enter the unit through connections on the back panel. They are filtered, and their pressure is measured and reduced to a working pressure. The incoming flow is then directed to two flow-control valves. (Note that in the Dräger Dura and the E-4, these flow-control valves are high-pressure electromagnetic servo valves.) The function of these valves is controlled by the microprocessor, which uses information from the settings on the front panel, internal flow, pressure transducers, and the action of the valve itself to control the flow to the patient. These valves regulate the amount of pressure and flow and the flow waveform of the gas delivered depending on the selected modes and settings. The valves also control the FiO_2 based on the set value, and the changes are instantaneous. From the flow-control valve, gas is directed to the patient.

A variety of pressure and flow transducers monitor internal gas flow, the output from the unit, and the gas return from the patient through the expiratory valve.

CONTROLS AND ALARMS

A number of controls, monitors, and alarm settings are available on the Dräger E-4. Basically, the E-4 uses a single rotary knob, several hard touch pads on the side the computer screen, and the touch-sensitive soft knobs (cyber knobs) and soft pads (cyber pads) on the computer screen (see Figure 10-31).

Peripheral Controls

Several controls used during normal operation of the ventilator are located on both sides of the screen. Those on the left side of the screen include the following: NEBULIZER, SUCTION 100% O_2, INSPIRATORY HOLD, PRINT, and several blank keys for future upgrades. These controls are reviewed in the discussion of special functions later in this section.

On the immediate right side of the computer screen are touch pads that are used to select several operations. These pads include the following:

1. MODE SETTINGS
2. ALARM LIMITS
3. VALUES MEASURED
4. SPECIAL PROCEDURE
5. A blank key (for future upgrades)
6. CALIBRATION
7. CONFIGURATION

The function of each will be covered as the various controls and alarms are described.

Three more touch pads and the rotary knob are to the right of these touch pads. These touch pads include an information key (i), a FREEZE control to freeze graphic waveforms, and a MAIN SCREEN pad for selecting standard menus to appear on the computer screen.

The knob can be rotated and pressed to select numerical values for parameters and activate the new parameters,

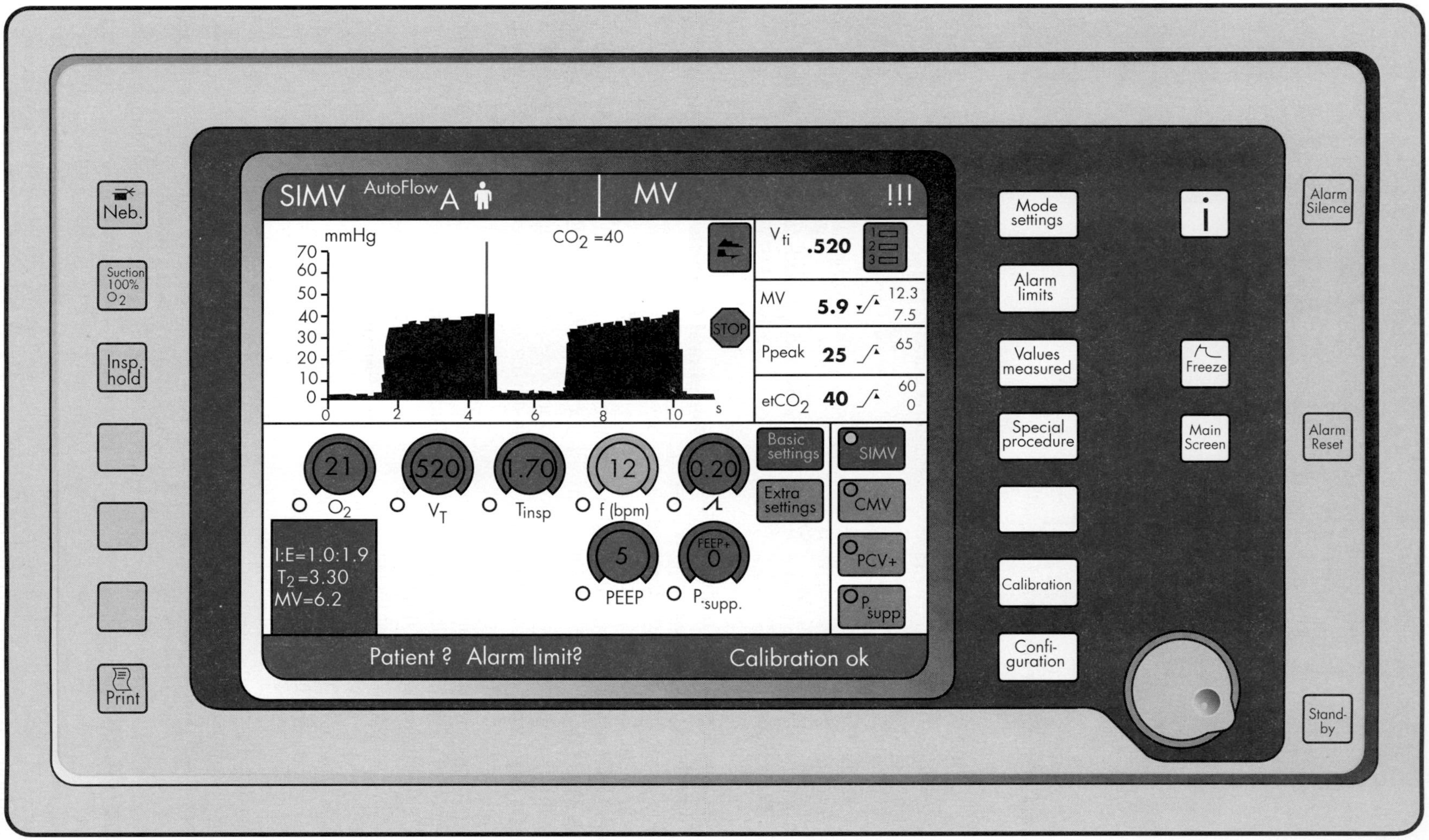

Figure 10-31 (continued) **B,** the front panel of the Dräger E-4 ventilator showing the touch pad controls, the rotary knob, and the screen in a standard ventilating mode.

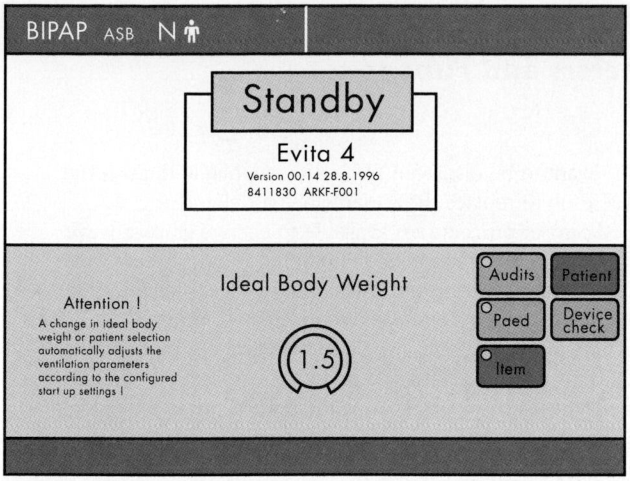

Figure 10-32 The screen during ventilator start-up on the Dräger E-4 version 2.n with Neoflow. (Redrawn from Dräger Corp., Telford, Penn.)

TABLE 10-4

Ranges for parameters on the Dräger E-4

Tidal volume	
Adult	0.1 to 2 L
Pediatric	20 to 300 mL
Neonate	3 to 100 mL
Flow	
Adult	6 to 120 L/min (to 180 L/min with Autoflow)
Pediatric	6 to 30 L/min (to 60 L/min with Autoflow)
Neonate	0.25 to 30 L/min
Neonate continuous flow	6 L/min
Variable ranges for all patients	
Respiratory rate	0 to 100 breaths/min 0 to 150 breaths/min with Neoflow
Inspiratory time	0.1 to 10 sec
Inspiratory pressure (set)	0 to 80 cm H_2O
Maximum pressure limit	0 to 100 cm H_2O
Percent oxygen	21% to 100%
PEEP	0 to 35 cm H_2O
Trigger Sensitivity	1 to 15 L/min
Recommended trigger sensitivity for neonates	0.3 to 5 L/min
Pressure support	0 to 80 cm H_2O
Rise time for PS	0 to 2 seconds

respectively. It can also be used to move the cursor (vertical line) on the screen when it appears under certain functions.

On the far right side of the front panel are the following additional touch pads:

1. ALARM SILENCE (2 minutes)
2. ALARM RESET
3. STAND-BY (for switching between the stand-by and the operating modes)

Overview of Stand-by Controls

After the POWER switch is turned on, the unit runs a series of self-tests and a signal can be heard. Once the tests are complete, the screen asks you to select ADULT, PEDIATRIC, or NEONATE (E-4 upgraded version 2.n software) by touching the desired soft pad (cyber pad) and entering the ideal body weight (IBW) of the patient (Figure 10-32). The available volumes and flows are different for each type of patient (Table 10-4). To set the IBW, touch the screen soft knob for IBW, which highlights the knob and changes its color to yellow. Rotate the dial knob to set the actual numerical value, which appears inside the screen soft knob. When the desired IBW appears, push the knob to set the selected value, which changes the soft knob from yellow to green to show that it has been set. These same actions (touching [soft knob or pad], turning [rotary knob], and pushing [rotary knob]) are how most controls are set. The manufacturer refers to this sequence as "touch, adjust, confirm."

The unit requests the patient's IBW because the unit is programmed at the factory to automatically begin ventilation using CMV with factory-set parameters. The factory default V_T is 7 mL/kg, based on the IBW of the patient. The respiratory rate is based on Radford's nomogram for the $\dot{V}_E$ of a person that size.[2] The mode and parameters may be reconfigured, but you also can do a standard ventilator set-up and select the mode and other appropriate parameters.

To have the unit automatically start ventilating a patient with programmed (configured) parameters, simply push the rotary knob. To set the unit up more specifically, touch the STAND-BY soft key and hold it down for about 3 seconds until the unit displays "Stand-by Activated." The gas is shut off, but all adjustments can be made. Press the MODE SETTINGS soft pad and make the desired settings. Touch the STAND-BY soft pad again, and the unit begins ventilation.

(Note that the programmed values can be changed by "configuring" the unit so that some other mode and parameters are available as soon as the unit is turned on [see the discussion of configuration in this section and Box 10-38].)

Because of the design of the E-4 unit, the control knobs that appear on the screen vary for each mode of ventilation selected. For example, if you wish to use the SIMV mode in volume ventilation, only the controls that are active in

BOX 10-38

Configuring the Ventilator, or Setting Parameters and Functions into Memory on the Evita-4

As with many computer programs, the Dräger E-4 microprocessor permits the operator to set a certain mode and its parameters. The operating manual provides a detailed description of each adjustment that can be made during configuration of the unit. A few examples are provided here.

To access the configuration function, press the configuration touch pad. The computer screen lists a menu of parameters or variables that you can select, including values, curves, trends, sound, screen, ventilation, and system defaults. To adjust any available screen, touch the desired soft pad. For example, if you wish to change the VALUES MEASURED screen, touch the VALUES soft pad to bring up a menu of current available values (e.g., MV, Pplat, C, R, and f).

To replace one value with another, touch the appropriate soft pad to highlight the value to be deleted. A column of all the available measured and calculated variables appears to the left. Using the dial knob, select (highlight) the variable you want to be displayed. When it is highlighted, push the dial knob to replace the variable being deleted.

A similar procedure is available to change graphic waveforms, data trends, ventilation parameters, and system defaults. System defaults allow the unit to access specific external computer ports, such as the port that connects to a printer. System defaults also lets you select computer variables, such as baud rate and parity check bits. System defaults provide a way to change the date, time, and language on the screen or the desired units of measurement (e.g., mbar [millibars] vs. cm H_2O).

If you want to change the ventilation mode and the parameters that automatically appear when the unit is turned on, you must enter an access code. This code is usually known by the individuals in the department who have the authority to change this set function (e.g., the clinical specialist or the department head).

that mode appear on the screen. For this reason, it is easier to discuss the various controls as their uses or the specific modes are discussed. The available ranges for control variables are listed in Table 10-5. If you go beyond the range of normal ventilation for a parameter, the knob stops adjusting as you turn it. A message appears at the bottom of the screen telling you what needs to be done to continue. For example, if you select a respiratory rate of 4 breaths/min in SIMV, and T_I (inspiratory time) is set at 1 second, the knob will freeze and the message at the bottom will read "I:E < 1:3 confirm," followed by an icon for the rotary knob. When you press the knob, the SIMV rate will go down to 4 breaths/min with a T_I of 1 second.

TABLE 10-5

Commonly measured and displayed parameters on the Dräger E-4

Parameter	Definition	Range
Ppeak	peak pressure	0 to 99 cm H_2O
Pplat	plateau pressure	0 to 99 cm H_2O
Pmean	mean pressure	0 to 99 cm H_2O
PEEP	positive end expir. press.	0 to 99 cm H_2O
Pmin	minimum pressure	0 to 99 cm H_2O
MV	minute ventilation	0 to 99 L/min
MVspn	spontaneous MV	0 to 99 L/min
f	total frequency	0 to 150 breaths/min
fspn	spontaneous frequency	0 to 150 breaths/min
fmand	mandatory frequency	0 to 150 breaths/min
V_{TE}	exhaled tidal volume	0 to 3999 mL
V_{Ti}	inhaled tidal volume	0 to 3999 mL
Fio_2	fractional inspired O_2	15% to 100%
T	temperature	18 to 51° C
R	resistance	cm H_2O/L/sec
C	compliance	mL/cm H_2O

Monitors and Alarms

In every mode of ventilation, the E-4 provides monitored parameters at the top of the screen. There may be a graphic on the left side. On the top right are current values, such as O_2%, Ppeak, Pplat, and MV (minute ventilation). Although these are the variables most commonly selected, they can be changed by the institution per the standards of the clinical site. Box 10-39 describes the selection of ventilator parameters for display.

Measured Values

The VALUES MEASURED touch pad brings up a screen that displays values being measured or calculated by the unit (see Table 10-5 and Figure 10-33), such as FiO_2. The ventilator has a built-in oxygen analyzer and does an automatic oxygen calibration every 24 hours. The unit can optimally include a mainstream carbon dioxide analyzer that provides information on end-tidal carbon dioxide ($etCO_2$), CO_2/time, and single-breath CO_2 (CO_2/volume). Calculated values include carbon dioxide production ($\dot{V}_{CO2}$), deadspace (V_D), and V_D/V_T measurements. The analyzer is normally taken out of the circuit and calibrated before use. There is a special block built into the ventilator that al-

BOX 10-39

Selecting Displayed Parameters

The E-4 allows graphed and digitally displayed information to be viewed. Available graphs include pressure, flow, volume, or end-tidal CO_2 graphed per unit of time. Any two graphs may be selected by touching the green soft (cyber) pad at the top right of the curve, and then touching the particular curve.

On the top right, digital measurements are displayed in three groups of four. Scroll through these measurements by touching the green soft pad at the top right of the measurements. O_2, V_T exhaled, MV, and f (frequency) are the most common. Pressures (Ppeak, Pplat, PEEP, and mean airway pressure) are the most common for Screen 2. End-tidal data is often placed on Screen 3.

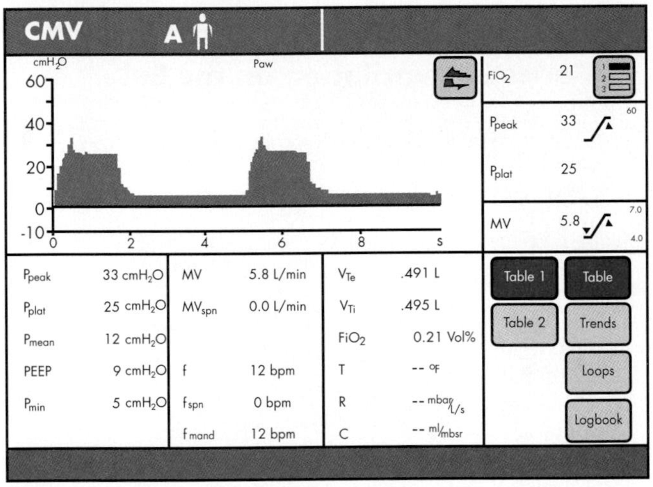

Figure 10-33 Example of a VALUES MEASURED screen on the Dräger E-4 ventilator. (Redrawn from Dräger Corp., Telford, Penn.)

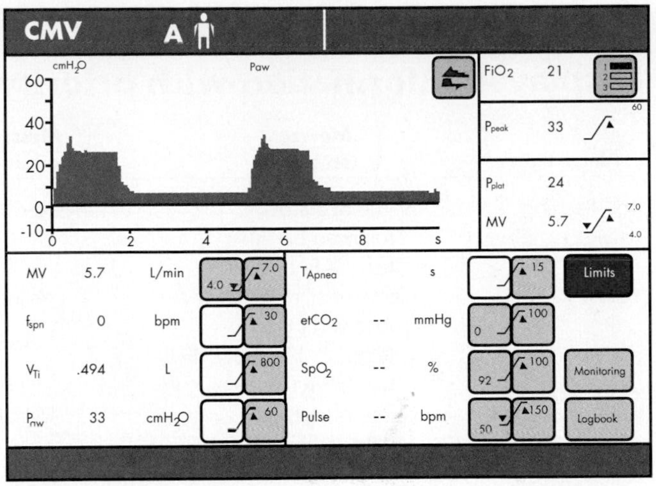

Figure 10-34 The ALARM PARAMETER screen on the Dräger E-4. (Redrawn from Dräger Corp., Telford, Penn.)

TABLE 10-6

Alarm ranges for the Dräger E-4

Parameter	Range
Minute ventilation	High MV 0.5 - 41 L/min Low MV 0 - 40 L/min
High fspn*	0 to 120 breaths/min
High V_{Ti}*	30 to 4000 mL
High Paw	10 to 100 cm H_2O
Apnea time	15 to 60 seconds
High end-tidal CO_2 ($etCO_2$)†	0 to 100 mmHg
Low $etCO_2$†	0 to 99 mmHg
Nonadjustable O_2% alarm	
O_2% <60%	upper O_2% alarm is +4% lower O_2% alarm is −4%
O_2% >60%	upper O_2% alarm is +6% lower O_2% alarm is −6%

*No lower alarm limit available.

†Only available when CO_2 analyzer (capnograph) is added.

lows zero and reference calibration of the carbon dioxide analyzer (see the operator's manual for instructions).[1]

Alarms

Alarms can be set by pressing the ALARM LIMITS soft pad, which provides a screen display allowing adjustment of the available alarm values (Figure 10-34). For example, to set the HIGH RATE alarm, touch the soft pad (cyber pad) adjacent to the respiratory rate (fspn). The soft pad changes from green to yellow. Using the rotary knob, set the desired high rate; the number appears inside the soft pad. Press the dial knob to activate the new setting; the soft pad changes back to green. Table 10-6 lists the ranges for the adjustable alarms. The limits for O_2% are automatically set by the ventilator (see Table 10-6). The automatic alarm limit for low airway pressure is the set PEEP value plus 5 cm H_2O. For example, if PEEP is 5 cm H_2O, the low pressure limit is 10 cm H_2O and is not adjustable. When the upper Paw alarm limit is reached, an audio/visual alarm is activated and inspiratory flow delivery stops and the expiratory valve opens, dropping pressure to baseline. This alarm is functional in all modes of ventilation and is similar to the upper pressure limit on most ventilators. However, the P_{PEAK} alarm is not to be confused with the Pmax pressure limit. The Pmax limit is not an alarm, but actually changes the way a breath is delivered during CMV, SIMV, and MMV ventilation. For this reason, Pmax is reviewed under the discussion of modes of ventilation.

TABLE 10-7

Displayed information with priority alarms on the Dräger E-4

Alarm light	Message* (on screen)	Message (background color)	Audio	Alarm level
Red flashing	Name of alarm followed by "!!!" (e.g., "APNEA!!!")	Red	Five tones; repeated twice every 15 seconds	Warning; top priority
Yellow flashing	Name of alarm followed by "!!" (e.g., "O_2 PRESSURE HIGH!!")	Yellow	Three tones; repeated every 30 seconds	Caution; medium priority
Yellow constant	Name of alarm followed by "!" (e.g., "FAN MALFUNCTION!!")	Yellow	Two tones; occurs only once	Advisory; low priority

*Appears in the upper right corner of the screen.

There are basically three levels of alarm indicators on the E-4, as follows:

1. WARNING (top priority)
2. CAUTION (medium priority)
3. ADVISORY (low priority)

The function of each of these is listed in Table 10-7. Once an alarm has been activated, the audible tone can be silenced with the ALARM SILENCE touch pad. The LED appears on the ALARM SILENCE pad when the audible alarms are inactive and is functional for 2 minutes. Once the problem is corrected, the alarm is turned off by touching the ALARM SILENCE soft pad (LED off). Medium- and low-priority messages do not need to be acknowledged once the problem is solved, but high-priority messages must be acknowledged by the operator to verify that the problem has been resolved by pressing the ALARM RESET touch pad. The message leaves the screen and is stored in memory. (Note that access to the LOGBOOK function is available on the ALARM LIMITS and the MEASURED VALUES screens to recall any stored, top-priority alarm messages.)

Examples of low-priority alarms include AIR SUPPLY LOW, FLOW MONITORING OFF, and INSPIRATORY HOLD INTERRUPTED. Examples of medium-priority alarms are AIR SUPPLY PRESSURE TOO HIGH, CHECK SETTINGS, and PRESSURE LIMITED. Examples of top-priority alarms are numerous. A few examples are APNEA, DEVICE FAILURE, and LOW O_2 supply. The operator's manual provides a list of all alarms.[1] After any top-priority alarm, the operator must be absolutely certain that the patient is being ventilated. (Note that when a MIXER INOP. alarm occurs, the blender is defective and the manufacturer advises that the patient be manually ventilated and the unit removed from service until repaired by a service representative.)

BOX 10-40

Modes of Ventilation on the E-4

CMV (continuous mandatory ventilation, an A/C mode)
SIMV
SIMV+PSV
PCV+
PCV + PS
PSV
APRV
MMV
MMV/PSV
Apnea ventilation
Autoflow
PPS* (proportional pressure support)
Neoflow*

*Available on the upgraded version of the Dräger E-4.

MODES OF VENTILATION

Modes of operation available on the E-4 are listed in Box 10-40.

Standard Settings of Ventilator Modes

When the ventilator is first turned on, the standard mode that is programmed (configured) is CMV (i.e., an A/C mode using volume ventilation). The institution purchasing the unit can change this by reconfiguring the unit. (To change the start-up mode, press CONFIGURE, then press the VENTILATION soft pad; enter the access code; touch MODES, select the desired start-up mode with the dial knob; and activate it by pressing the dial knob.) The operator's manual provides a full description of configuring the start-up modes and alarm settings.

If the operator wants to change the mode of ventilation, pressing the VENTILATION soft pad provides a screen that lists the available modes. When the new mode soft pad is pressed, the parameters that can be set in that mode appear on the screen, and the mode soft pad turns yellow. Parameters are set very similarly to the way in which alarm parameters are set. Touch the parameter soft knob that you want to change, V_T, for example. The soft knob changes from green to yellow. Turn the rotary knob to obtain the desired numerical value, which appears in the center of the soft knob. Then press the rotary knob to activate this setting. The old mode continues to operate until the new setting has been selected. When it is selected, the new mode soft pad changes to black. Inactive modes appear green.

The Dräger E-4 provides flow triggering in all modes of ventilation. The flow trigger level is set by performing the following:

- Touching the EXTRA SETTINGS soft pad
- Touching the FLOW TRIGGER soft pad
- Touching the FLOW soft knob
- Dialing in the desired flow triggering value using the rotary knob
- Pressing the rotary knob activate the newly set flow trigger value

Trigger sensitivity can only be turned off in CMV, but should probably never be turned off. PEEP/CPAP and O_2% can be selected in any mode. (Note that if the power fails or STANDBY is selected, the settings that were in effect before the interruption are again in effect when the unit is reactivated.)

Continuous Mandatory Ventilation (CMV)

The CMV mode is an A/C volume ventilation mode. The operator sets V_T, FLOW, f, T_I, and desired alarm settings. Breaths are patient- or time-triggered, volume-targeted, and time-cycled. All breaths deliver the set V_T. Flow to the patient is restricted to the flow setting value. If the flow is high and the V_T is delivered before T_I is achieved, the inspiratory valve closes (the expiratory valve is already closed), and the breath is held. This can be identified by an inspiratory pause pressure in the pressure/time graph and flow returning to zero on the flow/time graph (Box 10-41 and Figure 10-33). (Note that an inspiratory pause may also be identified by touching the I TIME or FLOW soft pad. When the pad is yellow, a blue "**smart window**" appears at the bottom left of the screen and displays the I:E ratio, T_E, and pause time. As the variable selected is changed, the new calculated values are displayed. For example, if the flow is decreased and T_I shortened, the pause time decreases.)

The high peak pressures that occur with volume ventilation can be avoided by using the Pmax pressure limit function. When Pmax is used, the pressure and flow delivery characteristics of the unit change (see the following discussion and Figure 10-27 and Box 10-42).

> **BOX 10-41**
>
> **Decision Making & Problem Solving**
>
> You are setting up a patient on CMV with the Dräger E-4. The settings are as follows: V_T = 0.5 L; f = 10 breaths/min; flow = 60 L/min; T_I = 2 sec; and the waveform is constant. Answer the following questions
>
> 1. What is the I:E ratio?
> 2. How long does it take the ventilator to deliver the volume?
> 3. If delivery time is shorter than the selected T_I, when does inspiration end?
>
> See Appendix A for the answers.

Pmax Pressure Limit Function

Pmax operates in CMV, SIMV, and MMV modes. To configure Pmax, access CONFIGURE, then VENTILATION; enter the access code; touch MODES, and then PMAX. When Pmax is operational, the unit will guarantee the set V_T but limit the pressure delivered during the breath. The pressure in the circuit rapidly reaches the maximum pressure setting (Pmax), inspiration continues for the set inspiratory time (time-cycled), but the amount of pressure in the circuit does not go above this setting. Flow rises rapidly at the start of inspiration, and plateaus at the set value. It remains at the set value until the set Pmax is reached, at which point flow descends, maintaining the Pmax pressure throughout T_I (see Figure 10-27). The V_T will remain constant at the set value as long as flow drops to zero before the end of inspiration (i.e., a inspiratory hold). If flow does not drop to zero for the pressure being provided by the unit, the volume cannot be delivered and a VOLUME NOT CONSTANT alarm is activated.

It is recommended that the AutoFlow be used with this and any other volume mode so that patient flow is not restricted. When AutoFlow is used, it takes over the task of setting both INSP. FLOW and PMAX, and these screen soft knob controls are no longer displayed (see the discussion of AutoFlow later in this section).

SIMV and SIMV with Pressure Support Ventilation (SIMV + PSV)

As described in Chapter 9, SIMV provides a maximum number of mandatory breaths and allows the patient to breathe spontaneously between them. Spontaneous breaths can be provided using pressure support. Mandatory

BOX 10-42

Pmax: Pressure-Limit Function

Pmax was the concept behind the first Evita ventilator. The manufacturer now believes that the Autoflow function is superior to Pmax and should be the option of choice for pressure reduction. In Pmax, you may manually adjust it to within 3 cm H_2O of the plateau. In Autoflow, the E-4 automatically brings Ppeak equal to or close to the P_{plat}, as timing allows. In Autoflow, the exhalation valve floats, but in Pmax it is closed. The manufacturer recommends that the Pmax be kept off in machine configuration.[3]

breaths can be patient- or time-triggered, volume-targeted, and time-cycled. Pressure-support breaths are described in the discussion on pressure support in this section. In the SIMV mode, Pmax or AutoFlow can also be used. The flow trigger ensures synchronous triggering of a mandatory breath with patient effort.

The function of SIMV on the E-4 is similar to its function on the Dräger Evita (see the discussion of the SIMV mode in the modes of ventilation section in the part of this chapter on the Evita).

PCV +

Pressure-control ventilation in the Dräger E-4 is referred to as PCV+ and can be set in CMV and SIMV modes. Regardless of the setting, however, the patient can breathe spontaneously between mandatory breaths, which means that the unit really always operates as SIMV. The patient can also breathe spontaneously during inspiratory flow delivery (see Figure 10-35). Mandatory breaths are patient- or time-triggered, pressure-targeted, and time-cycled.

The operator sets a minimum respiratory rate and a flow trigger. Time triggering is determined by the set rate, and patient triggering by the set flow trigger. Pressure during a mandatory breath is equal to the PINSP pressure setting.

During PCV+, the unit functions as follows. When it is time for a mandatory breath and the patient makes an inspiratory effort, a mandatory breath is delivered. During this time, the set pressure is held relatively constant, but the patient can still breathe spontaneously by receiving flow on demand (see Figure 10-35). Spontaneous breaths that occur between mandatory breaths can be assisted with pressure support by setting the desired pressure-support level (PCV + PS). An elevated baseline (PEEP/CPAP) can also be set.

The RISE TIME control is used in this mode to slow flow and pressure delivery by using the soft knob with the symbol for an ascending ramp below it on the computer screen. PRESSURE RISE is adjustable from 0 to 2 seconds and represents the amount of time it takes the ventilator to achieve the

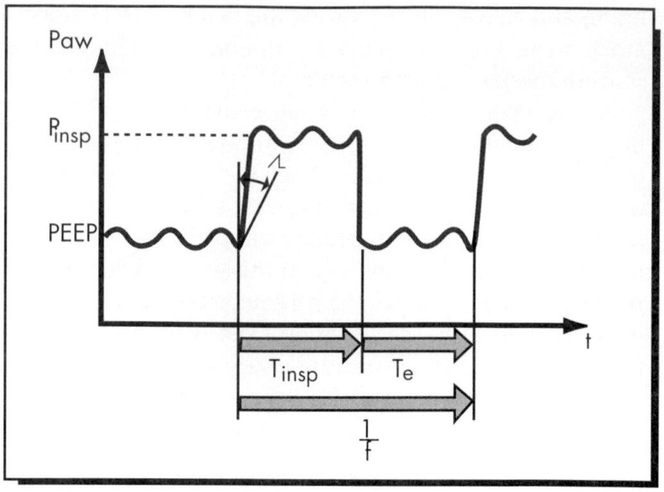

Figure 10-35 The pressure/time curve for a spontaneously breathing patient on PCV+. (*Pinsp* = inspiratory pressure setting; *Tinsp* = inspiratory time setting, and *Te* = expiratory time based on the total cycle time [TCT = 1 min/f, or 60 sec/f].)(Redrawn from Dräger Corp., Telford, Penn.)

set pressure from the beginning of inspiration. A rapid rise is appropriate for a patient with a high peak inspiratory flow. A slow rise is more appropriate for a small pediatric patient with less of a high flow demand. In most clinical settings, the default time of 0.2 seconds is adequate; it is seldom necessary to go above 0.4 seconds. If rise time is being used, it will affect both mandatory and PS breath delivery.

Because V_T and $\dot{V}_E$ may vary in this mode, the operator needs to set $\dot{V}_E$ alarm limits carefully. As with SIMV volume ventilation, apnea ventilation can be on during this mode as well, but Pmax and AutoFlow are not active during this mode because breath delivery is already pressure-targeted, and the unit controls these functions.

Pressure-Support Ventilation (PSV)

The E-4 can provide PSV during SIMV, PCV+, MMV, and spontaneous (CPAP) ventilation. The target pressure is set using the PSUPP. soft knob, which indicates the pressure above PEEP that will be delivered during a PS breath. PS breaths are patient-triggered, pressure-targeted, and flow-cycled (25% of peak for adults; 6% of peak for pediatric and neonatal settings). Patient triggering can be based on the flow trigger or the volume trigger when inspired volume exceeds 25 mL (12 mL in pediatric mode and 1 mL/32 msec for the neonatal setting)—whichever occurs first. Whenever PSV is active, the PRESSURE RISE TIME control is also functional.

If the patient actively exhales or fights the ventilator during the start of a PS breath, inspiratory flow ends. This is detected by the flow going to zero or less than zero. Inspiratory flow will also time cycle at 4 seconds (1.5 for pediatric patients, but adjustable with the T_I control in neonatal patients). Prolonged T_I most commonly occurs if a leak is present. If the time-cycling criteria occur for three consecutive breaths, an alarm is activated to warn of a possible leak in the system.

Continuous Positive Airway Pressure (CPAP)

Spontaneously breathing patients often benefit from breathing at elevated baseline pressures (CPAP), which increases functional residual capacity (FRC). CPAP is available on the E-4 and can be provided with or without PSV. Simply turn the PSV level to 0 cm H_2O using its soft knob, and set the PEEP soft knob to the desired CPAP level (cm H_2O) if you wish to use CPAP alone.

Airway Pressure-Release Ventilation (APRV)

APRV is a mode of ventilation in which two levels of CPAP are set. It operates very much like PCV+, except that the "expiratory" interval is very brief in comparison (see Figure 10-30). After selecting the APRV soft pad, the upper pressure level is set using P_{high}, and the lower level is set using P_{low}. The unit also times the length of both pressure levels. T_{high} is the length of time that high pressure is provided, and T_{low} is the length of time that low pressure is provided. Both are intended for use with spontaneously breathing patients (see Chapter 9). The RISE TIME control can be used to taper the pressure change from P_{low} to P_{high}, but the length of rise time cannot be longer than the set T_{high} time. Apnea back-up ventilation is recommended when using this mode.

Mandatory Minute Volume Ventilation (MMV) and MMV with Pressure Support (MMV/PSV)

Mandatory minute volume ventilation (MMV) is set by selecting that soft pad and then setting the MMV you want the patient to accomplish using the V_T, FLOW, f, and T_I settings. A pressure-support level should be set to ensure that the patient has adequate spontaneous V_Ts. As described in Chapter 9, with MMV the patient can breathe spontaneously and contribute all of the $\dot{V}_E$ with only PSV or CPAP with no mandatory breaths; or the patient might contribute only a portion of the $\dot{V}_E$. The difference between the spontaneous and the set $\dot{V}_E$ is provided by mandatory breaths at the set volume. Pmax or AutoFlow can be used in MMV. (Note that it is important to set the HIGH RATE alarm to protect the patient from rapid shallow breathing that would result in an equivalent $\dot{V}_E$ but would also increase work of breathing and provide an inadequate alveolar ventilation.)

Apnea Ventilation

Apnea ventilation supplies volume ventilation with a set respiratory rate and V_T in case the patient becomes apneic in any of the following modes: SIMV, PCV+, CPAP, and APRV. If the patient stops breathing for the length of time set on the APNEA ALARM control, the alarm is activated and apnea ventilation begins. To set apnea ventilation, touch the EXTRA SETTINGS soft pad, then the APNEA VENT. soft pad, and then the ON soft pad. Set the desired volume and rate using the V_{TApnea} and f_{Apnea} soft knobs on the APNEA VENTILATION screen. When these parameters are set, press the dial knob for activation. The baseline pressure, O_2%, trigger sensitivity, and other alarm parameters remain as they are in the current mode.

AutoFlow

AutoFlow is a dual mode of ventilation similar to PRVC and VS in the Servo 300 ventilator. Use of AutoFlow provides pressure-targeted breaths with volume guarantee whenever volume ventilation (CMV, SIMV, MMV) is simultaneously selected (see Chapter 9). AutoFlow also alters the function of the inspiratory and expiratory valves, allowing patients to receive whatever inspiratory flow they demand—up to 180 L/min in any volume mode regardless of the volume settings. In addition, it makes the expiratory valve more interactive with the patient. For example, if the patient coughs or breathes during the set inspiratory time of a mandatory breath, the expiratory valve system allows the patient to inhale and exhale freely while maintaining the inspiratory pressure. There is little build-up of resistance and pressure in the circuit. In AutoFlow, the circuit pressure rarely builds to the upper Paw alarm limit.

When AutoFlow is in use, the unit calculates the system compliance (C) and resistance (R) and establishes the minimum pressure needed to deliver the set volume.

To access AutoFlow, do the following:

- Select EXTRA SETTINGS on the screen
- Touch the AutoFlow ON soft pad
- Press the rotary knob to confirm that AutoFlow should be activated

In AutoFlow the unit takes over the function of PMAX PRESSURE LIMIT and INSP. FLOW, and the soft knobs are deleted from the screen. When AutoFlow is started, the ventilator delivers a volume-targeted mandatory breath and measures the plateau pressure during that breath. The plateau pressure is used as the starting ventilating pressure for AutoFlow (Figure 10-36). The unit delivers plateau pressure, measures delivered volume, and calculates system C and R. If the delivered volume is lower than the set volume, it increases pressure delivery. If the delivered volume is too high compared to the set volume, it decreases pressure delivery. Pressure change between breaths is never greater than 3 cm H_2O. Volume delivery may also be higher than the set value if the patient is actively inspiring. If the operator wants to avoid exceeding a specific V_T, the V_{Ti} UPPER LIMIT alarm can be used for this purpose. If the alarm is exceeded once, an advisory alert ("!") occurs

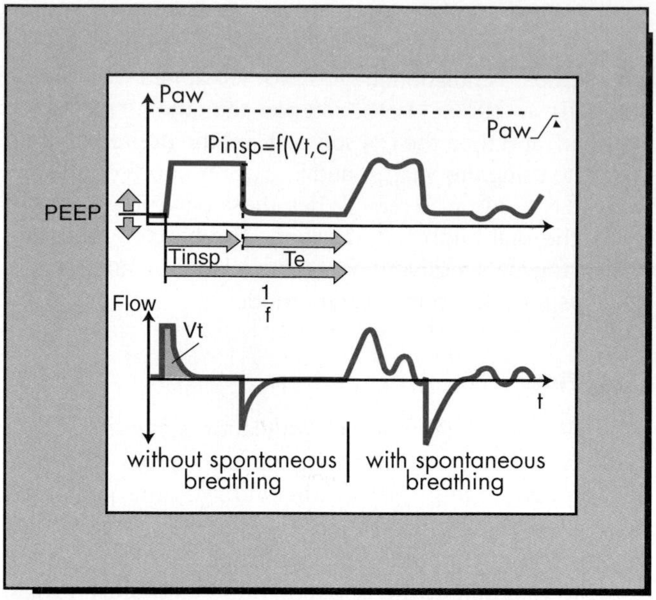

Figure 10-36 AutoFlow with a pressure-controlled, volume-guaranteed breath without spontaneous breathing (*left*). Flow drops to zero, and pressure delivery equilibrates with the pressure in the lungs. V_T has been delivered. During the second breath (*right*), the patient is spontaneously breathing during the plateau portion of the mandatory breath and afterward during the expiratory phase. (Redrawn from Dräger Corp., Telford, Penn.)

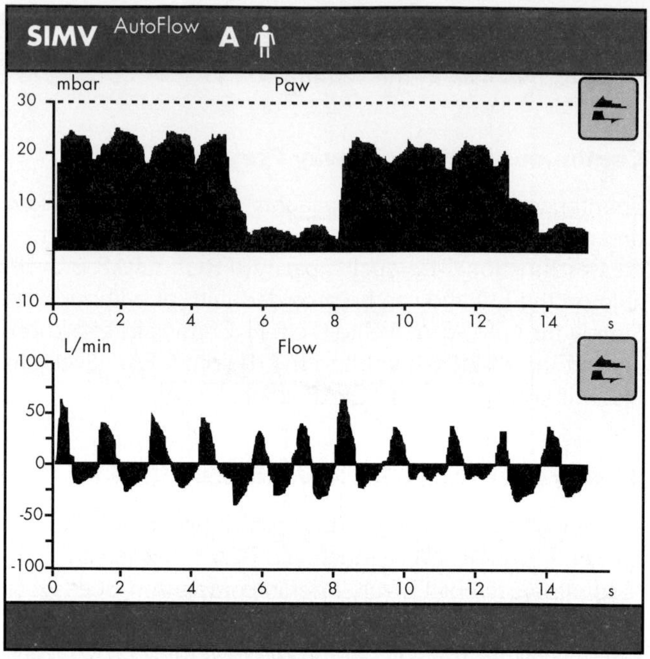

Figure 10-37 Volume-oriented SIMV with AutoFlow. Spontaneous breathing is possible in all phases. (Redrawn from Dräger Corp., Telford, Penn.)

and V_T delivery is limited. If the alarm is exceeded three times the following occurs:

1. A warning alarm is activated ("!!!," in red) with the message "exceeding $V_{ti} \times 3$."
2. V_T delivery is limited to the value of the V_{Ti} upper-limit setting for all breaths.
3. The ventilator goes into exhalation and drops airway pressure to the set baseline (set PEEP) if necessary for all breaths.

During spontaneous patient inspiratory efforts between mandatory breaths, the unit delivers whatever flow the patient demands. The patient can also breathe during the plateau phase of a mandatory breath (Figure 10-37). Inspiratory pressure is limited by the upper Paw limit setting minus 5 cm H_2O.

When AutoFlow is used, there are several types of breath patterns that can occur, as follows:

1. If V_T is delivered and flow drops to zero before the unit time-cycles out of a mandatory inspiration, the ventilator ensures that the patient can breathe spontaneously during the remaining inspiratory time. During this time, however, the pressure being delivered by the unit is maintained.
2. If the patient breathes in and out during a mandatory breath, the plateau delivery stays constant and does not fluctuate significantly. Flow is provided as needed to meet patient demand. The expiratory valve opens during spontaneous exhalation to avoid pressure build-up and resistance to exhalation while still maintaining plateau pressure (Figure 10-38).
3. If inspiration ends before flow drops to zero, the volume will be delivered, but the pressure may be higher than the true plateau. The unit may have to step up pressure and flow to deliver V_T in a short T_I. The clinician may want to increase T_I to decrease pressure, but sometimes the pressure does not decrease (Box 10-43).[3]

It is strongly recommended that AutoFlow be activated whenever a spontaneously breathing patient is being ventilated—regardless of the volume mode chosen, CMV, SIMV, and MMV.

Proportional Pressure Support (PPS)[4]

Proportional pressure support (PPS) is a proportional assist ventilation mode (described in Chapter 9) that is available on the upgrade of the Evita-4 ventilator (Software version 2.n). (Note that the company is currently awaiting FDA approval of PPS, but it is expected soon.) PPS provides a positive feedback system of respiration; that is, the more patients inspire, the more pressure they receive. The amount of pressure provided is based on the volume assist and flow assist set by the operator, which will be explained later in this section.

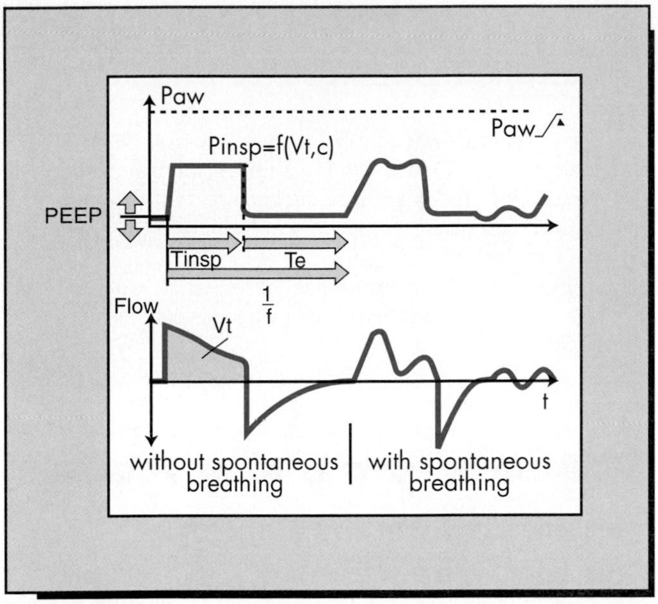

Figure 10-38 AutoFlow with a pressure-control breath in which flow does not drop to zero before inspiration ends. The set pressure does not equilibrate with the lungs. V_T delivery is lower because T_I was not long enough to deliver the pressure. Remember that this pressure is calculated to be what is required based on system C and R to deliver the set V_T. (Redrawn from Dräger Corp., Telford, Penn.)

Key things to remember with PPS include the following:

1. There is no support if there is no inspiratory effort from the patient. Therefore the patient must have an adequate inspiratory effort and ventilatory drive.
2. It is important to set MINIMUM $\dot{V}_E$ and APNEA alarms, as well as APNEA BACK-UP VENTILATION in case the patient quits breathing. UPPER PAW and UPPER V_T alarm limits are also set to protect against high pressures and volumes.
3. This is a positive-feedback system. The more actively patients inspire, the more assistance they receive from the unit, and vice-versa.
4. There must be no leaks in the system (cuffs, connections, or bronchopleural).

When inspiration is strong during PPS, the unit supports the patient with a high pressure. With shallow, less forceful breaths, the unit provides a lower pressure. The amount of assistance provided during PPS is separated into the elastic (compliance) and the resistive components. Using VOL ASSIST, the operator decides how much work the unit will support for the elastic portion of the work of breathing. Using FLOW ASSIST, the operator determines how much work is provided by the unit to overcome resistive work.

To set PPS, the operator should perform the following procedure:

- Touch the PPS soft pad on the ventilator screen (standard screen for setting up ventilator modes)
- Touch the VOL ASSIST soft knob

BOX 10-43

Decision Making & Problem Solving

A patient on AutoFlow has the following ventilator settings and monitored parameters: mode = SIMV; V_T (set) = 0.65 L; f = 12 breaths/min; inspiratory pressure = 20 cm H_2O; T_I = 2 seconds; upper pressure limit = 30 cm H_2O.

The patient has done well on these settings for the past 4 hours. During the next hour, however, the respiratory therapist notices that inspiratory pause time (i.e., time when flow is zero) has become progressively shorter, and eventually there is no pause. Flow never goes to zero before the end of inspiration; inspiratory pressure is now 25 cm H_2O. What do you think the therapist should do in this situation?

See Appendix A for one possible answer.

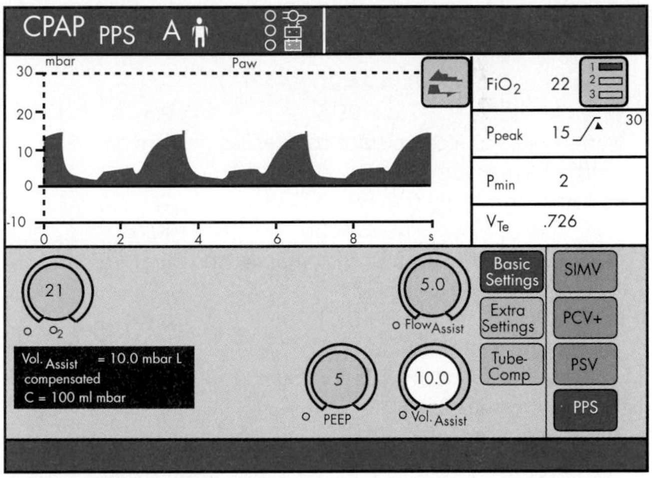

Figure 10-39 The screen during PPS on the Drager Evita 4 (version 2.n). (Redrawn from Dräger Corp., Telford, Penn.)

- Set the desired value using the dial knob
- Press the dial knob for activation
- Touch the FLOW ASSIST soft knob and set the desired value using the dial knob (Figure 10-39)
- Press the dial knob for activation

The range of values for volume assist and flow assist are listed in Table 10-8. For example, if 10 cm H_2O/L is set, the unit compensates for the elastic work of breathing with a compliance of 100 mL/cm H_2O (Box 10-44). If 5 cm H_2O/L/sec is set for the flow assist, the unit will compensate for a resistance of 5 cm H_2O/L/sec (see Box 10-44). The ventilator calculates the amount of airway pressure it needs to provide for both the volume and flow assist portions of the breath.

PPS has the following limits: maximum Paw is equal to the upper Paw alarm limit minus 5 cm H_2O; maximum inspiratory V_T is equal to the upper alarm limit for V_{Ti};

TABLE 10-8

Proportional pressure support ranges of available settings on the E-4 with upgrade (version 2.n)

	Flow assist (cm H_2O/L/sec)	Increment (cm H_2O/L/sec)
Adult	0 to 30	0.5
(corresponds to a resistance compensation of 0 to 30 cm H_2O/L/sec)		
Pediatric	0 to 30	0.5
	30 to 100	5.0
(corresponds to a resistance compensation of 0 to 100 cm H_2O/L/sec)		
Neonatal	0 to 30	0.5
	30 to 300	5.0
(corresponds to a resistance compensation of 0 to 300 cm H_2O/L/sec)		

	Volume assist (cm H_2O/L)	Increment (cm H_2O/L)
Adult	0 to 24.9	0.1
	25 to 99.5	0.5
(corresponds to a compliance compensation of infinity to 10 mL/cm H_2O)		
Pediatric	0 to 99	1.0
	100 to 1000	10.0
(corresponds to a compliance compensation of infinity to 1 mL/cm H_2O)		
Neonatal	0 to 30	0.5
	30 to 300	5.0
(corresponds to a compliance compensation of infinity to 0.5 mL/cm H_2O)		

maximum T_I is limited to 4 seconds (1.5 seconds in pediatric patients; the neonatal setting is adjusted by the clinician with the T_I control [E-4 with Neoflow]). This is a new mode of ventilation in the United States, so its effectiveness will be evaluated as the results of its use in clinical studies are made available.

Neoflow[5,6]

Neoflow is an upgraded mode of ventilation that has been added to the Evita 4 ventilator, which allows it to be adapted for neonatal use (patient weight from 0.5 to 6 kg). Neoflow requires the installation of a flow sensor that attaches to the wye connector of the patient circuit, between the end of the endotracheal tube and the wye connector of the patient circuit. The other end is attached to the back of the ventilator unit. The flow sensor must be calibrated when first used and then at least once every 24 hours (see the operator's manual).

BOX 10-44

Calculating Compliance with PPS

The setting for volume assist is a pressure/volume measurement of elastance (cm H_2O/L). It is the inverse of compliance. In this example, if elastance = 10 cm H_2O/L; compliance = 1 L/10 cm H_2O, or 0.1 L/cm H_2O, or 100 mL/cm H_2O.

Flow assist is a measurement of resistance, where $R = \Delta P/\text{flow}$. The setting for flow assist is cm H_2O/(L/sec).

TABLE 10-9

Specifications for Neoflow on the Dräger E-4

Parameter	Range
Frequency	0 to 150 breaths/min
V_T (inspiratory)	3 to 100 (max 2000) mL
Inspiratory pressure	0 to 80 cm H_2O
PEEP/CPAP	0 to 35 cm H_2O
PCV	0 to 80 cm H_2O
Trigger	0.3 to 15 L/min

When the unit is turned on and the screen displays the stand-by mode, the operator selects the NEO. soft pad for neonatal ventilation. In the neonatal mode, the unit can provide volume ventilation; AutoFlow; apnea back-up ventilation; pressure support with assisted spontaneous breathing (ASB); continuous base flow; and measurements of circuit leaks, airway pressure, and breath triggering (Table 10-9).

Flow Monitoring During Neonatal Ventilation

The addition of the flow sensor allows flow monitoring at the airway during neonatal ventilation. The unit is still functional if the sensor fails and cannot be replaced immediately. The flow sensor can be deactivated if a large leak is present. If flow monitoring is deactivated, however, neither volume ventilation nor patient-triggered breaths are possible. $\dot{V}_E$ cannot be monitored without the neonatal flow sensor.

Continuous Base Flow in Neonates

With the addition of Neoflow, the Evita 4 offers a continuous base flow of 6 L/min. Because the flow is continuous, the infant has the opportunity to obtain flow on demand. As soon as the patient begins inspiration, the unit delivers additional flow to maintain the baseline, thus keeping flow compatible with the patient's needs.

Measurement of Leakage Flow in Neonatal Ventilation

The leakage flow that normally occurs around uncuffed endotracheal tubes in infants can be monitored with the flow sensor of the Evita 4 ventilator. The unit displays minute ventilation leakage (MVleak) on the front of the unit. MVleak represents the difference between inspiratory and expiratory flow averaged over time and displayed as a percentage of the delivered inspired minute volume. The unit assumes that any gas that does not flow back through the sensor from the patient must have escaped through a leak around the endotracheal tube and out through the patient's upper airway. The unit automatically corrects V_T (inspiratory and expiratory) and flow values based on its calculation of the leak.

Trigger Response in Neonates

The neonatal flow sensor detects the patient's inspiratory effort and is responsible for triggering any assisted breaths or patient-initiated gas flow from the unit. To avoid incorrect triggering due to leaks around the endotracheal tube, the E-4 takes into account the flow sensor signal (inspiratory flow) and the calculated leakage flow (MVleak). A trigger range of 0.3 to 3 L/min is recommended for neonatal ventilation.

AutoFlow in Neonates

Autoflow as a volume entity with the Evita 4 is only available in neonates with the flow sensor. When the sensor is attached, Autoflow is always active in CMV, SIMV, and MMV modes. Without the sensor, the ventilator will not volume ventilate, but will provide time-cycled, pressure-targeted ventilation and allow for spontaneous breathing throughout inspiration and expiration.

It is important to set the UPPER PAW ALARM limit so that if the patient's lung characteristics change or there is a sudden change in leakage, the patient will be protected from high pressures. When Autoflow is initiated in neonates with the flow sensor attached, the unit provides two test breaths, first with a Paw of +5 cm H_2O and then with a Paw equal to 75% of that required to deliver the set volume. The third breath is at a pressure determined to be appropriate to achieve the set V_T.

Volume Ventilation in Neonates

Volume ventilation can be provided with CMV, SIMV, and MMV modes. When these are selected, AutoFlow is automatically active, allowing the patient to breathe spontaneously at any time.

Apnea Ventilation in Neonates

As in adult ventilation, the operator selects an apnea time. If this time is exceeded, an alarm is activated, and the ventilator switches to back-up ventilation. Unlike adult or pediatric back-up ventilation, apnea ventilation in the neonatal mode is pressure-controlled ventilation. The operator selects apnea frequency (f_{Apnea}) and pressure above PEEP (P_{Apnea}). The I:E ratio is fixed at 1:2, and the FiO_2 and PEEP levels remain the same.

The unit will also switch to back-up ventilation if a volume ventilation mode is in use and the flow monitor is either switched off or fails to monitor flow. In this situation, the pressure applied is the last mean pressure measured during a mandatory breath. T_I, f, O_2%, and PEEP remain the same.

Pressure Support (PS), or Assisted Spontaneous Breathing (ASB) in Neonates

Pressure support is also referred to as assisted spontaneous breathing (ASB) in some of the Dräger literature. As with adult and pediatric ventilation, PS is available with SIMV, MMV, and PCV+ modes, as well as for strictly spontaneous breathing. The pressure rise control is also operational. Maximum inspiratory time should also be set when using PS.

SPECIAL FUNCTIONS

There are a variety of features on the Dräger E-4, some of which are similar to other ICU ventilators and others that are unique to this unit. These functions are reviewed here.

Sigh (Intermittent PEEP)

The E-4 provides sigh breaths in a format similar to the Evita. Sigh breaths are accomplished by increasing PEEP in the CMV mode. As with a sigh breath, the intended purpose of intermittent PEEP is to open up or keep areas of the lung likely to become atelectatic open. PEEP is increased to the set cm H_2O selected by the operator, which is added to the set PEEP for two breaths every 3 minutes (see Figure 10-25). Intermittent PEEP can be selected by touching the EXTRA SETTING soft pad on the screen and is set like other parameters. During the sigh interval, the VOLUME NOT CONSTANT alarm is deactivated. Because intermittent PEEP increases the baseline, it is advisable to appropriately set the Pmax pressure limit to avoid overdistention of the lungs during regular breath delivery (see Figure 10-25).

Intrinsic PEEP

An estimate of the amount of auto-PEEP as well as an estimate of the trapped volume in a patient can be determined by using the intrinsic PEEP (PEEPi) function. These measurements can only be performed as long as no patient activity occurs during the measurement.

To perform an auto-PEEP measurement, select the SPECIAL PROCEDURE touch pad. From the computer screen, touch the PEEPi soft pad. The maneuver is performed automatically, and the waveform display is frozen. On the screen, values for PEEP(set), PEEPi, and trapped volume (Vtrap) are shown. Using the dial knob and the screen cursor, you can select to view the auto-PEEP level at any time on the graph of pressure/time. The PEEPi values appear above the waveform.

Occlusion Pressure

Measurements of occlusion pressure ($P_{0.1}$) are used to evaluate a patient's neuromuscular drive.[5] At the beginning of inspiration, the ventilator occludes the inspiratory and expiratory valves at 0.1 second after the beginning of inspiratory flow. The pressure measured at that time is displayed. This procedure can be automatically performed by selecting the SPECIAL PROCEDURES touch pad, the $P_{0.1}$ soft pad, and the START soft pad. The value for occlusion pressure is shown on the screen. The normal value is from −3 to −4 cm H_2O. Values below −6 cm H_2O may indicate impending exhaustion and respiratory muscle fatigue that may lead to respiratory failure in patients with chronic obstructive pulmonary disease (COPD). As with PEEPi, the waveform is frozen on the screen. Using the rotary knob and screen cursor the specific value for pressure from the pressure/time curve can be viewed at precise moments during the maneuver.

Special-Function Touch Pads

As mentioned previously, there is a set of touch pads to the left of the screen on the front panel of the E-4. Their function is explained here.

Neb Touch Pad

The nebulizer touch pad (NEB) switches on the nebulizer gas source and functions during adult ventilation only. Gas only flows through the nebulizer outlet during inspiration and automatically maintains the set $\dot{V}_E$ and approximates the set O_2%.

When the nebulizer is activated, the LED on the touch pad appears with a screen message: "Nebulizer on." The nebulizer continues to operate for 30 minutes or until the pad is touched again. Following its use, a "flow calibration" message appears, showing that the nebulizer is off and the flow transducer is being automatically cleaned and recalibrated to preserve accuracy (Box 10-45).

The expiratory flow sensor is a heated wire (see Chapter 7). To protect the sensor during the use of nebulized medications, a filter placed in-line before the sensor may be helpful.

Suction 100% O_2

The SUCTION 100% O_2 touch pad is used to provide 100% O_2 for 3 minutes. When pressed, the LED on the pad is lit and the message "O_2 enrichment 180 s" appears at the bottom of the screen. The SUCTION 100% O_2 control functions similarly to that on the Evita (see the discussion of this function in the section on the Evita). During the 3-minute suction interval, the LOW $\dot{V}_E$ alarm is turned off (Box 10-46). For 2 minutes thereafter, 100% O_2 is provided and the alarms are reactivated. (Note that if the patient is not disconnected after the 100% O_2 control is activated, you must touch the pad again to reactivate the alarm, or an undetected disconnect may occur.)

Inspir Hold

The INSPIR HOLD touch pad provides an inflation hold maneuver when pressed and held down for as long as the inspiratory pause is desired (maximum of 15 seconds). When activated, either the current inspiration is held, or a new mandatory breath is delivered and the inspiration is held. It functions in all modes except CPAP if a pressure support level is not set.

BOX 10-45

Clinical Note: Caution During Nebulization

1. Do not use a heat moisture exchanger (HME) during nebulization because it reduces medication delivery and may increase airway resistance by depositing medication on the HME.
2. Do not use filters on the nebulizer outlet because they may increase resistance and impair ventilation.

BOX 10-46

Decision Making & Problem Solving

Clinical note on suctioning:

1. If the patient is not disconnected after the SUCTION 100% O_2 pad is pressed, the unit continues to ventilate the patient in the set mode but uses 100% O_2. After 3 minutes, the O_2 program is terminated and the alarms are reactivated.
2. To stop "suction 100% O_2", press the pad again. The LED will flash for 15 seconds and normal operation resumes. The oxygen enrichment cannot be restarted until the flashing stops.

Some institutions use closed-suction catheter systems and do not disconnect the patient prior to suctioning. Do you think that the clinician should still disconnect the patient to activate the oxygen enrichment function?

See Appendix A for comment.

Print

The PRINT function allows the microprocessor to print if a compatible printer is attached.

Special Upgrades with Software Update 2.n

The Dräger E-4 has a software update version 2.n that includes the following few special features.

Compliance Compensation

The E-4 now provides compensation for volume lost due to tubing compressibility. The unit adds the volume needed to compensate for the volume lost and subtracts this added volume from the measured expiratory volume to give a close measurement of the volume actually exhaled by the patient. The resistance and compliance of the patient circuit are determined when the patient circuit is changed (stand-by mode) with the AIRTIGHT CHECK soft pad.

Support During Hose Change

When a patient circuit is changed, it is possible for the ventilator to check the hose for leaks by using the stand-by mode (selecting the AIRTIGHT CHECK soft pad). In addition, the resistance and compliance of the circuit are also measured in order to provide compliance compensation for the volume lost due to tubing compliance (see the previous discussion of compliance compensation).

Automatic Tubing Compensation (ATC)

As a part of the breathing support package (software update version 2.n), an automatic tube compensation (ATC) feature has been added to the E-4 to compensate for the airway resistance associated with small artificial airways. ATC can be used with the PPS mode of ventilation, as well as with all other modes of ventilation. In CMV, SIMV, and MMV, tube compensation is active during expiration after a mandatory breath and during spontaneous breathing phases.

This ventilator function regulates airway pressure at the tracheal level (Box 10-47). When it is selected, the ventilating pressure during all breaths compensates for the resistance associated with varying size endotracheal tubes. This compensation depends on the direction of air flow. The airway pressure is increased during inspiration and decreased during expiration. (Note that the expiratory portion can be switched off if the operator only wants to compensate for the inspiratory portion.) The pressure can be increased to a value equal to the upper Paw alarm limit minus 5 cm H_2O or reduced to a minimum of 0 cm H_2O.

To set the tube compensation function, the following should be performed:

1. During stand-by, select the TUBE COMP. soft pad.
2. Touch either the ET TUBE or the TRACH. TUBE soft pad, depending on the type of artificial airway in use.
3. Use the ID 0 soft knob to set the size of the tube's inner diameter (with the dial knob) and confirm it by pressing the dial knob.
4. Use the COMP. soft knob and the dial knob to set the percentage of compensation provided. For example, a reading of "70" inside the COMP. soft knob provides 70% compensation for the artificial airway.

BOX 10-47

Calculation of the Tracheal Pressure on the Evita-4 Upgrade (version 2.n)

The Dräger E-4 (2.n software version) calculates and displays tracheal pressure based on a mathematical equation

$$P_{trachea} = Paw - K_{tube} \times Flow^2$$

where $P_{trachea}$ is the pressure in the trachea, *Paw* is the pressure at the wye connector of the patient circuit, K_{tube} is the tube coefficient (listed in the operating manual), and *Flow* is the patient flow (inspiratory flow is >0, and expiratory flow is <0). An example of a tube coefficient is 6.57 cm $H_2O/L^2/seconds^2$ for an endotracheal tube with an inner diameter (ID) of 8.0 mm.

For pressure support the equation is as follows:

$$\Delta Paw = Comp. \times K_{tube} \times Flow^2$$

where ΔPaw = pressure support at the tube, *Comp.* = degree of compensation (0% to 100%), K_{tube} = tube coefficient, and *Flow* is patient flow.

VENTILATOR GRAPHIC WAVEFORMS

The graphics monitor with the E-4 is part of the main computer screen during standard operation. Additional waveforms can be viewed simultaneously, and different waveforms may be displayed during its normal function (see Box 10-39; Box 10-48). Timed graphics can be frozen by pressing the FREEZE touch pad on the right side of the unit's front panel. A more specific measured numerical value for a given time on any graph can be viewed by positioning the cursor on the computer screen and rotating the dial knob to the desired time on the curve. The value is shown on the screen above the waveform. The graph can be unfrozen by pressing FREEZE a second time.

The E-4 can also display trends of data. Select MEASURED VALUES and then TRENDS. In this setting, you can "zoom in" or "zoom out" to narrow or widen the time frame for the data trend by selecting those soft pads. Again, you can change the parameters being viewed or trended by touching the waveform icon. This function can also be analyzed by using the cursor with a link to the logbook.

BOX 10-48

Waveform Display on the Dräger E-4

1. Select the STANDARD PAGE computer screen by pressing the MAIN SCREEN touch pad. In the right field, four measured values are displayed. In the left field, two waveforms are displayed.
2. To select waveforms, touch the icon on the computer screen at the top right of the waveform area that looks like two tiny waveforms (Figure 10-31). Touch the screen key that indicates the waveform you desire.
3. To select loops, touch the VALUES MEASURED touch pad. The computer screen displays several selections on the lower right corner. Touch the LOOPS soft pad on the screen. Two different loops appear on the lower left part of the screen. To change the loop parameters, touch the waveform icon between them.

TROUBLESHOOTING

The alarms and monitored information sections offer a great deal of assistance for solving the majority of problems that might occur with the E-4. In addition, the operator's manual contains a troubleshooting section that alphabetically lists all the alarm messages, gives their priority level, provides common causes, and recommends remedies. For additional information of Dräger products check their web site: www.draeger.com.

Review Questions

(See Appendix A for answers.)

1. Proportional pressure support (PPS) is similar to which one of the following modes of ventilation described in Chapter 9?
   a. airway pressure-release ventilation
   b. pressure-regulated volume control ventilation
   c. pressure-support ventilation
   d. proportional assist ventilation
2. AutoFlow on the E-4 is similar to which mode on the Servo 300?
   a. PRVC
   b. pressure augment
   c. APRV
   d. VAPS
3. When the patient actively inspires during proportional pressure support, the E-4:
   a. increases its support
   b. maintains a constant pressure
   c. slows flow delivery
   d. allows the patient to breathe spontaneously from a steady baseline pressure
4. Which of the following are accurate descriptions of the function of AutoFlow?
   I. AutoFlow allows spontaneous inspiratory flows up to 180 L/min.
   II. AutoFlow regulates inspiratory pressure delivery to achieve the set V_T.
   III. AutoFlow fixes flow delivery at the set flow value.
   IV. It allows the patient to cough without significant build-up of pressure in the circuit.
   a. I only
   b. II only
   c. II and III only
   d. I, II, and IV only
5. During PCV+ ventilation with the E-4, the patient can breathe spontaneously at any time during a mandatory breath, even during the expiratory portion of the breath—true or false?
6. The Pmax pressure limit function of the E-4 is an upper airway pressure alarm—true or false?
7. The function of Neoflow on the E-4 is to provide flow triggering—true or false?
8. Describe the controls on the front panel of the Dräger E-4 ventilator.
9. Explain how to change the numerical value for a parameter, such as V_T, with the E-4.
10. An audible 5-tone alarm is heard, and a red area is present at the top right corner of the E-4 computer screen. Inside the red area is a message that reads "High frequency!!!" What priority level is this alarm, and what does it indicate?

References

1. Evita 4: Intensive care ventilation operating instructions 90 28 676-GA 5664.510, ed 1, Telford, Penn., 1996, Dräger, Inc., Drägerwerk AG.
2. Pilbeam SP: Mechanical ventilation: physiological and clinical applications, ed 3, St Louis, 1998, Mosby.
3. Lear, GF: Personal communication, August 1998.
4. Breathing support package proportional pressure support PPS, tube compensation, ATC, supplement to the instructions for use of the Evita 4 as from Software version 2.n 90 28 825-GA 5664.520 e, ed 1, Telford, Penn., 1996, Dräger, Inc., Drägerwerk AG.
5. E-4 plus option NeoFlow NI 5664.515e/117D, Telford, Penn., 1997, Dräger, Inc.
6. NeoFlow: neonatal mode, supplement to the instructions for use of the Evita 4 as from software version 2.n ED 2077947.97, ed 2, Telford, Penn., 1997, Dräger, Inc., Drägerwerk AG.

Dräger Evita 2 Dura

OUTLINE

LEARNING OBJECTIVES

Upon completion of this section, the reader should be able to:

1. Discuss the function of each control on the front panel of the Dräger Evita 2 Dura.
2. Compare the set-up of a ventilator mode on the Dräger Evita 2 Dura to that on the E-4.
3. Assess an alarm situation, describe its priority level, and suggest a possible cause and solution.
4. Describe the special functions available on the Dura.
5. Compare and contrast the modes on the Dräger Evita 2 Dura.

The Dräger Evita 2 Dura[1] is a modification of the Evita 2, a ventilator that was never marketed in the United States. The Evita 2 Dura is another in a series of three ventilators that includes the Evita and the E-4. All are manufactured by Drägerwerk in Lubeck, Germany and represented in the United States by the Dräger corporation, although these units will soon be manufactured in the United States. There are a number of similarities between the units that will be mentioned as they are described.

The front panel is divided into two main sections (Figure 10-40). The right side contains a majority of the ventilator settings touch pads and a primary control knob, which is called the dial knob. Settings are displayed in individual LCD windows in this section. The left side contains a screen. The Evita 2 Dura uses either a high-contrast black and white or an optional color computer (LCD) screen. Although similar to the E-4, the Evita 2 Dura has a larger number of touch pads on the front panel. There are images or icons on the computer screen. All of the dials and knobs used to control the unit are discussed later in this section.

Below the front operating panel are the connections for the main inspiratory and expiratory lines, the expiratory valve, and the nipple connector for the nebulizer line (see Figure 10-40). The expiratory flow sensor is to the left of the expiratory valve. On the far right side, below the unit's main control knob (dial knob), is a cover that protects the oxygen sensor and the ambient air filter.

POWER SOURCE

The Evita 2 Dura normally uses air and oxygen at high pressure (ranging from about 40 to 87 psig) as pneumatic power sources. A standard AC 120-volt outlet is used to power the microprocessor and electrical components. The unit can also operate with a single gas source, such as an air compressor; but this will alter the oxygen delivery capabilities. The ON/OFF switch is on the back panel of the unit.

INTERNAL MECHANISM

The Evita 2 Dura has the same internal pneumatic components as the Evita 4 (see the discussion of internal mechanisms in the section on the E-4).

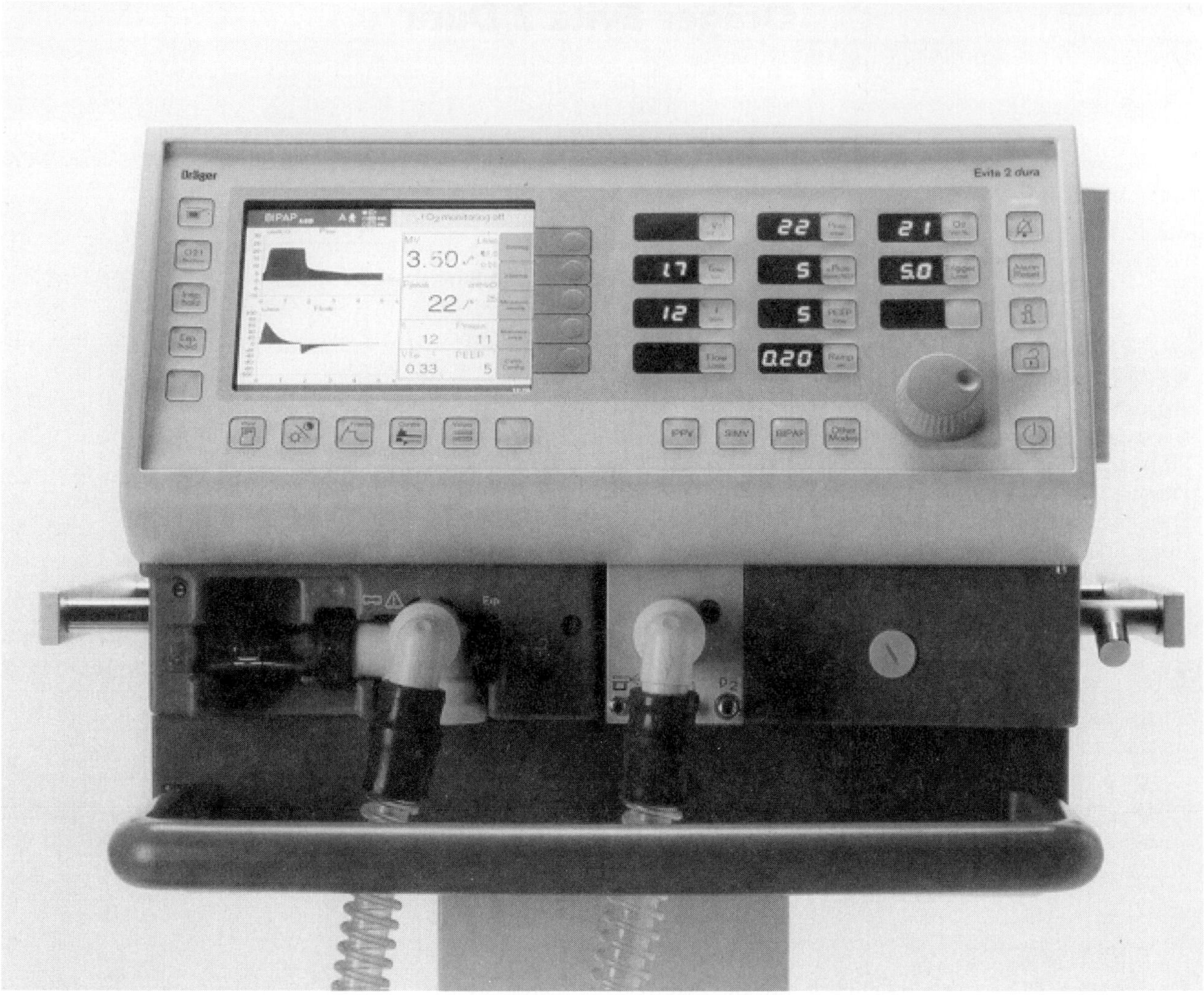

Figure 10-40 The Evita 2 Dura. (Redrawn from Dräger Corp., Telford, Penn.)

Controls and Alarms

The controls, monitors, and alarms are similar to those on the E-4. The Evita 2 Dura uses a single control knob or dial knob, several hard touch pads alongside the computer screen, and the touch-sensitive soft knobs and soft pads of the computer screen (see Figure 10-40).

Peripheral Controls

Several controls used during the normal operation of the ventilator are located around the screen (see Figure 10-40 and Figure 10-41). Those to the left of the screen include the NEBULIZER, SUCTION 100% O_2 ENRICHMENT, and INSPIRATORY and EXPIRATORY HOLD. These are reviewed under the discussion of special functions in this section.

Below the computer screen are the following controls:

1. PRINTER to print material when the unit is attached to a compatible printer.
2. A touch pad with a symbol of a sun and new moon to set the screen backlighting bright or dark.
3. FREEZE screen touch pad for freezing waveforms.
4. WAVES key with symbols of waves on the touch pad to display a different pair of waveforms.
5. VALUES touch pad for displaying different combinations of measured values.
6. Blank touch pads for future use.

To the immediate right of the computer screen is a column of keys touching the side of the screen. When a menu screen appears, a column of items appears adjacent to these touch pads on the right of the screen. For example, Figure 10-42 shows the following list in the currently active screen: settings, alarms, measurements, maneuvers, and calibration configuration. The operator can touch MEASUREMENT, for example, and the unit will display a screen of all measured values in the current mode. Box 10-49 lists the specific functions for these touch pad controls.

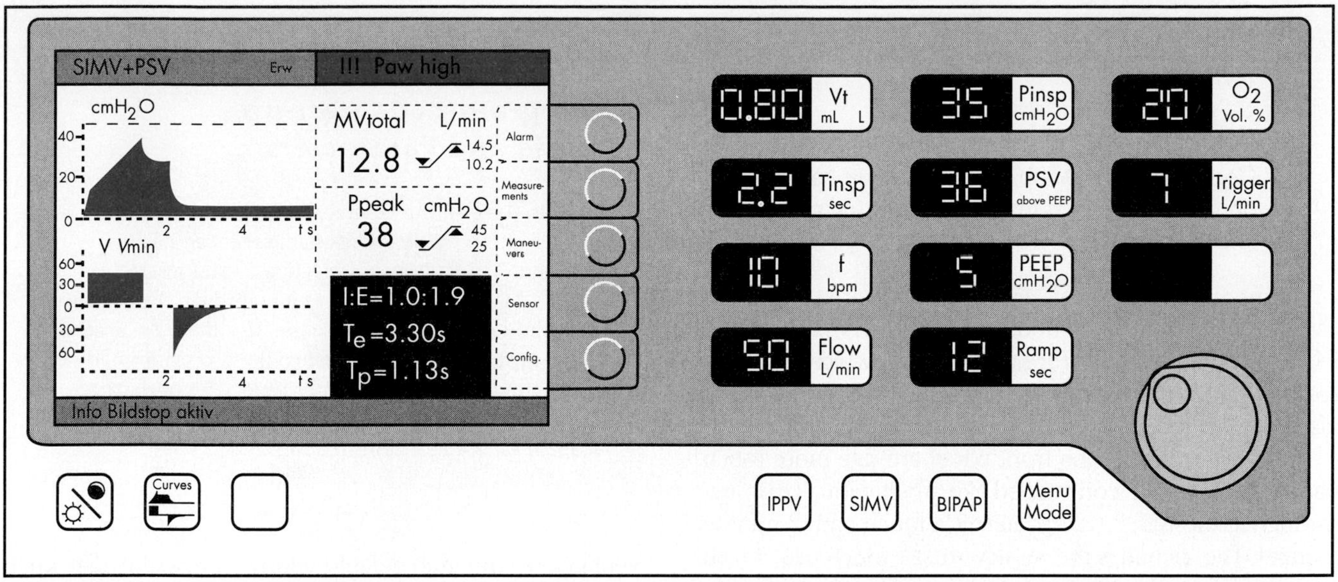

Figure 10-41 The front panel of the Dura, showing a typical monitoring screen and digital displays of the set parameters. (Redrawn from Dräger Corp., Telford, Penn.)

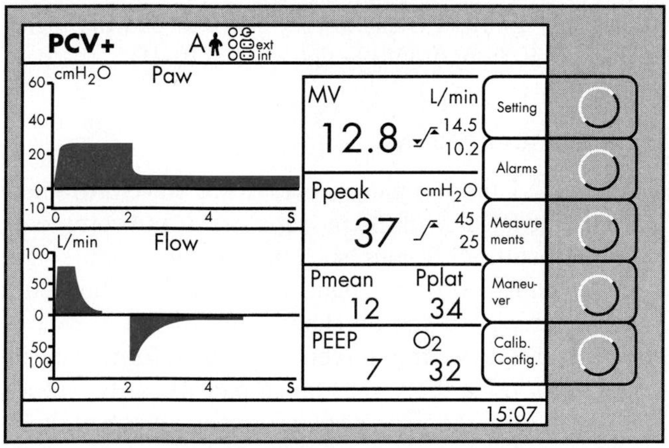

Figure 10-42 A close-up of the monitoring screen, showing the touch pads adjacent to the right side of the screen. (Redrawn from Dräger Corp., Telford, Penn.)

To the right of the screen and its adjacent keys are three columns of touch pads used to adjust several parameters (see Figure 10-41). These pads include the following:

1. Tidal volume (V_T; in milliliters or liters)
2. Inspiratory time (T_{insp}; in seconds)
3. Respiratory rate (f; in breaths/minute)
4. Flow (in liters/minute)
5. Inspiratory pressure (P_{insp}; in centimeters of water), for the pressure-control mode
6. Pressure support (P_{supp} above PEEP; in centimeters of water)
7. PEEP (in centimeters of water)
8. Pressure rise time (Ramp; ranges from 0.0 to 2.0 seconds), which adjusts the rate of rise in pressure

BOX 10-49

The Specifications for the Menu Keys at the Right Edge of the Evita 2 Dura Screen

ADDITIONAL SETTINGS is used for:

- Programming the OTHER MODES touch pad with one of the following available modes: CPAP/PSV, MMV, or other added options.
- Setting back-up ventilation parameters.
- Setting intermittent PEEP and the sigh control available during CMV ventilation.

ALARMS is used for:

- Displaying measured values with their alarm limits.
- Setting alarm limits.

MEASURED VALUES is used for displaying all measured values in the current mode. OPTIONS allows for the selection of lung mechanics maneuvers, loops, and any optional or additional controls added to the unit.

CALIBRATION/CONFIGURATION allows the following functions to be performed:

- Automatic calibration of O_2 or flow sensors.
- Turning monitor functions on/off.
- Setting audible alarm volume, screen contrast, date and time, language, measurement units, and configuring external interfaces under VENTILATOR.
- Selecting two of the six available measured values for display.
- Selecting two sets of waveforms for display.
- Setting the default start-up ventilator parameters, alarm limits, and mode.

at the beginning of a breath and is active for breaths during PCV+ and PS and when Autoflow is on

9. Oxygen percent (O_2%)
10. Trigger sensitivity (Trigger; in liters/minute)
11. Control or dial knob, which can be rotated and pressed to select numerical values for parameters and activate the new parameters, respectively

Immediately below this area are four more touch pads used to select ventilator mode screens (CMV, SIMV, and PCV+) and a touch pad for MENU MODE, which brings up a menu screen. The ventilator modes are explained in the discussion of modes of ventilation later in this section.

To the far right of the front panel are five more touch pads. The first is an icon shaped like a bell with a cross line through it; this is the ALARM SILENCE touch pad (2-minute silence). The second is the ALARM RESET touch pad, which resets or acknowledges alarm messages. The third is the information key, i. The fourth touch pad is a lock-shaped icon that can lock the controls to prevent inadvertent or unauthorized changing of ventilator settings. The fifth touch pad allows the unit to be placed in the standby mode. To place the unit in standby and stop ventilation, press and hold down the STANDBY touch pad for about 3 seconds, then press the ALARM RESET pad. To switch back to ventilation, press and release the STANDBY touch pad.

System Tests and Calibration

Before the unit is turned on and connected to a patient, a series of tests and calibrations is performed. First, the patient wye connector is connected to its "park" bracket on the right side of the ventilator. After the POWER switch is turned on, the unit runs a series of self-tests (for about 10 seconds). Once the tests are completed, press and hold the STANDBY touch pad to switch the unit to standby. Silence any alarms with the ALARM RESET pad. Once the unit is in standby, additional tests can be performed by pressing the CHECK menu touch pad (on the right side of the screen) and following the instructions as they are provided by the unit.[1]

If the CHECK calibration has been performed before the ventilator is brought to the ICU for use, then the Evita 2 Dura simply has to be turned on, and the self-tests run. After 30 seconds, the unit will automatically begin ventilation based on the programmed default parameters, alarms and mode. During these 30 seconds, however, the operator can select another mode and other parameters and activate these settings by pressing the dial knob (Box 10-50). Before it begins operation, the screen requires you to select ADULT or PEDIATRIC patient. Rotate the dial knob to choose the desired patient size, and press it to make a choice. The available volumes and flows are different for each type of patient. These values and other available parameter ranges are the same in the Dura as in the E-4 (see Table 10-4). To start ventilation with the default settings, press the dial knob again; ventilation begins immediately. The main screen is then displayed. Figure 10-42 shows an example of the computer screen during patient ventilation. The digital displays adjacent to the parameter touch pads display the selected setting. For example, next to the V_T touch pad the digital window will show the V_T setting (Figure 10-41).

BOX 10-50

Changing the Default (Programmed) Start-up Mode and Parameters

As with the E-4, the Evita 2 Dura can have the automatic start-up mode and its parameters and alarms changed. This is done by selecting CALIBRATION/CONFIGURATION, and proceeding through the selection of desired options, such as mode, V_T, and f. An access code must be entered to change these programmed default settings. Usually the clinical specialist or department head has the access code. (See the operator's manual for additional instructions.)[1]

Monitors and Alarms

The Evita 2 Dura normally provides two waveform selections on the left side of the monitor screen and commonly viewed measured values such as airway pressure and minute ventilation on the right (Figure 10-42). The values normally displayed can be changed by using the VALUES touch pad below the screen. The waveform can be changed by using the WAVES touch pad. These two touch pads bring up additional sets of information that have been programmed into the unit. In addition, these selections can be changed using the configuration function so that any of the measured or calculated parameters and waveforms can be displayed as the operator chooses.

Measured Values

To view measured values, touch the VALUES MEASURED touch pad to bring up a screen displaying a variety of values being measured or calculated by the unit, similar to those available with the E-4 (see Table 10-5 in the section on the Evita 4), including the MVleak measurement. With the measured values screen, a bar graph appears on the left that continually shows airway pressure.

Alarms

Alarms can be set by pressing the ALARM LIMITS touch pad on the right side of the screen, which provides a window allowing available alarm values to be adjusted (Figure 10-43). There is a diagonal line that is the symbol for alarm setting. The down arrow on this line indicates the lower

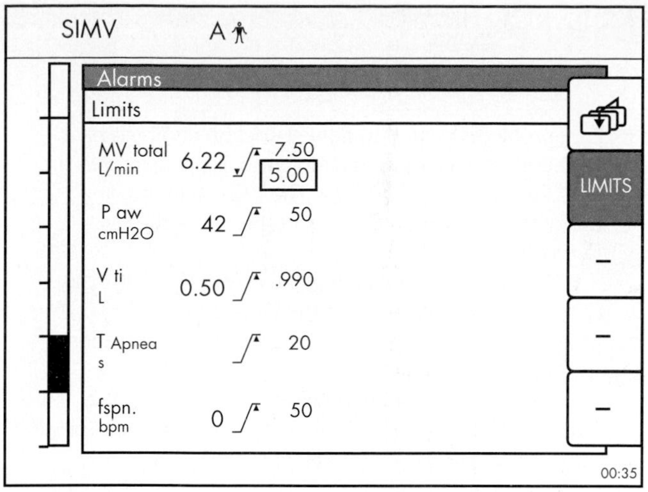

Figure 10-43 The alarm screen on the Evita 2 Dura. (Redrawn from Dräger Corp., Telford, Penn.)

BOX 10-51

Decision Making & Problem Solving

A respiratory therapist is trying to set the high respiratory rate alarm on the Dura. After using the cursor and the dial knob to select "fspn bpm," the desired value appears next to the alarm symbol on the screen. This, however, does not set the new alarm value. What is the problem?

See Appendix A for the answer.

alarm limit and the up arrow the upper alarm limit. For example, to set the HIGH RATE alarm, use the cursor and the dial knob to select FSPN BPM for spontaneous rate breaths/min alarm. Turn the dial knob to establish the desired HIGH RATE; the number appears next to the alarm symbol. Press the dial knob to activate the new setting. The adjustable alarms for $\dot{V}_E$, upper airway pressure, apnea time, high V_T, and high respiratory rate are the same as on the E-4 (see Table 10-6). The automatic alarm limit for low airway pressure is the set PEEP value plus 5 cm H_2O. For example, if PEEP = 5 cm H_2O, the low pressure limit is 10 cm H_2O and is not adjustable. See Box 10-51 for an example problem related to alarm settings.

As with the E-4, the P_{peak} alarm is not to be confused with the Pmax pressure limit that is available on the Evita 2 Dura. The Pmax limit is not an alarm and is reviewed in the discussion of modes of ventilation later in this section.

The same three levels of alarm priority in the E-4 are used in the Evita 2 Dura. Table 10-7 lists and describes these alarms. Once an alarm has occurred, it can be silenced with the alarm silence touch pad.

BOX 10-52

Modes of Ventilation on the Evita-2 Dura

CMV: Continuous mandatory ventilation
SIMV: Synchronized intermittent mandatory ventilation
MMV: Mandatory minute volume ventilation
CPAP: Continuous positive airway pressure
Psupp: Pressure support
PCV +: Pressure-control ventilation
APRV:Airway pressure release ventilation
Apnea ventilation
Independent lung Ventilation

When an alarm event occurs, exclamation points ("!," "!!," or "!!!") appear on the black and white monitor at the upper right corner of the unit. On a color monitor, a red or yellow light flashes, the color determined by the alarm priority level. In addition, an alarm message is displayed at the upper right corner of the computer screen, providing information on the type of alarm limit that has been exceeded. If a low- or medium-priority alarm occurs and the problem is corrected, the alarm (lights, message, and sound) switches off. Warning messages ("!!!"), however, must be acknowledged by pressing the alarm reset touch pad. The sound is discontinued on a high-priority alarm, and the color returns to blue. The alarm wording is removed with the reset pad.

MODES OF VENTILATION

Modes of operation available on the Evita 2 Dura are listed in Box 10-52.

Standard Settings of Ventilator Modes

When the ventilator is first turned on, one of the following three types of patient ventilation will take place within 30 seconds:

1. If a system check has been performed, the default mode programmed into the unit becomes active.
2. If system checks have not been run since the unit was turned off, the ventilator automatically starts using the patient mode last used and the previously selected parameters. (Note that in this phase, the operator can change the ventilator settings to the default parameters by pressing the dial knob.)
3. If the operator wants to change the mode of ventilation at the start time and does not want to use the default values, a new mode and appropriate parameters can be selected. After this is performed and the dial knob is pressed to confirm the new variables, the new mode is operational.

New parameters and modes can be selected when a ventilation mode is not currently active. A new parameter is adjusted by pressing the touch pad. For example, pressing the V_T pad allows selection of V_T. The LED on the V_T pad flashes, indicating that it can be changed. Turn the dial knob until the appropriate V_T value appears in the digital window next to the touch pad. Once the desired value appears, press the dial knob to confirm selection of that value. If more than 30 seconds passes before the dial knob is pressed, the original value remains active. (Note that once the range limit of a parameter is reached, the indicated value does not change. A message appears at the bottom of the screen describing the problem and a possible solution.) To activate the mode keys, press and hold the key for about 3 seconds, or press the key once and then press the dial knob. The selected mode immediately becomes active.

If a mode besides the one set on the screen is desired, pressing the OTHER MODES key provides the option of selecting whatever has been programmed into the unit. To prevent unauthorized changes, press the lock touch pad. When its LED is lit, the parameter keys and ventilation mode keys are protected from being changed. To unlock, simply press the LED again.

Trigger Sensitivity

The Evita 2 Dura provides flow triggering in all modes of ventilation. The flow trigger level is set by performing the following:

- Touching the TRIGGER touch pad
- Turning to the desired flow-triggering value using the dial knob
- Pressing the dial knob to activate the newly set flow-trigger value

Trigger sensitivity can only be turned off in CMV, but probably should never be turned off. (Note that to deactivate flow triggering, the value should be turned to <0.3, or >15 L/min; the display will show "–.") PEEP/CPAP, and O_2% can be selected in any mode, but if the power fails or STANDBY is selected, the settings that were in effect before the interruption are in effect when the unit is turned on again.

Continuous Mandatory Ventilation (CMV)

The CMV mode is an A/C volume ventilation mode. The operator sets V_T, FLOW, f, T_I, and desired alarm settings. Breaths are patient- or time-triggered, volume-targeted, and time-cycled. All breaths deliver the set V_T. Flow to the patient is restricted to the flow setting value. If flow is high and V_T is delivered before T_I is achieved, the inspiratory valve closes (the expiratory valve is already closed) and a breath hold occurs. This can be identified by an inspiratory pause pressure in the pressure/time curve and by the flow returning to zero on the flow/time curve. This is similar to the function of the E-4 (see Figure 10-34). See Box 10-53 for a note on Autoflow and Pmax related to mode setting.

BOX 10-53

Autoflow and Pmax During SMV

Any problems related to flow restriction and high peak pressures, as well as most problems with pause time can be corrected using Autoflow. The understanding and use of Autoflow is paramount in the use of the Evita 2 Dura and the E-4.

Pmax is a system that originated with the first Evita and is not recommended in the Dura and E-4. Pmax pressure limit is also called pressure-limited ventilation (PLV) by the manufacturer.

The functions of Autoflow or Pmax with the E-2 Dura are the same as with the E-4 ventilator. For a description of AutoFlow and Pmax, see the appropriate discussions in the section on the Dräger E-4 ventilator.

SIMV and SIMV with Pressure Support Ventilation (SIMV + PSV)

SIMV provides a minimum number of mandatory breaths and allows the patient to breathe spontaneously between the mandatory breaths (see Chapter 9). Spontaneous breaths can be provided using pressure support. Mandatory breaths can be patient- or time-triggered, volume-targeted, and time-cycled. Pressure-support breaths are patient-triggered, pressure-limited, and normally flow-cycled (see the later discussion of PS in this section). In the SIMV mode, Pmax or AutoFlow can also be used. Setting the respiratory rate (f) to zero turns the unit to spontaneous ventilation, and provides the selected CPAP.

The flow trigger ensures synchronous triggering of a mandatory breath with a patient effort. The function of SIMV is similar in the Dura, the Evita, and the E-4 (see the discussion of SIMV in the section on the Evita ventilator in this chapter).

Pressure-Control Ventilation Plus (PCV+)

Pressure control ventilation in the Dräger Evita 2 Dura is called "PCV+," "PCV+ with P_{supp}," and BiPAP by the manufacturer. The patient can breathe spontaneously at any time—even during the inspiratory inflation cycle. Due to the open expiratory valve system, the unit is similar in function to a high-flow CPAP device. Mandatory breaths are patient- or time-triggered, pressure-targeted, and time-cycled.

The operator sets a minimum respiratory rate, inspiratory pressure above PEEP (ΔP), and a flow trigger. The PCV+ mode in this ventilator is always an SIMV-based mode. That is, the patient can breathe spontaneously during the **expi-**

ratory time. When f is 0, the patient is on CPAP, the spontaneous breathing mode. The PRESSURE RISE TIME control can be used in this mode to slow flow and pressure delivery during a pressure breath. Pressure rise is normally set from 0.0 to 0.5 sec (range: 0.0 to 2.0 seconds) and represents the amount of time it takes the ventilator to achieve the set pressure from the beginning of inspiratory flow delivery.

Spontaneous breaths that occur between mandatory breaths can be assisted with pressure support by setting the desired pressure-support level (PCV+ with P_{supp}).If pressure rise is being used, it will affect both mandatory and PS breath delivery. PEEP and FiO_2 can be set when desired. The function of PCV+ of the Dura is identical to that mode on the E-4 (see Figure 10-35).

Because V_T and $\dot{V}_E$ may vary in this mode, the operator must carefully set $\dot{V}_E$ alarm limits. As with SIMV volume ventilation, apnea ventilation is effective during this mode, as well, but activation of Pmax and Autoflow is not necessary during this mode because breath delivery is already pressure-targeted with the unit controlling these functions.

Pressure-Support Ventilation (PSV)

The E-2 Dura can provide PSV during SIMV, PCV, and spontaneous (CPAP) ventilation. To place the Dura in CPAP/PS, the following steps are performed:

- Either go to a rate of 0 in SIMV or to the SETTINGS key pad
- Then go to the OTHER MODES key pad
- Select CPAP/PS as the other mode
- Activate it by either pressing the OTHER MODES key pad at the mode selections and holding it for 3 seconds or touching the OTHER MODES keypad and pressing the rotary dial for confirmation

The target pressure is set by touching the PS key pad in the parameter selection keys. PS breaths are patient-triggered, pressure-targeted, and flow-cycled (25% of peak for adults, 6% of peak for pediatric patients). Patient triggering is based on the flow trigger. Whenever PSV is active, the PRESSURE RISE TIME control is also functional.

If the patient actively exhales or fights the ventilator during the start of a PS breath, inspiratory flow ends. This is detected by the flow going to zero or less than zero during the early portion of inspiration.

Inspiratory flow during PSV will also time-cycle at 4 seconds (1.5 seconds for pediatric setting). Prolonged T_I most commonly occurs if a leak is present. Apnea ventilation is available when PSV is selected.

Continuous Positive Airway Pressure (CPAP)

CPAP is available on the E-2 Dura by selecting SIMV, PCV+, or APRV modes and setting the respiratory rate to zero. It is set in the same manner as pressure support. Set the desired CPAP level (in centimeters of water) if you wish to use CPAP alone. Set PS above PEEP if you want to assist spontaneous breaths with pressure support. Apnea ventilation is available when CPAP is selected.

Mandatory Minute Volume Ventilation (MMV) and MMV with Pressure Support (MMV/PSV)

As described in Chapter 9, a patient can breathe spontaneously with MMV and contribute a portion of the overall $\dot{V}_E$. The difference between the spontaneous $\dot{V}_E$ and the set $\dot{V}_E$ is provided by mandatory breaths at the set volume. Autoflow or Pmax can be used in MMV ventilation.

MMV is made operational by pressing the SETTINGS key and then the OTHER MODES key. Highlight the MMV setting on the screen by rotating the dial knob, and then press the dial knob to activate the setting. To switch modes, press and hold the OTHER MODES control for 3 seconds. (Note that you can also highlight the desired selection and press the dial knob for confirmation.) MMV then becomes the active mode. The operator selects V_T, flow (not necessary with Autoflow), f, T_I, trigger sensitivity, FiO_2, and PEEP level. PRESSURE RISE TIME can be used to taper pressure and flow delivery during PSV. The use of this sloping feature in the Dura is the same as described with the Evita.

The frequency of a mandatory breath is determined by the level of spontaneous breathing. If the patient is providing sufficient spontaneous $\dot{V}_E$, no mandatory breaths occur. If spontaneous $\dot{V}_E$ falls below what the ventilator anticipates based on the set $\dot{V}_E$, however, mandatory breaths occur when the balance between set and spontaneous $\dot{V}_E$ becomes negative. The program for MMV ventilation is designed to allow for irregular patterns of spontaneous breathing with occasional short apnea intervals, and permits these irregularities without allowing too long to pass with no breathing—either spontaneous or mandatory.

Apnea Ventilation

Apnea ventilation provides volume ventilation with a minimum respiratory rate in case the patient becomes apneic in any of the following modes: SIMV, PCV+, CPAP, and APRV (an upgrade feature). If the patient stops breathing for the length of time set on the apnea alarm control, the alarm is activated and apnea ventilation begins.

To set apnea ventilation, touch the SETTINGS touch pad, using the dial knob select the APNEA VENT. soft pad on the screen. Select and set the desired volume and rate using V_{TApnea} and f_{Apnea} on the screen using the dial knob. The baseline pressure, O_2%, trigger sensitivity, Autoflow, and other alarm parameters will remain as they are in the current mode if apneic ventilation becomes active.

If an apneic ventilation alarm occurs, apneic ventilation can be canceled by pressing the ALARM RESET touch pad. The unit continues to function in the original ventilation mode.

Airway Pressure-Release Ventilation (APRV)

APRV is a mode of ventilation that can be added to the Evita 2 Dura as an optional feature. It functions similar to the APRV mode in the Evita and the same as that in the Evita and the E-4 (see the section on the E-4 and also Figure 10-30). (Note that APRV timing and pressure ranges have been expanded on the Dura and on the E-4 compared with those on the Evita ventilator.)

APRV is set in the following way:

1. Press the SETTINGS touch pad
2. Press the OTHER MODES touch pad
3. Select APRV on the screen by rotating the dial knob
4. Confirm by pressing the dial knob

The initials *APRV* appear in the upper right corner of the screen. The ventilator parameters are set in the same way, (i.e., by using the dial knob to adjust the number values and pressing it to confirm the new value).

An upper pressure level is set using P_{high} and a lower using P_{low}. The unit also times the length of both pressure levels. T_{high} is the length of time that high pressure is provided, and T_{low} is the length of time that low pressure is provided. Pressure rise can taper the slope from the low-pressure to the high-pressure level. The length of the pressure rise time, however, cannot be longer than the set T_{high} time. (Use of APRV is further explained in Chapter 9 and in other references[2] so it is not repeated here.) Box 10-54 presents a comparison of APRV and PCV+.

Apnea back-up ventilation is recommended when using this mode. For Apnea ventilation select SETTINGS, VENTILATION; then APNEA VENT. (dial knob); and choose the desired V_{TAPNEA} and f_{APNEA} with the dial knob.

BOX 10-54

Decision Making & Problem Solving

What is the primary difference between the APRV mode and the PCV+ mode on the Evita-2 Dura?

See Appendix A for the answer.

SPECIAL FUNCTIONS

The additional features on the Dräger E-2 Dura are similar to the same features on the E-4.

AutoFlow

AutoFlow is the same feature available with the E-4 ventilator that can be added to the Evita 2 Dura as a special feature with the ventilator plus upgrade and functions in the same manner. To select AutoFlow on the E-2 Dura, press the SETTINGS touch pad and then the AUTOFLOW screen pad using the dial knob. When the mode is operating, a black dot appears in the upper left corner of the AUTOFLOW screen soft pad.

AutoFlow is available during CMV, SIMV, and MMV. It is strongly recommended that it be activated whenever a spontaneously breathing patient is being ventilated—regardless of the chosen mode. It allows for flow on demand and more rapid response of the inspiratory and expiratory valves. (Note that the function of AutoFlow in the Dura is identical with that in the E-4. For complete details of its operation, review the discussion of Autoflow in the section on the E-4.)

Independent Lung Ventilation

As with the E-4, independent lung ventilation (ILV) can be programmed into the unit so that it can be coupled with another Dräger E-2 Dura or E-4. Used together, these ventilators can be employed for ILV in patients who are intubated with a double-lumen endotracheal tube. ILV synchronizes the function of the two units so that breath delivery to both lungs can occur simultaneously. ILV requires that the units be connected by appropriate cables. ILV set-up is reviewed in the operator's manual and is not covered here.

Sigh (Intermittent PEEP)

As in the Evita and the E-4, the intermittent PEEP function on the E-2 Dura provides sigh breaths by increasing PEEP in the CMV mode (see Figure 10-25). Starting and setting intermittent PEEP increases end-expiratory pressure by the set value for intermittent PEEP for two consecutive mandatory breaths every 3 minutes.

Intermittent PEEP can be activated by touching the SETTINGS key and using the dial knob to select intermittent PEEP, as is done with other parameters. During the sigh interval, the VOLUME NOT CONSTANT alarm is inactivated. Because intermittent PEEP increases the baseline, it is advisable to set the upper pressure limit appropriately to avoid lung overdistention during regular breath delivery. Figure 10-25 shows the pressure/time graph of intermittent PEEP.

Intrinsic PEEP

An estimate of the amount of auto-PEEP present in a patient as well as an estimate of the trapped volume can be determined using the intrinsic PEEP (PEEPi) function. This is an added (optional) function. These measurements can only be performed when no patient activity occurs during the measurement.

To perform an auto-PEEP measurement, press the MANEUVER menu key, select PEEPi, and use the dial knob to select START soft pad on the screen. To start the measurement, press the dial knob. The maneuver is performed automatically, and the waveform display is frozen. Values for PEEP (set), PEEPi, and trapped volume (Vtrap), are shown on the screen. Using the dial knob and screen cursor, the auto-PEEP level at any time on the graph of pressure/time can be viewed. The PEEPi values appear above the waveform.

Occlusion Pressure

Measurement of occlusion pressure (P 0.1) is an added option to the Evita 2 Dura that functions the same way as in the E-4. This procedure can be automatically performed by selecting the MANEUVER menu touch pad, then the P 0.1 screen value (dial knob), and then the START screen soft pad using the dial knob. To start the measurement, press the dial knob. The maneuver is automatically performed, and the value for occlusion pressure is shown on the screen.

Carbon Dioxide Monitoring

Carbon dioxide monitoring (single-breath carbon dioxide analysis [$SBCO_2$]) can also be added to the Evita 2 Dura with the addition of the end-tidal carbon dioxide ($etCO_2$) option. As with the E-4, values for $etCO_2$, CO_2 production, and dead space can be analyzed, calibrated, and displayed. Dead space is measured as series dead space, a function of mechanical, not physiologic, dead space.

Special Function Touch Pads

As mentioned previously, there is a set of touch pads to the left of the screen on the front panel of the E-2 Dura. Their functions are explained here.

Nebulizer Touch Pad

The NEBULIZER control functions during any adult or pediatric ventilatory mode. Pressing the NEBULIZER touch pad turns the nebulizer gas source on, displays a nebulizer symbol and message on the screen, and lights the LED on the touch pad. Gas only flows through the nebulizer outlet during inspiration in the adult settings. In adult modes, it automatically maintains the set $\dot{V}_E$ and very closely approximates the set O_2% (±4%). During pediatric ventilation, nebulization is continuous and available during pressure-targeted modes of ventilation: PCV+, CPAP, PSV, and APRV, as well as in all volume modes to which Autoflow is added.

The nebulizer continues to operate for 30 minutes or until the pad is touched again. After its use, a "flow calibration" message appears to indicate that the nebulizer is off and the flow transducer is being automatically cleaned and recalibrated to ensure accurate measurements.

O_2 Increase Suction

The 100% O_2 SUCTION touch pad is used to provide 100% oxygen for 3 minutes in adults and uses the set O_2% plus 25% in pediatric ventilation. When pressed, the LED on the pad is lit and the message "O_2 enrichment 180 s" appears at the bottom of the screen. This function operates in the same manner on the Dura as it does on the Evita and the E-4 and is described in the section on the Evita ventilator.

Inspiratory Hold

The INSPIR HOLD touch pad provides an inflation hold maneuver when pressed. When held down, it provides an inflation hold for as long as the pause is desired, up to a maximum of 15 seconds. When activated, either the current inspiration is held, or a new mandatory breath is delivered and the inspiration held. It is functional in all modes except CPAP if a pressure-support level is not set.

Expiratory Hold

An expiratory hold maneuver can be performed using the EXP. HOLD touch pad. This manually prolongs the expiratory phase for as long as it is pressed, up to 15 seconds. It can be used to estimate end-expiratory pressure during any mode of ventilation. (When the MEASUREMENTS screen is up, you can press the EXP. HOLD key and have the patient perform an MIP maneuver; the value is displayed as the minimum pressure value at the start of the next breath.)

VENTILATOR GRAPHIC WAVEFORMS

The graphics monitor on the Dräger E-2 Dura is part of the main computer screen during standard operation. Additional waveforms can be viewed simultaneously, and different waveforms can be displayed during normal function. Trends and loops can be added as options to the E-2 Dura package.

TROUBLESHOOTING

Press the i (information) touch pad to access on-screen help on operating the ventilator or troubleshooting. The alarms and monitored information sections provide a great deal of assistance for solving the majority of problems that might occur with the Dura. In addition, the operator's manual contains a troubleshooting section that alphabetically lists all the alarm messages, tells their priority level, gives common causes, and recommends remedies. For additional information on Dräger products, check their web site: www.draeger.com.

Review Questions

(See Appendix A for answers.)

1. Which of the following components are present on both the Evita 2 Dura and the E-4?

I. a single-dial knob control
II. a screen for viewing waveforms (graphics)
III. touch pads for selecting variables and alarms
IV. mode-selection touch pads
a. I and III only
b. II and IV only
c. I, II, and III only
d. I, II, III, and IV

2. The function of the control or dial knob is to:
I. change the numerical value of a selected parameter
II. activate new parameters
III. move the cursor (vertical line) on the screen
IV. turn the unit on and off
a. I only
b. II and IV only
c. I, II, and III only
d. II, III, and IV only

3. During patient ventilation, PIP is 20 cm H_2O and baseline pressure is 5 cm H_2O. What is the low airway pressure alarm value?
a. 5 cm H_2O
b. 10 cm H_2O
c. 15 cm H_2O
d. cannot be determined from the information given

4. The nebulizer function during pediatric ventilation is only operational during:
a. volume-targeted ventilation (Autoflow inactive)
b. Neoflow function
c. pressure-targeted modes of ventilation
d. independent lung ventilation

5. An audible tone occurs and 3 exclamation points ("!!!") appear in the upper right corner of the Dura. Which of the following statements is true?
I. This is a low priority alarm.
II. A message will appear on the screen describing the alarm condition.
III. This is a warning message (high-priority) that must be acknowledged by the operator.
IV. This alarm will automatically reset once the problem has been corrected.
a. I and II only
b. II and III only
c. III and IV only
d. II, III, and IV

6. The EXP. HOLD touch pad can prolong the expiratory phase up to 15 seconds—true or false?

7. As in the E-4 ventilator, the Evita 2 Dura requires you to select either neonatal, pediatric, or adult patient before selecting additional parameters—true or false?

8. The LED on the V_T touch pad flashes, indicating that the value can be changed—true or false?

9. Describe what occurs during an alarm situation on the Evita 2 Dura.

10. Explain the function of the Pmax setting on the Evita 2 Dura compared with that on the E-4.

References

1. Evita 2 Dura intensive care ventilator operating instructions, software 3 n, 90 28 961, Telford, Penn, 1997, Drager Inc.
2. Pilbeam SP: Mechanical ventilation: physiological and clinical applications, ed 3, St Louis, 1998, Mosby.

Hamilton AMADEUS

OUTLINE

LEARNING OBJECTIVES

Upon completion of this section, the reader should be able to:

1. Describe the function of each control, alarm, and monitor parameter on the Hamilton Medical AMADEUS ventilator.
2. Explain the function of the flow trigger.
3. List the value for the expiratory base flow when the flow trigger value is given.
4. Calculate T_I, pause time, T_E, and I:E ratio when given the settings on the % CYCLE TIME control.
5. Compare the volume modes with the pressure modes of ventilation in terms of triggering, limiting, and cycling features and volume and pressure delivery.
6. Troubleshoot a problem when an alarm indicator is lit.

POWER SOURCE

The Hamilton AMADEUS[1-4] is produced by Hamilton Medical, Inc. (Figure 10-44). It requires a standard 115-volt AC electrical outlet and normally uses air and oxygen high-pressure gas sources (29 to 86 psig) for operation. It is a pneumatically powered, microprocessor-controlled ventilator that is used to manage pediatric and adult patients.

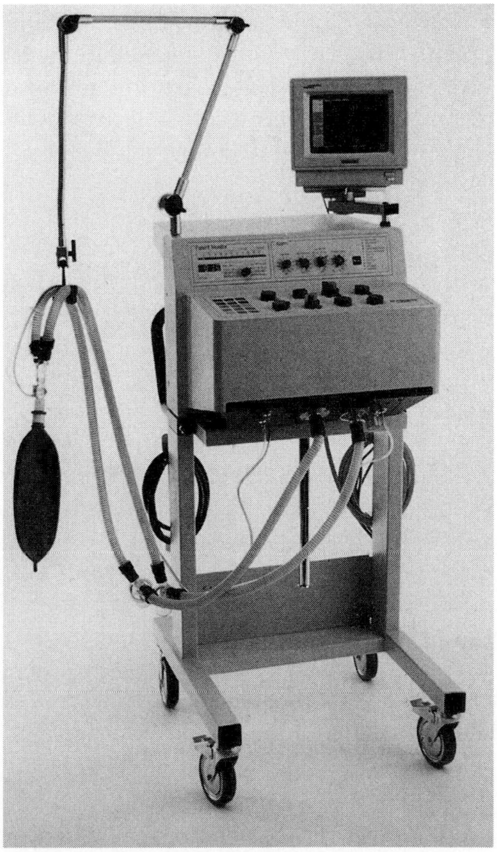

Figure 10-44 The Hamilton AMADEUS. (Courtesy Hamilton Medical, Inc., Reno, Nev.)

INTERNAL MECHANISMS

Air and oxygen sources enter through high-pressure lines connected in the back of the unit and individually pass through separate filters and solenoids (Figure 10-45). Gas flow from these electronic solenoids is monitored and blended in an electronic mixer to match the desired FIO_2. A differential pressure transducer monitors the flow generated while the gases leave this mixing area. Gases are delivered to an 8-L aluminum reservoir that is pressurized up to 350 cm H_2O. When the reservoir is filled to maximum pressure, the differential pressure transducer shuts down the flow of the blended gases. There is a pressure-relief valve on the reservoir set for 400 cm H_2O to avoid overpressurization. The advantage of the reservoir is that it permits the ventilator to provide high peak inspiratory flows to 180 L/min, thus doubling the rate of source gas mixing that occurs at levels up to 90 L/min. Gas passing

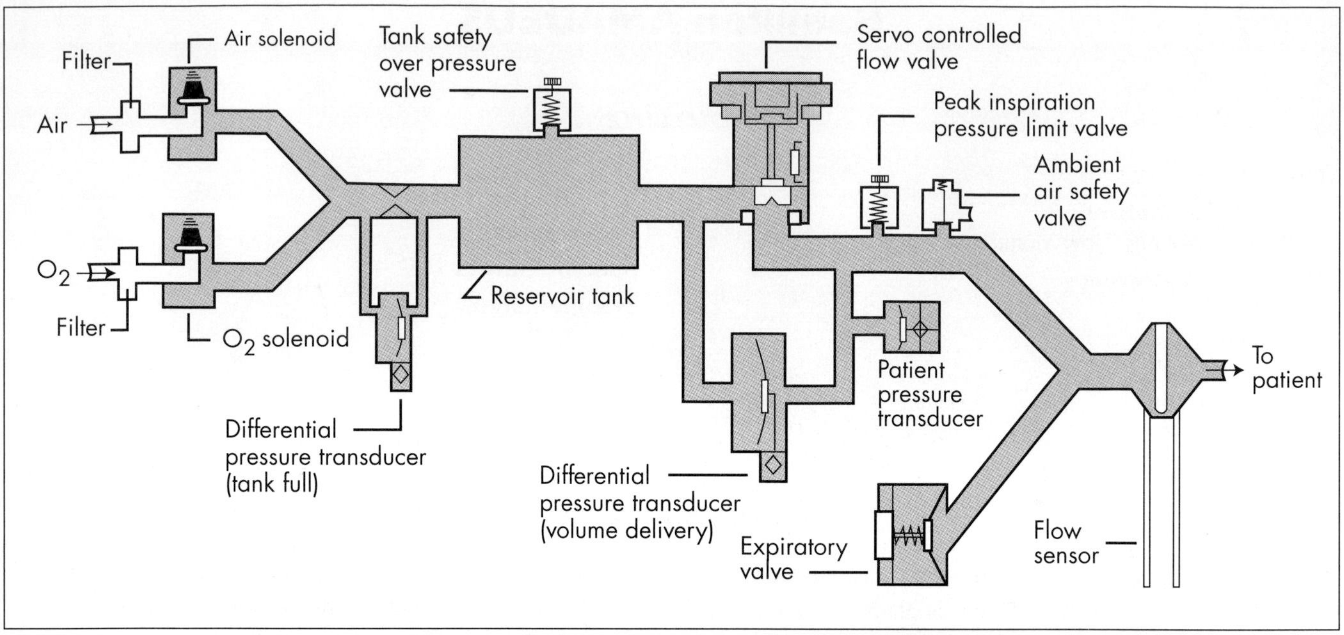

Figure 10-45 Schematic of the internal mechanisms of the AMADEUS; see text for explanation.

from the reservoir is directed to the patient through a servo-controlled flow valve made up of an electromagnetically actuated plunger, a position sensor, and a differential pressure transducer (see Chapters 7 and 9). The motion of this valve is governed by the ventilator's electronic control processor, which takes information from the control panel about what it measures as flow demand and establishes how the gas will be delivered by the flow control valve. This ensures accurate volume and flow delivery to the patient.

After leaving the reservoir, the gas passes through a pressure-release valve set at about 120 cm H_2O. Located with the overpressure valve is an antisuffocation valve, which opens if there is an emergency to allow the patient to breathe room air. There is also an oxygen-sensing fuel cell in this area through which the inspiratory flow of gas passes before entering the main inspiratory line of the patient circuit. After gas is delivered to the patient, it leaves the patient during exhalation and passes through the main expiratory line and finally through the expiratory valve (see Figure 9-75 and Figure 10-45). The expiratory valve contains a large silicon diaphragm with a big metal plate in the center to help stabilize the diaphragm. The action of the expiratory valve is governed by an electromagnetic plunger, which closes the valve during inspiration and controls the resistance through the valve on expiration in order to control the selected PEEP/CPAP levels.

Proximal Pressure/Flow Monitoring Sensor

One of the unique features of the Hamilton Medical ventilators (AMADEUS, VEOLAR, and GALILEO) is the variable orifice pneumotachograph, also called the flow sensor, that is placed at the patient's wye connector (Figure 10-46). The function of pneumotachographs is explained in Chapter 7. The flow sensor of the Hamilton ventilator allows flows to be monitored directly at the patient's airway, eliminating the need to correct for compressed gas trapped in the patient circuit. This flow sensor, along with pressure transducers within the ventilator, gathers information for display in the monitoring section (see the following discussion of controls and alarms).

Controls and Alarms

The AMADEUS ventilator has a front panel that is divided into two sections. The top section contains monitors and alarms, and the lower section contains the operating controls (Figure 10-47).

Control Panel

The control panel has two rows of knob controls across the middle right side of the front and a set of 15 touch pads on the left side (see Figure 10-47).

The top row of control knobs contains RATE, V_T, % CYCLE TIME (INSPIRATORY PLATEAU), and PRESSURE SETTING for pressure control. The RATE control(0.5 to 120 breaths/min) has a shaded area. The area of lower rates (0.5 to 5 breaths/min) is not available in A/C, PCV, or CMV modes (see the discussion of modes of ventilation later in this section). The TIDAL VOLUME control can be adjusted from 20 to 2000 mL. The % CYCLE TIME control independently controls T_I, T_E, and pause time as percentages of TCT.

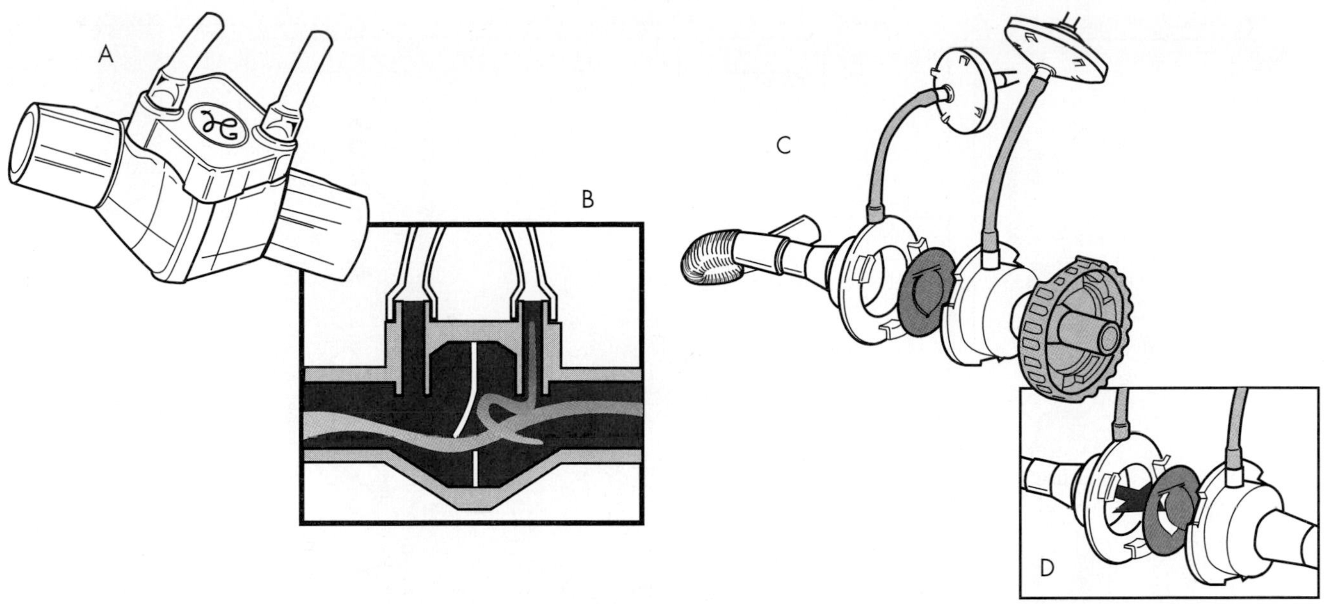

Figure 10-46 **A,** the variable orifice pneumotachograph used to measure flows at the patient wye connection on Hamilton ventilators. **B,** a cross-section through the pneumotachograph, or flow sensor. **C,** a line drawing of assembled components. **D,** a drawing that shows displacement of the diaphragm during gas flow.

Because it is designed differently than most ventilators, the % CYCLE TIME control deserves more explanation. This control knob contains two dials: one that is dark blue and sets T_I as a percentage of TCT, and one that is light blue and sets inspiratory pause time as the remaining percentage of TCT. As long as these two dials are kept together, their total equals the T_I. For example, if T_I is set at 30%, this represents the total inspiratory cycle time, so the expiratory time will be 70%. The I:E ratio can be calculated from this: $T_I = 30\%$, $T_E = 70\%$, so I:E = 1:2.33. If a space exits between the tip of one dial and the tip of the other, the space between becomes a pause time. For example, if T_I is 20%, and pause (light blue dial) is set at 30%, the 10% gap becomes a pause time equal to 10% of TCT (Box 10-55). Pause time is considered part of T_I. The sum of T_I and pause time cannot exceed 80% of the TCT.

As with most other ventilators, pause is most often used to obtain a reading of plateau pressure to determine lung compliance. The T_I and T_E settings affect the delivery of flow during inspiration. Short T_I times increase the flow rate. In other words, the ventilator must deliver flow more quickly to get the selected V_T to the patient in the time provided for inspiration. Conversely, long T_Is give slower peak flows. The actual peak flow can be viewed in the monitoring section (Box 10-56).

Finally, the last control in this row is the PRESSURE-CONTROL knob, which sets the inspiratory pressure during pressure-control ventilation (ranges from 5 to 100 cm H_2O, or off). The higher pressures on this control are highlighted to warn the operator that these are considered very high ventilating pressures.

The second row of control knobs consists of the following: PRESSURE TRIGGER, PEEP/CPAP (PINSP [SUPPORT]), OXYGEN, and FLOW TRIGGER (see Figure 10-47). The PRESSURE TRIGGER control allows for pressure-triggered breaths (−1 to −10 cm H_2O, or off) when the FLOW TRIGGER control is off. When FLOW TRIGGER is on, an internal setting of −3 cm H_2O acts as a back-up to the flow trigger. The PRESSURE TRIGGER setting is the amount of pressure below baseline that must be generated by patient effort in order to trigger a breath.* The PEEP/CPAP, PINSP (SUPPORT) control contains two control dials. The dark blue control sets the PEEP/CPAP level (0 to 50 cm H_2O), and the light blue control determines the inspiratory pressure for pressure-support breaths and is the difference between the set peak pressure (PIP) and PEEP. For example, if the dark blue pointer is at 10 cm H_2O, and the light blue pointer is at 20 cm H_2O, then PEEP is 10 cm H_2O, pressure support is 10 cm H_2O, and PIP is 20 cm H_2O.

The OXYGEN CONTROL sets the desired oxygen percentage. The ventilator has a built-in oxygen analyzer that measures inspired oxygen levels and displays this value in the monitor section. The FLOW TRIGGER control sets the flow (in liters/minute) that the patient must draw from the expiratory base flow in order to flow-trigger a breath. The flow is measured by the flow sensor at the patient wye connector. The expiratory base flow in liters/minute is twice the flow trigger setting. It is only present at the end of expiration because it is delayed at the beginning of exhalation to allow the patient to complete the expiratory phase without an increase in resistance.

*The pressure trigger is PEEP compensated.

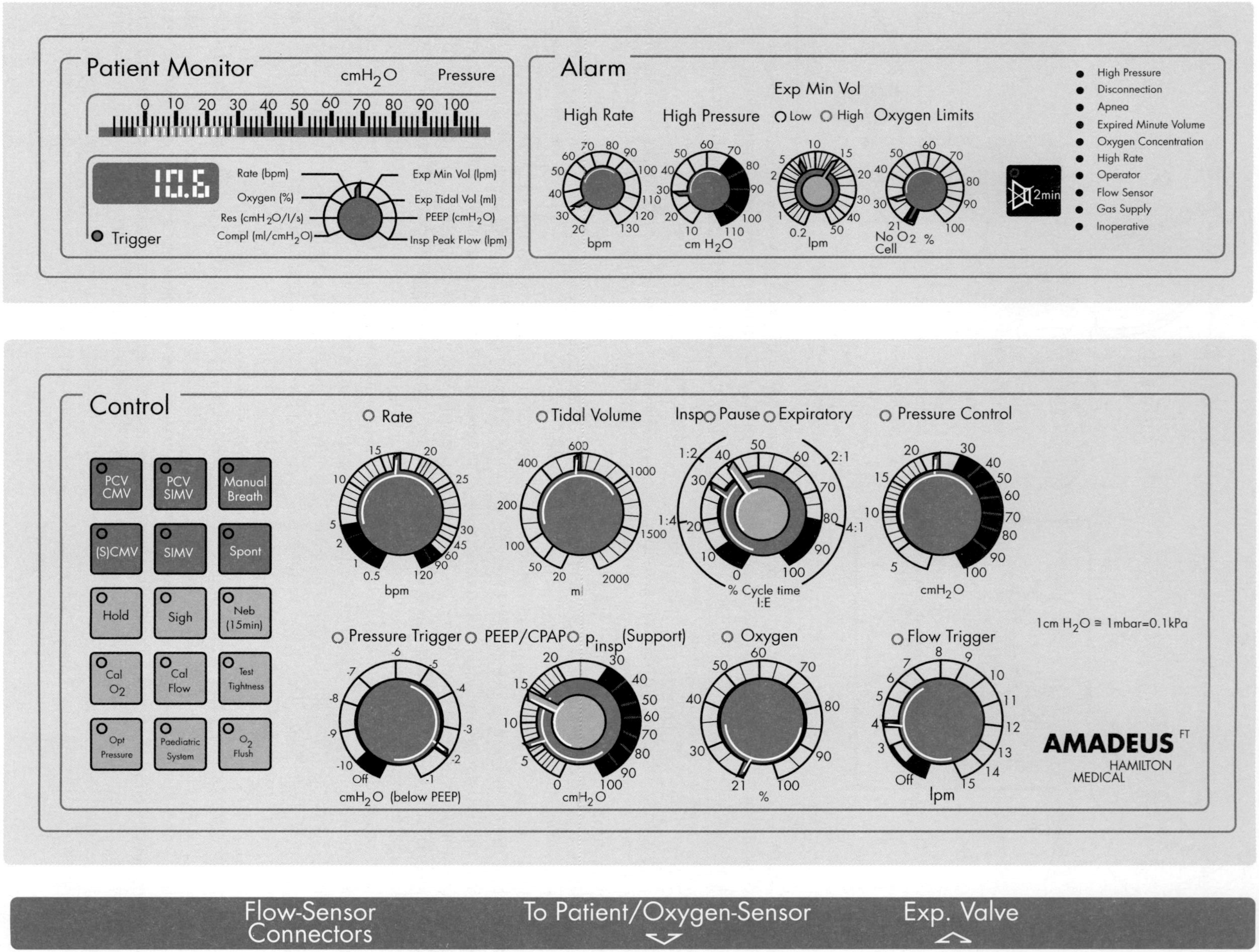

Figure 10-47 The AMADEUS front panel; the bottom section contains the controls, and the top section contains the monitors and alarms.

BOX 10-55

Decision Making & Problem Solving

The respiratory therapists sets the % CYCLE TIME control on the AMADEUS as follows: T_I is 30% (tip of dark blue control at 30%) and 45% (tip of light blue control at 45%). What is the inspiratory pause time as a percentage of TCT? What percent of TCT is the T_E?

See Appendix A for the answers.

BOX 10-56

Decision Making & Problem Solving

A respiratory therapist is adjusting the controls for volume ventilation on an AMADEUS. V_T is set at 0.7 L, and rate at 10 breaths/min. The desired I:E ratio is 1:4. What setting should be selected on the % CYCLE TIME control?

See Appendix A for the answer.

A flow trigger level of 5 to 6 L/min is recommended for most patients. Patients with minimal inspiratory effort may benefit by levels set at 3 to 4 L/min, which may also be more appropriate for pediatric patients. For patients with high inspiratory flow demands or with an air leak, a setting of 8 L/min or more may be more appropriate. Flow triggering is available in all modes of ventilation. Even when flow triggering is not selected, a base flow of 4 L/min is present during the end-expiratory phase to provide flow to patients as soon as they begin to make an inspiratory effort.

The left side of the control panel contains the touch pad controls. The first two rows consist of the modes of ventilation that are reviewed in the discussion of modes of ventilation later in this section. There is one exception to this: the MANUAL BREATH control, which activates a mandatory breath based on T_I, FiO_2, flow pattern, and set volume for volume modes (including spontaneous) or set pressure for PCV.

The HOLD control is for delivery of an inspiratory or expiratory hold. Inspiratory hold pressure can be used to calculate compliance. Expiratory hold pressure provides an estimate of auto-PEEP. To read the value, turn the selection switch in the monitoring panel to PEEP and press the HOLD touch pad during the expiratory phase of a patient's breath. The SIGH control delivers a sigh breath equal to 1.5 times the V_T setting using the inspiratory time and flow waveform selected. Sighs are delivered every 100 accumulative breaths (spontaneous or mandatory) when this control is activated. SIGH is only available in volume ventilation modes, not in PCV modes.

The next row contains calibration and testing functions. CAL O_2 initiates calibration of the oxygen cell. For 2 minutes, 100% oxygen flows through the circuit and allows the oxygen sensor to recalibrate. This procedure only needs to be performed if the monitored value for oxygen is >5% in value different from the selected O_2%. CAL FLOW, when selected, activates calibration of the flow sensor and displays the word "CAL" in the display window. When CAL FLOW is pressed, the flow sensor must be removed from the wye connector, turned around, and placed back in the wye connector. The microprocessor will zero and calibrate the sensor on the expiratory side, which takes about 30 seconds. When the process is complete, the display window shows "Turn," signaling you to turn the flow sensor back to its original position. The flow sensor calibration then calibrates the flow sensor on the inspiratory side, which takes another 30 seconds.

When the TEST TIGHTNESS control is pressed, the leak test procedure is started. Once pressed, the operator occludes the patient wye connector and observes the pressure bar graph. Normally, little or no pressure drop occurs. If a rapid pressure drop occurs, a large leak is present, which will trigger an audio/visual alarm indicating that an unacceptably large leak is present and considered unsafe for patient use. The leak should be found and corrected and the tightness test repeated.

The final row contains three additional functions. OPT PRESSURE switches the pressure monitor to the optional pressure connection port transducer. An optional pressure reading can be obtained by using a small-bore tube attached externally to the nipple adapter below the front panel near the patient circuit connectors. When this is used, the pressures in the monitor section reflect pressures measured through this port when the touch pad marked OPT PRESSURE is activated.

PEDIATRIC SYSTEM changes the calibration and pressure regulation function of the microprocessor to accommodate patient circuits that are less than 22 mm in diameter. O_2 FLUSH increases the delivered FiO_2 to 1.0 for 5 minutes, unless it is activated a second time. This is useful before suctioning a patient.

Monitor and Alarm Panel

The upper section of the operating panel contains monitored information and the alarm controls (see Figure 10-47). The PATIENT MONITOR section contains a dynamic bar graph that gives a visual indication of peak airway pressure in 2-cm H_2O increments and PEEP. The highest value during inspiration (Ppeak) remains lit until the next mandatory inspiration. The monitor section also has an eight-position selection knob that lets the operator look at any of the following: compliance (milliliters/centimeters of water),

BOX 10-57

List of LED Alarm Indicators on the Alarm Panel

High pressure
Disconnection*
Apnea
Expired minute volume
Oxygen concentration
High rate
Operator*
Flow sensor*
Power*
Gas supply*
Inoperative

*Nonadjustable alarms

resistance (centimeters of water/liter/sec), OXYGEN PERCENTAGE, RATE (total breaths/minute, spontaneous plus mandatory), EXPIRED $\dot{V}_E$ (in liters/minute), EXPIRED V_T (in milliliters), PEEP (in centimeters of water), and INSPIRATORY PEAK FLOW (in liters/minute). Once selected, the real time value is displayed in the digital display window. Just below the digital window is a small indicator (trigger) that lights when the machine senses a patient inspiratory effort sufficient to trigger a breath.

The alarm section contains five operator adjustable alarms, eleven LEDs, and an ALARM SILENCE touch pad (see Figure 10-47). The alarms include: HIGH RATE (20 to 130 breaths/min), HIGH PRESSURE (10 to 110 cm H_2O), HIGH/LOW $\dot{V}_E$ (0.2 to 50 L/min), and LOW/HIGH OXYGEN LIMITS (18% to 100%). The HIGH/LOW $\dot{V}_E$ control contains two dials for setting high and low $\dot{V}_E$ alarm limits. The eleven diodes illuminate when a set or built-in alarm parameters has been violated (Box 10-57). The adjustable alarms have already been reviewed; nonadjustable alarms have been set. A DISCONNECTION alarm indicates that the patient has become disconnected from the ventilator. The APNEA alarm activates if no flow is detected by the proximal flow sensor for 20 or 40 seconds, depending on the setting of the option switches (see the discussion of special features later in this section). The OPERATOR LED lights when the person operating the ventilator has set a unallowable parameter, such as when the RATE control is set in the shaded area (<5 breaths/min) and the current mode is A/C.

A FLOW SENSOR indicator means that the flow sensor has either been placed on backwards, needs calibration, or its tubing is kinked. The POWER LED illuminates when electrical power has been interrupted. The GAS SUPPLY LED means that one or both of the high-pressure source gases has fallen to a pressure <29 psig. The INOPERATIVE LED means that an internal microprocessor error has occurred, and the patient needs to be manually ventilated until the ventilator can be replaced. Sometimes turning the ventilator off and then on again can correct some problems. If the problems are more complex than this, the ventilator should be immediately taken out of service and a company representative contacted.

BOX 10-58

Decision Making & Problem Solving

A respiratory therapist is switching a patient from A/C to PCV ventilation. After touching the PCV touch pad, the therapist monitors the next breath and discovers it is a volume breath and is not being delivered as a pressure breath. What could be the problem?

See Appendix A for the answer.

MODES OF VENTILATION

When a mode of ventilation is selected, the LED on that touch pad is illuminated. The touch pad must be pressed for 2 seconds before a change occurs to prevent accidental mode changes. Green LEDs adjacent to the knobs for specific controls (e.g., V_T) illuminate when the control is active in the mode selected. For example, the V_T LED illuminates when the A/C mode is selected, but not for the PCV mode (Box 10-58).

Pressure-Control Ventilation

Pressure-control ventilation is labeled PCV/CMV on the AMADEUS. It is a patient- or time-triggered, pressure-targeted, time-cycled mode of ventilation. During PCV, the PRESSURE CONTROL knob determines the inspiratory pressure level, including PEEP. It is active in either PCV/CMV or PCV/SIMV.

SIMV with Pressure-Control Ventilation

PCV/SIMV, as it is called, provides SIMV ventilation with pressure-targeted breaths. Pressure is set using the PRESSURE CONTROL setting. These breaths are time- or patient-triggered and time-cycled. Between mandatory (or assisted) breaths at the set pressure, the patient can breathe spontaneously from the set baseline. Spontaneous breaths can also be pressure-supported (PSV), in which case they are flow-cycled (see the discussion of pressure support later in this section). Inspiratory support pressure for PS breaths is set using the light blue dial of the PEEP/CPAP PRESSURE SUPPORT control.

Assist/Control

The A/C touch pad activates A/C (patient- or time-triggered) volume-targeted ventilation. Breaths are time-cycled out of inspiration. The controls for RATE and V_T establish the minimum rate and the set volume delivery. The % cycle control determines the I:E ratio and any pause setting desired. PEEP/CPAP (dark blue control) can also be used to provide a positive-pressure baseline.

SIMV

The control labeled SIMV provides volume-targeted SIMV ventilation. Mandatory or assisted breaths are patient- or time-triggered, volume-limited (targeted) and time-cycled. Spontaneous breaths occur from baseline and may include pressure support.

Spontaneous

In the spontaneous mode the ventilator provides flow to the patient to maintain the baseline pressure. Spontaneous breaths can be assisted with pressure support, and CPAP may also be added.

PSV is always patient-triggered (pressure or flow). During PSV, a rapid gas flow is directed into the patient circuit as soon as inspiration is detected. The ventilator reaches and sustains the target pressure until gas flow drops to approximately 25% of peak flow. The following section describes how the percentage amount at which flow cycling occurs can be changed (see the description of Option 6 in the following discussion of special features).

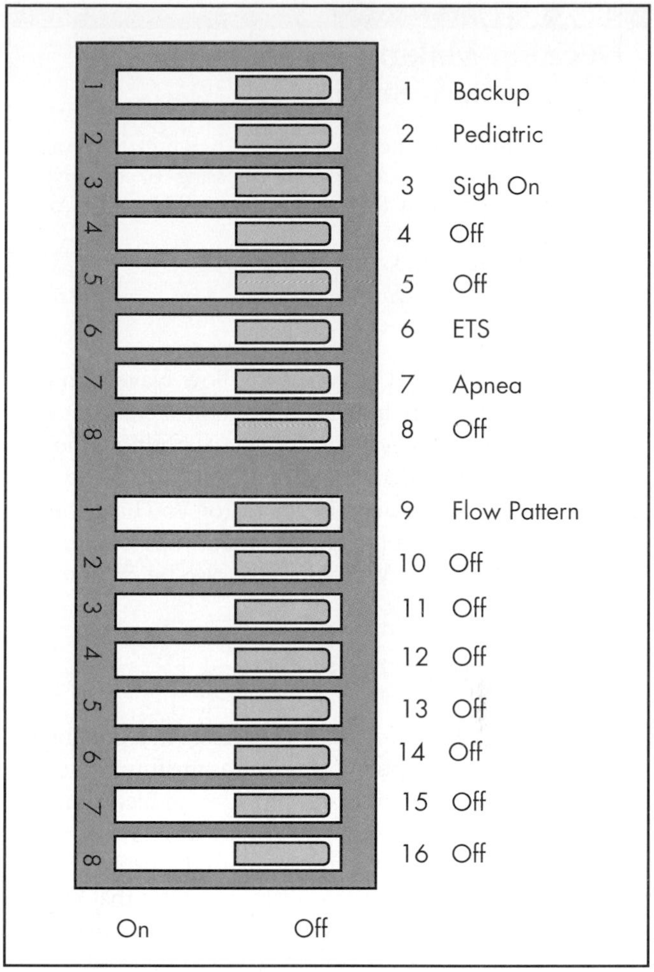

Figure 10-48 DIP (option) switches on the back panel of the AMADEUS; see text for explanation.

SPECIAL FEATURES

In the back of the ventilator are 16 option switches or DIP (dual in-line package) switches that are used to access optional functions and must be set before the ventilator is turned on. The microprocessor identifies which switches are on and off when it boots-up. It performs this search only once, during the first second after the ventilator is turned on. The option (DIP) switches function similarly in the Hamilton VEOLAR to those in the AMADEUS. The operating manual gives a list of DIP switch functions, which are reviewed here (Figure 10-48).

OPTION 1 programs the unit to switch to back-up ventilation if apnea is detected. During spontaneous ventilation and SIMV, the apnea back-up mode is the A/C mode. The back-up V_T is the set value. The back-up rate is 15 breaths/min for SIMV and is the set rate when the spontaneous ventilation mode is active. T_I is the % cycle time set.

OPTION 2 activates the pediatric system touch pad. If this switch is not turned on, the PEDIATRIC touch pad on the control panel will not activate pediatric application of the controls.

OPTION 3 activates the SIGH touch pad. Unless this switch is on, the SIGH touch pad is not operational on the front panel.

OPTIONS 4, 5, 8, and 10 to 16 are either used by service personnel or can be programmed for future functions.

OPTION 6, which is also called the expiratory trigger sensitivity (ETS) switch, determines when inspiration ends during pressure support or spontaneous breathing based on end-inspiratory flow termination. For example, in the OFF position, a spontaneous or PS breath flow cycles at 25% of peak inspiratory flow. In the ON position, the operator can select flow cycling at one of the following settings: 12%, 18%, 31%, or 37% of peak flow. The desired optional percent flow cycle must be selected and set at the time of installation. Some clinicians favor lower cycling percentages for small pediatric patients. Patients with COPD may benefit from higher percentage settings.

OPTION 7 controls the apnea detection time. In the OFF position, the apnea interval is 20 seconds. In the ON position, the timer is set at 40 seconds.

BOX 10-59

Decision Making & Problem Solving

A respiratory therapist is to add sigh breaths to the AMADEUS, but repeated pressing of the sigh touch pad fails to set this control. What could be the problem?

See Appendix A for the answer.

OPTION 9 (8 is OFF) governs the flow waveform during volume ventilation. In the OFF position, a constant (rectangular) waveform is present. In the ON position, the factory set waveform (descending ramp, to 50% of peak) is active. Before installation of the ventilator, you have the option of selecting a descending ramp that drops flow to zero instead of 50%. A sine waveform can also be chosen.

TROUBLESHOOTING

The AMADEUS has three microprocessors that continually monitor each other's operation as well as the function of the unit. A technical error message provides an alert, but you must evaluate the problem to determine if it can be solved, or if the ventilator must be changed and the problem diagnosed. The software contains a series of tests that can be used to troubleshoot virtually any problem that might occur. These tests are explained in the service manual.

Sometimes tears or holes in the silicone expiratory valve diaphragm cause problems (i.e., circuit leaks and potential problems maintaining the PEEP/CPAP levels). Running the tightness test will detect the problem.

The AMADEUS flow sensor is always calibrated before connecting the machine to a patient. Difficulty in the calibration procedure may be due to a problem with the flow sensor, so be sure it is positioned correctly and that there is nothing wrong with it. If the sensor is malfunctioning, it can be replaced quickly. During operation, the flow sensor must be maintained. Because the flow sensor is located so close to the patient, you should watch for build-up of secretions or moisture in the connecting tubes or the device itself. The unit provides a purge flow of 0.6 to 1.0 mL/sec through the connections of the flow sensor to minimize moisture problems in this part.

Occasionally, there are minor problems with the unit not starting up as expected when it is turned on. This may be because of the position of the DIP or option switches, so their position should be checked prior to turning the unit on (Box 10-59).

Additional information about the company can be obtained by checking the company's web site: www.hammed1.com. Solutions to most problems can be found in the operator's manual.

Review Questions

1. The advantage of the aluminum reservoir inside the AMADEUS is its ability to provide flows up to:
   a. 90 L/min
   b. 150 L/min
   c. 180 L/min
   d. 240 L/min
2. The PEEP/CPAP, PINSP (SUPPORT) control is set with the dark blue knob at 8 cm H_2O, and the light blue knob is set at 25 cm H_2O. The pressure-support level provided to the patient is:
   a. 8 cm H_2O
   b. 17 cm H_2O
   c. 25 cm H_2O
   d. It cannot be determined from this information
3. PCV and A/C volume ventilation have which of the following features in common?
   I. patient triggering (flow or pressure)
   II. time cycling
   III. pressure-targeted breaths
   IV. time triggering
   a. I only
   b. I and II only
   c. III and IV only
   d. I, II, and IV only
4. The oxygen monitor shows a measured oxygen level of 30% while the set value is 40%. Which of the following is the most appropriate procedure to perform in this situation?
   a. analyze the inspired gas using a separate oxygen analyzer
   b. use the CAL O_2 control to calibrate the oxygen cell
   c. turn the set oxygen up to 50% to offset the difference
   d. contact a qualified technician from Hamilton Medical
5. The factory set waveform is the constant (rectangular) waveform—true or false?
6. OPTION 3 activates the SIGH control—true or false?
7. A flow trigger of 3 L/min is set on the AMADEUS. What is the base flow during exhalation?
8. The following ventilator parameters are set on the Hamilton AMADEUS: Mode = A/C, V_T = 0.5 L, rate = 10 breaths/min, T_I% = 25%, and Pause % = 10%. What is the total cycle time? What is the pause time, as well as the total inspiratory time and expiratory time? What is the I:E ratio?
9. The FLOW SENSOR indicator in the alarm section is activated. What might be possible causes of this alarm?

10. The respiratory therapist wants to change the flow waveform from constant to descending ramp. Where is the control for this function and how can this be accomplished?

References

1. Hamilton Medical: AMADEUS, Order No 610414, Reno, Nev., 1994, Hamilton Medical Corp.
2. Hamilton Medical: AMADEUS: study guide, Part #56061-SG, Reno, Nev., 1994, Hamilton Medical Corp.
3. Hamilton Medical: AMADEUS: users guide, Part No 56061-UG, Reno, Nev., 1994, Hamilton Medical Corp.
4. Pilbeam SP: Mechanical ventilation. In Burton GG, Hodgkin JE, and Ward JJ, editors: Respiratory care: a guide to clinical practice, ed 4, Philadelphia, 1997, Lippincott.

Hamilton VEOLAR^{FT}

OUTLINE

LEARNING OBJECTIVES

Upon completion of this section, the reader should be able to:

1. Describe the function of each control, alarm, and monitor parameter on the Hamilton VEOLAR^{FT}.
2. Calculate peak inspiratory flow from ventilator settings.
3. Explain the set-up of both the MMV and the PCV modes of ventilation.
4. Compare the set-up of PCV on the VEOLAR with that on the AMADEUS.
5. Discuss the function of the HOLD control.

POWER SOURCE

The Hamilton VEOLAR^{FT} is marketed by Hamilton Medical, Inc.(Reno, Nev) (Figure 10-49).[1-4] It requires a standard 115-volt AC electrical outlet and normally uses air and oxygen high-pressure gas sources for operation (ranging from 29 to 116 psig). It is a pneumatically powered, microprocessor-controlled ventilator used in the management of pediatric and adult patients. Because of the similarities between the VEOLAR^{FT} and the AMADEUS, only the differences between them are emphasized here.

INTERNAL MECHANISM

The basic internal mechanisms of the VEOLAR^{FT} are similar to the AMADEUS (see the discussion of internal mechanisms in the previous section on the AMADEUS and Figure 10-45). As in the AMADEUS, the VEOLAR^{FT} uses a variable-orifice pneumotachograph, which is placed at the patient's wye connector, to monitor flow, volume, and pressure (see Figure 10-46).

CONTROLS AND ALARMS

The VEOLAR^{FT} ventilator has a front panel that is divided into three sections. The top two sections are for patient monitoring and alarms, and the lower section contains the controls (Figure 10-50).

Control Panel

The control panel has two rows of control knobs and a set of eight touch pads (left side). The first row of knobs includes

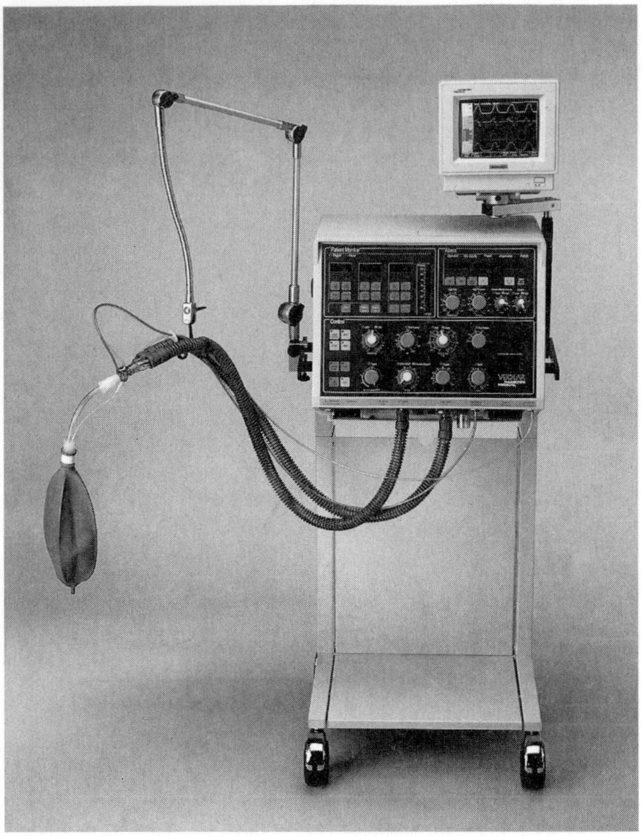

Figure 10-49 The Hamilton VEOLAR. (Courtesy Hamilton Medical Corp., Reno, Nev.)

RESPIRATORY RATE (fSIMV and fCMV), V_T, and % CYCLE TIME (inspiration, pause, and expiration).

Two respiratory frequencies are controlled by the rate knob: CMV and SIMV frequency. The light blue knob adjusts the rate in the CMV mode (from 5 to 120 breaths/min). This setting is also important because it determines the TCT for a mandatory breath. For example, if rate is 10 breaths/min, TCT is (60 sec)/(10 breaths/min), thus 6 seconds. It is active in A/C, SIMV, PCV, sigh, and apnea back-up ventilation. The dark blue knob sets the rate in SIMV (0.5 to 60 breaths/min). It is active in SIMV, PCV-SIMV, and apnea back-up. Suppose that you have the following set parameters:

- SIMV rate = 4 breaths/min
- CMV rate = 10 breaths/min (TCT = 6 seconds)

A mandatory breath occurs no more than every 15 seconds because the rate is set at 4 breaths/min. A complete mandatory breath time is 6 seconds; the patient has the remaining 9 seconds to breathe spontaneously.

The TIDAL VOLUME control can be adjusted from 20 to 2000 mL. The % CYCLE TIME knob is a dual knob similar to the respiratory rate control that independently determines T_I, T_E, and pause time as percentages of TCT. (See Box 10-60 for an example and Boxes 10-55 and 10-56 for practice problems.) The last control in this row is the FLOW PATTERN control, which provides six different options (seven in older models) for inspiratory waveforms during volume ventilation (see Figure 10-50). Inspiratory flow patterns and peak flow are explained in Box 10-61.[1,2]

The second row of control knobs consists of the following: PRESSURE TRIGGER, PEEP/CPAP, and PINSP (SUPPORT), OXYGEN, and FLOW TRIGGER, which have the same function as the identical controls on the AMADEUS.

The left side of the control panel contains the touch pad controls. The first set of four are MODE controls. The modes are reviewed in the discussion of modes of ventilation later in this section. The second set of touch pads contains the control for a fifth mode of ventilation, PCV. Also in this set of controls are touch pads for MANUAL, FLUSH, and NEBULIZER. The MANUAL touch pad delivers a manually triggered mandatory volume- or pressure-targeted breath based on the control panel settings. The FLUSH control allows for a rapid change in FiO_2 by flushing the system with 60 L/min of fresh gas, based on the selected oxygen percentage setting.

The NEBULIZER control activates the nebulizer system. Blended gases at the set FiO_2 are diverted from the internal pressurized reservoir to the nebulizer connector, which is a small nipple connector below the front panel near the other patient circuit connectors. It provides gas flow for 15 minutes, unless the NEB control is pressed again. The nebulizer gas flow slightly increases V_T delivery.

Monitor and Alarm Panel

The upper section of the operating panel contains monitored information and alarm controls (see Figure 10-50). The left side contains monitored information, and the right side contains alarm information and controls.

In the left section, directly under the words "Patient Monitor," are two lights. The TRIGGER light illuminates when the ventilator detects a patient's inspiratory effort, resulting in gas flow to the patient. The PAUSE light indicates that an inspiratory pause of at least 0.2 seconds is occurring.

The remainder of the patient display area contains three digital display windows and a vertical pressure bar graph. The operator can select the information seen in each display window. By pressing the appropriate touch pad below the window, the operator selects the variable to be displayed. When it is selected, the LED on the pad illuminates. For example, if the operator presses INSP. FLOW, the numerical value in the digital window will be the inspiratory peak flow in liters/minute.

The left window can display the following:

1. Peak inspiratory flow (INSP FLOW, in liters/minute) for a mandatory or spontaneous breath
2. Mean airway pressure (PMEAN, in centimeters of water)
3. Oxygen percentage measured by the built-in oxygen analyzer (O_2 %)
4. Lung compliance (C, milliliters/centimeters of water)

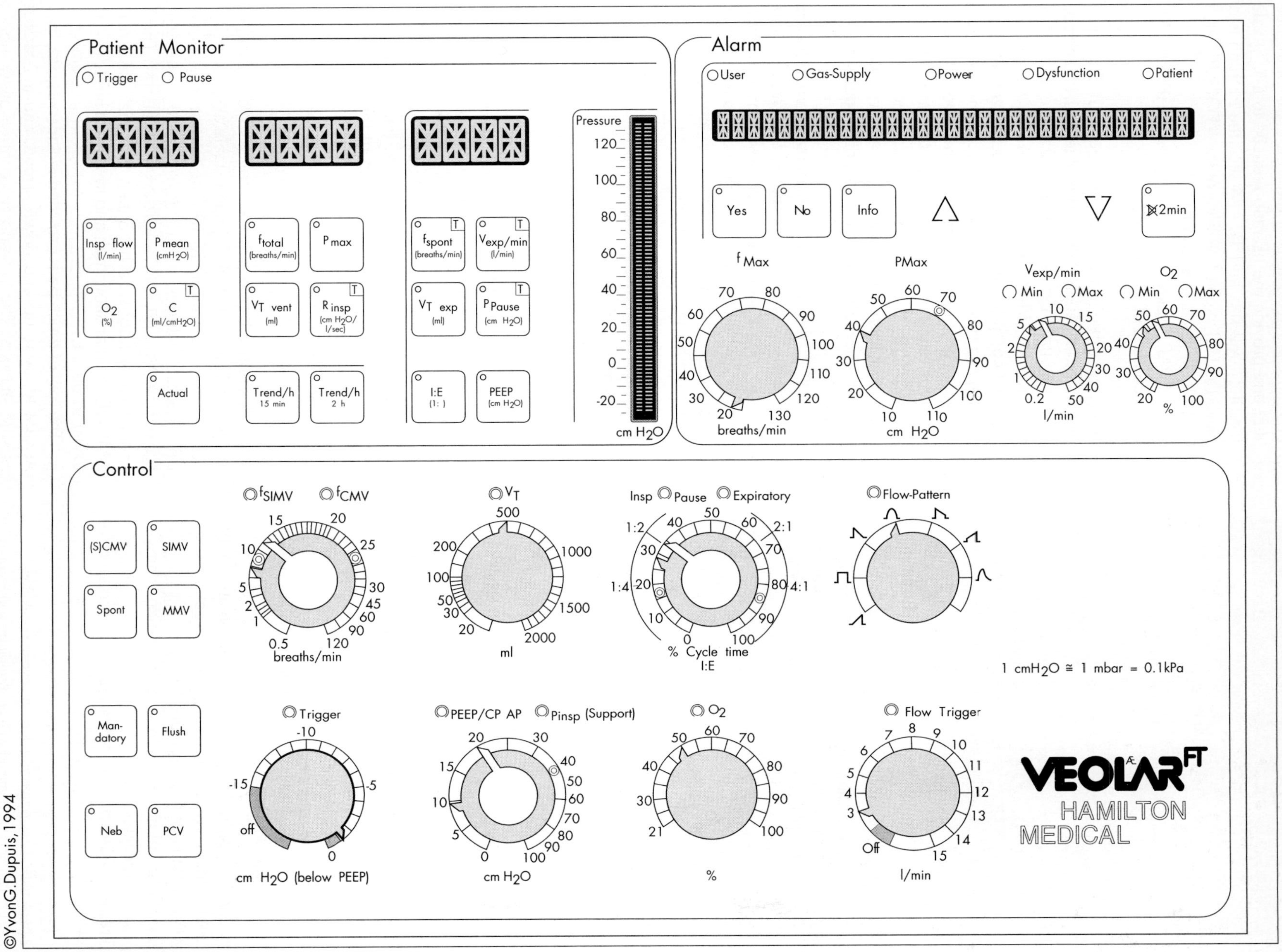

Figure 10-50 The operating panel of the Hamilton VEOLAR^{FT}. (Courtesy Yvon Dupuis.)

BOX 10-60

% Cycle Time Control

On the % cycle time, the dark knob sets T_I for mandatory breaths. T_I is set as a percentage of TCT. For example, if TCT is 6 seconds (rate = 10 breaths/min) and $\%T_I$ is set at 20%, 20% of 6 seconds is 1.2 seconds (T_I).

The light knob sets the point where inspiratory pause ends. For example, $\%T_I$ is 20%, and TCT is again 6 seconds. T_I is 1.2 seconds.

Pause (light knob) is set at 30%. Pause time = 30% −20% = 10% of TCT. Pause is 0.6 seconds.

Total $T_I = T_I$ + pause = 1.2 seconds + 0.6 seconds = 1.8 seconds.

The resulting I:E ratio can be read on the outside scale of the % CYCLE TIME knob.

A plateau pressure reading of at least 10% of the TCT is necessary to determine compliance (and also airway resistance). To obtain a plateau, simply separate the T_I% and T_E% dials on the % CYCLE TIME control.* The percent difference between the two is the % pause based on TCT. When the pause LED flashes, this gives a plateau pressure measurement that the computer can use to calculate compliance and resistance. (Be sure to return the % CYCLE TIME dials to their original position.)

The central display window can provide information on the following:

1. Total respiratory rate (fTOTAL, in breaths/minute)
2. Maximum pressure, or peak inspiratory pressure (PMAX, in centimeters of water)
3. Ventilator tidal volume (i.e., the volume that leaves the ventilator during a mandatory breath) (V_T VENT, in milliliters)
4. Airway resistance, calculated from the pressure change during inspiration and the average flow during inspiration (RINSP, in centimeters of water/liter/second)

A plateau pressure reading (minimum 10%) is also needed for the computer to calculate resistance.

The right window in the patient monitor area provides the following information:

1. Spontaneous respiratory rate (fSPONT, in breaths/min)
2. Expired minute volume measured at the patient's airway ($\dot{V}$EXP/MIN, in liters/minute)
3. Expired tidal volume measured at the patient's airway (V_T exp, in milliliters)
4. Inspiratory pause pressure (PPAUSE, in centimeters of water)†

*It is best to increase T_E% so that you don't change the peak flow.

†Pause pressure can only be obtained with an inspiratory pause control during a mandatory breath in SIMV or CMV modes.

5. I:E ratio (Earlier versions of the VEOLAR[FT] are labeled "I:E" and provide the I:E ratio reduced to a 1:__ value. [i.e., if T_I = 2 sec. and T_E = 4 sec., the I:E ratio is displayed as 1:2]; Newer versions of the VEOLAR[FT] are labeled INSP TIME, in seconds)
6. PEEP/CPAP display the baseline pressure (PEEP/CPAP, in centimeters of water).

There are three more touch pads beneath the first two patient monitor panels. When the blue pad is pressed, it displays the current measured (actual) value of the parameter selected. When the TREND/H 15 MIN LED is pressed, the computer estimates a trend of what it expects to see over the next 15 minutes based on the last hour of readings for fSPONT, $\dot{V}$ EXP/MIN, C, and RINSP.

When TREND/H 2H is selected, the computer predicts a trend for the next two hours based on the last hour of calculations for the same parameters. Both touch pads automatically go back to current readings after 10 seconds.

The VEOLAR[FT] obtains monitoring information from the flow sensor at the patient's airway and from the internal pressure transducer. It uses the flow sensor at the patient's wye connector to determine expired volume and $\dot{V}_E$. Because of its location at the patient's airway, these volumes are the actual exhaled volumes and do not include volume compressed in the patient circuit. The value for expired $\dot{V}_E$ is based on the last eight breaths (updated breath-by-breath) and displayed in liters/minute. The volume that actually leaves the ventilator is monitored by the integral servo-control valve. These values can be monitored and displayed in the monitor panel.

The internal pressure transducer, which is similar to that on the AMADEUS (see Figure 10-45), monitors peak, mean, and PEEP pressures, which can all be displayed in the monitor panel. Mean pressure is calculated based on the last eight breaths and updated every breath. The pressure manometer is a lighted, bar graph display vertically mounted in the central part of the upper panel. An optional pressure monitoring feature is also available and is described in the discussion of special features later in this section.

The alarm section contains adjustable control alarms, a row of control touch pads, a display window, and five LEDs (see Figure 10-50). The adjustable alarm specifications are listed in Table 10-10. The bottom row of control knobs includes HIGH RATE, HIGH PRESSURE, HIGH/LOW $\dot{V}_E$, and LOW/HIGH OXYGEN LIMITS. The $\dot{V}_E$ and OXYGEN knobs each contain two dials (as on the AMADEUS) that allow high and low alarm limits ($\dot{V}_E$ and O_2%) to be set.

The row of touch pads provided include YES, NO, INFO, ALARM RECALL, up and down arrows, and a 2-MINUTE ALARM SILENCE. The YES and NO controls allow input to be given to the computer in response to messages in the

BOX 10-61

Flow Patterns and Flow Rate of the VEOLAR^{FT}

Flow Patterns of Waveforms

The current six flow patterns include the following:

1. Constant (rectangular or square)—flow remains constant during inspiration.
2. Full descending ramp—flow begins at the highest value and decreases to zero when the V_T has been delivered.
3. Sine—flow begins and ends at zero; at midinspiration, flow is most rapid; at this point, one half of the V_T has been delivered.
4. 50% descending ramp—flow begins at a high value and falls linearly to 50% of the initial flow, at which point all the V_T has been delivered.
5. 50% ascending ramp—flow starts at a low value and increases to twice the initial flow, at which point all the V_T has been delivered.
6. Modified sine—similar to sine where flow begins slow, but here it accelerates more rapidly to a high value, at which time about 1/3 of the V_T has been delivered; flow then descends to zero at end-inspiration.

The pure ascending ramp was omitted from the updated version because clinical research did not support its usefulness. (Note that if T_I is set at less than 0.5 seconds, the delivered flow waveform will always be constant, regardless of the flow waveform setting.)

Inspiratory Flow Rate

The patient monitor can display the peak flow measured by the servo-control valve. You can also calculate inspiratory flows from the set V_T, T_I, and flow pattern (flow = V_I/T_I).

For example, given the following settings:

- V_T = 1.0 L
- Rate = 15 breaths/min (TCT = 60 seconds/15 = 4 seconds)
- %T_I = 25% seconds (T_I = %T_I × TCT = 0.25 × 4 seconds; T_I = 1 second)
- Waveform = constant

Flow = 1.0 L/1 second, or 60 L/60 seconds = 60 L/min.

Affect of Flow Pattern on Peak Flow

- For the full descending pattern, the peak flow is twice that of the constant flow.
- For the 50% descending or ascending flow patterns, peak flow will be 1.33 times that of the constant flow.
- For the sine wave, peak flow is 1.57 times that of the constant flow.

TABLE 10-10

Alarm specifications for the VEOLAR^{FT}

Alarm	Range
High rate	20-130 breaths/min
High pressure	10-110 cm H_2O
Low expiratory $\dot{V}_E$	0.2-50 L/min
High expiratory $\dot{V}_E$	0.2-50 L/min
Low O_2 %	18%-103%
High O_2 %	18%-103%
Apnea	20 or 40 seconds
Fail to cycle	25 seconds
Disconnection	two breaths (sensed by flow sensor)
V_T mismatch	three breaths (flow sensor vs. setting error)
Flow out of range	flow exceeds 180 L/min

message window. INFO, which is called ALARM RECALL on newer versions, can bring up information and alarm events during multiple alarm conditions. The up and down arrows can be used to give information to the computer during calibration, option set-up, and programming of modes (e.g., MMV and PCV). The ALARM SILENCE control quiets the audible alarms for 2 minutes when pressed; the LED on the pad illuminates. If pressed a second time, the alarms can reactivate. This control can also be used to prevent back-up ventilation from activating. For example, if the operator wants to disconnect the patient from the ventilator for some reason, this would normally cause several alarm conditions, as well as trigger apnea ventilation. By pressing the ALARM SILENCE button, apnea back-up ventilation is prevented for 2 minutes.

A display window is also located in the alarm section. A written message of an active alarm appears in this window. When more than one alarm is active, the operator can bring up alarms chronologically by pressing the INFO or the ALARM RECALL pad. When an important datum is available, such as "Flow Sensor Calibration Needed," this LED flashes. A continuously lit LED indicates that data or alarm information are available. Pressing the pad accesses the information, which is displayed for 10 seconds. Information available besides alarm data include:

1. Patient circuit = pediatric
2. Flow sensor cal needed
3. Apnea back-up on
4. Apnea time = 40 sec
5. No O_2 cell in use
6. Sigh on

The five diodes at the top of the alarm panel illuminate when one of these alarm parameters has been violated. These alarms include USER (OPERATOR), GAS SUPPLY, POWER, DYSFUNCTION (INOPERATIVE), and PATIENT. The USER or OPERATOR LED lights when the person operating the unit must take some action (e.g., reconnect the patient to the ventilator). The GAS SUPPLY LED means that one or both of the high-pressure source gases has fallen to a pressure below 29 psig. The POWER LED lights when electrical power has been lost. The DYSFUNCTION or INOPERATIVE LED means that an internal microprocessor error has occurred, and a technical fault number appears in the window. The PATIENT alarm is often caused by the patient (e.g., during a cough, which triggers a HIGH-PRESSURE alarm as well). When GAS SUPPLY, POWER, or DYSFUNCTIONAL (INOPERATIVE) alarms occur, the ALARM SILENCE button cannot silence the audible alarm, and the internal ambient valve opens to allow for spontaneous ventilation.

Nonadjustable alarms are also available and provide messages in the display window of the alarm panel. The nonadjustable alarms are listed in Box 10-62.

BOX 10-62

Nonadjustable Alarms on the VEOLAR^{FT}

Loss of PEEP
Apnea
Failure to cycle
Failure to set trigger
Flow out of range
Circuit disconnection from either the ventilator's or the patient's side of the flow sensor
Mismatch of inspiratory or expiratory V_Ts (flow sensor measurements vs. control setting of output)
Flow sensor in wrong direction
Low pressure for air or oxygen supplies or both
Low internal reservoir pressure
Inappropriate or absent power
Various internal technical failure alarms

Modes of Ventilation

The VEOLAR has the following modes available: A/C, SIMV, spontaneous (including pressure support), MMV, PCV, and SIMV/PCV. When a mode of ventilation is selected, the touch pad must be pressed for 2 seconds before a change occurs to prevent accidental mode changes. The LED on that touch pad then illuminates. Green LEDs adjacent to the knobs for specific controls (e.g., V_T) illuminate when the control is functional. For example, the LED for V_T illuminates when the A/C mode is selected, but not for PCV mode.

Assist/Control

The A/C mode is a patient- or time-triggered, volume-targeted, time-cycled ventilatory mode. The controls for RATE and V_T establish the minimum rate and set volume delivery. The % CYCLE CONTROL determines the I:E ratio and any pause setting desired. Trigger sensitivity is set to allow patient triggering. (Note that there are 0.2 seconds after expiratory flow begins during which the patient cannot trigger another breath. This helps prevent breath stacking.) PEEP/CPAP (dark blue control) can also be used to provide a positive-pressure baseline.

Synchronized Intermittent Mandatory Ventilation (SIMV)

The SIMV control provides volume-targeted SIMV ventilation. Breaths are patient- or time-triggered and time-cycled. Spontaneous breaths occur from baseline between mandatory breaths and may include pressure support. As with the A/C mode, there is a brief (0.2-second) period at the end of inspiration of a mandatory breath during which another mandatory breath cannot be triggered. It is important to set both the CMV rate, which establishes inspiratory flow rate, and the SIMV rate to determine maximum mandatory breath rate delivery (Box 10-63).

Spontaneous

In the spontaneous mode, the ventilator provides flow to the patient to maintain the baseline pressure and the capacity to continuously monitor the patient. It also provides an apnea back-up ventilation mode. Spontaneous breaths can be assisted with pressure support. CPAP may also be added along with sigh breaths, if desired.

Pressure-Support Ventilation (PSV)

PSV is available for spontaneous breaths in spontaneous ventilation, PCV, PCV-SIMV, SIMV (volume targeted), and MMV. Breaths are always patient-triggered (pressure or flow). The mode is set by using the dual PEEP/CPAP

BOX 10-63

Effects of CMV Rate and % Cycle Time in SIMV

While setting up SIMV ventilation, the initial CMV rate should be 15 breaths/min and the % T_I should be 33% to allow adequate flow for most patients. Setting CMV high increases the peak flow, but does not affect the maximum set SIMV rate. You should not set the CMV lower than 15 breaths/min in the SIMV mode unless *very* slow flows are desired, which is unlikely.

and PRESSURE-SUPPORT control. The dark blue dial sets the baseline pressure, and the light blue dial sets the maximum inspiratory pressure above PEEP/CPAP. The amount of PS is the difference between the two settings.

During PSV, a rapid gas flow is directed into the patient circuit as soon as inspiration is detected. The ventilator reaches and sustains the target pressure until gas flow drops to about 25% of the peak flow. The percentage at which flow cycling occurs can be changed (see the discussion of OPTION 6 in the special functions section on the AMADEUS). If a leak is present that prevents flow from dropping to the flow-cycling value, inspiratory flow will end after 3 seconds. If the patient circuit is disconnected, a LOW INTERNAL PRESSURE alarm may occur because the unit increases flow to try to maintain the set PS level. Because this cannot be done, the internal reservoir will lose pressure, and the alarm will sound.*

Minimum Minute Ventilation (MMV)

Minimum minute ventilation (MMV) is a patient-triggered, pressure-targeted, minute-volume–guaranteed mode of ventilation. As described in Chapter 9, this mode is a servo-controlled mode of ventilation used for weaning patients from ventilatory support. This control is normally set at a value less than that provided during regular ventilation (A/C or SIMV). When the patient's exhaled $\dot{V}_E$ drops below the set MMV level, the ventilator provides increased levels of pressure-support ventilation to spontaneous breaths until the exhaled $\dot{V}_E$ is maintained at the set MMV level.

To better understand how MMV operates on the VEOLAR, the set up of this mode is reviewed. First, press the MMV touch pad. In the display window of the alarm panel, a flashing message appears: "X L/min." Use the up or down arrows in the alarm panel to set the desired MMV (in liters/minute), and press YES when you have the desired value. The unit then switches to MMV. It is also appropriate to set an inspiratory pressure level with the PRESSURE-SUPPORT control that will achieve an acceptable V_T for the patient and reduce work of breathing.

As the patient initiates a pressure-supported breath, the ventilator monitors the patient's exhaled volumes, rate, and pressure-support level for eight breaths (updated breath-by-breath). If the predicted $\dot{V}_E$ is more than the level set on the MMV control, the ventilator does not interfere with the operation of the unit or the patient's breathing. If the predicted exhaled $\dot{V}_E$ based on these calculations falls below the set MMV, the ventilator begins to increase the PS level in increments of 1 cm H_2O. Any changes in pressure can be observed by watching the peak pressure display in the patient monitor section. As a result of pressure changes, each patient-initiated breath receives slightly more pressure, and thus more volume, until the minimum acceptable $\dot{V}_E$ and the MMV level are achieved. As the patient improves and the $\dot{V}_E$ becomes higher than the set MVV, the pressures decrease in increments of 1 cm H_2O.

There are safety limits of pressure within which the ventilator must operate. It cannot go below the set pressure-support level (plus PEEP). The absolute minimum is PEEP + 5 cm H_2O. It cannot go higher than the high-pressure setting, which should be set at 10 cm H_2O above the initial pressure-support value that provided an acceptable starting V_T.*

Another safety feature is that the ventilator will not increase the PS level by more than 30 cm H_2O to a maximum of 50 cm H_2O (PS + PEEP). No mandatory breaths occur during MMV unless an apnea ventilation option is set and apnea is detected, at which time the apnea back-up ventilation mode initiates. Box 10-64 provides an example situation of the use of MMV on the Hamilton VEOLAR.

Pressure-Control Ventilation

PCV is a patient- or time-triggered, pressure-targeted, time-cycled mode of ventilation. It is available for A/C (PSV-CMV) or SIMV (PCV-SIMV) breathing patterns. In PCV, setting T_I, pause time, and T_E is the same as in A/C.

In order to establish PCV on the VEOLAR, select the PCV touch pad. When this is activated (LED lights), a message will appear in the display window of the alarm section: "PCV-CMV PCV-SIMV," one of which will be flashing. Use the YES and NO touch pads to select the desired option.

After this, the message display window provides a number (flashing) that is equal to the PEEP setting plus 20 cm H_2O. For example, if PEEP is 10 cm H_2O, the window will read 30 cm H_2O. Use the up or down arrows in the alarm section to increase or decrease the desired pressure value for

*When you need to disconnect a patient on PSV, you should turn off PS first.

*Be sure to set a high rate alarm so that you will be alerted if the spontaneous rate becomes too high.

BOX 10-64

Decision Making & Problem Solving

A respiratory therapist sets an MMV level of 6.0 L/min on a patient. Initial settings and monitored values are as follows:

- PS = 12 cm H_2O
- PEEP = 5 cm H_2O
- V_T exhaled = 0.6 L
- Respiratory rate (f) = 12 breaths/min
- $\dot{V}_E$ exhaled = 7.2 L
- Alveolar ventilation ($\dot{V}_A$)= 5.4 L/min

$[(V_T - V_D) \times f]$, where V_D = 150 mL

The patient develops a pleural effusion, exhaled V_T drops to 0.3 L, and respiratory rate increases to 18 breaths/min. Exhaled $\dot{V}_E$ drops to 5.4 L/min, and the patient's $\dot{V}_A$ has also dropped to 2.7 L/min.

$$(0.30 - 0.15) \times 18 = 2.7$$

How will the ventilator respond to this situation? What is an important alarm to set when using MMV?

See Appendix A for the answers.

PCV. For example, for PCV = 20 cm H_2O and PEEP = 5 cm H_2O, scroll down to a value of 25 cm H_2O. Remember the value of the peak value setting includes PEEP and the PC pressure level. In this example, the target pressure in PCV is 20 cm H_2O plus 5 cm H_2O of PEEP, or 25 cm H_2O (Ppeak).

Once the desired pressure is set, chose the YES touch pad to activate the PCV mode. The minimum PCV level is the baseline pressure (PEEP) plus 5 cm H_2O. To change the pressure, use the up or down arrows, and then push YES to activate. Pressing NO returns the key pad to the current setting so the operator can read the peak pressure above PEEP. Box 10-65 provides an important clinical note about this mode.

SIMV with Pressure-Control Ventilation

PCV-SIMV provides SIMV ventilation with pressure-targeted breaths. Settings are established in the same way as with PCV, except that PCV-SIMV is selected instead of PCV. Between mandatory breaths at the set pressure, the patient can breathe spontaneously from the set baseline. Spontaneous breaths can also be pressure-supported (PSV), in which case they are flow-cycled (see the discussion of pressure support earlier in this section). Pressure for PS breaths is set using the light blue dial of the PEEP/CPAP-PRESSURE-SUPPORT control.

It is advisable to use graphic monitoring whenever possible. The VEOLAR^{FT} and AMADEUS can both connect to the Hamilton LEONARDO computer graphics package (Figure 10-51).

BOX 10-65

Important Clinical Note

Because of variable V_Ts during pressure ventilation such as PCV and PSV, the clinician should set high and low $\dot{V}_E$ and high rate alarms carefully to provide an alert if the patient's lung condition changes. The high-pressure alarm control should also be set 5 to 10 cm H_2O above the value in the windows. Just because the ventilator is in the PCV mode does not mean the pressure cannot be exceeded. If the patient coughs, for example, pressure increases. The high-pressure alarm control prevents circuit pressure from exceeding its set value (10 to 110 cm H_2O). If the set level is reached, inspiration ends. (Note that this control also adjusts a mechanical pressure-release, which is automatically set 10 cm H_2O above the high-pressure alarm setting. If the pressure continues to rise for any reason (e.g., patient coughing), pressure is released through a separate outlet.)

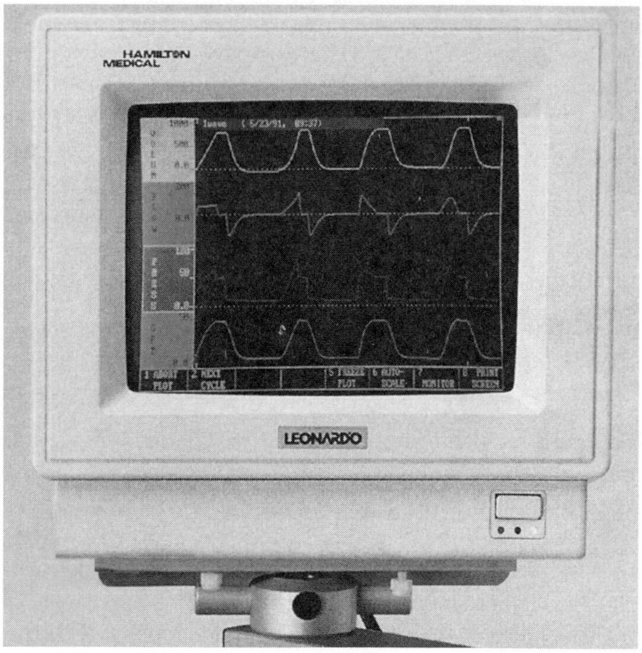

Figure 10-51 The Hamilton Leonardo Graphics Display Screen/Monitor. (Courtesy Hamilton Medical Corp., Reno, Nev.)

SPECIAL FEATURES

A hinged panel or drawer just below the control panel on the right side of the ventilator contains several other controls (Figure 10-52).

Additional Controls

These include an optional PRINT control; an unused control for future options; an ALARM VOLUME control; a CAL-

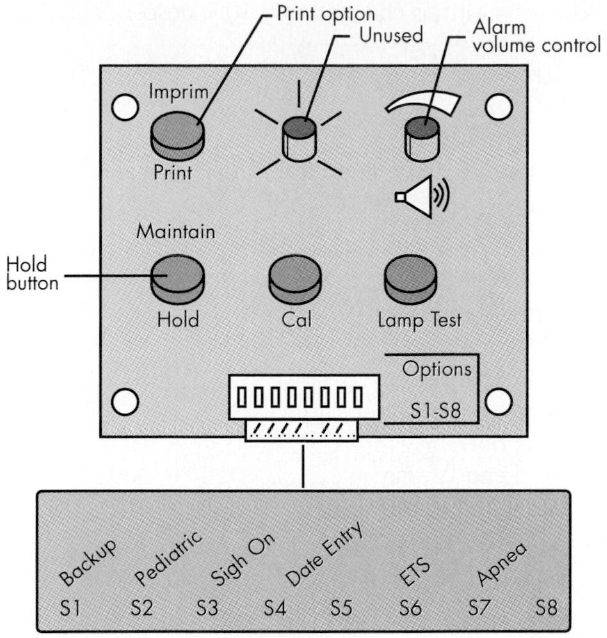

Figure 10-52 The additional controls under the front panel of the Hamilton VEOLAR^{FT}; see text for further explanation. (Courtesy Hamilton Medical Corp., Reno, Nev.)

IBRATION button, which initiates calibration (performed before patient use); a LAMP test, which illuminates the lamps on the control panel; and a HOLD control, which can measure a patient's plateau pressure, auto-PEEP, and spontaneous maximum inspiratory pressure (MIP) (i.e., negative inspiratory force [NIF]) (Box 10-66).

DIP Switches

In addition to these controls, there are eight option or DIP switches that are used to access optional functions and must be set before the ventilator is turned on. The microprocessor identifies which switches are on and off when it boots-up and performs this search only once and that is during the first second after the ventilator is turned on. The option (DIP) switches function similarly in the VEOLAR^{FT} as in the AMADEUS. For a description of AMADEUS options, see the discussion of special features in the section on the AMADEUS.

The following are the options for the VEOLAR:

1. OPTION 1 programs the unit to switch to apnea back-up ventilation if apnea is detected. Apnea is determined to be present if no flow is detected by the flow sensor for 20 or 40 seconds, or when the exhaled $\dot{V}_E$ is <1 L/min. When apnea is present, the VEOLAR^{FT} switches to a back-up mode, and an alarm is activated (Box 10-67).
2. OPTION 2 is the pediatric selection.
3. OPTION 3 is sigh.
4. OPTIONS 4, 5, and 8 are for service personnel and must be in the OFF position.
5. OPTION 6 is ETS (expiratory trigger sensitivity).
6. OPTION 7 is the apnea time control. To select 20 seconds, use the OFF position. The ON position is for 40 seconds.

BOX 10-66

The Function of the Hold Control on the VEOLAR^{FT}

When HOLD is pressed during exhalation, it stops the delivery of the next breath (i.e., the valve closes when inspiratory flow is detected) and keeps the exhalation valve closed for measuring end-expiratory pressure or auto-PEEP. To read this value, select the PEEP touch pad in the monitoring section. The HOLD button can also be used to estimate a patient's maximum inspiratory pressure (MIP). Again, press HOLD during expiration. When the expiratory valve closes (beginning of inspiratory flow), the PEEP display acts as a scrolling pressure manometer. The MIP is the most negative value seen. Pressing HOLD during inspiration closes the expiratory valve at the end of inspiration and provides a reading of plateau pressure.

BOX 10-67

Back-up Ventilation on the VEOLAR^{FT}

The type of ventilation provided during apnea back-up ventilation depends on which mode was functioning when the condition occurred. If the mode is set on spontaneous (with or without CPAP or PSV) or MMV ventilation, the ventilator switches to SIMV. If the mode is SIMV, then the ventilator switches to A/C. If the mode is PCV-SIMV, the ventilator switches to PCV (A/C form). The back-up V_T or pressure (PCV) is the set value. The back-up rate is either the fCMV rate or the fSIMV rate (rate control knobs).

Optional Pressure Measurement

The VEOLAR^{FT}, similar to the AMADEUS, can allow you to monitor an additional pressure port for things such as measuring pressures above the carina. The small connection for the optional pressure sensor, if installed, is below the front panel in the right corner where the tubing connections are. This pressure can only be used for monitoring and does not affect any functions. You can choose internal or optional pressure monitoring by using the installed option switch designed for that purpose. In the OFF position, internal pressure is used for all functions. In the ON position, the internal pressure sensor is used for control purposes, and the optional sensor is used for information presented in the patient monitor section. The microprocessor only looks at this switch when the unit is turned on, so it must be in the desired position beforehand. Using this sensor requires that a small-bore tube with filter be attached externally to the nipple adapter located below the front panel near the patient circuit connectors. This is then connected to the desired measurement port, for example, on a special endotracheal tube to measure pressures above the carina.

TROUBLESHOOTING

Occasionally the operator has problems starting normal ventilator operation once the POWER switch is turned on. This may be because of the position of the DIP or option switches, the function of which should be checked before the POWER switch is turned on (see Box 10-59).

The VEOLAR^{FT} has two microprocessors that continually monitor each other's operation, as well as the function of the unit. A behavioral error will give a technical error message to alert the operator that the ventilator must be changed and the problem diagnosed. The software contains a series of tests that can be accessed with the help of the service manual and can be used to troubleshoot virtually any problem that might occur.

The expiratory valve diaphragm is a metal disc that seals the system during normal operation. Sometimes a bent or malformed disc causes problems, which could include circuit leaks or difficulty maintaining PEEP/CPAP levels. The miniature pneumotachograph or flow sensor is located so close to the patient that you should watch for build-up of secretions or moisture in the connecting tubes or in the sensor itself. A purge flow of 0.5 mL/min through the sensor lines helps to maintain their patency. The VEOLAR^{FT} also autocalibrates the sensor every 20 minutes while the unit is operating to avoid any problems.

Additional information can be found in the operator's manual and by checking the company's web site: www.hammed1.com.

Review Questions

(See Appendix A for the answers.)

1. The peak inspiratory flow is 60 L/min during delivery of a breath using a constant flow waveform. If the flow waveform is changed to a 50% descending ramp, what will be the peak flow?
   a. 60 L/min
   b. 80 L/min
   c. 90 L/min
   d. cannot be determined from the information given
2. Which of the following controls has two functions (dual knobs)?
   I. rate (breaths/min)
   II. tidal volume
   III. flow pattern
   IV. minute ventilation alarm
      a. I only
      b. I and IV only
      c. II and III only
      d. III and IV only
3. During the initial setting of an SIMV rate of 5 breaths/min, appropriate CMV rate and % cycle time settings include:
   a. CMV = 15 breaths/min; % Cycle Time = 33%
   b. CMV = 10 breaths/min; % Cycle Time = 50%
   c. CMV = 8 breaths/min; % Cycle Time = 25%
   d. CMV = 5 breaths/min; % Cycle Time = 33%
4. A patient is being assisted with the spontaneous mode on the VEOLAR^{FT} with 5 cm H_2O of CPAP and PSV of 10 cm H_2O when the LOW INTERNAL PRESSURE alarm activates. What is the most likely cause of this alarm?
   a. an endotracheal tube cuff leak
   b. an inappropriately set alarm limit
   c. a loss of high-pressure gas source
   d. a patient disconnection
5. When using the MMV or PCV modes of ventilation on the VEOLAR^{FT}, the operator must use which of the following?
   I. the message window in the alarm section
   II. the YES or NO touch pads
   III. the up and down arrows
   IV. the PCV INSPIRATORY PRESSURE knob
      a. I and II only
      b. II and IV only
      c. I, II, and III only
      d. I, II, III, and IV
6. The AMADEUS flow sensor monitors flow and volume at the airway while the VEOLAR^{FT} monitors flow, volume, and pressure—true or false?
7. The function of the FLUSH control on the VEOLAR^{FT} is to provide 100% oxygen to the patient circuit—true or false?
8. Using the NEBULIZER control affects the FiO_2 and the V_T on the VEOLAR^{FT}—true or false?

9. The following settings are being used on the VEOLAR: rate = 15 breaths/min, the percent inspiratory time (I%) = 25%. Calculate the percent expiratory time (E%), TCT, T_I, T_E, and I:E.

10. How do you use the hold control to obtain a reading of end-expiratory pressure (auto-PEEP)?

References

1. Hamilton Medical: VEOLAR operating manual, Reno, Nev., 1992, Hamilton Medical Corp.
2. Hamilton Medical, VEOLAR study guide, Part #51061-SG, Reno, Nev., 1994, Hamilton Medical Corp.
3. Hamilton Medical, VEOLAR users guide, Part No 51061-UG, Reno, Nev., 1994, Hamilton Medical Corp.
4. Pilbeam SP: Mechanical ventilation. In Burton GG, Hodgkin JE, and Ward JJ, editors: Respiratory care: a guide to clinical practice, ed 4, Philadelphia, 1997, Lippincott.

Hamilton GALILEO

OUTLINE

LEARNING OBJECTIVES

Upon completion of this section, the reader should be able to:

1. Describe the function of the two knobs on the front of the GALILEO ventilator.
2. Explain how to select a ventilator mode and the parameters for that mode.
3. Explain how to select the alarm screen and set the alarms.
4. Compare the addition of APV to standard PCV.
5. Discuss how the microprocessor selects V_T, $\dot{V}_E$, and rate values for a patient receiving ASV.
6. Describe the method the ventilator uses when starting ASV.
7. Assess a patient case representing one of the three common scenarios that describes the function of ASV to determine how the ventilator will function.
8. Troubleshoot a problem when an alarm indicator is activated.
9. Describe back-up ventilation in the GALILEO.

The GALILEO is manufactured in Switzerland by Hamilton Medical, Inc. and was first introduced in the United States in December of 1997. It is marketed by Hamilton Medical Inc., of Reno, Nevada. The unit is currently intended for use with adult and pediatric patients (weighing ≥3.0 kg). The addition of the ALADDIN neonatal ventilation package allows it to be adapted to neonatal ventilation.*

*This option is expected to be released soon.

POWER SOURCE[1]

The GALILEO is a microprocessor-controlled unit that requires high-pressure gas and electricity for power. It normally operates from air and oxygen outlets (pressure range from 29 to 87 psi). An additional external compressor can be purchased as an option and can provide the required gas power

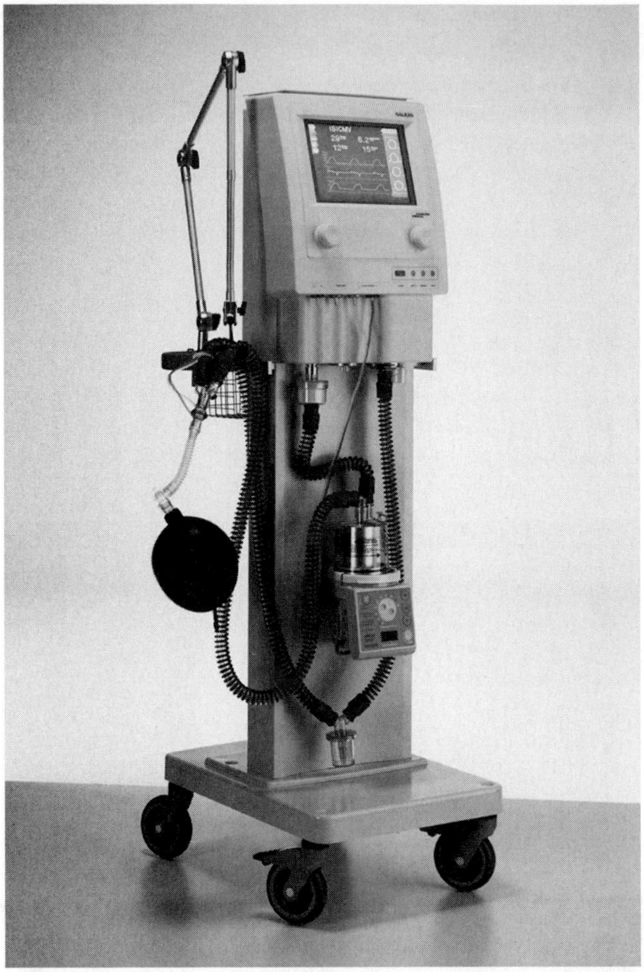

Figure 10-53 The Hamilton GALILEO. (Courtesy Hamilton Medical Corp., Reno, Nev.)

source if no others are available. A 110-volt standard electrical outlet can provide the electrical power needed to operate the unit (range from 100 to 240 volt, alternating current). The main power ON/OFF switch is on the back panel.

The patient circuit has a proximal airway sensor that uses a variable-orifice differential pressure transducer to monitor and measure flow, volume, and pressure at the proximal airway. The pressure transducer is the same as that used in the AMADEUS and the VEOLAR. The expiratory valve uses a variable-orifice expiratory threshold resistor that is also similar to those in the AMADEUS and the VEOLAR. The GALILEO has a built-in galvanic fuel cell for analyzing and monitoring delivered oxygen concentrations.

Four small nipple connectors are close to the normal patient circuit main outlet and inlet (Figure 10-53). The two right adapters connect to the proximal airway pressure transducer. The next connector will power a small-volume nebulizer from a 15 psi independent compressor built into the ventilator. Using the nebulizer results in a small increase in volume delivery, but does not affect FiO_2. The far left connector is for an auxiliary pressure line (Paux) that provides the option for adding an additional pressure monitor line for measurements such as carinal pressures or esophageal pressures. The auxiliary pressure line in the GALILEO is comparable to the optional (opt) pressure line in the VEOLAR and the AMADEUS.

Internal Function

Two medical gas sources, air and oxygen, enter the internal circuit where their pressures are reduced. If one source becomes unavailable, the unit switches to the remaining gas source but remains operational. This affects FiO_2 delivery, however. During normal operation, the gases are blended at the set FiO_2 and stored under pressure in an internal reservoir tank that holds up to 8 liters under pressures up to 350 cm H_2O. This allows for an uninterrupted gas flow, even at moments of high flow demand. After exiting the reservoir tank, gas is directed to a electromagnetic flow control valve that is a reengineered version of the one in the VEOLAR and the AMADEUS. The flow control valve governs the pattern of gas delivery to the patient and is under the control of the microprocessor unit. Modes and parameters selected by the operator are monitored, along with information received from the proximal airway monitor. This information governs the function of the flow control valve, the expiratory valve, and similar internal operating mechanisms.

Controls and Alarms

The control panel for the GALILEO is a very simple design. It uses two knobs for controlling the color-active matrix computer screen. The right knob is called the C (control) knob and the left is called the M (monitor) knob (see Figure 10-53). These knobs allow the operator to scan, select, and control all variables for operating and monitoring the ventilator.

MODE, CONTROL, and ALARM are visible as a menu on the right side of the screen during normal operation (Figure 10-54). As you scroll through the terms using the C knob, each term is highlighted in yellow. Once the desired term (option) is highlighted, it is selected when the C knob is pushed. For example, if MODE is the option chosen and knob C is pushed, the unit opens a window displaying the ventilator mode screen listing all of the modes that can be selected (Figure 10-55). Select the desired mode by rotating knob C through this menu until the desired mode is highlighted. Push knob C to select the mode. You then must choose the CLOSE option on the same menu to verify the selection and automatically open the CONTROLS window.

Each mode has its own CONTROLS window that contains only the parameters that can be adjusted in that

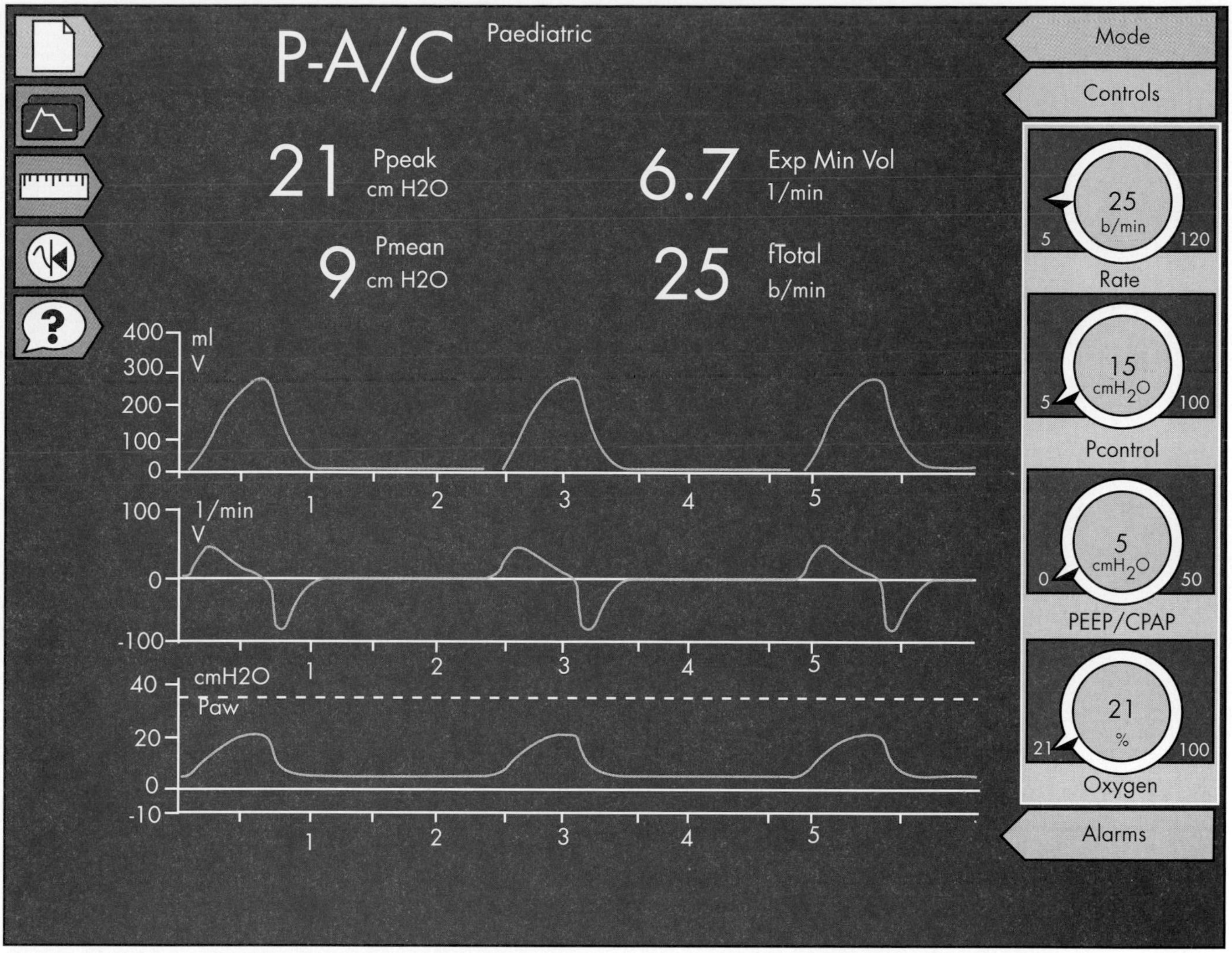

Figure 10-54 The normal operating window for P-A/C ventilation.

mode. Initial default settings are displayed for the specific mode, so select and adjust all the variables you want to change. Figure 10-54 shows the control window for P-CMV mode (shown as P-A/C). The controls appear on the screen as icons (drawings) of ventilator knobs. For example, in pressure ventilation using A/C, you have control over parameters such as PCONTROL, RATE, PEEP, O_2%, and %I TIME. Just as with mode selection, you must scroll through each parameter icon. When the desired control knob is highlighted, select it by pushing control knob C. The icon then changes to red. Once red, change the numerical value of the parameter by rotating knob C either clockwise (to increase) or counterclockwise (to decrease). If, for example, the PRESSURE icon (knob) is highlighted red, turning knob C can change its value from 5 cm H_2O to 100 cm H_2O. Once the desired value is selected, it can be confirmed by pushing knob C. A selected control knob automatically deactivates after 15 seconds if the operator does nothing to change it (Box 10-68).

After the operator has chosen all the control parameters, the CLOSE icon must be selected to confirm and activate the ventilator mode and parameters. The window (control window) showing parameters for that mode disappears, and the new mode becomes active. The control window must be closed before the new mode becomes active.

Depending on the mode selected, from two to four parameter knob icons remain in a column on the right side of the screen. These icons display the parameters most often changed or manipulated in that mode of ventilation. For example, in the P-A/C (P-CMV) mode, RESPIRATORY RATE, PCONTROL, PEEP/CPAP, AND O_2% appear (see Figure 10-54). This way the control window does not have to be reopened to make common changes. Box 10-69 summarizes the general rules for using knob C.

Configuration of T_I, Peak Flow, or I:E

The GALILEO allows the user to program a basic function into the unit. This function relates to the cycling of a breath

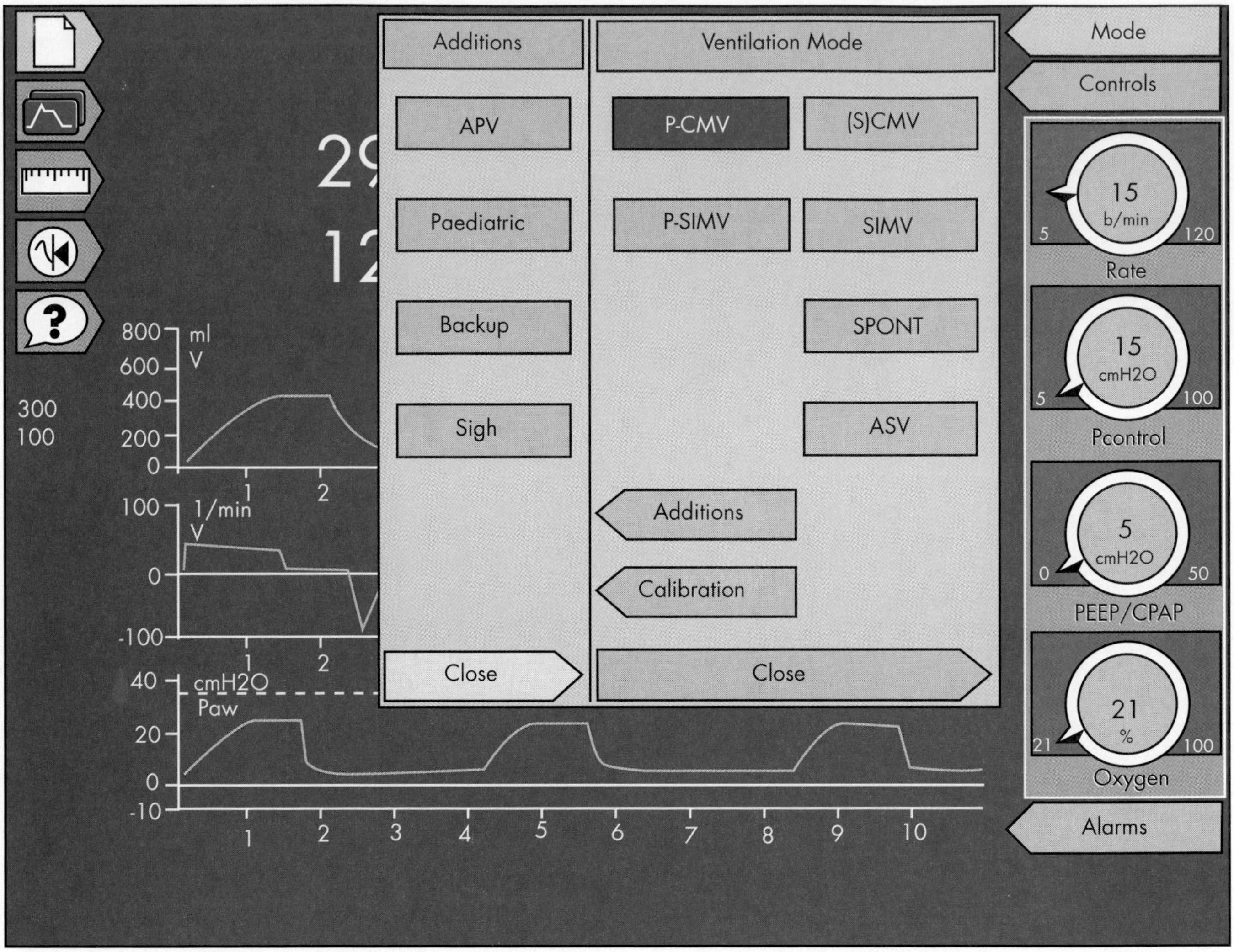

Figure 10-55 The Hamilton GALILEO window showing mode selections.

BOX 10-68

Activating the New Mode

Once any control menu has been chosen, the operator has a 30-second time limit. If knob C is not used and no selections are made within that time, the normal operating menu returns. In this way, the operator is not required to close a menu if no action is taken.

This rule also holds true for changing a parameter during ventilation. Suppose a respiratory therapist changed the set rate from 8 to 10 breaths/min. If she did not confirm the change, the change would not take place even though the numerical value on the rate icon went from an 8 to a 10. Without CLOSE being activated, the ventilator screen returns to 8 breaths/min after 30 seconds, and the rate actually never changes.

BOX 10-69

General Rules for Using Control Knob C

Knob C is rotated to either highlight something on a menu or to change the numerical value of a parameter. It is pushed to select (activate) the highlighted option.

Operating controls that are yellow can be selected. Controls change from yellow to red when they are selected (by a push of Knob C) and are then active (i.e., the operator can change their numerical values). Once the desired value appears on the screen near the active icon, pushing C again locks in that value.

The general rule is: rotate to locate, push to select, rotate to desired value, and push to confirm.

in volume ventilation modes. The operator can choose any of the following three options:

1. T_I
2. PEAK FLOW
3. I:E RATIO

Notice that each of these relates to the timing of breath delivery. For example, individuals who are used to ventilating patients with a set T_I would select the T_I option.

This programming option is only available during the start-up of the unit. You must press the M knob when the ON switch is turned on. The configuration screen appears and allows you to select one of the three options. Once a choice is made and confirmed, the selected parameter becomes the control that appears on the normal operating screens.

For example, if T_I is selected, mandatory breaths are time-cycled regardless of the mode. If peak flow is selected, volume-targeted breaths in A/C and SIMV have their inspiratory flow determined by the peak flow setting, and in this case, T_I would be based on peak flow and tidal volume. (Note that if peak flow is chosen, T_I still operates in PCV (P-A/C) and SIMV pressure-targeted (P-SIMV) modes. Mandatory breaths in these modes remain time-cycled.) If I:E is selected, the I:E ratio remains constant in all volume modes, regardless of changes in flow or pause time (Box 10-70).

BOX 10-70

Decision Making & Problem Solving

Answer each of the following questions in relation to breath cycling.

1. The GALILEO is configured to keep T_I constant. The respiratory therapist is using volume-targeted A/C ventilation. The V_T is 0.5 L, rate is 10 breaths/min, and T_I is set at 25%. Calculate the T_I and the inspiratory flow (assume constant flow pattern).
2. Assume that the rate is increased to 12 breaths/min, but that V_T and T_I are the same as in the previous question. What is the new T_I and the new flow?
3. In this example, the GALILEO is configured to keep peak flow constant at the set peak flow during volume ventilation.
   - The respiratory therapist is using volume-targeted SIMV with a rate set at 15 breaths/min, and a V_T of 0.8 L. The peak flow is set at 60 L/min. What is the T_I?
   - The therapist switches the mode to P-SIMV. What is the new T_I?
4. The GALILEO is configured for I:E constant. The respiratory therapist is using PCV or P-A/C. I:E is 1:3, rate is 15 breaths/min, and Pcontrol is set at 15 cm H_2O.
   - What is the T_I?
   - What is the peak flow?
   - Imagine that an inspiratory pause of one-half second is added. Does the pause increase the T_I when the unit is configured for a constant I:E ratio? How would using a pause affect breath delivery in this case?

See Appendix A for the answers.

Adjustable Control Parameters

Knob C provides access to several adjustable control parameters for each mode of ventilation (Box 10-71).[2] Once all the necessary control parameters have been selected and confirmed, the CONTROL PARAMETER menu is closed and the normal operating screen reappears.

Alarms

When ALARMS is selected on the operating screen (controlled by C knob), the ALARM menu appears on the screen (Figure 10-56). Alarms can be automatically set by the ventilator. The operator simply selects and activates the term AUTO from the ALARMS menu. The computer is programmed to provide high and low alarm defaults for all available options in each mode.* You may choose to manually adjust high and low alarms to whatever value desired within the available range. The alarms appear on the menu as bar graphs. Selecting a particular alarm, such as low V_T, illuminates that bar graph (orange) to tell you it has been selected. Pushing knob C activates the selected alarm, changing it to red. Once activated, turning knob C allows the alarm value to be adjusted to the desired numerical value. Pushing knob C when the desired number is present sets and confirms the alarm value.

For each alarm bar graph there is also a green horizontal line that appears on the graph (see Figure 10-56) that indicates the actual value measured for that parameter. Suppose that the HIGH-PRESSURE LIMIT alarm is selected, the green line shows the actual measured pressure value that is occurring for each breath. To the left of the green line, the numerical value for pressure also appears (green). This information is available whenever you are in the alarm menu so that you can visually adjust your alarm range around the current value and also know the set value of each alarm parameter.

When multiple alarms occur, the alarm with the highest priority is always displayed on the screen as a written message across the bottom of the screen and remains on as long as the condition persists. When the condition is

*Values for these are currently available from the manufacturer.

BOX 10-71

Adjustable Control Variables for the Hamilton GALILEO

Rate Control

Sets the mandatory respiratory rate and determines the TCT for the mandatory breath.

Tidal Volume Control

Sets the desired volume delivery for a mandatory breath.

Pressure Control (Pcontrol)

Determines inspiratory pressure above baseline during inspiration for a mandatory pressure breath (e.g., pressure-targeted breaths in A/C and SIMV modes (range: minimum of PEEP + 5 cm H_2O, maximum of 100 cm H_2O).

Maximum Pressure Limitation

Sets the maximum pressure above baseline during adaptive support ventilation (ASV) and adaptive pressure ventilation (APV) modes.

Pressure Support (Psupport)

Establishes the pressure above baseline delivered during inspiration for PSV.

PEEP/CPAP Control

Adjusts the amount of positive baseline pressure that is applied to the patient's airway in all modes of ventilation.

Oxygen Control

Adjusts the percentage of inspired oxygen delivery.

I:E Control

Fixes the I:E ratio for mandatory breaths. This ratio is based on the relationship of the set rate, Ti/%Ti, and Pause/Tip, which establish the time cycling of a mandatory breath. Patient triggering can shorten T_E and modify the I:E ratio for that breath, but it does not change the set value (see Box 10-70).

Ti/%Ti Control

Determines the time allotted to deliver V_T. Ti/%Ti + inspiratory pause determines I:E ratio.

Inspiratory Pause (Pause/Tip) Control

Keeps the exhalation valve closed for the set time following V_T delivery.

Peak Flow Control

Sets peak flow delivery for volume-targeted breaths. Peak flow plus inspiratory pause determines the I:E ratio when the unit is configured for peak flow.

Flow Pattern (Flow-P) Control

Allows the selection of the desired inspiratory gas flow pattern during volume ventilation (four patterns available: constant, full ascending and descending ramps, 50% ascending and descending ramps, and sine).

Flow Trigger/Pressure Trigger/Trigger Off ($V'_{TR}/\Delta P_{TR}$/Trigger Off) Control

Allows the operator to adjust how sensitive the unit is to patient inspiratory effort. The measurement is performed at the proximal flow sensor (differential pressure transducer) located at the wye connector. An automatic leak compensation is linked with flow trigger. The flow trigger is linked to the expiratory base flow to initially satisfy flow demand by the patient.

Percentage Minute Ventilation (%MinVol) Control

Used to set the minimum $\dot{V}_E$ delivered by the ventilator. Total target $\dot{V}_E$ is calculated as 0.1 L/min/kg IBW for adults and 0.2 L/min/kg for infant/pediatric patients.

Ideal Body Weight (Body Wt) Control

Allows the operator to enter the patient's IBW in kilograms.

Target Volume (Vtarget) Control

Sets the desired (targeted) V_T delivered during a mandatory pressure-controlled breath in the APV addition.

Pressure Ramp (Pramp) Control

Determines the rise time of pressure delivery during pressure-targeted breaths (either pressure control or pressure support).

Expiratory Trigger Sensitivity (ETS) Control

Allows the operator to adjust the percentage of peak flow at which a pressure-support breath will flow-cycle (i.e. end-inspiration). The range is 10% to 40% of measured peak inspiratory flow, in increments of 5%. For example, suppose peak flow during PSV is 100 L/min. If the operator sets ETS at 10%, inspiration will end when flow drops to 10 L/min.

corrected, the alarm event is stored into memory in a file called the info buffer and can be recalled or pulled up later. When more than one alarm condition occurs at the same time, the highest priority alarm is displayed, but the operator can check what other alarms are active by selecting the alarm buffer, which is an icon that looks like a balloon with a bell inside. It will list up to six alarm conditions in order of occurrence and give the date and time of each alarm.

If an alarm condition occurred and is corrected, it is stored into memory also. An icon with an "i" inside a balloon that appears on the lower left screen is the info buffer file for alarms that can provide a list of the six most recent

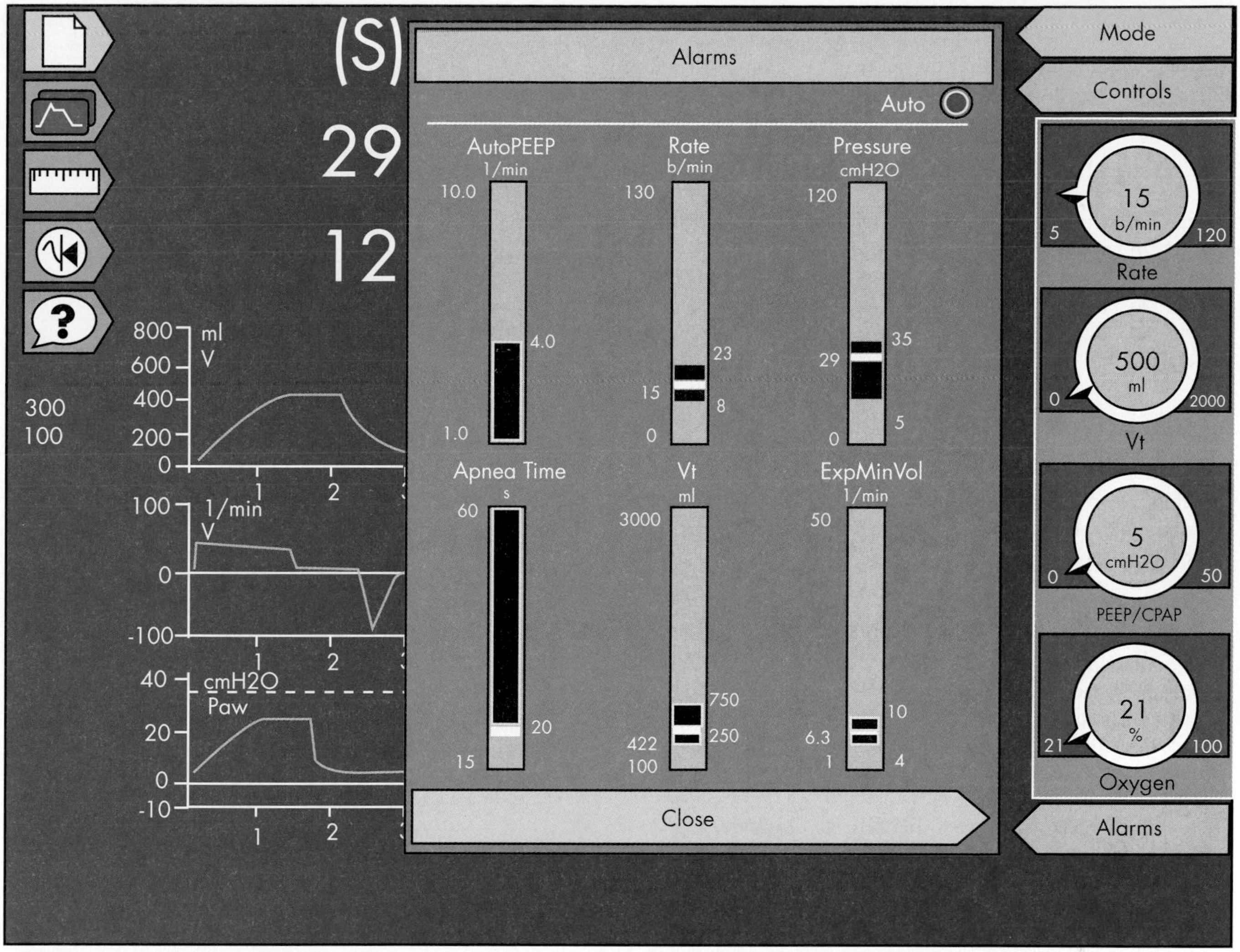

Figure 10-56 The alarm window on the GALILEO.

alarms. It is visible only if there is an alarm event in memory. Once viewed, the alarms are listed for a period of 30 seconds and then cleared from memory.

Different priority alarms give different sounds, which helps the practitioner distinguish those requiring immediate attention from those that are less critical. Using the ventilator and listening to the various alarms helps the operator learn the different audible signals.

Adjustable and nonadjustable alarms are listed in Table 10-11. Box 10-72 lists user-attention messages for the GALILEO.

Upper Pressure Limit (Pmax)

Because of its importance in ventilator function, the HIGH-PRESSURE alarm and its setting are worth reviewing. It is common for respiratory therapists to set an upper pressure limit 5 to 10 cm H_2O above the peak ventilating pressure. This should be set for all modes—pressure- or volume-targeted. For example, in PCV the set pressure may be 40 cm H_2O, but what happens if the patient coughs? The pressure can rise above 40 cm H_2O (assuming that the high-pressure alarm is set above the PCV level). For safety purposes, always set the HIGH-PRESSURE LIMIT 5 to 10 cm H_2O above the ventilating pressures. When high pressure is reached, inspiratory flow ends and the expiratory valve opens.

In the GALILEO, the HIGH-PRESSURE LIMIT (Pmax) also serves another function when adaptive support ventilation (ASV) or adaptive pressure ventilation (APV) are selected (see the discussion of modes of ventilation in this section). During the use of ASV or APV, the ventilator will not deliver pressures any higher than the upper pressure limit minus 10 cm H_2O (Pmax − 10 cm H_2O). Pressures can become higher than Pmax − 10 cm H_2O in the circuit if, for example, the patient coughs, but they can *never* go higher than the upper pressure limit setting (see the pressure bar graph in Figure 10-56 and "pressure" in Figure 10-57).

TABLE 10-11

Alarm specifications for the GALILEO

Adjustable alarms

Alarm system	Range
Low/high minute ventilation	0 to 50 L/min
Low/high pressure	0 to 110 cm H_2O
Low/high V_T	0 to 3000 mL
Low/high rate	0 to 130 breaths/min
Apnea time	15 to 60 seconds
Air trapping	1 to 10 L/min end expiratory flow

Nonadjustable alarms

High pressure during sigh
Pressure not released
Oxygen and air supply low
Internal pressure low
Check flow sensor tubing
Disconnection on ventilator side
Disconnection on patient side
Oxygen concentration (high/low)
No O_2 cell in use
O_2 cell defective
Turn the flow sensor (placed in the wrong direction)
Oxygen supply, air supply (less that 28 psig)
Loss of PEEP (3 cm H_2O below baseline for 10 seconds)
Check settings (inappropriately set)
Loss of power supply
Ventilator inoperative

Monitoring

During normal operation, four parameters are always displayed on the screen: PEAK PRESSURE, MEAN AIRWAY PRESSURE, EXPIRED MINUTE VOLUME, and TOTAL RESPIRATORY RATE. In addition to these, several monitoring options appear on the upper left side of the screen (Figure 10-58) that are controlled by the M knob on the left side of the front panel (see Figure 10-53). The five main options appear as small icons. One is a piece of paper, one is an *i* for information, one is a graph, one is a hand inside a stop sign, and one is a question mark.

When the sheet of paper icon is selected, its menu displays three icons: a single sheet of paper, two sheets of paper, or a pressure icon (Paux/Paw). Selecting the single sheet of paper gives you information on the basic parameters being measured and calculated (9 main parameters), including peak pressure, V_T, PEEP/CPAP level, $\dot{V}_E$, total respiratory rate, mean airway pressure, percentage of oxygen, static compliance, and inspiratory airway resistance. Selecting the single sheet of paper icon lists the monitored parameters that are measured and calculated breath-to-breath but are not constantly displayed on the standard screen.

BOX 10-72

User Attention Messages

Flow sensor calibration needed
O_2 cell calibration needed
Check trigger
Check % MinVol/Pmax
Check rate
Check V_T
Check PEEP/Pcontrol
Check Psupport/Pcontrol
Check PEEP/Psupport,
Check I:E
Check rate/T_I
Check V_T/T_I
Check T_I
Check %Ti
Check peak flow
Check Vtarget/Pmax
Check pause
Check flow pattern
Check Pramp
Check controls for sigh
Nebulizer inactive
Power alarm

If the message, "TECHNICAL FAULT" appears and is followed by a number, the ventilator is experiencing technical difficulties and needs to be replaced. The manufacturer's service engineer should be called and given the number of the technical fault.

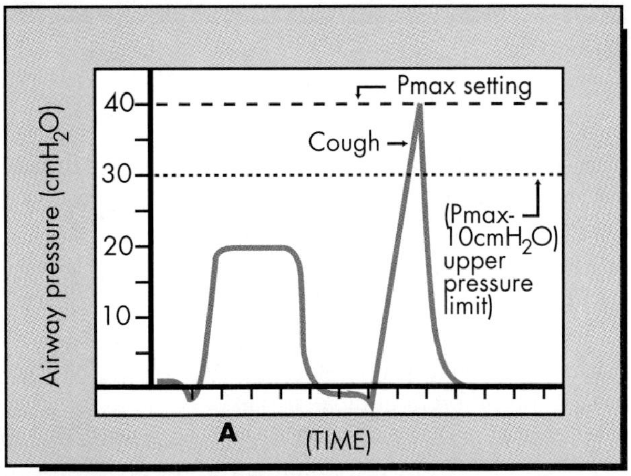

Figure 10-57 A pressure/time graph showing the Pmax pressure setting (*dashed line*), the upper pressure limit (Pmax minus 10 cm H_2O), and a normal breath delivery during P-A/C + APV (**A**) and during a cough.

The double sheet of paper icon gives expanded monitoring of a total of 27 parameters, including pulmonary mechanics, pressure-time products, rapid shallow breathing index, I:E ratio, T_I, T_E, work of breathing (WOB), and time constants. Paux and Paw are also available under this icon

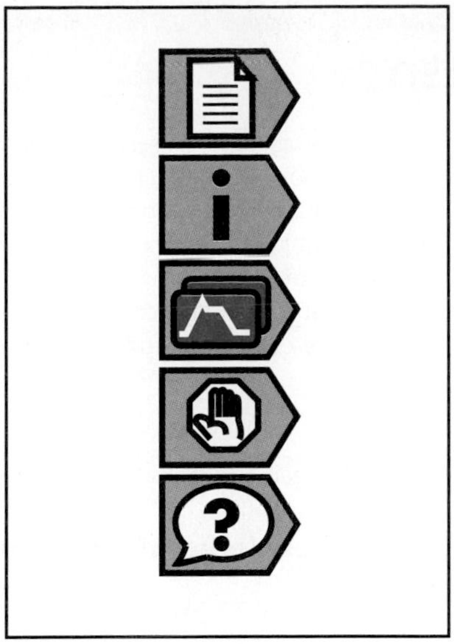

Figure 10-58 Monitor options on the GALILEO.

and provide monitored information on pressures measured from either the auxiliary pressure sensor connector or the standard pressure measurements made with the flow sensor located at the wye connector (Paw). Recall that there is a small nipple connector (Paux) that allows a pressure monitor other than the one at the patient wye connector to be used. For example, the operator may want to monitor transpleural pressure using an esophageal balloon or carinal pressure using a special endotracheal tube or tube adapter. The user is advised to contact the manufacturer to find out the most appropriate auxiliary pressure monitoring equipment to use with the GALILEO.

The "i" icon is an information (help) menu. The waveform main icon for the monitoring menu pulls up a menu for selecting pressure, flow, and volume/time graphs as well as the following loops: pressure/volume, flow/volume, and flow/pressure. In the LOOPS menu, you can also choose Paux or Paw vs. volume so that you can observe total pressures compared with volume and pressures in the airway or in the esophagus vs. volume.

The next icon (stop sign with a hand inside) allows selection of end-inspiratory and end-expiratory hold. Selecting the desired function results in the ventilator automatically performing the function. For example, in the inspiratory hold maneuver, it waits until the next inspiratory breath delivery to activate the hold. (Note that the ventilator will provide up to a 10-second hold for either inspiration or expiration unless the operator stops the function by selecting it again.)

There is an icon marked "?" on the left side of the screen. Under the "?" menu, the operator can select BASIC or EXPERT. Chosing BASIC allows one graphic waveform to be displayed on the normal operating screen. Selecting EXPERT allows you up to three graphic waveforms to be shown at one time on the main screen. Besides allowing for BASIC/EXPERT, this icon allows the selection of ASV. The ASV menu provides information about adaptive support ventilation. For example, in the ASV mode, the screen provides the target values for rate, V_T, $\dot{V}_E$, and inspiratory pressure above PEEP and displays actual measured V_T, rate, and $\dot{V}_E$. The target values can only be provided if the operator has selected ASV and completed the necessary setup (see ASV in the discussion of modes of ventilation in this section).

Real Time Monitoring

The parameters measured by the proximal flow sensor and those calculated by the microprocessor are listed in Box 10-73.

Front Panel Touch Keys

At the lower right corner of the control panel are four touch controls. The red ALARM touch pad silences the audible portion of the alarm system for 2 minutes. It can be reactivated by touching it again. The highest priority alarms cannot be silenced with this control; that is, the audible alarm for the following cannot be silenced:

1. Loss of source gas pressure
2. Loss of electrical power
3. An internal technical error that can be life-threatening or cause catastrophic problems.

The next touch pad is the 100 % O_2, which provides 100% oxygen for 5 minutes. This is useful in procedures such as oxygenation before suctioning. If pressed a second time, the set oxygen percent is quickly resumed.

The MANUAL touch pad delivers a manually-triggered mandatory (pressure or volume) breath. To avoid auto-PEEP after a manual mandatory breath, the unit waits until it recognizes a period of 0.2 seconds of no expiratory gas flow. The fourth touch pad is a PRINT pad, which when pressed can print the current computer screen when the ventilator is connected to a compatible printer.

MODES OF VENTILATION

The modes of ventilation currently available for the GALILEO are listed in Box 10-74. A back-up rate is available whenever apnea is detected during any mode of ventilation. The following section reviews each mode.

Assist/Control (A/C)

This is a standard A/C volume-targeted mode that offers time- or patient-triggering (flow or pressure). The breath can be time- or volume-cycled. The term *volume-cycling* is used here to mean inspiration ends when the measured flow and time are calculated to have delivered the set volume (see Box 10-70). The parameters that can be adjusted

BOX 10-73

Parameters Monitored and Calculated in the GALILEO

Pressures*

Peak pressure (Ppeak), minimum pressure (Pminimum), plateau pressure (Pplateau), PEEP/CPAP pressure, and mean airway pressure (Pmean, calculated value).

Flows*

Inspiratory (Insp Flow) and expiratory (Exp Flow) flows.

Volumes*

Expiratory Tidal Volume (VTE)

Measured as exhaled air from the patient at the proximal airway pressure monitor.

Expired Minute Volume (ExpMinVol)

Measured at the airway; is the sum of eight consecutive measured breaths extrapolated to 1 full minute and updated after each breath.

Leakage Volume (VLeak)

This is the difference between inspired and expired V_T measured at the patient's airway.

Breath-to-Breath Measurement

Time

I:E ratio expressed as 1:X for normal I:E ratios and X:1 for inverse ratios, where *X* is the relative expiratory time for a measured breath and is updated with each breath. (Minimum is 1:9, and maximum is 4:1.)

fTotal† is the sum of spontaneous and mandatory breaths. fSpont† is the sum of only spontaneous breath frequency.

T_I is the actual inspiratory time (in seconds) for a mandatory breath, measured from the beginning of inspiration to the end of inspiratory pause. For a spontaneous breath, it is measured from the beginning of inspiration until the ETS (flow-cycling) criteria are met.

T_E is the actual expiratory time in seconds; it is the time between the beginning of exhalation and the start of inspiration.

Oxygen

Measured inspiratory oxygen concentration.

Calculated Parameters (other than mean airway pressure)

Rinsp‡ (inspiratory airflow resistance) and Rexp‡ (expiratory airflow resistance) result from the patient's airway and the endotracheal tube and are measured in all modes and types of breaths.

Cstat (static lung-thorax compliance) is calculated using exhaled V_T (in liters) and measured pressures (in centimeters of water).‡

RCInsp (inspiratory time constant) and RCExp (expiratory time constant) are calculated from peak expiratory flow and volume.

WOBInsp (inspiratory work of breathing), auto-PEEP, $P_{0.1}$ (occlusion pressure), PTP (inspiratory pressure-time product), and RSB (rapid shallow breathing index) are other calculated parameters.

*Breath-to-breath measurement.

†Measured for 8 consecutive breaths and extrapolated to one minute. Updated after each breath.

‡Calculated using least squares fit.[2]

in this mode are similar to other ventilators and include V_T, rate, peak flow, or $\%T_I$ or I:E, flow pattern, sensitivity (pressure or flow triggering), $O_2\%$, and PEEP/CPAP.

BOX 10-74

Modes of Ventilaton

Assist/Control
SIMV
Spontaneous (CPAP and PSV)
Pressure control ventilation (P-A/C)
P-A/C + adaptive pressure ventilation (P-A/C + APV)
SIMV pressure-targeted (P-SIMV)
P-SIMV (+ APV)
Adaptive support ventilation (ASV)
Back-up ventilation

Synchronized Intermittent Mandatory Ventilation (SIMV)

As with most ventilators, the SIMV mode can be time- or patient-triggered and volume-targeted. Inspiration is time- or volume-cycled as in A/C. Breaths can be delivered with an elevated baseline (PEEP/CPAP). The patient can breathe spontaneously between mandatory breaths. PSV can be added to spontaneous breaths (see the discussion of the spontaneous mode in this chapter). Box 10-75 lists parameters that can be selected on the control menu and adjusted by the operator in SIMV when this mode is activated.

BOX 10-75

Parameters that Can Be Adjusted by the Operator in SIMV (Volume or Pressure Ventilation)

Respiratory rate
V_T or Pressure (Pcontrol above PEEP)
PEEP/CPAP
O_2%
I:E ratio or %T_I or peak flow in volume ventilation
Flow or pressure trigger ($V'_{TR}/\Delta P_{TR}$)
Pressure support (for spontaneous breaths)
Flow pattern and pause (in volume ventilation)
Pressure ramp (P_{ramp}; in pressure control and pressure support only)
Expiratory trigger sensitivity (ETS; in PSV only)
Target volume (in APV)

In the GALILEO during SIMV, the mandatory breaths have a maximum TCT of 4 seconds, which is equal to a set rate of 15 breaths/min. If the rate is set higher, the TCT is shorter. For example at 20 breaths, the TCT is 3 seconds. If the rate is lower than 15 breaths/min, (e.g., 10 breaths/min [TCT = 6 seconds]), the TCT for a mandatory breath is still 4 seconds. A time of ≤4 seconds is used as a trigger window for the mandatory breath. If there is no triggering inside this 4-second window, a mandatory breath is delivered (time-triggered) at the end of the 4 seconds. If you are in a time-cycled mode, the T_I is also determined by the 4-second time frame. For example, in SIMV with a T_I set at 25%, T_I is 1 second. At a T_I of 50%, it will be 2 seconds. (Note that expiratory time may vary. If a patient triggers a breath, this can shorten the T_E, so the TCT is shortened as well.)

Spontaneous Mode (CPAP and PSV)

The spontaneous mode is used when the patient can breathe spontaneously but still requires some support (i.e., CPAP, PSV, or monitoring with alarms). The operator can adjust pressure support, CPAP, % O_2, triggering (flow- or pressure-), pressure ramp (PSV), and expiratory trigger sensitivity (ETS for PSV only). The ventilator provides flow to meet patient demand, while maintaining the desired baseline pressure and pressure support. In the GALILEO, PSV is set above the PEEP/CPAP level. For example, if the clinician wants 10 cm H_2O of pressure support and the patient is receiving 5 cm H_2O of CPAP, the operator sets PSV at 10 cm H_2O. The pressure during inspiration will reach 15 cm H_2O (PS + CPAP). Inspiratory time cannot exceed 3 seconds in the spontaneous mode. The ventilator provides 2 cm H_2O of pressure support within the system, even when PSV is set at zero. This is provided to reduce the work required by the patient to initiate flow from the demand system.

Another important feature of pressure-support ventilation that the GALILEO offers the user is the ability to adjust the flow percentage at which the unit cycles out of inspiration. Commonly a value of 25% of peak flow is used as the cycling flow in PSV. The GALILEO is preprogrammed to flow cycle at 25% of peak for adults and 15% of peak for pediatric patients, but allows this value to be adjusted from 10% to 40% of peak flow. The control for this function is called the expiratory trigger sensitivity (ETS). For example, if the peak flow during a pressure-support breath is 100 L/min, and ETS is set at 30%, a PS breath will end inspiration when flow decreases to 30 L/min. As a safety back-up, inspiratory flow cannot exceed 3 seconds in case there is a leak in the system. The GALILEO will also cycle out of a PS breath if the pressure reaches more than 2 cm H_2O.

Whenever pressure-targeted breaths are selected with either PSV or PCV the GALILEO allows you to adjust the slope or rise (ramp) of the pressure curve P_{ramp}. The P_{ramp} determines the amount of time it takes from the very beginning of inspiratory flow until the set pressure is reached. The pressure curve can be tapered so that pressure does not abruptly enter the upper airway. P_{ramp} is available in PSV, PCV, PCV + APV, and ASV.

Pressure-Control Ventilation (P-A/C)

PCV is also referred to as pressure-targeted assist/control (P-A/C) in the GALILEO. In P-A/C, the ventilator is time- or patient-triggered (flow or pressure), and the breath is pressure-targeted at the set pressure-control level and time-cycled out of inspiration. V_T varies with T_I, set pressure, patient effort, and changes in the patient's lung conditions. For this reason, it is especially important to set exhaled $\dot{V}_E$ alarm levels. As with PSV, the $P_{control}$ value is added to PEEP. For example, if $P_{control}$ is set at 15 cm H_2O, and PEEP is 10 cm H_2O, the maximum pressure generated by the ventilator during inspiration will be 25 cm H_2O. In this example, it is advisable to set the upper pressure limit (Pmax) between 30 and 35 cm H_2O to limit the amount of pressure that could build up in the circuit if the patient coughs or forcibly exhales. The amount of pressure control cannot be set lower than 5 cm H_2O above the baseline pressure (PEEP).

Pressure-Control Ventilation Plus Adaptive Pressure Ventilation (P-A/C + APV)

The operator can also select APV when using pressure control (P-A/C + APV). On the upper portion of the screen, "P-A/C^{APV}?" is displayed. With this selection the operator sets a target volume (VTarget) instead of a target pressure. This is a servo-control mode. Through the automatic control of inspiratory pressure and flow, the specified target volume is applied with the lowest pressure profile possible with the current lung conditions. If exhaled V_T is less than the set value (VTarget), pressure adjusts upward to deliver the desired volume. If V_T is more than VTarget, pressure is reduced.* Maximum pressure is determined by the upper pressure alarm limit setting (Pmax). The upward adjustment in pressure that is performed by the ventilator to correct V_T cannot exceed Pmax − 10 cm H_2O. The amount of pressure control cannot be set lower than 5 cm H_2O above the baseline pressure (PEEP). When the ventilator has to go beyond these pressure limitations to achieve VTarget, audible and visible alarms occur and a message appears at the bottom of the screen telling you that the ventilator has now reached "pressure limitations." The ventilator reaches and maintains pressure at the upper limit, and the breath time-cycles out of inspiration. The target volume cannot be delivered with the current setting for Pmax. The clinician must then decide either to reduce the target V_T or increase Pmax, depending upon the patient's condition.

BOX 10-76

Decision Making & Problem Solving

A patient is being set up on P-A/C + APV on the GALILEO. The ventilator parameters are as follows: rate = 10 breaths/min, T_I = 1.5 seconds, PEEP = 5 cm H_2O, Pmax = 35 cm H_2O, Fio_2 = 0.5, Vtarget = 0.6 L.

A ventilating pressure of 25 cm H_2O is required to deliver the target volume for this patient. A few breaths after the mode is initiated, the respiratory therapist hears an audible alarm and sees a message indicating that ventilation is on "Pressure Limitation." What changes should the therapist make?

See Appendix A for the answers.

Pressure Control/SIMV (P-SIMV)

The GALILEO can provide SIMV using pressure-targeted mandatory breaths (P-SIMV). This mode is very similar to conventional SIMV. Breaths are patient- or time-triggered and time-cycled, but in this case pressure-targeted. V_Ts vary depending on the set pressure, T_I, patient lung characteristics, and any patient effort that might be present. As with volume-targeted SIMV, spontaneous breaths can be given a positive-pressure baseline (PEEP/CPAP) and also aided with the use of pressure support.

Pressure Control/SIMV Plus Adaptive Pressure Ventilation (P-SIMV + APV)

P-SIMV can also be altered using the APV function. At the top of the screen "P-SIMV^{APV}?" appears. In P-SIMV + APV, mandatory breaths are still pressure breaths, but they become volume-targeted (set Vtarget). The ventilator adjusts pressure delivery during these mandatory breaths in order to achieve the volume target using the lowest possible inspiratory pressure. This is similar to P-A/C + APV (see the previous discussion of this mode). The primary difference is that a patient can breathe spontaneously between mandatory breaths at the set baseline and pressure-support level (Box 10-76).

Adaptive Support Ventilation (ASV)

ASV is a servo-controlled technique that functions using pressure-targeted breaths to assure a chosen target ventilation, while establishing protective lung strategies. It adapts to the changing capabilities and lung conditions of the patient. The GALILEO automatically adapts its performance to the patient's demands—from full support to CPAP. The more work the patient is able to perform, the less the ventilator provides. It can ventilate the patient through the acute stage process to a successful wean.

ASV is such a new approach to ventilation that an explanation of its operation is divided into several different sections:

1. Setting up the ventilator for ASV
2. Ventilator programming to establish respiratory parameters
3. Initial test breaths
4. Variations in breath delivery

Setting up the Ventilator for ASV

Ideally, when respiratory therapists or physicians initially establish ventilation in a patient, they calculate initial settings based on a predicted $\dot{V}_E$, rate, and V_T. These predictions are usually calculated from equations that have been established through clinical research that use parameters such as ideal body weight (IBW); patient height and sex; and any abnormal conditions that may be present.[3] For example, $\dot{V}_E$ may be based on body surface area calculated from patient weight and height and adjusted for abnormal body temperature.[3]

In ASV, the ventilator calculates $\dot{V}_E$ and divides it into optimal targets for respiratory rate and V_T. The ventilator performs a series of calculations based on information provided by the practitioner. Input data include: IBW, %$\dot{V}_E$, inspiratory pressure, PEEP/CPAP, % O_2, pressure or flow trigger sensitivity, pressure ramp, and ETS. The first three are important to establish $\dot{V}_E$, f, and V_T delivery. PEEP/CPAP and oxygen percentage help patient oxygenation. Trigger sensitivity adjusts the ease of breath triggering, and pressure ramp and ETS tailor PS breaths.

*Pressure changes are made in increments of 1 cm H_2O.

BOX 10-77

Otis's Formula

Total respiratory frequency (f)

$$f = \frac{\sqrt{1 + 4\pi^2 RCe\left(\frac{\dot{V}_E - f \times V_D}{V_D}\right)} - 1}{2\pi^2 RCe}$$

Here RCe = expiratory time constant; $\dot{V}_E$ = minute ventilation; V_D = deadspace volume.

The Galileo estimates dead space as 1 mL/pound IBW using Radford's nomogram.

BOX 10-78

Decision Making & Problem Solving

Problem 1:
An adult patient has an IBW of 60 kg. The operator sets $\dot{V}_E$ at 100%. What will be the $\dot{V}_E$ established by the ventilator for the patient?
Problem 2:
If an infant has an IBW of 5 kg, and the operator sets the $\dot{V}_E$ at 50%, what will be the $\dot{V}_E$ delivery for the infant by the ventilator?

See Appendix A for the answers.

Ventilator Programming to Establish Respiratory Parameters

The ventilator is programmed to calculate and deliver overall minute ventilation using pressure targeted breaths. It uses a combination of P-SIMV (time-triggered breaths) and PSV breaths (any patient-triggered breaths). It bases f, V_T, and $\dot{V}_E$ on the equations and limitations placed on those parameters that are programmed into the microprocessors. For example, rate is calculated using Otis's least work of breathing equation (Box 10-77).[4-8]

The ventilator sets $\dot{V}_E$ based on the set percentage $\dot{V}_E$ (%$\dot{V}_E$) and the following constants:

100% $\dot{V}_E$ = 100 mL/min/kg (0.1 L/min/kg) in adults and
200 mL/min/kg (0.2 L/min/kg) in infants

For example, a baby with an IBW of 10 kg and a $\dot{V}_E$ setting of 100% would have a predicted and a set minimum $\dot{V}_E$ of 2000 mL/min, or 2 L/min. In this example, suppose that the infant has an elevated body temperature. You should increase the $\dot{V}_E$ to compensate for the elevated metabolism.[3] You might set the $\dot{V}_E$ to 110% of that predicted. (The available range is 10% to 350% of predicted.) You must remember to set the desired percentage of predicted $\dot{V}_E$ you want to occur.

For another example, suppose an arterial blood gas sample reveals that a patient's initial 100% $\dot{V}_E$ setting results in mild hypocapnia. You might reduce the $\dot{V}_E$ to 90% to reduce the amount of ventilation provided and allow $PaCO_2$ to rise toward normal (Box 10-78). In addition to $\dot{V}_E$, the GALILEO calculates V_T based on its internal equation for V_T, and upper and lower limits (lower $V_T = 2 \times$ dead space [V_D]; upper $V_T = 10 \times V_D$). For example, a person with an IBW of 150 lbs has a predicted V_D of 1 mL/lb IBW (150 mL). The V_T range for this person would be 300 mL to 1500 mL. In addition, the internal equation for V_T looks at patient lung characteristics, which change with differences in disease pathology. For example, pulmonary edema results in reduced lung compliance. Low lung compliance is associated with a body's response of a higher rate and lower V_T. The ventilator makes an effort to reduce work of breathing by providing a rate and a V_T that reflects the patient's lung condition (lung compliance [C] and airway resistance [R]), but stays within its limitations (Table 10-12).

TABLE 10-12

Safety limits in ASV

Parameter	Value
Minimum pressure	PEEP + 5 cm H_2O
Maximum pressure	PMax setting − 10 cm H_2O
V_T minimum	4.4 mL/kg IBW (2 × V_D)
V_T maximum	22.0 mL/kg IBW (10 × V_D)
Minimum mandatory rate	5 breaths/min
Maximum mandatory rate	60 breaths/min
Minimum T_I	RCe, or 0.5 seconds
Maximum T_I	2 × RCe, or 3 seconds
Minimum T_E	2 × RCe
Maximum T_E	12 seconds

RCe = expiratory time constant

The ventilator is constantly analyzing T_I, T_E, total rate, inspired $\dot{V}_E$, expiratory time constant (RCe), R, C, and ventilating pressures (Box 10-79).[2] It uses all this information, plus the input from the operator to establish an appropriate breathing pattern that at all times tries to reduce the work of breathing and balance the patient's spontaneous and mandatory breaths.

Initial Test Breaths

The GALILEO assesses the patient by providing five test breaths (pressure breaths), starting at a minimum pressure just above baseline and gradually increasing the pressure. During the test breaths, the ventilator performs its measurements and calculations of V_T, f, C, R, and time constants. From these measurements, the ventilator can assess

BOX 10-79

Static Compliance and Airway Resistance

The calculation of static compliance by the GALILEO does not require that the operator select an inspiratory pause (inflation hold) to get a static pressure reading. The static compliance is calculated mathematically using the least squares fit method. The unit performs 200 measurements/second of flow, pressure, and volume then does a linear regression calculation to estimate static compliance and airway resistance. The analysis of pressure, flow, and volume is based on a mechanical model of the respiratory system.[2]

the elastic and resistive workload and establish the optimum breath pattern (i.e., the ventilatory pattern that represents the least work of breathing for the patient). Table 10-12 lists the safety limits autoprogrammed by the unit to avoid complications associated with mechanical ventilation, including auto-PEEP, lung tissue injury associated with excessive volume (volutrauma) and excessive pressure (barotrauma), apnea, and tachypnea.

Variation in Breath Delivery

The ventilator begins to deliver the optimum breathing pattern using pressure-targeted breaths.* It adjusts inspiratory pressure and mandatory rate to achieve a given minimal $\dot{V}_E$ based on Figure 10-59. All parameters are sampled 200 times/sec. If compliance, resistance, or spontaneous breathing efforts change, ASV measures these changes and readjusts the inspiratory support and rate to maintain protective lung strategies. It allows the patient to resume spontaneous breathing when able. Remember that although the mode provides a minimum selected $\dot{V}_E$, patients can achieve a higher $\dot{V}_E$ if they so choose.

Three common scenarios can occur that help to describe the function of ASV.

1. If the patient is not spontaneously breathing, P-SIMV breaths are delivered. The ventilator provides the % $\dot{V}_E$ set. Breaths are time-triggered and pressure-targeted to achieve the desired volume, as well as time-cycled. As lung conditions change, the pressure level is adjusted between minimum and maximum to deliver the calculated V_T with the least amount of pressure.

   If the patient assists a breath after having been apneic, the ventilator delivers a PS breath at the same pressure used for the pressure-controlled breath. This is logical because the ventilator has calculated this pressure to be that which is required to deliver the optimal V_T.

*These breaths are like pressure-control breaths but are also volume-targeted to achieve the optimum calculated V_T.

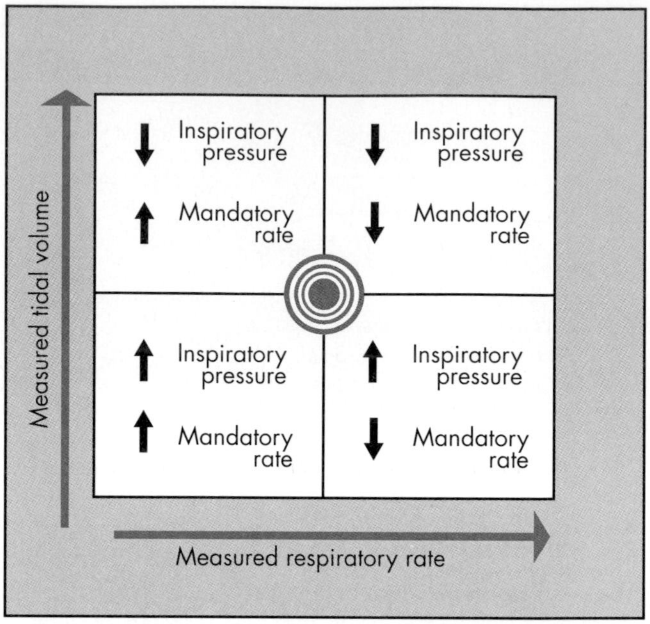

Figure 10-59 An illustration of ASV. If measured frequency (f) is greater than target f, mandatory f is decreased, and vice-versa. If measured V_T is greater than target V_T, PIP is decreased, and vice-versa. (Redrawn from Hamilton Medical, Reno, Nev.)

2. If the patient is providing some—but not all—of the work of breathing, patient-triggered breaths are pressure-support breaths. Time-triggered breaths are pressure-control breaths. The ventilator calculates the difference between the spontaneous breathing rate and volume delivery, and the calculated rate (missing breaths) and volume delivery. The missing breaths are provided as added (time-triggered) pressure-controlled breaths designed to achieve the desired V_T.
3. If the patient is spontaneously breathing and triggering all breaths, they will be pressure-support breaths with pressure adjusted to maintain optimum volume.

To try and summarize ASV, it is a servo-controlled mode of ventilation that delivers pressure breaths targeted to achieve the desired, calculated volume. Time-triggered breaths are in PCV, and patient-triggered breaths are in PSV. The ventilator continually monitors patient lung characteristics and breathing patterns and calculates an optimum V_T with required pressure delivery and rate to optimize ventilation and minimize patient work of breathing. Patients may be completely controlled when first connected to the ventilator, but as they begin to recover and are able to spontaneously breathe, fewer mandatory breaths are required. Eventually patients breathe with only pressure-supported breaths. The ventilator continues to monitor all parameters and adjust its performance as needed.

Mode Additions

In addition to the modes previously described, you can select ADDITIONS from the mode menu.

Additions

Several additional options are listed under additions. APV is under this section (see the discussion of modes of ventilation in this chapter). The PEDIATRIC option adapts the ventilator to infants weighing from 3 to 30 kg and switches standard controls and alarms to a range appropriate for infant/pediatric ventilation.

Two final items available under the ADDITIONS menu are SIGH and NEBULIZER. A sigh breath can be applied every 100 breaths and increases the V_T for volume-targeted breaths by 50% of the set value and increases inspiratory pressure by 5 cm H_2O with pressure-targeted breaths. The HIGH PRESSURE DURING SIGH alarm occurs if the peak pressure limit is reached during a sigh breath.

Activating the nebulizer causes the internal nebulizer compressor to deliver gas flow to the nebulizer line for 30 minutes, unless it is manually turned off before that time. If the set peak flow for volume-targeted breaths is less than 20 L/min, the nebulizer turns off.

Back-up Ventilation

BACK-UP VENTILATION also appears under the ADDITIONS menu and is available in all modes but is actually not necessary in ASV. The operator has the opportunity to select the desired BACK-UP VENTILATION (ADDITIONS menu) and APNEA TIME (ALARMS window). If the apnea time is exceeded, the back-up apnea rate becomes active, and the ventilator uses A/C as its mode. Breath delivery is either volume- or pressure-targeted. The ventilator uses whatever pressure or volume value is set when the apnea event occurs. Back-up ventilation is automatically stopped, and the original mode resumed if the patient starts to breathe spontaneously.

To prevent back-up ventilation from occurring when the patient is disconnected for suctioning or a similar procedure, press the ALARM SILENCE touch pad. This prevents back-up ventilation from becoming active for 2 minutes. In addition, whenever you change the ventilator mode or perform ventilator calibration procedures, back-up ventilation is automatically suppressed for 30 seconds.

GRAPHICS

The graphics available on the GALILEO are available by using knob M and were discussed in the previous section on controls and alarms.

TROUBLESHOOTING

The monitor and alarm system for the GALILEO provide an important part of the troubleshooting if the ventilator alarms or alerts. When a technical message occurs, the operator must record the number indicated with the message and then contact Hamilton Medical technical support about the problem. Any ventilator with a technical error problem should immediately be removed from service and replaced by another unit. At this time, the GALILEO has just begun its clinical use in the United States. For this reason, limited personal experience with this unit prevents any other comments that may be pertinent about troubleshooting. For more information about the company see its web site at: www.hammed1.com.

Review Questions

See Appendix A for answers.

1. To select and set a specific ventilator control on the GALILEO, which of the following should be performed?
   I. Scroll through screen options or ventilator parameters using knob C.
   II. Select a highlighted option (parameter) by pressing knob C.
   III. Once an icon is red, rotate knob C to change the numerical value.
   IV. Press knob C to select the newly set value.
   a. III only
   b. I and IV only
   c. II and III only
   d. I, II, III, and IV

2. Which of the following options can be configured as a cycling mechanism in volume ventilation?
   I. T_I
   II. Peak flow
   III. TCT
   IV. I:E
   a. I and IV only
   b. II and III only
   c. I, II, and IV only
   d. II, III, and IV only

3. An apneic patient is being ventilated with ASV on the GALILEO. Which of the following best describes the breath delivery in this situation?
   a. time-triggered, pressure-targeted breaths that are volume guaranteed
   b. flow- or pressure-triggered PS breaths that are volume guaranteed
   c. pressure-triggered, volume-targeted breaths with a constant flow delivery
   d. time-triggered, volume-targeted breaths with a constant flow delivery

4. Expiratory trigger sensitivity functions by which of the following?
   a. flow-triggering inspiration
   b. pressure-triggering the expiratory phase
   c. flow-cycling PS breaths at a specified flow
   d. limiting the maximum airway pressure during expiration

5. In PCV, the set pressure for breath delivery is also the maximum pressure that can be reached in the circuit—true or false?
6. Once all desired parameters are set for a specific mode, you must select the CLOSE icon to confirm and activate the new mode—true or false?
7. Explain how a ventilator parameter such as V_T is adjusted on the Hamilton GALILEO.
8. When the viewing screen is in the alarms menu, how do you determine the actual (current) value for airway pressure?
9. If the patient's IBW is entered as 50 kg and the $\dot{V}_E$ support is set at 100%, what will be the $\dot{V}_E$ delivery in an adult?
10. Compare the setting of PSV and PEEP levels during spontaneous ventilation on the VEOLAR with that on the GALILEO.

References

1. Operating manual: GALILEO, 610 175/00, Reno, Nev., 1997, Hamilton Medical.
2. Lotti GA, et al: Respiratory mechanics by least squares fitting in mechanically ventilated patients: applications during paralysis and during pressure support ventilation, Intensive Care Med 21:406, 1995.
3. Pilbeam SP: Mechanical ventilation: physiological and clinical applications, ed 3, St Louis, 1998, Mosby.
4. Radford EP, Ferris BG, and Kriete BC: Clinical use of a nomogram to estimate proper ventilation during artificial respirations, N Engl J Med 251:877, 1954.
5. Otis AB, Fenn WO, and Rahn H: Mechanics of breathing in man, J Appl Physiol 2:592, 1950.
6. Brunner JX , et al: Simple method to measure total expiratory time constant based on the passive expiratory flow-volume curve, Crit Care Med, 23(6):1117, 1995.
7. Laubscher TP, et al: The automatic selection of ventilation parameters during the initial phase of mechanical ventilation, Intensive Care Med, 22:199, 1996.
8. Laubscher TP, et al: Automatic selection of tidal volume, respiratory frequency and minute ventilation in intubated ICU patients as startup procedure for closed-loop controlled ventilation, International J of Clin Monitoring and Computing, 11:19, 1994.

Nellcor Puritan Bennett Adult Star

OUTLINE

Power Source

Internal Mechanisms

Testing
- Tubing Compliance Compensation

Controls and Alarms
- Pressure Bar Graph
- Ventilation Settings Screen
- Patient Status Screen
- Graphic Monitoring Screen
- Messages
- Alarms

Modes of Operation
- Assist/Control
- SIMV
- CPAP
- Pressure Support
- Pressure-Control Ventilation
- Graphic Displays
- Special Features

Troubleshooting

LEARNING OBJECTIVES

Upon completion of this section, the reader should be able to:

1. Describe the internal mechanisms of the Adult Star.
2. Discuss the function of the controls on the control panel.
3. Explain how to select and change ventilator settings.
4. Recommend a solution to an alarm situation.
5. List the modes of ventilation.
6. Compare data in ventilator settings and patient status screens with graphic displays on the graphic monitor screen.
7. Solve a problem related to an error message that is presented on the screen.
8. Calculate inadvertent PEEP (auto-PEEP) levels given total PEEP and extrinsic PEEP.

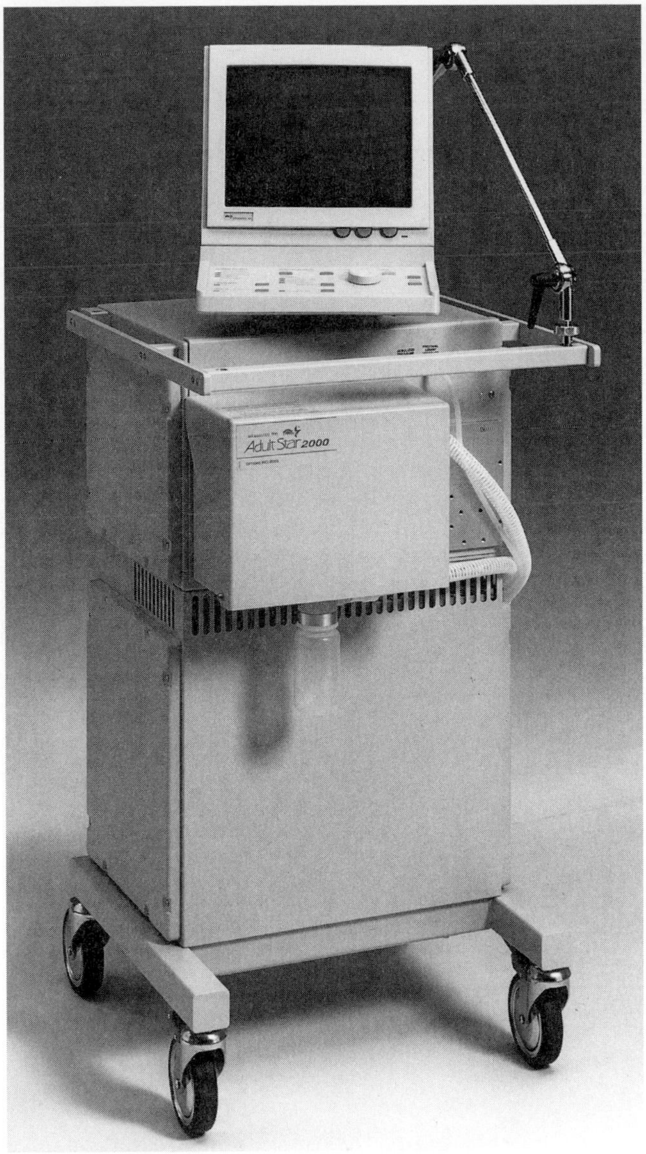

Figure 10-60 The Adult Star ventilator. (Courtesy Nellcor Puritan Bennett Corp., Pleasanton, Calif.)

The Adult Star[1,2] ventilator has two models, the 1500 and the 2000. The Adult Star 1500 is the basic model, and the 2000 comes equipped with additional features, such as a graphic monitor package, printer and analog interfaces, nebulizer function, and software for measuring respiratory mechanics. Figure 10-60 shows the Adult Star 2000 model, which is the focus of this discussion. These units are designed for pediatric and adult use primarily in acute care settings.

POWER SOURCE

The Adult Star is electrically and pneumatically powered and microprocessor-controlled (five microprocessors). It requires a standard electrical outlet (107- to 132-volt AC at 60 Hz) to operate the microprocessor and electronic components. The system has both a main ON/OFF switch on the rear of the ventilator and an ON/OFF switch at the left rear of the control panel. Both must be on for the unit to operate. Leaving the main switch on when the machine is not in use and keeping the unit plugged into a wall outlet charges the internal battery.

The pneumatic system normally uses two high-pressure gas sources (30 to 90 psi, air and oxygen) to power the pneumatic circuit, but it can run from a single gas source, such as the optional air compressor (piston-driven) that is housed in an enclosed wheel base (see Figure 10-60). This, of course, alters FiO_2 delivery.

INTERNAL MECHANISMS

The Star ventilator uses its five microprocessors for the following functions:

1. Main processor
2. Analog/digital (A/D) processor
3. Two stepper motors
4. Graphics processor

The main processor controls the pneumatic system through a direct input/output (I/O) interface with the two microprocessors that govern the flow-control valves that are stepper motor-controlled proportioning valves (see Chapter 9 for an explanation). The main processor receives information from several sources, including the pressure and flow transducers, the output control valve, and the front panel settings. Using this information, it controls triggering, flow delivery, cycling, and alarm functions.

The A/D processor converts analog signals to digital signals for the other microprocessors. The graphics system operates the graphics waveform display and the interfaces to the graphics screen.

In the pneumatic system, air and oxygen enter the unit through connections on the back panel, after which they are reduced to 6.5 to 7.5 psi before entering the internal flow-control valves for air and oxygen (proportional valves) (Figure 10-61). The stepper motors that drive these valves establish the flow, volume, and O_2% delivery to the patient. From these valves, gas flows through a flow transducer, which is a pneumotachometer device that measures flow and provides feedback to the main processor. From here, gas enters the patient circuit.

Part of the gas from the input gas sources is directed to the large-diameter, pneumatically controlled expiratory valve. Pressure against this valve helps determine PEEP levels. An expiratory flow transducer (pneumotachometer), similar to the inspiratory flow transducer, is distal to the expiratory valve (see Figure 10-61).

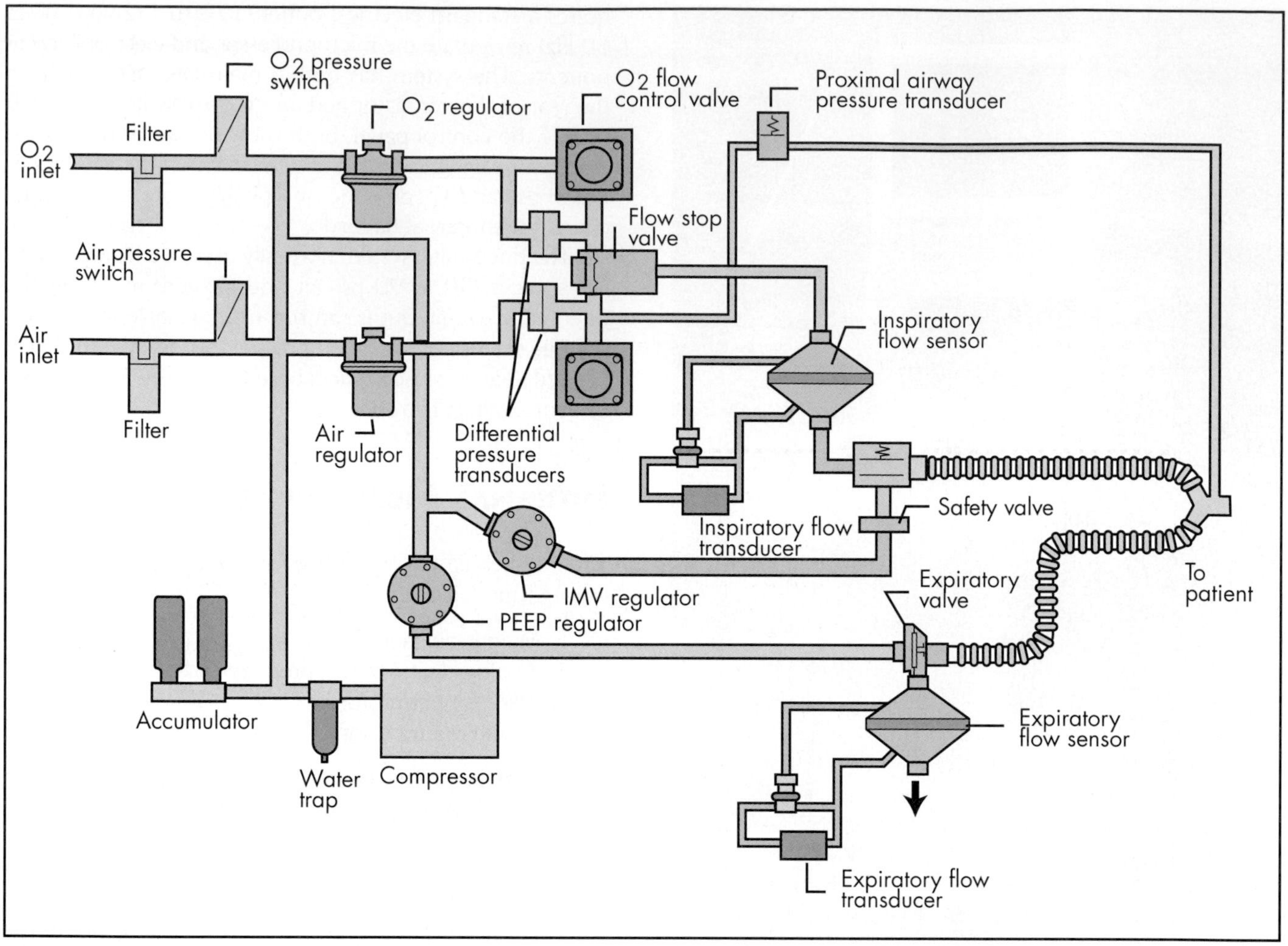

Figure 10-61 The internal components of the Adult Star ventilator control circuit. (Courtesy Nellcor Puritan Bennett, Pleasanton, Calif.)

Testing

As with all microprocessor-controlled ventilators, when the unit is turned on, it runs through a series of self-tests before it can be connected to a patient. More extensive testing can also be performed by holding down the VISUAL RESET and ALARM SILENCE buttons when turning on the machine. After about 5 seconds, the screen displays the ADULT STAR PERFORMANCE, SAFETY, AND DIAGNOSTICS TEST screen. You can select either DIAGNOSTICS or a QUICK TEST. Move the cursor to the desired test and press ENTER to have the ventilator make the selection. Diagnostic tests help assess ventilator and performance capabilities and are not be reviewed here. We will briefly outline the quick test. Box 10-80 lists the 14 tests performed during the quick test.

After selecting QUICK TEST, disconnect the test lung or patient from the ventilator, move the cursor to YES and press ENTER. You must cap the patient wye connector and press ENTER again to begin the test. If the unit fails any of the 14 tests, you can choose to rerun the test, abort the test,

BOX 10-80

Tests Performed During Quick Test on the Adult Star

Pressure transducer comparison test
Patient circuit leak test
Patient circuit compliance test
One-way valve leakage test
Airflow delivery test
Exhaled flow measurement test
Oxygen flow delivery test
Safety valve pressure-relief test
Redundant safety valve pressure test
PEEP test
Exhalation filter test
Ventilator inoperative test

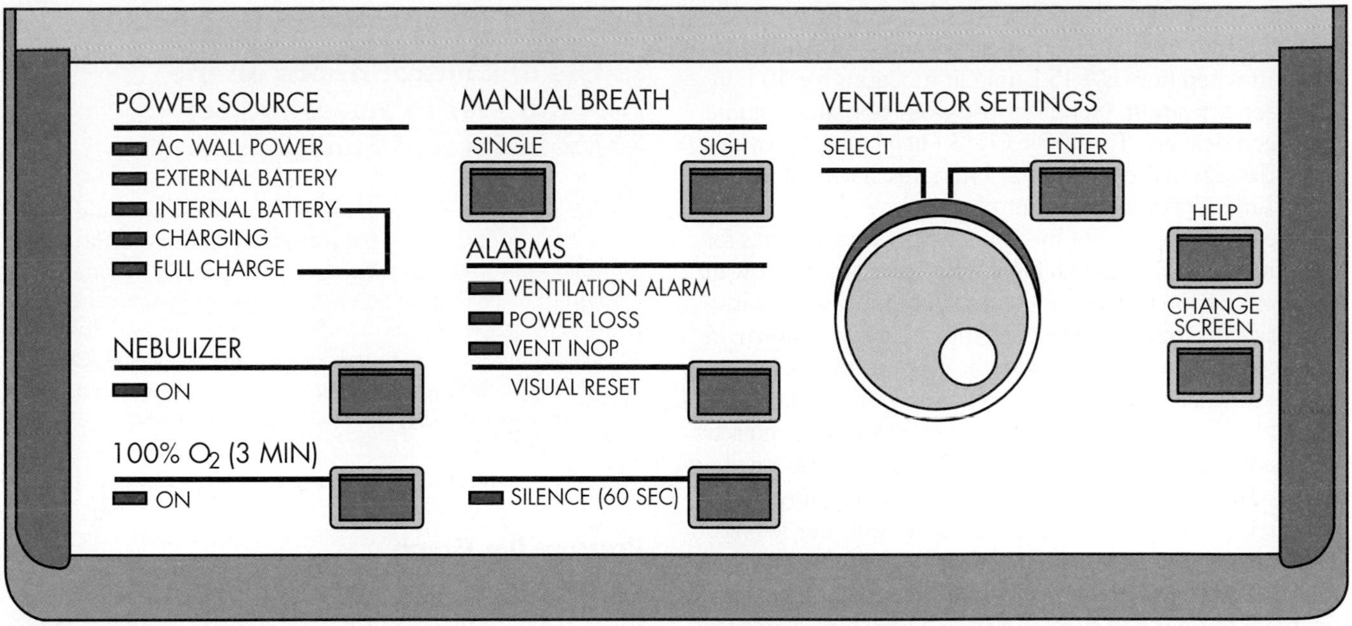

Figure 10-62 The control panel of the Adult Star ventilator. (Courtesy Nellcor Puritan Bennett Corp., Pleasanton, Calif.)

or proceed to the next test. The final step is the VENT. INOP. test, in which the machine simulates a ventilator inoperative situation to verify that this safety function works. After the ventilator declares VENT.INOP., you are asked to verify that the VENT. INOP. light is on. At this point you can print out the results if you wish. Otherwise, to exit, clear the VENT. INOP. condition (ALARM RESET) and turn the ventilator off using the ON/OFF switch. Simply turn the unit back on if you wish to restart it for use.

Tubing Compliance Compensation

Loss of volume due to tubing compliance can be compensated for in the Adult Star (Software 219.2 and higher).[2] The DIAGNOSTICS TESTS menu allows for the selection of this option. Simply select and enter COMPLIANCE COMPENSATION from the DIAGNOSTICS TEST menu. After its selection, press the HELP button to choose between YES (compensate) and NO (don't compensate). The help button toggles between the two choices. Your selection is automatically placed in memory.

Circuit compliance is measured during the quick test. (Be sure you have it checked with the new patient circuit in place and a filled humidifier before you use the tubing compensation feature.) Once it is operational, the ventilator automatically increases V_T delivery based on peak pressure. In addition, the exhaled V_T display automatically decreases the measured V_T by the amount added to compensate volume delivery. However, the graphics display for flow and volume provide the actual flow and volume reading. Therefore the digital display and the graphic display differ slightly.

BOX 10-81

Power Source Indicators

AC Wall Power

Illuminates when the machine is plugged into a wall outlet.

External Battery

Lights when a 12-volt battery is used for power (e.g., during patient transport).

Internal Battery and Charging

Light up when the internal battery is being recharged.

Full Charge

Light turns on when the internal battery is at 90% of full charge.

CONTROLS AND ALARMS

Figure 10-60 shows the Star front panel, which consists of two parts. There is a CRT (cathode ray tube) screen for display of menus, controls, and information, as well as a control panel (Figure 10 62). The control panel has three main sections. On the left are indicators of the power source, the nebulizer control, and the 100% O_2 control. (Older versions of the Adult Star control panel have the ON/OFF switch on the left side of the panel, but otherwise are similar in design to the current panel.) The power source indicators located on the left of the control panel are described in Box 10-81.

The NEBULIZER control provides 8 L/min of flow from the nebulizer outlet during mandatory and spontaneous inspiration when flow is ≥15 L/min. It functions for 30 minutes after activation. Nebulizer use does not alter volume or oxygen delivery. The 100% O_2 (3-MIN) control provides 100% oxygen to the patient for 3 minutes. It can be turned off by simply pressing the control again.

The central portion of the panel has manual controls for triggering mandatory or sigh breaths and an alarm panel with a SILENCE button (60 second), a RESET button (visual alarms), and indicators for alarm types (see the discussion of alarms in this section). The panel on the right contains the main controls for the machine: SELECT knob and an ENTER button. The SELECT knob rotates clockwise and counterclockwise and acts like a computer mouse to highlight different areas on the screen. The ENTER button activates highlighted areas. Box 10-82 reviews the procedure for selecting ventilator settings.

There is also a HELP button and a SCREEN CHANGE button. The HELP button brings up additional information regarding settings and suggestions for alarm corrections for the screen that is displayed. The screen change button gives access to the three main menu screens, as follows:

1. Screen 1—Ventilator Settings
2. Screen 2—Patient Status
3. Screen 3—Graphic Monitoring

All three screens have a VENTILATOR SETTING section, a PATIENT STATUS section, an ALARM LIMITS STATUS section, and a message window, each of which is reviewed here.

BOX 10-82

Use of Control Knobs on the Adult Star to Select and Set Variables and Functions

All ventilator parameters and alarms are set using the SELECT knob. The knob is rotated until the cursor (a yellow bar) backlights (highlights) the variable or function to be changed. The ENTER button is then pressed to activate the selected variable. The knob is again rotated until the desired function or numerical value for a variable is displayed. Pressing the ENTER button again accepts and activates the new value or function.

Pressure Bar Graph

Both Screens 1 and 2 have a bar graph showing airway pressure (−20 to 120 cm H_2O). The pressure bar graph shows real time pressures measured through the proximal pressure line. To the left of the pressure bar are indicators for the current settings of high inspiratory pressure (HIP), low inspiratory pressure (LIP), and low PEEP/CPAP (LOP) alarms.

Ventilation Settings Screen

Screen 1, the VENTILATOR SETTINGS screen, displays operator-set parameters and alarm thresholds (Figure 10-63).

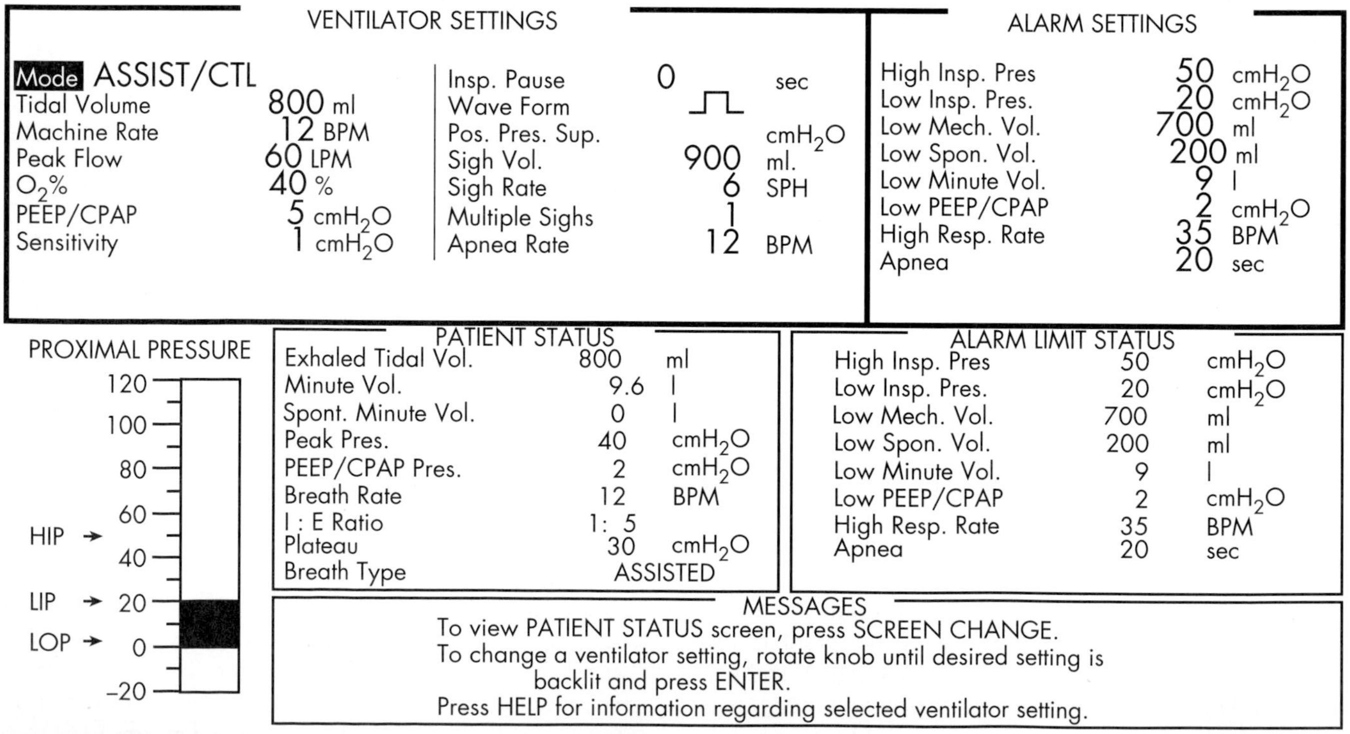

Figure 10-63 The ventilator settings screen for volume ventilation on the Adult Star. (Courtesy Nellcor Puritan Bennett Corp., Pleasanton, Calif.)

Ventilator settings can be made either from this screen or the GRAPHICS screen. Table 10-13 provides a list of available parameters and their ranges that you can change and provides addition information about alarm status and monitored information. Figure 10-63 shows information provided on Screen 1 with volume ventilation; Figure 10-64 shows the display for PCV.

Patient Status Screen

Screen 2, the PATIENT STATUS screen, lists measured patient information (Table 10-14 and Figure 10-65). The pressure values displayed are measured through the proximal pressure line connected to the patient wye. The expired volumes are measured at the expiratory flow sensor. This screen is automatically displayed during normal ventilator operation if no changes are made for 60 seconds.

Graphic Monitoring Screen

Screen 3, the GRAPHIC MONITOR screen, gives graphically displayed information on the left portion of the screen (Figure 10-66). You can also make ventilator setting changes from this screen by moving the yellow bar (cursor) into the VENTILATOR SETTING section of the screen, highlighting the desired option, and pressing ENTER.

Box 10-83 provides an exercise in problem solving related to the graphics presented in Figure 10-66.

TABLE 10-13

Available parameters and ranges on the Adult Star

Parameters	Ranges
V_T	100 to 2500 mL (50 to 2500 mL with the pediatric ventilation option)
Respiratory rate	0.5 to 80 breaths/min (0.5 to 120 breaths/min with the pediatric ventilation option)
Peak flow	10 to 120 L/min (10 to 160 L/min breaths/min with the pediatric ventilation option)
O_2 %	21% to 100%
PEEP/CPAP	0 to 30 cm H_2O (0 to 50 cm H_2O optional)
Sensitivity	−0.5 to −20 cm H_2O
Inspiratory pause	0 to 2.0 seconds
Waveforms	constant, sinusoidal, ascending and descending ramps
Pressure support	0 to 70 cm H_2O (above PEEP)
Sigh volume*	100 to 2500 mL
Sigh rate*	0 to 20 sighs/hour
Multiple sighs*	1 to 3 sighs per sigh event

*The sigh function works in all modes except CPAP and PCV, but a manual sigh breath can be delivered in CPAP.

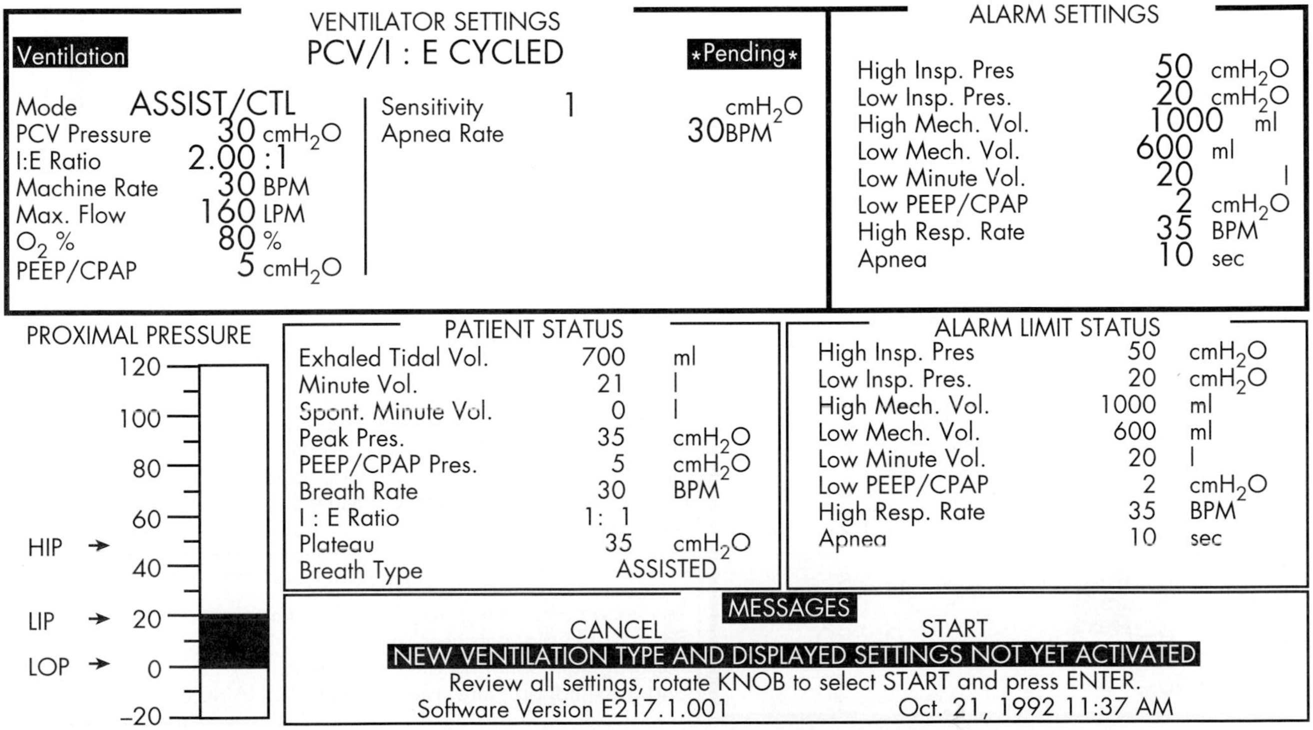

Figure 10-64 The ventilator settings screen for pressure-control ventilation on the Adult Star. (Courtesy Nellcor Puritan Bennett Corp., Pleasanton, Calif.)

TABLE 10-14

Monitored parameters in the Adult Star

Parameter	Range
Exhaled V_T (updated breath by breath)	0 to 2500 mL
$\dot{V}_E$ (last minute)	0 to 99.9 L/min
Spontaneous $\dot{V}_E$ (last minute)	0 to 99.9 L/min
Peak pressure	0 to 120 cm H_2O
Mean airway pressure	0 to 120 cm H_2O
PEEP/CPAP	0 to 30 cm H_2O (0 to 50 cm H_2O optional)
Plateau pressure	0 to 120 cm H_2O
Breath rate	0 to 150 breaths/min
I:E ratio	99.9:1 to 1:99.9
Breath type	assisted, controlled spontaneous, sigh

Messages

The message window is available in any screen and provides information about the current software in use, altitude setting, date, time, and general information about making ventilator changes.[1] Figures 10-63 through 10-66 show examples of different messages.

Alarms

All three screens provide information about alarm settings and status. Alarm settings are the values you set for adjustable alarms (Table 10-15). Table 10-16 provides information about nonadjustable alarms.

The ALARM LIMIT STATUS screen lists information about current or recent alarm conditions. If one or more alarm thresholds are violated, the screen visually highlights the affected alarms. Sometimes alarm conditions occur, but are corrected. For example, a high-pressure alarm may be triggered for a single breath, but not occur again. Inactive alarms (i.e., alarm conditions that have been corrected) are represented by an "X" or an asterisk "*." The X indicates the first alarm condition; the * indicates subsequent alarms. These symbols are to the left of the condition that occurred, thus allowing you to determine which alarm occurred in your absence. Pressing VISUAL RESET clears these indicators, although they automatically clear after 5 minutes if the condition is corrected—even if reset is not pushed.

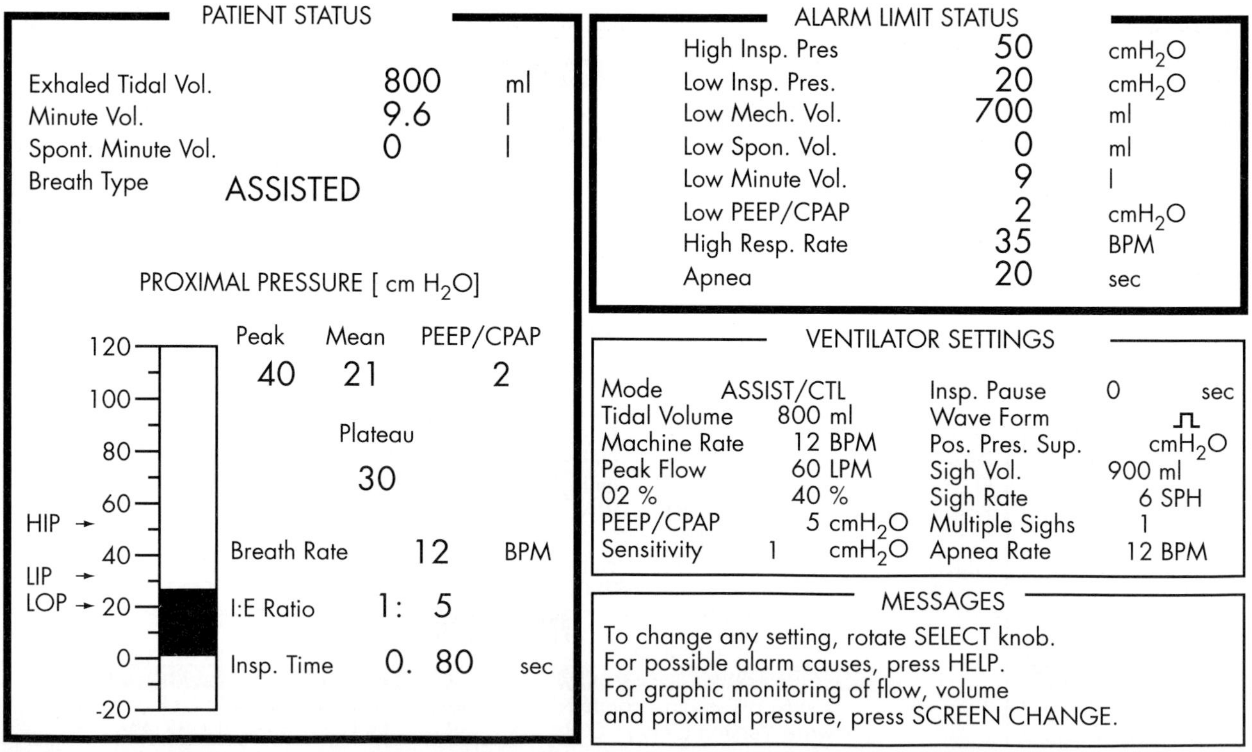

Figure 10-65 The patient status (monitoring) screen on the Adult Star. (Courtesy Nellcor Puritan Bennett Corp., Pleasanton, Calif.)

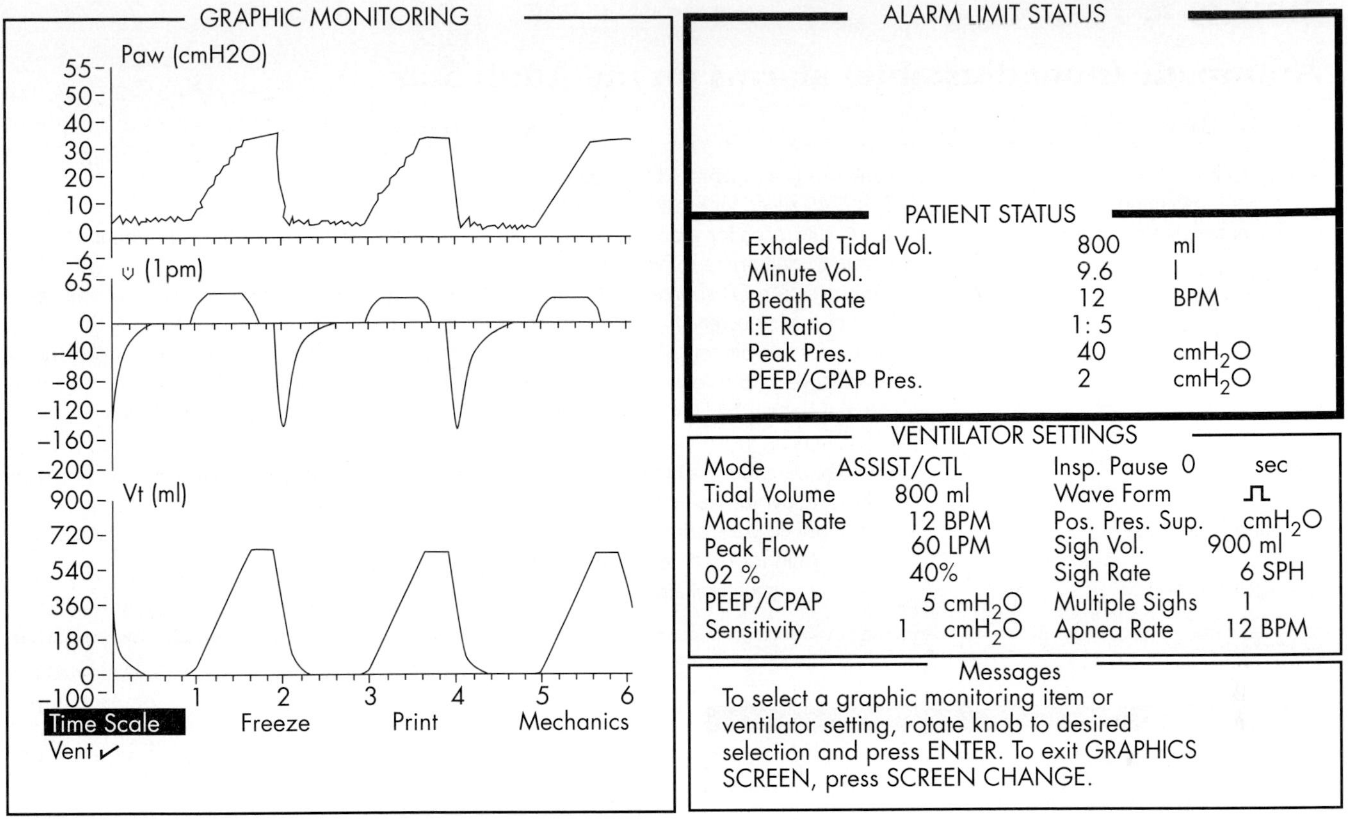

Figure 10-66 The graphic display screen on the Adult Star. (Courtesy Nellcor Puritan Bennett Corp., Pleasanton, Calif.)

BOX 10-83

Decision Making & Problem Solving

Figure 10-66 provides three waveforms on the left and ventilator and patient data on the right. Assuming that the two represent the same event, what inconsistencies do you see between the data listed and the graphs shown?

See Appendix A for the answers.

Alarms and warnings that merit more discussion are LOW V_T, HIGH PEEP/CPAP, APNEA, INVERSE I:E RATIO, POWER LOSS, and VENT.INOP.

Low V_T Alarm

The LOW V_T alarm activates if the last V_T is less than the alarm setting *and* the LOW-PRESSURE alarm is on *or* the average of the last 4 breaths is less than the set low V_T alarm. A LOW SPONTANEOUS V_T alarm activates if two of four spontaneous breath V_Ts *and* the average of the last four spontaneous breath V_Ts are both less than the low V_T setting.

High PEEP/CPAP

A HIGH PEEP/CPAP alarm sounds if baseline pressure is more than 10 cm H_2O above the set PEEP level for ≥2 seconds, or if baseline pressure fluctuates 5 to 10 cm H_2O above the set baseline for more than 5 seconds. Box 10-84 shows an example situation with a HIGH PEEP alarm.

TABLE 10-15

Adjustable alarm settings for the Adult Star

Alarm settings displayed on Screens 1 and 2	
Alarm	**Range**
High inspiratory pressure	10 to 120 cm H_2O
Low inspiratory pressure	3 to 60 cm H_2O
Low mechanical volume	0 to 2500 mL
Low spontaneous volume	0 to 2500 mL
Low minute volume	0 to 60 L/min
Low PEEP/CPAP	0 to 25 cm H_2O
High respiratory rate	0 to 90 breaths/min
Apnea time	5 to 60 seconds

Apnea Alarm

The APNEA alarm activates when the set apnea time passes without inspiration being detected. Apnea time can be adjusted from 5 to 60 seconds. If an apnea rate is set (0.5 to 80 breaths/min), the ventilator automatically switches to

TABLE 10-16

Automatic (nonadjustable) alarms on the Adult Star

Alarm	Activating factor
Airway leak	Leak >6 L/min when PEEP is set
Insufficient inspiratory time	T_I < 240 msec for mandatory breath
Insufficient expiratory time	T_E < 200 msec for mandatory breath, or < 260 msec for PSV breath; machine limits rate to guarantee minimum T_E
Low-pressure oxygen	High-pressure O_2 source < 30 psig with O_2% set at >21%; ventilator switches to air for pneumatic power
Low-pressure air	High-pressure air source <30 psig and no internal compressor available, or compressor pressure <16 psig; ventilator switches to 100% O_2 for pneumatic power
Low battery	Internal battery has <4 min of power available; requires a 120-volt AC or 12-volt DC source
High PEEP/CPAP	Average baseline >10 cm H_2O above set PEEP/CPAP, or baseline fluctuates 6 to 10 cm H_2O above set value for >5 seconds; safety valve opens
Exhalation valve leak	Expiratory flow transducer measures flow >10% of set peak inspiratory flow; must be >4 L/min for 60 msec; reseat expiratory valve diaphragm
Obstructed tube	Gas flow or proximal airway pressure lines obstructed

BOX 10-84

Decision Making & Problem Solving

A respiratory therapist hears an alarm on the Adult Star ventilating an ICU patient. He notes that the high PEEP alarm is visually highlighted. The patient is not in any distress, and breath sounds are equal bilaterally. On examining the patient circuit, he notes water in the proximal pressure line. Could this be the cause of the problem?

See Appendix A for the answer.

apnea ventilation. The apnea rate must be set at a value greater than or equal to the set rate.

Inverse I:E Ratio Warning

When using IRV, the following warning message appears on the screen for 10 seconds: "WARNING: When using inverse I:E ratios, air trapping may occur. Perform Auto-PEEP measurements frequently to assure Auto-PEEPs are acceptable." In reality, auto-PEEP is rarely acceptable.

Power Loss Alarm

When the internal battery is nearly depleted of power, a LOW BATTERY alarm sounds for 4 to 5 minutes as a warning. When the internal battery is depleted and there is no AC power, a POWER LOSS alarm occurs.

Ventilator Inoperative Alarm

If a major problem occurs with the microprocessors, the ventilator is placed into VENT.INOP. (ventilator inoperative) status. Audio and visual signals are activated, and the expiratory and internal safety valves open to allow a spontaneously breathing patient access to room air. The message "Vent.Inop" occurs on the screen, and the VENT.INOP. LED on the control panel lights. The error code responsible for the event appears on the screen. The patient should be immediately ventilated by another method, and the unit taken out of service until it can be repaired.

MODES OF OPERATION

There are four modes normally available in the Adult Star: A/C, SIMV, CPAP, and pressure support. PCV can be added as an option. The first two lines of information on the VENTILATOR SETTINGS screen describe the breath type (volume or pressure) and the mode (Box 10-85). The mode listing includes A/C, SIMV, and CPAP. Box 10-86 describes the steps of setting a mode of ventilation. (When changing from volume ventilation to PCV and vice-versa, machine and apnea rates do not carry over, but remain as set in the last ventilation type (i.e., PCV or volume ventilation).

Assist/Control

In assist/control, breaths are patient- or time-triggered, volume-targeted, and volume (flow) cycled. (Note that in volume-targeted ventilation, the ventilator cycles out of inspiration when it determines that the set volume has been delivered based on the set peak flow, flow waveform, and inspiratory time. Thus it can be called volume- or flow-cycling [see Chapter 9].)

BOX 10-85

Types of Breaths Displayed on the Ventilator Settings Screen

Volume cylced: volume-targeted ventilation
PCV/time-cycled: pressure-targeted, time-cycled ventilation
PCV/I:E cycles: pressure-targeted, I:E ratio-cycled ventilation

BOX 10-86

Setting Modes of Ventilation

To Select a New Mode

1. Select VENTILATION from the ventilator setting screen. (Note that modes cannot be changed from the graphic monitor screen.)
2. Press ENTER and select the desired mode.
3. Press ENTER; the screen will display "Pending" and the following message: "Ventilation will continue in the previous VENTILATION type and ventilation MODE with the previous ventilator and alarm settings until the procedure is completed."
4. Review and adjust variables and alarms as needed.
5. After alarm adjustments (alarm setting window), highlight START and press ENTER (within the "Messages" window). You must choose START, or the changes will not be entered.
6. Press ENTER to begin ventilation with the new mode. The "Pending" screen is replaced with the regular "Ventilator Settings" screen.
7. To cancel a "Pending" screen, do one of the following:
   - Press CANCEL and ENTER
   - Do not rotate the SELECT knob for 60 seconds
   - Press the SCREEN CHANGE button

SIMV

In SIMV, mandatory breaths are patient- or time-triggered, volume-targeted, and volume-cycled. Spontaneous breaths are maintained at the set baseline and can be assisted with pressure support. Spontaneous breaths are pressure-triggered, pressure-limited, and pressure-cycled—unless PSV is selected, in which case they are flow-cycled. Normally, the patient triggers and receives a mandatory breath. After breath delivery, the patient breathes spontaneously without receiving another mandatory breath. Following the spontaneous period, the next mandatory (SIMV) period occurs. A patient effort in this period triggers another mandatory breath. If the ventilator does not sense a patient effort during this SIMV period, a mandatory breath is delivered at the beginning of the next period. The machine continues to deliver mandatory breaths at the set rate until it senses a patient effort, and the cycle repeats itself.

CPAP

In CPAP, breaths are pressure-triggered, pressure-limited, and pressure-cycled. Spontaneous breaths can be assisted with pressure support, in which case they become flow-cycled. When CPAP is in use (spontaneous mode), an internal demand valve controls the inspiratory pressure by trying to maintain the set baseline pressure. Whenever the PEEP/CPAP control is set >0 cm H_2O, the machine compensates for leaks up to 22 L/min (7 L/min with the pediatric ventilation option). If a leak >6 L/min is detected, an alarm is activated to alert the operator of its presence.

Pressure Support

With the Adult Star, the pressure-support mode is referred to as positive-pressure support (PPS) and is available to assist spontaneous breaths in SIMV and CPAP modes. PSV is patient-triggered and pressure-targeted, and normally terminates inspiration when the flow drops to 4 L/min. However, it also cycles out of inspiration when pressure is more than 3 cm H_2O above the set pressure level, or when T_I is more than 3.5 seconds.

Pressure-Control Ventilation

PCV is available as an added option to the Adult Star. It can be used with the A/C or SIMV modes. Mandatory PCV breaths are patient- or time-triggered, pressure-targeted (5 to 100 cm H_2O), and time-cycled. The set pressure is above the set PEEP. For example, if pressure is set at 15 cm H_2O and PEEP is at 5 cm H_2O, PIP is 20 cm H_2O. The maximum sum of PCV and PEEP cannot exceed 110 cm H_2O. In PCV, sigh breaths are not available.

Cycling in PCV

Time cycling is provided during PCV in one of two ways. Either T_I is constant (PCV time-cycled), or the I:E ratio is constant (PCV I:E ratio-cycled). Box 10-87 describes the two cycling mechanisms. PCV also pressure cycles out of inspiration if airway pressure exceeds the high pressure limit.

Minimum Expiratory Time in PCV

In PCV, T_E cannot be less than 200 msec. If the expiratory time is less than 200 msec, the INSUFFICIENT EXHALATION TIME alarm activates. The ventilator slows the respiratory rate in order to lengthen T_E to a minimum of 200 msec. As a result, the delivered and the set rates differ.

Maximum Flow in PCV

With the Adult Star, you actually set a maximum flow control (MAX.FLOW) in the PCV mode. This control determines

BOX 10-87

T_I and I:E Constants in PCV and the Display of I:E Ratio

T_I Constant

If T_I is selected as the constant in PCV (0.24 to 5.0 seconds), inspiration ends when T_I has elapsed. If the respiratory rate changes, the I:E ratio varies. For example, if the rate is 10 breaths/min and the T_I is 2 seconds, the I:E is 1:2. If the rate is increased to 12 breaths/min with the same T_I, the ratio becomes 1:1.5.

PCV with T_I constant is available in the following modes:

- A/C
- SIMV
- SIMV + PSV
- CPAP
- CPAP + PSV

In the last two modes (CPAP and CPAP + PSV), PCV time-cycled breaths are delivered only when the apnea back-up mode is activated or when a manual breath is delivered.

I:E Ratio Constant

If I:E is set as the constant, the T_I and T_E change when the rate is changed. The available range is 1:499 to 4:1. T_I is determined by the I:E setting and the rate, based on the following equation:

$$T_I = (60/f) \div (I + E),$$

where *f* is respiratory rate.

For example, if the rate is set at 10 breaths/min and I:E at 1:2, T_I will be 2 seconds $(60/10) \div (1+2) = 2$ sec. T_E is also determined by the ventilator and in this case is: 6 seconds − 2 seconds = 4 seconds.

(Note that the I:E ratio as a constant in PCV can *only* be used in the A/C mode. All breaths are mandatory. Because both T_I and T_E are machine-determined, this method of ventilation is not intended for patients with spontaneous breathing efforts. The ventilator will respond to a patient effort, however, so sensitivity must be set.)

I:E Ratio Display

The displayed, calculated I:E ratio is established as follows: I = 1 when $T_I \geq T_E$. For example, if T_I = 2 seconds, and T_E = 4 seconds, I:E = 1:2. E = 1, when $T_I \leq T_E$. For example, if T_I = 4 seconds, and T_E = 2 seconds, I:E = 2:1.

BOX 10-88

Decision Making & Problem Solving

A patient is being ventilated with the PCV time-cycled mode on the Adult Star. The pressure is set at 40 cm H_2O, T_I is at 0.5 seconds, max.flow is at 80 L/min, and the low-pressure alarm is at 30 cm H_2O. The respiratory therapist hears the low-pressure alarm and notices that during inspiration the set pressure is not reached and the machine cycles into exhalation before inspiratory flow has dropped to zero (Figure 10-67). The desired V_T is 0.8, but the exhaled V_T is only 0.4 L. What can the therapist do to correct this situation?

See Appendix A for the answer.

the maximum flow delivered during a mandatory pressure-targeted breath. When MAX.FLOW is set at ≤160 L/min, the slope of the inspiratory pressure curve changes from a sharp, rapid rise to a slower rise to set pressure. The pressure/time curve becomes sloped at the beginning of inspiration.

Both T_I and MAX.FLOW must be set sufficiently high or the set pressure may not be reached during inspiration. Box 10-88 and Figure 10-67 provide an appropriate problem-solving exercise.

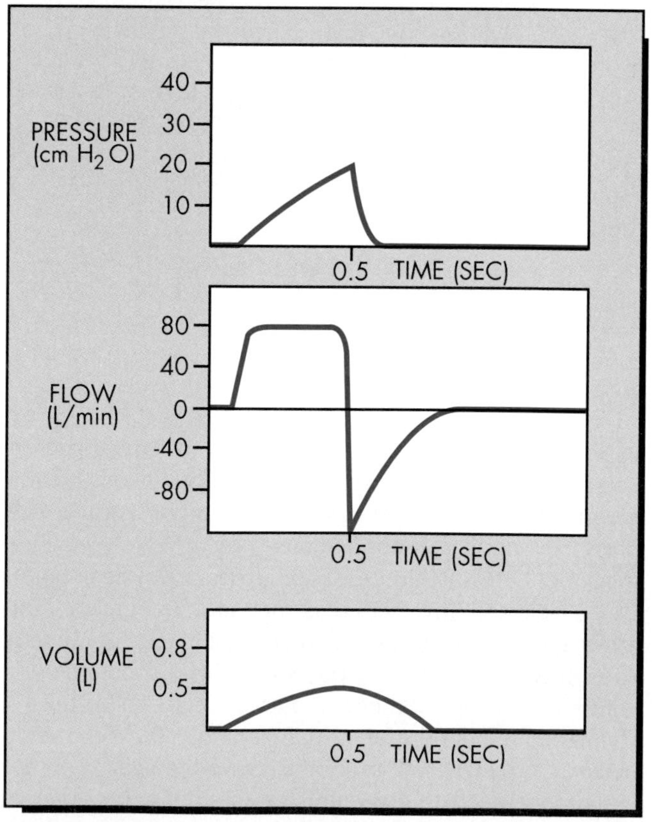

Figure 10-67 The pressure/time, flow/time, and volume time curves are shown for a patient being ventilated with the Adult Star (see Box 10-88).

BOX 10-89

List of Respiratory Mechanics Measurements for the Adult Star

1. Flow/volume and pressure/volume loops
2. Static mechanics
   - Static compliance (Cstatic or C_S)
   - Static inspiratory resistance (Rstatic or R_S)
3. Auto-PEEP
   - Auto-PEEP (actually measures total PEEP)
   - Inadvertant PEEP
4. Dynamic mechanics
   - Dynamic compliance (Cdynamic or C_D)
   - Inspiratory resistance (Rinsp or Ri)
   - Expiratory resistance (Rexp or Re)
   - Pressure at 100 msec ($P_{0.1}$)
5. Slow vital capacity (slow VC)
6. Negative inspiratory force (NIF)

PCV and Volume Alarms

It is advisable to set both HIGH and LOW V_T alarms and HIGH PRESSURE alarms during PCV. A HIGH V_T alarm might occur if a patient actively inspires, achieving a larger volume than before. If a patient's lung condition improves, then a set pressure may deliver a higher V_T. When a HIGH V_T alarm occurs, inspiration does not end until it is time-cycled out of inspiration. A low V_T may indicate a worsening of C or Raw or a leak in the system.

It is very important to set the high-pressure limit during PCV. If the patient actively exhales or coughs during inspiration, for example, and the high-pressure limit is reached, inspiration ends. The expiratory valve opens to vent excessively high airway pressures.

Graphic Display Screens

Waveforms for pressure/time, flow/time, and volume/time appear on Screen 3 (GRAPHIC MONITORING screen). You can change the sweep speed or horizontal axis to 6, 12, or 24 seconds using the TIME-SCALE function (Figure 10-66). There is also a FREEZE function.

Special Features

A RESPIRATORY MECHANICS SOFTWARE option for the Adult Star allows a variety of values to be measured and calculated (Box 10-89). It is accessed from the GRAPHICS MONITOR screen. Once in Screen 3, select the MECHANICS option and press ENTER. From the LUNG MECHANICS window (Figure 10-68), you can select and activate the desired value to be measured just as on any ventilator setting. (Note that leak compensation is suspended during all respiratory mechanics measurements except dynamic compliance and resistance.)

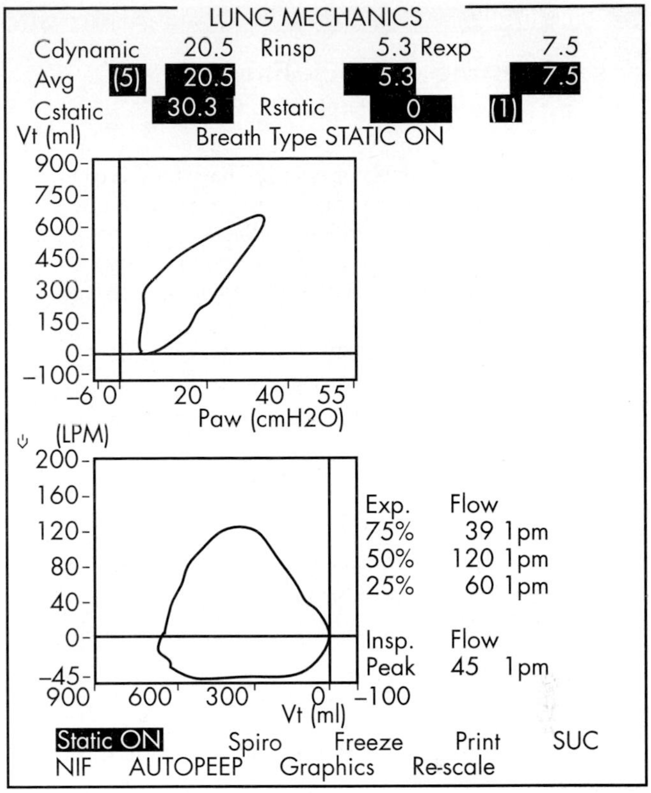

Figure 10-68 An example of a respiratory mechanics screen. (Courtesy Nellcor Puritan Bennett Corp., Pleasanton, Calif.)

Flow/Volume and Pressure/Volume Loops

These loops can be accessed once the mechanics feature has been activated. Simply select the LOOPS option and press ENTER. You can change the scale to the desired units using RE-SCALE, just as in the normal graphics screen.

Static Mechanics

During a static mechanics maneuver, the ventilator automatically uses a constant flow pattern and requires a stable inspiratory plateau reading after delivery of a mandatory volume breath. STATIC ON is selected to perform this maneuver. Static compliance and static inspiratory resistance are reported on the screen. Three different breaths are measured. The NUMBER in parentheses is the number of study breaths tested. A question mark appearing on the screen means that a stable pressure plateau could not be obtained for a test breath, so the breath measurement may be inaccurate. Finally, an average of all three breaths is displayed. Again, a question mark appears if a static plateau was not obtained for one of the three breaths.* When STATIC ON is activated, this test is performed every 15 minutes. You must turn the function off if you do not want it run every 15 minutes. Box 10-90 provides a clinical note on checking plateau pressures for calculating static compliance.

*For results to be accurate, the patient cannot make respiratory efforts during the procedure.

BOX 10-90

Performing a Quick Pause Maneuver to Check C_S

If your Adult Star ventilator does not have the Respiratory Mechanics software option, and you need to obtain a plateau pressure reading to calculate C_S, there are two ways to do it. One way is to set an inspiratory pause. The disadvantage of this is that you have to turn it off after you are finished.

Another way is to obtain a quick check of pause pressure, by doing the following:

1. From the screen, scroll to PAUSE, highlight it, and press ENTER.
2. Spin the SELECT knob with a quick spin.
3. The screen will flash the message, "0.5 sec × 3 breaths."
4. Press ENTER, and the unit performs a pause pressure measurement of three breaths.

Auto-PEEP

As mentioned in Chapter 9, you can detect the presence of auto-PEEP when a flow/time curve shows flow failing to return to baseline (zero) before the next ventilator breath begins. Besides using ventilator graphics to establish the presence of trapped air (auto-PEEP), the Adult Star has an auto-PEEP option (available with the RESPIRATORY MECHANICS package) that measures auto-PEEP levels.

To perform this measurement, the machine briefly closes the expiratory valve while the inspiratory flow is at zero when a mandatory breath is due. The mandatory breath is delayed for 0.2 to 2.0 seconds until the measure of a static expiratory plateau pressure is recognized. The total PEEP with the Adult Star is called AUTO-PEEP, but actually includes extrinsic (set) PEEP and inadvertent PEEP (usually called auto-PEEP). To determine inadvertent PEEP levels, the ventilator subtracts the set-PEEP from the (total) PEEP. Auto-PEEP can only be done when a time-triggered breath occurs because patient breathing efforts interfere with the measurement. Box 10-91 describes how this measurement is performed.

Dynamic Mechanics

Dynamic mechanics do not require a breath hold or an inspiratory plateau. They are performed on volume-targeted breaths that are patient- or time-triggered.* Calculated values of dynamic compliance and inspiratory and expiratory resistance are displayed as an average of the last eight breaths, and are updated every breath. The number of study breaths is in parentheses on the screen.

*These mechanics cannot be measured in CPAP, PSV, or PCV.

BOX 10-91

Auto-PEEP Measurement

1. Select and enter Auto-PEEP from the menu choices.
2. The auto-PEEP screen is displayed with the auto-PEEP choice highlighted.
3. Press ENTER.
4. The sequence is activated and the display message changes from "Standby" to "In Progress."
5. When measured respiratory rate is ≤6 breaths/min, the maneuver is performed on three successive time-triggered breaths.
6. When the measured respiratory rate is >6 breaths/min, the maneuver is performed on the next time-triggered breath after every three breaths (spontaneous or mandatory) until three tests have been run.
7. To stop the measurement, press ENTER and select STANDBY.
8. Auto-PEEP (total PEEP) and inadvertent PEEP are displayed after each breath. If a static pressure plateau is not obtained, a question mark is displayed after the last value measured to indicate its probable inaccuracy.
9. The average value of the three readings is displayed 5 seconds after the last test breath. A question mark follows any breath that did not satisfy static pressure conditions.

Slow Vital Capacity

A SLOW VC test is available when you choose SELECT and SVC from the menu. (Note that PSV is suspended during a slow VC and during NIF tests.) To begin the test, press ENTER; the display message changes from STANDBY to IN PROGRESS. When a slow VC maneuver is in progress, the CPAP mode is automatically used by the ventilator to avoid excessively high pressures that could occur if the ventilator delivered a mandatory breath. If no patient breath is detected within 20 seconds, the test automatically ends.

Just as with any test of VC, the patient must be coached through the procedure. The test ends after three breaths are studied. The best of the three efforts then replaces the last breath (after about 5 seconds). A flow/volume loop of the last maneuver is displayed along with the best VC. The volume scale of the graph can be rescaled just as with other graphic displays.

Negative Inspiratory Force

Negative inspiratory force (NIF), which is also commonly called maximum inspiratory pressure (MIP)[3] can be performed when the RESPIRATORY MECHANICS option is available. As with the slow VC maneuver, the patient must be coached through the procedure. Just as in other tests described above, press SELECT and enter NIF from the menu.

Once the maneuver starts, the patient cannot inspire or expire through the patient circuit and the apnea mode and PSV are suspended. The CPAP mode is automatically activated, just as in slow VC measurement. Both NIF and $P_{0.1}$ (also called P_{100}) are measured at the same time. (Note that $P_{0.1}$ is the most negative pressure the patient generates against a closed system 100msec after the start of an inspiratory effort.) To begin NIF testing, press and hold the ENTER button. The display message changes to IN PROGRESS. The test ends after 20 seconds, and the patient can again breathe from the circuit with the normal settings. To end the test before the 20-second maximum, simply release the ENTER button. NIF and $P_{0.1}$ are displayed on the screen. There is also a graphic display of the patient's airway pressure/time waveform (Figure 10-69).

As with all the respiratory mechanics tests, the screen provides all the needed instructions to perform the test right on the screen, making this option very simple to use (see Figure 10-69).

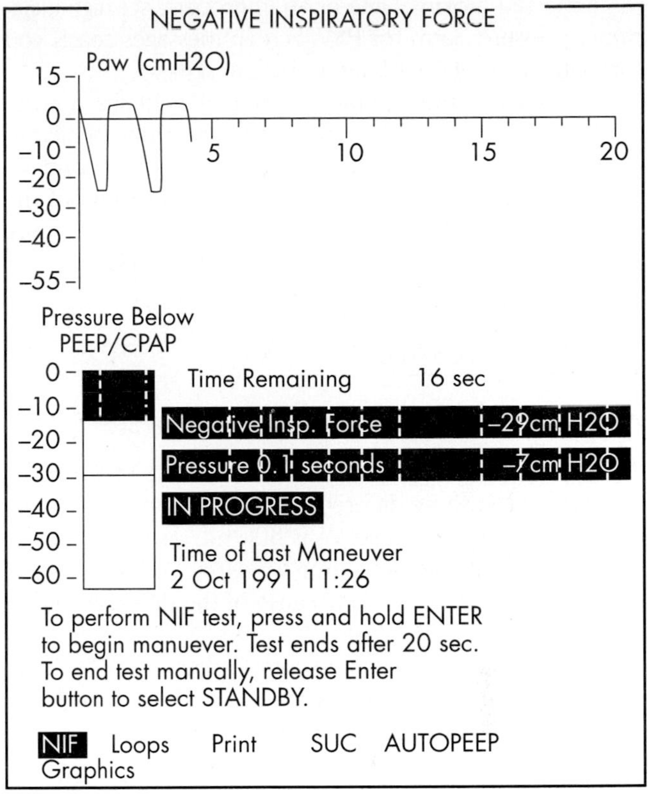

Figure 10-69 An example of an NIF maneuver on a respiratory (lung) mechanics screen. (Courtesy Nellcor Puritan Bennett Corp., Pleasanton, Calif.)

TROUBLESHOOTING

In addition to the various monitored parameters and alarms available, the screen on the Adult Star provides information about possible causes that may have activated many alarm situations. This directly assists you in determining causes of problems. For example, suppose the OBSTRUCTED TUBE alarm (audio and visual) was on. Possible causes could be an obstruction or kink in either the patient circuit or the proximal airway pressure line. It could also be caused by a

TABLE 10-17

Warning messages that appear on the Adult Star

Warning message	Possible cause	Corrective action
Internal pressure transducer detects over-pressure condition	• Obstruction or disconnection of proximal pressure line • Main inspiratory line of patient circuit kinked or obstructed	Reconnect line or clear obstruction or kink
Airway leak >6 L/min (may compromise spontaneous and assisted breaths)	Patient circuit is leaking	Check circuit for leaks, especially at connections (e.g., water traps and filters)
Pressure did not reach PPS + PEEP level in 5 seconds	Patient circuit is leaking	Check circuit for leaks, especially at connections (e.g., water traps and filters)
Delivered V_T exceeds 3 L	Patient circuit is leaking	Check circuit for leaks, especially at connections (e.g., water traps and filters)
Air compressor won't start	Circuit breaker for compressor may be open, or A/C line voltage too low	• Check circuit breaker • Check wall voltage • Turn ventilator off and back on • Contact qualified service representative

disconnected proximal line or an improperly set high inspiratory pressure alarm for PSV. Screen messages coach you through checking your lines and alarm settings.

In addition, the operator's manual contains a troubleshooting section of common alarm situations (similar to those reviewed in Chapter 9) with possible causes and solutions. The warning messages listed in this section of the manual are provided in Table 10-17 because they are more specific to the Adult Star than most other ventilators.

Review Questions

(See Appendix A for answers.)

1. The volumes displayed on the GRAPHICS MONITORING screen show different numerical values. The digital readout of exhaled V_T is 800 mL, as is the set V_T. However, the volume/time waveform shows a V_T of 860 mL. The most likely cause of the difference is:
   a. a patient circuit leak
   b. a correction for tubing compliance
   c. the expiratory flow sensor is out of calibration
   d. there is water in the proximal pressure line
2. A LOW-PRESSURE OXYGEN alarm is activated. Assuming the Adult Star is still connected to a wall high-pressure air source, which of the following will occur?
   a. the ventilator continues to function from the air source
   b. the ventilator switches to VENT.INOP, and the safety valve opens
   c. the internal compressor turns on, and its pressure is used to power the internal oxygen lines
   d. the ventilator switches to the back-up mode of ventilation
3. Which of the following statements is true about nebulizer function in the Adult Star 2000?
   I. An external flowmeter must be used to provide nebulized medications.
   II. Flow through the nebulizer outlet only occurs during inspiration when flow is $\geq$15 L/min.
   III. The amount of flow alters V_T delivery but not O_2%.
   IV. The nebulizer function must be turned off when the treatment is finished.
   a. I only
   b. II only
   c. I and IV only
   d. II, III, and IV only
4. The control that is used to select options on the CRT screen is called the:
   a. mouse
   b. cursor
   c. SELECT knob
   d. ENTER button
5. Which of the following are adjustable alarms on the Adult Star?
   I. HIGH INSPIRATORY PRESSURE
   II. LOW SPONTANEOUS VOLUME
   III. HIGH PEEP/CPAP
   IV. AIRWAY LEAK
   V. APNEA TIME
   a. I and III only
   b. II and V only
   c. III and IV only
   d. I, II, and V only
6. A warning message reads "Pressure did not reach PPS + PEEP level in 5 seconds." The cause of this alarm is:
   a. an obstruction in the proximal airway pressure line
   b. a kink in the expiratory line of the patient circuit
   c. a leak in the patient circuit
   d. a compressor failure
7. An Adult Star being used for an apneic patient has the PCV option. To ventilate the patient using a constant I:E ratio, a respiratory therapist should select which two of the following?
   I. A/C mode
   II. PCV I:E ratio cycling
   III. PCV time cycling
   IV. SIMV mode
   a. I and II only
   b. II and III only
   c. II and IV only
   d. III and IV only
8. Sigh breaths are available in PCV—true or false?
9. You can display loops as well as waveforms on the normal GRAPHICS MONITORING screen—true or false?
10. From which screen or screens can you make changes to ventilator settings on the Adult Star?

References

1. Adult Star Ventilator 2000/1500 operating instructions, PN 9910405 Rev B 9/95, San Diego, 1995, Infrasonics, Inc.
2. Model 2000/1500 Adult Star operating instruction manual addendum for ventilators with software level 219.2, PN 9930274 Rev B 3/95, San Diego, 1995, Infrasonics, Inc.
3. Pilbeam SP: Mechanical ventilation. In Burton GG, Hodgken JE, and Ward JJ: Respiratory care: a guide to clinical practice, ed 4, Philadelphia, 1997, Lippincott.

Nellcor Puritan Bennett 740

OUTLINE

LEARNING OBJECTIVES

Upon completion of this section, the reader should be able to:

1. Describe the internal mechanisms involved in breath delivery.
2. Explain how ventilator and alarm settings are made.
3. Assess an alarm situation and identify the probable cause.
4. Identify messages that appear in the message window.
5. Compare POST with SST.
6. Define the function of the various keys in the ventilator settings and patient status sections.
7. Interpret flashing vs. constantly lit indicators in the ventilator status section.
8. Explain the function of all modes of ventilation available on the 740, including apnea ventilation.
9. Identify functions that can be accessed through the MENU key.
10. Describe the appropriate corrective action when the VENT.INOP. alarm is activated.

The Nellcor Puritan Bennett 740 ventilator[1,2] is a relatively simple and inexpensive machine that is adaptable for pediatric and adult use in subacute, as well as in acute care settings (Figure 10-70). Its lightweight, electrically powered design allows it to be used readily in patient transport.

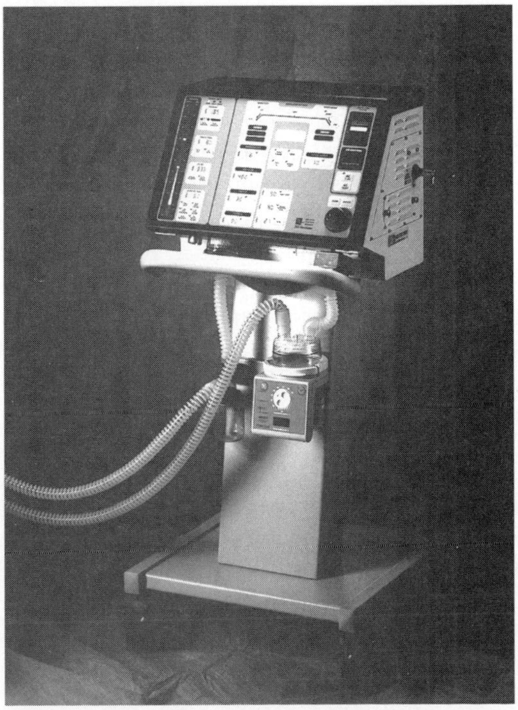

Figure 10-70 The Nellcor Puritan Bennett 740 ventilator. (Courtesy Nellcor Puritan Bennett Corp., Pleasanton, Calif.)

POWER SOURCE

The 740 is an electrically powered, microprocessor-controlled ventilator that does *not* require high-pressure gas to function. It normally uses a standard 120-volt AC outlet (100 to 240 volt, 50 to 60 cycles), but can also use the 2.5-hour internal battery or an optional 7-hour external battery. If an FiO_2 above 0.21 is needed, the unit must be connected to a 50-psi (40 to 90 psi) oxygen source. The power ON/OFF switch is on the back panel of the machine, and the high pressure connector is on the right side.

When the ventilator is first turned on, the message window shows "POST running . . . ," and "PM Due:xxx." POST is the power-on self-test that checks the essential system functions and must be completed before the unit will operate. (If an ABNORMAL RESTART alarm occurs, the unit

BOX 10-92

Short Self-Test (SST) on the 740 Ventilator

1. Run the SST every 15 days, between patients, and when the patient circuit is changed.
2. Be sure a patient is not connected to the ventilator.
3. Turn the ventilator on. (If it's already on, turn it off and on again.)
4. Press MENU and select SST.
5. Follow the instructions as they appear in the message window.
6. The ventilator runs the POST test.
7. Select the humidifier type: HME (heat moisture exchanger), dual heated wire (humidifier with heated wire on the expiratory limb or both inspiratory and expiratory limbs), and no heated wire (conventional humidifier without a heated wire circuit on the expiratory limb) when instructed.
8. Select the tubing type (adult or pediatric) when instructed.
9. Select the ET tube size. Enter the millimeter tube size when instructed. The pressure (flow) rise time is automatically adjusted based on the tube size.
10. When each test run during SST is displayed, press one of the following: ACCEPT, CLEAR (to repeat), RESET (to restart SST), and ALARM SILENCE (2 minutes) to stop the current test and skip to the end of SST.
11. When the last test is completed, the message "SST finished testing" is displayed along with the overall SST result.
12. Unblock the patient wye and press ACCEPT, and the ventilator reruns POST. After this, it is ready for ventilation.

may be running on AC, but the battery is low.) The PM DUE message gives you the number of hours until a routine maintenance check is due. After you turn on the unit, the manufacturer recommends that you let it warm up (run) for 10 minutes before connecting it to a patient so that the flow sensors respond more readily.

There is a more extensive test called the short self-test, or SST. You should run SST and test alarms before using the unit on a patient (Box 10-92).

When the ventilator is not in use, it is appropriate to store the unit in the standby mode between patient uses. The standby mode is a waiting state during which the ventilator maintains its settings and the battery charges, thus assuring it will be charged for the next use.* Box 10-93 provides instruction on entering the standby mode. Remember, *never* put the ventilator in the standby mode when a patient is connected.

*To keep the battery charged, the ventilator must be plugged into an AC outlet and the power switch must be on.

BOX 10-93

Entering the Standby Mode

1. Turn the ventilator on. If it is already on, turn it off and on again.
2. Press MENU and use the CONTROL knob to select STANDBY.
3. Press ACCEPT. The message window displays "Is pt disconnected? ACCEPT to proceed."
4. With the patient disconnected, press ACCEPT. The message window displays the confirmation message: "In standby mode. Clear to exit."
5. To exit, press CLEAR, and the POST will run.

BOX 10-94

Decision Making & Problem Solving

Because the 740 uses a linear drive piston, only one flow waveform is produced during volume ventilation. What is that waveform?

See Appendix A for the answer.

Internal Mechanism

Information from the control panel is processed by a microprocessor and stored in the ventilator's memory. A second microprocessor responsible for breath delivery uses this information to control and monitor the pattern of gas flow to the patient.

The 740 uses a frictionless, linear drive piston that eliminates the need for a blender, compressor, or wall air system. The piston/cylinder system is designed with a very thin gap (about as thick as a sheet of paper) between the piston and the cylinder wall to reduce friction between the piston and the wall and allow for a faster response than a sealed system. Understandably, a small amount of gas leaks through the gap between the piston and the cylinder. The software program compensates for this minimal leak, assuring accurate volume ventilation. During expiration, the continuous forward motion of the piston is regulated and maintained to compensate for the leak and maintain set PEEP levels (Box 10-94).

Room air enters the ventilator through an air intake filter (Figure 10-71). If the O_2% setting is more than 21%, oxygen is also injected from the oxygen high pressure inlet. The pressure from the oxygen source is reduced to a more appropriate working level and mixed with the incoming air. During exhalation, the backward motion of the piston draws blended air and oxygen at the desired O_2% into the piston housing. When inspiration begins,

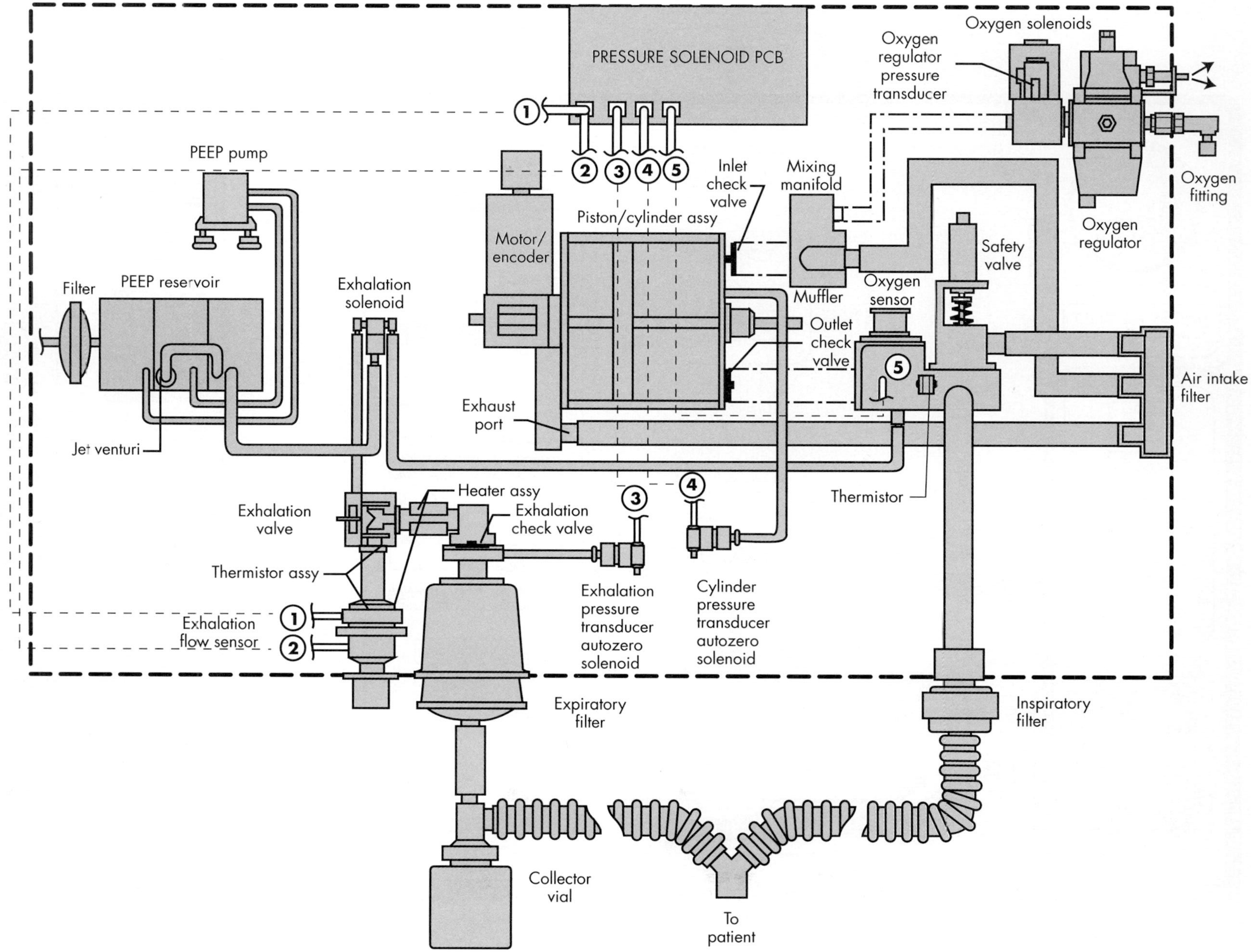

Figure 10-71 The internal pneumatic components of the Nellcor Puritan Bennett 740. (Courtesy Nellcor Puritan Bennett Corp., Pleasanton, Calif.)

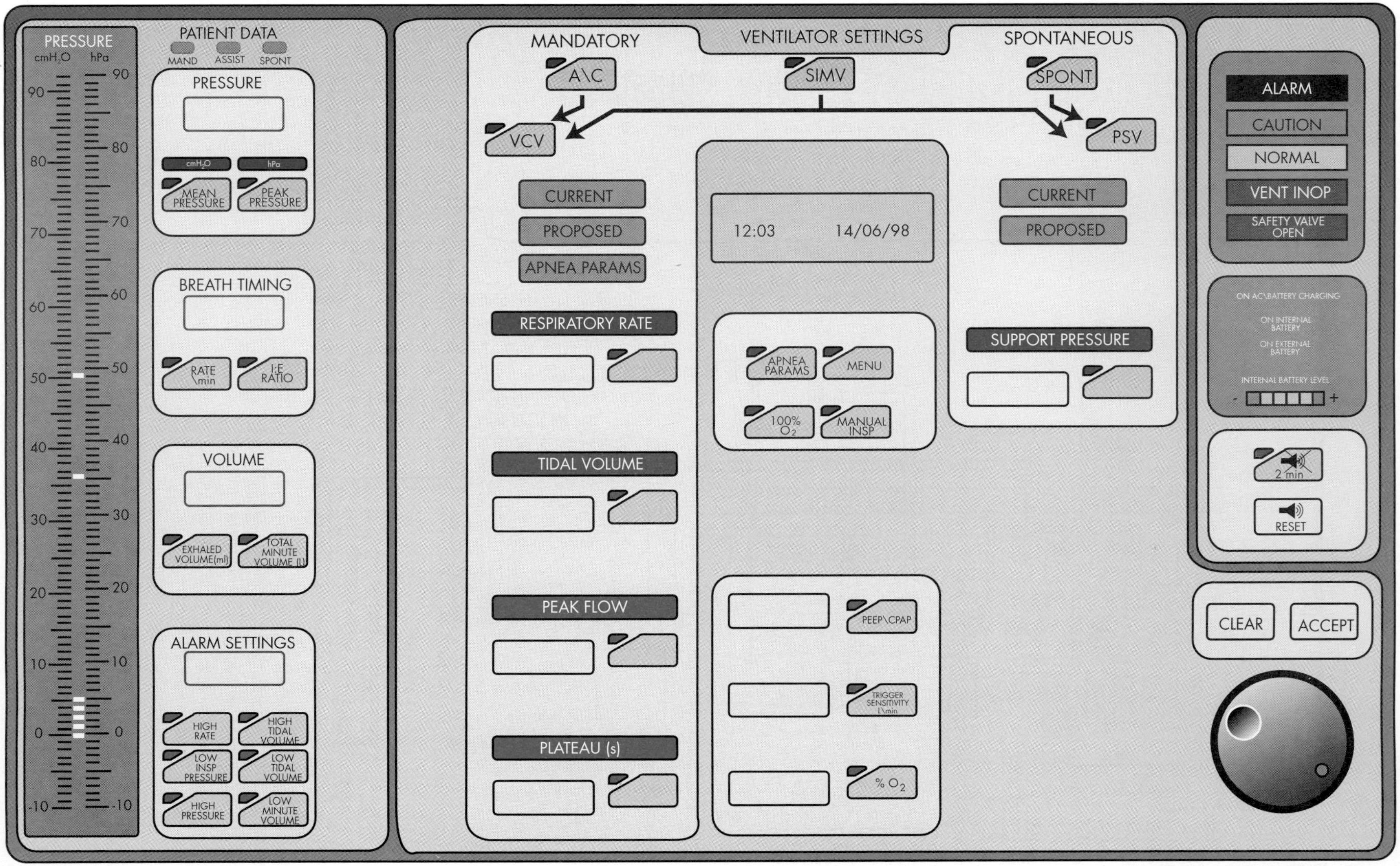

Figure 10-72 The front panel of the Nellcor Puritan Bennett 740.

the forward motion of the piston sends the gas past a galvanic oxygen sensor, a safety pressure-relief valve, a temperature thermistor, and finally into the patient circuit. (Note that while O_2% is monitored, it is not displayed.)

CONTROLS AND ALARMS

The front panel of the 740 is grouped into the following three sections (Figure 10-72):

1. The VENTILATOR SETTINGS section allows you to select the mode of ventilation, breath type, oxygen percentage, apnea parameters, and menu functions.
2. The PATIENT DATA section displays monitored airway pressure information, breath timing, volumes, and current alarm settings.
3. The VENTILATOR STATUS section displays the current ventilator parameters and status including alarms, battery conditions, alarm silence, and alarm reset.

In general, to set controls and alarms, you follow three simple steps. First, touch the control pad or touch key of the parameter you wish to change. Then rotate the CONTROL knob to change the setting of the parameter and press the ACCEPT key to apply the new setting (Box 10-95).

Ventilator Settings

Within this section are controls for selecting the mode and basic parameters for ventilation.

Mode and Breath Selection Keys

The touch keys labeled A/C, SIMV, SPONT., VCV (volume-control ventilation), and PSV (pressure-support ventilation) govern the mode of ventilation and breath delivery and are described later in this section.

Parameter Settings

RESPIRATORY RATE (3 to 70 breaths/min) sets the guaranteed respiratory rate in A/C and SIMV. The TIDAL VOLUME control (40 to 2000 mL) determines mandatory breath delivery in A/C and SIMV. PEAK FLOW (range 3 to 150 L/min) delivers a constant flow of gas at the set rate during a mandatory breath. Inspiratory time is determined by V_T, flow, and rate. PLATEAU (0.0 to 2.0 sec) provides an inspiratory pause at the end of a mandatory breath.

Pressure Support

The PSV control (0 to 70 cm H_2O) sets pressure delivery for spontaneous breaths above the PEEP/CPAP baseline.

PEEP/CPAP

This control sets the baseline between 0 and 35 cm H_2O and establishes the minimum pressure maintained during both inspiration and expiration.

BOX 10-95

Changing Ventilator and Alarm Settings[1]

1. Touch a setting key; the key lights, the selected setting flashes, and the message window shows the current setting.
2. Turn the knob to adjust the setting.
3. Repeat steps 1 and 2 for every setting you want to change. Press CLEAR to cancel the most recent setting.
4. Press ACCEPT to apply the new setting. The key lights turn off, and the new settings are displayed. The message window reads: "Setting(s) accepted."

Trigger Sensitivity (L/min)

The 740 uses flow triggering to initiate all breaths. The TRIGGER SENSITIVITY control (1 to 20 L/min) establishes the trigger level. Unlike most ventilators, the 740 does not require a base flow to measure flow changes in order to provide flow triggering. The microprocessor monitors flow coming from the piston. If the patient's inspiratory flow exceeds the flow trigger level set by the user, inspiration begins.

% O_2

The %O_2 is adjustable from 21% to 100%, but requires that a high-pressure oxygen source be connected to the unit.

Additional Ventilator Settings

Table 10-18 provides the key or indicator name and the specific function of each control. The MENU key is worth a more extensive discussion.

Menu Key. The MENU key can be used at any time to view active and reset alarms, to run the short self test (SST), change alarm volume, enter the standby mode, and view and change other information. Table 10-19 summarizes the menu functions. Information for the MENU key is presented in the message window. (Note that the first item of information in the message window is always reserved for displaying any high-priority active or autoreset alarm.) Menu information is displayed in the second line in the message window.

To access items in the menu, touch MENU, use the CONTROL knob to select the desired item, and press ACCEPT to enter the new menu function. To exit the menu, press CLEAR, which also cancels the current function or display setting, or press any ventilator or alarm setting key. These actions cancel any change that was in progress but not completed.

TABLE 10-18

Additional ventilator settings on the Nellcor Puritan Bennett 740

Key/indicator	Specifies	Range
	Spontaneous (PSV) settings	
Support pressure	Pressure above PEEP maintained during spontaneous inspiration. Support pressure is terminated when inspiratory flow falls to 25% of peak inspiratory flow or 10 L/min—whichever is lower. Maximum T_I is 3.5 sec for adults, 2.5 sec for pediatric patients.	0 to 70 cm H_2O (0 to 0.7 kPa); Accuracy: ± (3 + 2.5% of setting) cm H_2O
	Common settings	
PEEP/CPAP	Positive end-expiratory pressure/continuous positive airway pressure. Minimum pressure maintained during inspiratory and expiratory phases.	0 to 35 cm H_2O (0 to 3.5 kPa); Accuracy: ± (0.6 cm H_2O + 10% of setting)
Trigger sensitivity (L/min)	Inspiratory flow required to trigger the ventilator to deliver a breath.	1 to 20 L/min
% O_2	Percentage of inspired oxygen of the gas delivered to the patient. (Note that it may take several minutes for the O_2 % to stabilize.)	21% to 100%; Accuracy: ± 3% full scale
	Other keys, knobs, and indicators	
100% O_2	Switches the O_2 % to 100% for 2 min, then returns to the current O_2 % setting. The 2-min interval restarts every time you press 100% O_2.	
MENU	Allows you to view active and reset alarms, run SST, enter standby mode, enable or disable O_2 % alarm limits, and view and change other information.	
APNEA PARAMS KEY	Allows you to select settings for apnea ventilation. The apnea interval is fixed at 20 seconds. Apnea ventilation can only become active during the spontaneous mode.	
MANUAL INSP	Delivers one mandatory breath to the patient according to the current apnea parameters (in spont.). You can deliver a manual inspiration at any time during the exhalation phase of a breath, except during apnea ventilation.	
CLEAR	Pressing CLEAR before accepting a setting cancels the proposed setting. Pressing CLEAR does not cancel accepted settings. Pressing it twice returns the ventilator to its previous state.	
ACCEPT	Makes changes to settings effective. If you don't press ACCEPT within 30 seconds of proposing a new setting, the user interface returns to its previous state.	
Knob	Adjusts the value of a setting or selects a menu option. A setting value that flashes means that the knob is linked to that setting. Turning the knob clockwise increases the value, and turning it counter-clockwise decreases the value.	
CURRENT	Lights when the ventilator is operating according to the displayed settings, or during apnea ventilation. (There is one indicator for mandatory breaths, and one for spontaneous breaths.)	
PROPOSED	Lights when you propose a mode or breath type, or you are setting apnea parameters. Once a proposed setting is accepted, it becomes effective at the next breath.	
APNEA PARAMS (indicator)	Lights when apnea ventilation is active. Lights with proposed indicator when you are setting apnea parameters, and both indicators turn off once apnea parameters are accepted.	
Message window	Shows up to four lines of information (20 characters per line). First line is reserved for the highest priority active or autoreset alarm. Second line gives information about the menu function or settings, alarm silence time remaining, or current date and time. Third and fourth lines are reserved for other messages.	

Courtesy Nellcor Puritan Bennett, Carlsbad, Calif.

Patient Data

The PATIENT DATA section of the keyboard allows you to view information on pressure, measured volume, rate, and alarm settings. To the far left, a PRESSURE LED bar graph provides immediate readings of airway pressure. The highest sustained double bar of the pressure graph represents the HIGH-PRESSURE LIMIT setting. The next double bar down is the CURRENT PEAK PRESSURE, which is only displayed during exhalation. LEDs on this bar graph rise and fall synchronously with circuit pressure. Also within this section are monitoring indicators for regular ventilation parameters and common alarms. Table 10-20 lists patient data indicators or keys along with the function and range of each.

TABLE 10-19

Menu function summary

MENU option	Function
More active alarms	Lists other active alarms in order of priority. (The highest priority active alarm is always displayed on the first line of the message window.) Turning the knob displays other active alarms. The ALARM RESET key clears (erases) this list. CLEAR returns to menu options.
Autoreset alarms	Lists alarms that have autoreset since ALARM RESET key was last pressed. Turning the knob lists other autoreset alarms. The ALARM RESET key clears (erases) this list. CLEAR returns to menu options.
SST	Begins short self-test (SST).
Alarm volume	Sets the loudness of the audible alarm. You can adjust the volume level from 1 to 5 (5 is the loudest), then return to menu options. You can adjust the alarm volume even when the alarm silence is active. CLEAR returns to menu options without making any change.
Date and time set	Sets date and time. CLEAR returns to menu options.
Standby mode	Places the ventilator in a non-ventilating waiting state.
Battery info	Displays the estimated operational time remaining on the internal and external batteries until they need recharging. (Available only when ventilator is operating on battery power.) CLEAR returns to menu options.
Software revision	Displays the version of software installed in the ventilator. CLEAR returns to menu options.
O_2 alarm info	Allows you to enable or disable the oxygen sensor. CLEAR returns to menu options without making any change.
Service summary	Allows you to view estimates of oxygen sensor life remaining, internal battery operational time remaining, and the time until the next preventive maintenance is due.

(Courtesy Nellcor Puritan Bennett, Carlsbad, Calif.)

Ventilator Status

At the top right of the front panel, there is a section showing the current operating conditions of the ventilator, which are briefly described here.

Alarm

The ALARM light flashes in red to indicate a high-priority alarm and gives an audible signal pattern of three beeps, then two beeps that repeats. It is steadily lit when an alarm condition existed but was self-corrected (i.e., autoreset). The message window displays the alarm type that was present.

Caution

The flashing yellow CAUTION light indicates a medium-priority alarm. It repeats a sequence of three beeps, and is lit steadily when the condition corrects itself (autoreset).

Normal

During normal operation, the NORMAL light is constantly green.

Ventilator Inoperative

A ventilator inoperative condition is serious. The safety valve opens while an alarm sounds so a patient can spontaneously breathe room air. A trained individual must run the EST test, and the ventilator must pass before it can be used on a patient. The discussion of special features in this section describes the VENT. INOP. condition in more detail.

Safety Valve Open

A red indicator shows you that the safety valve is open. This may indicate a ventilator inoperative condition or an obstructed patient circuit. If possible, the message window will display the cause and give the time that has elapsed since the last breath. If the condition is corrected and the VENT. INOP. indicator is off, press the ALARM RESET key to resume ventilation.

Table 10-21 lists additional ventilator status keys and indicators.

Alarms

Within the PATIENT DATA section are the common alarms for HIGH RATE, HIGH and LOW PRESSURE, LOW $\dot{V}_E$, and HIGH and LOW V_T (see Table 10-20). The VENTILATOR STATUS section uses color indicators to specify the type of alarm occurring (i.e., high- or medium-priority). If the active alarm is an adjustable alarm, its key light also flashes and the

TABLE 10-20

The patient data section with indicators, functions, and ranges

Key/indicator	Function	Range
	Pressure	
MEAN PRESSURE	Shows the calculated value of ventilator breathing circuit pressure over an entire respiratory cycle. Updated at the beginning of each breath.	0 to 99 cm H_2O (0 to 9.9 kPa) Accuracy: ± (1 + 3% of reading) cm H_2O
PEAK PRESSURE	Shows the pressure measured at the end of inspiration (excluding plateau, if any). Updated at the beginning of each expiratory phase. (Default pressure display.)	0 to 140 cm H_2O (0 to 14 kPa) Accuracy: ± (1 + 3% of reading) cm H_2O
	Breath timing	
RATE/MIN	Shows the calculated value of the total respiratory rate, based on the previous 60 seconds or eight breaths (whichever interval is shorter). Updated at the beginning of each breath. (Default breath timing display.) The calculation is reset (and display is blank) when ventilation starts, when apnea ventilation starts or autoresets, and when you press the ALARM RESET key.	3 to 199 breaths/minute Accuracy: ± (0.1 + 1% of reading)/minute
I:E RATIO	Shows the ratio of measured inspiratory time to measured expiratory time. Updated at the beginning of each breath.	1:99.9 to 9.9:1 Accuracy: ± (0.1 + 2%)
	Volume	
EXHALED VOLUME (mL)	Shows the patient's measured expiratory tidal volume for the just-completed breath. Corrected to BTPS and compliance-compensated. Updated at the beginning of each inspiration. (Default volume display.)	0 to 9 L Accuracy: ± (10 mL + 10% of reading)
TOTAL MINUTE VOLUME (L)	Shows the patient's measured expiratory minute volume, based on the previous 60 seconds or eight breaths (whichever interval is shorter). Updated at the beginning of each breath. The calculation is reset when ventilation starts, when apnea ventilation starts or autoresets, and when you press the ALARM RESET key.	0 to 99 L Accuracy: ± (10 mL + 10% of reading)
	Alarm settings	
HIGH RATE	An active alarm indicates that measured respiratory rate is higher than the alarm setting.	3 to 100 breaths/minute Accuracy: ± (0.1 + 1% of setting)/minute
LOW INSP PRESSURE	An active alarm indicates that monitored circuit pressure is below the alarm setting at the end of inspiration. Inactive in spontaneous mode.	3 to 60 cm H_2O (0.3 to 6 kPa) Accuracy: ± (1 + 3% of setting)
HIGH PRESSURE	An active alarm indicates that two consecutive breaths were truncated because circuit pressure reached the alarm setting.	10 to 90 cm H_2O (10 to 90 kPa) Accuracy: ± (1 + 3% of setting)
LOW MINUTE VOLUME	An active alarm indicates that monitored minute volume is less than the alarm setting, based on an eight-breath running average.	0 to 50 L Accuracy: ± (10 mL + 10% of setting)
HIGH TIDAL VOLUME	An active alarm indicates that exhaled volume for three out of four consecutive breaths was above the alarm setting.	20 to 9000 mL Accuracy: ± (10 mL + 10% of setting)
LOW TIDAL VOLUME	An active alarm indicates that exhaled volume for three out of four consecutive breaths was below the alarm setting.	0 to 2000 mL Accuracy: ± (10 mL + 10% of setting)

TABLE 10-20 (cont'd)

The patient data section with indicators, functions, and ranges

Key/indicator	Function	Range
	Other indicators	
Bar graph	Shows real-time pressures in centimeters of water (cm H_2O) or hectopascals (hPa). An LED shows the current high pressure alarm setting. During exhalation, LEDs show the peek pressure of the last breath.	−10 to 90 cm H_2O (−1 to 9.0 kPa) Resolution: 1 cm H_2O (1 kPa)
MAND	Lights at the start of each breath to indicate that a ventilator- or operator-initiated mandatory breath is being delivered.	Not applicable
ASSIST	Lights at the start of each breath to indicate that a patient-initiated mandatory breath is being delivered.	Not applicable
SPONT	Lights at the start of each breath to indicate that a patient-initiated spontaneous breath is being delivered.	Not applicable

Courtesy Nellcor Puritan Bennett, Carlsbad, Calif.

TABLE 10-21

Additional ventilator status indicators

Key/indicator	Color	Function
ON AC/BATTERY CHARGING	Green	Lights when the ventilator is running on AC power and the battery is charging.
ON INTERNAL BATTERY	Yellow	Flashes when the ventilator is running on the internal battery.
ON EXTERNAL BATTERY	Yellow	Flashes when the ventilator is running on the external battery.
INTERNAL BATTERY LEVEL	Green	Shows the relative charge level of the internal battery.
2 min	Yellow	Alarm silence: Silences the alarm for 2 minutes from the most recent key press.
RESET	Not applicable	Alarm reset: Clears all alarm indicators, cancels the alarm silence period, and resets the patient data displays. If the condition that caused the alarm still exists, the alarm reactivates. Cancels apnea ventilation, if active. Reestablishes previous settings and ventilation resumes, unless the ventilator is inoperative.

Courtesy Nellcor Puritan Bennett, Carlsbad, Calif.

message window is blank. (Note that an alarm setting can be changed even while the alarm is active.) The message window also shows additional alarm messages for both clinical and technical alarms. Table 10-22 lists the messages that appear for and the causes of common clinical alarms. Table 10-23 lists the technical alarm messages. When more than one alarm is or has been active, you can view these in the message window using the MENU function.

When the alarm condition corrects itself, the alarm will autoreset, and the ALARM or CAUTION indicators light steadily. The alarm condition that occurred is added to the autoreset alarm list, which can be accessed using the MENU function.

Pressing ALARM SILENCE quiets the audible portion of the alarms for 2 minutes. If a new alarm condition occurs within the 2 minutes, the alarm sounds again. (Note that pressing ALARM SILENCE during normal operation (no alarms) gives you 2 minutes to perform bedside procedures without the audible alarm sounding. If an alarm occurs, the ALARM or CAUTION indicators flash, and the message window displays a message about the alarm.) Using the ALARM RESET key clears all alarm indicators and cancels the 2-minute alarm silence.

MODES OF OPERATION

There are three basic modes of ventilation in the 740 ventilator: A/C, SIMV, and spontaneous, each of which has a touch pad control on the front panel. In the A/C and SIMV

TABLE 10-22

Clinical alarm messages

Message	Meaning
APNEA	No patient effort detected for 20 seconds
CONTINUOUS	High pressure in circuit has not dropped below high pressure setting (SVO)
DISCONNECT	Exhaled $V_T \leq 15\%$ of set V_T for four breaths; resets if exhaled $V_T > 15\%$
HI EX TIDAL VOLUME	Exhaled $V_T > V_T$ set for 3 of 4 consecutive breaths
HI RESP RATE	Measured rate > high rate alarm set
HIGH PRESSURE	Circuit pressure > high pressure limit setting for two breaths; inspiration ends, and exhalation valve opens for each breath with excessive pressure
LOW EX TIDAL VOLUME	Measured $V_T <$ low V_T alarm set for three of four consecutive breaths
LOW EX MINUTE VOLUME	Measured $\dot{V}_E <$ set $\dot{V}_E$ alarm
LOW INSP PRESSURE	Circuit pressure < set low-pressure alarm during inspiration; active in A/C and SIMV modes only
O_2 % HIGH	Measured O_2 % > 10% of set O_2 % for ≥ 30 seconds
O_2 % LOW	Measured O_2 % < 10% of set O_2% for ≥ 30 seconds
OCCLUSION	Patient circuit, inspiratory and/or expiratory filters occluded; ventilator detects abnormal differences in measured inspiratory and expiratory pressures; safety valve opens and ventilation is suspended
SETUP TIME ELAPSED	30 seconds or more have passed since you pressed a key or turned the control knob during power-on

TABLE 10-23

Technical alarm messages

Message	Meaning
AIR INTAKE ABSENT	Missing air intake filter
AIR INTAKE BLOCKED	High resistance on air intake filter
BAT NOT CHARGING	Battery voltage not increasing
CONTACT SERVICE	Ventilator service required
DELIV GAS HI TEMP	Room air temperature high
DELIV GAS LOW TEMP	Room air temperature low
EXH CCT HI TEMP	Differential pressure sensor temperature high
EXH CCT LO TEMP	Differential pressure sensor temperature low
FAN FAILED ALERT	Fan not operational or fan filer blocked
HI BBU TEMP ALERT	Internal power supply temperature high
HI SYS TEMP ALERT	Internal temperature of ventilator high
LOSS OF AC POWER	AC power disconnect
LOSS OF POWER	AC power lost and batteries are low
LOW EXT BATTERY	Low external and internal battery power
LOW INT BATTERY	Low internal battery power
LOW O_2 SUPPLY	O_2 line pressure low
REPLACE O_2 SENSOR	O_2 sensor missing or reading out of range*
SPEAKER FAILURE	Main alarm speaker failed
SWITCH INT BATTERY	Power source has switched to internal battery

*This message will not appear if O_2 alarm is disabled.

modes, mandatory breaths are volume-targeted. When either A/C or SIMV is selected, the vcv pad LED lights, indicating that breaths are volume-targeted. Spontaneous breaths can be assisted with PS in either the SIMV or the spontaneous mode.

During ventilation, the current mode key is lit and settings are displayed. To change the mode, perform the same procedure as changing a setting. Select the mode by pressing the desired key. All of the available settings in that mode flash. For every flashing setting key, you must touch the key—and adjust the setting if necessary—before the new mode can be applied (see Box 10-95). Pressing ACCEPT after all entries are completed activates the new mode.

Assist/Control

In A/C, the ventilator delivers volume-targeted breaths that are labeled as vcv breaths on the control panel. Breaths are patient- or time-triggered, volume-targeted, and volume-cycled. T_I can be extended by adding a plateau.

SIMV

In SIMV, mandatory breaths are patient- or time-triggered, volume-targeted, and volume-cycled. Spontaneous breaths are flow-triggered, pressure-targeted, and pressure-cycled unless PS is added (see the discussion of pressure support in this section). Breath timing is based on what the manufacturer describes as a breath period (Tb), which is divided into the mandatory interval (Tm) and the spontaneous period (Ts) (Figure 10-73, *A*). When the breath period begins, the ventilator enters the mandatory interval, during which

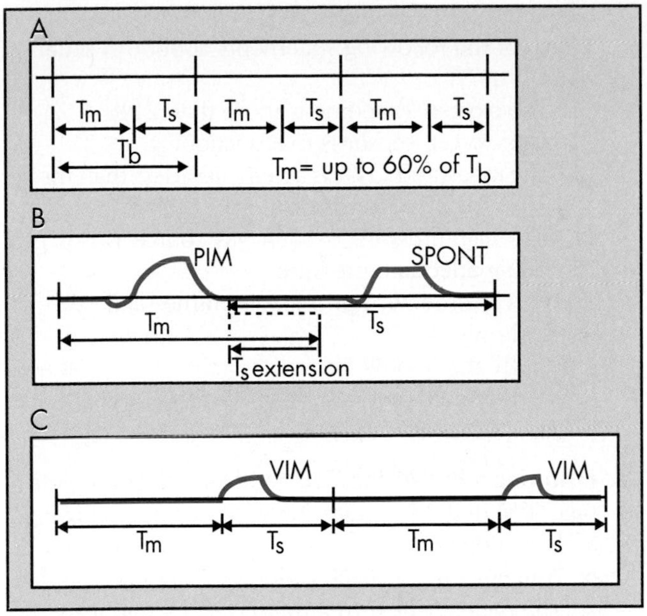

Figure 10-73 Timing of SIMV breaths. (Courtesy Nellcor Puritan Bennett Corp., Pleasanton, Calif.)

the patient can trigger a mandatory breath. After breath delivery, the mandatory interval ends and the spontaneous period begins and continues to the end of the breath period (*B*). If the patient triggers a breath during the spontaneous period, the ventilator delivers a spontaneous breath based on the PS setting. The ventilator remains in spontaneous period until the breath period ends, then it reenters the mandatory interval and a new breath period. If the patient does not trigger a breath during the mandatory interval, a time-triggered mandatory breath is delivered at the beginning of the spontaneous period, when the mandatory interval is over (*C*).

Spontaneous

During spontaneous ventilation, the patient can breathe spontaneously from a zero baseline or from CPAP. Breaths are flow-triggered, pressure-limited, and pressure cycled. In addition, spontaneous breaths may be assisted using PSV.

Pressure Support

With PSV selected, patient-triggered spontaneous breaths in either the spontaneous or the SIMV mode receive the set pressure above PEEP/CPAP during inspiration. Breaths are patient-triggered, pressure-targeted, and flow-cycled. Inspiration normally ends when flow drops to 10 L/min or 25% of peak inspiratory flow—whichever is lower. If pressure at the patient wye increases to 3 cm H_2O above the set PS level, inspiration ends as well. In addition, flow also stops if T_I exceeds 3.5 seconds (2.5 seconds with pediatric patient circuits). Box 10-96 provides a problem solving exercise related to setting up a ventilator mode.

BOX 10-96

Decision Making & Problem Solving

You are setting up the A/C mode for a patient who will be ventilated with the 740. After selecting all of the settings you want to change, you notice that the TIDAL VOLUME key is flashing. What does this indicate, and what should you do?

See Appendix A for the answer.

GRAPHIC DISPLAY SCREENS

Although the use of graphics features is valuable in patient monitoring, it is not an inexpensive feature to add to a ventilator. Nellcor Puritan Bennett has not added a graphics monitor package to the 740, but this has helped to keep its market price lower than most microprocessor ventilators currently designed for acute care use.

SPECIAL FEATURES

Two features come standard with the 740: apnea ventilation and the ventilator inoperative condition. Although, the following two features may be added in the future, pending FDA approval. That is, the unit will have an option to deliver pressure-targeted, as well as volume-targeted breaths in the A/C and SIMV modes. It will also have an option for proportional assist ventilation. The upgraded options will be available for the 740 or sold as a package called the 760.

Apnea Ventilation

Apnea back-up ventilation is an emergency mode of ventilation only available in the spontaneous mode. It is triggered when the 20-second apnea time elapses without a patient-detected breath. Apnea parameters can only be viewed or changed when the ventilator is in the spontaneous mode. Box 10-97 outlines the procedure for setting apnea ventilation.

Ventilator Inoperative Condition

If a hardware failure or a critical software error occurs that could compromise safe ventilation of the patient, a ventilator inoperative condition occurs. The VENT. INOP. indicator light illuminates, a high-priority alarm sounds, and the safety valve opens (SVO), allowing the spontaneously breathing patient access to room air. The ventilator must be turned off and another means of patient ventilation established immediately. When the unit is turned on again, a

BOX 10-97

Setting Apnea Parameters

1. While the ventilator is in the spontaneous mode, press APNEA PARAMS. The APNEA PARAMETER key lights steadily.
2. The following key lights flash for apnea settings: RESPIRATORY RATE, TIDAL VOLUME, and PEAK FLOW. The message window displays "Apnea setup. Select a setting."
3. Each flashing light control must be touched. If necessary, adjust the setting as well. For example, touch the TIDAL VOLUME key; it now lights steadily. Use the knob control to change the volume setting if desired and touch ACCEPT to have the new apnea V_T accepted.
4. Once all settings are set, press ACCEPT again to apply the new apnea settings. The message window will read "Setting(s) accepted."
5. If you press CLEAR before the settings have been accepted, the parameter is not updated. The APNEA PARAMS key flashes. The message window shows: "All setup canceled. Update apnea."

trained individual must run an EST to establish the cause of the problem and correct it.

The ventilator remains in the SVO state until a POST verifies that the power levels to the ventilator are acceptable and that the microprocessors are functioning correctly. The ventilator settings must then be confirmed.

TROUBLESHOOTING

The message window and alarm package available with the 740 help to troubleshoot the majority of problems that may occur. The operator's manual provides more detail about the technical and clinical alarm conditions if special problems arise.

As with microprocessor-operated medical equipment, the Nellcor Puritan Bennett 740 may be susceptible to certain transmitting devices such as cellular phones, walkie-talkies, cordless phones, and pagers. The radio frequency emissions from these devices are additive, so the ventilator must be located a sufficient distance from these to avoid interruption of its operation.

Review Questions

(See Appendix A for answers.)

1. During ventilation of a patient with the 740, the message window reads "O_2% Low" and "Low O_2 Supply." The red alarm indicator is flashing, and an audible pattern of three beeps, then two beeps repeats. Which of the following statements about this situation is(are) true?
   I. The oxygen % setting is more than 21%
   II. The oxygen sensor is malfunctioning
   III. The measured O_2% is at least 10% less than the set O_2% for 30 seconds or more
   IV. The high-pressure oxygen gas source is not providing adequate pressure
   V. This is a medium-priority alarm message
   a. I only
   b. III and V only
   c. II and IV only
   d. I, III, and IV only
2. Following a POST, the 740 ventilator gives the message "PM due 24," indicating which of the following?
   a. It is midnight
   b. A maintenance check is due in 24 hours
   c. The patient's next treatment is in 24 minutes
   d. The patient has been on the ventilator for 24 hours
3. An SST should be run under which of the following conditions?
   I. every 15 days
   II. when a new patient is to be started
   III. when the patient circuit is changed
   IV. after any alarm situation
   a. II only
   b. I and III only
   c. I, II, and III only
   d. I, II, III, and IV
4. Which of the following functions would you activate before suctioning a patient?
   I. STANDBY mode
   II. ALARM SILENCE
   III. 100% O_2
   IV. CLEAR
   a. I only
   b. II only
   c. III and IV only
   d. II and III only
5. You return to a patient's bedside who is being ventilated with a 740 and notice that the alarm indicator is illuminated steadily in red. The message window reads "HIGH PRESSURE," and no alarm is sounding. Which of the following statements is true?
   a. inspiration has ended because high pressure was reached
   b. the inspiratory line is occluded
   c. an autoreset of the HIGH-PRESSURE alarm has occurred
   d. the patient needs suctioning
6. The modes of ventilation on the 740 include which of the following?

I. PSV
II. A/C volume ventilation
III. PCV
IV. SIMV volume ventilation
a. II and III only
b. III and IV only
c. I, II, and IV only
d. I, II, III, and IV

7. When the ventilator is not in use, it should be kept plugged in and turned off—true or false?
8. Apnea ventilation works in all modes on the 740—true or false?
9. Flow triggering of all breath types is available on the 740—true or false?
10. A 20 second interval of apnea has occurred with a patient receiving three mandatory breaths/min in the SIMV mode on the 740. Will the apnea ventilation mode begin? If not, why?

References

1. 740 Ventilator System operator's manual, G-060143-00 Rev. B 0697, Pleasanton, Calif., 1997, Nellcor Puritan Bennett.
2. 740 Ventilator System pocket guide, A-AA2213-00 Rev.A (06/97), Pleasanton, Calif., 1997, Nellcor Puritan Bennett.

Nellcor Puritan Bennett 7200

OUTLINE

LEARNING OBJECTIVES

Upon completion of this section, the reader should be able to:

1. Compare the POST, QUEST, and TEST functions.
2. Describe the steps in setting normal operating parameters, such as tidal volume and respiratory rate.
3. Solve a problem related to an error that has occurred when setting a parameter.
4. Explain the selection of functions and options on the front panel.
5. Given total and extrinsic PEEP, calculate an auto-PEEP level after the auto-PEEP maneuver.
6. Identify the type of breath delivery based on the LED activated in the patient data section of the front panel.
7. Determine the actual volume delivered to the patient circuit based on set V_T, PIP, and tube compliance (C_T).
8. Assess an error message related to the I:E ratio.
9. Recommend low V_T and apnea time settings when SIMV is the mode of ventilation.
10. Discuss the use of constant T_I and constant I:E ratio in PCV.
11. List the three emergency modes of ventilation and the circumstance under which they occur.
12. Describe the respiratory mechanics options available.
13. Identify an error message when static mechanics are performed.
14. Solve a problem related to the setting of flow triggering in the Flow-by version 2.0.

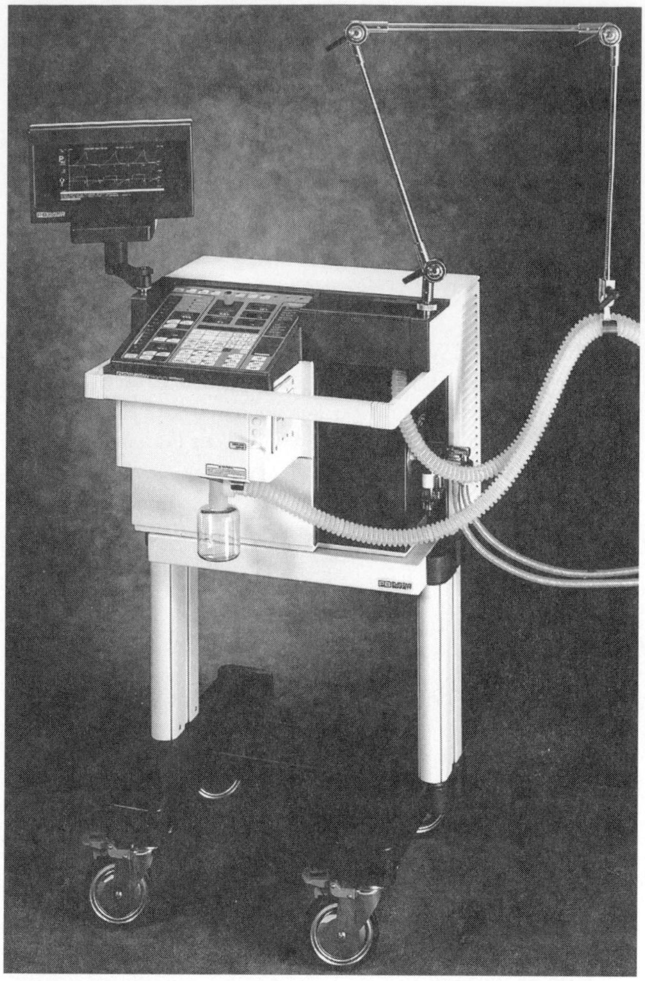

Figure 10-74 The Nellcor Puritan Bennett 7200 and graphics monitor. (Courtesy Nellcor Puritan Bennett Corp., Pleasanton, Calif.)

The Nellcor Puritan Bennett 7200[1,2] was one of the first ventilators to provide microprocessor control of its electrical functions (Figure 10-74). It was originally released in the early 1980s and has since gone through a series of upgrades, which included two different front control panel changes to improve ease of use. The third and current front panel version is the one described throughout this section. The 7200 is intended for pediatric and adult patient use in the acute care setting.

Power Source

The unit requires both pneumatic and electrical power sources to operate. It normally uses air and oxygen high-pressure sources (35 to 100 psi) for pneumatic functions, but it can also operate from a single gas source or a high-pressure compressor. The latter two options will, of course, alter oxygen delivery. A standard 115-volt AC 60 Hz outlet provides the electrical power source.

Internal Mechanism

The internal mechanism is shown in Figure 10-75. The air and oxygen sources flow through inlet filters to regulators (*A* and *B*), which reduce and balance pressure to 10 psi (about 700 cm H_2O). The gases are then conducted through flow transducers (*D* and *E*) to the electrically operated, microprocessor-controlled proportional solenoid (metering) valves (*F1* and *F2*). These valves regulate the amount and pattern of gas flow to the patient based on settings and microprocessor control. The crossover solenoid (*C*) powers the PEEP control using air or oxygen, depending on which is available.

As gas passes from the solenoid valves, it flows through the following:

1. A pressure transducer (*G*), which acts as an internal barometer
2. A safety/check valve that serves two functions:
   - as an overpressure-relief valve (*H*) that opens at 140 cm H_2O
   - as an antisuffocation (safety) valve (*I*) that opens during the start up self-test and if pneumatic or electric power is lost

Gas flow to the expiration valve is controlled by a solenoid (*J*). During a mandatory breath, this solenoid opens, allowing gas to be directed through the expiratory line and closing the expiratory valve (*K*). During expiration, the expiratory solenoid (*J*) closes and gas flows from the PEEP regulator (*L*) and the PEEP Venturi (*M*) to the back of the expiratory valve. This produces the set level of PEEP/CPAP during expiration.

There are two differential pressures transducers: one measures PEEP (*N*), and one measures airway pressure (*O*). Exhaled patient air passes through the expiratory flow transducer (*P*), which provides information for measuring and calculating V_T and $\dot{V}_E$, as well as monitors and provides some alarm functions.

Controls and Alarms

The three front panels designed for the 7200, beginning with its original design in the 1980s and progressing to the most recent version in 1994 (shown in Figure 10-76), are divided into three basic sections, as follows:

1. VENTILATOR SETTINGS (controls)
2. PATIENT DATA (monitoring information)
3. VENTILATOR STATUS (alarm information)

Box 10-98 describes the function of each section. Although the positioning of these controls has changed somewhat, the overall design stayed consistent. Table 10-24 lists the specifications for the updated (enhanced) version of the 7200.

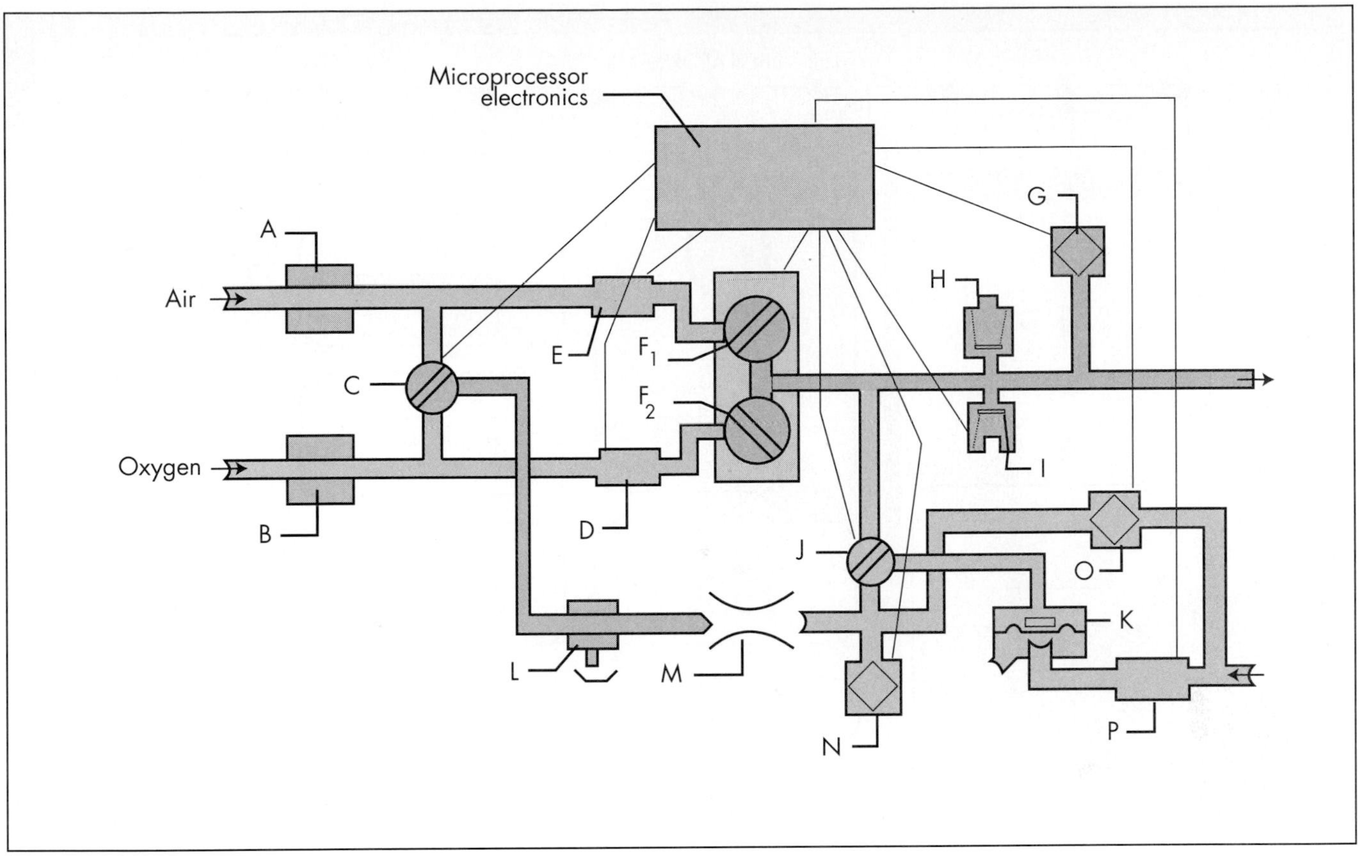

Figure 10-75 The Nellcor Puritan Bennett 7200 interval schematic. (From Pilbeam SP: Mechanical ventilation. In Burton GG, Hodgkin JE, and Ward JJ, editors: Respiratory care: a guide to clinical practice,ed 4, Philadelphia, 1997, Lippincott.)

Self-Test

When the ventilator is first turned on (power switch on the left side), the microprocessor starts the POST. It usually lasts about 5 seconds, depending on the version used. Like most microprocessor-controlled ventilators, the 7200 must complete these essential tests before it becomes functional. POST actually runs in the following situations:

1. When the ventilator is turned on
2. When EST is run
3. When power is interrupted
4. When ongoing checks detect a system error

After POST, all previous ventilator settings are recalled from memory and activated (Box 10-99). If POST fails, the back-up ventilation mode becomes operational. (The discussion of special functions later in this section provides an explanation of back-up ventilation.) In addition, the message window gives all error codes that need to be recorded for the service representative. A replacement ventilator should be provided as soon as possible.

Two additional ESTs, called QUEST and TEST, can also be selected. (Note that no EST or POST should be run while the ventilator is connected to a patient.) The quick extended self test (QUEST) executes 26 tests and takes about 2 minutes. To run QUEST, press the EST button on the side panel and ENTER on the front panel, then ENTER again when the window reads "PAT TUBING OFF-ENTER." (This instruction is to ensure that you are not trying to ventilate the patient while the test is being run.) You then follow the instructions provided in the display window as they appear. QUEST should be run whenever the patient circuit is changed.

The total extended self-test (TEST) executes 60 tests and takes about 3 to 5 minutes. It is part of the normal maintenance procedure and is routinely performed by biomedical personnel. As with QUEST, it is accessed by pressing the EST and ENTER buttons After the "PAT TUBING OFF-ENTER" instruction, press ENTER, and in response to "QUICK EST," press the key labeled "++" and then ENTER. As with QUEST, you then simply follow the instructions sequentially displayed in the window. (Note that the explanation for canceling EST and responding to error messages is beyond the scope of this text and is really intended for ventilator maintenance. The reader is referred to the operator's manual if these procedures are required.)

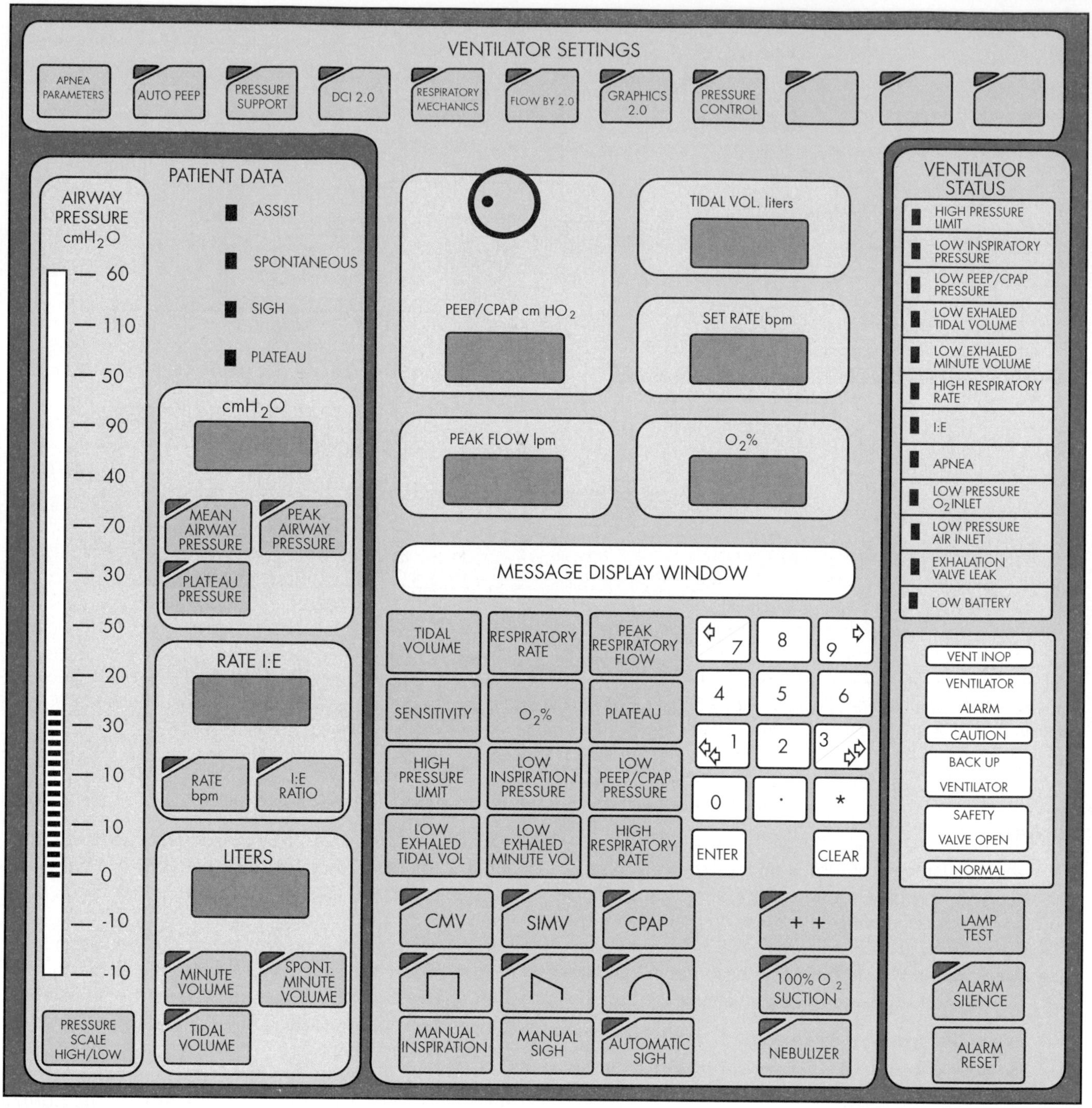

Figure 10-76 Third-generation control panel for the enhanced 7200 ventilator. (Courtesy Nellcor Puritan Bennett Corp., Pleasanton, Calif.)

Initial Start-up

After the machine is turned on and the POST is completed, the message "Review Apnea Params" appears in the window to remind you to check apnea parameters appropriate for the patient and the mode selected (see the discussion of special functions later in this section). Also check automatic sigh parameters to be sure they are set as desired for the new patient because old values stored in memory will become operational. The operation of sigh is described in the discussion of additional control parameters in this section. In addition, look at the PEEP control because it may have been set on the last patient and not returned to the zero position after use.

General Setting of Parameters

The ventilator is operated using the touch pads on the front panel. With the exception of the PEEP/CPAP control knob, all parameters are set using these function keys.

BOX 10-98

Description of Keyboard Sections

Patient Data Section

Displays monitored patient information, such as pressure, volume, rate, I:E ratio, and breath type.

Ventilator Settings Section

Contains the keys that allow you to set values for specific parameters and alarms. It contains a message window that displays values for set parameters and allows selection of special functions, such as manual inspiration, manual sigh, and 100% O_2 suction. Use of the ++ key in this section, along with the numeric key pads, provides access to supplemental functions, such as pressure control and flow-by. (Note that some of these functions are also available by pressing the labeled keys at the top of the front panel [see Figure 10-76].)

Ventilator Status Sections

Contains 12 alarm indicators and six status display indicators that notify you if there is an alarm condition. Three key pads additionally allow for testing of the front panel lights, such as ALARM SILENCING, ALARM RESET, and LAMP TEST.

To view the set value for any parameter, press the appropriately named function key. There are some function keys that display the parameter value at all times, including the following:

- TIDAL VOLUME
- RESPIRATORY RATE
- PEAK INSPIRATORY FLOW
- SENSITIVITY
- O_2%

There are also function keys for alarm variables. These are reviewed in the discussion of monitors and alarms in this section.

When you press a key pad, the current set value for that variable appears in the message display window on the central portion of the panel. Changing the value requires several steps, which are outlined in Box 10-100 and can be followed using the algorithm in Figure 10-77.

Ventilator Settings

Establishing appropriate settings includes setting breath parameters and additional control parameters.

Breath Parameter Keys

The V_T control is functional in volume-targeted modes (CMV and SIMV) and provides a range of 0.10 to 2.5 L. The range for respiratory rate is adjustable from 0.5 to 9.9 breaths/min in increments of 0.1 breaths/min and from 10 to 70 breaths/min in increments of 1.0 breaths/min. The RATE control functions in CMV, SIMV, and PCV. The PEAK INSPIRATORY FLOW (10 to 120 L/min) only operates during volume ventilation.

Breaths are volume-cycled during volume ventilation; that is, a breath ends when the ventilator determines that the flow provided over a specific time has delivered a specific volume (V_T = flow × inspiratory time).* If a flow is selected that cannot deliver the set volume within a time that provides an acceptable I:E ratio, a message reads "DECR RESP RATE FIRST." The ventilator microprocessor knows that reducing the rate allows a longer T_I. Of course, increasing the flow also solves the problem and will not change $\dot{V}_E$. Box 10-101 provides a list of situations in which this message occurs, and Box 10-102 provides an exercise for calculating the volume, rate, and flow that would result in an error message.

Pressure sensitivity (0.5 to 20.0 cm H_2O) is adjusted with the key pad and numerical controls. However, flow triggering is also available when the flow-by function is selected. Flow-by and flow triggering in the 7200 are described in the discussion of special functions in this section. The available % O_2 ranges from 21% to 100%. There is no built-in oxygen analyzer to test the FIO_2 delivery.

Use of the PLATEAU control closes the inspiratory and expiratory valves at the end of inspiration for the amount of time selected (from 0.0 to 2.0 seconds). This is only functional during a volume breath. The inspiratory phase is increased by the set amount; see Box 10-101 for the error message.

Additional Control Parameters

In addition to the variables and settings already described, there are three more areas of the front panel (Figure 10-76) where functions can be set and settings monitored:

1. The lower central portion of the front panel, below the ALARM function keys and the numerical pad
2. A row of controls across the top of the panel
3. A set of display screens that show current settings

The controls directly below the alarm function keys are discussed first. The first three functional keys are used for selecting CMV, SIMV, and CPAP. Press the desired key pad and then press ENTER to activate a new mode (see the discussion of modes of ventilation in this sections).

Next are the three function keys that determine the flow waveform in volume-targeted breaths. The available waveforms are constant (rectangular), descending ramp, and sine wave. The amount of flow delivered during each type of waveform is determined by the peak flow setting. For example, with a constant (rectangular) waveform selection, the flow is constant at the value set on the peak flow control. For a descending ramp, the starting flow is the peak flow setting,

*This can also be called flow cycling; see Chapter 9.

TABLE 10-24

Specifications for the Nellcor Puritan Bennett 7200 microprocessor ventilator

Modes
A/C (CMV) (volume control)
A/C (CMV) (pressure control)
SIMV (volume control)
SIMV (pressure control)
SIMV (volume control) + PSV
SIMV (pressure control) + PSV
CPAP (with PSV)
CPAP (without PSV)

Breath type	Range
Breath type–mandatory	
Volume control	
Volume (mL)	100-2500
Rate (breaths/min)	
A/C (CMV)	0.5-70
SIMV	0.5-70
Peak inspiratory flow (L/sec)	10-120
Flow waveform	Square, descending ramp
Plateau (sec)	0-2.0
Inspiratory hold (sec)	0.0-2.0
Pressure control	
Inspiratory pressure (above PEEP) (cm H_2O)	5-100
Inspiratory time (sec)	0.2-5
Rate (breaths/min)	
A/C (CMV)	0.5-70
SIMV	0.5-70
I:E ratio	1:9.0-4:1
Breath type–spontaneous	
Pressure support (cm H_2O)	10-70
PEEP/CPAP (cm H_2O)	0-45

Common parameters	
Oxygen percentage	21-100
Inspiratory trigger	
Pressure (below PEEP, cm H_2O)	0.5-20
Flow (L/min)	1-15

Other featured parameters/functions
Manual inspiration
Manual sigh
Automatic sigh
100% oxygen suction (2 min)
Nebulizer
Apnea interval and ventilation
Flow-by (flow-triggering)
Clock/calendar set
Auto-PEEP
Digital communications interface
Respiratory mechanics
Graphics
Trending
Pulse oximeter
Display screen
Metabolics (integrated)

Alarm indicators
High and low pressure
Apnea
I:E ratio
Power loss
Exhalation valve leak
Low volume
Low exhaled minute volume
Ventilator inoperative
Low pressure oxygen/air inlet
High rate
Low CPAP/PEEP
Low battery

From Pilbeam SP: Mechanical ventilation. In Burton GG, Hodgkin JE, and Ward JJ: Respiratory care: a guide to clinical practice, ed 4, Philadelphia, 1997, Lippincott.

and the ending flow is 5 L/min. For a sine curve, the flow begins and ends at 5 L/min, and the flow rises to the peak flow setting at the middle of inspiration.

Since breaths are volume-cycled in the 7200, changing the peak flow and/or the waveform also changes the I:E ratio. To keep the I:E ratio the same when changing a waveform from constant to descending, the peak flow is doubled. When changing from constant to sine, the peak flow setting must be increased to 1.5 times the current setting.

The next function pads are MANUAL INSPIRATION, MANUAL SIGH, and AUTOMATIC SIGH. Selecting MANUAL INSPIRATION delivers a breath based on the selected parameters. MANUAL SIGH delivers a sigh breath based on the settings selected for automatic sigh. Pressing the AUTOMATIC SIGH function key allows the operator to select sigh parameters. The display window requests entry of sigh parameters, which are described in Box 10-103.

Below the numeric key pads are three more function keys, as follows:

1. ++
2. 100% O_2 SUCTION
3. NEBULIZER

BOX 10-99

Back-up Memory Battery

The memory that contains previous set parameter values is powered by batteries. This helps prevent loss of information if electrical power is interrupted (e.g., the machine is accidentally unplugged while in use). If the battery fails, the message "1401 ERR" tells you that the 7200 is using the default parameters that are programmed into the read-only memory (ROM) of the microprocessor. The operator should review all settings immediately, per the following list of default parameters:

Mode CMV
Constant flow waveform
V_T of 0.5 L
Rate of 12 breaths/min
Flow of 45 L/min
Sensitivity of -3 cm H_2O below baseline
100% O_2
High-pressure limit of 20 cm H_2O
Low-pressure limit of 3 cm H_2O
Apnea interval of 20 seconds

The following functions are off or disabled: 100% O_2 suction, sigh, nebulizer, low PEEP/CPAP alarm, low V_T alarm, Low $\dot{V}_E$ alarm, and low rate alarm.

BOX 10-100

Changing the Value of a Parameter

To change the value of any variable (e.g., tidal volume), do the following:

1. Press the key pad with the variable on it.
2. Press the desired numerical value using the number keys located below the message window.
3. Press the ENTER key to place the new value in memory.

An acceptable setting is confirmed by two beeps. If the entry is outside the range of the parameter, four beeps will sound and the display screen displays an error message: "INVALID ENTRY." For example, a tidal volume of 3.0 L is outside the range of the unit (see Table 10-29) and therefore invalid. You must press CLEAR and try again.

If it takes more than about 20 to 30 seconds for you to make the change, the unit reverts back to the previous setting. (Note that the new setting is never changed until the ENTER key is pressed.)

The ++ key allows you to select certain functions and options and operates like a computer menu. When you press it, the number of the last function selected appears in the window (Table 10-25). To scroll to the desired option, press the ++ key to go forward or the * key to go backward. Another way to access a specific function is to press the numbers representing the desired option and then ENTER. Once an option or function is selected, follow the directions in the message window. For example, apnea parameters are Option 1. The message "1 APNEA PARAMETERS" appears. Pressing ENTER when that message appears results in the message, "APNEA INT XX SEC." Use the NUMBER keys to set the desired apnea time interval and again press ENTER. Then the next window appears, so follow the directions again. This continues until all the necessary parameters have been selected and "UPDATE PARAMS-ENTER" is displayed. Pressing ENTER updates all the selected apnea parameters and activates them.

Selecting the 100% O_2 SUCTION key causes the ventilator to deliver 100% O_2 for 2 minutes prior to patient suctioning. The message window flashes to indicate that delivered oxygen is different than the set value (as long as the set O_2 is $<100\%$). Choosing this option does not deactivate alarms, so if the patient is disconnected for suctioning, alarms will occur (e.g., low pressure alarm).

The NEBULIZATION key allows a gas flow at the set O_2% to exit the nebulizer connector for 30 minutes after it is activated. It automatically turns off the flow-by function and only works during inspiratory flow when the flow is greater than 10 L/min (mandatory or spontaneous breaths). Box 10-104 lists conditions when the nebulizer function is suspended. If the nebulizer function is suspended, the NEBULIZER key's light goes off, and the key does not work. However, the 30-minute clock continues to run. When the condition has been corrected, nebulizer flow resumes.*

The top row of controls in the ventilator setting section was added to the most recent version of the 7200 (enhanced key board) and allows direct access to many of the functions and options listed under the ++ key. By pressing one of these keys, the display window immediately accesses that function. You simply follow the directions for setting up or operating the selected option, just as you would if you had accessed the function through the ++ key. (Note that some of the key selections allow access to more than one function, such as the respiratory mechanics option.) The controls in this row include the following:

1. APNEA PARAMETERS
2. AUTO-PEEP
3. PRESSURE SUPPORT
4. DCI 2.0
5. RESPIRATORY MECHANICS
6. FLOW-BY 2.0
7. GRAPHICS 2.0
8. PRESSURE CONTROL

*If flow-by was used prior to giving a nebulizer treatment, be sure to turn it back on.

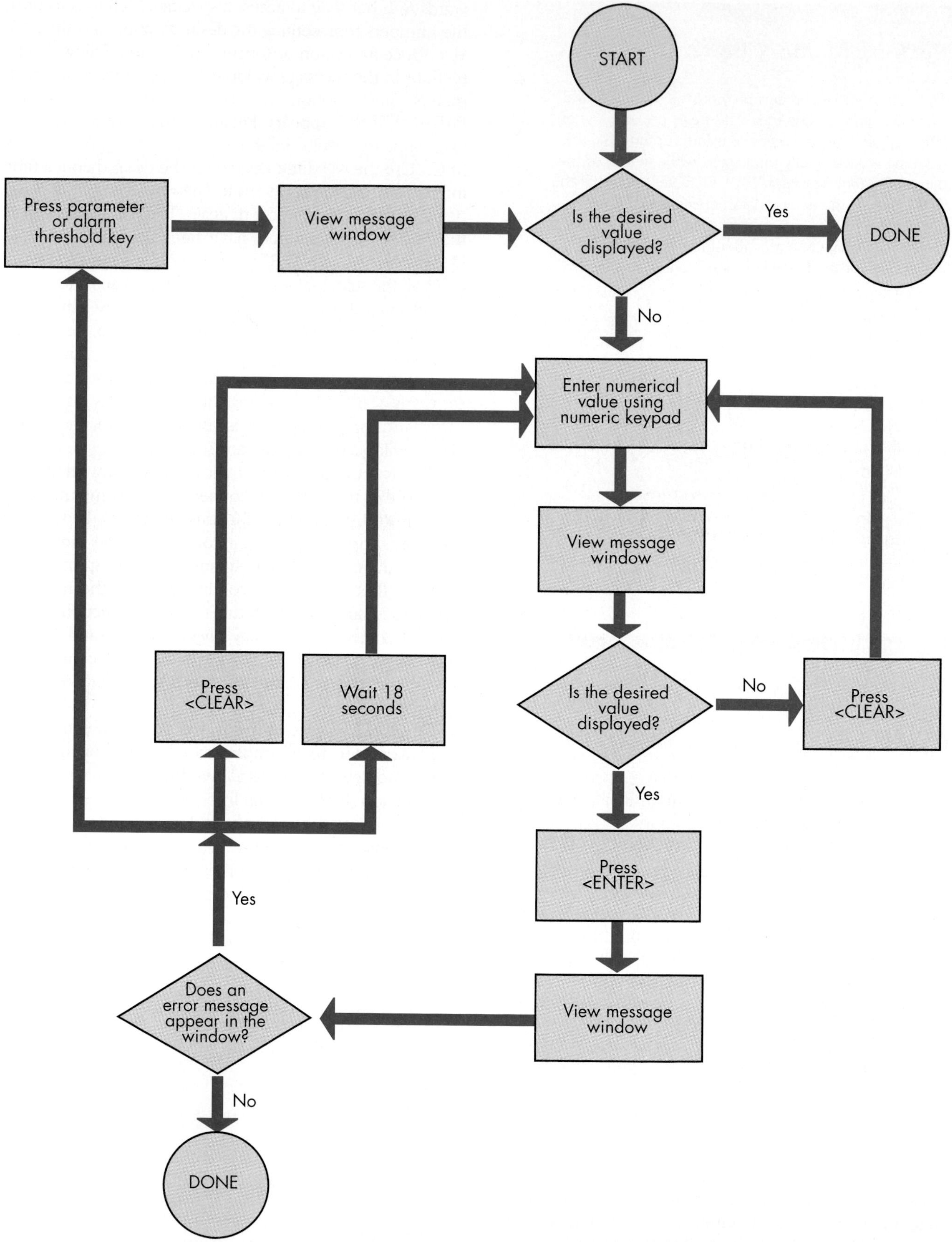

Figure 10-77 An algorithm for viewing and changing ventilator parameter values. (Courtesy Nellcor Puritan Bennett Corp., Pleasanton, Calif.)

BOX 10-101

Message: "DECR RESP RATE FIRST"

This message appears when a new value for V_T, peak inspiratory flow, or plateau or flow waveform is selected that results in lengthening the T_I to ≥75% of TCT based on the rate setting. Therefore the ventilator gives preference to T_I to lengthen TCT, so it is suggested that you reduce the rate. Of course, you could also increase inspiratory flow, alter the plateau time, or change the waveform pattern.

(Note that during PCV, T_I can be ≥80% of TCT to allow for inverse ratios up to 4:1 in this mode.)

BOX 10-102

Decision Making & Problem Solving

A respiratory therapist selects the following settings on the 7200 ventilator during a laboratory test with the machine: V_T = 1.0 L, rate = 20 breaths/min, flow = 30 L/min, and flow waveform = constant. Will the "DECR RESP RATE FIRST" message appear with these settings?

See Appendix A for the answer.

BOX 10-103

Sigh Parameters

After pressing the AUTOMATIC SIGH key, follow the instructions in the message window.

Sigh TV (tidal volume)—0.1 to 2.5 L
Sigh HIPL (high-pressure limit)—10 to 120 cm H_2O
Sigh Events—1 TO 15 (corresponds to a sigh every 4 to 60 minutes)
Multiple Sighs—1 to 3 sighs per event.

Once all new entries are complete, press enter when the window message is "UPDATE PARAMS-ENTER." This updates the sigh parameters. Finally, press ENTER when the window reads "AUTO SIGH ON-ENTER" to complete the entries and turn on the automatic sigh function.

To clear the sigh function, press the AUTOMATIC SIGH function key. When "AUTO SIGH OFF-ENTER" appears in the window, pressing the ENTER key turns off the sigh function.

TABLE 10-25

List of ++ key options and functions for the Nellcor Puritan Bennett 7200

Number	Function or option
Function 1	Apnea ventilation*
Function 2	Clock-calendar reset
Function 3	Patient data
Function 4	Auto-PEEP
Option 10	Pressure support
Option 20	Digital communications interface (DCI)
Option 30/40	Respiratory mechanics*
Option 50	Flow-by (flow trigger)*
Option 60	Graphics
Option 80	Pressure-control ventilation
Option 90	Pulse oximetry

*Covered in the discussion of special functions in this section.

BOX 10-104

Conditions when Nebulizer Function is Suspended

1. Excessive nebulizer flow—checked every eight breaths; "NEB DISCONNECT" is in the display window; excessive flow can be caused by leaks or disconnects in the nebulizer tubing.
2. During apnea and disconnect ventilation.
3. When the Respiratory Mechanics/Monitoring option is selected.
4. If low oxygen or air inlet pressure alarms occur.
5. If you select any combination of peak flow and O_2% that yields less than 10 L/min through the solenoid supplying the nebulizer circuit, the microprocessor senses the low flow and deactivates the solenoid supplying the nebulizer. The light on the nebulizer key remains lit.

(NOTE: If Flow-by is on, it is turned off when the nebulizer is activated. Be sure to turn Flow-by back on when nebulization is complete.)

1, 5, and *6* are covered in the discussion of special functions later in this section. *3* and *8* are included in the discussion of modes of ventilation, and *7* is reviewed in the discussion of ventilator graphic waveforms. Of the remaining keys, two blank touch keys for future upgrades appear on the right, and the two remaining keys, AUTO-PEEP and DCI 2.0, provide additional special functions.

The AUTO-PEEP key is Function 4 and is now a standard feature on every enhanced 7200 ventilator (7200ae, 7200spe, and 7200e). It is used to estimate end-expiratory pressures. The unit measures total PEEP at end-exhalation and estimates auto-PEEP by subtracting the set (extrinsic) PEEP from the total PEEP.

The DCI (digital communications interface) function provides data reports that including things such as data logs, chart summary reports, ventilator status reports, and host reports.

Finally, the top central portion of the ventilator setting section has digital display screens for showing the values of the current settings of the following parameters:

1. PEEP/CPAP (in centimeters of water)
2. Tidal volume (in liters)
3. Set rate (in breaths/minute)
4. Peak flow (in liters/minute)
5. O_2%

Monitors and Alarms

The Nellcor Puritan Bennett 7200 has two main sections for providing information about monitored values and alarm displays. The monitored values are provided in the PATIENT DATA section of the front panel, and the alarm display is in the VENTILATOR STATUS section. Alarms are set using the control pads for the alarms in the lower portion of the VENTILATOR SETTING section just below the key pads that control breath delivery. The patient data section is reviewed first, then setting of alarms is discussed, and then monitoring of alarm information in the ventilator status section is presented.

Monitors: Patient Data Section

The PATIENT DATA section of the front panel includes monitoring displays for the following:

1. BREATH TYPE
2. PRESSURES
3. RATES
4. I:E RATIO
5. VOLUMES

Each of these sections provides calculated or measured patient information that is digitally displayed. All of these displays are blank during a POST. Measured data is obtained from sensors for flow, pressure, and temperature (both inspiratory and expiratory). The microprocessor uses the measurements to calculate and display the information.

Breath Type

Small LEDs at the top right of the patient data section light depending on the type of breath delivery. There is an LED for a patient ASSIST when the patient triggers a mandatory breath, an LED for a SPONTANEOUS breath, one for a SIGH breath, and one to indicate that a PLATEAU maneuver is being performed. If a mandatory breath is time-triggered, no light illuminates.

BOX 10-105

Pressure Monitoring on the 7200 Ventilator

1. Mean airway pressure—airway pressure averaged over all measurements made during an entire breath (I + E) for mandatory or spontaneous breaths; updated and displayed at the end of each subsequent breath cycle; negative values reported as zero.
2. Peak airway pressure—measures peak airway pressure at the end of inspiration for a mandatory breath.
3. Plateau pressure—measures plateau pressure. The ventilator reads the average of the last four pressure sample measurements made during a plateau and displays this average at the end of a plateau; otherwise, display window is blank.
4. PEEP/CPAP—displayed continuously on the right of the patient data panel on the enhanced key board; based on the amount of pressure applied to the ventilatory side of the exhalation valve multiplied by the area ratio. (Note that the area ratio is computed every time a self-test is run. The value, however, changes little.)

Pressures

On the left side of the section is a dual-scale, pressure-reading bar graph that displays airway pressure in centimeters of water. The other available selections require that you press the desired variable from the three available and then displays its value in the pressure window. The three available pressures are shown in Box 10-105, along with the measurement for PEEP/CPAP.

Respiratory Rates and I:E Ratio

You can select either the measured respiratory rate or the I:E ratio to be displayed. Respiratory rates (in breaths/minute) are digitally displayed in the assigned window. Rates are read as the average rate of breathing calculated for a patient's 10 previous breaths (spontaneous or mandatory). The I:E ratio is only for mandatory breaths and is the actual measured value displayed as "1:X.X." For example, an I:E of 1:4 is a normal value, and a reading of "1:0.5" represents an inverse ratio of 2:1. The X.X term is calculated by dividing the time for exhalation by the time for inhalation ($X.X = T_E/T_I$). (Note that T_E is calculated by subtracting T_I from the TCT, where *TCT* is the TCT measured from beginning of inspiration to the end of exhalation. The end of exhalation is not simply the end of expiratory flow (which may have occurred before this) but is also considered the beginning of the next breath.) During

BOX 10-106

I:E Ratio

The set value for I:E may not equal the actual value if the set value is based on a volume-targeted breath using volume flow and rate or on a pressure-targeted breath using T_I and rate. For example, during SIMV or CMV, the I:E ratio may vary even though the ventilator settings do not change if the patient triggers a breath during the T_E.

CPAP, the I:E ratio displayed is the one retained from the last mandatory breath delivered (Box 10-106).

Volumes

The digital display in the volume window provides readouts of measured values in liters for V_T, $\dot{V}_E$, and spontaneous $\dot{V}_E$. Simply select which value you want to be displayed. These values are corrected to BTPS (body temperature, ambient pressure, saturated) as well as for tubing compliance. (Note that this discussion is exclusive to the enhanced [newest] keyboard and does not apply to the basic keyboard. On the basic keyboard, the exhaled volume is displayed on an analog meter, but this reading is not corrected for BTPS or tubing compliance. As a result, the analog volume reading and the digital volume reading (corrected for both) differ on the basic keyboard.)

Spontaneous V_T is displayed on a breath-by-breath basis. The mandatory breath V_T displayed is usually an average of eight breaths. If a breath is 50 mL different than the average volume for the eight mandatory breaths, the digital display only shows that breath—not the average.

Both mandatory and spontaneous $\dot{V}_E$ are based on an eight-breath projected running average or a 1 minute sample, whichever occurs first.[1] The mandatory and spontaneous $\dot{V}_E$ are calculated separately at the end of each complete breath, and are also displayed at the end of a breath.*

Correction for Compressible Volume

The 7200 compensates for volume that is compressed in the patient circuit so that the amount of air reaching the patient's lungs is very close to the value for V_T delivery set by the operator (Boxes 10-107 and 10-108).

Setting of Alarms

Setting the alarm limits is done similarly to setting the ventilation parameters (see Box 10-100 and Figure 10-77). Table 10-26 provides a list of the key pad alarms and ranges. (Note that the low inspiratory pressure alarm parameter only applies to mandatory breaths.)

*When spontaneous $\dot{V}_E$ is used, the type of breath is displayed on the large graphics window.

BOX 10-107

Compensation for Compressible Volume

During an extended self-test (EST), the 7200 determines the compliance of the patient circuit. Whenever a mandatory volume-targeted breath is delivered, the machine measures PIP and increases or decreases the delivered volume of the next breath to ensure that the set V_T is the volume that reaches the patient's lungs. This is accomplished by holding T_I constant when based on V_T and flow settings, but slightly increasing flow delivery to increase volume delivery.

Each exhaled volume is corrected as well. The microprocessor simply subtracts the volume added during inspiration from that measured during exhalation at the expiratory valve. Thus the exhaled volume reading is also corrected so that it shows the amount that is theoretically delivered to the patient's lungs. This amount is theoretical because any leaks in the system affect delivered volumes. Box 10-108 provides a sample problem.

BOX 10-108

Decision Making & Problem Solving

A patient is being ventilated on the 7200 with a set V_T of 0.6 L, a constant (square) flow pattern, and a flow of 60 L/min. The tubing compliance (C_T) was calculated during the last EST as 2 mL/cm H_2O, and the PIP for the last breath was 30 cm H_2O. What will be the amount of volume added to the delivered breath? What will be the exhaled V_T reading, assuming that there are no leaks?

See Appendix A for the answers.

When alarm limits are violated, the following three events generally occur:

1. An audible alarm is activated
2. A visual indicator and the ventilator alarm display in the ventilator status section flash
3. A message appears in the message window to describe the alarm condition. If the alarm condition is corrected by the next breath, the audible alarm is silenced, but the CAUTION light is continuously lit, and the appropriate LED indicator changes from flashing to continuous. These are turned off by touching the ALARM RESET key pad. The advantage here is that if you are away from the ventilator when an alarm condition occurs, the data from the event is kept for later reference. Box 10-109 gives two exceptions to this general condition, and Box 10-110 provides a troubleshooting exercise.

TABLE 10-26

Permissible ranges for alarm thresholds

Alarm	Range
High-pressure limit	10 to 120 cm H_2O
Low inspiratory pressure	3 to 99 cm H_2O
Low PEEP/CPAP pressure	0 to 45 cm H_2O
Low exhaled V_T	0.00 to 2.50 L
Low exhaled $\dot{V}_E$	0.00 to 60.0 L/min
High respiratory rate	0 to 70 breaths/min

BOX 10-109

Low Battery and I:E Ratio Alarms

When either a low battery or an I:E event condition occurs, the ventilator lights the corresponding alarm indicator but does not light the alarm display or provide an audible alarm. Each alarm resets to a normal display when corrected.

BOX 10-110

Decision Making & Problem Solving

A patient is being ventilated with the 7200 ventilator using volume ventilation. The mode is switched from CMV to SIMV. The mandatory V_T is 0.7 L, and the rate is set at 5 breaths/min. The spontaneous rate is 10 breaths/min, and spontaneous V_T is 0.4 L. The low V_T alarm keeps activating even though it is set at 0.6 L and there are no leaks in the circuit. What is the problem?

See Appendix A for the answer.

Events that reduce supply gas make the ventilator inoperative or severely compromise its ability to function. For example, if both gas supplies are lost, an audible alarm sounds, SVO illuminates, and the valve opens. In addition, both the LOW AIR and LOW O_2 LEDs flash. The opening of the safety valves provides a source from which a spontaneously breathing patient can receive room air.

If the microprocessor systems find a major fault that prevents safe ventilator operation, the following two red alarm indicators flash:

1. VENTILATOR INOPERATIVE
2. SAFETY VALVE OPEN

If the gas system is still working but the electronics are not, the red BUV (back-up ventilator) indicator flashes, and an

TABLE 10-27

Types of alarms and events that occur with the 7200

Type of alarm	Triggering event
High pressure limit*	Measured peak airway pressure > set limit; ends inspiration and opens exhalation valve
Low inspiratory pressure	Airway pressure < set minimum for one mandatory breath cycle
Low PEEP/CPAP pressure	Airway pressure is ≤ the set minimum for > 1 sec, or 5 L/min of gas flow is delivered during a spontaneous breath
Low exhaled V_T	In CMV, value for mandatory breaths (4-breath running average) < set; in SIMV and CPAP, value for spontaneous breaths (4-breath running average) < set
Low exhaled minute volume	Sum of minute volume for mandatory and spontaneous breaths < set minimum (based on 8-breath projected running total, or on a 1-minute sample, whichever comes first)
High respiratory rate	Breath rate > set maximum (for 10-breath running average)
I:E	Length of mandatory inspiration including plateau time > 50% of length of total breath cycle
Apnea	No exhalation detected during set apnea time
Low-pressure O_2 inlet*	Pressure at O_2 inlet ≤ 35 psig, O_2 % set > 22%
Low-pressure air inlet*	Pressure at air inlet ≤ 35 psi when connected to wall outlet or < 7.5 psi when connected to compressor
Exhalation valve leak	Volume of gas measured by exhalation valve sensor during inspiration is > 10% of the delivered V_T or 50 mL, whichever is greater
Low battery	Internal battery power is not adequate to provide 1 hour of audible alarm and battery back-up memory

*Minute ventilation and/or oxygenation may be seriously affected if one of these alarm conditions persists.

audible alarm sounds. This provides back-up ventilation as is presented in the discussion of special functions in this section. The section on special functions describes the indicators for the various alarm conditions.

Ventilator Status

The ventilator status display has three basic sections: the top provides an LED display of any current or recent alarms (Table 10-27); the second section contains the ventilator status display (Table 10-28); and the bottom section has three touch pads (LAMP TEST, ALARM SILENCE, and ALARM RESET). Pressing LAMP TEST and ENTER initiates a test that checks lamps, displays, and meters that are located on the front panel, as well as the audible alarm and the remote alarm if installed. In addition, it cancels the alarm silence function. The ALARM SILENCE key quiets audible alarms for 2 minutes to allow for undisturbed bedside procedures. It also cancels displays of self-test error messages. The ALARM RESET clears all alarm indicators, initiates a battery test, and also, like the lamp test, cancels alarm silence.

TABLE 10-28

Function of the alarm summary display

Display	Function
Ventilator inoperative	Red display. When lit, the microprocessor has determined that the ventilator is not functional due to a system fault. Coincides with illumination of safety valve open display. Back-up ventilation is not provided.
Ventilator alarm	Red display. Signals that an alarm has been triggered and has not autoreset. Usually, one or more of 12 indicators flashes to identify it.
Caution	Yellow display. Signals than an alarm was activated and automatically reset. Steady illumination of one or more of the 12 indicators identifies the alarm that was active.
Back up ventilator	Red display. Lights when the back-up ventilator (BUV) emergency mode is active. When the ventilator is in BUV, factory-preset breath parameters are used.
Safety valve open	Red display. When lit, the patient circuit is opened to room air and the patient breathes unassisted by the ventilator. The ventilator enters this mode when all connected gas supplies are lost, POST is running, a system fault is detected, or AC power is lost. Safety valve open is employed temporarily during POST and is canceled after POST is completed successfully.
Normal	Green (or blue) display. When lit, the ventilator is operating within acceptable ranges and no alarm conditions exist. If an alarm is reset with the ALARM RESET key, this display lights instead of the caution display.

Courtesy Nellcor Puritan Bennett, Carlsbad, Calif.

MODES OF VENTILATION

The 7200 offers three primary modes of ventilation: CMV, SIMV, and CPAP (spontaneous), as well as two optional modes: PCV and PSV. The touch keys for CMV, SIMV, and CPAP are on the lower central portion of the front panel. CMV and SIMV are commonly selected to provide volume ventilation, but if PCV is in use, these key pads also establish breath triggering and pattern for pressure ventilation. That is, you can have PCV that is A/C (CMV) or PCV in the SIMV mode.

Continuous Mandatory Ventilation (CMV)

CMV is an A/C mode of ventilation in which breaths are patient- or time-triggered, volume-targeted (PCV not set), and volume-cycled. Press the CMV pad once, then select the desired V_T, flow, respiratory rate, flow waveform pattern, trigger sensitivity, and alarm thresholds. Pressing the CMV pad a second time activates the new mode.

Synchronized Intermittent Mandatory Ventilation (SIMV)

In SIMV, mandatory breaths can be patient- or time-triggered and are volume-targeted (PCV not set) and volume-cycled, as in CMV. Spontaneous breaths are patient-triggered. With the added option of PSV, spontaneous breaths can be assisted with the selected pressure level. Box 10-111 and Figure 10-78 describe the synchronization of mandatory breaths with spontaneous breaths. Box 10-112 provides an exercise in problem solving related to the SIMV mode.

Spontaneous/Continuous Positive Airway Pressure (CPAP)

The CPAP mode is a purely spontaneous mode. All breaths are patient-triggered and can be at a zero baseline or at a positive baseline (CPAP). They can also have PSV added.

BOX 10-111

Synchronization of SIMV and Spontaneous Breaths on the 7200 Ventilator

Whether a patient-triggered breath is mandatory or spontaneous is determined by when the patient effort occurs in the SIMV cycle. The SIMV cycle is composed of two phases, as follows:

1. Patient-initiated mandatory phase (PIM phase)
2. Spontaneous phase

In the PIM phase, patient-triggering results in a mandatory breath. After breath delivery, the PIM phase ends and the spontaneous phase begins. In this phase, patient-triggering results in a spontaneous breath. At the end of the spontaneous phase, the SIMV cycle ends and the next one begins with a new PIM phase. For example, with a rate of 10 breaths/min, the SIMV cycle is 6 seconds long. A PIM breath could occur at anytime during the 6 seconds. Once the patient triggers the breath and the mandatory breath is delivered, the remainder of the time can be spent in spontaneous ventilation.

If no PIM breath is triggered, the spontaneous phase never begins and PIM continues through the next SIMV cycle. At the start of the next SIMV cycle (12 seconds later in this example), the ventilator time-triggers a mandatory breath (see Figure 10-78). If no patient effort is detected, mandatory breaths follow the beginning of each subsequent SIMV interval.

BOX 10-112

Decision Making & Problem Solving

A patient on SIMV has been successfully ventilated for 24 hours at a rate of 2 breaths/min with the 7200 ventilator. Suddenly, the patient becomes apneic. How long could the patient remain unventilated?

See Appendix A for the answer.

Pressure Control Ventilation (PCV)

PCV is an added option (80) that can be accessed with either of the following two ways:

1. By pressing the PCV pad at the top of the front panel
2. By activating Function 80 under the ++ key (Box 10-113).

PCV provides pressure-targeted mandatory breaths in the CMV and SIMV modes. Table 10-29 lists the range of variables available in PCV. This option allows you to select either T_I or the I:E ratio as a constant based on respiratory rate (Option 82). Because the selection of these can be confusing the first time they are used, a detailed explanation is given in Table 10-30. Usually when an inverse ratio is desired, a constant I:E is set. With normal I:E ratios, it may be more appropriate to set T_I constant. When you change the respiratory rate, a message appears to remind you which parameter (I:E or T_I) is currently constant. Box 10-114 gives an example of initiating PCV and selecting T_I or I:E as constant.

Unlike with other modes of ventilation, during PCV or PCV apnea ventilation, the message window provides a continuous sequence of messages to inform you that PCV—not volume-targeted ventilation—is in use. The messages are preceded by an asterisk and, in general, list the following:

1. Mode
2. Pressure
3. T_I
4. I:E ratio

The 7200 even provides for pressure-targeted mandatory breaths in apnea ventilation when PCV is the operating mode (see apnea ventilation in the discussion of special functions in this section). Option 81 is the apnea ventilation option for PCV and has parameter ranges similar to those for normal PCV. An apnea interval of 10 to 60 seconds is available, although setting an interval >20 seconds is unusual.

Error messages that can occur in PCV, their causes, and possible solutions are listed in Table 10-31. It is very important to set the upper pressure limit in PCV. Although the selected inspiratory pressure is the maximum that can be provided by the ventilator, if the patient coughs, circuit pressure can rise above this value. Just as in volume ventilation, if airway pressure is greater than or equal to the upper pressure limit, inspiration ends.

The plateau function is not operational during PCV. An inspiratory pause can be obtained by increasing T_I (see Chapter 9). Sighs are also not operational during PCV.

Pressure Support Ventilation (PSV)

PSV (Option 10) provides pressure-targeted, spontaneous breaths in the SIMV and CPAP modes. PS breaths are patient-triggered, pressure-targeted (1 to 70 cm H_2O in newer version; 1 to 30 cm H_2O in earlier version), and flow-cycled (≤5 L/min). As a safety back-up feature, PSV also cycles out of inspiration when airway pressure is 1.5 cm H_2O above PSV + PEEP, or if T_I is ≥5 seconds.

The pressure setting in PSV is added to the CPAP level. For example, if CPAP is 5 cm H_2O and PSV is 10 cm H_2O, PIP is 15 cm H_2O. PSV is set by selecting the PRESSURE SUPPORT key pad at the top of the front panel or by selecting Option 10 using the ++ key. Then follow the instructions in the message window to select desired settings. (Note that PSV cannot be used when older versions of

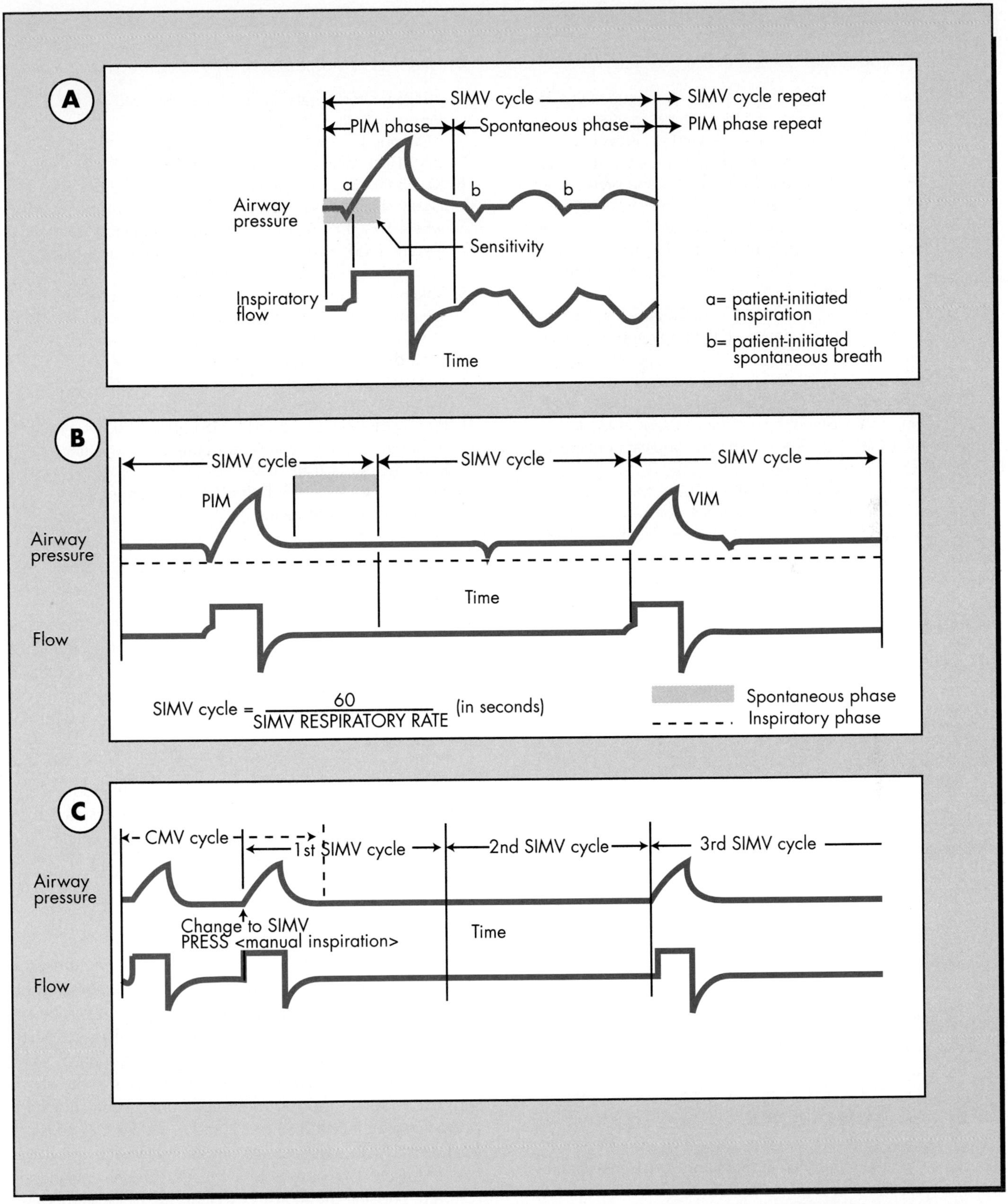

Figure 10-78 Breath patterns during SIMV on the Nellcor Puritan Bennett 7200. **A,** an adequate inspiratory effort that triggers a mandatory breath and is followed by a spontaneous phase. **B,** no adequate inspiratory effort is sensed; two SIMV cycles pass, and a time-triggered mandatory volume-targeted breath (VIM) occurs. **C,** the switch from CMV to SIMV; the ventilator automatically begins timing the first SIMV cycle (any time remaining from the CMV cycle is ignored). (Courtesy Nellcor Puritan Bennett Corp., Pleasanton Calif.)

BOX 10-113

Initiating Pressure-Control Ventilation

1. Press the PRESSURE CONTROL key (at the top of the front panel) or the ++ key, and then press 80 and ENTER.
2. "80 PCV" appears in message window; press ENTER.
3. "INSP PRESS YYY CMH$_2$O" appears; enter the desired pressure value for mandatory breaths and press ENTER.
4. "<I>E X.XX/XXX" appears. *<I>* indicates that the inspiratory component may be changed if desired. Select the desired value and press ENTER. The message "<I>/E Y.YY/XXX" appears, indicating *Y.YY* as the new inspiratory component.
5. Press enter and "I/<E> Y.YY/XXX" appears. *XXX* is the expiratory component. If the inspiratory component is anything but 1, *<E>* must be 1. If you try to enter something other than 1, T_I is automatically changed to 1. (Note that the numerical values entered for I and E components cannot be less than 1.0. For example, rather than 1:0.25, 4:1 is entered; you cannot type in 0.25.
6. The I:E ratio displayed in the message window appears as "X.XX/1.00 (IRV)" or "1:X.XX" for normal I:E ratios. The Patient Data display for I:E, however, is calculated using monitored data and is *always* displayed as "1/XX" for normal ratios and IRVs.
7. <E> must be ≤9. If <E> is >9, the message "E >9 SET INSP TIME" appears to indicate you have set E >9.
8. Key in the desired expiratory component and press ENTER. The message becomes "I/<E> Y.YY/YYY," where *Y.YY/YYY* represents the new I:E ratio. Press ENTER. "INSP TIME X.XX" is the T_I (in seconds) based on the requested I:E ratio and the set rate.
9. Values that result in an I:E ratio >4:1 cause the message window to read "DECR RESP RATE FIRST" or "CHANGE RR-I/E-IT."
10. Press ENTER. The message "NEW I/E = Z.ZZ/ZZZ" appears if you changed the I:E ratio, with *Z.ZZ/ZZZ* being the new ratio based on T_I and rate.
11. Press ENTER. "UPDATE PARAMS-ENTER" asks you to press ENTER again if you want to use the new settings. Press CLEAR to cancel.
12. Press ENTER. "REVIEW FUNCTION 81" appears to prompt you to update the PCV apnea parameters under function 81.

TABLE 10-29

Range of parameters for PCV

Pressure control ventilation parameter	Range	Increment
Inspiratory Pressure	5.0 to 100 cm H_2O	1 cm H_2O
I:E Ratio	(4≥I≥1, 9≥E≥1) (one component must be 1)	0.1 for each component
Respiratory rate	0.5 to 9.9 bpm	0.1 bpm
	10 to 70 bpm	1 bpm
Inspiratory time	0.20 to 5.00 sec	0.02 sec
O_2	21% to 100%	1%

Courtesy Nellcor Puritan Bennett, Carlsbad, Calif.

Flow-by [Option 50] are activated, but it is functional with Flow-by version 2.0.)

SPECIAL FUNCTIONS

There are a wide variety of options and functions available for the 7200, several of which have already been discussed. A few more important features, including the following, are presented here:

1. Three emergency modes of ventilation: apnea ventilation, backup ventilation, and disconnect ventilation
2. Respiratory mechanics and Flow-by

Whenever certain alarm conditions occur or the ventilator detects certain faults or system errors, the ventilator automatically starts one of the three emergency ventilation modes. When apnea or disconnect ventilation occur, the ventilator uses the operator-selected parameters set for apnea ventilation.

Note that because the PEEP/CPAP control is not part of the electronics, it is active at its current setting during any emergency mode of ventilation. Because the displays may not be functioning properly, you should not change the PEEP setting during an emergency mode.

Apnea Ventilation

Whenever an apneic period exceeds the set apnea time, the ventilator initiates apnea ventilation using the apnea parameters set by the operator (Table 10-32). These can be set for either volume- or pressure-targeted ventilation. When the unit is in CMV or SIMV, apnea ventilation has no low inspiratory pressure alarm. "Alarm" illuminates in the alarm summary display, and the message "Apnea Ventilation" appears. Only the ALARM SILENCE and ALARM RESET keys are operational. The machine will reestablish ventilation if the patient triggers two consecutive breaths. Once ventilation is restored, pressing the RESET key clears alarm indicators.

Backup Ventilation

Backup ventilation (BUV) occurs whenever POST detects an error, the ongoing checks detect three system errors

TABLE 10-30

Choosing the constant parameter of T_I or I:E in PCV

Operator action	Message window response	Comments
Select Option 82 Press ENTER	82 PCV I/E CONSTANT CONSTANT IT-PUSH CLR	The I:E ratio is being held constant. Press CLEAR to hold T_I constant, or press ENTER to keep I:E ratio constant.
Press CLEAR	82 PCV I-T CONSTANT	The T_I is now held constant when set respiratory rate is changed.
	–or–	
Select Option 82 Press ENTER	82 PCV I-T CONSTANT CONSTANT IE-PUSH CLR	T_I is being held constant. Press CLEAR to hold the I:E ratio constant, or press ENTER to keep T_I constant.
Press CLEAR	82 PCV I/E CONSTANT	The I:E ratio is now held constant when set respiratory rate is changed.

NOTE: Messages may differ slightly on the 7202 display. Press * at any point in the sequence to review the previous parameter or message. Press the ++ key at any point in the parameter set-up to exit the function.

Courtesy Nellcor Puritan Bennett, Carlsbad, Calif.

BOX 10-114

Decision Making & Problem Solving

Here are two example problems about changing the rate in PCV:
Problem 1—In PCV on the 7200, the rate is set at 10 breaths/min and the I:E ratio is 1:1. What is T_I? Assuming T_I is constant, and the rate is changed to 15 breaths/min, what will the new I:E be?

Problem 2—If the ratio rather than T_I is constant (1:1), and the rate is increased from 10 to 15 breaths/min, what will be the new T_I?
See Appendix A for the answers.

within 24 hours, or the AC voltage is <90% of the rated value. Audible and visible alarms occur, and the pneumatic system of the unit is controlled by an analog circuit that is separate from the microprocessor systems. BUV uses the following factory-preset parameters to ventilate the patient:

1. Rate = 12 breaths/min
2. V_T = 0.5 L (whether volume or pressure ventilation was previously set)
3. Constant flow delivery at 45 L/min
4. Current PEEP setting
5. 100% O_2 (if available)
6. High-pressure limit about 30 cm H_2O above PEEP

The BUV indicator lights in the alarm summary section. All other displays are blank, and all functions except the PEEP/CPAP are nonfunctional. If BUV occurs, provide another means of ventilating the patient as soon as possible and have the ventilator serviced.

In pediatric patients, the patient is protected from excessive volume or pressure provided by BUV by two factors. First, small endotracheal tubes increase resistance to inspiratory flow. Second, the pressure limit of about 30 cm H_2O prevents pressures from getting too high.

Disconnect Ventilation

Whenever the microprocessor detects inconsistencies in airway pressures, PEEP, and gas delivery pressure in the pneumatic system, the DISCONNECT emergency mode activates.[1] Tubing disconnects or plugged tubing can cause these conditions. The machine uses the apnea ventilation setting, but the sensitivity setting is not recognized. When DISCONNECT VENTILATION activates, the following alarm indicators are turned on:

1. ALARM (in alarm summary display)
2. HIGH PEAK PRESSURE
3. AIRWAY PRESS DISCONN (in message window)

Only the ALARM RESET and ALARM SILENCE keys are operational. DISCONNECT VENTILATION does not automatically reset itself. After the problem that caused the alarm is corrected, you must press RESET to restore the ventilator to its previous state.

If something prevents the 7200 from initiating an emergency ventilation mode, the safety valve opens to allow a spontaneously breathing patient access to room air.

Respiratory Mechanics

The Nellcor Puritan Bennett 7200 can measure, calculate, and display the following respiratory mechanics when Options 30 and 40 have been purchased:

TABLE 10-31

Error messages provided in PCV on the 7200

Error message	Explanation	Operator action
CHANGE I/E/ FIRST	This message appears when a change in set respiratory rate would cause a T_I of less than 0.2 second or more than 5 seconds (and Function 82 is holding I:E ratio constant).	Change the I:E ratio through function 80, change the respiratory rate, or change parameter control through Function 82.
CHANGE PF/TV/RR	This message appears when changing from PCV to volume ventilation and the current settings fail the I:E ratio check.	Check for the appropriate peak flow, V_T, or respiratory rate before changing to volume ventilation. Check also waveform and plateau settings.
DECR INSP TIME FIRST	This message appears when a change in set respiratory rate would cause the I:E ratio to exceed 4:1 (and Function 82 is holding T_I constant).	Decrease T_I, change the respiratory rate, or change parameter control through Function 82.
CHANGE RR-I/E-IT	This message appears when a change in the set I:E ratio causes the ventilator to calculate an invalid T_I.	Change the I:E ratio, T_I, or respiratory rate.
DECR RESP RATE FIRST	This message appears when a change in T_I would result in the I:E ratio exceeding 4:1.	Decrease the set respiratory rate or change T_I.
E>9 SET INSP TIME	This message appears when the requested expiratory component is greater than 9 for the set I:E ratio. To achieve a larger expiratory component, set the T_I.	Enter an expiratory component less than 9. Or, change the T_I to achieve an expiratory component greater than 9.

Courtesy Nellcor Puritan Bennett, Carlsbad, Calif.

TABLE 10-32

Parameter ranges for volume- and pressure-targeted apnea ventilation

Range of selection	Default value
For both	
Apnea interval: 10 to 60 seconds	20 seconds
Breath rate: 0.5 to 70 breaths/min	12 breaths/min
Oxygen percentage: 21% to 100%	100%
For volume ventilation	
Tidal volume: 0.1 to 2.5 L	0.5 L
Peak flow: 10 to 120 L/min	45 L/min
For pressure ventilation	
	Default to volume settings
Inspiratory pressure: 5 to 100 cm H_2O	
Inspiratory time: 0.5 to 50 seconds	
I:E ratio: 1:9 to 3:1 (4:1 in PCV)	

Courtesy Nellcor Puritan Bennett, Carlsbad, Calif.

1. Maximum inspiratory pressure (negative inspiratory force)
2. Vital capacity
3. Airway resistance (static and dynamic)
4. Compliance (static and dynamic)
5. Peak flow (spontaneous)

Maximum inspiratory pressure (MIP), which is called negative inspiratory pressure (NIP) on the 7200, measures the maximum negative pressure generated by the patient against an occluded airway during a 3-second interval. The maneuver ends when the patient begins to exhale and MIP (NIP) is displayed.

The vital capacity function does not measure forced vital capacity, but slow vital capacity. Before the patient begins a maximal inhalation, the message window must read "VC MNVR ACTIVE." The maneuver is successful and vital capacity is displayed when the patient begins a breath after the vital capacity-maneuvered breath.

Activation of a static mechanics maneuver causes the ventilator to deliver a volume-targeted breath with a constant flow, followed by a plateau measurement. Calculated values for Raw and C_S are displayed in the message window at the beginning of the next breath (Box 10-115). The dynamic mechanics for C and Raw measured during active

BOX 10-115

Static Mechanics Measurements

If a message followed by an asterisk appears in the display window after a static mechanics measurement (e.g., "SM CMP 40* RES 23*"), then a stable plateau was not obtained during the maneuver. Accuracy of these values depends on whether airway pressure stabilizes during inflation hold and the exhaled values fall to zero (baseline) at the end of the breath cycle.

Blank displays mean that the calculation was out of acceptable range (CMP [compliance], 0 to 500 mL/cm H_2O; RES [resistance], 0 to 100 cm H_2O).

TABLE 10-33

Recommended base flow and flow sensitivity settings for the 7200

Base flow setting	Range of allowed flow sensitivity
5 L/min	1 to 3 L/min
6 to 9 L/min	1 L/min to 1/2 of base flow set
20 L/min	1 to 15 L/min

flow delivery are determined by sampling the instantaneous values for pressure, volume, and flow at numerous intervals during inspiration for a mandatory breath. Using the equation of motion discussed in Chapter 9, the microprocessor determines and calculates the various values.

Peak spontaneous flow (Option 41) is measured, calculated, and displayed (in liters/minute) for spontaneous breaths. You can select either an eight-breath average or have the most recent breath displayed.

Flow and Flow-By Triggering

Flow-by (version 1.0) was first introduced as a method to provide a continuous air flow past the upper airway, similar to a continuous-flow IMV circuit (see Chapter 9). In order to accomplish mandatory breath triggering with the flow-by feature, the manufacturer had to make the unit flow- rather than pressure-triggered. In addition, the original version of flow-by (version 1.0) was only active in CPAP and SIMV and only when pressure support was not selected.

It is now known that flow-by actually reduces the work of breathing associated with breath triggering.[2] With continuous flow in the patient circuit, fresh gas is available to patients as soon as they begin to inspire. This reduces the delay between the patient's demand for flow and the beginning of flow from the internal flow valve.

BOX 10-116

Range of Flow-Trigger Variables

In flow-by version 1.0, the flow sensitivity or trigger range is 1 to 10 L/min. In flow-by version 2.0, the range is 1 to 15 L/min. The minimum base flow for both is 5 L/min, and the maximum is 20 L/min. If the base is set too high, it can cause inadvertent PEEP and increase airway pressures.

The introduction of flow-by version 2.0 made flow-triggering available in all modes of ventilation, including PSV.

To operate flow-triggering when flow-by is selected, first select FLOW-BY using the ++ key and selecting Option 50 or by pressing the FLOW-BY function key on the top row of controls on the front panel. You are prompted by the message window to set the base flow and the flow trigger level.

The base flow is the continuous gas flow present in the patient circuit. During mandatory inspiration and during inspiration in PSV, the base flow is suspended. At the beginning of exhalation, the base flow is always 5 L/min—regardless of the base flow set. This eliminates resistance to exhalation when it begins. The manufacturer has programmed the 7200 to require base flow to be about twice the flow trigger or flow sensitivity setting (Table 10-33). For example, if a flow trigger of 4 L/min is selected, a base flow of 8 L/min would be appropriate. Base flow is monitored by the expiratory flow transducer. When the base flow drops by the trigger flow amount, inspiration begins (Box 10-116). The lower settings for flow sensitivity require less work for the patient to trigger a breath. For example, triggering is easier with a trigger of 1 L/min than it is at a trigger of 3 L/min. During flow triggering, the manufacturer recommends the following settings:

1. 1 L/min for small patients (<25 kg)
2. 2 L/min for patients between 25 and 50 kg
3. 3 L/min for large patients (>50 kg)

Because flow-triggering is so sensitive, the operator needs to watch for auto triggering.

Flow-by is not available during nebulization. The older version of flow-by must be turned off during nebulization and then reactivated after the treatment. With the newer versions (2.0), the unit automatically switches to pressure-triggering when nebulization is activated, but the operator has to restart flow-by when nebulization is complete.

VENTILATOR GRAPHIC WAVEFORMS

The graphics 2.0 option allows the operator to select several waveforms to be viewed during ventilation (Figure 10-76) and provides the following monitoring capabilities:

BOX 10-117

Systems Evaluated to Verify Proper Function of the 7200 Ventilator

1. Microprocessor and associated electronics during POST program
2. Pressure and flow transducers
3. Expiratory valve
4. Patient circuit
5. PEEP regulator
6. BUV
7. Safety valve with associated over pressure relief

1. Waveforms (Function 60), including scalars and loops
2. Trending waveforms (Function 61)
3. A curser for trending curves
4. Freeze/print (Function 62) to freeze a waveform on the screen or print it with an attached compatible printer
5. Changing of patient number and room (Function 3)
6. "Plethysmogram" is another available waveform but requires Option 90: pulse oximetry

The waveforms menu allows two waveforms or loops to be displayed at one time (e.g., the scalars pressure, flow, and volume per unit time, and the loops pressure/volume and flow/volume). Selecting the ++ key and Option 60 accesses the graphics package. You can also press the GRAPHICS 2.0 key at the top of the front panel. The bottom of the graphics screen allows you to review your choice of curve selections and the directions for selecting those choices. Option 61 brings up the trending menu on the graphics screen with appropriate directions for setting up trending plots. Currently, there are 39 parameters available for trending, including regularly measured values such as V_T and rate, and added options including the pulse oximeter and the metabolic monitor.

TROUBLESHOOTING

The alarms and monitors on the 7200 provide a wide variety of methods to solve and detect problems. In addition, the extensive series of self tests and the continuous automatic testing verify the functional readiness of every subsystem of the ventilator, including those items listed in Box 10-117.

One problem occasionally encountered by clinicians operating the 7200 is auto-triggering. You have to carefully balance trigger sensitivity with patient effort. On one hand, you do not want to have the patient making excessive effort to trigger the unit, but on the other hand you don't want auto-triggering to occur due to leaky circuits or slight dips in pressure when PEEP is set at moderately high levels.

Another note of caution is indicated when slow SIMV rates are set. First, when you switch from CMV to SIMV, you should give a manually triggered breath. This prevents any delay that might occur with mandatory breath delivery. Then be sure that apnea time and low V_T alarm limits are set appropriately (see the discussion on SIMV earlier in this section).[1]

As with most medical equipment that is microprocessor controlled, the use of walkie-talkies, portable cellular phones, and other transmitting devices may interfere with their operation. Manufacturers are aware of this problem and have begun devising methods to protect against it. However, unless you are sure about the equipment, avoid the use of such devices.

Review Questions

(See Appendix A for answers.)

1. A respiratory therapist accidentally unplugs the 7200 ventilator being used for a patient in the ICU. Besides activating alarms, the ventilator will:
   a. continue to ventilate the patient using the current settings and be powered by the internal battery
   b. stop functioning
   c. continue to ventilate the patient using the default ventilator settings in memory
   d. continue to ventilate the patient using disconnect parameters
2. A respiratory therapist changes the respiratory rate from 10 to 15 breaths during volume ventilation with the 7200. An error message appears in the display window: "DECR RESP RATE FIRST." How can the therapist maintain the new $\dot{V}_E$ and correct the error message?
   a. increase the peak flow setting
   b. decrease the set V_T
   c. add a plateau time
   d. change to pressure-control ventilation
3. A patient is switched from CMV to SIMV with a rate of 4 breaths/min. After about 30 seconds, an alarm sounds and apnea ventilation begins. Which of the following is(are) true?
   I. The patient did not trigger a mandatory breath.
   II. The apnea period is probably set at 30 seconds.
   III. Switching from CMV to SIMV resulted in a delay in mandatory breath delivery.
   IV. The respiratory therapist should have given a mandatory breath after the switch to avoid the alarm condition.
   a. I only
   b. II only
   c. III and IV only
   d. I, II, III, and IV

4. A respiratory therapist has set a peak flow of 80 L/min and selected the descending flow waveform. At the beginning inspiration, what will be the actual flow delivered to the patient?
   a. 160 L/min
   b. 120 L/min
   c. 100 L/min
   d. 80 L/min

5. When changing from a constant (rectangular) to a descending ramp waveform on the 7200, what happens to the T_I?
   a. increases
   b. decreases
   c. stays the same

6. A patient is being ventilated with SIMV at a rate of 3 breaths/min. Set V_T is 0.75, spontaneous V_T is 0.35 L, and spontaneous rate is 10 breaths/min. Low V_T is set at 0.65 L, and apnea time is 20 seconds. Based on this information, which alarm is likely to activate?
   a. APNEA alarm
   b. LOW V_T alarm
   c. LOW PRESSURE alarm
   d. LOW RATE alarm

7. A respiratory therapist wants to perform weaning measurements using the 7200 ventilator. Which of the following are available under the respiratory mechanics option (Options 30 and 40)?
   I. forced vital capacity
   II. maximum inspiratory pressure
   III. static compliance
   IV. rapid shallow breathing index
   a. I and II only
   b. II and III only
   c. II, III, and IV only
   d. I, II, III, and IV

8. The 7200 microprocessor detects inconsistencies in airway pressure, PEEP measurements, and the gas delivery in the pneumatic system. Which of the following will occur?
   a. apnea ventilation begins
   b. back-up ventilation begins
   c. disconnect ventilation begins
   d. alarms activate, but regular ventilation continues

9. During PCV, the following parameters are set: pressure = 20 cm H_2O; T_I = constant at 1.0 second; rate = 10 breaths/min; mode = CMV; and PEEP/CPAP = 0 cm H_2O. What will be the I:E ratio if the rate is decreased to 6 breaths/min and the patient does not trigger additional breaths?
   a. 1:5
   b. 1:6
   c. 1:9
   d. cannot be determined with the information given

10. With the 7200, what flow trigger and base flow would you set for a 34 kg patient?

References

1. Nellcor Puritan Bennett Corp.: 7200 series microprocessor ventilator operator's manual, Carlsbad, Calif., 1993, Nellcor Puritan Bennett Corp.
2. Pilbeam SP: Mechanical ventilation. In Burton GG, Hodgkin JE, and Ward JJ: Respiratory care: a guide to clinical practice, ed 4, Philadelphia, 1997, Lippincott.

Newport Breeze E150

OUTLINE

LEARNING OBJECTIVES

Upon completion of this section, the reader should be able to:

1. Describe the internal mechanisms of the ventilator.
2. Explain the setting of controls and alarms.
3. Assess a problem associated with trigger sensitivity and recommend a solution.
4. Solve a problem related to the use of the low CPAP alarm.
5. Describe the available modes of ventilation.
6. Discuss the timing of mandatory and spontaneous breaths during SIMV.
7. Compare a manual breath (inflation) delivered in volume control with one delivered in pressure control.
8. Describe the effects of using the nebulizer function on normal volume delivery.
9. Identify a situation in which the pressure-relief valve is in operation.
10. List and discuss the various alarms violations.

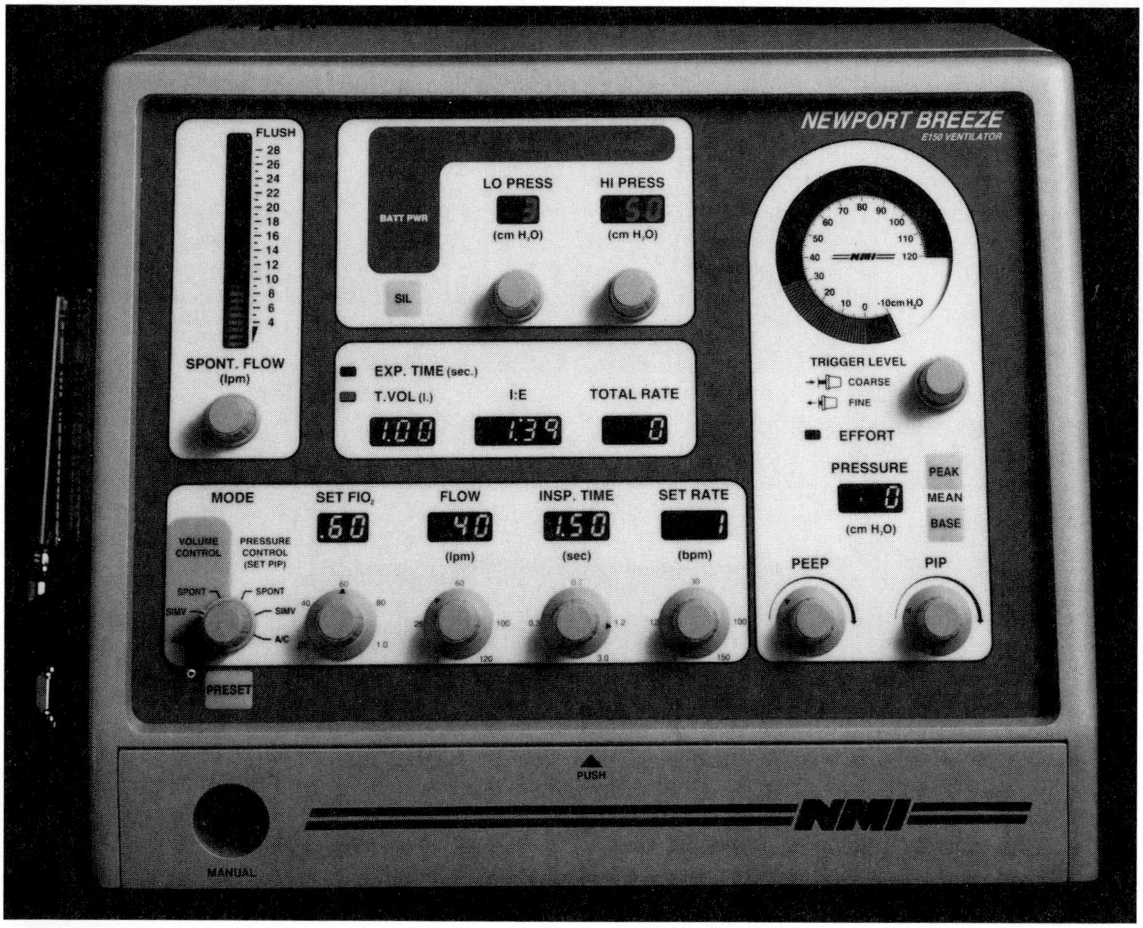

Figure 10-79 The Newport Breeze E150 ventilator. (Courtesy Newport Medical Instruments, Inc., Newport Beach, Calif.)

The Newport Breeze E150 is a general purpose ventilator that can be used for neonatal, pediatric, or adult patients (Figure 10-79).[1] The Duoflow system permits mandatory and spontaneous inspiratory gas flows to be controlled separately.

Power Source

This microprocessor-controlled ventilator is both pneumatically and electrically powered. It requires high-pressure air/oxygen gas sources (35 to 90 psi, optimum of 50 psi) and a standard AC electrical outlet (100 to 240 volts). The ON/OFF power switch is behind a drop-down door on the lower section of the front control panel. When the power switch is turned on, a temporary alarm sounds. This is followed by a brief self-test.

There is an internal battery that normally charges when the unit is plugged into an AC power source, usually a standard wall outlet. The internal battery acts as a back-up source of electrical power during power outages or if the AC power cord is disconnected. When fully charged, the battery lasts up to 1 hour.

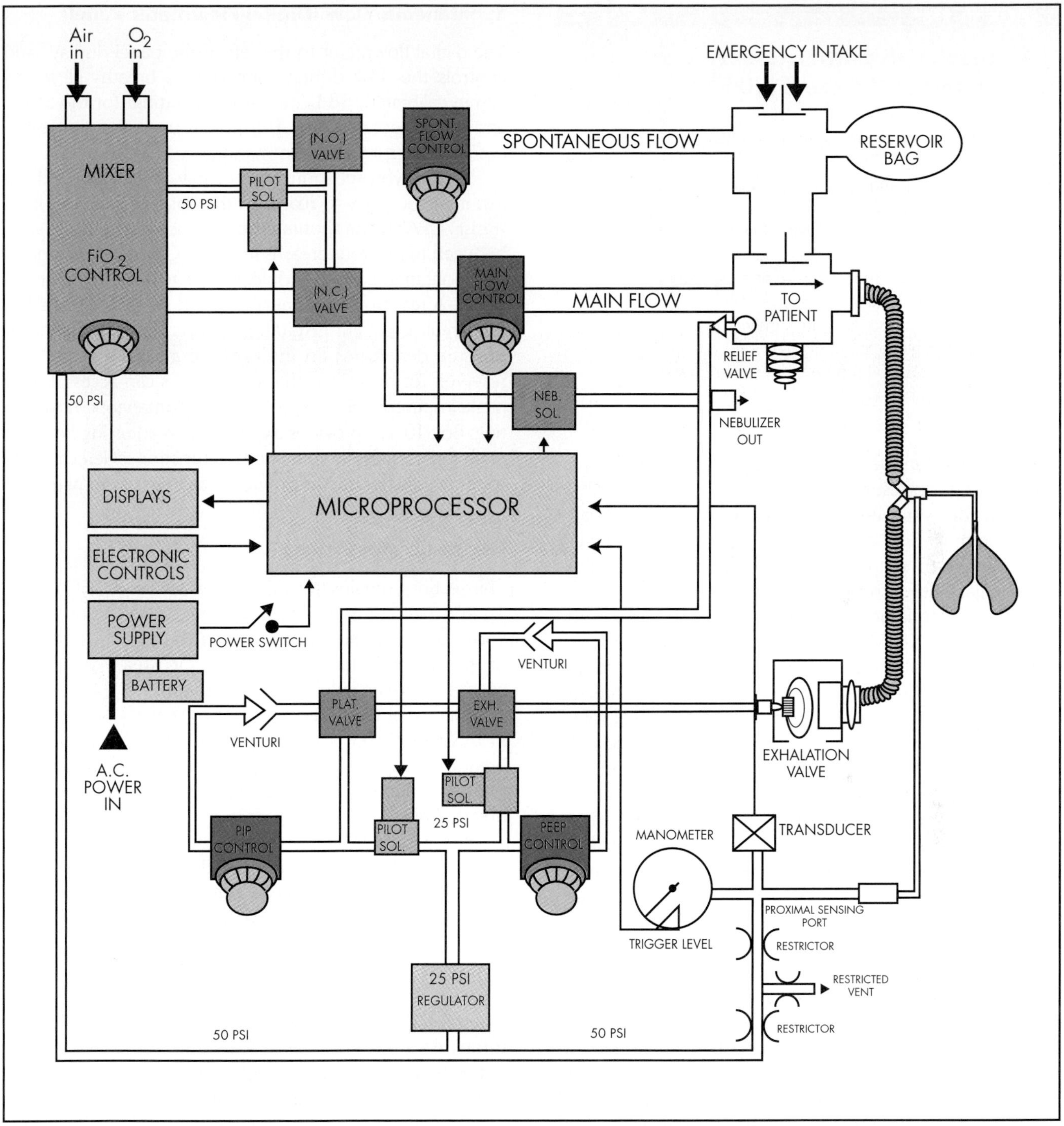

Figure 10-80 A pneumatic diagram of the Newport Breeze E150. (Courtesy Newport Medical Instruments, Inc., Newport Beach, Calif.)

The air and oxygen high-pressure hoses are connected to the back of the unit. The Breeze E150 operates from a single gas source if one becomes disabled, but this may affect the percentage of oxygen delivered. (If both gas sources fail, the spontaneously breathing patient can obtain room air through the internal emergency intake valve, which requires an inspiratory effort of about -2 cm H_2O.) There is no built-in internal oxygen analyzer, but an optional one is available. FiO_2 should be checked regularly by the operator.

An optional flowmeter that can be added to the side of the unit can be used to supply mixed gas for either a resuscitation bag or an external small-volume nebulizer.

INTERNAL MECHANISMS

The internal mechanisms are shown in Figure 10-80. High-pressure air and oxygen enter the ventilator through a

BOX 10-118

Control Valves that Govern Gas Flow in the Breeze E150

1. A spontaneous to mandatory flow-switching pilot solenoid valve
2. Spontaneous and mandatory inspiratory control pneumatic interface valves
3. Spontaneous and mandatory flow-regulating needle valves
4. Mandatory breath inspiratory and expiratory pressure-switching valves
5. Inspiratory (pressure control only) and expiratory pressure-regulating needle valves
6. A mushroom balloon type of exhalation valve

mixer (blender) inside the back of the unit. The mixer regulates inlet gas pressures, then blends the gases to the set O_2%. Blended gas then flows to two separate internal pathways: the main flow circuit and the spontaneous flow circuit. A series of control valves (listed in Box 10-118) governs the gas output from these circuits.

When a mandatory breath is triggered, this activates the pilot solenoid valve, which generates a pneumatic signal that opens the normally closed (n.c.), mandatory (main) inspiratory control, pneumatic interface valve. Gas is then directed from the blender through the mandatory flow-regulating needle valve into the patient circuit. If volume-targeted A/C, A/C plus sigh, or SIMV modes are selected, the mandatory breath trigger also causes an electronic signal, resulting in complete closure of the mushroom/balloon-style exhalation valve during inspiration. If pressure-targeted, A/C, or SIMV is selected, the mandatory breath trigger causes an electronic signal that allows the set PIP control to determine the maximum pressure in the patient circuit by establishing the pressure in the exhalation valve.

During mandatory breath exhalation, the spontaneous inspiration pneumatic interface valve is turned on and the main flow off. The PEEP solenoid valve causes the set PEEP level to be established at the patient circuit exhalation manifold. In the Breeze E150, as in the Wave E200 (without compass monitor), there is an externally mounted expiratory valve that must be connected to the exhalation valve small nipple-connector outlet to function.

Controls and Alarms

The front panel of the Newport Breeze E150 is visually divided into five distinctive sections: a flowmeter, an alarm and indicator panel, a digital display panel, a breath control panel, and a pressure control panel (Figure 10-81). The controls that govern breath delivery are reviewed first, and then the monitor and alarm sections are discussed.

Spontaneous Flow (Digital Flowmeter Panel)

The digital flowmeter to the left of the panel displays and controls the flow during spontaneous breaths (1 to 28 L/min calibrated, 58 L/min at flush setting) for the SIMV and spontaneous modes. This flow is used also to stabilize baseline pressure between mandatory breaths in A/C.

In A/C, you set spontaneous flow at 4 L/min and adjust it as necessary to maintain the baseline pressure level (PEEP/CPAP). The spontaneous flow is only operational in between mandatory breaths in the A/C and SIMV modes.

Spontaneous flow should be set to meet patient demand. A reservoir bag is available and should be added to the circuit if patient inspiratory efforts result in significant pressure deflections on the pressure gauge. It serves as a reservoir for mixed gas that the patients can access if their peak inspiratory flow exceeds the spontaneous flow setting. Box 10-119 provides an exercise in adjusting flow settings. If an electronic ventilator malfunction is detected, the spontaneous flowmeter provides gas flow to the patient.

Breath Control Panel

This section contains the adjustments for mode, FiO_2, flow, T_I, and rate controls. The MODE SELECTOR knob allows you to select either volume-targeted (VOLUME CONTROL) or pressure-targeted (PRESSURE CONTROL) ventilation. Modes are reviewed later in this section.

FiO_2 varies from 0.21 to 1.0. The FLOW CONTROL knob in this section sets the constant gas flow for mandatory breaths (3 to 120 L/min). T_I ranges from 0.1 to 3.0 seconds, and the mandatory rate setting varies from 1 to 150 breaths/min.

Pressing the PRESET touch pad (membrane switch) below the mode control causes the digital displays to illuminate, showing set parameters. This is useful if you want to switch from a spontaneous to a mandatory ventilator mode.

Pressure Display Panel

Use of the pressure display relies on pressure sensing through a proximal airway pressure line connecting the outlet on the lower right side of the ventilator to an adapter at the wye connector in the patient circuit. This line is purged with gas flow to reduce the risk of line obstruction from water or contaminants. Use of a bacterial filter in this line is also advised. Pressures are measured internally through an integral pressure transducer.

Pressure Gauge

An electronic pressure gauge at the top of this panel displays measured airway pressures (-10 to 120 cm H_2O). It is a backlit liquid crystal display (LCD) that lights in green to indicate the current pressure changes at the airway, peak pressure for the breath, baseline pressures, and trigger sensitivity setting.

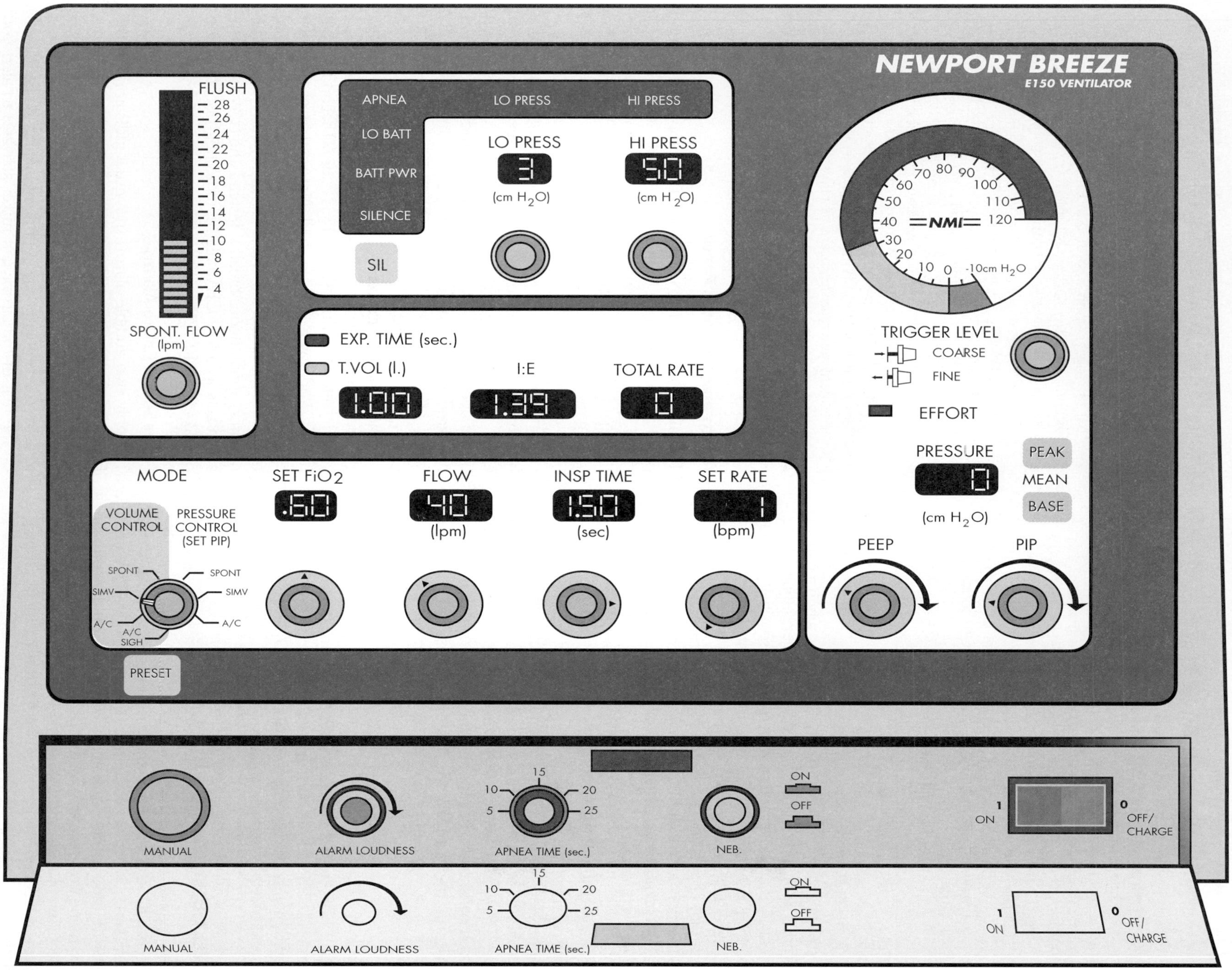

Figure 10-81 The front panel of the Newport Breeze E150.

BOX 10-119

Decision Making & Problem Solving

Problem 1—During SIMV ventilation of a patient on the Breeze E150, the respiratory therapist notes that the pressure gauge dips to -8 cm H_2O during the inspiratory phase of spontaneous breaths. What should the therapist do to correct this problem?

Problem 2—A patient is on 10 cm H_2O of CPAP on the Breeze E150 ventilator. The respiratory therapist notices that the airway pressure is 10 cm H_2O during inspiration but rises to 15 cm H_2O during expiration. What should the therapist do to correct this problem?

See Appendix A for the answers.

Trigger Level and Effort Indicator

A small visual indicator, EFFORT, illuminates when a patient effort is detected. This is based on the trigger setting. There is a knob that allows adjustment of trigger sensitivity (about -10 to + 60 cm H_2O). Coarse adjustment brings the trigger level within 5 cm H_2O of the desired setting. Fine adjustment allows you to set the trigger to respond to minimal patient effort without resulting in auto-triggering. Box 10-120 explains some additional information on setting trigger sensitivity.

Digital Pressure Indicator

You can read peak, mean, or baseline airway pressure (in centimeters of water) in a digital PRESSURE display window. Peak or baseline pressure readings can be displayed for 30 seconds by pressing either the PEAK or the BASE touch pads. After 30 seconds, the digital display automatically returns to mean pressure. (By pressing the PRESET touch pad, you can return the display to mean pressure at any time.)

PEEP and PIP Controls

The PEEP control adjusts baseline pressure from 0 to 60 cm H_2O. PIP adjusts pressure delivery during pressure-targeted mandatory breaths (0 to 60 cm H_2O) and is additive to the baseline or PEEP setting.

Data Display Panel

This panel displays the calculated V_T (liters) when the Breeze E150 is set to deliver volume-targeted breaths and displays T_E when set to deliver pressure-targeted breaths. The I:E ratio is the calculated value based on the settings for mandatory breaths. If the I:E ratio becomes inverse, the colon in the ratio flashes. When the maximum I:E ratio is exceeded (maximum is 4:1), the entire T_I display flashes.

BOX 10-120

Trigger Sensitivity on the E150

If the knob is in the coarse position when the ventilator is turned on, the trigger level will be from -10 to + 60 cm H_2O. Its precise value depends on the position of the knob.

If the trigger knob is pushed in for the fine-tuning position when the machine is turned on, the trigger level will be from -5 to -10 cm H_2O, depending on the knob position.

If the EFFORT light will not illuminate, check to be sure you have adjusted the trigger to reflect the baseline pressure setting. If the trigger level is set very close to baseline pressure, but the patient effort does not cause the light to illuminate, you may want to reduce the spontaneous flow setting. With too much flow in the circuit, the ventilator may not sense the patient effort. Also check for circuit leaks. With too little flow, you may see the patient generate significant negative pressures in order to breathe spontaneously.

Alarm and Indicator Panel

The alarm and indicator section at the top of the front panel allows you to set both a HIGH-PRESSURE (10 to 120 cm H_2O) and a LOW-PRESSURE (3 to 99 cm H_2O) alarm. If the HIGH-PRESSURE alarm setting is exceeded, the ventilator goes into the expiratory phase. The LOW-PRESSURE alarm activates if the proximal airway pressure fails to exceed the LOW-PRESSURE alarm setting during a mandatory breath. The LOW-PRESSURE alarm also serves as a low CPAP alarm in the spontaneous mode (see the discussion of the apnea alarm later in this section). Indicators within this same panel illuminate for APNEA, LOW and HIGH PRESSURE, LOW BATTERY, BATTERY POWER, and ALARM SILENCE (60 seconds).

The apnea alarm receives its information from the PATIENT TRIGGER EFFORT indicator in all modes. The APNEA TIME INTERVAL control (5, 10, 15, 30, or 60 seconds) is behind a drop-down door in the lower section of the front control panel. If this control is set at 5 seconds during spontaneous ventilation, the trigger level indicator no longer monitors spontaneous breaths. Instead, the LOW-PRESSURE alarm acts as a low CPAP alarm, indicating disconnection or leaks (Box 10-121).

Power Source Failure Alarms

The only two audible alarms (no visual indicator) on the E150 are the GAS SUPPLY SOURCE FAILURE and the POWER FAILURE alarms. If one gas supply is lost or the inlet gas pressure drops too low, a pneumatic crossover valve opens to allow the ventilator to continue operating. A reed alarm on the rear of the air/oxygen mixer activates to alert you

BOX 10-121

Setting a Low CPAP Alarm

In the spontaneous mode, only a low CPAP alarm is available in place of the apnea alarm. To set the CPAP alarm, place the apnea alarm delay in the first position (5-second). This inactivates the apnea alarm and activates the low CPAP alarm. Then set the low-pressure alarm just below the CPAP level (about 2 cm H_2O below). If the pressure in the patient circuit drops below the low CPAP alarm level for 4 seconds, the LO PRESS alarm is activated.

of the condition. O_2% delivery to the patient may vary in this situation. If both pressurized gas sources fail, the ventilator alerts you with a continuous audible alarm.

When the internal battery goes into operation, an alarm sounds every 5 minutes and the BATT PWR indicator lights. When only about 15 minutes of battery power remain, a quick pulse alarm activates, and the LOW BATT indicator lights. If an electrical or mechanical failure is detected, a continuous alarm sounds.

MODES OF VENTILATION

Using the MODE selector knob, choose either volume- or pressure-targeted ventilation. With either of these you can choose A/C, SIMV, or spontaneous modes. You can also choose volume-targeted A/C with sigh. If you are in the spontaneous mode, you can check existing settings by pressing the PRESET(below the MODE control switch).

Volume-Targeted Breaths

Volume-targeted mandatory breaths are available in A/C, A/C plus sigh, and SIMV.

Assist/Control

In the A/C volume-targeted mode, breaths are patient- or time-triggered, volume-targeted, and time-cycled. Mandatory flow delivery is constant at the set value. V_T delivery is determined by the flow and T_I settings. For example, if the flow is set at 60 L/min, and T_I is 1.0 seconds, V_T is 1.0 L. The I:E ratio is based on respiratory rate and T_I. Continuing with this example, if the rate is 10 breaths/min, TCT is 6 seconds (60 sec/[10 breaths/min]). T_I is 1 second, T_E is 5 seconds, and the I:E ratio is 1:5.

Assist/Control with Sigh

This mode functions like regular volume-targeted A/C, except that a sigh breath equal to 1.5 times the V_T is delivered every 100 breaths. During a sigh breath, T_I is extended to 1.5 times the set T_I.

BOX 10-122

Decision Making & Problem Solving

You are setting A/C, pressure-targeted breaths for a patient being ventilated by the E150. Settings are as follows: rate = 12 breaths/min, T_I = set at 0.5 sec, flow = 30 L/min, PIP = 30 cm H_2O. During inspiration, you notice that the pressure rises slowly during inspiration and peaks at 27 cm H_2O. What is causing the problem of achieving the target pressure delivery?

See Appendix A for the answer.

Synchronized Intermittent Mandatory Ventilation (SIMV)

During volume ventilation in the SIMV mode, mandatory breaths are the same as described previously. Spontaneous breaths are from the spontaneous flow source, which is described later in this section.

Pressure-Targeted Breaths

Pressure-targeted mandatory breaths are available in A/C and SIMV modes.

Assist/Control

Mandatory breaths are patient- or time-triggered, pressure-targeted, and time-cycled. Pressure during inspiration is based on the PIP setting. The PIP control determines the pressure in the exhalation valve, which in turn determines the maximum pressure in the patient circuit. Flow output from the ventilator is provided at the mandatory flow setting in the form of a square wave, but flow entering the airway tends to be more of an exponential descending waveform.

The length of inspiration is based on the T_I setting. As you would expect, volume and flow delivery to the patient vary just as lung mechanics do. The fact that maximum available flow is based on the *flow* setting is slightly different from many adult ventilators. For example, if you set a low flow value, it takes longer for the ventilator to achieve the set PIP. On the other hand, a high flow setting achieves the set PIP more quickly, functioning similarly to the slope or rise control on other products. A steeper slope or faster rise is equivalent to a higher flow, and a slower slope or slower rise is equivalent to a lower flow. Ideally, the flow should be set to achieve the fastest pressure rise possible in order to attain the most volume delivery during the early part of inspiration. Box 10-122 provides a problem along these lines.

SIMV

SIMV can have either volume- or pressure-targeted mandatory breaths. Mandatory breath delivery for each breath type was described previously.

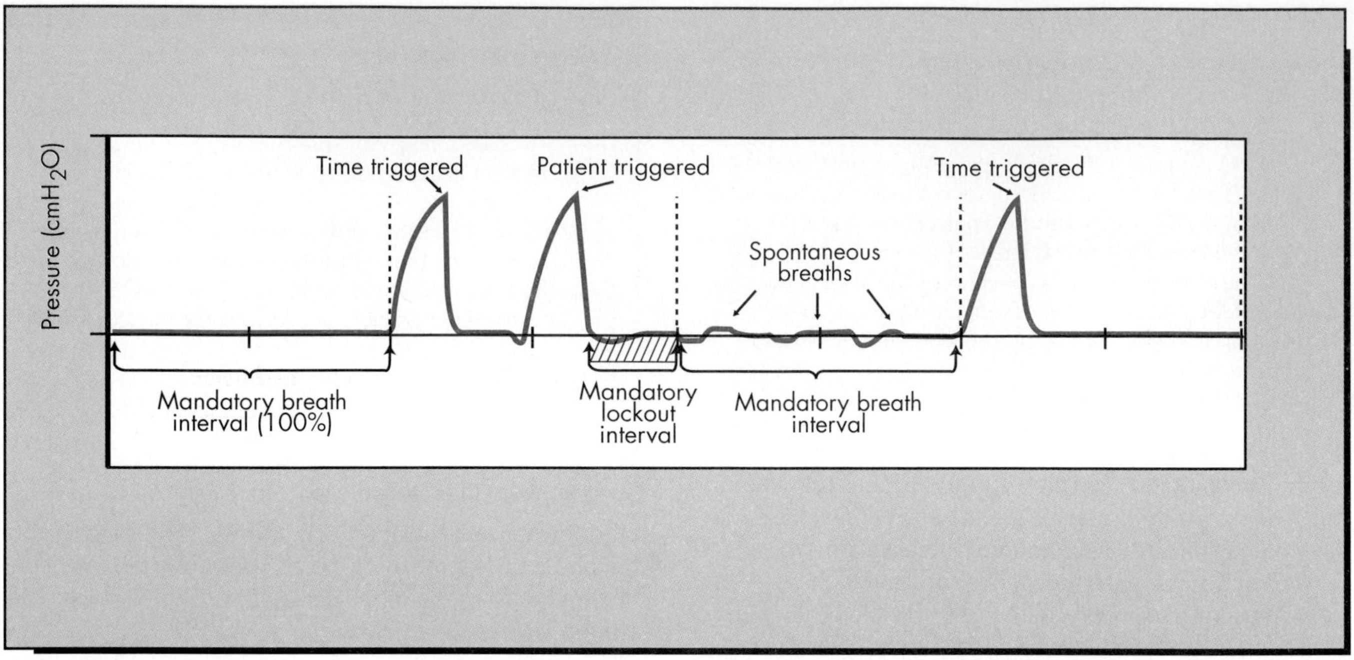

Figure 10-82 The timing of mandatory and spontaneous breaths in SIMV with the Breeze E150; see text for explanation.

Spontaneous breaths receive their flow based on the flow set on the spontaneous flowmeter on the front panel with the reservoir bag acting as a mixed gas reservoir accessible to the patient. (Note that the flowmeter must be turned on in SIMV and spontaneous modes to provide gas flow to the patient during spontaneous breathing efforts.) The mandatory breath rate is set by the RATE control. Both breath types are synchronized with a patient's spontaneous efforts based on the sensitivity setting. Figure 10-82 shows how mandatory breaths are timed.

The mandatory breath interval (MBI) is 60 seconds/(set breaths/min). For example, if the rate is 20 breaths/min, the MBI is 3 seconds. No patient effort was detected in the first MBI in Figure 10-82. Therefore at the beginning of the next MBI, a time-triggered mandatory breath is delivered. During the next MBI after the time-triggered breath, a patient triggers a mandatory breath. The patient can breathe spontaneously during the remaining time of the MBI. In the third MBI, a mandatory breath is not delivered because the patient received one in the second MBI. In the fourth MBI, a time-triggered breath is delivered because a complete MBI has just preceded it with no patient-triggered mandatory breath (Box 10-123).

Spontaneous

In the spontaneous mode, the patient receives air exclusively through the spontaneous flowmeter and reservoir bag. You can use the SPONTANEOUS setting under either the VOLUME or PRESSURE controls. The only difference will be in how a manual breath is delivered, which is included in the discussion of special features later in this section.

BOX 10-123

A Mandatory Breath Lockout Interval in SIMV with the Breeze E150 Ventilator

Whenever a mandatory breath is patient-triggered during SIMV, a mandatory breath lockout interval is activated. This limits the mandatory breath rate to the set rate. Note the second mandatory breath interval (MBI) in Figure 10-82. The lockout interval starts at the end of inspiration of a patient-triggered mandatory breath. A time-triggered breath is not delivered at the beginning of the third MBI because a patient-triggered breath occurred in the preceding interval. The patient can breathe spontaneously during the lockout interval.

Graphic Display Screens

Newport offers the Navigator Graphics Monitor for viewing and printing graphic data. This monitor can be purchased in addition to the regular ventilator and is included in the section on the Newport Wave in this chapter.

Special Features

A few special features that have controls behind a drop-down door in the lower section of the front control panel are described here. In addition, the function of the pressure relief valve is reviewed here.

Lower Control Panel

The MANUAL BREATH DELIVERY control on the left allows you to manually trigger a positive-pressure inflation in any mode. When you press this button, gas is delivered based on the mode (pressure or volume) and the current settings. FiO_2 remains the same. (Note that manual breaths are also described by the manufacturer as manual inflations because they deliver an inspiration.)

In all modes, on the volume side of the MODE control switch, a manual breath is delivered at the mandatory flow setting until one of the following occurs:

1. You stop pushing the button
2. The HIGH-PRESSURE alarm is violated (cycles into exhalation)
3. The maximum time limit (2 seconds) elapses

In all modes, on the pressure control side of the MODE switch, a manual breath delivers a pressure-targeted inflation using the set mandatory flow and PIP settings. It ends based on the three criteria just listed.

You can deliver as many as 150 manual inflations per minute. (Note that if the pressure-relief valve setting is reached before the high-pressure alarm limit during a manual inflation, the pressure will plateau but inspiration will not end [see the following section].)

The ALARM LOUDNESS control next to the MANUAL control adjusts the sound level of audible alarms.

The nebulizer control (NEB) provides gas flow through the nebulizer outlet with the same FiO_2 as main flow gas. It delivers approximately 6 L/min in addition to the flow provided during regular ventilation. This volume is added to the digital volume display so its reading is accurate for volume delivered from the ventilator. If you are using a T_I <0.4 seconds, you may want to use an external flowmeter because there is not enough time for nebulization through the nebulizer outlet itself.

The APNEA ALARM TIME control has settings for 5-, 10-, 15-, 30-, and 60-second apnea intervals. It is active in all modes and alerts you when the specified apnea interval elapses without a time or patient trigger breath being detected.

Pressure-Relief Valve

On the back panel of the E150 is a pressure relief valve that limits pressure delivery through the patient circuit during any mode, but does not end inspiration. It is adjustable from 0 to 120 cm H_2O. Clockwise rotation of the knob increases the pressure limit; counterclockwise rotation lowers it. During normal operation, it is set at a value above the high-pressure alarm setting as a safety pop-off device.

To set the pop-off pressure prior to patient use, turn the high-pressure alarm limit to 120 cm H_2O. Set the mode selector to volume-controlled, A/C. Press the manual control and watch the pressure gauge. Rotate the pressure-relief valve until the pressure plateaus at the desired value for pop-off or relief pressure.

TABLE 10-34

Additional examples for troubleshooting on the Newport E150 Breeze

Problem	Possible cause(s)
Inaccurate FiO_2 delivery	Faulty analyzer, problems with mixer
Reservoir bag deflates during a spontaneous inspiration	Spontaneous flow too low, leak in circuit or bag
Ventilator stops cycling	Blown fuse, electrical malfunction, gas source failure
Airway pressure dips below selected PEEP/CPAP pressure first, before stabilization	Faulty exhalation valve or diaphragm, or spontaneous flow does not meet patient's demand
Pressure builds too slowly during manual inflation	Flow setting too low, or leak in circuit

TROUBLESHOOTING

The operator's manual contains a table of common problems and their causes and solutions. In addition to the alarms and indicators already discussed, it also gives hints on solving other problems. Table 10-34 lists a few of the problems presented in the manual.

Because this unit is microprocessor-controlled, you need to be cautious with radio frequency-emitting devices, such as cellular phones, pagers, and walkie-talkies. These types of devices should not be used in the vicinity of the ventilator.

Review Questions

(See Appendix A for answers.)

1. A respiratory therapist has initiated ventilation on a patient using the A/C mode on the Breeze E150. The patient appears to be struggling to get a breath. The therapist notes that the pressure gauge is indicating pressures of -10 cm H_2O and the EFFORT indicator does not illuminate before mandatory breath delivery. What could be causing this condition?
   a. spontaneous flow is set too low
   b. the ventilator is in the control mode
   c. trigger sensitivity is not set correctly
   d. inspiratory flow is set too low

2. You are delivering aerosolized medications to a ventilated patient using the nebulizer control. Although the volume is set at 0.5 L, you note that the V_T display reads 0.53 L. What is the most likely cause of this difference?
   a. use of the nebulizer function
   b. a leak in the patient circuit
   c. an error in the inspiratory flow transducer
   d. an increase in the patient's spontaneous rate
3. You have initiated volume ventilation on a patient using the E150 and note that the pressure only rises to 10 cm H_2O. It then plateaus at this value for the length of inspiratory delivery. V_T is set at 0.8 L. No alarm is sounding. What is the most likely cause of this problem?
   a. the HIGH PRESSURE LIMIT alarm is being reached and the alarm is silenced
   b. the ventilator is set for pressure-targeted—not volume-targeted—ventilation
   c. the pressure-relief valve is set at 10 cm H_2O and is limiting inspiratory pressure
   d. there is a large leak in the inspiratory line
4. A patient is being supported in the spontaneous mode with 10 cm H_2O of CPAP at an FiO_2 of 0.5. A LOW PRESS alarm activates. The pressure gauge reads 3 cm H_2O. The low-pressure alarm is set at 5 cm H_2O. Which of the following is true about this situation?
   I. Circuit pressure has been lower than the low CPAP pressure alarm setting for 4 seconds.
   II. The APNEA alarm is not available because a low CPAP alarm has been set.
   III. There is a small leak in the circuit or around the patient airway.
   IV. The gas sources have failed.
   a. I and III only
   b. I and IV only
   c. II and IV only
   d. I, II, and III only.
5. Which of the following modes of ventilation are available on the Breeze E150?
   I. A/C volume-targeted
   II. pressure-control ventilation
   III. pressure-support ventilation
   IV. spontaneous
   V. mandatory minute ventilation
   a. I and V only
   b. II and III only
   c. I, II, and IV only
   d. I, II, IV, and V only
6. A plateau pressure during volume ventilation is achieved using what feature on the E150?
   a. inspiratory plateau time
   b. pressure-relief valve
   c. PIP setting
   d. HIGH-PRESSURE alarm limit
7. A high-pitched continuous reed alarm sounds during patient ventilation. This indicates which of the following?
   a. the internal battery is charged and being used as a power source
   b. one of the high-pressure gas sources has lost pressure
   c. the measured FiO_2 has exceeded the set FiO_2 by 5% for 30 seconds
   d. the pressure-relief valve has been activated
8. Use of the nebulizer feature increases volume delivery during volume ventilation—true or false?
9. V_T delivery during volume ventilation is based on the V_T control setting—true or false?
10. A respiratory therapist observes a patient's chest wall movement and notes inspiratory efforts. However, the EFFORT indicator does not illuminate. As a result, mandatory breaths are all time-triggered. How can the therapist change the ventilator settings to achieve better sensing of patient effort?

References

1. The Newport Breeze E150 ventilator: operating manual, OPR150, rev. B, Newport Beach, Calif., 1993, Newport Medical, Inc.
2. Pilbeam SP and Payne FR: Mechanical ventilators. In Burton GG, Hodgkin JE, and Ward JJ, Respiratory care: a guide to clinical practice, ed 4, Philadelphia, 1997, Lippincott.
3. Miller, Cyndy: Personal communication, Aug 1998.

Newport Wave E200

OUTLINE

LEARNING OBJECTIVES

Upon completion of this section, the reader should be able to:

1. Name the power sources required to operate the ventilator.
2. Describe the internal components.
3. Explain the function of the controls on the front panel.
4. Identify an alarm situation and suggest a possible cause and solution.
5. Assess a problem associated with using bias flow and trigger sensitivity during spontaneous ventilation and recommend a solution.
6. Solve a problem related to use of the LOW-PRESSURE alarm.
7. Describe the available modes of ventilation.
8. Explain the function of the NEBULIZER control.
9. Compare the setting of pressure-targeted modes with that of volume-targeted modes.
10. Identify a situation when the pressure-relief valve operating.

The Newport Wave E200[1-3] is a general-purpose ventilator designed for use in neonatal, pediatric, and adult patients (Figure 10-83). Two additional accessories can be added to enhance ventilator capabilities: the Compass Expiratory Monitor and the Navigator Graphics Monitor. The Wave is most often purchased with the Compass Monitor. Air compressors are also available to power this unit.

POWER SOURCE

The E200 WAVE is a microprocessor-controlled pneumatically and electrically powered ventilator. It requires high-pressure air and oxygen gas sources (35 to 90 psig, optimum of 50 psig) and a standard AC electrical outlet (100 to 240 volt).

The air and oxygen high-pressure hoses are connected to the back of the unit. The E200 operates from a single gas source if one become disabled, but this may affect oxygen delivery. (Note that if both gas sources fail, the spontaneously breathing patient can obtain room air through the internal emergency intake valve. This requires an inspiratory effort of about -2 cm H_2O. In such a situation the patient should be immediately ventilated by another method.)

The electrical ON/OFF power switch is on the back panel of the machine. When the power switch is turned on, a temporary audible alarm sounds. This is followed by a brief self-test.*

INTERNAL MECHANISMS

Internal mechanisms are shown in Figure 10-84. Source gases (air and oxygen) enter the internally mounted gas mixer. Blended gas leaving the mixer (28 psig) enters an accumulator tank and is pressurized to 2 atm. The accumulator helps provide a high gas flow source to meet the patient's peak inspiratory flow needs during spontaneous breathing—with or without pressure support. From the accumulator tank, flow is directed to the high-speed servo-control valve, which is also called a metering valve. This valve is an electromagnetic poppet valve. Its function is controlled by a microprocessor, which establishes the pattern of flow to the patient based on ventilator settings on the control panel. From the servo-control valve, gas is

*When you turn the ventilator off, push the ALARM SILENCE button to silence the alarm that results.

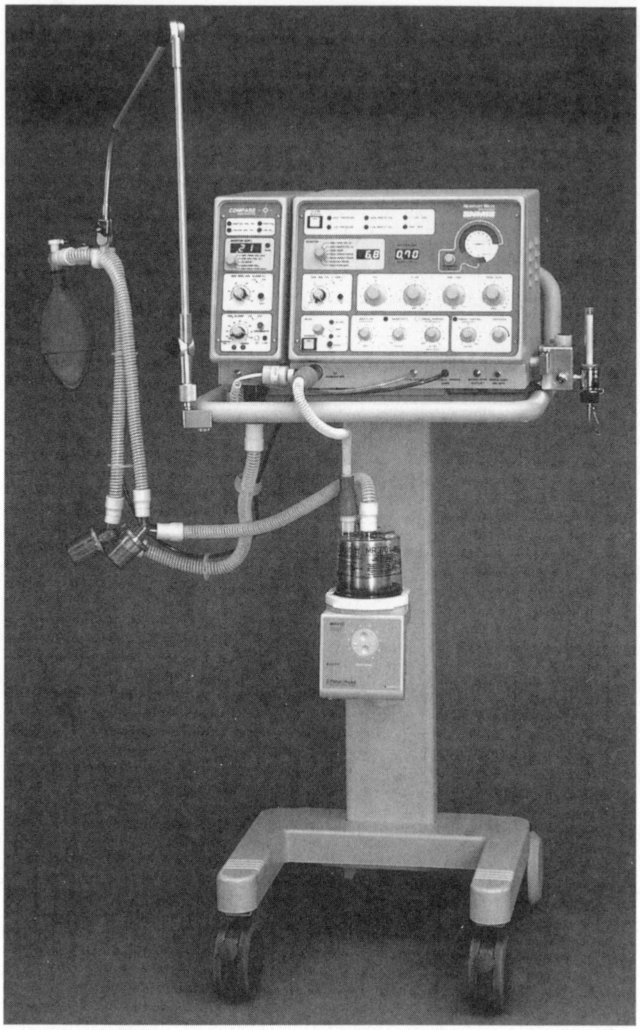

Figure 10-83 The Newport Wave E200 ventilator. (Courtesy Newport Medical Instruments, Inc., Newport Beach, Calif.)

directed through a flow sensor, which is a differential pressure transducer, and then on to the patient.

If the optional Compass monitor is not in use, the expiratory valve is mounted externally and is connected to the main unit's exhalation valve connector by a small-bore tube. The exhalation valve is a balloon diaphragm. The internal pressure on the balloon is determined by gas from the main flow manifold or by the flow from the PEEP control valve. Pressure in the exhalation valve is monitored by an electronic pressure transducer.

CONTROLS AND ALARMS

The Wave E200 has most controls on the front of the machine, but a few are on the back panel. The front panel controls are examined first here.

The front panel is divided into several sections (Figure 10-85). The top portion contains monitors, alarm indicators, and the high- and low-pressure alarm settings. The central portion houses the controls for ventilator settings and the $\dot{V}_E$ alarm control. The bottom section includes the connectors to the patient circuit and the nebulizer control button. Adjacent to many of the controls are LEDs that light to alert you to the activated control.

Ventilator Settings Section

Mode

At the left of the bottom row is the control for selecting a VENTILATOR MODE (spontaneous, SIMV, A/C, and A/C + sigh). There is a manual inflation (manual breath) button in this section as well. Pressing the MANUAL button delivers gas flow at the set flow value for as long as the button is pressed (maximum 3.8 seconds). Pressure is limited to the pressure-relief valve setting, or, if pressure control is engaged, the set pressure target—whichever is lower. If the inflation causes the airway pressure to reach the upper pressure limit alarm setting, the unit cycles into exhalation.

Bias Flow

Bias flow (0 to 30 L/min) provides flow in the circuit during the expiratory phase. It washes out any exhaled carbon dioxide, making fresh gas immediately available when the patient inhales. In addition, it reduces the ventilator's response time for pressure-triggering a breath.

Immediately after delivery of a breath (either mandatory or spontaneous), there is a brief period of no bias flow. The absence of bias flow at this time allows the patient to exhale without added resistance. When pressure in the circuit is within 2 cm H_2O of baseline, the bias flow resumes at the flow rate set. (Note that any time airway pressure is elevated more than 2 cm H_2O above baseline, there is no bias flow.)

A recommended starting level for bias flow on adult patients is 2 to 5 L/min. The adult range is marked in green. For neonatal and pediatric patients, start at 2 to 3 L/min. Observe the infant's spontaneous respirations on the pressure gauge. The pressure should fluctuate about 1 cm H_2O above and below baseline as the infant breathes. In general, it is recommended that the least amount of bias flow possible be used. If it is set too high, it is more difficult for a patient effort to be detected by the trigger sensor.

Sensitivity

The sensitivity setting adjusts the airway pressure change required for a patient to trigger a mandatory or spontaneous breath (-5 to 0 cm H_2O). It is also used to detect all breaths for monitoring. The total rate count is displayed in the monitor section. (Note that if a patient effort is not detected by the trigger sensitivity, it will not be counted into the monitored total rate, and the inspiratory V_T and the $\dot{V}_E$ will not be measured and displayed. If the Compass mon-

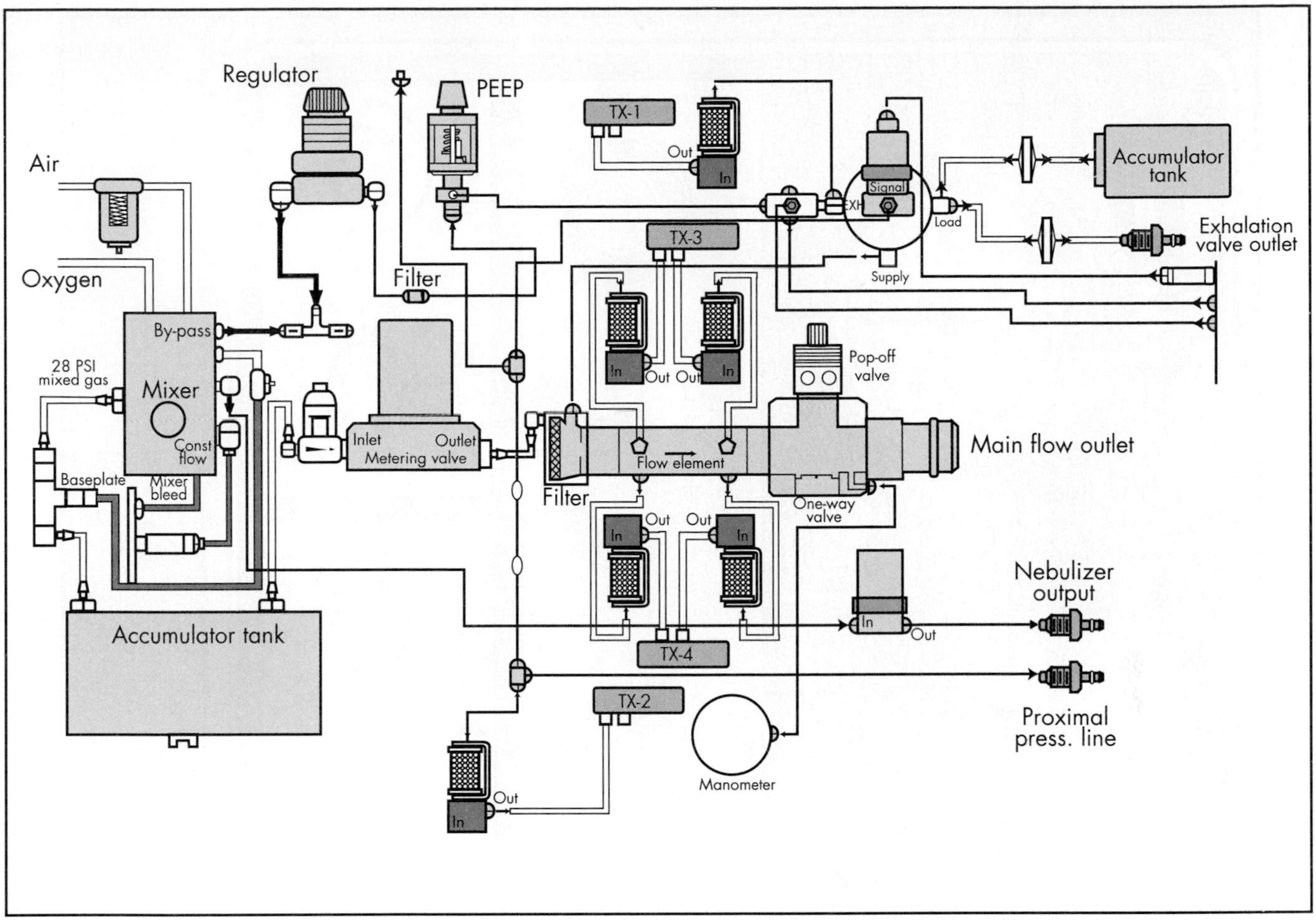

Figure 10-84 The internal circuit of the Newport Wave E200. (Courtesy Newport Medical Instruments, Inc., Newport Beach, Calif.)

itor is in use and the expiratory V_T and the $\dot{V}_E$ are not measured and displayed, the bias flow is set too high or the sensitivity trigger setting is set too low.

Sometimes patients have leaks around the endotracheal tube, such as occurs in uncuffed infant tubes. In this situation it is recommended that you increase the bias flow to help compensate for the leak and stabilize the baseline pressure. First, however, the integrity of the patient circuit should be confirm by performing a leak check. Sometimes, even when the patient circuit is not leaking, but a small airway leak is present, the ventilator appears to auto-trigger, and the baseline pressure may be unstable. In this situation, set the trigger sensitivity to -0.5 cm H_2O and increase the bias flow in 1 L/min increments until the auto-trigger condition ceases. A severe leak may require that you make the ventilator less sensitive to auto-triggering by reducing the trigger sensitivity to a more negative value.

Pressure Support (Spontaneous)

Use of this pressure setting provides PSV for spontaneous breaths in the spontaneous and SIMV modes. Pressure support in the Wave E200 offers automatic inspiratory slope control, as well as a self-adjusting, variable breath termination (cycling-off criteria). The pressure range settings can be up to 60 cm H_2O, or off. This pressure is additive to the baseline or PEEP/CPAP level (see the discussion of modes in this section).

Pressure Control (Mandatory)

This control adjusts the pressure provided during inspiration for pressure-targeted mandatory breaths. The pressure ranges from 0 to 75 cm H_2O, or is off. Whenever the PC control is activated, all mandatory breaths in A/C and SIMV are pressure-targeted. (When mandatory flow is set to the maximum level during PC, the unit automatically manages the inspiratory slope of all mandatory breaths [see the discussion of modes in this section].)

PEEP/CPAP

The baseline pressure is adjusted using the PEEP/CPAP control. Because it is not numbered, you have to watch the pressure displayed in the monitor window to view the selected baseline level. Baseline pressure ranges from 0 to 45 cm H_2O.

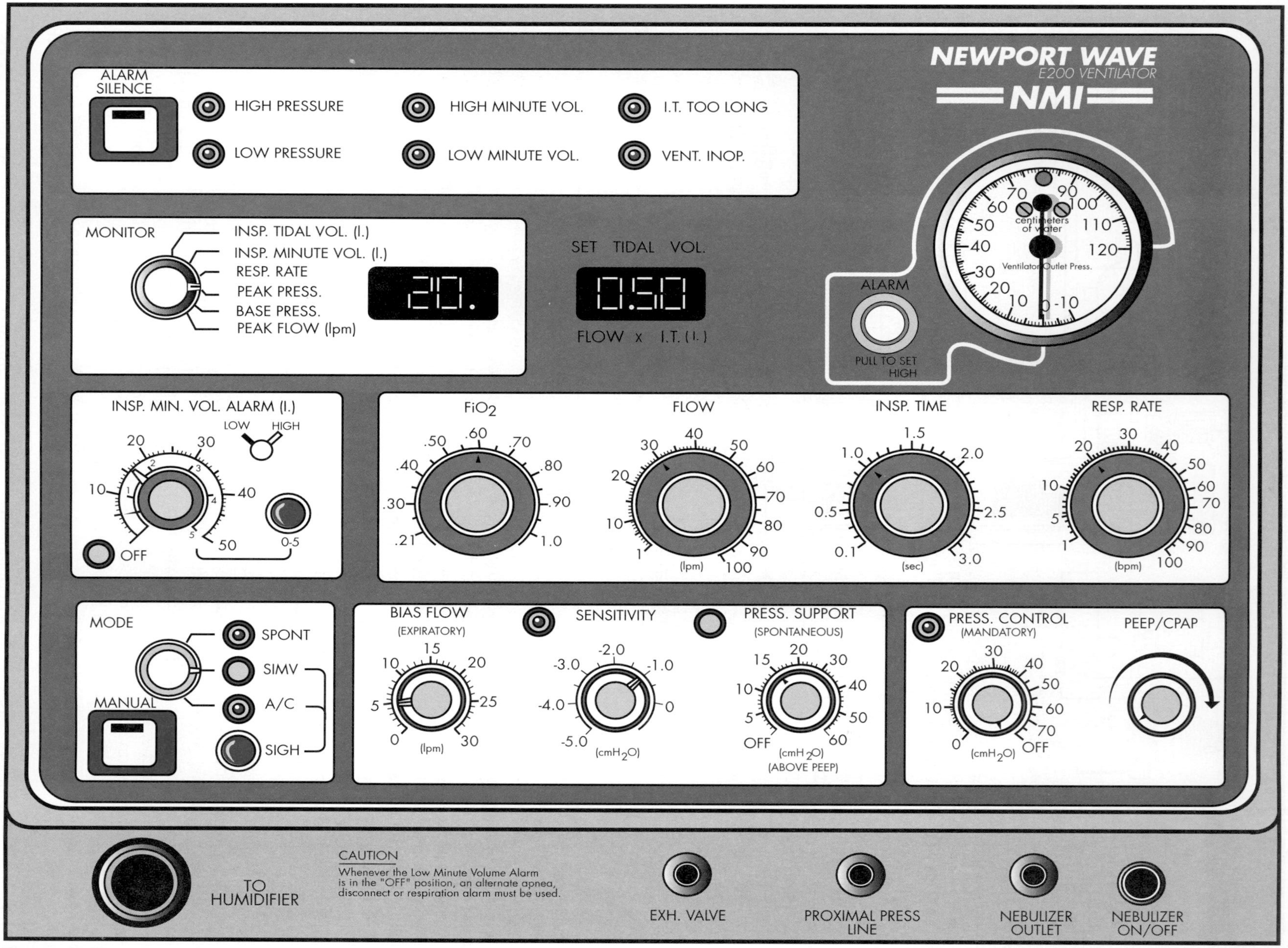

Figure 10-85 The front control panel of the Newport Wave E200.

BOX 10-124

The Inspiratory Minute Volume Alarm

This alarm is based on the rate of volume delivered from the ventilator, not including bias flow. When the bias flow is on, the LOW MIN. VOL alarm may sound if the patient's efforts do not cause the Wave to trigger because it will not measure any volume. For the alarm to work effectively, bias flow should be set as low as possible or at about 2 to 3 L/min.

For example, suppose the bias flow is set at 15 L/min, and the patient is in the spontaneous mode with a CPAP level of 10 cm H_2O. With so much flow passing, if the patient's efforts do not cause enough pressure drop to meet the trigger sensitivity setting, the ventilator will not "see" the patient's V_T and, therefore the low $\dot{V}_E$ may be violated.

BOX 10-125

Decision Making & Problem Solving

The following are the pressures and pressure alarms set on the Wave for a patient receiving volume ventilation:

- Peak pressure = 30 cm H_2O
- PEEP = 10 cm H_2O
- High-pressure alarm = 40 cm H_2O
- Low-pressure alarm = 25 cm H_2O
- Trigger sensitivity = -0.5 cm H_2O (below baseline)

The low-pressure alarm activates. You note the pressure gauge reads 7 cm H_2O during exhalation, and peak pressure is now 28 cm H_2O. The sensitivity trigger light flickers on, even though the patient does not appear to be inhaling. What do you think is causing the pressure drop? Why has the low-pressure alarm activated?

See Appendix A for the answer.

Inspired Minute Volume Alarm

This control is the first one on the left in the next row of the ventilator setting section. You can adjust for both HIGH and LOW $\dot{V}_E$ alarms (in liters/minute). It is a double knob control with the higher (white) indicator setting the high $\dot{V}_E$ and the lower (black) setting the low $\dot{V}_E$ alarm. This control has two possible ranges. With the 0-5 button unlit (i.e., not pressed) the range is from 0 to 50 L/min. When the 0-5 button has been pushed and is green, the range is from 0 to 5 L/min. See Box 10-124 for further explanation of this alarm. EXPIRATORY $\dot{V}_E$ alarms are located on the Compass monitor.

The HIGH $\dot{V}_E$ alarm can detect a leak or a disconnection in the patient circuit if the baseline pressure is set to a positive value. When proximal pressure drops due to a leak or disconnection and the drop in pressure repeatedly activates the trigger, the measured inspiratory $\dot{V}_E$ may increase in comparison with the patient's actual $\dot{V}_E$.

The low $\dot{V}_E$ alarm can be used to detect apnea when the spontaneous ventilation mode is in use or obstructions occur in the airway during pressure-targeted ventilation.

FIO_2

Oxygen delivery can be adjusted from 0.21 to 1.0. You should check the delivered oxygen concentration via the oxygen analyzer included in the optional Compass monitor or by using another oxygen analyzer.

Flow

The flow (1 to 100 L/min) provides a constant gas flow at the set value during volume ventilation and sets the maximum flow available during pressure-targeted mandatory breaths. It is recommended that the flow be set to the maximum (100 L/min) during pressure-targeted ventilation so that the Wave's microprocessor can automatically adjust the inspiratory rise (slope) during mandatory breath delivery.

Inspiratory Time

Mandatory breaths, either pressure- or volume-targeted, are time-cycled. The T_I setting ranges from 0.1 to 3.0 seconds.

Respiratory Rate

This control sets the rate for mandatory breath delivery in either A/C or SIMV modes. Rate ranges from 1 to 100 breaths/min.

Alarms and Monitors

In addition to the $\dot{V}_E$ alarm already reviewed, the top panel also has a HIGH- and LOW-PRESSURE alarm control located adjacent to the pressure gauge (-10 to 120 cm H_2O). The HIGH- and LOW-PRESSURE alarm settings are indicated by lit green segments on the pressure gauge. (Note that the LOW-PRESSURE alarm segment turns dark when its set value is exceeded by the current airway pressure level.) Rotating the knob to its normal position sets the LOW- and HIGH-PRESSURE alarms in tandem. To set only the high alarm, pull the knob out before rotating it. If the pressure does not exceed the low pressure setting during a mandatory inspiration, an audio/visual alarm occurs. (Note that the low-pressure alarm is also violated if the airway pressure drops below the sensitivity pressure setting for 3 seconds in any mode or for half of T_E for two consecutive breaths in the SIMV mode, whichever is shorter. Box 10-125 presents a problem about this situation.)

The pressure displayed on the pressure gauge must reach the high-pressure alarm setting for this high-pressure

TABLE 10-35

Alarm indicators on the E200 Wave

Alarm	Triggering condition
High pressure	Airway pressure exceeds set high-pressure alarm setting
Low pressure	Airway pressure does not achieve low-pressure alarm setting during a mandatory breath
High $\dot{V}_E$	Measured inhaled $\dot{V}_E$ exceeds set high $\dot{V}_E$ alarm
Low $\dot{V}_E$	Measured inhaled $\dot{V}_E$ is lower than low $\dot{V}_E$ alarm
T_I too long	T_I has exceeded setting based on I:E ratio limit setting of switch on back panel (manufacturer uses "IT" to abbreviate inspiratory time)
Vent. Inop.	Microprocessor has detected a malfunction. The ventilator goes into exhalation. (Sometimes turning the unit off and then back on allows it to reset. If it does not, find another machine to ventilate the patient and call a service representative.)

alarm to occur.* When patient circuit pressure reaches the set value, the ventilator cycles into exhalation. For the high-pressure alarm, the pressure is measured near the main flow outlet port just inside the ventilator. If a HIGH-PRESSURE alarm event occurs and the patient circuit pressure does not drop to at least 5 cm H_2O above baseline, no more mandatory breaths are delivered. An additional safety feature is the pressure-relief valve, which is reviewed in the discussion of special features later in this section.

At the top left corner of the front panel is a section containing an ALARM SILENCE button (60 seconds) and six LED indicators. Conditions resulting in illumination of these indicators are listed in Table 10-35.

Figure 10-85 shows a rotating knob with a list of measured and calculated parameters as well as a digital display window. Box 10-126 lists each parameter.

There is a window in the central portion of the E200 that displays the set V_T during volume-targeted breaths. This is based on flow and T_I settings and is not a measured value. The measured inspiratory V_T is displayed in the monitor window and the measured expiratory V_T is displayed in the monitor window of the optional Compass monitor.

Circuit Connections and Nebulizer Control

On the panel just below the main front panel are the connections for ventilator output to the humidifier, the exhalation valve line connector, the proximal airway pressure monitoring line (receives purged gas to reduce obstruction), and the nebulizer drive line connector. Each connection is color-coded and sized differently to avoid accidental interconnection of lines. The NEBULIZER control is on the far right side.

*There are some built-in AUTOMATIC HIGH-PRESSURE alarms as well.

BOX 10-126

Monitored Parameters

Measured Values

Inspired tidal volume (0 to 9.99 L)
Inspired minute volume (0 to 99.9 L/min)
Respiratory rate (0 to 999 breaths/min)
Peak airway pressure (0 to 120 cm H_2O)
Base pressure (0 to 120 cm H_2O; measured at the exhalation valve)
Peak inspiratory flow (0 to 999 L/min; spontaneous and mandatory)

Calculated Value

Mean airway pressure (0 to 120 cm H_2O)

Nebulization

Turning on the NEBULIZER control results in about 6 L/min (15 psi) of gas coming from the nebulizer drive line outlet during each mandatory volume-targeted inspiration. The NEBULIZER control does not function with PSV, PCV, or spontaneous breaths.

While the nebulizer is on, the flow from the ventilator is reduced by the amount delivered through the nebulizer drive line. This is to keep actual V_T and $\dot{V}_E$ delivery constant. You must remember to turn off this control when the treatment is finished. It also turns off when the ventilator is turned off.

Back Panel Controls

Back panel controls are described in Box 10-127. Two additional, nonadjustable alarms are the MIXER alarm, which sounds continuously if the air and/or oxygen inlet gas pressure drops below 31 psig, and the POWER SUPPLY alarm. If the AC power is lost or disconnected, this alarm is continuous for 5 minutes. If the unit is turned off, a continuous alarm sounds that may be silenced with the ALARM SILENCE button.

Modes of Operation

Modes of ventilation available on the E200 include A/C, SIMV (either volume- or pressure-targeted), and spontaneous (including PSV).

BOX 10-127

Back Panel Controls

Inspiratory Pause Control

Can be set at 0% (off), 10%, 20%, and 30% of T_I. (Note that during a pause, T_I for the Wave is constant at the value set on the front panel. Therefore using inspiratory pause does not increase T_I, but encroaches on the time during which inspiratory flow occurs. As a result, flow actually increases over the set value, and peak pressures may increase.)

I:E Ratio Switch

Allows I:E ratios of up to 3:1 or limits I:E ratios to 1:1 before alarming.

Audible Alarm Volume Control

BOX 10-128

Decision Making & Problem Solving

You are attending a patient being ventilated by the Wave E200. Current settings are as follows: mode = A/C, flow = 60 L/min, T_I = 0.75 sec, pressure control = off, rate = 10 breaths/min, FIO_2 = 0.5, bias flow = 4 L/min, and PEEP = 5 cm H_2O. Current blood gases are: pH = 7.38, $PaCO_2$ = 44 mm Hg, and PaO_2 = 56 mm Hg.

The physician wants to improve oxygenation and asks you to increase T_I in order to increase mean airway pressure. How would you respond to this request?

See Appendix A for the answer.

Volume-Targeted Ventilation

During volume ventilation, V_T is determined by the set flow and T_I. For example, if the flow is set at 80 L/min (1.33 L/sec) and the T_I is 1.0 seconds, V_T is 1.33 L. This value appears in the SET TIDAL VOLUME display. The I:E ratio is based on respiratory rate and T_I. For example, if the rate is 20 breaths/min, TCT is 3 seconds (60 sec/[20 breaths/min]). If T_I is 1 sec, T_E is 2 sec, and the I:E ratio is 1:2. Box 10-128 gives an example of a problem related to V_T adjustment on the Wave.

Pressure-Targeted Ventilation

If the PRESSURE control knob is not turned off, mandatory breath delivery is pressure-targeted. The SET TIDAL VOLUME digital display will read "—." As you would expect, flow is delivered in a descending, exponential manner as pressure at the airway increases toward the set value. Volume delivery varies with patient lung characteristics and patient effort. Real time V_T and $\dot{V}_E$ can be monitored. (If there is a slight leak in the circuit during pressure ventilation, the leak supplement function activates to help compensate and accomplishes this so that a pressure-targeted breath is delivered as expected. The unit simply increases flow to try and maintain the set pressure. However, be sure to carefully monitor and assess the patient, as well as ventilator parameters.)

The maximum available flow during PCV is based on the flow setting. If you set a low flow value, it takes longer for the ventilator to achieve the set PIP. A high flow setting achieves the set PIP more quickly. As mentioned, for best results set the highest flow value and allow the microprocessor to adjust the rise time or sloping. (The manufacturer calls this automatic slope control.)

If you choose to set flow manually, be sure it is set high enough to achieve the set pressure before the end of inspiration. In addition, as T_I is increased along with flow, the amount of time that the pressure plateaus during inspiration increases (see Chapter 9). This will increase mean airway pressure.

High-Pressure Alarm in Pressure Ventilation

When pressure is set on the PRESSURE control dial, an automatic HIGH-PRESSURE alarm limit is set at 10 cm H_2O above that value and terminates inspiration when exceeded. If pressure fails to fall to ≤5 cm H_2O below baseline during exhalation, no additional mandatory breaths are delivered. (Note that in PCV, an obstruction of the endotracheal tube cannot be detected by the HIGH-PRESSURE alarm system during inspiration. An obstructed tube does not require much flow to achieve the pressure, so there would not be a HIGH-PRESSURE alarm. An obstructed tube is detected as a drop in the $\dot{V}_E$ and activates the LOW $\dot{V}_E$ alarm. However, a HIGH-PRESSURE alarm is activated if the patient tries to actively exhale during inspiration.)

Low-Pressure Alarm in Pressure Ventilation

During pressure-targeted ventilation (pressure control set), an automatic LOW-PRESSURE alarm is set at half of the set pressure value. If the airway pressure does not exceed this value during inspiration, it activates. It also activates if the airway pressure falls and remains below the trigger sensitivity pressure setting for 3 seconds in any mode or half of the expiratory time for two consecutive breaths in the SIMV mode—whichever is shorter. This usually indicates a leak in the circuit.

Assist/Control

In A/C, breaths are patient- or time-triggered, volume- or pressure-targeted, and time-cycled. All breaths are mandatory.

Synchronized Intermittent Mandatory Ventilation[3]

In SIMV, mandatory breaths are patient- or time-triggered, volume- or pressure-targeted, and time-cycled. Spontaneous breaths are patient-triggered, pressure-limited, and pressure-cycled. PSV can be added to spontaneous breaths.

In SIMV, mandatory breaths are synchronized with patient's spontaneous efforts based on the sensitivity setting. Figure 10-82 shows how mandatory breaths are timed. The mandatory breath interval (MBI) equals 60 seconds/(set breaths/min). For example if the rate is 20/min, the MBI is 3 seconds. In the first MBI in Figure 10-82, no patient effort was detected. Therefore at the beginning of the next MBI, a time-triggered mandatory breath is delivered. During the next MBI after the time-triggered breath, a patient triggers a mandatory breath. The patient can breathe spontaneously throughout the remaining time of the MBI. In the third MBI, a mandatory breath is not delivered because the patient received one in the second MBI. In the fourth MBI, a time-triggered breath is delivered because a complete MBI has just preceded it with no patient-triggered mandatory breath (see Box 10-123).

Sigh

The Wave E200 can provide sigh breaths in either volume- or pressure-targeted ventilation. The sigh function is selected by pressing the small green button next to the mode selector (active, lit; inactive, unlit). A sigh breath is given every 100 breaths when it is selected. For volume-targeted ventilation, the V_T delivered during a sigh breath is 1.5 times the set V_T. For pressure-targeted ventilation, the set peak pressure is achieved, just as with a normal breath. However, for either volume- or pressure-targeted ventilation, T_I during a sigh breath is 1.5 times the set T_I. The HIGH-PRESSURE alarm limit does not change for the sigh breath. You may want to take this into account when setting this alarm and the sigh function.

Spontaneous

In the spontaneous ventilation mode, you adjust bias flow, FIO_2, PEEP/CPAP, pressure support, and sensitivity. The patient breathes gas provided by either the bias flow control and/or demand flow. The patient can also obtain gas at the set pressure when PSV is active. No mandatory breaths are delivered. If the patient's effort causes airway pressure to decrease by the amount set on the sensitivity control, the ventilator provides additional flow or pressure support. Once the breath is detected, the internal servo-control flow valve delivers whatever flow the patient demands or whatever flow is needed for pressure support, up to 160 L/min. For this reason, it is important to set the sensitivity appropriately so the patient's work of breathing is not increased (Box 10-129). Spontaneous breaths that are detected are counted and displayed by the rate monitor.

> **BOX 10-129**
>
> **Setting Bias Flow and Sensitivity in the Spontaneous Mode**
>
> It is very important to carefully adjust both bias flow and sensitivity in the spontaneous mode. The patient's inspiratory effort must exceed the sum of the pressure produced by the bias flow and the pressure required to trigger the sensitivity, or the internal flow valve will not open.

If a high bias flow is set, this may provide a substantial part of the patient's flow requirements. In this case, the pressure at the airway opening may not decrease. The potential problem with this is that the patient's efforts may not meet the trigger sensitivity setting, and the internal flow control valve will not open. No pressure support would be available. If this is a problem, the bias flow should be set lower.

Pressure support and/or demand flow work with bias flow to reduce the patient's work of breathing.

In the spontaneous mode, only the high-pressure alarm can be activated. When CPAP is applied, the LOW-PRESSURE alarm is automatically set based on the reading from the proximal pressure line. If the patient circuit pressure falls below the trigger sensitivity level for 3 seconds or longer, the LOW-PRESSURE alarm sounds.

Pressure Support

The PRESSURE-SUPPORT control adjusts the PSV level for spontaneous breaths in the spontaneous and SIMV modes. The LED lights when this mode is active. In either volume- or pressure-targeted SIMV mode, PSV is available in between mandatory breaths.

PS breaths are patient- (pressure-)triggered, pressure-targeted, and flow-cycled. The flow that ends inspiration in PSV is calculated by the microprocessor. This calculation is based on a formula using target pressure, maximum flow delivered, and time. The longer any PS breath lasts, the higher the percentage of peak flow required to end (cycle) the breath. Inspiratory flow during PSV also ends if one of the following conditions occurs:

1. V_T reaches 4.0 L
2. PIP is 2 cm H_2O > PSV pressure setting
3. T_I is longer than 3 seconds

Graphic Display Screens

The Navigator Graphics Monitor can be purchased as a separate unit and used with the Wave or the Breeze E150 ventilators. In addition to providing real time graphs of volume,

BOX 10-130

Procedure for Suctioning with the E200

1. Press and hold the ALARM SILENCE key for 3 seconds; beep will sound.
2. During the next 10 seconds, the alarm silence light is on, and the ventilator continues to function normally as it awaits for a circuit pressure change.
3. When airway pressure drops below the trigger sensitivity pressure during exhalation or when a low-pressure alarm condition occurs during a mandatory breath, the E200 switches into the suction stand-by mode.
4. In this mode, the following occur:
   - The LOW-PRESSURE alarm indicator flashes.
   - The alarm silence lamp remains lit for 60 seconds, after which the audible alarm sounds.
   - Bias flow is delivered through the circuit. When the high-range $\dot{V}_E$ alarm is set, flow is 20 L/min. When the low-range $\dot{V}_E$ alarm is set, flow is 10 L/min.
   - Pressure-targeted breaths (PC and PS) are disabled.
5. Reconnecting the patient and eliminating major leaks from the circuit cancels the suction standby mode and returns the ventilator to normal operation.

(Note that if suction standby is enabled by pushing the ALARM SILENCE button for 3 seconds, but the circuit is not disconnected, nothing happens. After 10 seconds, the alarm silence is canceled.)

flow, and pressure over time and loops for flow/volume and pressure/volume, it can also automatically perform measurements of compliance and resistance. It also monitors respiratory rate, inspiratory and expiratory $\dot{V}_E$, inspiratory and expiratory V_T, peak inspiratory and expiratory flows, inspiratory and expiratory times, leak percent, and dynamic compliance and resistance. Alarm functions are also available for respiratory rate, $\dot{V}_E$, PIP, and apnea.

SPECIAL FEATURES

A few special features are available with the Newport Wave E200 ventilator and are reviewed here.

Suctioning a Patient

The E200 has a special feature that allows you to place the ventilator into temporary standby for suctioning the patient. Box 10-130 lists the steps involved in this procedure.

Pressure-Relief Valve

On the side panel of the E200 is a pressure-relief valve that limits pressure delivery through the patient circuit during any mode, but does not end inspiration. This safety pop-off is adjustable from 0 to 120 cm H_2O. Turning the knob clockwise increases the pressure limit; turning it counterclockwise lowers it.

During normal operation you should set the pop-off pressure about 10 cm H_2O above the HIGH-PRESSURE alarm setting. Be sure to set this control prior to patient use. To do this, perform the following:

1. Make sure the PRESSURE control knob is set to the off position.
2. Set flow to a normal level for the patient to be ventilated.
3. Turn the high-pressure limit to 120 cm H_2O.
4. Occlude the patient wye connector.
5. Press the manual control and watch the pressure gauge.
6. Rotate the pressure-relief valve until the pressure plateaus at the desired value.
7. Return the ventilator controls to the proper settings.

Remote Alarm Silence

The E200 has a REMOTE ALARM SILENCE control, which is a long cable that connects to the back panel. You can use the button on the end of the cable to silence alarms for 60 seconds. This is helpful when suctioning the patient from the side of the bed opposite the ventilator.

Newport Compass Ventilator Monitor

A separate monitor unit, called the Compass, can be purchased and attached to the Wave to monitor expired gases. The unit can be mounted directly onto the left side of the Wave. The analyzer for FiO_2 can be hooked directly into the patient circuit or into the optional flush valve that mounts on the other side of the Wave E200. The Compass contains a heated, filtered exhalation system with its own exhalation valve. When it is in use, there is no need for the externally mounted valve. Instead, the expiratory valve drive line on the Wave is connected to a small connector near the bottom of the Compass. It provides alarms for HIGH- and LOW-EXPIRED $\dot{V}_E$, HIGH and LOW FiO_2, and monitors expired V_T, $\dot{V}_E$, I:E ratio, FiO_2 (analyzed), and expired peak flow.

TROUBLESHOOTING

In addition to the alarms, monitors, and indicators available, the operating manual contains additional tips on troubleshooting. There is also a laminated card containing this information that can be hung on the side of the ventilator. The Wave E200 performs self-zeroing on all sensors and transducers at timed intervals and whenever it is turned on, although it still may be possible for a component to require calibration. Malfunctions of electrical components or transducers can occur when such devices are out of calibration or failing. Keeping a regular maintenance schedule is essential to avoiding such problems. You should refer to the service manual in such circumstances or contact a service representative.

Because the Wave is microprocessor-controlled, avoid the use of radio frequency-emitting devices, such as cellular phones, pagers, and walkie-talkies, in the vicinity of the ventilator.

Review Questions

(See Appendix A for answers.)

1. The Wave E200 uses which internal flow delivery device?
   a. an electromagnetic poppet valve
   b. a stepper motor with a scissors valve
   c. a linear drive piston
   d. an internal bellows device
2. During volume ventilation of a patient on the E200, the airway pressure reaches the pressure limit set on the pressure-relief valve before it reaches the HIGH PRESSURE LIMIT alarm. Which of the following statements about this situation is (are) true?
   I. You should have set the pressure-relief valve higher than the HIGH-PRESSURE LIMIT alarm.
   II. An audible alarm will sound and the high-pressure alarm LED will illuminate.
   III. Pressure will plateau, but inspiration will not end.
   IV. Volume delivery will remain the same.
   a. I and III only
   b. II and IV only
   c. I, III and IV only
   d. I, II, III and IV
3. During PCV using the E200, you want to give a nebulized medication treatment to a patient. What should you do?
   a. select an external flowmeter to power the nebulizer and (while it is on) set the pressure relief valve 1 cm H_2O above set pressure
   b. until the treatment is finished, switch to a volume-targeted mode and use the pressure-relief valve to limit pressure
   c. connect the nebulizer line to the device and press the nebulizer button on the lower panel of the ventilator
   d. change the patient to another ventilator
4. When the use of sigh is selected, which of the following is (are) true?
   I. A sigh breath is delivered every 100 breaths.
   II. This can only be used in volume-targeted A/C.
   III. Sigh V_T is 1.5 times V_T set.
   IV. Sigh T_I is 1.5 times T_I set.
   a. I only
   b. II only
   c. III and IV only
   d. I, III, and IV only
5. You set the Wave E200 up for volume-targeted A/C ventilation. However, you notice that the pressure only rises to 10 cm H_2O, and the desired volume is not achieved. No alarms are active. What could be the problem?
   I. The PRESSURE control knob is not in the off position.
   II. There is water in the circuit.
   III. The pressure is being released through the pressure-relief valve.
   IV. The bias flow is set too low.
   a. I only
   b. IV only
   c. II and III only
   d. I and III only
6. You wish to use inverse ratio PCV on a patient being ventilated with the Wave. Rate is set at 12 breaths/min, and T_I is 2 seconds. You increase T_I to 3 seconds, and an audible alarm sounds. The IT TOO LONG LED illuminates. How can you solve this problem?
   a. reduce the flow instead of increasing T_I
   b. change the setting of the I:E RATIO switch on the back panel
   c. increase the pressure setting for PCV
   d. increase the bias flow to 10 L/min
7. You can set pressure- or volume-targeted SIMV with the Wave E200—true or false?
8. The Wave E200 requires both an electric and pneumatic power source to operate—true or false?
9. You notice the set V_T in the upper panel reads 0.7 L, and the inspired V_T in the monitor section reads 0.63 L. What is a possible cause of this discrepancy?
10. To calculate a patient's lung compliance, you set the plateau at 20% on the back panel of the Wave. You notice that the peak pressure has suddenly changed from 28 to 30 cm H_2O. What causes this change?

References

1. Newport Wave ventilator operating manual model E200, Version 1.5, 1993, Newport Beach, Calif., 1993, Newport Medical Instruments, Inc.
2. Pilbeam SP and Payne FR: Mechanical ventilators. In Burton GG, Hodgkin JE, and Ward JJ, Respiratory care: a guide to clinical practice, ed 4, Philadelphia, 1997, Lippincott.
3. Miller, Cyndy: Personal communication, Aug 1998.

Siemens Servo 900C

OUTLINE

Power Source
Internal Mechanisms
Controls and Alarms
Modes of Ventilation
- Volume Control
- Volume Control + Sigh
- Pressure Control
- Pressure Support
- Synchronized Intermittent Mandatory Ventilation
- SIMV + Pressure Support
- Continuous Positive Airway Pressure
- Manual

Troubleshooting

LEARNING OBJECTIVES

After reading this section, the reader should be able to:

1. Label the internal components on a diagram of the Servo 900C.
2. Explain the operation of each of the controls and alarms on the Servo 900C.
3. Given the ventilator control settings, calculate V_T, T_I, T_E, and I:E ratio during volume ventilation on the Servo 900C.
4. Estimate inspiratory flow during volume ventilation and SIMV when constant flow is selected and control settings are given.
5. Describe each of the modes of ventilation for the Servo 900C.
6. Indicate which control must be set for each mode.
7. Solve an alarm situation.

The Servo 900C ventilator[1-4] was released in the United States in 1981 and was designed for use in either infant, pediatric, or adult ventilation (Figure 10-86). It consists of a pneumatic section that sits over the electronic control section containing the operating controls and control panel and regulates gas flow to the patient.

POWER SOURCE

The Servo 900C requires a gas source and a standard electrical outlet for operation. It is pneumatically powered and electronically controlled, but does not use a microprocessor. It can be operated using either a high-pressure or a low-pressure gas source because both types of gas inlets are provided.

INTERNAL MECHANISMS

Internal mechanisms are shown in Figure 10-87. Compressed gases are blended to the desired FiO_2 and enter the ventilator through either the high-pressure or low-pressure inlet one-way valve, although both can be used simultaneously. The high-pressure unit is usually powered by a blender that connects to high-pressure air and oxygen. The low-pressure port can be used to operate the ventilator without a high-pressure gas source. It is also used to administer anesthetic gases. From the inlet port, gas passes through an oxygen analyzer (O_2 cell), a bacteria filter, and into a plastic, spring-loaded bellows (see Figure 10-87).

The spring-loaded bellows provides the working pressure and is capable of delivering pressures up to 120 cm H_2O into the patient circuit (Box 10-131). Tension on the spring is adjusted by using a control adjustment marked PRESET WORKING PRESSURE, as shown in Figure 10-88. Spring tension determines the operating pressure within the bellows. During inspiration, gas from the bellows is directed into the patient circuit by way of an inspiratory servo valve that is composed of an inspiratory flow transducer and a scissorlike valve controlled by a stepper motor (see Figure 9-16). Gas passes through the flow transducer, where it is measured, and flows into the main inspiratory line of the patient circuit. At the same time, the expiratory servo valve is closed. The expiratory valve movement is controlled by an electromagnetic solenoid (pull-magnet). During exhalation, the expiratory valve opens and the patient exhales freely through the main expiratory line.

CONTROLS AND ALARMS

The front control panel for the Servo 900C is divided into the an upper and lower portion (see Figure 10-88). The front adjustment screw on the pneumatic section is used to control the working pressure, which is set above the peak pressure required to ventilate the patient. On the face of the pneumatic unit is a manometer that provides a reading of the working pressure inside the bellows. The lower portion (control interface) contains the remaining primary operating controls, alarms, monitors, and the MODE setting control.

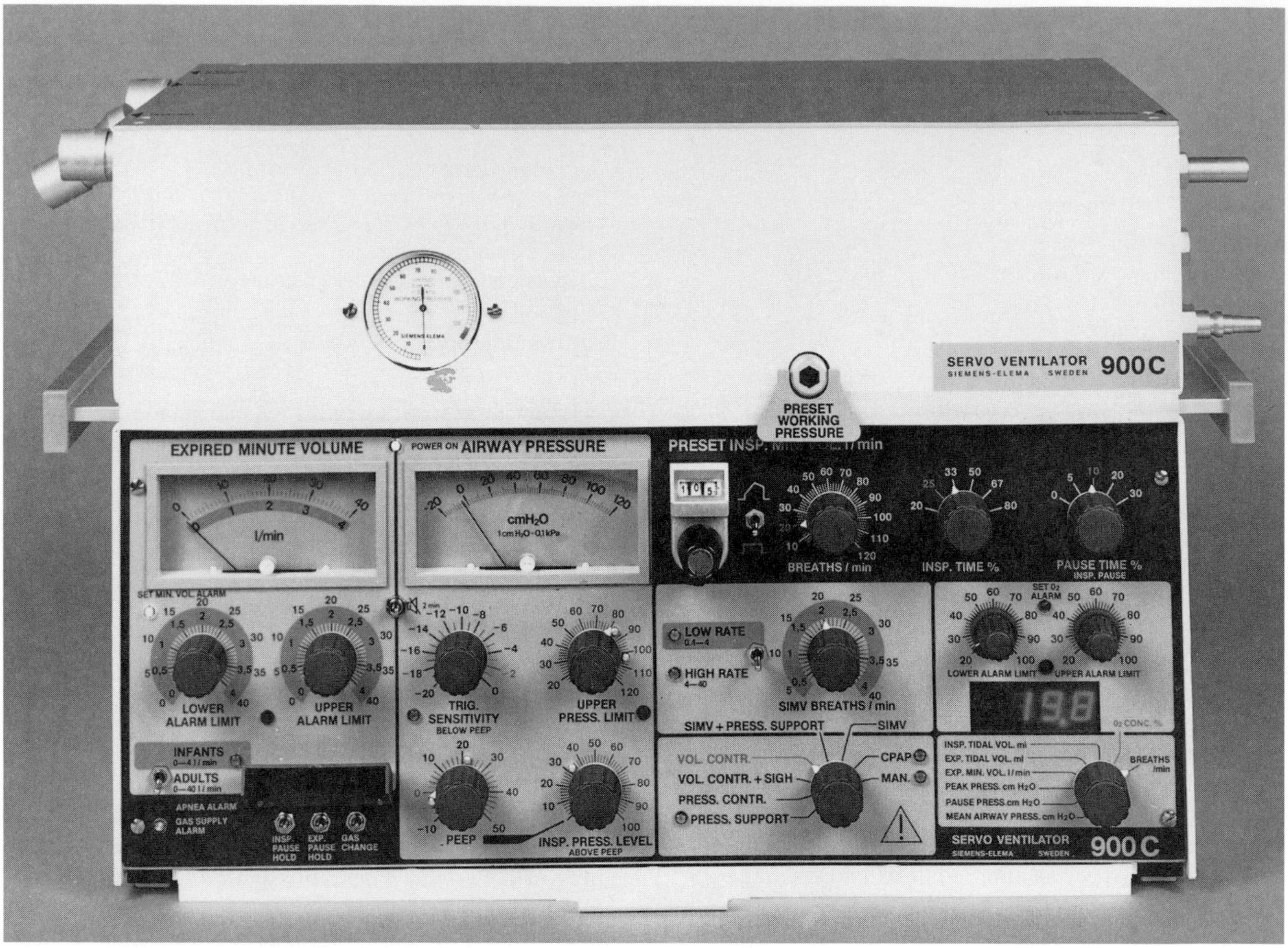

Figure 10-86 The Siemens-Elema Servo 900C. (Courtesy Siemens Medical Systems, Inc., Danvers, Mass.)

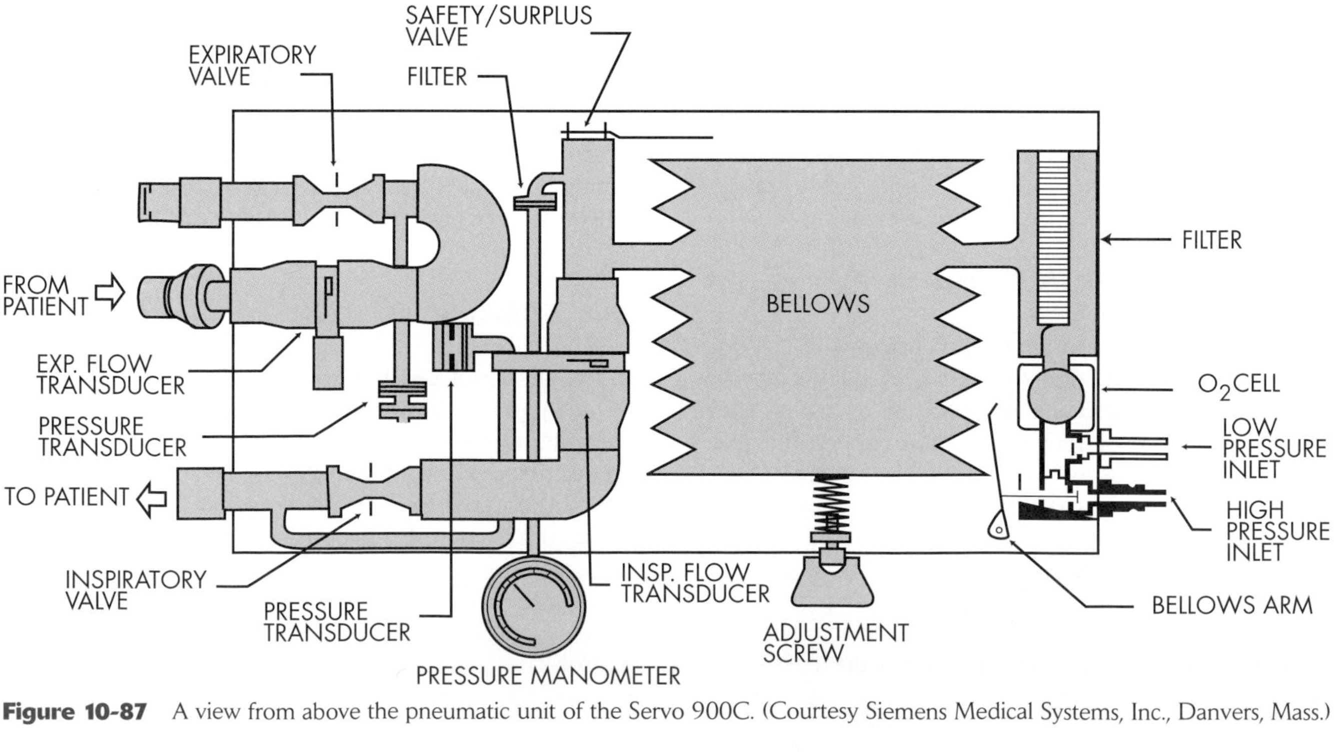

Figure 10-87 A view from above the pneumatic unit of the Servo 900C. (Courtesy Siemens Medical Systems, Inc., Danvers, Mass.)

BOX 10-131

Important Clinical Note

The bellows of the Servo 900C must have a pressurized gas source to fill and compress the spring, or the ventilator cannot operate. (see Chapter 9, Figure 9-13)

The left section of the control panel contains the HIGH- and LOW-$\dot{V}_E$ alarms, the EXPIRED $\dot{V}_E$ monitor, and several other alarms and indicators. At the lower left corner of the $\dot{V}_E$ monitor is a light that illuminates when the limits for the $\dot{V}_E$ alarm have not been set. At the upper right of the $\dot{V}_E$ monitor is a light indicator that activates when the electric power is connected and deactivates when power is disconnected (Box 10-132). The ALARM SILENCE button is located at the lower right corner of the $\dot{V}_E$ monitor. A switch at the lower left corner of the left panel governs the range of the $\dot{V}_E$ monitor settings. The adult settings for this switch range from 0 to 40 L/min; the infant settings range from 0 to 4 L/min (Box 10-133).

Three other alarm indicators are in this panel section: EXPIRED $\dot{V}_E$, APNEA, and GAS SUPPLY. The EXPIRED $\dot{V}_E$ alarm lights and sounds when the set alarm limits are exceeded (Table 10-36). The APNEA alarm gives an audio/visual signal if the time between two breaths (spontaneous or mandatory) is more than about 15 seconds. The GAS SUPPLY alarm indicates an inadequate source gas pressure to maintain ventilation.

In the lower left section of the control panel, under a small panel cover are three special function buttons: INSPIRATORY PAUSE HOLD, EXPIRATORY PAUSE HOLD, and GAS CHANGE. When the INSPIRATORY PAUSE button is depressed, both inspiratory and expiratory valves close at the end of the inspiration, but before exhalation begins, and remain closed until the button is released. The unit automatically delays the next mandatory breath, which provides a manually controlled inspiratory hold or pause maneuver for estimating plateau pressure. Depressing the EXPIRATORY PAUSE HOLD button closes both inspiratory and expiratory valves at the end of exhalation for a prolonged expiratory pause and allows measurement of end-expiratory pressures (auto-PEEP). Pressing the GAS CHANGE button opens both valves and allows the bellows to empty its volume through the patient circuit. Gas continues to flow from the gas inlet through the bellows and the circuit as long as the button is depressed (Box 10-134). This allows for a rapid change of the O_2%. For example, you could use this control to flush the circuit with the desired O_2% before connecting the patient to the ventilator. In this way, the O_2% in the circuit is at the desired value as soon as the patient is attached.

The airway pressure panel contains the pressure manometer for monitoring inspiratory gas pressure. Below this manometer are four knob controls. The top left control is TRIGGER SENSITIVITY BELOW PEEP, which establishes how much effort the patient must make to pressure-trigger inspiration. The UPPER PRESSURE LIMIT is the next control. It sets the maximum pressure that can occur during inspiration. If this value is reached, inspiration ends (pressure-cycling). The next control is the PEEP control, which establishes the positive pressure baseline. The control marked INSPIRATORY PRESSURE LEVEL ABOVE PEEP establishes the ventilating pressure for pressure-targeted ventilation in PCV and PSV. It is only functional when either of those modes is selected (i.e., pressure control, pressure support, and SIMV + pressure support).

The right side of the operating panel has a row of controls across the top used for establishing volume delivery and breath rate. The first control is the PRESET INSPIRATORY $\dot{V}_E$ (0.5 to 40 L/min). The front dial of this control is used to select the desired $\dot{V}_E$. Next to this is a STET switch to select either a constant flow pattern or what the manufacturer calls an accelerating inspiratory flow pattern. The flow patterns are only available during volume ventilation. To the right of the FLOW switch is the RATE control knob (in breaths/minute). The setting on this control and the $\dot{V}_E$ setting determine the V_T ($V_T = \dot{V}_E \div$ rate). The INSPIRATORY TIME % (20% to 80%) and the PAUSE TIME % (0% to 30%, or inspiratory pause) controls determine the length of inspiration. The sum of these two settings represents T_I. T_I cannot exceed 80% of the TCT when TCT is based on the breaths/minute setting (Box 10-135).

The $\dot{V}_E$ control and T_I % can be used to calculate inspiratory gas flow when the constant flow waveform is selected. Multiplying the $\dot{V}_E$ by (100% ÷ T_I%) equals the gas flow. Look at the following example:

- $\dot{V}_E$ is 10 L/min
- T_I % is 20%

$$10\text{ L/min} \times (100\% \div 20\%) = 10\text{ L/min} \times 5 = 50\text{ L/min}$$

What will happen if the T_I% is increased to 50%? Will the flow increase or decrease for the same $\dot{V}_E$? See the following equation:

$$10\text{ L/min} \times (100\% \div 50\%) = 10 \times 2 = 20\text{ L/min}$$

If T_I% is longer with the same $\dot{V}_E$, flow will be slower. Box 10-136 shows how using SIMV RATE control can help the clinician increase flow without changing V_T or $\dot{V}_E$.

Below the $\dot{V}_E$ and RATE settings is another set of controls. The first two controls are for setting the RESPIRATORY RATE during SIMV ventilation. On the right is the SIMV BREATHS/MIN knob, which is exclusively for controlling the respiratory rate in the SIMV mode. On the left is a toggle switch for selecting the range in which the SIMV BREATHS/MIN knob operates. In the up (LOW RATE) position, the rate ranges from 0.4 to 4 breaths/min. When it is

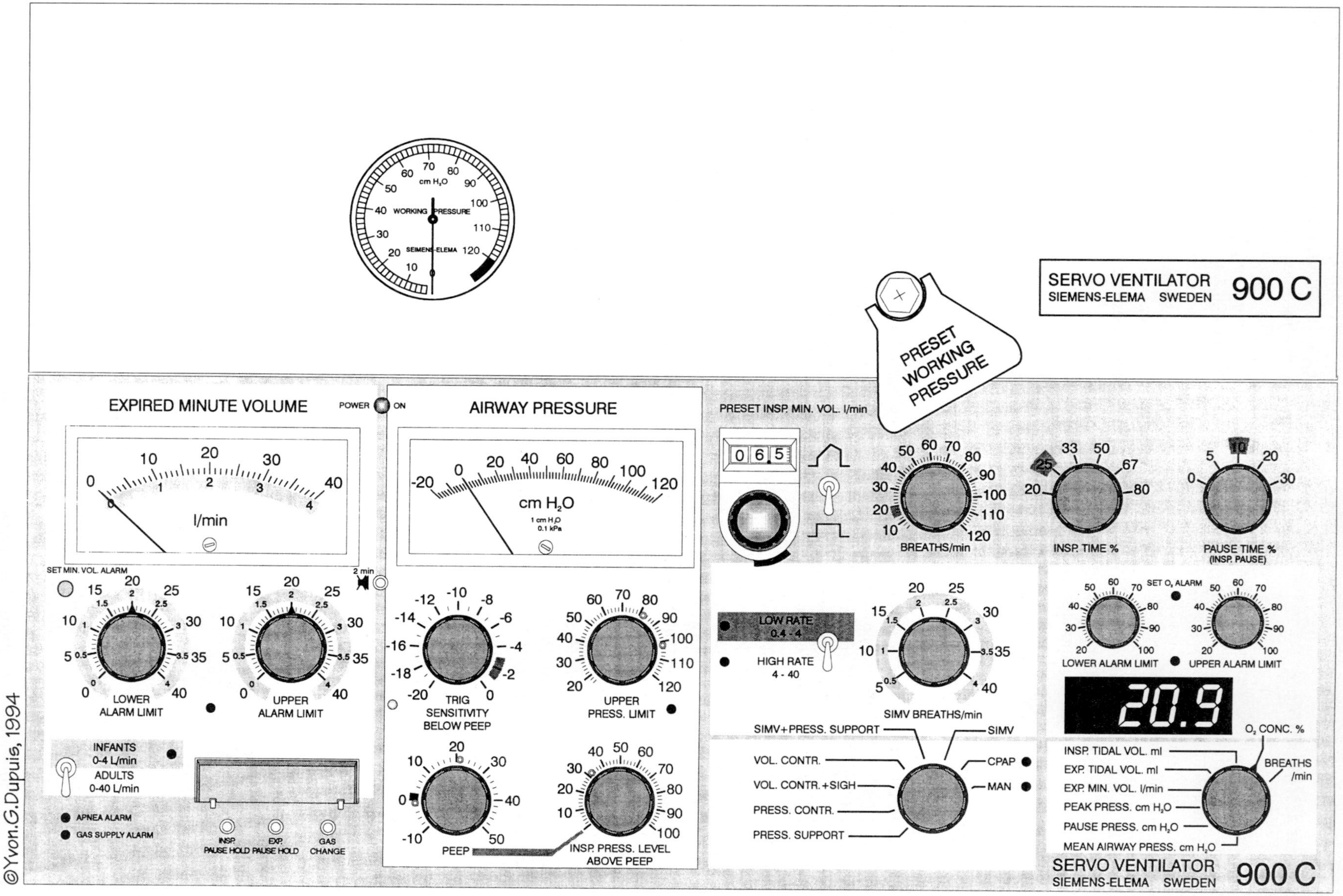

Figure 10-88 The control panel of the Servo 900C. (Courtesy Yvon Dupuis.)

BOX 10-132

Important Clinical Note

The green POWER ON light goes out if the ventilator is turned off (ON/OFF switch on back of ventilator) or if the electrical power is disconnected. An audible alarm occurs, as well. To stop the sound, the ALARM SILENCE button must be pushed and held down for several seconds. If nothing is done, the sound will eventually stop on its own (in 5 to 10 minutes).

TABLE 10-36

Alarm limits for the minute ventilation alarm on the Servo 900C

	Adult	Infant
Upper alarm limit	3 to 43 L/min	0 to 4.3 L/min
Lower alarm limit	0 to 37 L/min	0 to 3.7 L/min

BOX 10-133

Decision Making & Problem Solving

An audible alarm sounds during initiation of ventilation for an adult patient with the 900C. The clinician notices a visual alarm between the V_E setting controls; however, the rate and volume of ventilation seem appropriate for the patient (6 L/min), and the patient is being ventilated. Examination of the patient reveals that breath sounds are present with good chest wall excursion. What could be the problem?

See Appendix A for the answer.

BOX 10-134

Decision Making & Problem Solving

A patient will require hyperoxygenation prior to suctioning of the airway. What is a simple method for providing 100% oxygen to the patient through the ventilator?

See Appendix A for the answer.

BOX 10-135

Inspiratory Time and Total Cycle Time on the Servo 900C

T_I, T_E, and I:E are determined by the settings of the BREATHS/MIN, INSP.TIME %, and PAUSE TIME % controls.

Example

Suppose that the BREATHS/MIN control is set at 10, INSP. TIME % is 33%, and PAUSE TIME % is 0%.

$$TCT = 60 \text{ seconds/rate}$$
$$TCT = 60 \div 10 \text{ breaths/min, or 6 seconds}$$
$$T_I - TCT \times (\text{insp. time \%* + pause time \%*})$$
$$T_I = 6 \text{ seconds} \times 0.33^* = 2 \text{ seconds}$$
$$T_E = TCT - T_I = 6 \text{ seconds} - 2 \text{ seconds} = 4 \text{ seconds}$$
$$I{:}E = 1{:}(T_E/T_I) = 1{:}(4/2) = 1{:}2$$

Example

Suppose that BREATHS/MIN is set at 15, INSP. TIME % is 20%, and PAUSE TIME % is 10%.

$$TCT = 60 \text{ seconds/rate}$$
$$TCT = 60 \div 15 \text{ breaths/min, or 4 seconds}$$
$$T_I = TCT \times (\text{insp. time\%* + pause time \%*})$$
$$T_I = 4 \text{ seconds} \times 0.30 = 1.2 \text{ seconds}$$
$$T_E = TCT - T_I = 4 \text{ seconds} - 1.2 \text{ seconds} = 2.8 \text{ seconds}$$
$$I{:}E = 1{:}(T_E/T_I) = 1{:}(2.8/1.2) = 1{:}2.33$$

Example

Suppose the BREATHS/MIN is set at 12, the INSP. TIME % is 67%, and the PAUSE TIME % is 20%.

$$TCT = T_I + T_E \text{, or 60 seconds/rate}$$
$$TCT = 60 \div 12 \text{ breaths/min, or 5 seconds}$$
$$T_I = TCT \times (\text{insp. time \%* + pause time \%*})$$
$$T_I = 5 \text{ seconds} \times 0.87^* = 4.35 \text{ seconds}$$
$$T_E = TCT - T_I = 5 \text{ seconds} - 4.35 \text{ seconds} = 0.65 \text{ seconds}$$
$$I{:}E = 1{:}(T_E/T_I) = 1{:}(0.65/4.35) = 1{:}0.15 \text{ or } 6.7{:}1$$

In this example, how would the ventilator respond? What is wrong with this situation?

See Appendix A for the answer.

*Changed from a percentage to a fraction.

BOX 10-136

Adjusting Flow by Using the SIMV Rate

A patient is being ventilated in the volume-control mode with the 900C. The rate is set at 12 breaths/min, $\dot{V}_E$ is set at 6 L/min, $T_I\%$ is 20%, and pause % is 0%. The flow waveform is set on constant (rectangular). What is the V_T? What is the estimated inspiratory flow?

$$V_T = (6 \text{ L/min}) \div (12 \text{ breaths/min}) = 0.5 \text{ L}$$
$$6 \text{ L/min} \times (100\%/20\%) = 6 \text{ L/min} \times 5 = 30 \text{ L/min}$$

The patient has a high inspiratory flow demand, and the respiratory therapist must increase flow to the patient. $T_I\%$ is already at its shortest rate. How could this be done without changing $\dot{V}_E$?

The therapist could change to SIMV at the same rate (12 breaths/min). Then she could increase the breaths/min rate and the $\dot{V}_E$ settings to higher values that would still give a 0.5 L (500 mL) V_T. For example, 24 breaths/min at a $\dot{V}_E$ of 12 L/min provides a V_T of 500 mL (or 48 breaths/min at $\dot{V}_E$ of 24 L/min provides a V_T of 500 mL.

For these two examples, calculate the new flow:

$$\text{Example 1: } 12 \text{ L/min} \times (100\%/20\%) = 60 \text{ L/min}$$
$$\text{Example 2: } 24 \text{ L/min} \times (100\%/20\%) = 120 \text{ L/min}$$

Will these changes alter the rate or the $\dot{V}_E$? No. The rate is now established by the SIMV rate control, which is at the original rate of 12/min. V_T is still 500 mL. The parameters that have changed are the T_I, which changed the flow, and the mode, which is now SIMV. The guaranteed $\dot{V}_E$ is still the same.

(It could be argued that changing to SIMV may not be appropriate. A patient with a high inspiratory demand may also need a higher $\dot{V}_E$. The problem with switching to SIMV is that not every patient effort will be fully supported with a mandatory breath as with A/C.)

down (HIGH RATE position), the rate range is active, providing from 4 to 40 breaths/min. These two controls are active whenever an SIMV mode is selected (SIMV and SIMV + pressure support). In SIMV, the SIMV BREATHS/MIN control establishes the mandatory breath rate and must be set lower than the BREATHS/MIN control. If it is set higher, the ventilator defaults to the BREATHS/MIN control for rate and overrides the SIMV BREATHS/MIN setting. For example, if BREATHS/MIN is set at 10, and SIMV BREATHS/MIN is set at 12, the ventilator will deliver 10 breaths/min.

The MODE control knob on the lower panel of this section determines which mode is active. The eight available positions on this knob are included in the following discussion of modes of ventilation.

Finally, the far right section of the operating panel contains the control for the OXYGEN ALARM (upper and lower limits), and a digital window displaying various measured and calculated parameters. These parameters can be displayed by rotating the SELECTION knob just below the digital window, which allows the practitioner to view the following:

- Mean airway pressure (in centimeters of water)
- Pause pressure (in centimeters of water)
- Peak pressure (in centimeters of water)
- Expired minute volume (in liters/minute)
- Expired tidal volume (in milliliters)
- Inspired tidal volume (in milliliters)
- Oxygen percentage
- Breaths/minute

MODES OF VENTILATION

The Siemens Servo 900C can provide eight different modes of ventilation through its MODE selection switch (see Figure 10-88).

Volume-Control

A/C volume ventilation is available under the control marked VOL. CONTR. The inspiratory $\dot{V}_E$ is set as desired and the BREATHS/MIN control is set to the desired rate to establish the desired V_T. For example, if you set the $\dot{V}_E$ to 5 L/min and the rate to 12 breaths/min, the V_T will be 600 mL (V_T = [5 L/min] ÷ [12 breaths/min]).

The following additional parameters may also be set in A/C:

- Inspiratory time percentage
- Trigger sensitivity
- PEEP
- FiO_2
- Inspiratory pause

Breaths are patient- (pressure-) or time-triggered, volume-targeted, and time-cycled. For the rate just presented, let's set the INSP. TIME % at 33% and the FLOW WAVEFORM on constant. The TCT will be 5 seconds (60 seconds/12 breaths/min), and the T_I will be 33% of 5 seconds, or 1.65 seconds.

Volume Control + Sigh

Volume control plus sigh provides patient- or time-triggered, volume-targeted, time-cycled ventilation with a sigh breath every 100 breaths. The T_I and V_T are doubled for a sigh breath. When the MODE switch is moved to this setting, the sigh breath occurs on the second breath, giving the clinician an opportunity to evaluate peak pressure for a sigh breath.

Pressure Control

PCV provides patient- or time-triggered, pressure-targeted, time-cycled breaths. The INSPIRATORY PRESSURE control

BOX 10-137

Decision Making & Problem Solving

The following controls are set on the Servo 900C: inspiratory pressure = 14 cm H_2O, PEEP = 5 cm H_2O, breaths/min = 15, $\dot{V}_E$ = 15 L/min, and mode = pressure support.

(1) What is the V_T delivered to the patient? (2) What is the normal maximum pressure delivered during inspiration? (3) If the patient coughs during inspiration, at what point will inspiratory flow end? (4) Suppose a leak develops around the patient's endotracheal tube, and the flow never drops to the 25% level; what will cycle the breath and end inspiratory flow?

See Appendix A for the answers.

determines the pressure level above PEEP (baseline). Both working pressure and the upper pressure limit need to be set appropriately, as with any mode of ventilation. A breath will pressure cycle if the upper pressure limit is reached. This helps to avoid dangerously high pressures.

Pressure Support

PSV is patient- (pressure-) triggered, pressure-targeted, and flow cycled. As with pressure control, the target pressure is set using the INSPIRATORY PRESSURE control (above PEEP). The main difference between PCV and PSV is that when the flow decreases to about 25% of the peak flow measured during inspiration, PSV is flow-cycled out of inspiration. As a safety feature, inspiratory flow also ends if the airway pressure rises 3 cm H_2O above the set pressure or if T_I exceeds 80% of the TCT based on the set rate on the BREATHS/MIN control (Box 10-137).

Synchronized Intermittent Mandatory Ventilation

SIMV on the Servo 900C is similar to that on other ventilators. The rate is determined by the SIMV RATE control knob, which is set lower than the BREATHS/MIN knob. The BREATHS/MIN knob determines the time of a mandatory breath delivery. V_T is still determined by the $\dot{V}_E$ and the BREATHS/MIN rate settings. This mode is divided into different time frames (Figure 10-89), as follows:

1. An SIMV-cycle, which is the period of time between mandatory breaths (SIMV-cycle = 60 ÷ SIMV-rate setting)
2. An SIMV-period, which is the time allotted for each mandatory breath (SIMV-period = 60 ÷ BREATHS/MIN knob setting)
3. A spontaneous breathing period, which equals the SIMV-cycle minus the SIMV-period

For example, with the BREATHS/MIN knob set at 15 breaths/min and the SIMV rate is set at 6 breaths/min, the following are true:

- SIMV-cycle = 60/6 = 10 seconds
- SIMV-period = 60/15 = 4 seconds
- Spontaneous breathing period = 10 seconds − 4 seconds = 6 seconds

Figure 10-89 helps explain the spacing of breaths in SIMV. When the patient triggers a breath, the ventilator delivers a volume-targeted, time-cycled breath. The patient can then breathe spontaneously at the baseline pressure. The SIMV-cycle is timed from the beginning of the mandatory breath. When this time has elapsed, the ventilator waits for a patient effort during the SIMV period that follows. An effort sufficient to trigger a breath during this period will deliver the set volume. If the patient fails to take a breath during this period, the ventilator will time-trigger a mandatory breath.

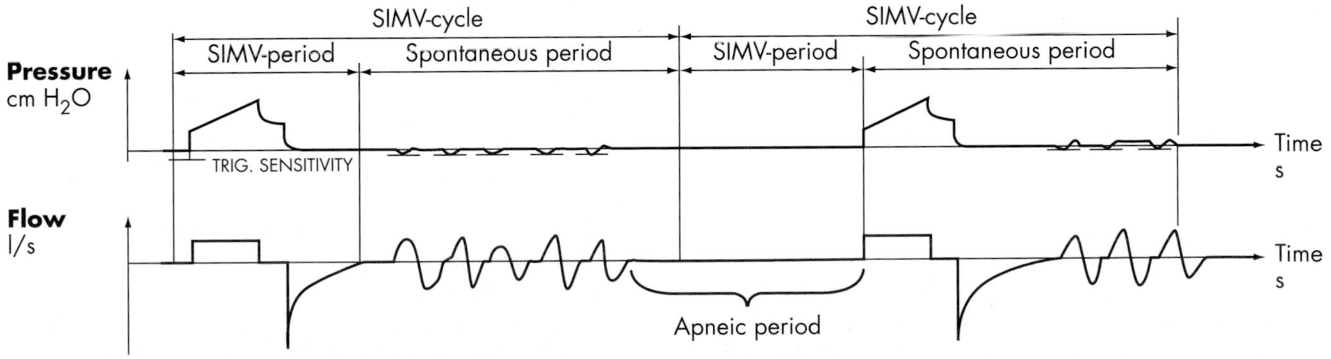

Figure 10-89 The SIMV cycle. (Courtesy Siemens Medical Systems, Inc., Danvers, Mass.)

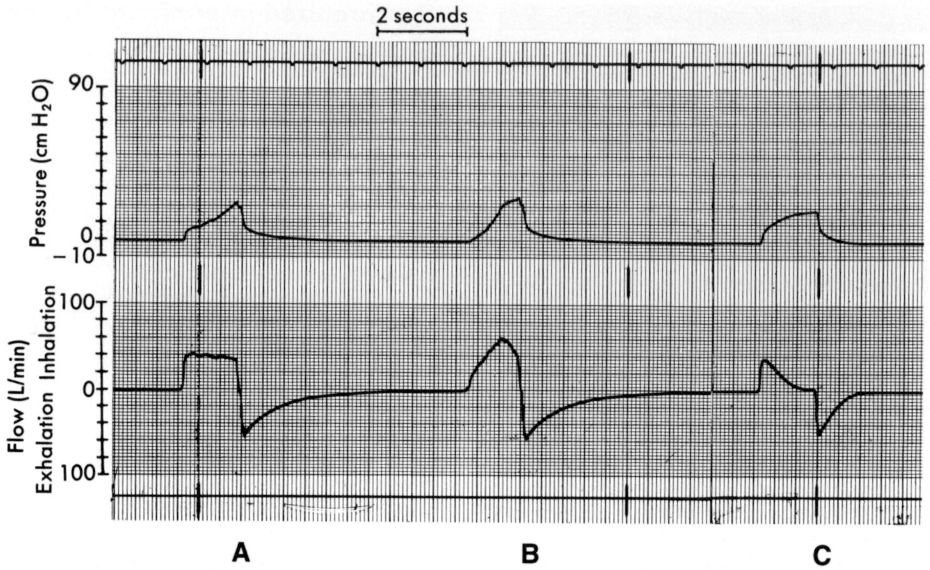

Figure 10-90 Flow and pressure patterns for the Servo 900B. Lung analog is set for 50 mL/cm H_2O compliance and 5 cm H_2O/L/sec resistance. **A,** the flow waveform is constant (rectangular). **B,** the flow waveform is a sine-wavelike pattern. **C,** working pressure is reduced to 20 cm H_2O, and the lung analog is set for 10 mL/cm H_2O compliance and 5 cm H_2O/L/sec resistance. Note the descending shape of flow curve with increased load and reduced working pressure. (Courtesy Siemens Medical Systems, Inc., Danvers, Mass.)

SIMV + Pressure Support

SIMV + pressure support is the same as SIMV described above except that spontaneous breaths are pressure-supported at the level indicated on the inspiratory pressure above PEEP control.

Continuous Positive Airway Pressure (CPAP)

CPAP is a purely spontaneous mode that provides the option of a positive-pressure baseline (0 to 50 cm H_2O).

Manual

The manual mode is generally restricted to use in the operating room in conjunction with an anesthetic bag and a manual ventilation valve (accessory equipment). The manual ventilation valve is attached to the ventilator's outflow port and connected to the inspiratory line of the patient circuit, similar to an anesthetic system. When circuit pressure rises above 4 cm H_2O during manual inflation, the expiratory valve closes and gas goes to the patient. When pressure drops below 4 cm H_2O during expiration, the expiration valve opens. When circuit pressure is less than 2 cm H_2O, demand flow fills the bag. The amount of flow into the bag is determined by the preset $\dot{V}_E$. The apnea alarm does not work in this mode. A patient can breathe spontaneously from the circuit as long as the inspiratory effort is great enough to open the valve (-2 cm H_2O).

Troubleshooting

The flow pattern on the 900C can only be maintained when adequate working pressure is set. Driving force can be reduced so that the peak pressure generated during a mechanical breath is nearly equal to the working pressure inside the bellows. Flow will then decrease or taper during inspiration, and V_T will be variable (Figure 10-90).

Use caution when reducing the breaths/min rate. As the rate drops, the V_T increases. For example, if the $\dot{V}_E$ is 5 L/min and the rate is 10 breaths/min, V_T is 0.5 L. Decreasing the rate to 6 breaths/min raises the V_T to 0.83 L. For this reason, it is usually advisable to reduce volume before rate when making a $\dot{V}_E$ change.

There is a troubleshooting section in the operating manual to help identify common problems. For additional information check the manufacturer's web site: www.siemens.vents.

Review Questions

(See Appendix A for answers.)

1. Which type of internal drive mechanism is used in the Servo 900C?
   a. linear drive piston
   b. proportioning valve
   c. spring-loaded bellows
   d. rotary drive piston

2. To estimate the auto-PEEP level with the Servo 900C, which control is used?
   a. T_I %
   b. PAUSE TIME %
   c. EXPIRATORY PAUSE HOLD
   d. GAS CHANGE

3. The inspiratory servo valve consists of which components?
   I. a scissorlike valve controlled by a stepper motor
   II. a bacterial filter
   III. an inspiratory flow transducer
   IV. an electromagnetic solenoid
   a. I only
   b. I and III
   c. II and IV
   d. III and IV

4. Where should the working pressure be set?
   a. 10 cm H_2O above PEEP
   b. 5 cm H_2O above the patient's plateau pressure
   c. 120 cm H_2O
   d. above the peak pressure for the patient

5. During ventilation in the SIMV mode, the therapist has set the SIMV rate at 10 breaths/min, but notes that the patient is receiving 8 mandatory breaths/min. The most likely cause of this is:
   a. the patient is triggering additional mandatory breaths
   b. the SIMV-RATE toggle switch is in the up position
   c. the BREATHS/MIN control set at 8 breaths/min
   d. the SIMV rate cannot go as high as 10 breaths/min

6. If the T_I % is set at 33%, the pause time is at 5%, and the rate is 10 breaths/min, what is the approximate T_I?
   a. 1.5 seconds
   b. 2.3 seconds
   c. 3.0 seconds
   d. 6.0 seconds

7. The 900C has a built-in oxygen analyzer—true or false?

8. If a patient becomes apneic during SIMV ventilation with a mandatory rate of 3 breaths/min, the APNEA alarm activates—true or false?

9. The $\dot{V}_E$ control is set at 12 L/min, the BREATHS/MIN at 12, flow is constant, and T_I % is 20% (inspiratory pause is 0%) during volume ventilation on the Servo 900C. What are the V_T, T_I, and inspiratory flow?

10. During pressure control on the Servo 900C, what control determines the inspiratory pressure, and does this value include the baseline pressure?

References

1. Mushin WW, et al: Automatic ventilation of the lungs, ed 3, Oxford, 1980, Mosby.
2. Siemens-Elema Servo Ventilator 900 operating manual, ME 461/5098.101,1974; and Servo Ventilator 900B preliminary supplement to operating manual, Solna, Sweden, 1974, Siemens-Elema AB.
3. Ingestedt S, et al: A servo-controlled ventilator measuring expired minute ventilation, airway flow and pressure, Acta Anaesthesiol Scand Suppl, 47:9, 1972.
4. MacGregor, Mike: Personal communication, March 1998.

Siemens Servo 300

OUTLINE

LEARNING OBJECTIVES

Upon completion of this section, the reader should be able to:

1. Label a diagram of the internal components of the Servo 300.
2. Explain the function of the controls on the operating panel of the Servo 300 and compare measured with set digital display values.
3. Recommend a safe method for changing rate and V_T settings on the Servo 300.
4. Assess an alarm situation and recommend an action to correct the problem.
5. Compare each of the modes of ventilation on the Servo 300, including a review of triggering and cycling mechanisms and breath delivery (volume vs. pressure).
6. Explain the use of the select parameter guide (SPG) for setting up controls when switching to a new mode of ventilation.
7. Describe the function of volume support, PRVC, and Automode.

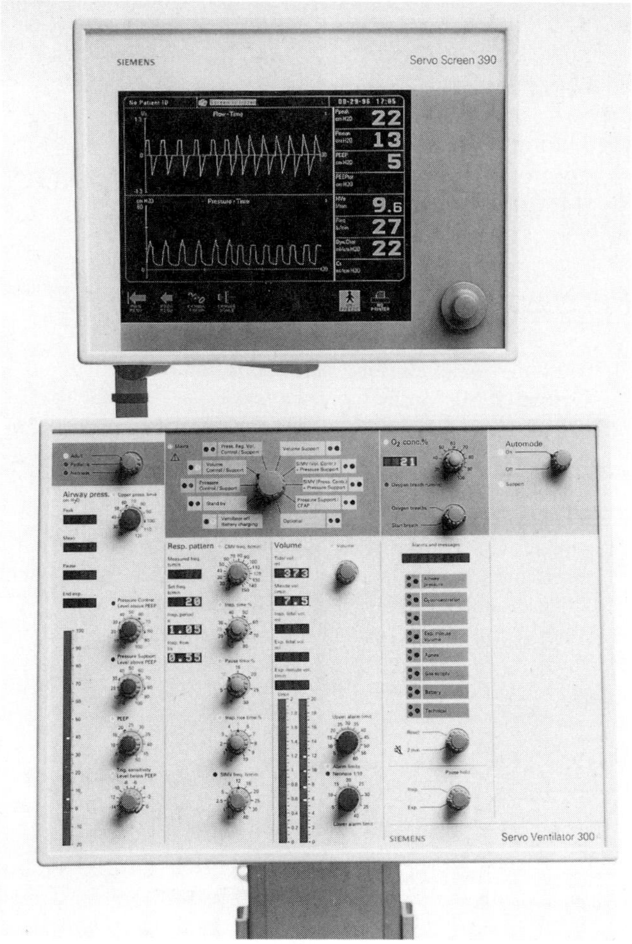

Figure 10-91 The Servo 300A with the graphics monitor on top. (Courtesy Siemens-Elema AB, Solna, Sweden.)

The Servo 300 Ventilator[1-3] is manufactured by the Siemens-Elema AB Medical Systems Corporation (Solna, Sweden) primarily for use in the ICU for neonatal, pediatric, or adult patients. It consists of two sections connected by a 2.9-meter cable. One section is the control or operating panel. The other is the patient unit, which connects directly to the patient circuit. The patient circuit consists of a main inspiratory and a main expiratory line.

The control panel contains the electronic circuits that control ventilator function (Figure 10-91). It also contains the touch pads and dials through which the operator selects specific patient settings. The control panel provides illuminated information about selected parameters (green digital display) and measured parameters (red digital display). The patient unit controls the flow of gas to the patient. Flow and pressure are continually measured within the patient unit and compared with the control panel and adjusted as needed. Practitioners often purchase the graphics monitor and an end-tidal carbon dioxide module as important additional items for monitoring patients.

Power Source

A standard 110- or 120-volt electrical outlet provides power to the display unit and the microprocessor-control unit. Two 50-psig (range from 29 to 94 psig) gas sources for air and oxygen are also normally used to power the Servo 300 and to provide the flow to the patient (single-circuit ventilator). (The unit can function with a single high-pressure gas source, but O_2% delivery may be altered.) This ventilator also contains two internal 12-volt batteries that provide back-up electrical power. The discussion of alarm features in this section reviews ventilator operation when either the electrical power or the gas supply fails.

The ON power switch is on the front panel at the top center of the ventilator control panel and is the same control that allows the operator to switch modes of ventilation (Figure 10-91). Switching to any of the ventilator modes activates the ventilator. Switching it from any mode back to the VENTILATOR OFF BATTERY CHARGING setting turns the ventilator off, but also activates an audible alert. In older models, the FAB (failure alarm box) alarm control was on the top, left side of the ventilator and was pressed to deactivate. In newer models, the FAB alarm is internal and does not require deactivation.

Internal Mechanisms

The flow delivery of gas to the patient is controlled by a high-performance, rapid-response (4 to 6 milliseconds) solenoid valve. Figure 10-92 shows the internal components of the Servo 300. The air and oxygen sources enter through separate gas inlets (*1* and *2*). They pass through bacterial filters and enter the gas modules where pressures are monitored (*3*). The two gas sources leave their respective modules and enter a mixing chamber, and pressure is again measured (*4*). Knowing the pressures within the modules and mixing chamber, the flow solenoid can determine the operation of the pin or needle valve that controls gas flow into the unit. The exiting gas is again measured for pressure (*5*) as it enters the inspiratory line (*6*). The inspiratory line houses a pressure release or a safety valve (120 cm H_2O maximum), the housing for the oxygen analyzer (*7*), and the main outlet for gas going from the ventilator to the patient (*8*).

The patient's expired gas passes into the ventilator through the connector for the main expiratory line (*9*), where expiratory gas flow (*10*) and pressure (*11*) are measured. (Note that patient circuit pressures are monitored by both the inspiratory (*5*) and the expiratory (*11*) pressure transducers. Transducers also monitor flow for flow triggering.)

Gas then passes through the expiratory valve (*12*), which helps control the phasing (inspiration/expiration) of a breath and the level of PEEP present in the expiratory line. The expiratory valve, also called a gate valve, contains a soft, compressible tube that passes between two rollers. These rollers float and come together to adjust resistance to expiration when PEEP is employed and also open and

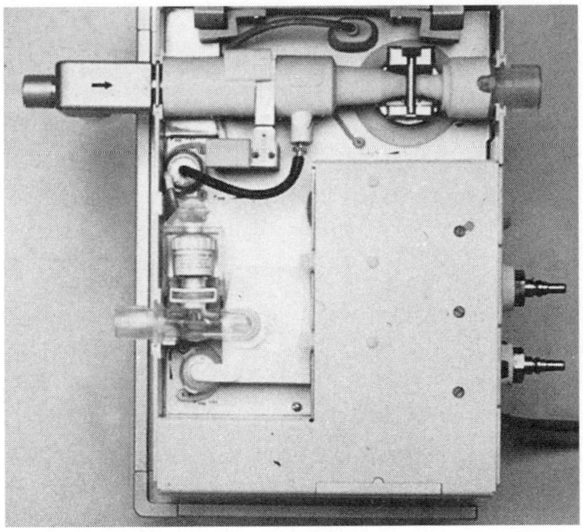

A

B

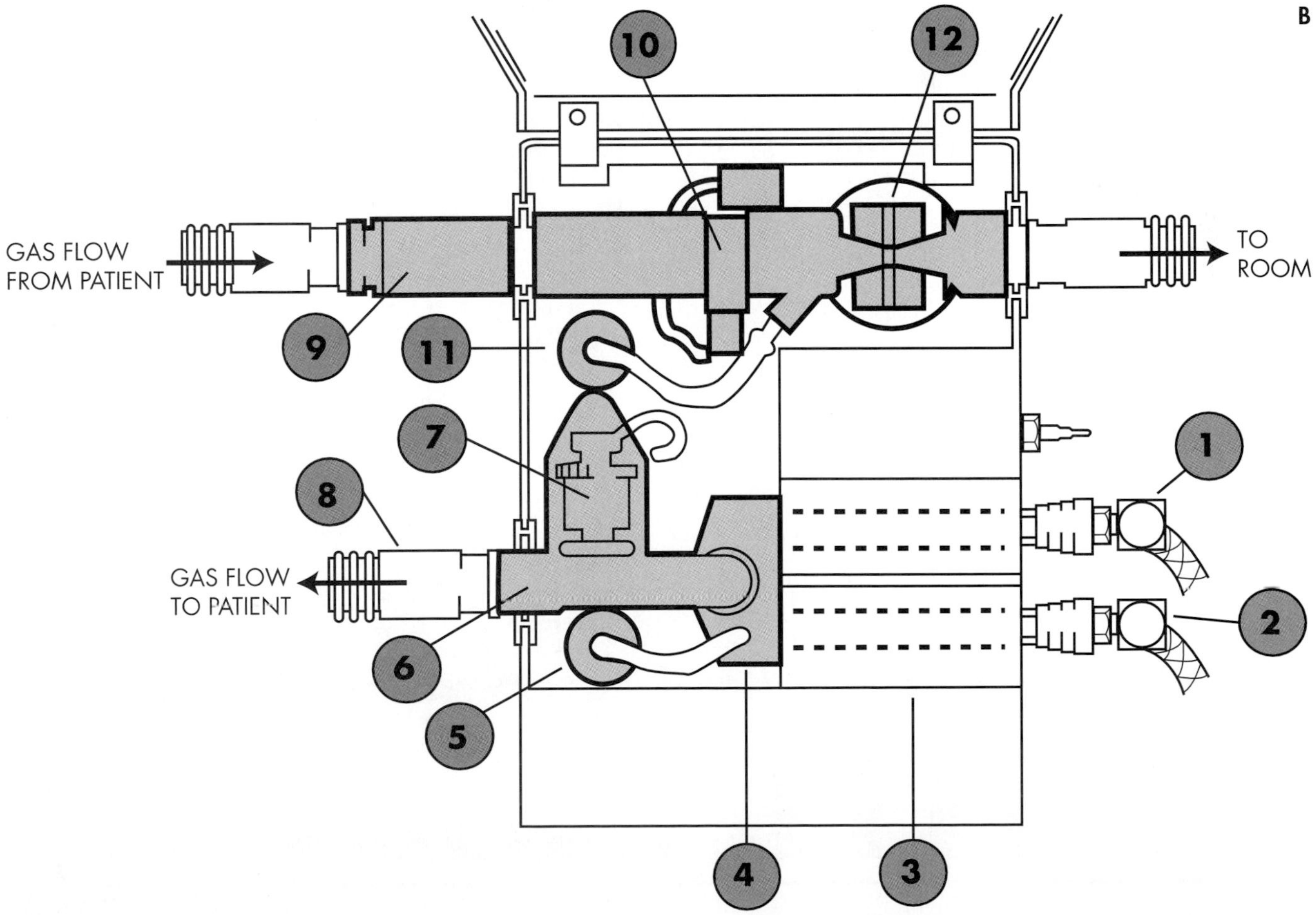

Figure 10-92 Internal components of the Siemens Servo 300. **A,** a photograph of the internal components. (Courtesy Siemens-Elema AB, Solna, Sweden.) **B,** a diagram of the internal components (see text for explanation).

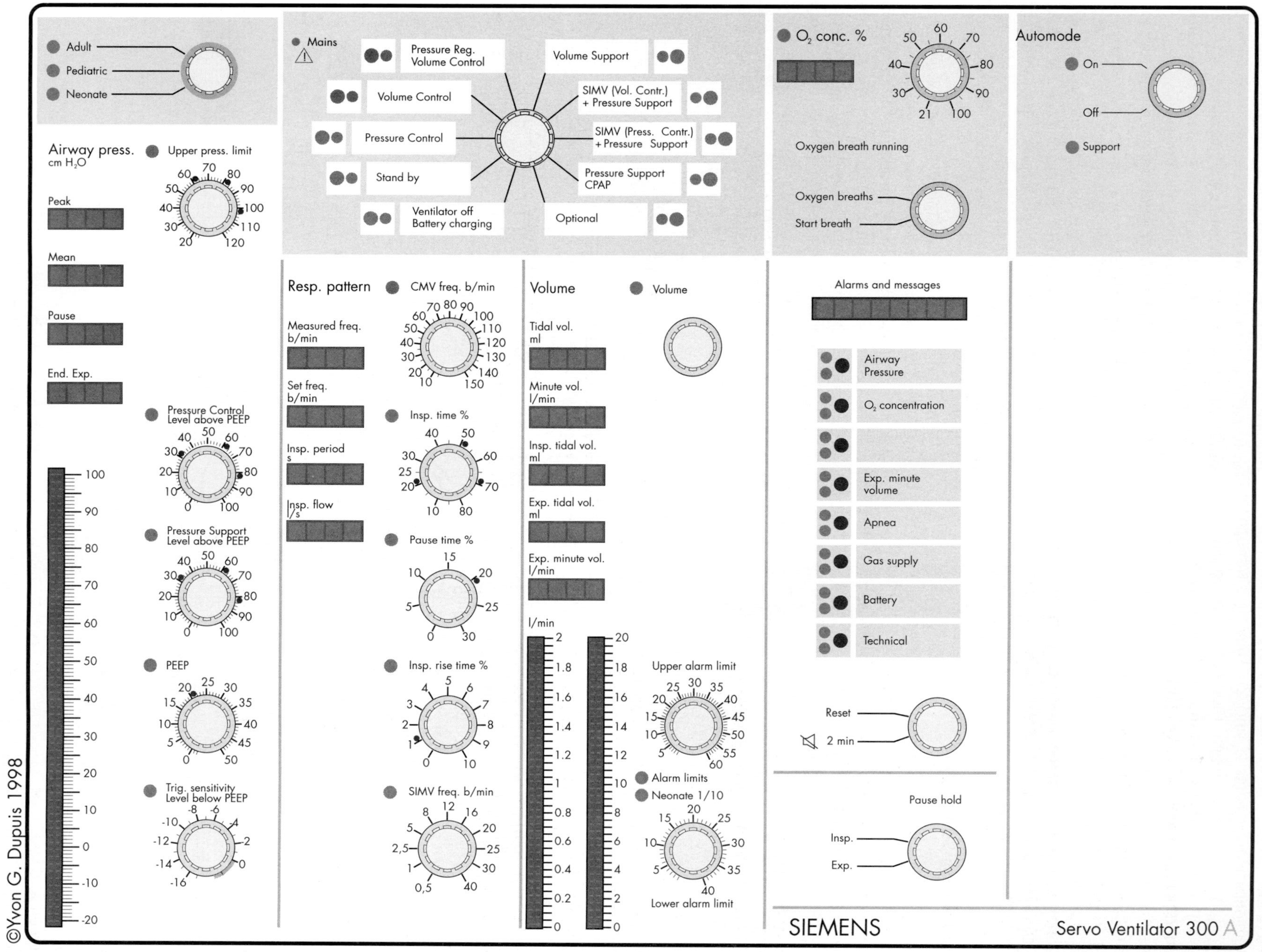

Figure 10-93 The front control panel of the Siemens Servo 300A. (Courtesy Yvon Dupuis.)

close to allow phasing of a breath. The gas then passes out of the ventilator through the expiratory one-way valve (*13*).

CONTROLS AND ALARMS

The control panel contains nine sections (Figure 10 93), which include the following: 1) PATIENT RANGE SELECTION, 2) AIRWAY PRESSURES, 3) MODE SELECTION, 4) RESPIRATORY PATTERN, 5) VOLUMES, 6) OXYGEN CONCENTRATION, 7) ALARMS, MESSAGES, and ALARM SILENCE/RESET, 8) PAUSE HOLD, and 9) AUTOMODE.

Patient Range Selection

The PATIENT RANGE SELECTION knob at the upper left corner lets the operator pick the appropriate patient size: ADULT, PEDIATRIC, or NEONATE. This selection affects several ventilator parameters (Table 10-37).

Airway Pressures

The left panel contains four pressure controls, one control for TRIGGER SENSITIVITY, four digital monitors of airway pressure, and a bar graph display of monitored pressure.

The four pressure controls are as follows:

1. UPPER PRESSURE LIMIT (16 to 120 cm H_2O)
2. PRESSURE-CONTROL LEVEL ABOVE PEEP (0 to 100 cm H_2O)
3. PRESSURE-SUPPORT LEVEL ABOVE PEEP (0 to 100 cm H_2O)
4. PEEP (0 to 50 cm H_2O)

The UPPER PRESSURE LIMIT is for patient safety and limits the maximum airway pressure in all modes of ventilation. If the upper pressure limit is reached during breath delivery, inspiration ends and an audible alarm activates. The PRESSURE CONTROL knob is active in two modes of ventilation: Pressure control and SIMV (press.contr.) + pressure support. The PRESSURE SUPPORT knob is active in three modes: pressure support, SIMV (vol.contr.) + pressure support, and SIMV (press.contr.) + pressure support. These are discussed in the following section on mode selection. PEEP sets pressure during exhalation in any mode currently available.

The TRIG. SENSITIVITY LEVEL BELOW PEEP is the knob that determines the patient effort required to trigger a breath and is active in all modes. It provides flow- or pressure-triggering. Pressure triggering is set by turning the knob counterclockwise to the indicated pressures (0 to -17 cm H_2O). This reduces the sensitivity, making triggering more difficult. The flow-triggering setting is indicated by the green and red (most sensitive) markings on the dial. With FLOW-TRIGGERING selected, a low flow of gas passes through the patient circuit only during the expiratory phase and is monitored by both the inspiratory and expiratory flow transducers. Flow-triggering of a breath occurs when the expiratory flow transducer measures a drop in flow (see Chapter 9). The set bias flow in the Servo 300 is based on the size of patient selected (ADULT, PEDIATRIC, or NEONATAL; see Table 10-37). For example, when ADULT is selected on the patient selection switch, 2 L/min flows through the circuit during exhalation. The flow-trigger range for an adult is 0.7 to 2 L/min, depending on where the operator sets the TRIGGERING SENSITIVITY dial. The closer to the red area, the less the amount of flow that must be removed and the more sensitive the triggering.

The airway pressure monitors provide illuminated red digital readouts of measured values for peak, pause, and

TABLE 10-37

Parameters and functions affected by patient range selections

Continuous flow through the circuit during exhalation	
Adult setting	2 L/min
Pediatric setting	1 L/min
Neonatal setting	0.5 L/min
Maximum inspiratory peak flow	
Adult setting	200 L/min
Pediatric setting	33 L/min
Neonatal setting	13 L/min
Maximum measured tidal volume	
Adult setting	3999 mL (range 0 to 4000 mL)
Pediatric setting	399 mL (range 0 to 400 mL)
Neonatal setting	39 mL (range 0 to 40 mL)
Apnea alarm time	
Adult setting	20 seconds
Pediatric setting	15 seconds
Neonatal setting	10 seconds
Flow trigger range	
Adult setting	0.7 to 2.0 L/min
Pediatric setting	0.3 to 1.0 L/min
Neonatal setting	0.17 to 0.5 L/min
Upper alarm limit—minute ventilation	
Adult setting	0 to 60 L/min
Pediatric setting	0 to 60 L/min
Neonatal setting	0 to 6 L/min
Lower alarm limit—minute ventilation	
Adult setting	0.3 to 40 L/min
Pediatric setting	0.3 to 40 L/min
Neonatal setting	0.06 to 4 L/min

end-expiratory pressures and a calculated value for mean pressure. PIP is the highest pressure reached during inspiration, as measured by the inspiratory pressure transducer. It is displayed on the pressure bar graph, which is described later in this section. The upper pressure limit uses this value for its operation, but the digital display value of PIP is the pressure measured by the expiratory pressure transducer. Mean pressure is a calculated value based on the pressure measured during each complete breath cycle (inspiration plus expiration). Pause pressure displays the pressure measured by the expiratory pressure transducer when a pause time is selected on the PAUSE TIME % control or when the manual inspiratory pause (INSP.) is held during inspiration long enough for a pause to occur. It can be activated whenever a mandatory volume or pressure breath occurs in SIMV or A/C modes. The end-expiratory pressure display shows the pressure at the end of each breath and is also measured by the expiratory pressure transducer. When an expiratory pause is manually activated, both the inspiratory and expiratory valves close and this window display shows the value for total PEEP ($PEEP_I$ + $PEEP_E$) as measured by the ventilator.

The airway pressure bar graph has flashing diodes of various colors, which monitor several pressure values. The diodes on the left side are red. The diodes on the right have different colors, depending on the pressure level. The right diodes are yellow for values less than 0 cm H_2O, green for values from 0 to 40 cm H_2O, yellow for values from 40 to 60 cm H_2O, and red for values from 60 to 100 cm H_2O. The upper pressure limit is indicated by four diodes (two on the left, two on the right) that flash when the pressure limit is reached or when it is set above 100 cm H_2O. The lower diodes on the bar graph indicate the pressure settings.

The actual airway pressure is shown by two side-by-side flashing diodes. The left one shows pressure measured by the inspiratory transducer and the right one shows that measured by the expiratory pressure transducer. Because they are measured at different places, you will see separations occurring between the two when they reflect pressure variations such as the rebound of pressure within the patient circuit or resistance to expiratory flow in the circuit. The value for the peak pressure digital display corresponds to the right illuminated diode (Figure 10-94). The pressure-control, the pressure-support, and the PEEP settings are shown by two diodes. If pressure support is set higher than pressure control, the diodes indicating both controls start flashing. PEEP is the lowest set of diodes because PC and PS are additive to the set PEEP value.

A patient-triggered breath is indicated on the bar graph by two red and yellow flashing diodes that appear on the bottom right.

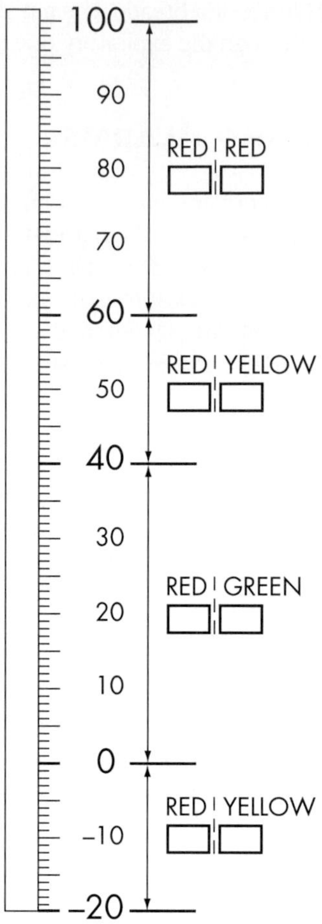

Figure 10-94 An airway pressure bar graph for the Servo 300 ventilator. (Courtesy Siemens-Elema AB, Solna, Sweden.)

Mode Selection

At the top center of the control panel is a rotating knob with nine different positions (see Figure 10-93). These include VENTILATOR OFF BATTERY CHARGING, STAND BY, PRESSURE CONTROL, VOLUME CONTROL, PRESSURE REG VOLUME CONTROL, VOLUME SUPPORT, SIMV (VOL.CONTR.) + PRESSURE SUPPORT, SIMV (PRESS.CONTR.) + PRESSURE SUPPORT, PRESSURE SUPPORT—CPAP, and OPTIONAL.

VENTILATOR OFF BATTERY CHARGING is the OFF position for the ventilator. Keeping the ventilator plugged into an electrical outlet with the knob in this position recharges the internal battery. The manufacturer recommends this as the best option for the ventilator when it is not in use. When the ventilator is in the STANDBY position, the electrical circuits are supplied with power and the expiratory flow transducer can warm to its operating temperature (104° F, 40° C). Patient settings can be selected for use while the ventilator is in STAND BY. The seven ventilator modes are described in the discussion of modes of operation later in this section. The OPTIONAL position of the mode knob has no function, but can be used to add future upgrades.

Respiratory Pattern Settings

Below the panel that contains the selection knob for the modes is a panel that controls the respiratory pattern and

BOX 10-138

Decision Making & Problem Solving

The respiratory therapist decides to use IRV on a patient who is difficult to oxygenate with the Servo 300 in volume control. The INSP. TIME % control is turned to 80%, and the PAUSE TIME % to 10%. The yellow light next to the PAUSE TIME % control begins to flash. What does this indicate?

See Appendix A for the answer.

digitally displays the selected and measured values. There are a total of five control knobs: CMV FREQ. B/MIN, INSP.TIME%, PAUSE TIME %, INSP.RISE TIME%, and SIMV FREQ.F/MIN. There are also four digital display panels: MEASURED FREQ. B/MIN, SET FREQ.B/MIN, INSP. PERIOD S, and INSP. FLOW L/S.

The control marked CMV FREQ. B/MIN sets the number of breaths/minute when volume control, pressure control, or pressure-regulated volume control are set on the MODE SELECTION knob (5 to 150 breaths/min). These are described as control modes by the manufacturer in relation to the new feature Automode, which is described in the discussion of ventilator modes later in this chapter. It is recommended that the CMV FREQ. B/MIN knob always be set appropriately for the patient being ventilated because it determines the TCT (breath cycle time) for all modes. The ventilator does not permit T_I to exceed 80% of this TCT. In addition, CMV FREQ.B/MIN is the back-up rate for volume support, if the patient becomes apneic.

INSP. TIME % determines the percentage of time spent providing inspiratory gas flow (10% to 80%) based on the TCT. All mandatory breaths in either volume- or pressure-control ventilation are time-cycled in either A/C or SIMV modes. PAUSE TIME % (0 to 30% of TCT) provides an inspiratory pause (no inspiratory gas flow) and increases the length of inspiration for a volume-controlled breath. The sum of inspiratory time and pause time can *never* exceed 80% of the total cycle time, as determined by the rate set on the CMV FREQ. B/MIN knob—regardless of the ventilator mode (Box 10-138). If the sum of these two settings exceeds 80%, the adjacent yellow indicator light flashes.

INSP. RISE TIME % determines the time (% of TCT) in which the flow or pressure will gradually rise to the set value in any mode of ventilation. INSP. RISE TIME % is considered a patient comfort feature in adults and a lung protective strategy in newborns because it prevents pressure overshoots. As long as the value is set above zero (ranges from 0% to 10% of TCT), the delivery of pressure and flow is tapered and does not instantly increase to the set value at the beginning of inspiration. Figure 10-95 shows how sloping affects pressure and flow delivery. At the zero setting there is no sloping, and pressure and flow rise rapidly. This can be uncomfortable for a patient and can cause oscillations or ringing in the patient circuit (see Figure 9-66). The maximum rise time setting of 10% gives the maximum time for tapering flow and pressure delivery as well as a more gradual rise to the set parameters.

SIMV FREQ. B/MIN determines the number of breaths per minute when either SIMV mode is selected (range: 0.5 to 40 breaths/min). It must be set at a value lower than the CMV FREQ. B/MIN control, or the ventilator will default to the frequency set on the CMV FREQ. B/MIN and the yellow light adjacent to the SIMV FREQ. B/MIN control will flash.

The display panels in this section provide information about the respiratory pattern. MEASURED FREQ. B/MIN indicates in red the total of all breaths (spontaneous and mandatory) measured by the ventilator. SET FREQ. B/MIN shows the set rate in green for A/C and SIMV modes. INSP. PERIOD S. provides the calculated T_I (in seconds) for mandatory breaths. INSP. FLOW L/S shows the calculated flow (in liters per second) based on the TCT, set volume, and T_I for mandatory volume breaths.

The TCT, flow (in liters/min), and the set I:E ratio can be obtained from the ventilator without manual calculations. Simply touch the pad next to the STANDBY setting, and immediately touch the touch pad next to the mode setting selected for the patient. (You don't have to press hard on these touch pads because they are light-sensitive, not touch- or pressure-sensitive.) This causes the digital display windows in this panel to read as follows:

1. SET FREQ. B/MIN will show "(t)s" alternating with a numerical display of the calculated TCT (in seconds).
2. INSP. PERIOD S will show "I:E" alternating with a numerical display of the set I:E ratio.*
3. INSP. FLOW L/S will show "/min" alternating with a numerical display of the calculated flow (in liters/minute). (This is only shown when volume ventilation modes are in use.)

In addition to these readings, the yellow light indicators adjacent to functional controls in the selected mode will flash. To return to the normal display function, touch the STANDBY touch pad again. The normal display will also resume if a minute passes without any operator intervention.

Volume Settings and Displays

The V_T and $\dot{V}_E$ are set using the VOLUME control, which is active during the following modes: volume control, pressure regulated volume control, volume support, and SIMV

*This is the set ratio and not a measurement of the I:E ratio. If the patient triggers a breath, this can shorten T_E and alter the set I:E ratio.

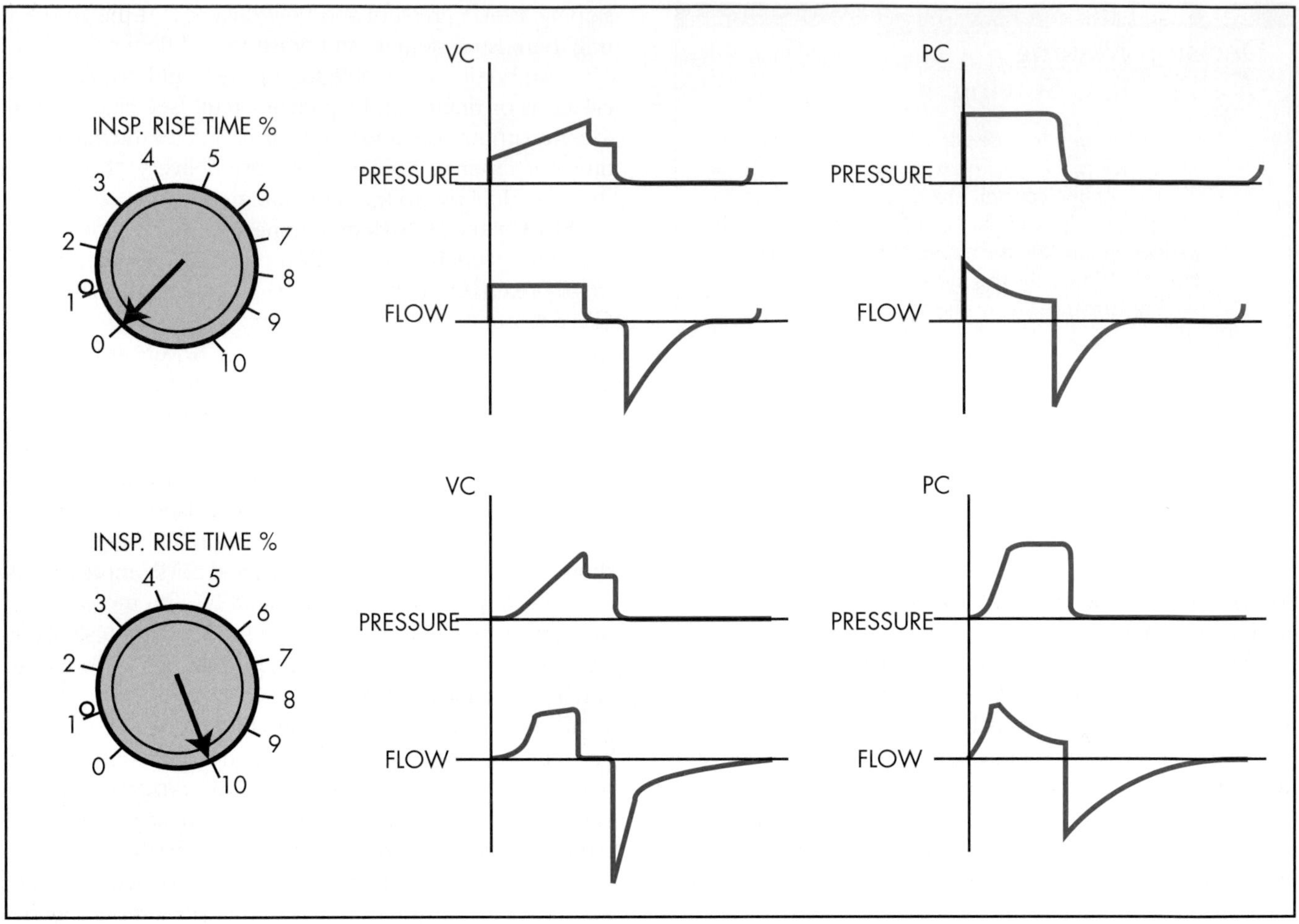

Figure 10-95 Inspiratory rise time percentage. During volume-control ventilation (*left curves*), flow is normally constant when the inspiratory rise time percentage is set at zero (*top left*). The use of inspiratory rise time tapers the beginning of the flow curve (*bottom left*). During pressure ventilation (*right curves*), flow is normally a descending ramp (*top right*). Use of an inspiratory rise time percentage above zero tapers the beginning of the flow curve (*bottom right*).

(Vol.Contr.) + pressure support. The available V_T range can vary depending on the size of the patient selected (see Table 10-37). All measured flows and set and indicated volumes are referenced to standard conditions (1013 mbar, 760 mmHg). To obtain a reading of ambient conditions, the operating manual provides the required conversion calculations and necessary tables. This provision might be significant at high altitude environments (e.g., 5,000 to 10,000 ft), and the reader is referred to the operator's manual.

There are two volume reading displays for the set values. TIDAL VOL. ML shows the set V_T (in milliliters) as a green digital number. MINUTE VOL. L/MIN shows the set $\dot{V}_E$ (in liters/minute; as a green number) for volume ventilation in A/C ("volume control") or SIMV ("SIMV [Vol.Contr.] + pressure support"). Also provided are values for $\dot{V}_E$ (green) in pressure-regulated volume control (PRVC) and volume support modes of ventilation.

Measured volumes are provided by the following three windows that give digital values illuminated in red:

1. INSP. TIDAL VOL. ML provides the volume of each breath as measured by the inspiratory flow transducer during delivery from the ventilator outflow port. Monitored range is 50 to 3999 mL for adult settings, 10 to 399 mL for pediatric settings, and 2.0 to 39 mL for neonatal settings. If the measured value exceeds the range for the patient size selected (see Table 10-37), the number flashes and an OVERRANGE alarm occurs (see the discussion of alarms later in this section).
2. EXP. TIDAL VOL. ML displays the volume measured by the expiratory flow transducer for each breath coming back through the ventilator's expiratory port connection. Monitored ranges are the same as those for inspired V_T. As with inspired volumes, if the value exceeds the set range, the number flashes. When no leaks

BOX 10-139

Important Clinical Note

The Servo is primarily a $\dot{V}_E$-based ventilator. This affects V_T delivery when the rate ("CMV freq.b/min") is adjusted. For example, suppose $\dot{V}_E = 5$ L/min ($V_T = 0.5$ L and f = 10 breaths/min). If you decrease f to 5 breaths/min, V_T will increase to 1.0 L to maintain $\dot{V}_E$. When you need to reduce the mandatory rate, it is recommended that you reduce the V_T (by 1/2 to 1/3) first.

BOX 10-140

Important Clinical Note

When "Oxygen Breaths" is activated, the following alarms are silenced for a maximum of 55 seconds:

- Oxygen alarm
- Expired $\dot{V}_E$ alarm
- Apnea alarm
- Technical alarm for overrange

are present, inspiratory and expiratory values are approximately equal.

3. EXP. MINUTE VOL. L/MIN indicates the measured exhaled $\dot{V}_E$ in red numbers. The display range is from 4.0 to 60 L/min for adults, 1.0 to 5.0 L/min for pediatric patients, and 0.20 to 1.50 L/min for neonatal patients (Box 10-139). (Expired $\dot{V}_E$ is calculated by using a digital low-pass filter of the expiratory flow with time constants: 10.5 seconds in adults, 4.9 seconds in pediatric patients, and 3.4 seconds in neonates.)

In this same section of the control panel are indicators and controls for the minute ventilation alarms. There are UPPER and LOWER MINUTE VOLUME ALARM controls, the scale of which varies depending on the patient range (due to size) selected (see Table 10-37). There is also a volume bar graph that provides indicators for various minute ventilation parameters. Colored diodes are red on the left side of the bar and green on the right. The set UPPER ALARM LIMIT is indicated by two red and two green diodes and is read at the lower two diodes. When the UPPER MINUTE VENTILATION LIMIT is set above 20 L/min, the lower two diodes start flashing. When the UPPER $\dot{V}_E$ alarm is exceeded, all four diodes flash. The monitored (measured) $\dot{V}_E$ is shown by one red and one green flashing diode. The set $\dot{V}_E$ is shown by one red and one green nonflashing diode. The measured $\dot{V}_E$ is superimposed on the set $\dot{V}_E$ when these values are equal. The LOWER $\dot{V}_E$ alarm limit is indicated by two red and two green diodes at the bottom of the volume bar graph. When the set lower alarm limit is violated, the diodes flash. (Note that the LOWER $\dot{V}_E$ alarm functions as the disconnect alarm. If the measured $\dot{V}_E$ falls below the lower alarm limit, the diodes flash.)

Oxygen Concentration

In the upper right section of the control panel is a control knob for adjusting the FiO_2 DELIVERY (0.21 to 1.0). UPPER and LOWER FiO_2 alarms are automatically set internally by the microprocessor at 0.06 (6%) above and below the selected FiO_2. The absolute minimum alarm limit is 0.18 (18%). There is a digital display of the set oxygen concentration. An internal oxygen analyzer continuously monitors oxygen delivery.

Near the OXYGEN control is a knob marked OXYGEN BREATHS/START BREATH. When the switch is turned to OXYGEN BREATHS, the ventilator provides 100% oxygen for 20 breaths or for 1 minute—whichever comes first, and switches back to the present oxygen delivery setting. A yellow indicator light labeled "oxygen breath running" lights when this control has been activated, and the display window reads "O_2 conc. %." This 100% oxygen delivery can be canceled by turning the switch to OXYGEN BREATHS again before 20 breaths or 1 minute has passed (Box 10-140).

The other side of this control knob is the START BREATH control, which is similar in some ways to the MANUAL BREATH control on other ventilators. When activated, a breath based on the set control values is delivered. In the SIMV mode, this activates a mandatory breath. It is important to allow the patient time to exhale before activating this breath delivery.

Alarms, Messages, and Alarm Silence/Reset

The ALARM section is on the right side of the PATIENT CONTROL panel. Small lights in this section are yellow or red. A steady yellow light indicates two possible conditions: either a high-priority alarm condition has been corrected, and the alarm condition has been stored in memory; or certain alarm limits have been overridden, and the alarm has been turned off manually. Another indicator is an audible caution (ticking) sound that occurs under a few special conditions and acts as a reminder to the user. For example, ticking occurs under the following conditions:

- The oxygen cell is disconnected.
- An error is detected in either a flow or a pressure transducer.
- The ventilator is placed in the stand-by mode.
- The ventilator is operating on battery power.
- Only one high-pressure gas source is being used.

A red flashing light and a sound signal a high-priority alarm condition requiring immediate attention. Table 10-38 lists the high-priority alarms in order of importance.

TABLE 10-38

All high alarm functions for the Servo 300 (in order of priority)

Technical errors—try restarting unit
Power failure test
Internal RAM (random access memory) test
Internal ROM (read-only memory) test
Internal CPU (central processing unit) test
Ref and timing micro module (MM) error
Mixer MM error
Panel MM error
Range switch error
Mode switch error

Operating error	Check function
Airway pressure	Airway pressure too high
Apnea	Apnea alarm
Expired $\dot{V}_E$	V_E too low/high
O_2 concentration	O_2 concentration too low/high
O_2 cell disconnect	O_2 sensor
No battery capacity left	No battery capacity
Limited battery capacity left	Limited battery capacity
High battery voltage	Internal battery voltage too high
Mains failure	Battery
Pressure transducer error	Check tubing
Power failure	Technical error (see operating manual)
O_2 potentiometer error	Technical error (see operating manual)
Out of gas	Check pneumatic power source
Gas supply air	Check pneumatic power source
Gas supply O_2	Check pneumatic power source
High continuous pressure	High continuous pressure
CMV potentiometer error	Technical error (see operating manual)
Servo Control Module (SCM)	Technical error (see operating manual)
	Microprocessor error
Overrange	Overrange: select pediatric/adult
Barometer error	Technical error (see operating manual)
Regulation pressure limited	Limited pressure

There are seven alarm indicators—eight in some versions (CO_2 concentration)—in this section of the control panel: AIRWAY PRESSURE, OXYGEN CONCENTRATION, EXPIRATORY MINUTE VOLUME, APNEA ALARM, GAS SUPPLY, BATTERY, and TECHNICAL. The message display window at the top of this panel provides information about a current or recent alarm. This window normally displays the measured oxygen concentration. If more than one alarm is active at a time, the highest priority alarm is displayed. The operator can display the alarm text for any of the seven alarm indicators by touching the light diode to the left of the desired alarm indicator. For example, if a yellow light next to an alarm indicator is constantly lit, a recent alarm condition for this parameter may have occurred. A message will appear in the display window showing the reason for the caution, but will alternate with the oxygen concentration reading. If more than one yellow light is present, the operator can sequentially select each illuminated light and check the alarm memory for that parameter. The lights can be turned off by using the RESET control or changing to another ventilatory mode.

Alarm conditions for the other seven parameters are listed in Table 10-39, which describes the more common causes for such conditions. Box 10-141 provides a historical note on one of the original alarms. Box 10-142 provides information about the safety switches on some of the control knobs.

Besides resetting visual alarms, the RESET/2 MIN control can be used to silence some high-priority alarms by turning it to the 2 MIN position for more than 2 seconds, thus providing 2 minutes of silence. If the knob is turned to RESET before the end of 2 minutes, the alarm sounds again. For example, before disconnecting a patient for suctioning or a similar procedure, turn the RESET/2 MIN control to 2 MIN. A short beep and the message "Alarms muted" indicate that the alarms are silenced. The audible alarms for MINUTE VENTILATION, OVERRANGE, and APNEA can be silenced for 2 minutes in this manner. (The HIGH-PRESSURE LIMIT alarm cannot be silenced with the 2 MIN. knob.)

Pause Hold

At the lower portion of the right section is a manual control used to provide an inspiratory or an expiratory pause. When an inspiratory pause is activated, the inspiratory and expiratory valves close at the end of inspiration, preventing expiratory gas flow. The valves remain closed until the INSPIRATORY PAUSE control is released or held for a maximum of 5 seconds, providing an opportunity to check plateau pressure during this pause time. When EXPIRATORY PAUSE is activated, the inspiratory and expiratory valves close at the end of exhalation, just when another mandatory breath would have occurred. The valves remain closed as long as the EXPIRATORY PAUSE control is activated or until it is held for a maximum of 30 seconds. This extended expiratory time allows expiratory pressure to be measured, which may facilitate estimation of the auto-PEEP level.

When a Servo 300 includes the available graphic monitor screen (see Figure 10-91), the INSPIRATORY and EXPI-

TABLE 10-39

Servo 300 alarm parameters, messages, and causes

Airway pressure	
"Upper Press. Limit"	Set upper pressure limit has been reached and inspiration ends.
"Airway Pressure Too High"	Airway pressure exceeds the upper pressure limit.
"Limited Pressure"	Inadequate pressure to deliver volume support or pressure-regulated volume control breaths.
"High Continuous Pressure"	Continuous pressure >15 cm H_2O plus PEEP level; continuous for more than 15 seconds.
Oxygen concentration	
"O_2 CONC TOO LOW/HIGH"	Fio_2 measured at above or below 0.6 of set Fio_2, or $Fio_2 < 0.18$; alarm inactive during and for 1 minute after oxygen breaths are activated.
"O_2 SENSOR"	Oxygen cell is not connected.
Expired $\dot{V}_E$	
(Must be set correctly for each patient size: adult, pediatric, neonatal.)	
"EXP MINUTE VOLUME TOO HIGH"	Expired $\dot{V}_E$ exceeds alarm setting.
"EXP MINUTE VOLUME TOO LOW"	Expired $\dot{V}_E$ is below alarm setting.
Apnea alarm	
"APNEA ALARM"	No breaths (spontaneous or mandatory) detected; Adult = 20 seconds, pediatric = 15seconds, neonatal = 10 seconds.
Gas supply alarm	
"AIR SUPPLY PRESSURE TOO LOW/HIGH AIR:X.X BAR O_2 X.X BAR"	Air supply is out of range. Ventilator defaults to use available gas source.
"O_2 SUPPLY PRESSURE TOO LOW/HIGH AIR:X.X BAR O_2 X.X BAR"	Oxygen supply is out of range. Ventilator defaults to use available gas source.
"AIR SUPPLY PRESSURE TOO LOW O_2 SUPPLY PRESSURE TOO LOW HIGH AIR:X.X BAR O_2 X.X BAR"	Both gas sources have failed. Internal safety valve and expiratory valve open so patient can breathe room air if able.
Battery	
If the main power source fails, the ventilator switches to battery power and this alarm activates (yellow light). The graphic screen turns off.	
"LIMITED BATTERY CAPACITY LEFT INTERNAL: X.X V"	High-priority alarm if voltage remaining ≤ 23 volts.
"NO BATTERY CAPACITY LEFT SEE OPERATING MANUAL"	Voltage ≤ 21 volts; cannot be silenced. At 18 volts, safety valve opens.
Technical alarms	
These are generally corrected by the technical staff. The alarm listed here can be corrected by the clinician.	
"CHECK TUBINGS"	Inspiratory/expiratory pressure difference ≥25%, or at least 5 cm H_2O for 20 seconds. Causes: disconnected pressure transducer tubings, transducer error, clogged bacterial filter, or any blockage in breathing system.

RATORY PAUSE controls can be used to have the microprocessor calculate a patient's static compliance (Cs). To perform this procedure, turn the INSPIRATORY PAUSE control until the graphic screen displays the message "Measuring Static Compliance" at the top center. Immediately switch from the INSPIRATORY to the EXPIRATORY PAUSE position for a few seconds and then release it. After a few seconds the calculated Cs value appears on the graphic screen. This calculation takes into account the PEEP level, but not the tubing compliance factor.

BOX 10-141

Historical Note

In the original version of the Servo 300, a separate back-up alarm was available that mounted on the left side of the ventilator and was called the failure alarm box (FAB). If there was a 24-volt power failure, or if the ventilator MODE CONTROL was turned to the VENTILATOR OFF position, this audible and visible (red) alarm was activated and *could not* be silenced until the button on the FAB was pressed. This alarm also activated briefly as a self-test when the ventilator was first turned on, but after a few seconds was silenced on its own. This failure alarm box prevented the electrical power from being disconnected or the ventilator from being turned off—either accidentally or deliberately—unless done by someone familiar with the FAB alarm who could silence it.

In newer versions of the Servo 300, the FAB alarm is incorporated internally and is self-tested when the unit is turned on. When the ventilator is turned off, this alert "chirps," and then is silenced automatically.

BOX 10-142

Descriptions of the Safety Features on the Servo 300

Measured values are shown as red digital displays. Set values are shown as green digital displays.

Yellow lights that are constantly illuminated indicate active controls that must be set by the operator in the selected mode. A flashing yellow light indicates that a control has been set incorrectly.

Safety catches are indicated by small black markings that appear on the number scale of certain control knobs or dials (e.g., UPPER PRESSURE LIMIT, PRESSURE-CONTROL LEVEL ABOVE PEEP, PRESSURE-SUPPORT LEVEL ABOVE PEEP, PEEP, INSP. TIME %, and O_2 CONC.). To turn a dial past a safety catch, the operator must push in the top of the knob while rotating it past the safety catch.

BOX 10-143

Steps of Using the Set Parameter Guide (SPG)

1. Before connecting the patient to the ventilator, use the MODE SELECTION switch to set the standby mode.
2. Touch the light diode next to the desired mode (e.g., next to the volume control). It will illuminate the controls or parameters to set for that mode.
3. Touch the light diode a second time; the first control parameter that needs to be set will flash, and the others will be off. For example, the light next to the PATIENT RANGE selection switch will flash, telling you to set that control.
4. Touch the light diode next to the mode (e.g., volume control) again, and the next control that needs to be set (e.g., upper pressure limit) will flash.
5. Continue setting controls when they flash and touching the light next to the desired mode until you have set all appropriate parameters.
6. Upon completion of the SPG, the ventilator will beep three times to indicate that you have completed the process. The mode is now ready to be operational or active.

(Note that if the patient is already connected to the ventilator and the clinician decides to use the SPG feature, any control that is active in the current mode of ventilation will be immediately changed. For example, a patient is in volume control with a rate of 12 breaths/min. The clinician uses SPG to switch the patient to SIMV at a rate of 12 breaths/min. If the CMV frequency knob is turned to 30 breaths/min so that it is higher than the SIMV frequency, the rate immediately goes to 30 breaths/min.)

MODES OF VENTILATION

The mode of ventilation is set with the MODE SELECTION switch. There are two ways in which appropriate settings for a mode can be made. First, if the patient is not yet connected to the ventilator, the patient settings can be selected (using the Set Parameter Guide [SPG]) while the mode selection switch is in the STANDBY position (Box 10-143). The second method of mode selection is commonly used when the patient is already being ventilated and you want to switch the mode. Touch the light diode to the left of the desired ventilator mode. The light next to the desired mode flashes, the parameters that are set for the desired mode illuminate, and those for the current active mode are turned off. When you touch the pad next to the desired mode a second time, the same sequence of the SPG, which essentially walks you through each control that needs to be set in the desired mode, can be followed. To actively change to the desired mode, turn the MODE control switch to the new mode. A word of caution needs to be added here because changing any parameter or control that is active in current mode takes effect immediately. To distinguish between the active and inactive controls, controls that are currently active flash rapidly, and those that will be active in the new mode flash at a normal speed. For example, the INSP. TIME % control adjusts T_I in both volume and pressure control.

Another example is that when changing the mode from volume to pressure control, T_I is increased as well. If you increase the time while following the SPG, the T_I in-

BOX 10-144

A Note of Caution

It is strongly recommended that whenever a patient is connected to a Servo 300 for the first time, all appropriate parameters should be selected from the start-up. For example, even if volume ventilation is going to be used, the appropriate inspiratory pressure for pressure control and pressure support settings must still be set. This way, even if the MODE switch is accidentally changed, the parameters appropriate for the patient will already be within a reasonable setting range and will pose no danger to the patient.

creases as soon as it is adjusted (i.e., changes don't wait for the new mode to be activated). Box 10-144 provides a word of caution.

The MODE selection switch has a left half and a right half. Modes on the left (PCV, VCV, and PRVC) are A/C modes and provide a clinician-selected volume or pressure for every patient breath. Modes on the right (VS, SIMV(VC) +PSV, SIMV(PV) +PSV, and PSV/CPAP) allow for spontaneous breaths. Not all patient-triggered breaths are mandatory.

Remember that regardless of the mode selected, there are certain things that are always true. Pressure cannot exceed the upper pressure limit setting. If it is reached, volume delivery is reduced. T_I cannot exceed 80% of TCT (based on the CMV frequency setting). Flow and volume delivery can vary if a patient's active inspiration drops pressure below the baseline. For example, during pressure ventilation, just as during pressure control, the flow pattern is commonly a descending flow curve, and flow and volume delivery can vary. During volume ventilation, flow is usually constant, and there is no control knob with which to select a particular inspiratory flow curve (e.g., constant flow or a descending flow waveform) during volume ventilation. The only control the operator has over the flow waveform is the sloping or tapering feature provided by the INSPIR. RISE TIME % control. The patient, however, can obtain as much flow as desired (up to 180 L/min) during any mode of ventilation when airway pressure drops below the baseline (PEEP setting). This results in a flow/time curve that varies depending on patient demand. Because a patient can obtain increased flow, volume can vary—even during volume ventilation. For example, using the volume control mode, the selected volume is normally delivered, and this represents a minimum volume. If the patient so desires, additional volume can be obtained with an active inspiration.

Each of the modes are reviewed with particular emphasis on some of the newer ventilatory methods available with the Servo 300.

Pressure Control

Pressure control allows patient- or time-triggering and provides pressure ventilation that is time-cycled based on the T_I %. Inspiratory pause cannot be used in this mode. Flow delivery usually follows a descending curve, and minimum respiratory rate is set with the CMV FREQUENCY control.

Volume Control

Volume control is patient- or time-triggered and provides volume-targeted ventilation with time-cycling. Flow delivery is normally constant. V_T is calculated based on CMV frequency and $\dot{V}_E$ settings, as follows:

$$V_T = V_E \div f.$$

Minimum respiratory rate is set with the CMV FREQUENCY control. T_I is determined by the INSPIRATORY TIME % and the PAUSE TIME % controls.

Pressure-Regulated Volume Control

Pressure-regulated volume control (PRVC) is a servo-control (closed-loop) mode of ventilation that is very similar to the pressure-control mode. Breaths are patient- or time-triggered, pressure-targeted, and time-cycled. The main difference is that the ventilator can guarantee volume delivery while still using pressure ventilation. It does this by constantly calculating system and patient compliance, volume delivery, and the pressure limits within which it has to operate. The following will explain how the Servo 300 performs its function in PRVC.

When PRVC is activated, the ventilator begins by giving a breath with an inspiratory pressure of 10 cm H_2O (5 cm H_2O on older models). It then measures the volume delivered and calculates system compliance. The next three breaths are delivered to provide a pressure that will deliver approximately 75% of the set V_T.* For each subsequent breath, the ventilator calculates compliance of the previous breath and adjusts the inspiratory pressure level to achieve the set V_T on the next breath (Figure 10-96). For example, suppose the set volume is 500 mL and the measured volume is 525 mL at a pressure of 23 cm H_2O (C = 22.8 mL/cm H_2O). In this case, the pressure might drop to 22 cm H_2O to deliver the 500 mL. The pressure is reduced until the set and the monitored volumes are the same. On the other hand, if the measured volume is too low, the pressure level is increased. The ventilator will not change the pressure more than 3 cm H_2O from one breath to the next. This protects the patient from large changes in pressure. The maximum pressure that can be delivered is equal

*The V_T is determined by the minute ventilation and rate settings, and is displayed in the V_T window.

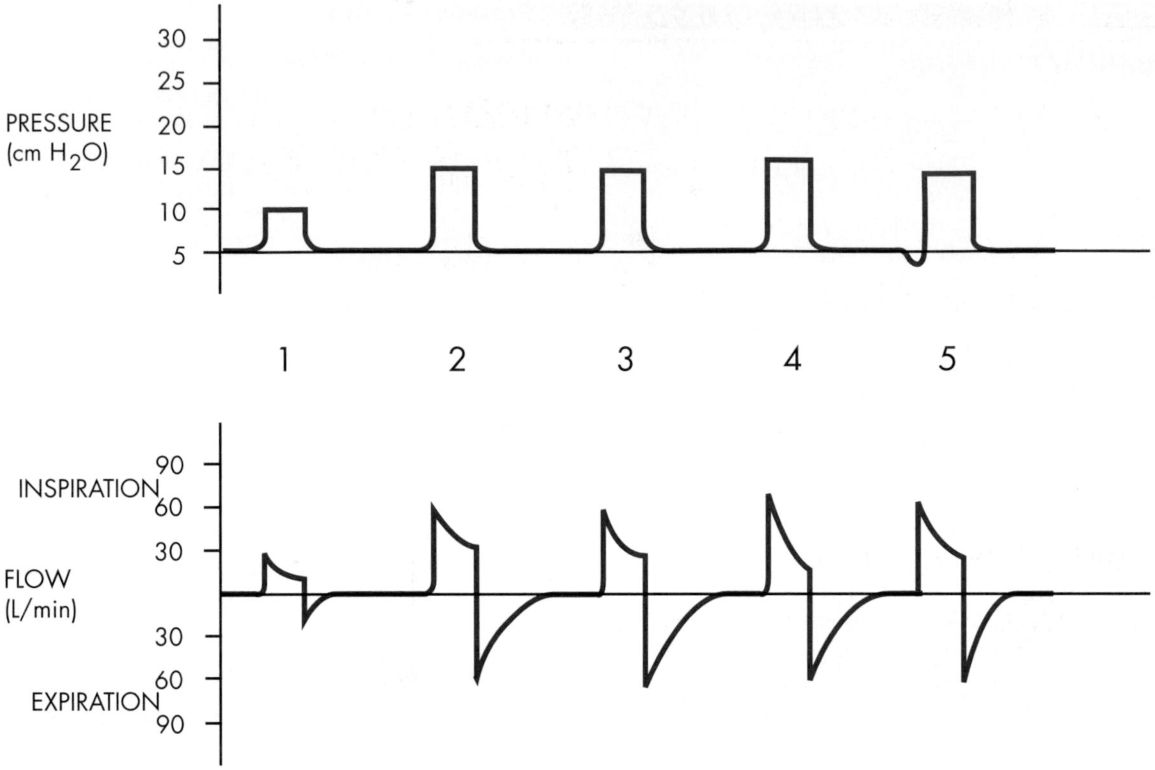

Figure 10-96 Test breaths in PRVC; see text for explanation.

to the upper pressure limit setting *minus* 5 cm H_2O. The minimum pressure limit is the baseline setting. If the pressure reaches the upper pressure limit − 5 cm H_2O, the message window will read "LIMITED PRESSURE," and an alarm sounds. The operator must then decide whether to increase the pressure to achieve the set V_T or to accept a lower V_T setting in order to prevent pressure from going too high.

One reason PRVC was designed was to provide the advantages of PCV, such as a descending flow ramp waveform to help improve gas distribution, an inspiratory flow rate that can vary with patient demand, and a limited pressure to prevent excessive pressures in the lungs. More important, however, PRVC provides another valuable feature: it guarantees a volume delivery. Suppose you are ventilating a patient with volume control and wish to switch to PRVC:

- Be sure the upper pressure limit is set appropriately. You might want to start at a value about 5 to 10 cm H_2O above the patient's current plateau pressure. This is a safe range and could be readjusted if necessary once PRVC is activated.
- As long as you don't want to change any other parameters (e.g., T_I, V_T, f, baseline pressure, or FiO_2), they can remain the same.
- Rotating the mode control switch to PRVC activates the mode, and the ventilator self-regulates within the parameters you have set.

As long as you are within safe limits for pressure and other parameters, the patient will be safe. Some respiratory therapists and physicians are currently hesitant to use PRVC in part because of the uniqueness of the concept and their reluctance to try something different. Undoubtedly, as clinical trials on this mode are evaluated, its use will reflect its success in managing ventilated patients.

Volume Support

Volume support (VS) is also a servo-control mode that might be considered the weaning counterpart to PRVC and volume control. It is a mode of ventilation that provides breaths that can best be compared to pressure-support breaths. That is, they are normally patient-triggered,

BOX 10-145

Decision Making & Problem Solving

A patient is on volume support; the rate is set at 12 breaths/min, and the minute ventilation is at 6 L/min. V_T is targeted at 500 mL. The ventilator is able to maintain this volume within the pressure limitations, but the patient's spontaneous rate drops. How will the ventilator respond to the drop in the patient's respiratory rate (to 8 breaths/min)?

See Appendix A for the answer.

pressure-targeted, and flow-cycled (5% of measured peak flow). The flow waveform is normally a descending-ramp-like curve. The primary difference is that like PRVC, a minimum V_T can be guaranteed. Also as in PRVC, the ventilator runs a series of test breaths beginning with one breath at 10 cm H_2O (5 cm H_2O in older models). It then gives three breaths at approximately 75% of the pressure calculated to deliver the V_T. Finally, the pressure is provided to give the appropriate volume. As with PRVC, breaths are constantly monitored, and pressure increases when the volume reading is low or decreases if the volume reading is high in increments of no more than 3 cm H_2O. Also as in PRVC, pressure can rise as high as the upper pressure limit setting minus 5 cm H_2O in order to deliver the set minimum volume. If the pressure reaches this limit, the message: "LIMITED PRESSURE" appears in the message window, and there is an audible alarm. Baseline pressure represents the minimum pressure level.

There are a few important differences between volume support and PRVC. First, there is no back-up rate in VS. If the patient becomes apneic, the ventilator automatically switches to PRVC, and the light diode next to that mode flashes. An alarm sounds, and the message window indicates that apnea has been detected. For this reason only spontaneously breathing patients who have intact respiratory centers should be placed on this mode. Another important difference has to do with the minute ventilation setting. The Servo 300 tries to maintain the minute ventilation that the operator has set on the ventilator. Box 10-145 provides an exercise with an example of how the ventilator responds in volume support.

Because volume-support breaths are really pressure support breaths, you might wonder why volume support is used. The reason, of course, is that you can guarantee a minimum volume delivery. If a patient is ready for pressure support, volume support is also appropriate. An advantage of VS is that you do not have to constantly adjust pressure levels, as sometimes occurs with PSV. The ventilator does it for you as the patient's condition changes. In addition, if the patient becomes apneic, the ventilator switches to a mode that provides continuous ventilation (e.g., PRVC).

BOX 10-146

Decision Making & Problem Solving

A patient on SIMV (vol. contr.) + pressure support has a set CMV frequency of 15 breaths/min and an SIMV frequency control setting of 3 breaths/min. What are the SIMV cycle time, the SIMV period, and the spontaneous period for these settings?

See Appendix A for the answers.

Synchronized Intermittent Mandatory Ventilation (SIMV Vol. Contr.) + Pressure Support

The SIMV (vol. control) + pressure support (SIMV vol. contr. + PSV) mode provides mandatory breaths similar to those in volume control. During SIMV, the mandatory rate and SIMV cycle time are determined in the following way. The SIMV FREQUENCY control must be set lower than the CMV frequency to correctly establish the desired SIMV mandatory breath rate. If it is not, the ventilator defaults to the CMV frequency setting, and the yellow indicator next to the CMV FREQUENCY control flashes. Cycling times are determined as follows: the SIMV cycle time is calculated by dividing the SIMV frequency into 60 seconds. For example, with the SIMV frequency set at 4 breaths/min, the SIMV cycle time is 15 seconds. The SIMV cycle time has two phases. The first phase is the SIMV period, and the second is the spontaneous period. The SIMV period equals the CMV frequency setting divided into 60. For example if the CMV frequency is set at 10, the SIMV period is 6 seconds. The spontaneous period is equal to the SIMV cycle time minus the SIMV period (e.g. 15 seconds − 6 seconds = 9 seconds).

When a mandatory breath is triggered, the SIMV cycle begins. After delivery of the mandatory breath, the patient has 9 seconds to breathe spontaneously without receiving a mandatory breath (spontaneous period). At the end of 9 seconds, the 6 second SIMV period begins. The patient has 6 seconds in which to make an inspiratory effort and get a mandatory breath. If the patient fails to take a breath, then a time-triggered breath occurs at the end of the 6 seconds. This is very much like SIMV in the Servo 900C (see Figure 10-89). Box 10-146 provides a problem related to SIMV.

SIMV (Press. Contr.) + Pressure Support

SIMV (press. contr.) + pressure support is SIMV in which mandatory breaths are pressure-control breaths. Pressure support can be added for spontaneous breaths. The only difference between SIMV (vol. contr.) and SIMV (press. contr.) is that mandatory breaths are volume-controlled in the former and pressure-controlled in the latter. The operator sets the pressure control level above PEEP.

TABLE 10-40

Control and support modes in Automode

Control mode		Support mode
Volume control	⟷	Volume support
Pressure control	⟷	Pressure support
Pressure-regulated volume control	⟷	Volume support

Pressure Support–CPAP

The pressure support–CPAP setting is intended for spontaneously breathing patients. Breaths are patient-triggered when spontaneous breaths can be detected at a set baseline pressure (0 to 50 cm H_2O). Pressure support can also be set for all spontaneous breaths and is added to the baseline pressure (pressure support level above PEEP). At PS greater than zero, inspiration is pressure-limited and flow-cycled at 5% of the measured peak flow. No minimum guaranteed rate or volume is provided in this mode.

Automode[2]

In late 1997 a new feature was introduced in the United States called Automode. The ON/OFF control for this mode is at the upper right corner of the updated operating panel (see Figures 10-91 and 10-93). This mode is designed to switch from a control mode to a support mode of ventilation if the patient triggers two consecutive breaths. The ventilator remains in the support mode as long as the patient keeps triggering breaths. Table 10-40 shows the control and support modes that are operational in Automode.

Automode works as follows. Suppose the patient is in the PRVC mode, and Automode is on. When the ventilator detects two consecutive patient efforts, it delivers one more PRVC breath on the second breath, and the next (third) breath is in volume support.

If the patient is in volume control and the same conditions occur, the ventilator switches to volume support in a similar fashion. The first volume-support breath in this situation (volume control to volume support) is delivered at a pressure level equal to pause pressure. If no pause time is set, the ventilator uses the following formula to determine the inspiratory pressure for volume support:

$$\text{set P} = [(\text{PIP} - \text{PEEP}) \times 0.5 + \text{PEEP}].$$

The ventilator does not run through the series of test breaths it normally performs when the MODE switch is turned to VOLUME SUPPORT.

If the patient is in pressure control with Automode and two patient efforts are detected, the switch to pressure support occurs on the third breath. The operator must have previously selected a pressure-support level above PEEP because that is the pressure that will be delivered by the ventilator when it switches to pressure support.

The purpose of Automode is to adapt ventilator status to a patient's spontaneous inspiratory efforts. The benefit of Automode obviously lies in its ability to monitor patient breathing effort. For this reason, it is essential that triggering sensitivity is set appropriately, and that auto-triggering is not occurring. Auto-triggering would be detected as a patient-initiated breath and might cause the ventilator to cycle into a support mode. There is a back-up safety feature if this occurs. If the ventilator does not detect a patient effort within a fixed time period while Automode is on, it switches from the support mode back to the control mode. In the adult setting, this time period is 12 seconds; in the pediatric setting, it is 8 seconds; and in the neonatal setting, it is 5 seconds.

At this time, Automode is a new feature of the Servo 300A. Additional clinical experience will help provide more information about its benefits and uses.

Graphics Display Screens

The graphics display screen provides the standard graphs for flow/time, volume/time, and pressure/time, in addition to several loops, including flow/volume and volume/pressure. From one to four different graphs can be viewed at any time. The right side of the graphic display has spaces for digital display of parameters, including peak pressure, mean pressure, dynamic compliance, and static compliance. Static compliance can be measured by using the PAUSE HOLD control and is described in the discussion of this control in this section. Data screens on which the operator can custom design the monitored parameters to be displayed are also available. An example of an available option is the I:E ratio, which is the actual value on this screen as measured by the ventilator.

A carbon dioxide analyzer module can be attached to the Servo 390 graphics screen to display capnographic waveforms and calculations, including end-tidal carbon dioxide, carbon dioxide production, and deadspace.

Troubleshooting

As noted earlier, whenever the mandatory breath rate is reduced in a volume-controlled mode, the V_T delivery is increased because the ventilator is designed to deliver a specific $\dot{V}_E$. It is recommended that the volume be reduced by about one-half before any large decrease in rate is performed.

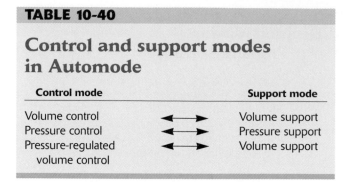

Because many of the safety features base their function on clinician-selected settings, it is advisable to set all available parameters and alarms prior to instituting ventilation on a patient. For example, the ventilator will never allow the T_I to exceed 80% of the TCT. This is the TCT based on the CMV frequency. The ventilator has many safety features to limit this type of error that were reviewed in the discussion of controls and alarms in this section.

The operating manual contains a section that reviews common alarms and associated problems. In addition, radio frequency interference (RFI) and electromagnetic frequency interference (EMI) can affect the function of medical devices using microprocessors. The Servo 300 is specially shielded to ensure protection against RFI and EMI interference. This shielding meets current safety standards.

SPECIAL FEATURES

The manufacturer has a module for the delivery and measurement of nitric oxide that is currently in use in Europe and may soon be available in the United States. Because of the ability to add to the microprocessor unit, adding new modes of ventilation as they are developed is always within the scope of future planning. For additional information, check the web site at: www.siemens.vents.

Review Questions

(See Appendix A for answers.)

1. As air and oxygen high-pressure gases enter the Servo 300, they pass to a:
   a. large pressurized reservoir
   b. pair of servo-controlled stepper motors
   c. mixing chamber
   d. spring-loaded bellows

2. The Servo 300 can be pressure- or flow-triggered in which of the following modes of ventilation?
   I. pressure control
   II. SIMV (vol. contr.)
   III. pressure support
   IV. PRVC
   a. II only
   b. I and IV only
   c. II and III only
   d. I, II, III, and IV

3. A patient is switched from volume control ventilation to SIMV (vol. cont.). The SIMV frequency is set at 9 breaths/min, but only eight mandatory breaths are being delivered. The yellow indicator next to the CMV frequency control flashes. The most likely cause of this condition is that:
   a. CMV RATE control is set at 8 breaths/min
   b. mode change was not activated correctly
   c. SIMV RATE control is out of calibration
   d. patient has become apneic

4. Which of the following modes will guarantee volume delivery using pressure-targeted breaths and has a minimum set respiratory rate?
   a. pressure-regulated volume control
   b. volume support
   c. Automode
   d. SIMV (press. contr.) + PS

5. An adult patient is being ventilated in volume support and becomes apneic. Which of the following will occur?
   I. The ventilator switches to PRVC.
   II. A light diode flashes next to the PRVC control.
   III. After 20 seconds, the APNEA alarm activates.
   IV. The ventilator will begin to ventilate the patient at the set rate.
   a. I only
   b. III only
   c. II and IV only
   d. I, II, III, and IV

6. A patient is in the pressure-support mode. The rate is set at 12 breaths/min. The patient's endotracheal tube cuff becomes deflated, and a leak develops, preventing flow-cycling. In this situation, what will end inspiratory flow?
   I. It will not end, but an APNEA alarm will sound.
   II. It will end after 4 seconds (80% of TCT).
   III. It will switch to PRVC, and the APNEA alarm will sound.
   IV. The circuit pressure reaches the upper pressure limit.
   a. II only
   b. I and III only
   c. II and III only
   d. I, II, and IV only

7. Digital display of values is in red for measured values and in green for set values—true or false?

8. Similar to the Servo 900C, the Servo 300 uses a stepper motor for an inspiratory flow valve—true or false?

9. Explain how the Servo 300 establishes appropriate ventilating pressures during PRVC to achieve the desired volume?

10. During volume-support ventilation, the following parameters are noted: upper pressure limit setting = 35 cm H_2O, set V_T = 0.6 L, PEEP = 10 cm H_2O, CMV frequency = 10 breaths/min. The pressure required to deliver the V_T rises to 30 cm H_2O. How will the ventilator respond to this situation? How would you respond to this situation?

References

1. Siemens Servo Ventilator 300, operating manual 6.0, s-171 95; Art. No.: 60 27 408 E313E, Solna, Sweden, Siemens-Elema AB.
2. Siemens Servo Ventilator 300A: Automode, Order No. 64 08 897 E315E, Solna, Sweden, 1997, Siemens-Elema AB.
3. MacGregor, Mike: Personal communication, March 1998.

Chapter Summary

This chapter reviews a significant number of currently used and newly released mechanical ventilators. The text for each was reviewed by manufacturing representatives (with the exception of the Adult Star*) as well as clinicians using these units in intensive care areas. If you look at the operating manuals for some of these machines, you will occasionally find discrepancies between the material there and the material in this chapter. Because of the addition of new options and the updating of software, it is not unusual for printed operating manuals to lag behind. In such situations, information taken directly from manufacturer representatives took precedent.

*The Adult Star was not manufactured after December 1998, so we were unable to have a company representative review this section.

Internet Resources

1. Dräger Inc.: http://www.draeger.com.
2. Hamilton Medical Inc.: http://www.hammed1.com
3. Nellcor Puritan Bennett: http://www.nellcorpb.com
4. Novametrics Medical Systems: http://www.novametrix.com
5. Pall Medical Inc.: http://www.pall.com
6. Sensormedics, Inc.: http://www.sensormedics.com
7. Siemens Medical Systems, Inc.: http://www.siemens.de
8. Bird Products Corp.: http://www.birdprod.com
9. Bear Medical Corp.: http://www.bearmedical.com

CHAPTER 11

CHAPTER OUTLINE

Infant and Pediatric Ventilators

Kenneth F. Watson and Michelle Lilley

CHAPTER LEARNING OBJECTIVES

Upon completion of this chapter, the reader should be able to:

1. Systematically review infant and pediatric ventilators.
2. Classify infant and pediatric ventilators.
3. List the modes of ventilatory support provided by each ventilator.
4. When given flow and inspiratory time (T_I), calculate the approximate tidal volume (V_T) delivered by a typical infant ventilator.
5. Describe noteworthy internal functions of infant and pediatric ventilators.
6. List and describe the controls, monitors, and alarm and safety systems for each infant and pediatric ventilator.
7. Describe the precautions and key troubleshooting points for each ventilator.

KEY TERMS

Accumulator
Amplitude
Analog Pressure Output Cable Outlet
Aneroid Manometer
Assist Back-Up
Background Flow Control
Back-Pressure Switch
Bias Flow
Check Valve
Circuit PEEP
Control Circuit
Demand-Flow System
Differential-Pressure Transducer
DIN Connector
Dump Valve
Electromagnetic
Electronic Pressure Switch
Exhalation Block
Expiratory Synchrony
Flow Interrupter
Gel-Cell Battery
Hertz
High-Frequency Jet Ventilator
Hi-Lo Jet Tracheal Tube
Illuminated Bar Graph
Impedance
Infrared Sensor
Jet Solenoid
Leak Compensation
Leak Makeup
Mechanical Oscillator
Mechanical Stop
Message Log
Micro-Controller Unit (MCU)
NCPAP Generator
Nickel Cadmium (NiCD) Battery
On/Off Locking Toggle Switch
Oscillating Quartz Crystal
Oscillator Subsystem
Overpressure-Relief Valve
Piston Assembly
Piston Centering
Polarity Voltage
Positive/Negative Pressure-Relief Valve
Proportioning Valve
Pulsation Dampener
Purge Valve
Rotary Baffle
Serial Output Connector
Soft Key
Square-Wave Driver
Subambient Relief Valve
Termination Sensitivity
Trough Pressure
Tracking-Relief Pressure Valve
Variable Inspiratory Variable Expiratory (VIVE)
Volume Limit

The Infant Ventilator

For almost 3 decades, infants have primarily been ventilated in the time-triggered, pressure-limited, time-cycled ventilation (TPTV) mode, which probably relates to the historical evolution of infant ventilators. Although no scientific evidence supports that TPTV is superior to volume control for infants, many clinicians have believed that TPTV reduces the risk of barotrauma.[1] Therefore, until recently, infant ventilators were designed to only provide TPTV and continuous positive airway pressure (CPAP). These ventilators were simple in design and incorporated many similar features.

Today, however, more precise patient monitors and sensors have made it possible to apply additional modes of ventilation (previously used only for adult and pediatric patients) to infants. Although infant ventilators have retained the basic design that enables them to provide TPTV and CPAP, many are more sophisticated models with unique features and additional options. For example, volume-limited ventilation and pressure support are now available on many models.

Most infant ventilators are designed to provide a continuous flow of an air/oxygen mixture into the ventilator circuit (Figure 11-1, *A*).[2] With this design, a positive-pressure breath results when the machine's exhalation valve closes, permitting the gas mixture to flow to the patient (*B*). When a preset pressure limit is reached during the inspiratory phase, pressure is maintained until the ventilator time-cycles into expiration (*C*). When the exhalation valve opens, the expiratory phase begins. As long as the exhalation valve is open, a constant flow of the gas mixture passes by the patient's airway and is available for spontaneous breaths.

If the pressure limit is reached in this type of ventilator, tidal volume (V_T) depends on flow, pressure limit, and inspiratory time (T_I) (Box 11-1). Changes in patient compliance and airway resistance, however, can affect tidal volume. For example, if a patient's compliance improves over a few hours and ventilator settings are not modified, the patient's lungs will accommodate flow from the ventilator over a longer time during the inspiratory phase, and peak pressure will be reached later in the inspiratory phase. Therefore the ventilator may deliver a tidal volume that is larger than desired. Inspiratory time and flow are set and digitally displayed on most TPTV ventilators. The calculation in Box 11-1 should be used to estimate the available tidal volume if the pressure limit is reached. If the pressure limit is reached early in the inspiratory phase, however, tidal volume could be substantially less than calculated.

Some ventilators use a **demand-flow system** to provide inspiratory gas for spontaneous breaths. This type of system delivers flow at a variable rate proportional to patient inspiratory flow. That is, the ventilator matches the patient's inspiratory flow. Some clinicians think that demand

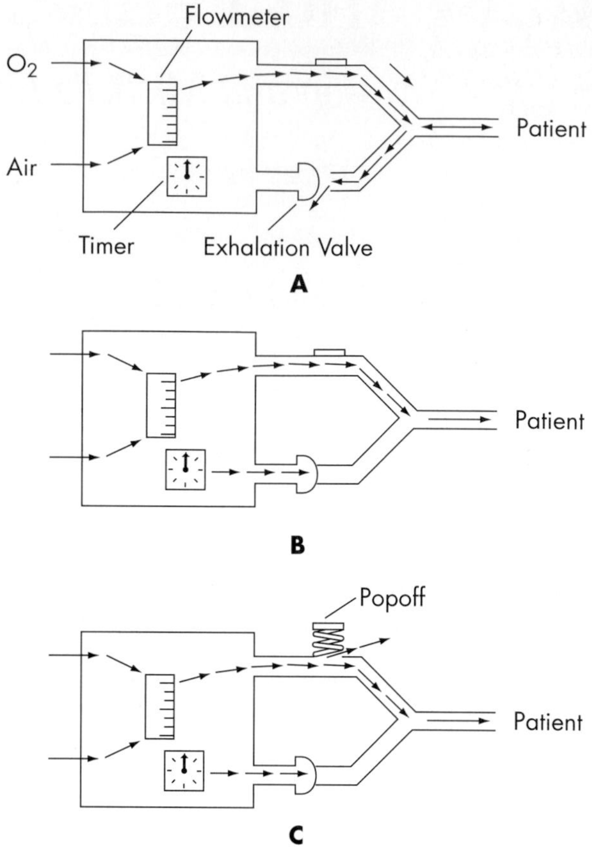

Figure 11-1 The typical continuous-flow ventilator circuit designed for time-triggered, pressure-limited, time-cycled ventilation (TPTV). **A,** spontaneous phase; **B,** inspiratory phase; **C,** pressure-limiting phase. (From Koff PB, Eitzman D, and Neu J: Neonatal and pediatric respiratory care, ed 2, St Louis, 1993, Mosby.)

BOX 11-1

Calculation of Maximum Available Tidal Volume for TPTV

$$V_T = \frac{\text{Inspiratory time (seconds)} \times \text{Flow (L/min)}}{60}$$

flow is advantageous to operator-selected continuous-flow systems because continuous-flow systems tend to produce resistance to expiration at the airway, which is commonly known as **circuit PEEP.** For patients whose ventilatory needs include high inspiratory flow but low end-expiratory pressure, the demand system eliminates the need to set a high continuous flow. Some patients may have highly variable ventilatory patterns, so the use of a demand system may ensure sufficient flow for transiently high inspiratory flow needs.

In a typical demand system, a minimum preset continuous flow is delivered by the ventilator. On spontaneous inspiration, the flow rate increases to maintain baseline pressure. When the ventilator delivers a mandatory breath, the flow rate increases to the value set on the FLOW RATE control knob.

With their improved flow-sensing capabilities, newer ventilators can distinguish between patient inspiratory flow and machine-generated flow, allowing the clinician to select the TPTV mode and adjust the ventilator to deliver patient-triggered mandatory breaths. This type of continuous-flow synchronized intermittent mandatory ventilation (SIMV) is possible even with small endotracheal tube (ET) leaks. Technically, the addition of SIMV to this mode means that it is no longer purely TPTV because triggering is determined by the patient—not by a time interval. Default triggering, however, is still according to a time interval. Flow-sensing capability has led to other advances, many of which are unique to a specific ventilator model. The ways in which flow-sensing applications have been developed are discussed with each ventilator that uses this technology.

The same flow-sensing technology that provides better ventilator-patient synchrony has enabled clinicians to use volume ventilation modes for infants. By closely monitoring inspired and expired tidal volume, ventilatory pressure, and waveforms, clinicians can better adjust ventilator settings according to physiologic changes. Compliance and airway resistance measurements are now possible. Providing the appropriate level of support, responding to physiologic changes more quickly, and weaning infants from the ventilator more effectively are greatly facilitated by some of the latest developments in infant ventilators.

Many clinicians prefer to use mechanical ventilators that are designed exclusively for infants and small children for infants; but manufacturers are starting to design models that are suitable for any patient size. Features such as flow-triggering and flow-cycling, short response times, volume monitoring, and low internal compressible volume are being incorporated into most new ventilator designs. Some hospitals today have even adopted a single ventilator model that can be used in both adult and neonatal intensive care units (ICUs).

ALADDIN INFANT FLOW NC CPAP SYSTEM

Hamilton Medical's ALADDIN Infant Nasal Cannula (NCPAP) System is designed to provide nasal CPAP to infants. Newer software also allows it to provide a flow of blended gas to oxygen hoods, cannulas, and bag/mask systems. The ALADDIN system consists of an electrically powered driver (Figure 11-2); a humidifier or a single-limb heated-wire delivery circuit; a CPAP generator with prongs; and a cap for fitting the prongs to the nose. The driver consists of a flowmeter, a blender with an FIO_2 control, a digital pressure bar graph, an alarm system, and a high-pressure–relief system. Any humidifier that accommodates standard temperature sensors and heated-wire connections can be used with this unit.[3]

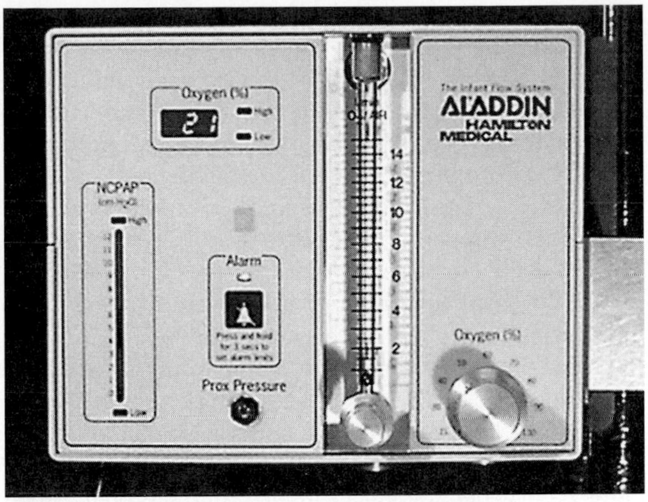

Figure 11-2 The ALADDIN Infant NCPAP System. (Courtesy Hamilton Medical, Inc., Reno, Nev.)

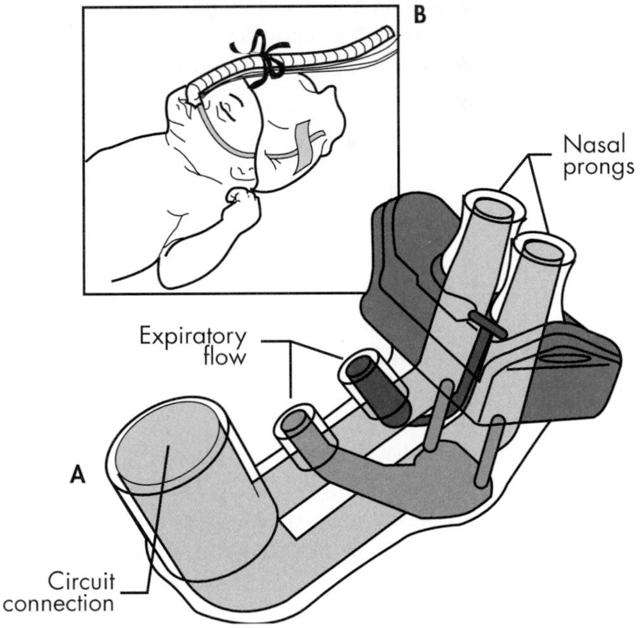

Figure 11-3 **A,** The infant flow generator used with the Alladin Infant Flow System. **B,** The infant flow generator mounting system.

Compressed air and oxygen from 50-psig sources are introduced into the back of the driver. If one source-gas pressure decreases to less than 30 psig, a shrill alarm is activated and can only be silenced by correcting the pressure drop or disconnecting both gas sources. Blended gas at a constant flow exits the driver, passes through the humidifier, and is carried to the ALADDIN **NCPAP generator** (Figure 11-3, *A*), which consists of two fluidic jets.

The geometric design of the jet delivery ports is amenable to the Coanda effect (see Chapter 9).

On inspiration, flow from the driver passes through the nasal prongs to the infant. If the infant's inspiratory flow is less than that delivered by the driver, however, excess flow is diverted from the prongs. On expiration, the expiratory flow pressure "flips" the direction of flow away from the prongs and through an expiratory port. Only a baseline amount of flow remains to maintain the set CPAP level. Diverting flow from the nasal prongs enables the infant to exhale through a low-resistance system.

Nasal prongs, which are made from a soft silicon-based elastomer, are available in four sizes. A mounting system incorporates a head cap, which is also available in four sizes, and two positioning straps, which attach to the two flanges of the nasal generator and are inserted into slits on the edge of the head cap (see Figure 11-3, *B*). The gas-delivery tube, the proximal airway pressure tube, and the exhalation tubing are positioned above the patient's head. The gas delivery and proximal pressure lines can be tied to the head cap with the cap ties. The infant can then be repositioned or held while the ALADDIN prongs stay in position.

Controls, Monitors, and Alarms

All controls are located on the ALADDIN driver, including an ON/OFF switch on the back panel, and the flowmeter, an O_2 % control, and an ALARM SILENCE/SET control on the front panel. A digital pressure manometer provides a dynamic display of airway pressure. Alarm conditions are audible as well as visually displayed on the front panel.

Power Switch

An ON/OFF power toggle switch is on the driver's rear panel. The ALADDIN driver has been released with various software versions. Microprocessor function may differ with each version because of programming changes. Immediately after the power to the driver is turned on, the version of the system software is displayed in the O_2 % window for 2 seconds. Clinicians should use the operator's manual specific to each software version.

Oxygen %

FiO_2 can vary from 0.21 to 1.0. The OXYGEN (%) knob is calibrated in 10% increments, but allows adjustments to be made in 1% increments. The set oxygen concentration is according to the knob's position. The digital display, which is also marked "oxygen (%)," is a reading from the unit's built-in oxygen analyzer. The clinician must calibrate this analyzer before each use by adjusting two potentiometers on the driver's left side panel: one while the OXYGEN (%) knob is set at 21%, and the other while the knob is at 100%.

An alarm system is incorporated into the analyzer's digital display. The microprocessor either sets alarm limits ±5% automatically within 2 minutes after driver start-up or when the ALARM keypad is pressed and held for 3 seconds. When the monitored FiO_2 falls outside of these limits, a red HIGH or LOW LED lights and an audible alarm sounds.

TABLE 11-1

Colors within the airway pressure bar graph indicating operational ranges for the ALADDIN Infant Flow System

Color	Pressure (cm H_2O)
Red	0
Yellow	1 to 3
Green	4 to 6
Yellow	7 to 12

Flowmeter

A non-back-pressure–compensated flowmeter adjustable to 15 L/min sets the driving flow to the patient. The flow setting also determines the CPAP level. A chart is available to guide the clinician in setting the flow for the desired CPAP level. Ideally, if prongs are sized and fitted correctly, a flow of 8 L/min will provide a CPAP level of 5 cm H_2O.

Pressure Manometer

The proximal pressure line of the delivery circuit attaches to the port on the front panel of the driver labeled "PROX PRESSURE." Proximal airway pressure is measured in centimeters of water and is displayed on the multicolored bar graph, which shows pressures from 0 to 12 cm H_2O. Bar graph colors indicate the operational ranges, as shown in Table 11-1.

Red LEDs above and below the bar graph light when pressure alarm limits are manually set and when they are violated. If alarm limits are not manually set (by pressing the ALARM keypad for 3 seconds), the driver's microprocessor sets them automatically within 2 minutes of the initial driver power-up.

Alarm Keypad/Alarm Limits

The ALARM keypad serves two functions. During an alarm condition, the audible alarm may be silenced for 30 seconds by touching the ALARM keypad briefly. This keypad is also used to set alarm limits. Once an infant is placed on the desired levels of CPAP and FiO_2, pressing and holding the keypad for 3 seconds sets the alarm limits. A green LED above the keypad lights when alarm limits have been set. HIGH- and LOW-PRESSURE and FiO_2 alarm conditions must persist for 15 seconds before audio and visual alarms are activated. If the pressure drops to

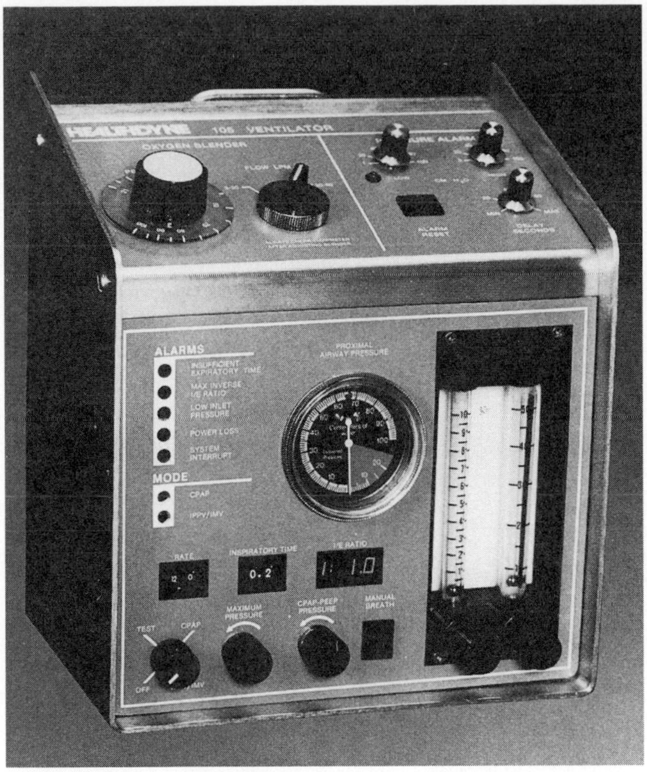

Figure 11-4 The Healthdyne 105 Infant Ventilator. (Courtesy Healthdyne, Inc., Marietta, Ga.)

zero or rises to the pop-off level, however, the alarm is activated immediately.

When alarm limits are set, audio/visual alarms activate when pressures rise more than 3 cm H_2O or fall below 2 cm H_2O from the baseline CPAP level. OXYGEN alarm limits are ±5% of the digitally displayed oxygen concentration.

Troubleshooting

The most common problem of the ALADDIN is leaks at the nose. In some cases, the nasal prongs may not be fitted at the correct angle; moving the straps to a higher or lower position can improve the fit. Improper cannula size also can result in leaks. Patient agitation is occasionally a problem in keeping the system properly fitted and delivering the desired level of CPAP.

In the case of OXYGEN alarms, recalibrating the oxygen analyzer usually resolves the problem. If frequent calibrations are necessary, the oxygen fuel cell may need replacing.

HEALTHDYNE 105 INFANT VENTILATOR

The Healthdyne 105 Infant Ventilator (Figure 11-4) is typical of many early designs that provided either TPTV with IMV or CPAP. It was originally intended for patients weighing less than 10 kg, but because it can generate up to 60 L/min flows, it can be used for pediatric patients. Some versions of the Healthdyne 105 permit the clinician to select either a high or low flow range.

The Healthdyne 105 is pneumatically powered and electronically controlled, and provides a continuous flow. Connections to external 50-psig air and oxygen sources and a 120-volt standard electrical outlet are required. Each gas passes through a **check valve** and then to individual reducing valves. The two gases are then directed to a dual **proportioning valve.** If one of the gas sources fails, however, additional check valves allow the remaining gas to crossover and provide pressure and flow requirements to the unit.

Ventilator controls are on panels at the top and front. A pass-over humidifier is available from the manufacturer, although other humidifiers approved for general-use may be used with this ventilator. Any standard infant circuit that includes a separate line for pressure monitoring can be used.

An external, pneumatically powered exhalation valve with a disposable diaphragm must be removed and disassembled for cleaning and disinfecting after each patient use. During reassembly, the diaphragm must be seated properly and the valve housing tightly screwed together. Most circuit leaks occur at the exhalation valve.

Controls

Mode Switch

The ventilator is turned on and off by the four-position MODE switch at the lower left corner (see Figure 11-4). When this control is turned one position clockwise, the TEST function is activated. All of the unit's visual indicators light, and the audible alarm sounds. The next two positions are the ventilator's modes: CPAP and IMV. An indicator lights to show the selected mode. If electrical power to the unit is interrupted, a battery-powered audible alarm sounds. This alarm can be silenced by either restoring electrical power or turning off the unit.

Inspiratory Pressure

Inspiratory pressure is adjustable to a maximum of 70 cm H_2O and is read from the proximal airway pressure manometer. The INSPIRATORY PRESSURE control is a needle valve that is turned counter-clockwise to increase pressure. On inspiration, the rate timer sends a 6-volt electric signal to a gas solenoid, which opens to allow a 30-psig gas source to flow through a restrictor that limits inspiratory pressure to 69 cm H_2O. The gas then flows to the inspiratory pressure needle valve, which reduces it to the set limit.

Turning the CPAP/PEEP control (also a needle valve) counter-clockwise adjusts end-expiratory pressure from 0 to 20 cm H_2O. During the expiratory phase of the breath cycle, a 30-psig gas source flows through a preset restrictor that limits PEEP/CPAP to 20 cm H_2O. The gas then flows to the PEEP/CPAP needle valve, which further reduces pressure to the desired level.

In addition to the PRESSURE LIMIT control (see the discussion of alarms later in this chapter for an explanation), the ventilator has a built-in **positive/negative pressure-relief valve.** If gas flow is interrupted and the patient attempts to take a spontaneous breath, this valve opens. The patient, however, must generate from -2 to -5 cm H_2O of pressure to open the valve.

Rate and Inspiratory Time

The mechanical rate and inspiratory time are adjustable using thumb wheels (see Figure 11-4). Turning the RATE thumb wheel in the IMV mode can increase the rate from 1 to 150 breaths/min. This control also sets the time interval at which electric current is sent to the inspiratory pressure solenoid. The INSPIRATORY TIME thumb wheel is adjustable from 0.1 to 4.9 seconds. At a given rate, the remaining part of the breath cycle is expiration. Because T_I is set by the clinician, the I:E ratio is determined by the T_I and ventilator rate settings. The I:E ratio is digitally displayed to the right of the thumb wheels. If an inverse I:E ratio $>$ 4:1 is set, the audio/visual MAXIMUM INVERSE I:E RATIO alarm is activated.

Manual Breath

A manual breath can be delivered with the ventilator set in either mode by pressing the MANUAL BREATH button. This button electronically activates a breath cycle at the set PIP, T_I, and FiO_2.

Flow

A flow selector on the top of the ventilator enables the clinician to choose flow ranges of 3 to 20 L/min or 20 to 60 L/min. Two Thorpe-tube flowmeters indicate flow for both spontaneous and mechanical breaths. Separate needle valves below each flowmeter control flow to them. The right flowmeter registers flow in increments of 10 to 50 L/min. The left flowmeter registers flow in 1 L/min increments, up to a total of 10 L/min. The total flow is the sum of both flowmeters.

Proximal Airway Pressure

An **aneroid manometer,** calibrated from 0 to 100 cm H_2O, indicates pressure at the airway. Both PIP and CPAP levels are adjusted and monitored with this manometer. Pressure is transmitted to the manometer from the proximal airway connection via small-diameter tubing. A low flow of dry blended gas constantly purges this tubing to keep it free of condensate.

Oxygen Blender

The OXYGEN BLENDER control adjusts FiO_2 from 0.21 to 1.0. It operates a dual-needle proportioning valve, which receives air and oxygen from the respective regulators and blends them to the desired percentage. Each gas is reduced to a pressure of 30 psig.

TABLE 11-2

Specifications for the Healthdyne 105 Infant Ventilator

Inspiratory time	0.1 to 4.9 seconds
Rate	1 to 150 breaths/min
Flow	0 to 60 L/min
Oxygen concentration	21% to 100%
Pressure limit	1 to 70 cm H_2O
PEEP/CPAP	0 to 20 cm H_2O
Audiovisual alarms	Insufficient T_E (<2 sec), maximum inverse I:E ratio (>4:1), low inlet pressure, power loss, system interrupt (ventilator malfunction), high pressure, and low pressure
Digital display	I:E ratio

Alarms

All alarms on the Healthdyne 105 are audio/visual. Red lamps on the front panel alert the clinician to the specific alarm condition cause. When an alarm condition is corrected, the audio and visual alarms reset automatically.

The HIGH- and LOW-PRESSURE alarm controls allow the clinician to set alarm limits for both PIP and PEEP/CPAP. Either pressure alarm is activated when a violation of the set alarm limits is sensed by the pressure switches connected to the proximal airway line. The ALARM DELAY lets the clinician set the amount of time to elapse before a HIGH- or LOW-PRESSURE alarm occurs. During active alarm conditions, the audible alarm can be silenced with the ALARM SILENCE button for the set delay period.

Additional audio/visual alarms indicate INSUFFICIENT EXPIRATORY TIME (T_E), MAXIMUM INVERSE I:E RATIO, LOW INLET PRESSURE, POWER LOSS, and SYSTEM INTERRUPT. Table 11-2 lists the specifications for the Healthdyne 105 infant ventilator.

Troubleshooting

Circuit leaks are a frequent problem with the Healthdyne 105 that, in many cases, can be traced to an incorrectly assembled exhalation valve. Other leaks at the exhalation valve may be caused by a defective diaphragm, which can be easily replaced. Some clinicians advocate applying powder to the exhalation valve diaphragm to make it seal tightly, but this practice is not recommended because the powder can become wet and potentially obstruct the ex-

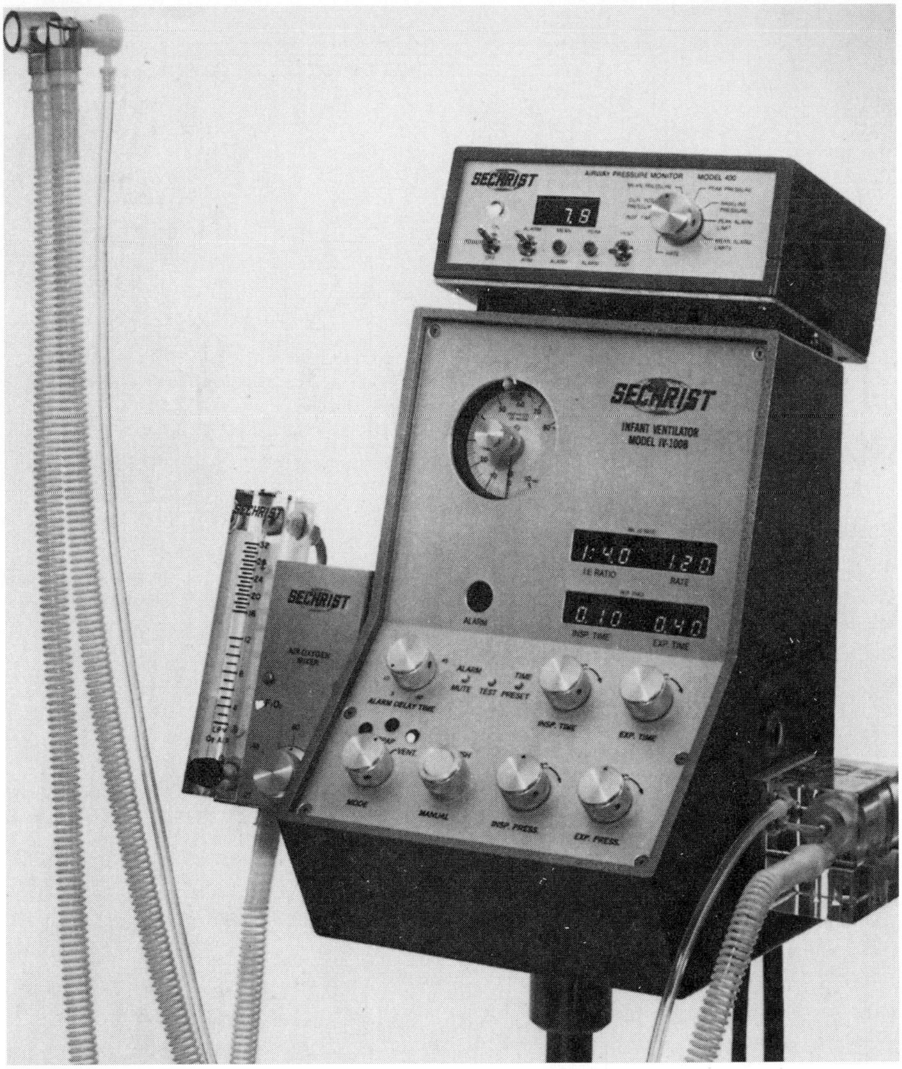

Figure 11-5 The Sechrist IV-100B Infant Ventilator with the optional Air/Oxygen blender and airway pressure monitor. (Courtesy Sechrist Industries, Inc., Anaheim, Calif.)

halation pathway. Powder can also prevent free movement of the diaphragm.

The ventilator should be checked for tightness by setting a low rate; obstructing the patient wye; and setting the flow at 3 to 4 L/min, the PIP to 80 cm H_2O, and the T_I to 3 seconds. If pressure rises to the approximate PIP setting and stays there for duration of T_I, circuit tightness is assured. If the manometer does not indicate the set PIP, the exhalation valve and the tubing connections should be checked for tightness before ventilator settings are returned to "safe" settings.

SECHRIST IV-100B AND IV-200 INFANT VENTILATORS

The Sechrist IV-100B and IV-200 Infant Ventilators (Sechrist Industries, Inc., Anaheim, Calif) (Figure 11-5) are pneumatically and electrically powered, electrically and fluidically controlled, continuous-flow ventilators. They provide time-triggered, pressure-limited, time-cycled ventilation and can function in the control mode (intermittent positive-pressure ventilation [IPPV]), the intermittent mandatory ventilation (IMV) mode (IPPV plus spontaneous breathing), or the CPAP mode.[4]

Noteworthy Internal Functions

The Sechrist ventilators use compressed air and oxygen at a 50-psig source. The pressure is reduced to 20 psig and supplies the **back-pressure switch** and OR/NOR gate. The back-pressure switch starts inspiration when the sensing line is occluded by the MANUAL control button or by the electrically controlled solenoid. The solenoid operates with signals from the microprocessor's timing system (Figure 11-6).

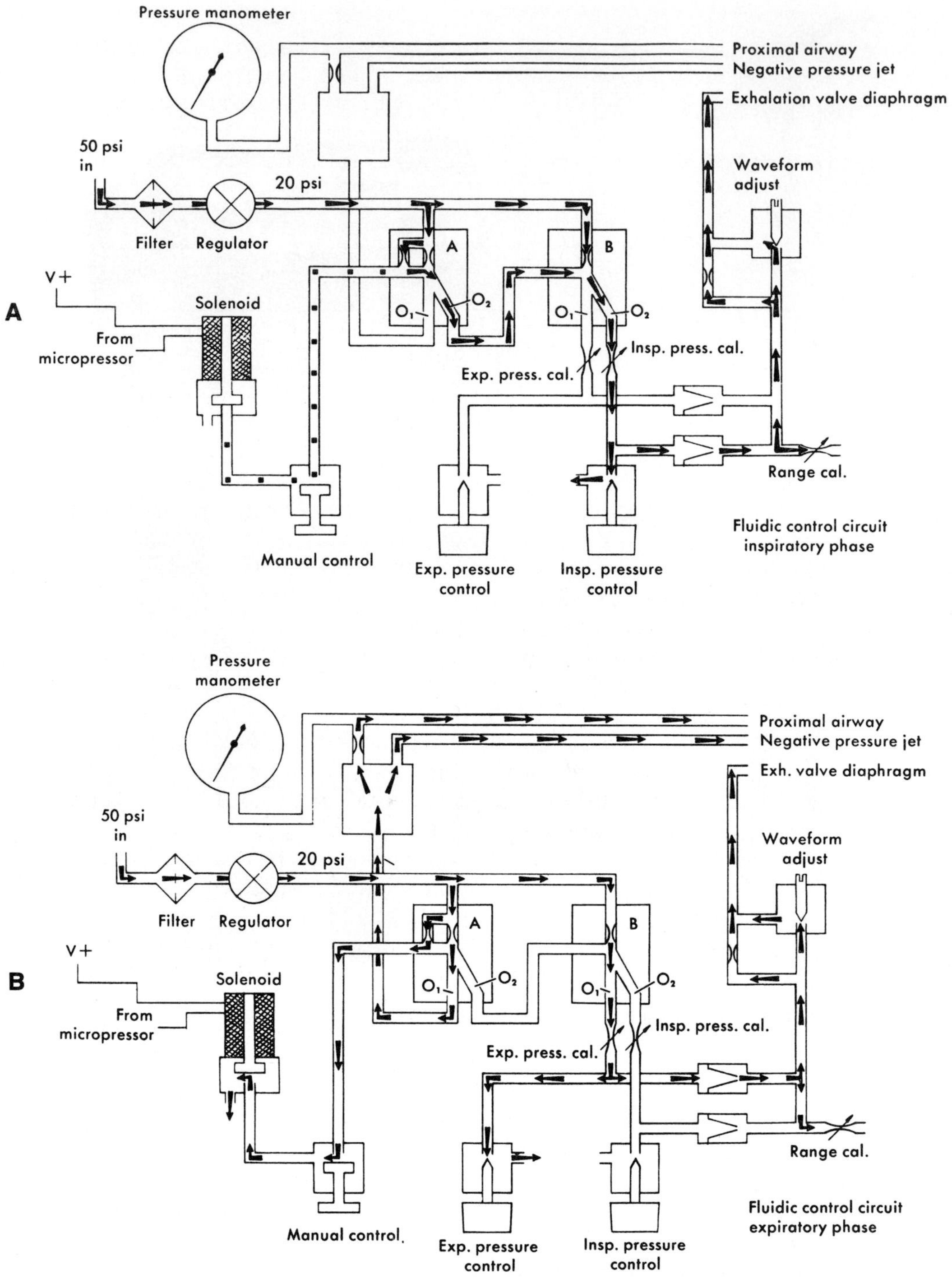

Figure 11-6 Functional flow diagram for the Sechrist IV-100B Infant Ventilator. **A,** inspiratory phase; **B,** expiratory and CPAP phases. (Courtesy Sechrist Industries, Inc., Anaheim, Calif.)

During the inspiratory phase, the back-pressure switch sends a pneumatic signal to the OR/NOR gate at *B* (see Figure 11-6 *A*), causing it to switch its output from O_1 to O_2. Gases flow from the OR/NOR gate through the inspiratory pressure calibration control, which is an internal needle valve. Some gas from this line vents past the inspiratory pressure control. Back pressure provided by this adjustable needle valve is then trapped in the exhalation valve diaphragm, which adjusts the maximum pressure in the patient circuit.

During the expiratory phase, the signal to the back-pressure switch is vented, and its output returns to O_1, allowing the OR/NOR gate to also return its output to O_1. The output of the OR/NOR gate then feeds the exhalation

TABLE 11-3

Specifications for Sechrist IV-100 Infant Ventilator

Inspiratory time	0.1 to 2.9 seconds
Expiratory time	0.3 to 30 seconds (0.3 to 60 sec for IV-100B)
Rate	2 to 150 breaths/min (1 to 150 breaths/min for IV-100B)
I:E ratio	10:1 to 1:300
Flow	0 to 20 L/min
Peak inspiratory pressure	7 to 70 cm H_2O
PEEP/CPAP	-2 to 15 cm H_2O
Oxygen concentration	21% to 100 %
Pressure alarm system delay time	3 to 30 seconds, or off
Trigger mechanism	Time

valve by way of the EXPIRATORY PRESSURE control. Output from the back-pressure switch now flows to two lines: to a negative-pressure jet in the exhalation valve block (to eliminate inadvertent PEEP) and (at a low flow of a few milliliters/minute) through the proximal airway sensing line (to prevent accumulation of condensation within the line).

Gases enter the patient circuit or a single flowmeter connected to a blender. The gases flow through the patient circuit continuously and exit at an exhalation valve. Continuous flow supplies the gas flow for spontaneous respiratory efforts.

Overview of Control and Alarm Panel (Sechrist 100-B)

Figure 11-7 shows the control and alarm panel of the IV-100B. The MODE selector knob is on the front bottom left panel and has two groups of modes: CPAP and VENT (IMV). A MANUAL control button to the right of the MODE selector knob allows the operator to manually trigger the ventilator into the inspiratory phase and is functional during both modes as long as a pneumatic source is connected to the ventilator—even during an electrical failure. The MANUAL control keeps the ventilator in the inspiratory phase for as long as it is pressed. Table 11-3 provides parameter specifications for the Sechrist IV-100 Infant Ventilator.

The rate is established by adjusting the INSPIRATORY TIME (0.1 to 2.9 seconds) and EXPIRATORY TIME controls (0.3 to 30 seconds). The ventilator breath rate ranges from 1 to 150 breaths/minute with the IV-100B and IV-200 Models. The timers are electronically controlled, and an **oscillating quartz crystal** provides accurate timing. T_I, T_E, rate, and I:E ratio are digitally displayed. These displays, however, are only for mechanical breaths and do not reflect any of the patient's spontaneous efforts.

The INSPIRATORY PRESSURE control knob on the front panel is used to set the maximum inspiratory pressure (7 to 70 cm H_2O). Pressure limit values can vary by 1 to 2 cm H_2O if the continuous flow changes significantly. Proximal airway pressure measurements are displayed on the pressure manometer. Ventilation is flow-controlled if the pressure within the patient circuit fails to reach the set pressure limit.

A secondary pressure-relief valve is in the flowmeter block outlet. This spring-loaded valve is generally set a few centimeters of water pressure higher than the INSPIRATORY PRESSURE LIMIT control as a back-up system and pops off to release gas pressure if the patient tubing is kinked or obstructed.

The EXPIRATORY PRESSURE control knob on the front panel is used to adjust the positive pressure maintained in the exhalation valve and patient circuit. The expiratory pressure setting ranges from −2 to +15 cm H_2O. Changing the amount of continuous flow can cause small changes in this pressure, usually about 1 to 2 cm H_2O, depending on the change in flow and the size of the patient circuit and its connectors. Pressures are monitored by the proximal pressure manometer.

Figure 11-5 shows the IV-100B with the Model 3500 Air-Oxygen Mixer attached. This mixer attaches to compressed air and oxygen at about 50 psig and matches the two gas pressures. A precision metering device is used to mix air and oxygen to the desired level. Oxygen concentrations from 21% to 100% are available with flow rates up to 40 L/min.

A single flowmeter is used to adjust the continuous flow into the patient circuit supplied by the 50-psig pressure. Adjustment of the flowmeter control which provides the potential for creating a square-wave flow pattern during a mechanical breath. If the exhalation valve is closed abruptly, the continuous flow enters the patient's lungs in a constant fashion. Flow continues until the pressure-relief valve level is reached or inspiration ends (time-cycling)—whichever occurs first. If the exhalation valve is closed slowly, the continuous flow ventilates the patient in somewhat of an accelerating fashion (ascending ramp) until the expiratory valve is fully closed. These changes in flow pattern to the patient change the pressure waveforms as well.

Alarm Systems

In the IV-100B, an **infrared sensor** is used to monitor movement of the mechanical pressure manometer's indicator needle. A thin red line on the pressure manometer is connected to a control knob and the infrared sensor and can be set within 0.5 to 1 cm H_2O of baseline pressure to detect pressure changes caused by patient breathing. A DELAY TIME control adjusts the time between needle movement detections; that is, if the needle does not pass by the infrared sensor at least once during each delay-time period, audio and visual alarms are activated. An

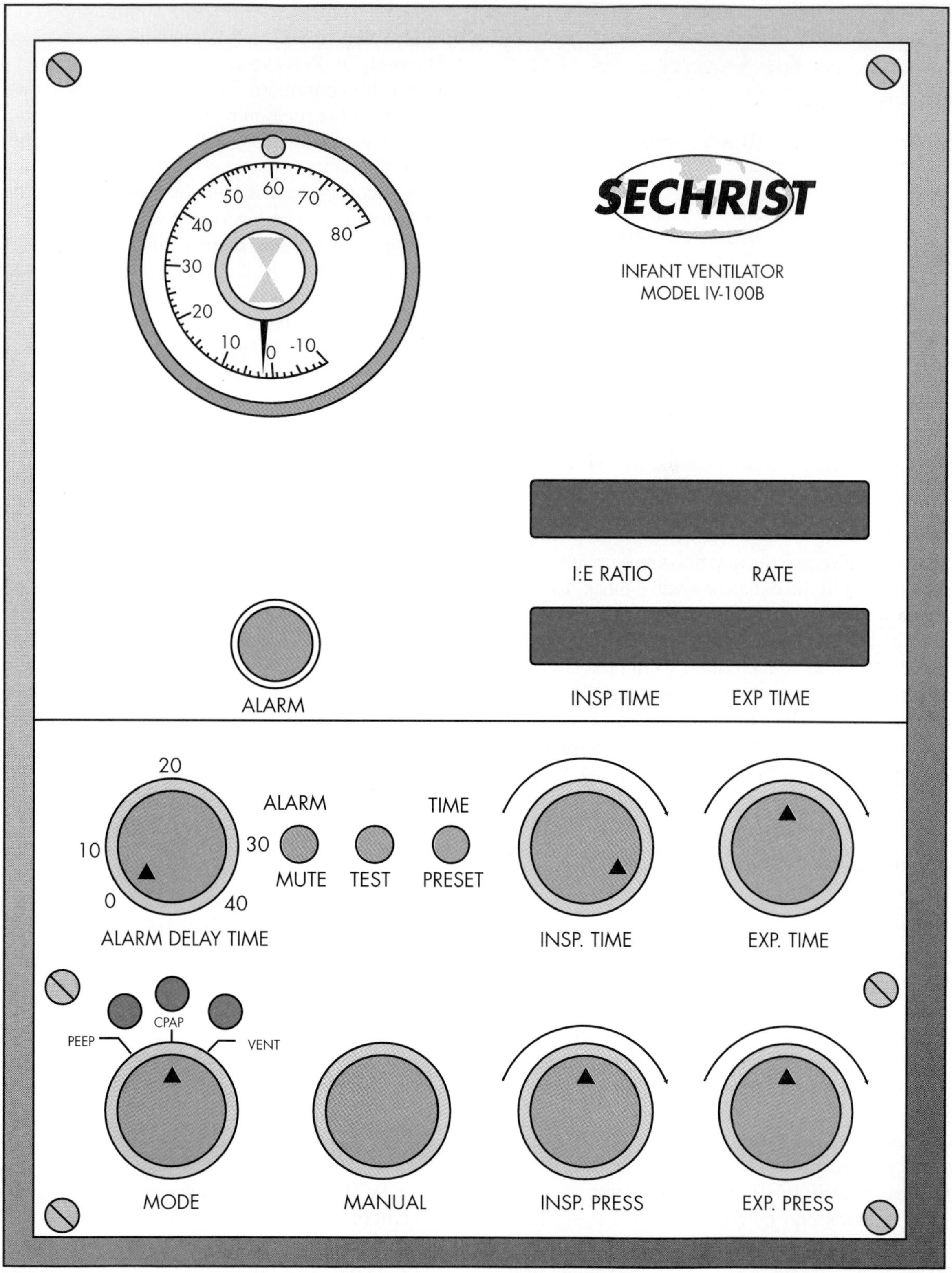

Figure 11-7 Control and alarm panel of the Sechrist IV-100B Infant Ventilator.

electronic manometer is standard on the IV-200 and optional on the IV-100B. The delay timer can be set from 3 to 30 seconds, and a RESET button can silence the audible alarm for 20 to 30 seconds or turn it off. The MODE switch must be in either the CPAP or the VENT position for the alarm system to function. This monitor can be used either during mechanical ventilation modes to detect leaks in or disconnection of the patient circuit or during spontaneous breathing (i.e., CPAP) to detect low rates or apnea.

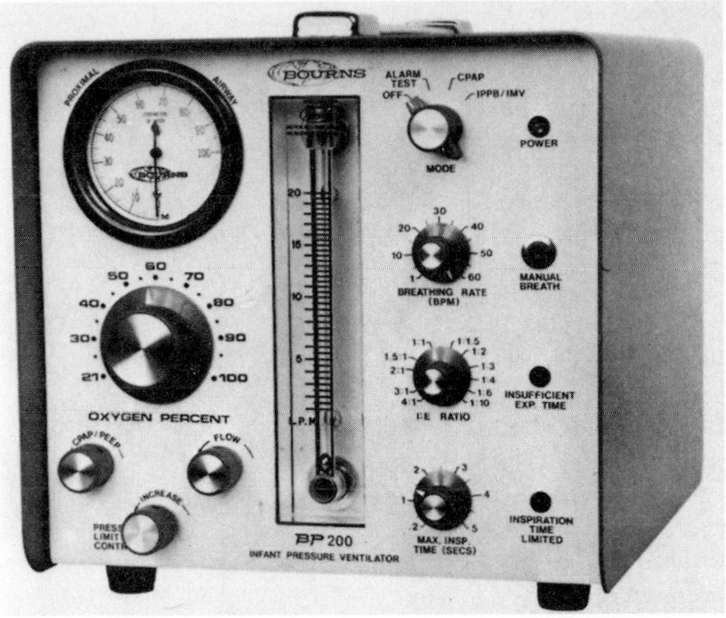

Figure 11-8 Bourns Bear BP 200 Infant Pressure Ventilator. (Courtesy Bourns Medical Systems, Inc., Riverside, Calif.)

A rechargeable battery can provide power to the sensor for continued monitoring of airway pressures in case of an electrical failure.

An alarm bypass system is incorporated into the air/oxygen mixer. If one gas source fails completely, or if there is a 30-psig difference between the air and the oxygen inlet pressures, the remaining or higher source gas supplies the ventilator and an audio alarm alerts the clinician.

Troubleshooting

Similar to many other ventilators, leaks in the circuit are the most common troubleshooting problem. The ventilator should be checked for tightness by setting a low rate; obstructing the patient wye; and setting the flow to 3 to 4 L/min, the PIP to at least 60 cm H_2O, and the T_I to 3 seconds. If pressure rises to the PIP setting and stays there for the duration of T_I, circuit tightness is assured. If the manometer does not indicate the set PIP, the tightness of the exhalation valve and the tubing connections should be checked.

BEAR BP 200

The Bear BP 200 (Bear Medical Systems, Inc., Riverside, Calif.) provides time-triggered, pressure-limited, time-cycled ventilation (TPTV) for infants weighing up to 10 kg (Figure 11-8). Operating only with continuous flow, it is pneumatically powered and electrically controlled and can be used in either the IMV or CPAP mode.[5]

To operate, the ventilator must be connected to external, 50-psig air and oxygen sources and a standard 120-volt outlet. Each source gas is monitored by an **electronic pressure switch** connected to an audible alarm. If either pressure drops to a critical level, the alarm sounds. The ventilator continues to operate if there is an interruption of one of the source gases. The FiO_2 of the remaining source gas is delivered until the pressure of the interrupted gas is restored.

A pass-over humidifier is available from the manufacturer, but other humidifiers and infant-ventilator circuits approved for general use can be used with this ventilator.

Controls, Monitors, and Alarms

Proximal Airway Pressure

An aneroid manometer, which is calibrated from 0 to 100 cm H_2O, indicates pressure at the airway and reflects pressure transmitted from the airway connection via small-diameter tubing (proximal pressure line). This part of the ventilator circuit connects to the unit in the back. Both PIP and CPAP levels are adjusted to the desired levels and monitored by this manometer.

Oxygen Percent

The OXYGEN PERCENT control, which is a precision metering device, adjusts FiO_2 from 0.21 to 1.0 and regulates the oxygen concentration by opening one source-gas outlet while closing another.

Mode Select

The ventilator is turned on with the MODE switch at the top right of the front panel (see Figure 11-8). The most counterclockwise position turns the power off. When this control is turned to the right, the POWER indicator illuminates. When this control is turned clockwise one position, the ALARM TEST is selected. The next two positions are the ventilator's modes: CPAP and IMV/IPPB. If electrical power to the unit is interrupted, the ventilator stops operating, and a battery-powered alarm sounds. This alarm can be silenced by restoring the electrical power or turning the unit off.

CPAP/PEEP

The CPAP/PEEP control adjusts end-expiratory pressure from 0 to about 20 cm H_2O. Turning this knob counter-clockwise increases the PEEP/CPAP level. PEEP and CPAP are determined by a flow of oxygen from a Venturi device that exerts pressure against the expiratory valve. Increasing the end-expiratory pressure level increases the flow from the Venturi. If CPAP is desired, it may be selected with the MODE switch. If PEEP is desired in the IMV mode, it is simply dialed in using the CPAP/PEEP knob. The expiratory pressure level is read from the proximal pressure manometer.

Pressure Limit

The PRESSURE LIMIT control is at the bottom left of the front panel. Turning this control counter-clockwise increases PIP from about 10 to 80 cm H_2O. Similar to the PEEP/CPAP level, the PIP is read from the proximal pressure manometer.

Flow

Continuous flow is set using the FLOW control. The same flow is delivered for both spontaneous and mandatory breaths. Flow can be increased from 1 to 20 L/min by turning this control counter-clockwise and is read from the flowmeter. Although this flowmeter is non-back-pressure–compensated, it is relatively accurate because its driving pressure is 10 psig.

Breathing Rate (BPM) and Manual Breath

The breath rate is adjustable with the BREATHING RATE (BPM) control. Turning this control clockwise in the IMV mode increases the rate from 1 to 60 breaths/min. Models built since 1981 deliver rates up to 150 breaths/min. The BREATHING RATE control is actually a timer that sets the TCT. The respiratory rate is not monitored by the ventilator; therefore the set breath rate must be manually counted.

A manual breath can be delivered in either mode by pressing the MANUAL BREATH button. This button electronically activates a breath cycle at the set PIP, T_I, and FiO_2.

I:E Ratio and Maximum Inspiratory Time

The I:E RATIO control divides the TCT into inspiratory and expiratory portions. This control is calibrated in I:E ratios from 4:1 to 1:10. Actual inspiratory time must be calculated (Boxes 11-2 and 11-3).

The MAX INSP TIME control overrides the I:E RATIO control setting to limit the inspiratory time. Turning the MAX INSP TIME control clockwise sets a limit on the T_I: from 0.2 to 5 seconds. In older models, the minimum setting of this control is 0.5 seconds. Specifications for the Bear BP 200 are listed in Table 11-4.

BOX 11-2

Calculation of Inspiratory and Expiratory Time

1. The ventilator rate is divided into 60 seconds to find the total cycle time.
   $(60 \div f = TCT)$
2. The *I* and E of the I:E ratio are added together.
   $(I + E = x)$
3. The sum of the I:E ratio is divided into the total cycle time.
   $(TCT/x = y)$
4. The *I* of the I:E ratio is multiplied by this number to find the inspiratory time.
   $(I \times y = T_I)$
5. The *E* of the I:E ratio is multiplied by this number to find the expiratory time.
   $(E \times y = T_E)$

BOX 11-3

Example of Calculation of Inspiratory and Expiratory Times

A BP 200 is set at a rate of 10 bpm at an I:E ratio of 1:3. Calculate the inspiratory and expiratory times.

1. $60 \div 10 = 6$-second TCT
2. $I + E = 4$
3. $6 \div 4 = 1.5$
4. $1 \times 1.5 = 1.5$-second T_I
5. $4 \times 1.5 = 4.5$-second T_E

Troubleshooting

The BP 200 rarely poses any troubleshooting problems except for occasional circuit leaks. The ventilator should be checked for tightness by setting a low rate; obstructing the patient wye; and setting the flow at 3 to 4 L/min, the PIP at 60 cm H_2O, and the T_I at 3 seconds. If pressure rises to the approximate PIP setting and remains there for the duration of T_I, circuit tightness is assured. If the manometer does not indicate the set PIP, the exhalation valve and the tubing connections should be checked. Then the ventilator settings should be returned to "safe" settings.

TABLE 11-4

Specifications for the Bourns BP200 Infant Pressure Ventilator

Rate	1 to 60 breaths/min (1 to 150 breaths/min for new units)
I:E ratio	4:1 to 1:10
Continuous flow	0 to 20 L/min
Maximum inspiratory time	0.5 to 5 sec (early units), 0.2 to 5 sec (new units)
Minimum expiratory time	Internally preset for 0.5 seconds (0.2 on new units)
PEEP	Up to 20 cm H_2O (approximately)
Pressure limit	10 to 80 cm H_2O (approximately)
Oxygen concentration	21% to 100%
Pressure manometer	0 to 100 cm H_2O
Audible alarms	Electric power failure; inadequate air/oxygen pressure
Visual indicators	Power pilot light (electric power is on); inspiration time limited (setting on maximum inspiratory time control reached); insufficient expiratory time (indicates preset internal time is not allowing exhalation to last over 0.5 seconds (or 0.2 seconds); air inlet pressure gauge; oxygen inlet pressure gauge

BEAR CUB INFANT VENTILATOR BP 2001

The Bear Cub BP 2001, which is shown in Figure 11-9 (Bear Medical Systems, Inc., Riverside, Calif.), provides time-triggered, pressure-limited, time-cycled ventilation (TPTV). Because its maximum flow capability is 30 L/min, the ventilator is suitable for infants weighing up to 30 kg. It is pneumatically powered and electrically controlled. IMV or CPAP are the standard modes, but flow-triggered SIMV is available with the addition of the Bear CEM Controller (Figure 11-10).[6]

To operate, the ventilator must be connected to external, 50-psig air and oxygen sources and a standard 120 volt electrical outlet. Each source gas is monitored by an electronic pressure switch that is connected to audio/visual alarms. If either of the pressures drops below 22.5 psig, the alarms are activated, although the ventilator continues to operate if one of the source gases is interrupted. The FiO_2 of the remaining source gas is delivered until the pressure of the interrupted gas is restored.

A pass-over humidifier is available from the manufacturer, although other humidifiers and infant ventilator circuits approved for general use may be used with this ventilator as well.

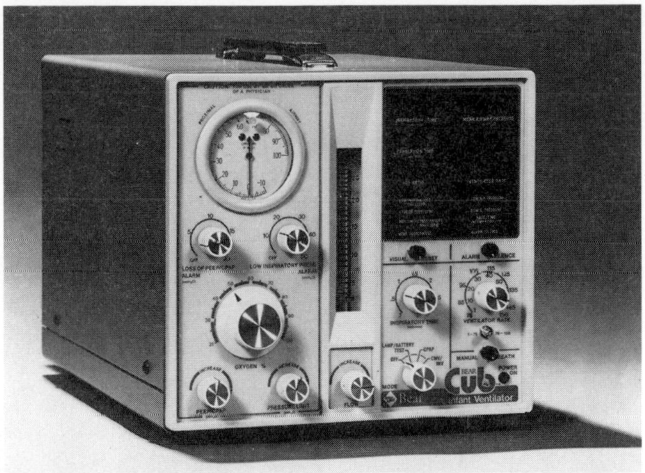

Figure 11-9 The Bear Cub BP 2001 Infant Ventilator. (Courtesy Bear Medical Systems, Inc., Riverside, Calif.)

Controls, Monitors, and Alarms

Proximal Airway Pressure

An aneroid manometer that is calibrated from 0 to 100 cm H_2O (see Figure 11-10) indicates pressure at the airway. Both PIP and CPAP levels are adjusted and monitored with this manometer. Pressure is transmitted from the airway to the manometer via small-diameter tubing. A 0.2 L/min flow of dry blended gas constantly purges this tubing to keep it free of condensate.

Loss of PEEP/CPAP and Low Inspiratory Pressure Alarms

Two controls beneath the airway pressure manometer set the LOW-PRESSURE alarm limits. The first control, the LOSS OF PEEP/CPAP alarm, is adjustable from OFF to 20 cm H_2O. If the PEEP or CPAP level falls below the level set by this control, an audio/visual alarm is activated. The second control, the LOW INSPIRATORY PRESSURE alarm, is adjustable from OFF to 50 cm H_2O. If the inspiratory pressure fails to meet or exceed the set limit, the audio/visual alarm is activated. When either alarm condition is corrected, the audio portion of the alarm is silenced, but the visual alarm remains until the VISUAL RESET button is pressed.

Oxygen %

The OXYGEN % control adjusts the FiO_2 from 0.21 to 1.0. This control, which is a proportioning valve, receives air and oxygen from the respective regulators. Each gas is reduced to a pressure of 17 psig. The proportioning valve regulates the oxygen concentration by opening one source-gas outlet while closing another according to the FiO_2 selected.

PEEP/CPAP and Pressure Limit

The PEEP/CPAP and PRESSURE LIMIT controls establish expiratory and inspiratory pressures. Turning the CPAP/PEEP control clockwise adjusts end-expiratory pressure

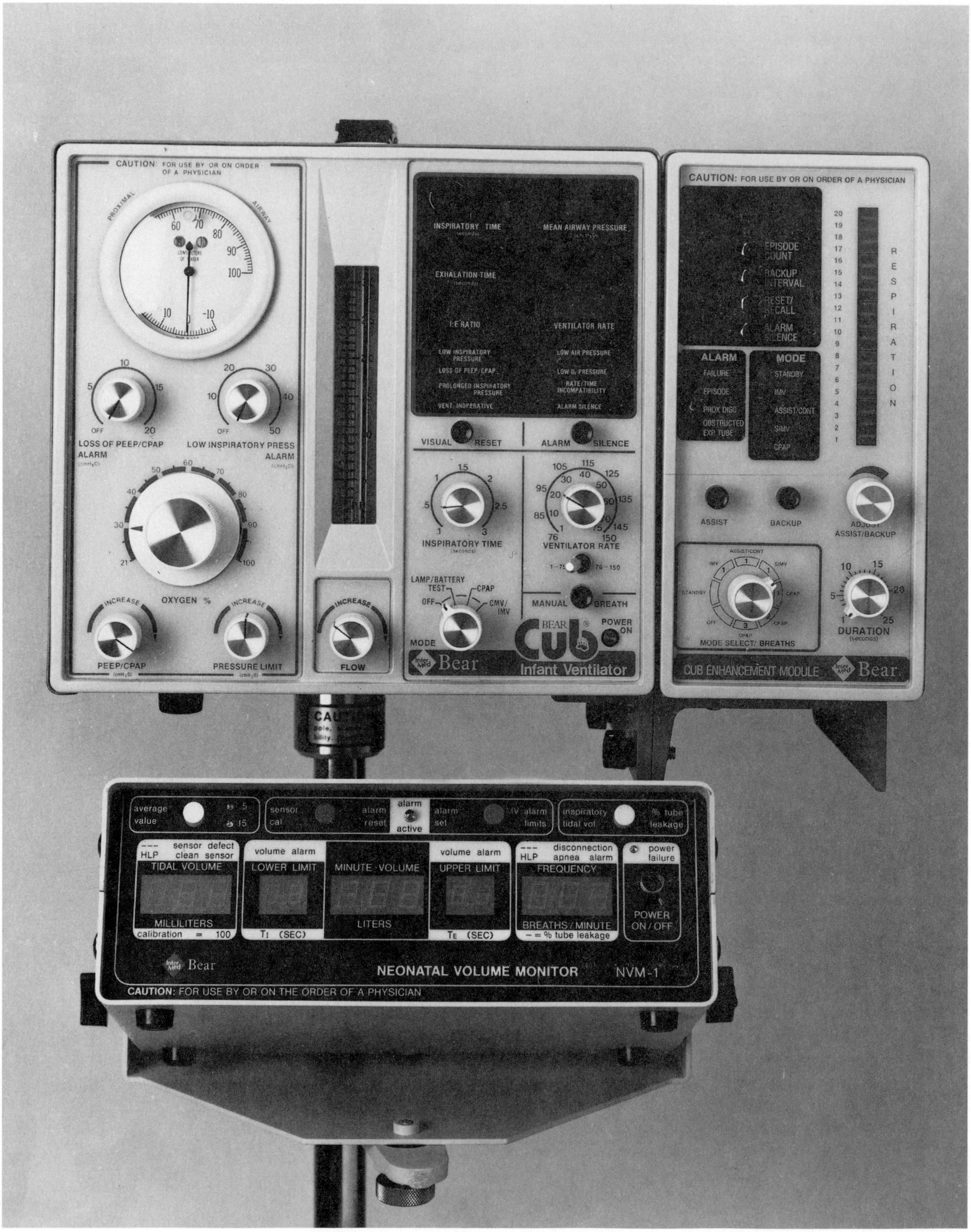

Figure 11-10 The Bear Cub BP 2001 with Bear CEM Controller. (Courtesy Bear Medical Systems, Inc., Riverside, Calif.)

from −2 to about 20 cm H_2O. Turning the PRESSURE LIMIT control clockwise increases PIP from 0 to 72 cm H_2O. Both the PEEP/CPAP level and the PIP are read from the proximal pressure manometer. A digital readout of mean airway pressure (MAP) is continuously displayed on the front panel.

The unit's exhalation valve is a jet/Venturi design. During the expiratory phase, a pressure balance is maintained between flow from the jet at the narrow end of the Venturi and resistance from a plunger at the wide end connected to the PEEP/CPAP control. The Venturi helps eliminate circuit PEEP.

The ventilator has several built-in safeguards against high pressure. A PROLONGED INSPIRATORY PRESSURE audio/visual alarm activates if inspiratory pressure remains 10 cm H_2O or more above the LOSS OF PEEP/CPAP alarm setting for 3.5 seconds.

An external safety pressure-relief valve is at the inspiratory connection of the patient circuit. This adjustable, spring-loaded valve serves as a back-up to the internal pressure limit system and also protects against excessive pressure increases due to inadvertent kinking or blocking of the expiratory limb of the patient circuit.

A second safety valve is built into the pressure-delivery system. This valve, the overpressure-relief and **subambient relief valve,** not only guards against extremely high pressure, but also provides a mechanism for the patient to breathe room air if gas flow to the ventilator is interrupted. If pressure within the ventilator circuit rises to 87 ± 4 cm H_2O, the **overpressure-relief valve** activates a pneumatic whistle alarm and immediately drops the pressure to 40 ± 15 cm H_2O. Also, if gas flow is interrupted, the subambient relief valve opens to room air if the patient generates a pressure of at least −2 cm H_2O.

Flow

A flowmeter in the center of the unit's control panel indicates the flow delivered for both spontaneous and mechanical breaths. Turning the FLOW control clockwise adjusts flow from 3 to 30 L/min. Although the flowmeter is non-back-pressure–compensated, it is relatively accurate because of a 17-psig driving pressure.

Visual Reset and Alarm Silence

After alarm conditions are corrected, the audible alarm self-silences. The visual alarm or alert, however, remains until the VISUAL RESET button is pressed. During active alarm conditions, the audible alarm can be silenced for 30 seconds by pressing the ALARM SILENCE button.

Inspiratory Time and Ventilator Rate

The INSPIRATORY TIME control is set independently of other controls on the Bear Cub 2001. Turning this control clockwise lengthens inspiratory time from 0.1 to 3.0 seconds. At a given rate, the remaining part of the breath cycle is expiration. The mechanical rate is adjusted with the VENTILATOR RATE control. Turning this control clockwise in the IMV mode increases the rate from 1 to 150 breaths/min. This control is a timer that sets the TCT. Because T_I is set by the clinician, the I:E ratio is determined by the INSPIRATORY TIME and VENTILATOR RATE settings. T_I, T_E, ventilator rate, and I:E ratio are digitally displayed on the front panel. If an inverse I:E ratio is set, a visual RATE/TIME INCOMPATIBILITY alert appears on the front panel.

Mode Select

Power to the ventilator is controlled with the MODE switch. The most counter-clockwise position of this control turns the power off. When this control is turned to the right, the POWER indicator lights. Turning this control one position clockwise selects the LAMP/BATTERY TEST. The next two positions are the ventilator's modes: CPAP and CMV-IMV. If electrical power to the unit is interrupted, a battery-powered alarm sounds. This alarm can be silenced by restoring electrical power or turning the unit off.

Manual Breath

A manual breath can be delivered in either mode by pressing the MANUAL BREATH button. This button electronically activates a breath cycle at the set PIP, T_I, and FiO_2.

BEAR CEM CONTROLLER AND NVM-1 MONITOR

The Bear Cub Enhancement Module (CEM), which is a microprocessor-controller, and the NVM-1 monitor (see Figure 11-10) are optional components of the Bear Cub 2001 that are no longer available from the manufacturer. Together, these additions can be used to provide patient flow triggering for either assist/control (A/C) or SIMV modes. They also provide enhanced monitoring capability. Moreover, the system can detect periods of reduced patient effort and apnea during spontaneous breathing. Depending on CEM settings, the device can signal the ventilator to supplement ventilation when it determines (through the NMV-1) that the patient's inspiratory efforts are either absent or insufficient.

Careful adjustment of the **ASSIST BACK-UP** setting is essential to proper application of the CEM. As the patient breathes spontaneously, an airway sensor sends flow data by the NVM-1 monitor to the CEM. The magnitude of the patient's inspiratory flow is reflected on a bar graph. Turning the ASSIST BACK-UP control clockwise increases the flow threshold that the patient's spontaneous inspiratory flow must exceed in order to trigger an SIMV or an A/C breath. The flow threshold also is displayed on an LED bar graph, alongside the patient's flow. Beneath the ASSIST BACK-UP control is the DURATION control, which sets the number of seconds in which the patient must generate an adequate

TABLE 11-5

Specifications for Bear Cub Infant Ventilator BP 2001

Rate	1 to 150 breaths/min
Inspiratory time	0.1 to 3.0 seconds
Flow	3 to 30 L/min
Oxygen concentration	21% to 100% (integral blender)
Pressure limit	0 to 72 cm H_2O
PEEP/CPAP	−2 to 20 cm H_2O
Audio/visual alarms	Low inspiratory pressure; loss of PEEP/CPAP; prolonged inspiratory pressure (10 cm above loss of PEEP/CPAP alarm setting for longer than 3.5 sec); ventilator inoperative (electronic failure); low oxygen pressure; low air pressure
Visual alerts	Rate/time incompatibility; alarm silence
Alarm silence	30 seconds
Digital displays	Inspiratory time; exhalation time; I:E ratio; ventilator rate; mean airway pressure

inspiratory flow (see Figure 11-10). If the patient's inspiratory flow does not exceed the threshold within the set duration, not only is triggering affected, but the CEM also activates an audio/visual alarm. If the CEM SELECT/BREATHS control is in either the A/C or SIMV modes, the CEM triggers the ventilator to deliver a mechanical breath.

The enhanced system can be used in the CPAP mode, and the number of back-up breaths can be set by the clinician. If patient effort is adequate during the set duration, up to three mechanical breaths can be delivered at the set ventilator rate.

The enhanced system can also be used just for monitoring (i.e., with no triggering of positive-pressure breaths). This is accomplished by selecting the STANDBY mode on the CEM. In this mode, the unit does not send triggering signals to the ventilator, which allows the spontaneously breathing patient to be monitored. The system alerts the clinician, however, when the patient's flow drops below the clinician-selected threshold. In all modes, the number of insufficient flow episodes in the past 60 or 120 minutes is displayed on the CEM front panel. The NVM-1 displays additional data, including minute volume ($\dot{V}_E$), V_T, and respiratory rate. Table 11-5 lists the specifications for the Bear Cub 2001 infant ventilator.

Troubleshooting

Checking for circuit tightness is accomplished with the same procedure as described for the BP-200. Other than checking for leaks and proper assembly of the exhalation valve housing, little troubleshooting is required.

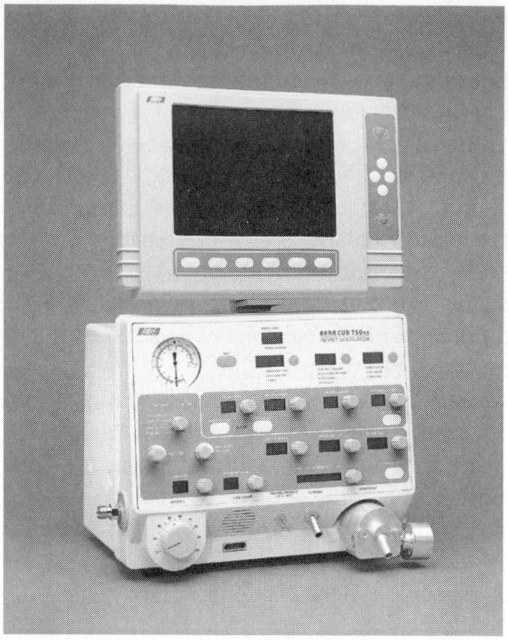

Figure 11-11 The Bear Cub 750vs Infant Ventilator. (Courtesy Bear Medical Systems, Inc., Riverside, Calif.)

BEAR CUB 750VS INFANT VENTILATOR

The Bear Cub 750vs is the latest infant ventilator from Bear Medical Systems, Inc. (Figure 11-11). Although this unit is designed for neonates, it can be used with pediatric patients weighing up to 30 kg. Like its predecessors, the 750vs is pneumatically powered and electrically controlled. Flow triggering, spontaneous rate, and machine/patient V_T monitoring are fully integrated into this model. Independent base and inspiratory flows, a **volume limit** feature, and an internal battery back-up are new features available with this ventilator.[7]

Two **micro-controller units (MCUs)** determine all of the ventilator's functions. One MCU is designated the controller, and the other is designated the monitor; each is assigned specific and duplicate tasks. The controller MCU receives information from the control settings as well as from signals given from the flow sensor, pressure transducer, and monitor MCU. In turn, the controller MCU tells the unit's components to operate. The monitor MCU reads information from all switches and potentiometers and monitors ventilator performance. It also receives data from the controller MCU. Each MCU monitors the performance of the other and can shut down the ventilator and trigger alarms if software or hardware errors are detected.

A key component of the unit's features is the flow sensor, which is a hot-wire anemometer consisting of two platinum hot wires. This sensor incorporates an electronic memory circuit, eliminating the need for calibration, and can determine flow in two directions. Designed to be placed at the patient airway, the sensor permits monitoring and display of patient V_T, T_I, and respiratory rate. It also provides patient flow-triggering and enables the VOLUME LIMIT control, which is explained later in this chapter. The percentage of endotracheal tube leak is calculated using the inspired and expired V_T measured by the flow sensor. The monitor MCU makes this calculation and displays it on the front panel. Use of the flow sensor is optional. If the clinician wants to use the ventilator without its monitoring and synchronization functions, the sensor can be removed.

Connections to both compressed air and oxygen are required for the ventilator to operate. An optional external air compressor (model 3600) is provided by the manufacturer. If one of the gas sources fails, a back-up system ensures continued operation with the remaining gas source. A source gas failure, however, alters the FiO_2. When the ventilator is connected to compressed air and oxygen and is in standby, blended gas is available from the auxiliary gas outlet. Gas flow to this outlet is set with the BASE FLOW control.

Patient circuits and humidification units are available from the manufacturer, although commercially available infant/pediatric circuits and humidifiers can be used if they meet manufacturer specifications.

Controls and Monitors (Figure 11-12)

PEEP/CPAP and Inspiratory Pressure

PEEP/CPAP is adjustable from 0 to 30 cm H_2O. INSPIRATORY PRESSURE can be adjusted to a maximum of 72 cm H_2O. Desired levels are set by rotating each control knob clockwise and observing the pressure on the analog manometer at end-expiration and peak inspiration.

The ventilator is designed for proximal airway pressure monitoring. A 1/8-inch internal diameter tubing is required to connect the proximal airway to the proximal pressure outlet of the ventilator. A flow of 100 mL/min continuously purges this tubing to prevent moisture accumulation and contamination of the tubing.

The exhalation valve consists of a seated diaphragm that operates as a pneumatic, servo-controlled regulator. Exhaled gas passes through the diaphragm and is vented to the atmosphere. PEEP/CPAP and PIP levels are regulated by a **differential-pressure transducer** (the control transducer). This transducer is electronically signaled to reference one level of pressure during a mechanical breath and another level during expiration. The control transducer is separated from the proximal airway transducer by the control diaphragm.

When the control pressure equals the set PIP during inspiration, the control diaphragm opens, pressurizing the exhalation valve diaphragm to maintain the PIP level until the set T_I elapses. When the control pressure drops to the set PEEP during expiration, the control diaphragm closes, allowing the exhalation valve to open until the PEEP level is reached. The control diaphragm opens enough to maintain the PEEP level during the expiratory phase.

The exhalation valve assembly incorporates a jet Venturi to eliminate or reduce circuit PEEP generated by the base flow. This Venturi allows for a PEEP/CPAP level of 0 cm H_2O at a base flow of 10 L/min and 4 cm H_2O at 20 L/min.

If PEEP/CPAP is set higher than the INSPIRATORY PRESSURE control, the PRESSURE SETTINGS INCOMPATIBLE alarm activates. When this occurs, the set PEEP/CPAP is maintained, but mechanical breaths are not delivered.

Rate

The VENTILATOR RATE control, which is adjustable from 0 to 150 breaths per minute, sets the number of mechanical breaths in the SIMV/IMV mode or the minimum number of breaths delivered in the A/C mode. The set number of breaths per minute is indicated by the LED to the left of the control.

Inspiratory Time

The INSPIRATORY TIME control is adjustable from 0.1 to 3.0 seconds. The set T_I (in seconds) is shown on the LED to the left of the control. If this control is set to deliver an inverse I:E ratio, the digital display flashes, and the SETTINGS INCOMPATIBLE alarm sounds. During the alarm condition, the ventilator limits the T_I to provide an I:E ratio of 1:1 at the set ventilator rate. Adjusting the INSPIRATORY TIME control to an I:E ratio of 1:1 corrects the alarm condition.

Volume Limit

The VOLUME LIMIT control, which is adjustable from 5 to 300 mL, sets a ceiling for the V_T delivered by mechanical breaths. If the set volume limit is reached, the ventilator terminates inspiration before the set T_I is delivered. The VOLUME LIMIT LED illuminates, and an indicator sounds to alert the clinician that the breath is volume- not time-cycled. To correct this condition, the clinician may either select a higher volume limit, decrease the T_I, or decrease the inspiratory pressure. During the alarm condition, the set T_I is not delivered, and the set inspiratory pressure may not be delivered as well (Box 11-4).

Base Flow and Inspiratory Flow

The background flow available to the patient for spontaneous breathing is set using the BASE FLOW control. The flow delivered to the patient during mechanical breaths is set using the INSPIRATORY FLOW control. Both of these

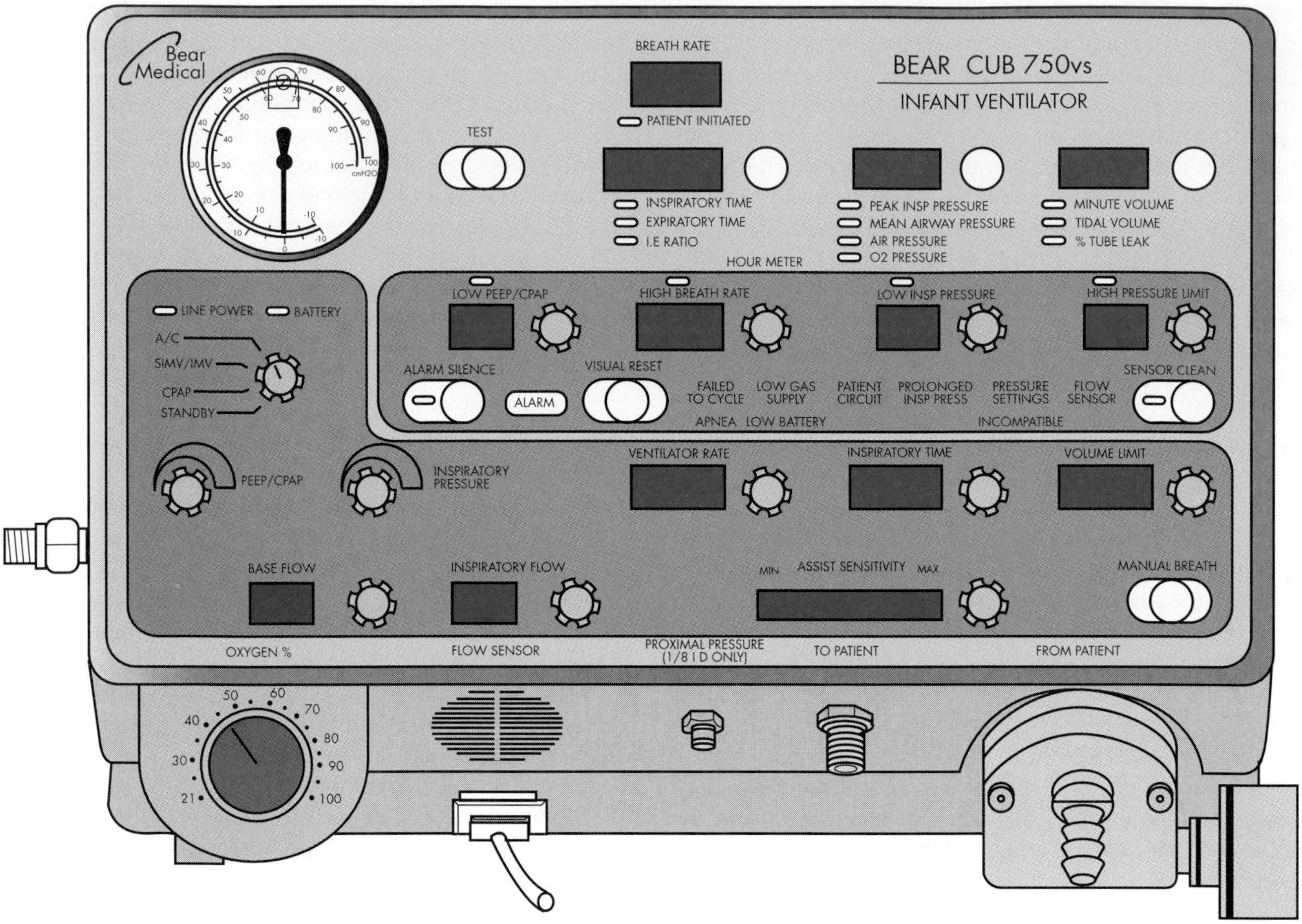

Figure 11-12 The Bear Cub 750vs Infant Ventilator control panel.

> **BOX 11-4**
>
> ### Flow and Pressure Limits Assigned to Volume Limit Settings
>
> The ventilator's microprocessor is programmed with flow and pressure limits for each volume limit setting. If the inspiratory flow setting is too high, the VOLUME LIMIT LED flashes, alternating with the message "E.FL." If the inspiratory pressure setting is too high, the VOLUME LIMIT LED flashes, alternating with the message "E.PL." If the flow sensor is disconnected or disabled, the VOLUME LIMIT LED displays dashes.

flows can be adjusted from 1 to 30 L/min, and both are regulated by individual flow-control valves. The two control valves are switched by a solenoid valve. Each control valve is connected to a potentiometer that provides signals to the monitor MCU. The ventilator's internal barometer calculates the flow setting for the barometric pressure. The calculated flow is then displayed on the front panel.

Insufficient or excessive flow settings result in an INCOMPATIBLE SETTINGS alarm. During this alarm condition, either the BASE FLOW or the INSPIRATORY FLOW display flashes, depending on which flow is inappropriately set. Adjusting the control(s) to a more appropriate flow corrects the alarm condition (Box 11-5).

Assist Sensitivity

The amount of inspiratory effort the patient must exert to trigger a mechanical breath is determined by the ASSIST SENSITIVITY control. This control, which is adjustable from 0.2 to 5.0 L/min, sets the minimum flow the patient must generate to trigger A/C or SIMV breaths. Also, in either the SIMV or CPAP mode, this control allows spontaneous breaths to be counted and displayed in the BREATH RATE window.

The flow sensor is essential to patient triggering and breath rate monitoring. If the sensor is disconnected, no flow is displayed by the ASSIST SENSITIVITY LED, and the patient is unable to trigger a breath.

BOX 11-5

Effect of Using Auxiliary Gas Flow on Base or Inspiratory Flow

The total flow capability of the 750vs is 30 L/min. When the auxiliary gas outlet is used, flow coming from the outlet added to the base or inspiratory flow (whichever is higher) represents the total flow output of the ventilator. When total flow exceeds 25 L/min, the actual base flow or inspiratory flow may be less than set. Therefore the clinician should be alerted to a potential decrease in base or inspiratory flow when high flows are used in the auxiliary gas outlet. For example, if base flow is set at 3L/min, inspiratory flow is at 10 L/min, and auxiliary flow is at 15 L/min, then total flow will be 25 L/min.

Manual Breath

The MANUAL BREATH button delivers a mechanical breath when pressed. Each manual breath is delivered at the set inspiratory time, inspiratory flow, and inspiratory pressure.

Auxiliary Gas Outlet

A 12-psi auxiliary gas outlet on the left side of the ventilator provides an additional flow of blended gas. This port is a spring-loaded DISS fitting to which an optional flowmeter (available from the manufacturer) can be added. (Standard flowmeters should not be used because they are calibrated to 50 psi.) Up to 8 L/min flows are available through this outlet. If electric power is disrupted, this valve is still functional and can be used with a manual resuscitator.

Oxygen %

The delivered oxygen concentration is adjusted with the OXYGEN % control, which regulates an internal air/oxygen blender.

Overpressure Relief

An external, mechanical overpressure-relief valve is located on the ventilator's back panel. This valve, which is adjustable from 15 to 75 cm H_2O, relieves excessive pressure in the inspiratory limb of the ventilator circuit.

This valve is not intended to be used as the ventilator's primary PIP control but as a safety valve instead. If this valve is set lower than the INSPIRATORY PRESSURE control, the unit's audio/visual HIGH-PRESSURE alarms will *not* alert the clinician to a high-pressure situation.

Alarms

Visual alarm indicators, which are all red LEDs, are in the middle of the front panel (see Figure 11-12) and include four adjustable alarms and nine fixed alarms. When an alarm condition occurs, both visual and audio alarms are activated. The audio alarm is intended to alert the clinician to an alarm condition, and the visual alarm indicates the specific problem. When an alarm condition is corrected, the audio part stops automatically, but the visual part continues to indicate the alarm condition until the VISUAL RESET button is pressed. With the exception of the FAILED TO CYCLE alarm, the audio part of an alarm can be silenced with the ALARM SILENCE button. The alarm is silenced for 60 seconds, unless the clinician cancels the silent period by pressing the button a second time. A control to adjust alarm volume levels is on the ventilator's rear panel. Adjustable alarms for the Bear Cub 750vs are described in Table 11-6; fixed alarms are listed in Table 11-7.

Special Features

A graphics display is available as an upgrade option on the Bear Cub 750vs. With this display, scalar pressure, flow, and volume waveforms can be viewed simultaneously. Loops and additional data can be displayed as well. A computer interface is also available, allowing a computer to be used in lieu of the graphics monitor. Three analog signals (representing pressure, flow, and breath phase) are generated by the ventilator for connection to an oscilloscope or strip-chart recorder.

Within the grouping of alarm indicators is a SENSOR CLEAR button (see Figure 11-12), which provides a way to help free the sensor wires of organic contaminants. When this button is pressed, an instantaneous 1-second increase in sensor-wire temperature occurs at the ventilator's next expiratory phase. Mucus and other debris clinging to the sensor wires burn off, reducing interference with the sensor's performance. This feature is useful because the clinician can sometimes avoid having to remove and clean or exchange the sensor when readings are erratic. Specifications for the Bear Cub 750vs are listed in Table 11-8.

Troubleshooting

An extensive troubleshooting guide is found in the ventilator's instruction manual. Leaks in the patient circuit cause most troubleshooting problems, but the ventilator's sophisticated alarm and diagnostic system facilitates the resolution of most troubleshooting issues.

Infrasonics Infant Star Ventilators

There are three versions of the Infrasonics Infant Star: the original version, the Infant Star 500, and the Infant Star 950. The original version was available as either a conventional ventilator or a conventional ventilator with high-frequency ventilation. The Infant Star 500 is an updated version of the original that is only available as a conventional ventilator. The Infant Star 950 offers all of the features of the 500, but also incorporates high-frequency ventilation. All versions can be used with the optional Star Sync, which enables patient triggering of IMV breaths.

TABLE 11-6

Adjustable alarms on the Bear Cub 750vs Infant Ventilator

Alarm	Adjustable range	Triggering condition
Low PEEP/CPAP	−5 to 30 cm H_2O	Measured proximal airway pressure falls below the set value for at least 60 milliseconds
High breath rate	3 to 255 breaths/min	Monitored value for breath rate exceeds alarm setting
Low inspiratory pressure	1 to 65 cm H_2O	Proximal airway pressure does not exceed set threshold during delivery of a mechanical breath
High pressure limit	10 to 75 cm H_2O	Proximal airway pressure exceeds set threshold

TABLE 11-7

Fixed alarms on the Bear Cub 750vs Infant Ventilator

Alarm	Triggering condition
Failed to cycle	Microprocessor detects an internal or external malfunction; once alarm condition is corrected, MODE SELECT switch must be turned to STANDBY position and then to the desired ventilatory mode
Low gas supply	Either air or oxygen inlet pressure (or both) decrease to below 24±2 psig
Patient circuit	Occlusion of inspiratory limb of breathing circuit; proximal sensing line disconnection
Prolonged inspiratory pressure	Proximal airway pressure stays above reference value (low PEEP/CPAP + 10 cm H_2O) for more than 3.5 sec
Settings incompatible	One or more of the following: Inspiratory time and ventilator rate settings incompatible (INSPIRATORY TIME and VENTILATOR RATE displays flash) Base Flow is incompatible with inspiratory flow (BASE FLOW and INSPIRATORY FLOW displays flash); note that some software versions allow the base flow setting to be about two times the inspiratory flow setting Volume limit setting is incompatible with flow and inspiratory pressure settings; if inspiratory flow setting is too high, VOLUME LIMIT LED flashes, alternating with "E.FL."; if inspiratory pressure setting is too high, VOLUME LIMIT LED flashes, alternating with "E.PL."
Pressure settings incompatible	Inspiratory pressure setting is less than PEEP/CPAP setting, or PEEP/CPAP setting is greater than inspiratory pressure setting
Flow sensor	Sensor malfunction or disconnection from ventilator
Apnea	Lack of breath initiation within set time period; apnea time period can be adjusted with control on the ventilator's rear panel; apnea time period is adjustable from 5 to 30 seconds in 5-sec increments When flow sensor is in use, apnea alarm activates when no flow is detected within set time period; when flow sensor is disconnected or disabled in the A/C or SIMV/IMV modes, apnea alarm activates if mandatory breaths are not delivered; when flow sensor is disconnected or disabled in the CPAP mode, apnea alarm is inactive
Low battery	Internal battery has about 5 minutes of power remaining before full discharge

Infrasonics Infant Star Neonatal Ventilator (Original Model)

Overview

The original Infant Star (Nellcor Puritan Bennett, Pleasanton, Calif.) (Figure 11-13, *A*) is electrically and pneumatically powered and microprocessor-controlled. It is time-triggered, time-cycled, and pressure-limited and is designed to provide either continuous flow or continuous plus demand flow.[8] The ventilator's pneumatic components are housed in a separate case, composing the base of the unit. On top of the ventilator is the electrical component module with all of the ventilator's electronic controls and indicators. This module rotates so it can be viewed at different angles.

Either AC power or an external DC battery can be used to power the ventilator. Because the unit's microprocessors require DC power, a transformer converts AC to DC power, protecting the ventilator from AC power surges. When the ventilator is connected to AC power, the

TABLE 11-8

Specifications for the Bear Cub 750vs Infant Ventilator

Rate	1 to 150 breaths/min
Inspiratory time	0.1 to 3.0 seconds
Inspiratory flow	1 to 30 L/min
Base flow	1 to 30 L/min
Volume limit	5 to 300 mL
Oxygen concentration	21% to 100%
Pressure limit	0 to 72 cm H_2O
PEEP/CPAP	0 to 30 cm H_2O
Audio/visual alarms	Low PEEP/CPAP, high breath rate, low inspiratory pressure, high pressure limit, failed to cycle, low gas supply, patient circuit, prolonged inspiratory pressure, settings incompatible, pressure settings incompatible, flow sensor, apnea, low battery
Monitors	Breath rate, breath type (patient-initiated), minute volume, tidal volume (exhaled), % tube leak, inspiratory time, expiratory time, I:E ratio, peak inspiratory pressure, mean airway pressure, air pressure, O_2 pressure, proximal airway pressure, hourmeter, test, battery
Alarm silence	60 seconds

battery is either being recharged or its full charge is being maintained. A completely discharged battery is fully recharged in 1 to 1.5 hours. A fully charged battery can power the ventilator for at least 30 minutes.

Compressed air and oxygen are required for the Infant Star to operate. These gases are blended and reduced to a 18-psig pressure source, which drives a series of solenoid valves to control gas flow to the patient. These solenoid valves work together to provide flow from 4 to 40 L/min (in 2 L/min increments) for spontaneous and mechanical breaths. These flow limits allow the ventilator to be used for infants weighing up to 10 kg.

High-frequency ventilation is an optional feature on the original Infant Star ventilator, but those units fitted with this option operate similarly to the Infant Star 950 (see the related discussion later in this chapter).

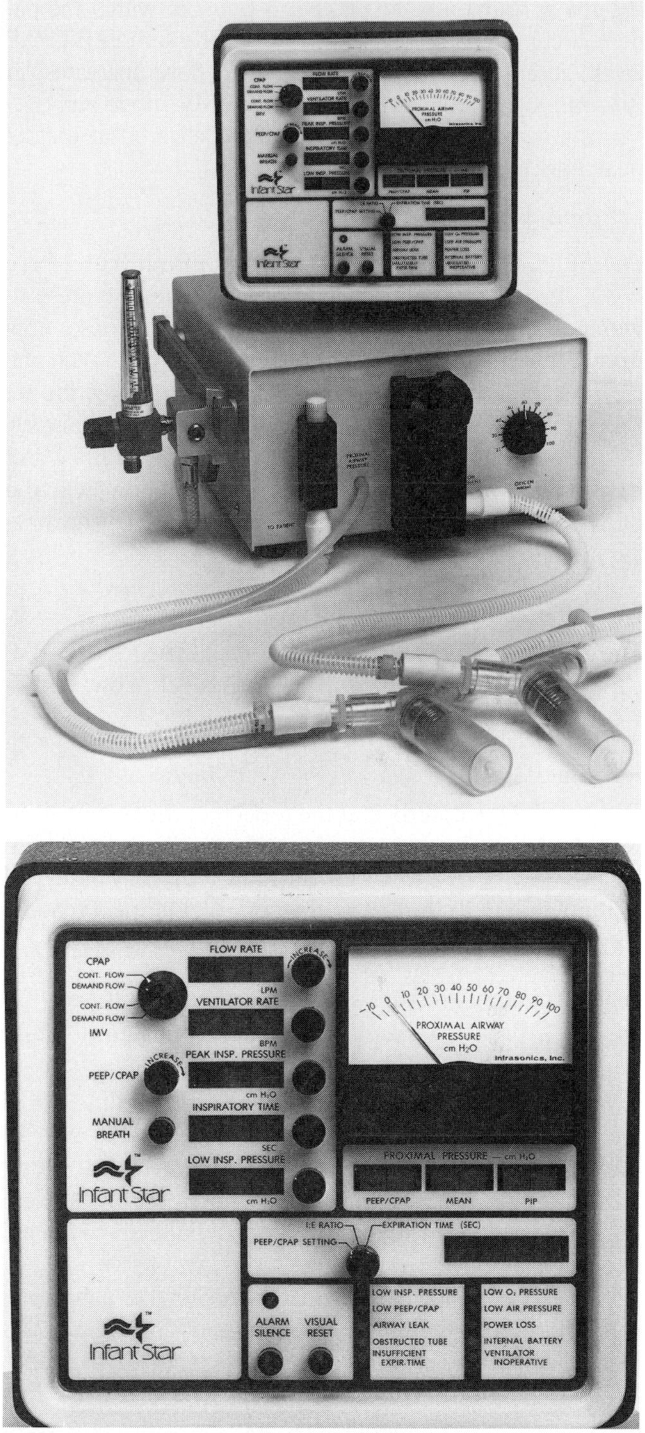

Figure 11-13 **A,** Infant Star Ventilator; **B,** control panel of an Infant Star Neonatal Ventilator. (Courtesy Infrasonics, Inc., San Diego, Calif.)

Controls (Figure 11-13, *B*)

Mode Selector

Using the four-position MODE selector switch, the clinician can select IMV or CPAP with either continuous or demand flow. When CONTINUOUS FLOW is selected, the set flow is delivered through the circuit during both a mandatory and a spontaneous breath. During spontaneous breathing, if pressure within the patient circuit drops below 1 cm H_2O of the set PEEP/CPAP level, flow is increased in 2 L/min increments up to 40 L/min. This enables the clinician to select low flows without limiting the patient's inspiratory flow demand. When DEMAND FLOW is selected, a background flow of 4 L/min is delivered continuously during spontaneous breathing. With DEMAND FLOW, if pressure within the patient circuit drops below 1 cm H_2O of the set PEEP/CPAP level during spontaneous breathing, flow increases in 2 L/min increments. When set in the IMV mode with DEMAND FLOW, mandatory breaths are delivered at the set peak flow in a decelerating flow pattern.

PEEP/CPAP

The PEEP/CPAP control is adjustable to from 0 to 24 cm H_2O. Turning this control clockwise increases the pressure within the exhalation valve diaphragm, which opposes flow from the expiratory limb of the patient circuit. With the knob to the left turned to the PEEP/CPAP setting, the set PEEP/CPAP level can be read on the lower digital display. Monitored PEEP/CPAP is displayed in the PEEP/CPAP monitoring window, the SELECTED DATA window (with the PEEP/CPAP setting), and the proximal airway pressure analog meter.

Manual Breath

The MANUAL BREATH control is beneath the PEEP/CPAP control and delivers a breath at the set PIP, flow, and T_I when pressed.

Flow Rate

The FLOW RATE control is at the top left of the proximal airway pressure meter. Adjusting this knob clockwise increases flow from 4 to 40 L/min. Flow is digitally displayed in the window to the left of the control. During a mandatory breath, the ventilator delivers the set flow.

Peak Inspiratory Pressure and Mean Airway Pressure

The PEAK INSPIRATORY PRESSURE (PIP) control is adjustable from 8 to 90 cm H_2O by turning the control clockwise. The set PIP is displayed in the window to the left of the control. Monitored PIP is displayed in both the PIP monitoring window and the PROXIMAL AIRWAY PRESSURE analog. Proximal airway pressure is monitored by an electric pressure transducer that is connected directly to the patient wye connector via tubing.

At the beginning of a mandatory breath, the exhalation valve closes and the set flow is delivered. Once the proximal airway pressure almost reaches the set PIP, the ventilator's microprocessor starts to reduce flow. If the PIP is reached, flow stops completely, and the exhalation valve stays closed until the set T_I lapses. If a leak is present, at least one solenoid valve delivers a sufficient gas flow to maintain the desired PIP for the duration of the T_I.

Mean airway pressure is displayed in the MEAN PRESSURE monitoring window. The microprocessor recalculates mean airway pressure every second and updates the visual display every 5 seconds.

Ventilator Rate, Inspiratory Time, and I:E Ratio

Turning the VENTILATOR RATE control clockwise increases the mechanical breath rate from 1 to 150 breaths/minute.

TABLE 11-9

Difference in set/measured pressure triggering for a low PEEP/CPAP alarm

PEEP/CPAP setting (cm H_2O)	Set/measured pressure difference triggering low PEEP/CPAP alarm (cm H_2O)
0 to 5	2
6 to 8	3
9 to 12	4
13 to 24	5

The ventilator rate is digitally displayed in the window to the left of the control. Below this control is the INSPIRATORY TIME control, which increases the T_I from 0.1 to 3.0 seconds when turned clockwise. The T_I is digitally displayed in the window to the left of this control. I:E ratio is determined by the ventilator rate and inspiratory time. Digital displays of the I:E ratio and T_E can be monitored with the SELECTED DATA switch at the lower center of the control panel. Although inverse I:E ratios are attainable, the ventilator's microprocessor does not permit T_E to be less than 0.2 to 0.3 seconds, depending on the rate control setting (see the following discussion of alarms).

Alarms

Alarm Silence/Visual Reset

The ALARM SILENCE button silences alarms for 60 seconds. Pressing this button a second time cancels the silence. An indicator light goes on during the silent period. After alarm conditions are corrected, the audible alarm stops sounding, although visual alarms are displayed until the VISUAL RESET button is pressed.

Low Inspiratory Pressure

The LOW INSPIRATORY PRESSURE audio/visual alarm, which is adjustable from 0 to 60 cm H_2O, is set at or slightly below the PIP setting. If a leak develops in the ventilator circuit or the ventilator fails to deliver the desired PIP, this alarm is activated. Each breath not reaching this setting triggers the alarm. When the alarm condition is corrected, the audible alarm stops.

Low PEEP/CPAP

The LOW PEEP/CPAP alarm is set automatically by the microprocessor and cannot be adjusted by the operator. If the measured PEEP or CPAP is lower than the set level over 25 seconds, this audio/visual alarm is triggered. The difference between the set and the measured pressure that triggers the alarm varies with the PEEP/CPAP setting. These pressure differences are listed in Table 11-9. It is important to note that the LOW PEEP/CPAP alarm may not be activated if there is an accidental extubation because backpressure produced by endotracheal tube resistance may prevent enough of a difference between measured and set PEEP/CPAP levels to trigger an alarm.

Airway Leak

A circuit leak that drops PEEP and activates demand flow may trigger the AIRWAY LEAK alarm. This alarm system can detect a leak smaller than one that would trigger the LOW PEEP/CPAP alarm. That is, the AIRWAY LEAK alarm activates if the leak is large enough to decrease the PEEP by 1 cm H_2O and cause the demand flow to increase 8 L/min or more above background flow for 4 seconds or longer. Some ventilators automatically detect and compensate for sizable leaks by increasing circuit flow. This feature is most useful in ventilator applications involving undersized, uncuffed artificial airways. Although the Infant Star compensates for leaks, it deems a leak larger than 13 L/min to be an alarm condition that must be corrected.

Obstructed Tube Alarms

If obstructions occur in the inspiratory or expiratory limbs of the ventilator circuit, audio/visual alarms are triggered and a message is displayed. For all of these alarms, the OBSTRUCTED TUBE LED flashes.

If proximal airway pressure rises 5 cm H_2O above the set PIP, inspiration immediately terminates, and an AAO1 visual alarm condition occurs. The message "AHI-PP-AO1" appears in the monitoring window, and the yellow OBSTRUCTED TUBE LED flashes. If proximal airway pressure rises 10 cm H_2O above the set PIP, inspiration immediately terminates, and an AAO2 alarm condition occurs. The exhalation valve and an internal safety valve open to reduce circuit pressure to ambient. "AHI-PP-AO2" is displayed in the monitoring window and is accompanied by an audible alarm.

If the expiratory tubing is blocked, an AAO3 alarm results. Normally, when the exhalation valve opens, pressure must fall to one-half the difference between PIP and PEEP settings within 300 milliseconds (200 milliseconds if rate is higher than 100 breaths/min). If this does not occur, the flow solenoid valves close, and the internal safety valve opens. "AHI-PP-AO3" is displayed, and an alarm sounds.

An AAO4 audio/visual alarm occurs if the proximal airway pressure exceeds the set PEEP/CPAP level by $\geq$6 cm H_2O for 5 seconds. When this occurs, the flow solenoid valves close, the internal safety valve opens, and the message "AHI-CP-AO4" is displayed.

If pressure within the ventilator circuit rises to 15 cm H_2O above the set PIP, an AAO5 audio/visual alarm results. This alarm condition is determined by the internal pressure transducer instead of by the proximal airway pressure transducer. Therefore it can even occur when the proximal airway pressure tubing is blocked or disconnected. The exhalation valve and the internal safety valve open.

For all of these alarm conditions, the visual or audio/visual alarms continue until the next mechanical breath. If the conditions that caused the alarm are corrected, the ventilator resumes normal operation, and the message display and the audible alarms terminate.

Insufficient Expiratory Time

An audio/visual alarm indicating insufficient expiratory time is activated when combined ventilator settings prevent a T_E of 0.2 or 0.3 seconds. When the rate setting is >100 breaths/min and the T_I is set so that T_E is less than 0.2 seconds, the alarm is activated. If the rate is set below 100 breaths/min, but the T_I is set so that T_E is less than 0.3 seconds, the alarm is also activated. In this alarm condition, the set T_I and a minimum T_E are maintained, resulting in a lower rate than that which is set. The RATE display flashes to indicate that the actual rate is less than that set. Once the alarm condition is corrected, however, the ventilator resumes normal operation. The yellow INSUFFICIENT EXPIRATORY TIME indicator flashes until the VISUAL RESET button is pressed.

Low Oxygen Pressure and/or Low Air Pressure

If either compressed gas pressure drops below 45 psig, the LOW OXYGEN PRESSURE and/or LOW AIR PRESSURE alarm is activated. An audible alarm sounds, and the yellow LOW OXYGEN PRESSURE and/or LOW AIR PRESSURE LED flashes. The ventilator continues to operate if only one gas source pressure drops, but FiO_2 varies. If both pressures drop, however, the internal safety valve opens.

Power Loss

The ventilator can be operated by an internal battery that can last at least 30 minutes when fully charged. At 5 to 10 minutes before complete battery discharge, the POWER LOSS and INTERNAL BATTERY LEDs start flashing and the audible alarm sounds. When the battery is fully discharged, the ventilator stops operating and the exhalation valve and internal safety valve open. The audio/visual alarm continues.

Internal Battery

When the ventilator is turned on but not connected to an A/C power source, the internal battery automatically powers the ventilator for at least 30 minutes. The yellow LED lights while the unit is operating on the internal battery, and no alarm sounds until the battery approaches full discharge.

Ventilator Inoperative

When the audio/visual ventilator INOPERATIVE ALARM is activated, flow through the solenoid valves stops and the internal safety valve opens. This alarm condition occurs if at least one of the following occurs:

1. The exhalation valve does not open for 3.5 seconds.
2. The exhalation does not close for 66 seconds in the IMV mode.
3. The microprocessor fails.

BOX 11-6

Using the External Pressure Limit as the Primary Inspiratory Pressure Control

Some clinicians advocate using the external pressure limit on the Infant Star as the primary pressure control in certain situations. For example, when a small-volume nebulizer is placed in-line, the additional flow can increase system pressure and activate the AO4 alarm. Some clinicians also recommend setting the PIP with the external pressure limit in patients who cough frequently or are fighting the ventilator.

If the external pressure limit is used to establish the PIP, the ventilator's inspiratory pressure control should be set 5 to 10 cm H_2O higher as a safety pop-off.

Safety-Relief Valve

A spring-loaded pressure-relief valve is located at the ventilator outlet. When the pressure set by this valve is reached, excess gas is vented to the atmosphere. Turning the valve clockwise increases relief pressure. This valve is intended to be used as a back-up safety valve in case the primary PIP control and the HIGH PRESSURE alarm system fail. Normally, the safety-relief valve is set at least 25 cm H_2O above the desired PIP. Exceptions to the way the valve is normally used are discussed in Box 11-6.

Additional Features

The original Infant Star incorporates additional features to enhance its operation. Alarm loudness can be adjusted with a **rotary baffle** on the unit's back panel. Although the ventilator does not incorporate a graphics monitor, an **analog pressure output cable outlet** allows connection to an oscilloscope or strip chart recorder. A **serial output connector** enables the ventilator to connect to a computer or cardiac monitor.

Connections are also available to add an external DC power source, a remote alarm, and the Star Sync interface (see the discussion of the Star Synch later in this chapter). Table 11-10 lists specifications for the Infant Star.

Troubleshooting

The exhalation valve diaphragm on the Infant Star must be turned in the proper direction and seated properly. The housing must be properly assembled and tightened. Circuit leaks are also common. The ventilator can be tightness-tested in the same way as the BP-200 and the Bear Cub. A "quick checkout" procedure is outlined in the ventilator's instruction manual, and should be used before placing the ventilator back into service after cleaning or when optimum performance is questioned.

TABLE 11-10

Specifications for Infant Star Neonatal Ventilator

Rate	1 to 150 breaths/min
Flow rate	4 to 40 L/min
Peak inspiratory pressure	8 to 90 cm H_2O
Inspiratory time	0.1 to 3.0 seconds
PEEP/CPAP	0 to 24 cm H_2O
Oxygen percent	21% to 100%
Monitors/displays	
I:E ratio	
Expiratory time	
Monitored PEEP	
Mean airway pressure	
Measured peak inspiratory pressure	
Alarms	
Alarm silence	60 seconds
Low inspiratory pressure	0 to 60 cm H_2O
Low PEEP/CPAP	varies with set PEEP/CPAP (see text)
Airway leak	
Obstructed tube conditions	AO1 to AO5 (see text)
Insufficient expiratory time	<0.2 to 0.3 seconds
Low oxygen inlet pressure	<40 psig
Low air inlet pressure	<40 psig
Power loss	5 to 10 minutes of battery use left
Ventilator inoperative conditions	various causes (see text)
Alarm intensity	rotary baffle

Infrasonics Infant Star 500 Ventilator

Overview

The Infant Star 500 (Figure 11-14) is electrically and pneumatically powered. All of its functions are controlled by dual microprocessors: one controls all of the unit's operations, and the other controls display information. Continuous operational checks between the two microprocessors ensure more dependable operation.[9] Like the original model, the ventilator's pneumatic components are housed in an updated case that makes up the base of the unit. The electrical component module with all of the ventilator's electronic controls and indicators is on top and rotates so it can be viewed at different angles.

The 500 is time-triggered, time-cycled, and pressure-limited. It is designed to provide continuous background

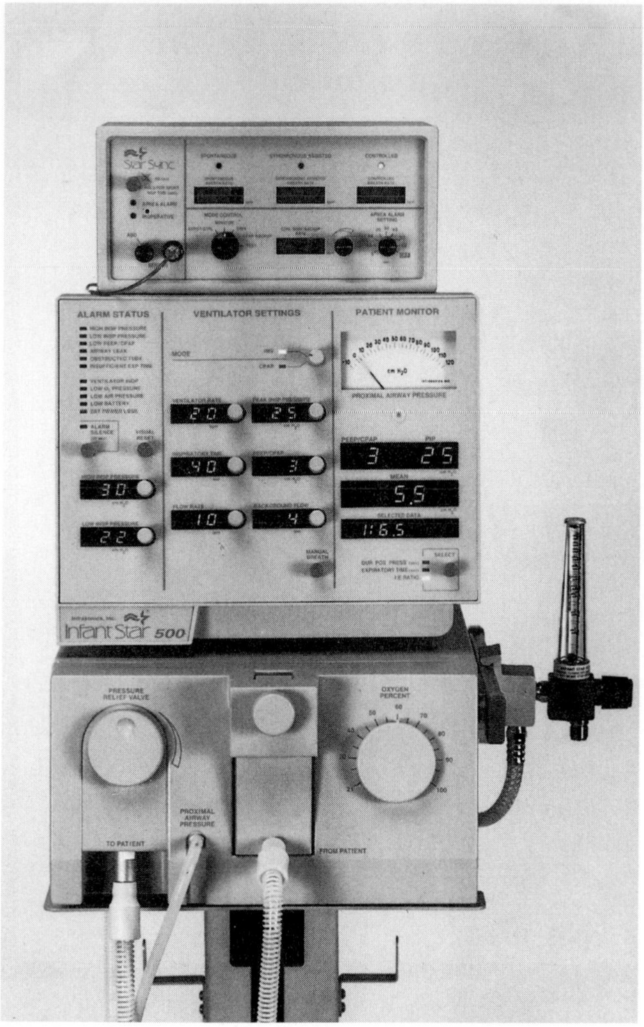

Figure 11-14 The Infrasonics Infant Star 500 Neonatal Ventilator. (Courtesy Infrasonics, Inc., San Diego, Calif.)

flow for spontaneous breathing. This background flow is supplemented by a demand system that provides additional flow to the patient if necessary.

The ventilator's POWER switch is located on the rear panel. Either AC power or an external battery can be used to power the ventilator. A fully discharged external battery can be completely recharged in 1 hour if the ventilator is turned off while connected to electrical power. If the ventilator is turned on, a discharged battery requires 1.5 hours to fully recharge.

Compressed air and oxygen are required for the Infant Star to operate. These gases are blended and reduced to an 18-psig pressure source, which drives a series of solenoid valves to control gas flow to the patient. These solenoid valves work together to provide flow from 2 to 32 L/min for background flow and from 4 to 40 L/min for mechanical breaths. (Both flows are provided in 2 L/min increments.) Flows up to 40 L/min are available from the demand-flow system for spontaneous breaths. These flow limit ranges differ slightly among software versions. The ventilator may be used in infants weighing up to 18 kg. A standard infant circuit and an approved humidifier can be used with the Infant Star 500.

Controls (Figure 11-15)

The front panel is organized into three sections from left to right: 1) the ALARM STATUS section; 2) the VENTILATOR SETTINGS section; and 3) the PATIENT MONITORING section, each of which is discussed here.

Alarm Status Section

The ALARM STATUS section features red LED indicators that light when alarm conditions occur. An audible alarm is also activated for all alarm conditions except EXT POWER LOSS. Because the battery always powers the ventilator and begins to discharge when AC power is interrupted, only a visual indicator is activated. If the battery is discharged, an audio/visual alarm activates immediately.

The ALARM SILENCE button silences the audible alarm for 60 seconds. Pressing the button a second time cancels the silent period. The ALARM SILENCE indicator light illuminates during the silent period. For certain alarm conditions (i.e., electrical and internal function failures), the audible alarm cannot be silenced.

After alarm conditions are corrected, the audible alarm stops. The LED corresponding to the alarm continues to be lit after alarm conditions are corrected until the VISUAL RESET button is pressed.

High Inspiratory Pressure

The HIGH INSPIRATORY PRESSURE alarm is activated when the PIP exceeds a set limit. This limit can be adjusted from 5 to 105 cm H_2O using the HIGH INSPIRATORY PRESSURE control. The pressure limit is digitally displayed in the window to the left of the control.

The limit should not be adjusted more than 15 cm H_2O above the PIP set for ventilation. If a limit greater than 15 cm H_2O is selected, the HIGH INSPIRATORY PRESSURE LED flashes and the microprocessor automatically sets the pressure limit to 15 cm H_2O above the set PIP.

When the pressure limit is activated, the exhalation valve opens and the inspiratory phase is terminated (pressure-cycled). The message "AHI PIP, AO1" appears in the PEEP/CPAP, PIP, and SELECTED DATA windows in the patient monitor section. The ventilator attempts to deliver the next breath at the appropriate timed interval and continues to sound the alarm and display the alarm message until the alarm condition is corrected.

Low Inspiratory Pressure

The LOW INSPIRATORY PRESSURE alarm is activated if a set minimum pressure is not reached during the inspiratory phase. This minimum pressure is selected using the LOW INSPIRATORY PRESSURE control. A digital display of the set

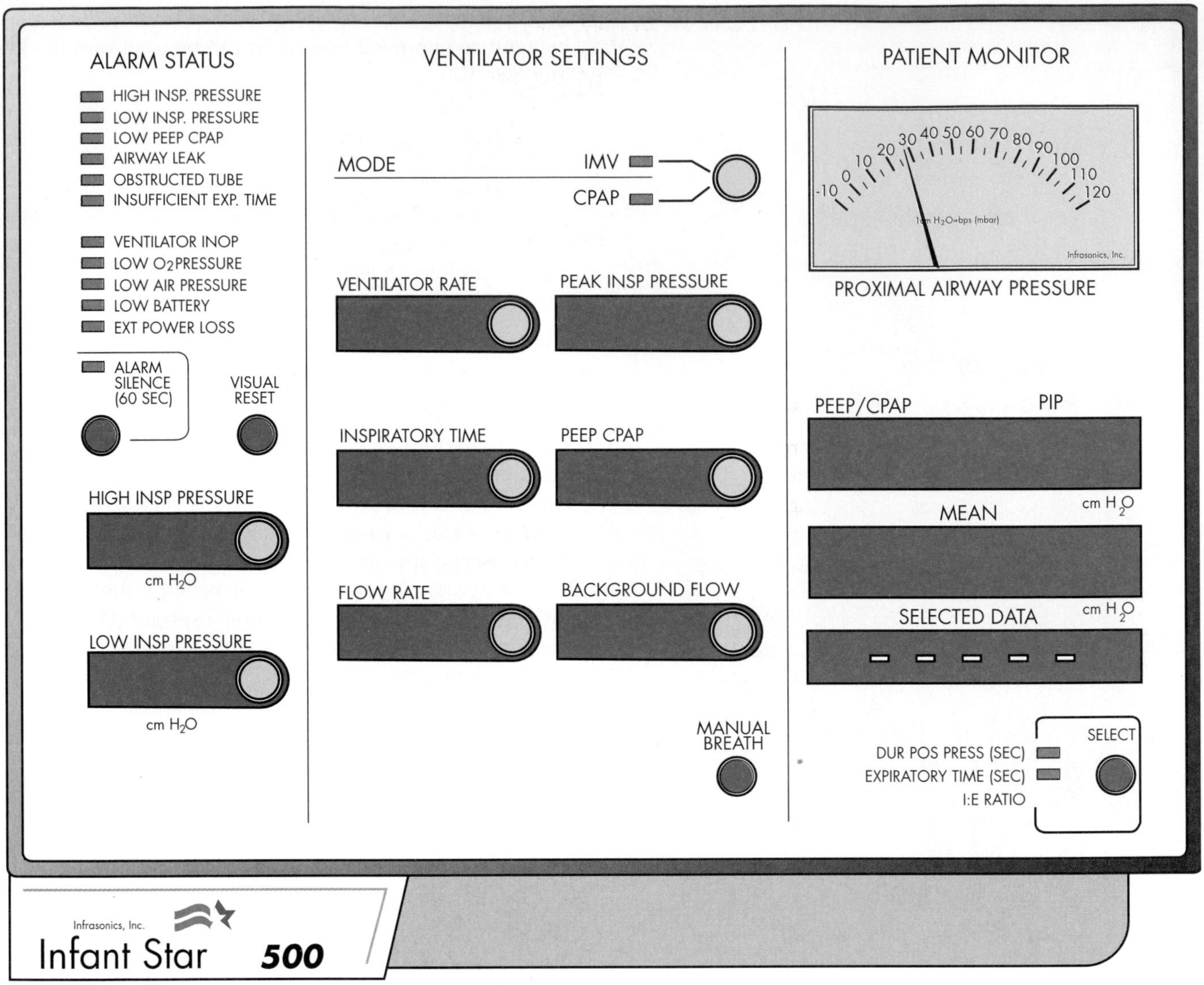

Figure 11-15 The Infrasonics Infant Star 500 Neonatal Ventilator control panel.

low inspiratory pressure appears in the window to the left of the control.

Adjustable from 3 to 60 cm H_2O, the LOW INSPIRATORY PRESSURE setting must be lower than the PIP setting. If a large leak develops in the ventilator circuit or the ventilator fails to deliver the desired PIP, this alarm is activated. This alarm is also activated if the LOW INSPIRATORY PRESSURE control or the pressure-relief valve is inappropriately set.

If the LOW INSPIRATORY PRESSURE control is turned fully counter-clockwise to 3 cm H_2O and the PEEP/CPAP is set higher than this, the ventilator automatically tracks the PEEP/CPAP level as the minimum inspiratory pressure. The alarm is not activated unless the PEEP level drops below 3 cm H_2O.

When the LOW INSPIRATORY PRESSURE alarm is activated, the ventilator continues to deliver the next breath at the appropriate timed interval. Each breath not reaching the low inspiratory pressure setting triggers the alarm (Box 11-7).

BOX 11-7

Decision Making & Problem Solving

An Infant Star 500 ventilator is operating with the following settings: PIP = 26 cm H_2O; PEEP = 4 cm H_2O; rate = 22 breaths/min; flow = 4 L/min; T_I = 0.6 seconds; low inspiratory pressure alarm = 23 cm H_2O. What alarm condition will be active?

See Appendix A for the answer.

Low PEEP/CPAP

The LOW PEEP/CPAP alarm is not adjustable by the operator but is set automatically by the microprocessor. If the measured PEEP or CPAP is less than the set level over 25 seconds, the alarm is triggered. The difference between the set and the measured pressure that triggers the alarm varies

TABLE 11-11

Difference in set/measured pressure triggering a low PEEP/CPAP alarm on the Infant Star 500 and 950

PEEP/CPAP setting (cm H_2O)	Set/measured difference triggering low PEEP/CPAP alarm
0 to 5	2
6 to 8	3
9 to 12	4
13 to 24	5

TABLE 11-12

Message displayed for obstructed tube alarm on the Infant Star 500 and 950

Message	Problem
HI PIP, AO2	Proximal airway pressure is 5 cm H_2O above high inspiratory pressure setting
HI PIP, AO3	Less than 50% pressure drop from PIP to PEEP during expiration
HI CPP, AO4	PEEP/CPAP is 6 cm H_2O higher than that set for 5 seconds
HI PIP, AO5	PIP at the outlet of the ventilator is 10 cm H_2O higher than high inspiratory pressure setting

with the PEEP/CPAP setting. These pressure differences are shown in Table 11-11.

Airway Leak

The AIRWAY LEAK alarm is activated when large leaks are detected in the patient circuit with ≥3 cm H_2O of PEEP or CPAP. Small circuit leaks are automatically compensated for by the ventilator's demand valve in order to maintain the set PEEP/CPAP. The valve accomplishes this by adding a compensatory flow called **leak makeup.** If this compensatory flow reaches 13 L/min above the background flow setting for 4 seconds or longer, however, the AIRWAY LEAK alarm is activated.

Obstructed Tube

If obstructions occur in the inspiratory or expiratory limbs of the ventilator circuit, the OBSTRUCTED TUBE alarm is activated. Specifically, the alarm is triggered if any of the following four conditions occur:

1. Proximal airway pressure rises 5 cm H_2O above the high inspiratory pressure setting.
2. PEEP/CPAP rises above the set level.
3. The expiratory circuit is partially or completely obstructed.
4. The internal pressure reading is 10 cm H_2O higher than the high inspiratory pressure setting.

When the OBSTRUCTED TUBE alarm is activated, one of four messages is displayed in the selected data window to alert the clinician to the reason for the alarm (Table 11-12).

For all of the OBSTRUCTED TUBE alarm conditions, either the exhalation valve or the internal safety valve opens. The audible alarm continues until the next mechanical breath. If the conditions causing the alarm are corrected, the ventilator resumes normal operation. The message display and the audible alarms also terminate.

Insufficient Expiratory Time

The INSUFFICIENT EXPIRATORY TIME alarm is activated when combined ventilator settings prevent a T_E of 0.2 or 0.3 seconds. When the rate setting is (>100 breaths/min and the T_I is set so that the T_E is <0.2 seconds, the alarm is activated. If the rate is set below 100 breaths/min but the T_I is set so that T_E is less than 0.3 seconds, the alarm is also activated. Until this alarm condition is corrected, the ventilator rate decreases to permit sufficient T_E. The VENTILATOR RATE display flashes, indicating that the set rate is not the actual rate.

Ventilator Inoperative

The VENTILATOR INOP alarm is activated when either microprocessor detects an electronics error. With this alarm condition, mandatory breath delivery stops, gas flow stops, and the internal safety valve opens. Patient spontaneous breathing of room air is possible through the internal safety valve. The audible alarm cannot be silenced.

When a VENTILATOR INOP alarm condition occurs, an error message appears in the selected data window. The message is a code that may be useful to service personnel. Before turning off the ventilator, the clinician should record this code.

Low O_2 Pressure

The LOW O_2 pressure alarm is activated if oxygen line pressure drops below 35 psig. When the alarm is activated, the ventilator will continue operating but delivers 21% oxygen. If the oxygen concentration is set above 80%, however, ventilator performance may be impaired.

Low Air Pressure

The LOW AIR PRESSURE alarm is activated if the compressed-air line pressure drops below 35 psig. When the alarm is activated, the ventilator continues operating but delivers 100% oxygen. If the oxygen concentration is set below 30%, however, ventilator performance may be impaired.

Low Battery

When the ventilator is turned on but not connected to an AC power source, the internal battery automatically powers the ventilator for at least 30 minutes. When the battery is 5 to 10 minutes from complete discharge, the LOW BATTERY and EXTERNAL POWER LOSS indicators start to flash alternately. The audible alarm sounds and cannot be silenced.

When the battery becomes completely discharged, the VENTILATOR INOP and the LOW BATTERY INDICATORS light and the alarm sounds. (Once again, the audible alarm cannot be silenced.) Mandatory breath and gas flow delivery stops, and the internal safety valve opens. Room air is available to the patient for spontaneous breathing through the safety valve.

External Power Loss

If electrical power is interrupted, the EXT POWER LOSS LED lights, but the ventilator continues to operate by the internal battery. No other alarms are activated, and no alarm sounds until the battery is almost discharged.

Ventilator Settings Section

The VENTILATOR SETTINGS section includes all of the unit's operational controls. Each setting is digitally displayed with green LEDs in a window to the left of the control.

Mode Selector

Modes on the Infant Star 500 are set using the two-position MODE selector switch. IMV and CPAP are available, and green LEDs indicate the mode selected.

When using the CPAP mode, only the BACKGROUND FLOW and the PEEP/CPAP controls are operational. The other controls should be set to back-up settings in case manual breaths are given or ventilation in the IMV mode is necessary.

Ventilator Rate

Adjusting the VENTILATOR RATE control clockwise increases the mandatory breath rate from 1 to 150 breaths/min. Adjustments can be made in one-breath increments to a rate of 60 breaths/min. From 60 to 130 breaths/min, adjustments can be made in two-breath increments. For rates from 130 to 150 (the maximum rate), only five-breath increments are possible.

Inspiratory Time and Flow Rate

The INSPIRATORY TIME control, when turned clockwise, increases the T_I from 0.1 to 3.0 seconds. The T_I is adjustable from 0.10 to 0.60 seconds in 0.01-second increments. From 0.60 to 1.0 seconds, the control is adjustable in 0.02-second increments. For T_Is from 1.0 to 3.0 seconds, the control is adjustable in 0.1-second increments.

The I:E ratio is determined by the ventilator rate and T_I. Although inverse I:E ratios are attainable, the ventilator's microprocessor does not permit T_E to be less than 0.2 to 0.3 seconds (see the discussion of alarm status later in this chapter).

Adjusting the FLOW RATE control clockwise increases flow (in 2-L/min increments) delivered during mechanical breaths from 4 to 40 L/min.

Peak Inspiratory Pressure

The PEAK INSPIRATORY PRESSURE (PIP) control is adjustable from 5 to 90 cm H_2O by turning the control clockwise. If the control is not adjusted to at least 5 cm H_2O above the PEEP/CPAP setting, the PIP display to the left of the control flashes.

At the beginning of a mechanical inspiration, the exhalation valve closes and the set flow is delivered. When proximal airway pressure almost reaches the set PIP, the ventilator's microprocessor begins to reduce flow until it stops. If PIP is reached, flow stops completely and the exhalation valve stays closed until the set T_I elapses. If a leak or spontaneous breathing is present, at least one of the solenoid valves delivers a gas flow sufficient to keep PIP above the T_I.

PEEP/CPAP

The PEEP/CPAP control is adjustable from 0 to 24 cm H_2O. Turning this control clockwise increases the pressure within the exhalation valve diaphragm, which opposes flow from the expiratory limb of the patient circuit.

After suctioning procedures or major changes in control settings, the measured PEEP/CPAP may be 2 to 3 cm H_2O above or below the set level. This also may occur after disconnecting and reconnecting the patient to the ventilator. Up to 30 seconds may be required for the pressure to stabilize.

Background Flow

The **BACKGROUND FLOW control** sets the flow available for spontaneous breathing in both CPAP and IMV modes. Turning this control clockwise adjusts the flow from 2 to 32 L/min (in 2-L/min increments). If patient flow demand or a leak reduces PEEP/CPAP by 1 cm H_2O, the demand system automatically provides additional flow, up to 40 L/min.

The BACKGROUND FLOW control sets flow independently from that selected for the mechanical inspiratory phase. This control enables the clinician to minimize circuit PEEP, or the amount of ba#k pressure that develops in the ventilator circuit due to gas flow. In many cases, a flow sufficient for spontaneous breathing can be set significantly lower than the flow necessary for a mechanical breath.

Manual Breath

The MANUAL BREATH button delivers a single breath at the set PIP and T_I. The button is operational in both IMV and CPAP modes.

Patient Monitor Section

The PATIENT MONITOR section of the Infant Star 500 front panel displays all monitored data in amber LEDs. A proximal airway pressure manometer also displays dynamic airway pressures. Airw!y pressure is transmitted to the ventilator's pressure monitoring transducer via tubing directly connected to the patient wye connector. Fixed digital displays show monitored levels of PEEP/CPAP, PIP, and

TABLE 11-13

Specifications for the Infant Star 500 and 950 Infant Ventilators

Rate	1 to 150 breaths/min
Inspiratory time	0.1 to 3.0 seconds
Inspiratory flow	4 to 40 L/min
Background flow	2 to 32 L/min
Rate	1 to 150 breaths per minute
Oxygen concentration	21% to 100%
Pressure limit	5 to 90 cm H_2O
PEEP/CPAP	0 to 24 cm H_2O
Alarms	High inspiratory pressure; low inspiratory pressure; low PEEP/CPAP; airway leak; obstructed tube conditions (see text); pressure; low air pressure; low battery; external power loss
Monitors	I:E ratio; expiratory time; monitored PEEP/CPAP; mean airway pressure; measured peak inspiratory pressure
Alarm silence	60 seconds
Audio/visual alarms	Low PEEP/CPAP; low inspiratory pressure; high pressure limit; failed to cycle; low gas supply; low battery
Monitors	Inspiratory time; expiratory time; I:E ratio; peak inspiratory pressure; mean airway pressure; air pressure; O_2 pressure; proximal airway pressure; hourmeter; test; battery
Alarm silence	60 seconds
HFV rate (950 model only)	2 to 22 Hertz
Amplitude (oscillatory pulse flow; 950 model only)	12 to 120 L/min

mean airway pressure. The PEEP/CPAP level is measured every 10 milliseconds and is updated every 200 milliseconds. The PIP is updated every breath. Mean airway pressure is measured every 5 milliseconds and is updated every 200 milliseconds.

A SELECTED DATA window digitally displays a choice of three additional data. By pushing the SELECT button, the clinician can toggle between the data choices, which are indicated by LEDs and displayed in the window. The DUR POS PRESSURE display indicates the amount of time the proximal airway pressure exceeds 1 cm H_2O above baseline during a mechanical breath. The EXPIRATION TIME display indicates the duration of the expiratory phase in seconds. The I:E RATIO display shows the relationship of the inspiratory phase to the expiratory phase. The inspiratory phase is always expressed as 1, and the expiratory phase is expressed in whole numbers and/or decimals. For inverse relationships, the expiratory phase is expressed in tenths.

Safety-Relief Valve

A spring-loaded pressure-relief valve is located at the ventilator outlet. When the pressure set by this valve is reached, excess gas is vented to the atmosphere. Turning the valve clockwise increases the relief pressure. This valve, which is adjustable from 5 to 120 cm H_2O, is intended to be used as a back-up safety valve in case the primary PIP control and the HIGH-PRESSURE alarm system fail. It is also used to limit the PIP during in-line aerosol therapy.

Additional Features

The Infant Star 500 incorporates an additional feature to enhance its operation. The unit's **exhalation block** is heated to 120° to 140° C to minimize condensation. With the cooling effect of the flow through the ventilator circuit, the block's temperature is reduced to 60° C.

Alarm volume level can be adjusted using a rotary baffle on the unit's back panel. Loudness can be regulated from approximately 72 to 88 decibels.

Although the 500 ventilator does not incorporate a graphics monitor, an analog pressure output enables it to be connected to an oscilloscope or strip-chart recorder. A serial output connector allows for connection to a computer or cardiac monitor. Ventilator settings and pressures can then be displayed with other patient data in a central location.

Connections are also available to add an external DC power source, a remote alarm, and the Star Sync, which is discussed later in this chapter. Specifications for the Infant Star 500 are included in Table 11-13.

Troubleshooting

To avoid system leaks, the exhalation valve must be properly assembled and tightened. Circuit leaks trigger LOW PEEP/CPAP and AIRWAY LEAK alarms. More complex troubleshooting problems are addressed in the ventilator's instruction manual.

INFRASONICS INFANT STAR 950 VENTILATOR

The Infrasonics Infant Star 950 (Figure 11-16) is almost identical in design to the 500 model. The 950, however, incorporates high-frequency ventilation, which can be used with or without conventional ventilation. Internally, the two models differ only in their high-frequency components. Because

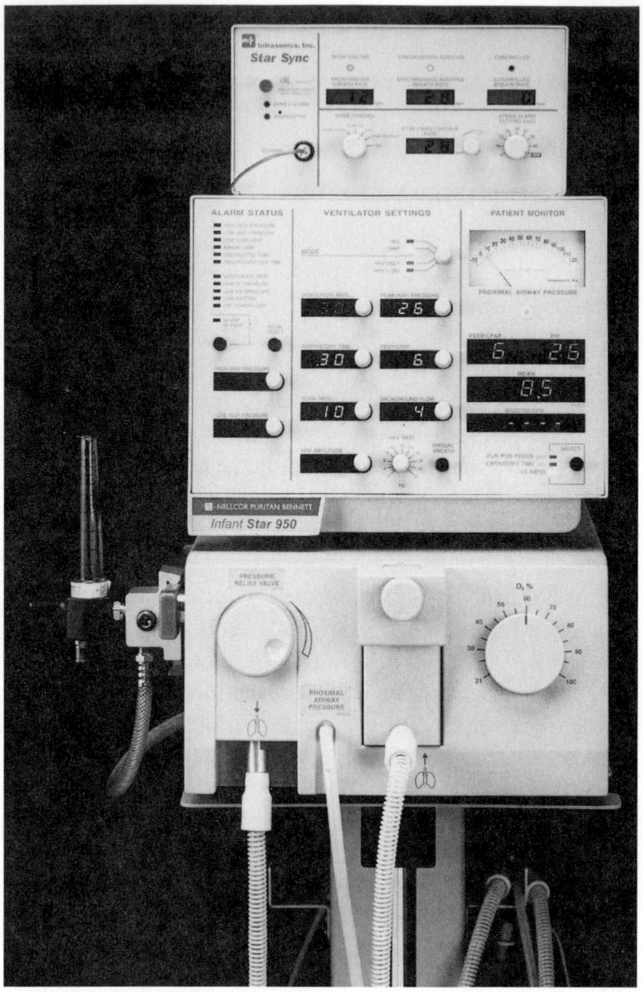

Figure 11-16 The Infrasonics Infant Star 950 Ventilator and Star Synch module. (Courtesy Nellcor Puritan Bennett, Pleasanton, Calif.)

the 950's alarms, controls, and monitors are similar to those of the 500, only the differences between the two units are discussed in the corresponding sections that follow.

Minimum compressed oxygen and air pressure for the Infant Star 950 is 45 psig rather than 35 psig as for the 500. Higher pressures are required to meet the additional gas flow demands of the high-frequency system.[10]

Standard infant ventilator circuits and humidifiers can be used with the 950 to provide conventional ventilation. If high-frequency ventilation is employed, however, a reusable Tygon circuit specifically designed for the ventilator is recommended. This circuit minimizes compliance and provides greater **amplitude** to high-frequency breaths. A Fisher-Paykel humidifier with a low compressible chamber is also recommended. If a continuous water feed system is not used, the chamber should be refilled to its maximum water level marking hourly.

The type of high-frequency ventilation provided by the 950 is comparable with a **mechanical oscillator,** which is a device that employs a diaphragm, piston, or plate to move gas bidirectionally (see Chapter 9). Although the Infant Star 950 also provides bidirectional flow, it is more accurately described as a **flow interrupter,** which is a type of pneumatic oscillator in which flow abruptly starts and stops at very high rates. The effect of flow interruption is the creation of pulses that can produce pressure swings at the patient's airway. These pressure swings provide the high-frequency amplitude.

Using proportioning valves, the 950 delivers high, instantaneous pressure pulses to the inspiratory limb. A jet Venturi within the exhalation valve assembly creates a negative pressure. Between the positive pressure pulses and the negative flow from the expiratory limb, an oscillator-like bidirectional gas flow is generated at the airway.

Controls (Figure 11-17)

The front control panel is almost identical to that of the 500 except that two additional modes are available, and there are also controls for amplitude and frequency. When using high-frequency modes, mean airway pressure is adjusted with the PEEP/CPAP control. There are no flow adjustments except for IMV breaths. Other aspects of the ventilator are identical to the 500 model, except that there is a key switch on the rear panel that enables HFV operation.

Mode

In addition to the IMV and CPAP modes, HFV ONLY or HFV + IMV can be selected. When in the HFV mode, conventional settings are dimly displayed and nonfunctional. Only mean airway pressure (adjusted with the PEEP/CPAP control), FIO_2, amplitude, and frequency can be adjusted. The MANUAL BREATH button is operational and delivers a conventional breath at the set flow, T_I, and PIP.

When in the HFV + IMV mode, all controls except BACKGROUND FLOW are operative. The BACKGROUND FLOW LED is dimly lit. In this mode, high-frequency oscillations are momentarily interrupted, and IMV breaths are delivered at the set rate, flow, T_I, and PIP.

HFV Rate and HFV Amplitude

The HFV RATE control adjusts the number of oscillations from 2 to 22 **Hertz;** 1 Hertz is equal to 60 cycles, or breaths, per minute. The HFV AMPLITUDE control varies the pressure of the oscillatory pulses (i.e., the oscillatory pulse pressure) from 0 to 160 cm H_2O. Although this control is technically a flow control, adjusting it affects the intensity of the pulses. Therefore it alters the ΔP, or the change from **trough pressure** to peak pressure that occurs with every oscillation around the baseline. As with other controls, green LED displays indicate control settings. Specifications for the Infant Star 950 are included in Table 11-13.

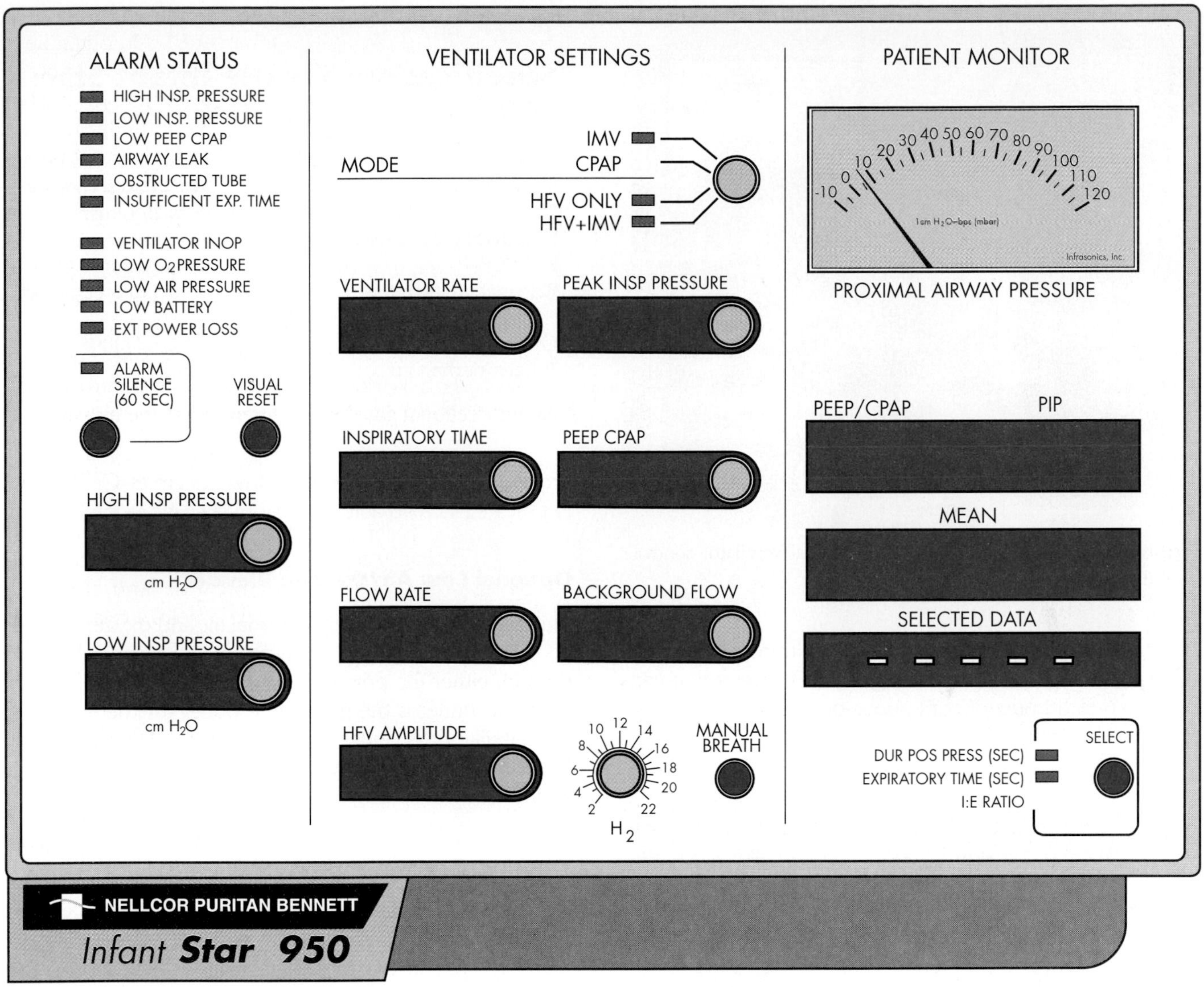

Figure 11-17 The Infrasonics Infant Star 950 Ventilator control panel.

INFANT STAR SYNCH

Patient triggering of SIMV or A/C breaths is available through the Infant Star Sync interface (see Figure 11-16). This unit, which can be attached to all Infant Star models, consists of the interface module and cable and a disposable abdominal capsule. Using **impedance** to detect abdominal movements, the Star Sync system is designed to signal the ventilator to deliver a breath when the patient initiates an inspiratory effort. The module also provides a digital display of spontaneous breaths, assisted breaths, unassisted breaths, and spontaneous T_I. An optional, time-adjustable APNEA alarm is also incorporated into the system.

Troubleshooting

In addition to the troubleshooting issues that occur in the Infant Star 500, the clinician should be aware of the effect of water in the circuit when operating the ventilator in the high-frequency mode. Large collections of water affect gas movement and may dampen oscillations. The effects of water condensation are usually reflected in undesired changes in the amplitude reading. The circuit should be checked for condensation before the AMPLITUDE control knob is readjusted.

INFANT STAR 100 NEONATAL VENTILATOR

The Infant Star 100 Neonatal Ventilator (Figure 11-18) is a time-triggered, pressure-limited, time-cycled, continuous-flow ventilator designed for either in-hospital or field transport of neonatal and pediatric patients. It is electrically powered with 120-volt AC and pneumatically powered by two external gas sources at 40 to 75 psig. It incorporates a

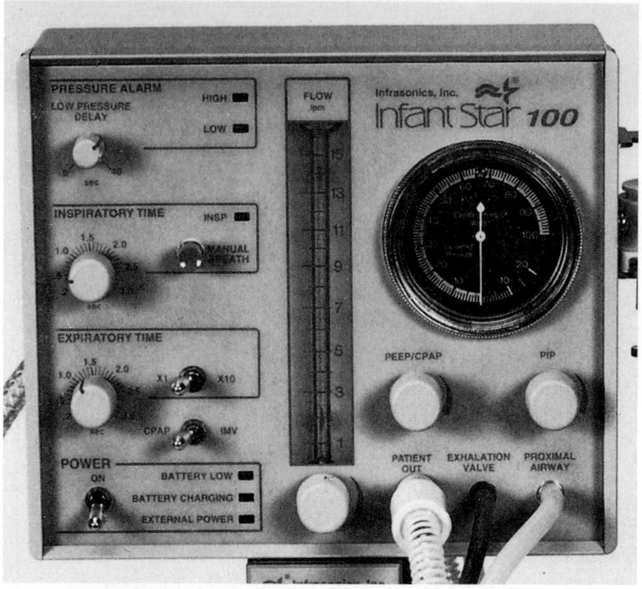

Figure 11-18 The Infant Star 100 Neonatal Ventilator control and alarm panel.

low bleed flow to conserve gas during transport and includes an internal rechargeable **gel-cell battery** that can provide 6 to 8 hours of continuous operation.[11]

Overview of Control and Alarm Panel

Figure 11-18 is a diagram of the control and alarm panel. The CPAP/IMV locking toggle selector switch is on the bottom of the front left panel. The control settings are: INSPIRATORY TIME (0.2 to 3.0 seconds), EXPIRATORY TIME (0.2 to 30 seconds), EXPIRATORY TIME ×1/×10 (multiplies T_E setting by one or ten), FLOW (1 to 15 L/min), PEEP/CPAP (0 to 20 cm H_2O), and PIP (0 to 60 cm H_2O). A proximal airway pressure gauge has a range of −20 to 100 cm H_2O. The inspiratory indicator (amber LED) illuminates during mandatory inspirations. The MANUAL BREATH button delivers a single mandatory breath in both modes. When the manual breath control is activated, the breath is based on the PIP, flow, and T_I settings. Table 11-14 lists parameter specifications for the Infant Star 100.

The **ON/OFF locking toggle switch** prevents accidental movement. The internal battery recharges automatically—even if the ventilator is off. The BATTERY LOW indicator sounds an alarm until the ventilator is connected to an external power source. The BATTERY CHARGING indicator lights until the battery is fully charged. A red LED illuminates when the ventilator is supplied by external power.

Alarms

The HIGH-PRESSURE alarm is a nonadjustable alarm with audio/visual indicators that activate when the proximal airway pressure exceeds 72 to 92 cm H_2O. The LOW-PRESSURE alarm is also preset with audio/visual indicators when the proximal airway pressure falls below 2.5 cm H_2O. The LOW PRESSURE DELAY is adjustable from 0 to 40 seconds.

TABLE 11-14

Specifications for the Infant Star 100 Neonatal Ventilator

Inspiratory time	0.2 to 3.0 seconds
Expiratory time	0.2 to 30 seconds
Flow	1 to 15 L/min
Peak inspiratory pressure	0 to 60 cm H_2O
PEEP/CPAP	0 to 20 cm H_2O
Rate (determined from T_I and T_E settings)	2 to 150 breaths/min
Oxygen concentration	21% to 100%
Trigger mechanism	Time

Optional Low Air/Oxygen Blender

This blender is supplied by external air and oxygen sources at 40 to 70 psig and delivers oxygen concentrations through either the primary or auxiliary gas outlet. The primary gas outlet is the gas source outlet for the ventilator. The auxiliary gas outlet supplies metered low flows (0 to 30 L/min) through a flowmeter. An audible alarm indicates a difference of 30 psig between the two gas sources.

Tracking-Relief Pressure Valve

The **tracking-relief pressure valve** automatically limits airway pressure and is inside the ventilator. If the set PIP is ≥10 cm H_2O, the pressure relief occurs at 10 to 15 cm H_2O above the set PIP. If the set PIP is <10 cm H_2O, the pressure relief occurs at 15 to 20 cm H_2O above the set PIP.

Infant Star 200 Neonatal/Pediatric Ventilator

The Infant Star 200 Neonatal/Pediatric Ventilator (Figure 11-19) is a time-triggered, pressure-limited, time-cycled, continuous-flow ventilator. It is electrically powered with 120-volt AC and pneumatically powered by two external gas sources at 40 to 75 psig. SIMV is available with a 9-pin **DIN connector** that provides communication between the Infant Star 200 and Star Sync patient-triggered interface.[12]

Overview of Control and Alarm Panel

The front panel comprises three sections: ALARM STATUS, VENTILATOR SETTINGS, and PATIENT MONITOR (Figure 11-18). The first section is the ALARM STATUS panel, which is located on the left side of the ventilator. The HIGH-PRESSURE

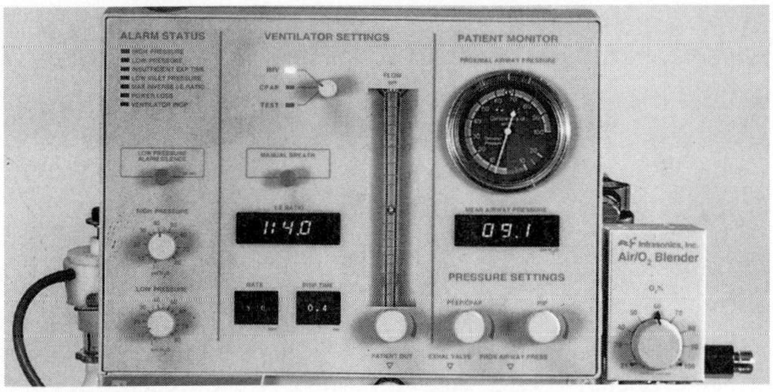

Figure 11-19 The Infant Star 200 Neonatal/Pediatric Ventilator control and alarm panel. (Courtesy Infrasonics, Inc., San Diego)

TABLE 11-15

Infant Star 200 Neonatal/ Pediatric Ventilator

Inspiratory time	0.1 to 2.9 seconds
Rate	0 to 150 breaths/min
I:E ratio	1:0.25 to 1:9.9
PEEP/CPAP	0 to 20 cm H_2O
Peak inspiratory pressure	0 to 70 cm H_2O
Flow	2 to 50 L/min
Trigger mechanism	Time or abdominal motion (Star Sync)

alarm has a range of 1 to 85 cm H_2O. The LOW-PRESSURE alarm has a range of 1 to 85 cm H_2O. The low pressure alarm silence is 60 seconds. The INSUFFICIENT EXPIRATORY TIME alarm is activated when the T_I and rate settings result in a T_E <0.2 seconds. The LOW INLET PRESSURE alarm is activated when the gas source is below 40 psi. The MAX INVERSE I:E RATIO ALARM is activated when the I:E ratio is > 4:1. The POWER LOSS alarm is activated when insufficient power is present. When the microprocessor detects a malfunction, the VENTILATOR INOP alarm is activated. The audible alarm intensity is adjusted with a rotary baffle, which muffles the alarm sound when rotated counterclockwise. A remote alarm output is available to connect an external alarm system. Table 11-15 provides parameter specifications for the Infant Star 200 Neonatal/Pediatric Ventilator.

The middle section is the VENTILATOR SETTINGS panel. The available modes of ventilation are IMV, CPAP, and TEST. The IMV and CPAP modes have continuous flow available for spontaneous respiratory efforts. The TEST mode verifies proper function of the monitoring LEDs and alarms, and all mandatory breaths cease during this mode. The FLOW CONTROL range is from 2 to 50 L/min. The flowmeter is calibrated in the following two ranges: from 2 to 12 L/min (in 1-L/min increments) and from 15 to 50 L/min (in 5-L/min increments). The VENTILATOR RATE range is from 1 to 150 breaths/minute (1-breath increments). The INSPIRATORY TIME range is from 0.1 to 2.9 seconds (0.1-second increments). The MANUAL BREATH button delivers a mandatory breath in all modes. The V_T delivered depends on the set flow, T_I, and PIP. The I:E ratio ranges from 1:0.25 to 1:9.9.

The third section is the PATIENT MONITOR panel. The pressure settings include PEEP/CPAP (0 to 20 cm H_2O) and PIP (0 to 70 cm H_2O). The monitored pressures are proximal airway pressure (−20 to 100 cm H_2O) and mean airway pressure (0 to 99.9 cm H_2O).

Optional Air/Oxygen Blender

This blender is supplied by external air and oxygen sources at 40 to 70 psig. The blender delivers oxygen concentrations through either the primary or auxiliary gas outlet. The primary gas outlet is the gas-source outlet for the ventilator. The auxiliary gas outlet supplies metered low flows (2 to 90 L/min) through a flowmeter. An audible alarm indicates a 30-psig difference between the two gas sources.

Tracking-Relief Pressure Valve

The tracking-relief pressure valve automatically limits airway pressure and is located inside the ventilator (as in the 100 model). If the set PIP is <10 cm H_2O, the pressure relief occurs at 10 to 15 cm H_2O above the set PIP. If the set PIP is >10 cm H_2O, the pressure relief occurs at 15 to 20 cm H_2O above the set PIP.

VIP BIRD INFANT/PEDIATRIC VENTILATOR

The VIP Bird Infant/Pediatric Ventilator (Bird Products Corp., Palm Springs, Calif.) (Figure 11-20) mechanically supports neonatal, infant, and pediatric patients with the most common ventilator modes. It is electrically powered by 115-volt AC and pneumatically powered by external compressed air and oxygen at 40 to 75 psig. The VIP Bird is microprocessor-controlled by three processors. Flow triggering and cycling can be accomplished by using the Bird Partner IIi volume monitor and infant flow sensor. The blender auxiliary output is located on the side of the ventilator for use with a nebulizer or hand-held resuscitator.[13]

Noteworthy Internal Functions

The Microblender mixes the two gases according to the set oxygen percentage. The blended gas then enters the 1.1-L **accumulator** (Figure 11-21). The accumulator reserves pressurized gas during the expiratory phase in order to meet the high inspiratory flow demands of a patient with maximum flow capabilities of 120 L/min. The gas exits the accumulator and enters a pneumatic regulator that sets the

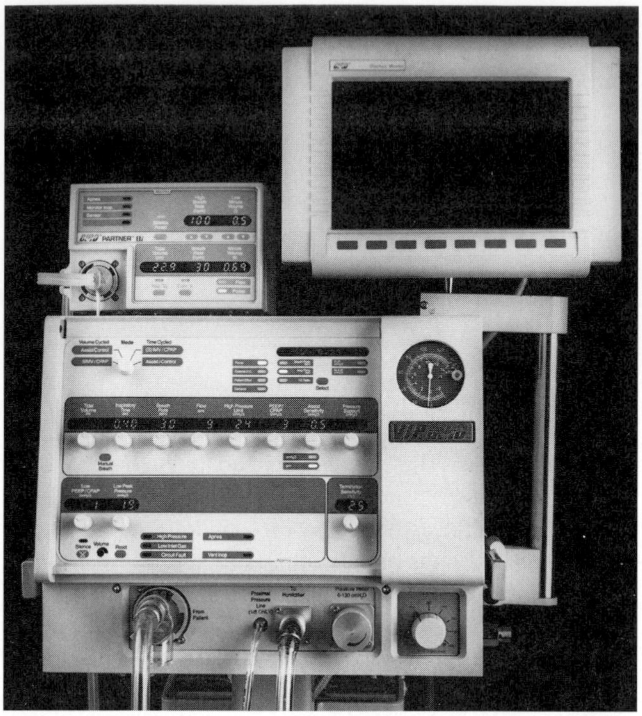

Figure 11-20 The VIP Bird Ventilator. (Courtesy Bird Products Corp., Palm Springs, Calif.)

flow-control valve driving pressure at 25 psig (see Figure 11-21). A **pulsation dampener** is between the regulator and flow-control valve and is used to stabilize pressure and maintain driving pressure to the flow-control valve. Gas flow is delivered to the patient by means of a flow-control valve (electromechanical device), and all gas from the patient is controlled by an exhalation valve (electromechanical device; see Chapter 9). The flow-control valve shifts the stepper motor's rotary motion to a linear motion, which is required to throttle flow through the variable poppet type of orifice. Delivered flow rates are determined by the system driving pressure and the diameter of the valve opening. Flow rates are unaffected by downstream patient circuit pressures (maximum level of 350 cm H_2O) with a system pressure of 25 psig.

Because of the possibility of inadvertent PEEP developing from the continuous flow (time-cycled modes) in the expiratory limb of the patient circuit during time-cycled pressure-limited ventilation, a jet Venturi is incorporated into the exhalation manifold. The **jet solenoid** controls the driving pressure to the exhalation valve jet Venturi and is controlled by the microprocessor. The jet solenoid is active when the flow rate control is set at $\geq$5 L/min with a PEEP of 0 to 5 cm H_2O, or when PEEP is set at zero and the flow is at any setting.[13]

A pneumatically driven safety valve is activated when a ventilator inoperative event or electrical power failure occurs and allows the patient to breathe room air. For example, if a pressure difference of 20 psig occurs between the air and oxygen sources, the gas source with the highest pressure is used by the ventilator, resulting in a delivered oxygen concentration of 21% or 100%.

Overview of Control and Alarm Panel

Figure 11-22 is a diagram of the control and alarm panel. The MODE selector knob is on the top left front panel and has two groups of modes. The volume-cycled (VC) modes are A/C and SIMV/CPAP. The time-cycled (TC) modes are A/C and (S)IMV/CPAP. The front panel control settings are: TIDAL VOLUME (20 to 995 mL); INSPIRATORY TIME (0.1 to 3.0 seconds); RATE (0 to 150 breaths/minute); FLOW (3 to 120 L/min for VC modes, and 3 to 40 L/min for TC modes); HIGH PRESSURE (3 to 120 cm H_2O for VC modes and 3 to 80 cm H_2O for TC modes; Box 11-8); PEEP/CPAP (0 to 24 cm H_2O); ASSIST SENSITIVITY (1 to 20 cm H_2O or off for VC modes, and 0.1 to 5.0 L/min or off only for TC modes with a neonatal flow sensor in use); and PRESSURE SUPPORT (0 to 50 cm H_2O). Table 11-16 lists parameter specifications for the VIP Bird Infant/Pediatric Ventilator.

The MANUAL BREATH control is on the control panel and provides an operator-initiated, controlled breath in all modes. Control displays that are illuminated are functional controls in a specific mode. Control displays that are dimmed are not functional controls in a specific mode. For example, the TIDAL VOLUME display is dimmed when the ventilator is in a time-cycled, pressure-limited mode. During CPAP, the INSPIRATORY TIME and HIGH-PRESSURE LIMIT displays remain lit and are functional during manual ventilation.

Directly below the control section is the alarm section which includes LOW PEEP/CPAP (−9 to 24 cm H_2O); LOW PEAK PRESSURE (3 to 120 cm H_2O, or off); HIGH PRESSURE; LOW INLET GAS; CIRCUIT FAULT; APNEA (inactive with continuous flow); VENT INOP; ALARM SILENCE (60 seconds); and RESET. An additional safety feature is the MECHANICAL PRESSURE-RELIEF knob (next to the oxygen concentration dial), which can be adjusted from 0 to 130 cm H_2O in all modes. Turning the MECHANICAL PRESSURE-RELIEF knob clockwise increases the value and counterclockwise decreases the value. The high-pressure limit should be set below the overpressure-relief valve setting in order for the high-pressure limit to activate (Box 11-9).

When the POWER switch (on the top left rear panel) is off, the VENT INOP alarm can be silenced by pressing the ALARM SILENCE button. The ALARM SILENCE button is on the front bottom left panel and silences the alarm for 60 seconds, unless the RESET button on the right is pressed.

Front panel digital displays include BREATH RATE (0 to 250 breaths/minute); INSPIRATORY TIME (0.05 to 60 seconds); I:E RATIO (1:0.1 to 1:60); PIP (0 to 120 cm H_2O); MEAN AIRWAY PRESSURE (0 to 80 cm H_2O); POWER (lit when power is on); EXTERNAL DC (lit when external DC power source is used); PATIENT EFFORT (lit when assist sensitivity is met); and DEMAND (lit when the demand system

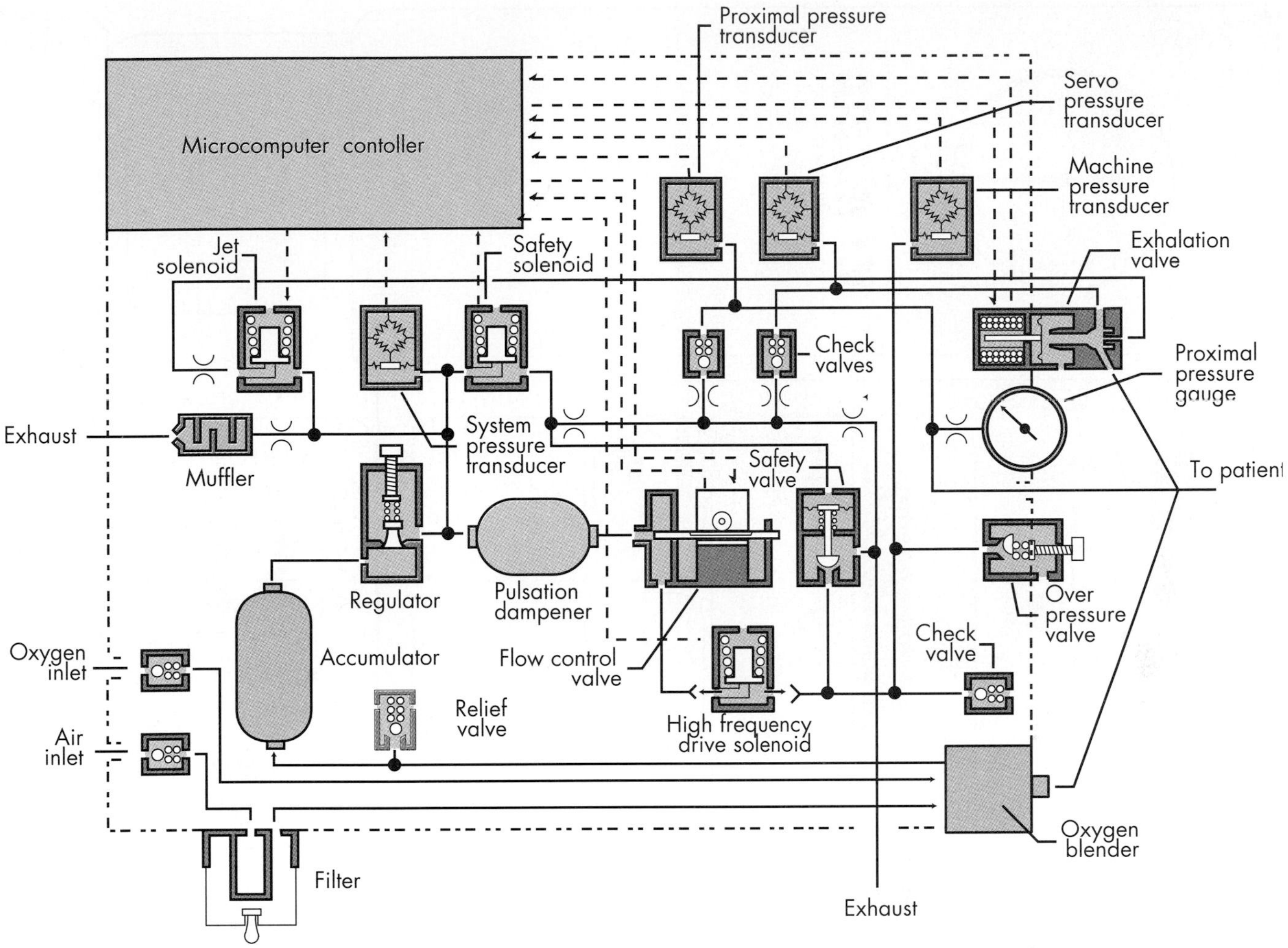

Figure 11-21 The VIP Bird 1.1-L accumulator and internal circuit. (Courtesy Bird Products Corp., Palm Springs, Calif.)

is triggered). The PATIENT EFFORT LED flashes when the patient's inspiratory effort exceeds the assist sensitivity setting. The DEMAND LED flashes when the demand flow system is triggered by spontaneous efforts, decreasing airway pressure 1 cm H_2O below the baseline pressure during time-cycled IMV. Airway pressures are displayed on a pressure gauge. In the IMV mode, only the mandatory breaths are displayed in the BREATH RATE display. The I:E RATIO LED flashes when there is an inverse I:E ratio.

Modes of Ventilation

Volume-Cycled Modes

In the A/C volume-cycled mode, inspiration is volume-targeted, flow-limited, pressure- or time-triggered, and volume-cycled. Inspiration can be pressure-cycled if the airway pressure reaches the HIGH-PRESSURE alarm setting. The operator sets the following parameters: V_T, breath rate, flow, high-pressure limit, PEEP/CPAP, and assist sensitivity.

In the SIMV/CPAP volume-cycled mode, mandatory breaths are volume-targeted, flow-limited, pressure- or time-triggered, and volume-cycled. Inspiration can be pressure-cycled if the airway pressure reaches the HIGH-PRESSURE alarm setting. Spontaneous respiratory efforts between mandatory breaths are pressure-targeted, pressure-triggered, pressure-limited, and pressure-cycled. Pressure support can be added to spontaneous efforts, which are then pressure-targeted, pressure-triggered, pressure-limited, and flow-cycled. The maximum demand flow available is 120 L/min for spontaneous and pressure-supported breaths. The operator sets the following parameters: V_T, breath rate, flow, high-pressure limit, PEEP/CPAP, assist sensitivity, pressure support (if desired), and pressure-support time limit.

Pressure support termination criteria are set up differently with the VIP Bird ventilator because of the varied patient population that can be ventilated with it. For example, if the unit fails to flow-cycle at 25% of peak flow because of an air leak around the artificial airway, this may result in excessive T_Is (some units time-cycle at 2 to 3 seconds). If the VIP Bird does not flow-cycle, it time-terminates based on the T_I setting. The termination criteria for the VIP Bird are based on delivered V_T ranges (Box 11-10). The pressure support display flashes when the breath is time-cycled.

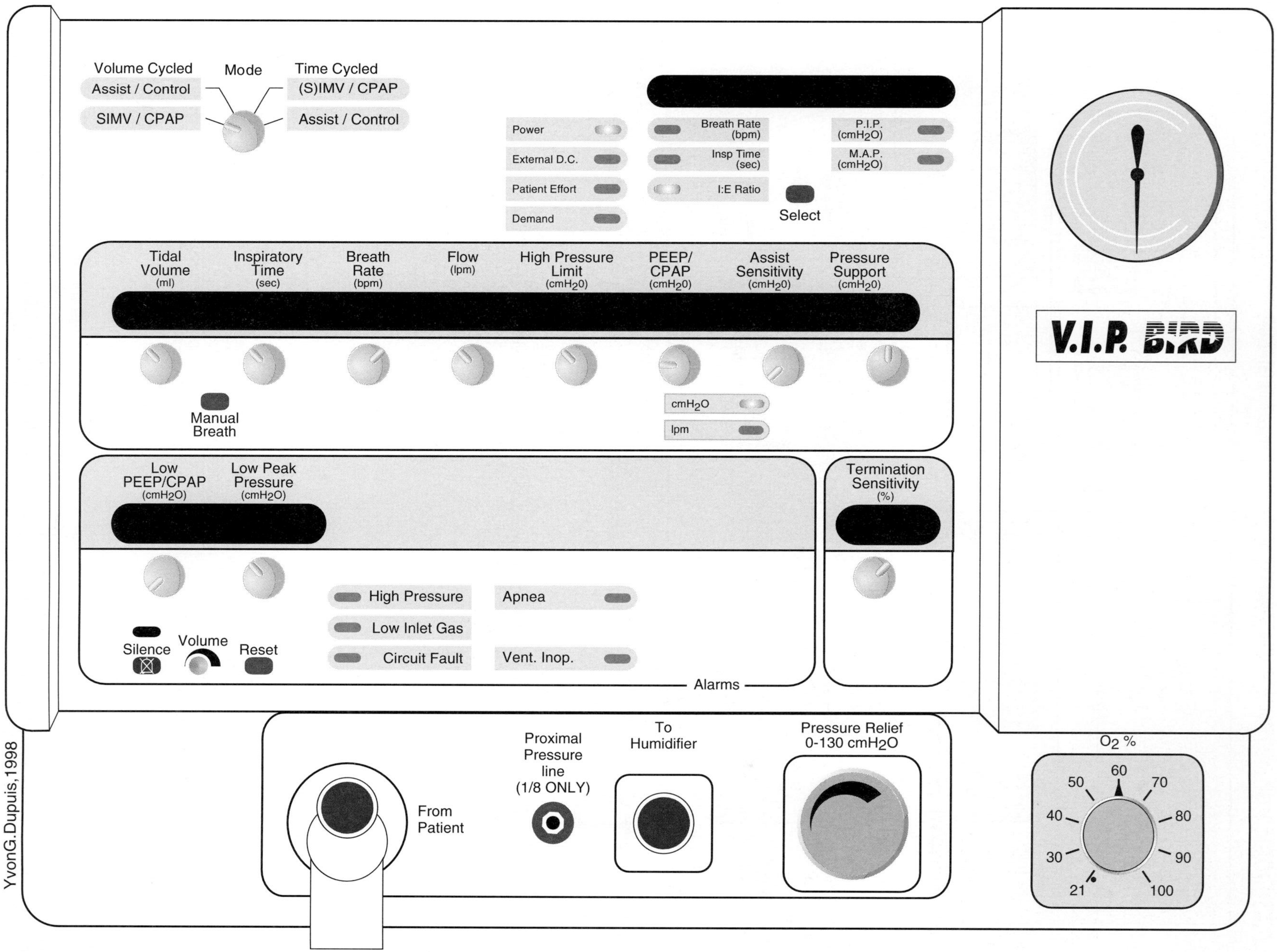

Figure 11-22 The VIP Bird Ventilator control and alarm panel. (Courtesy Yvon Dupuis.)

BOX 11-8

Decision Making & Problem Solving

The Infant Star 500 ventilator is set to operate at a rate of 78 breaths/min and a T_I of 0.5 seconds. What alarm condition will occur?

See Appendix A for the answer.

TABLE 11-16

Specifications for VIP Bird Infant/Pediatric Ventilator

Tidal volume	20 to 995 mL
Inspiratory time	0.1 to 3.0 seconds
Breath rate	0 to 150 breaths/min
Flow (TC modes)	3 to 40 L/min
Flow (VC modes)	3 to 120 L/min
Peak inspiratory pressure (TC modes)	0 to 80 cm H_2O
High pressure limit (VC modes)	3 to 120 cm H_2O
PEEP/CPAP	0 to 24 cm H_2O
Assist sensitivity (TC modes)	0.1 to 5.0 L/min, or off
Assist sensitivity (VC modes)	1 to 20 cm H_2O, or off
Pressure support	1 to 50 cm H_2O, or off
Trigger mechanism	Pressure (VC)/flow (TC)
Alarms	Low PEEP/CPAP; low peak pressure; high pressure; low inlet pressure; circuit fault; apnea; ventilator inoperative

Time-Cycled Modes

In the IMV time-cycled mode, mandatory breaths are pressure-targeted, time-triggered, pressure-limited, and time-cycled. In IMV, the operator sets the following parameters: breath rate, T_I, flow, high-pressure limit (PIP desired), and PEEP/CPAP. The continuous- and demand-flow systems support spontaneous efforts. Continuous flow is determined by the FLOW knob setting (0 to 15 L/min). Demand flow is available when spontaneous inspiration decreases the airway pressure 1 cm H_2O below the baseline pressure. The maximum level of demand flow is 120 L/min. CPAP is activated when the breath rate setting is zero.

In (S)IMV/CPAP (utilizing the Bird Partner IIi volume monitor with infant flow sensor), the mandatory breath is pressure-targeted, flow- or time- triggered, pressure-limited, and time-cycled. CPAP is activated when the breath rate setting is zero. In SIMV, the operator sets the following parameters: breath rate, T_I, flow, high-pressure limit, PEEP/CPAP, and assist sensitivity (L/min).

In the A/C mode (only available when a Partner Iii monitor with an infant flow sensor is used), inspiration is pressure-targeted, flow- or time- triggered, pressure-limited, and flow- or time-cycled. The patient receives the set pressure with every spontaneous respiratory effort. The breath rate setting acts as a back-up rate if respiratory effort is decreased. The operator sets the following parameters: breath rate, T_I, flow, high-pressure limit, PEEP/CPAP, assist sensitivity, and **termination sensitivity.**

The TERMINATION SENSITIVITY control is an additional feature that adjusts the flow termination point of the breath, preventing airtrapping and an inverse I:E ratio, therefore providing **expiratory synchrony.** It is only used with the A/C pressure-limited, time-cycled mode.

Termination sensitivity ranges from 5% to 25% of peak flow, or off. For example, a setting of 25% means that the breath will be terminated when the flow (measured at the proximal airway) decreases to 25% of the measured peak flow. If the flow fails to decrease to the set percentage (which might occur with a lower percentage setting and an air leak around the artificial airway), the breath is time-cycled. The termination sensitivity setting flashes to indicate that the breath is time-cycled. Airway graphics are helpful in evaluating patient/ventilator synchrony, and it is strongly recommended that they be used with this mode of ventilation (Box 11-11).

The ASSIST SENSITIVITY control is adjustable from 0.2 to 5 L/min with the infant flow sensor. By pressing the CONTINUOUS FLOW button on the Bird Partner IIi monitor, the

BOX 11-9

Function of the High-Pressure Control

The HIGH-PRESSURE LIMIT controls the set PIP in the time-cycled, pressure-limited modes. In the volume-cycled modes, it functions as a high-pressure limit.

BOX 11-10

Breath Termination Ranges According to Tidal Volume

5% of peak flow for a delivered V_T of 0 to 50 mL
5% to 25% of peak flow for a delivered V_T of 50 to 200 mL
25% of peak flow for a delivered $V_T > 200$ mL

BOX 11-11

Important Clinical Note

If the patient cannot self-regulate ventilation (e.g., has hiccups), the termination sensitivity should be turned off or the mode of ventilation changes until the situation resolves.

real-time flow signal can be evaluated by observing the continuous flow readout at end-exhalation. If the digital readout returns to zero, the assist sensitivity should be set at 0.2 L/min to provide optimal patient-triggering capabilities. If there is a leak (e.g., flow readout does not return to zero), adjust the assist sensitivity to 0.2 L/min above the digital readout. Adjusting the sensitivity above the leak avoids autocycling and requires that the patient only generate the flow difference between the leak and the assist sensitivity setting.

Graphics Displays

Airway graphics are an invaluable tool, allowing the clinician to monitor and adjust ventilatory strategies for each patient. An analysis of graphics also provides real-time and trend assessments of ventilator parameters and patient-ventilator interaction (see Chapter 9). The Bird Graphics Monitor is designed for use with the VIP Bird, the Bird 8400 STi, and the T-Bird ventilators (see Figure 11-21). It requires use of the Bird Partner or Bird Partner IIi monitor, which is portable and easily moved between ventilators (see the discussion of these monitors later in this chapter). A communication port is available for a printer. Compatible printers include the HP ThinkJet, Epson FX-850, and the HP DeskJet Series 300, 400, 500, and 600.

The graphics monitor displays real-time scalar waveforms for pressure, flow, and volume (vertical axis) plotted over time (horizontal axis). The WAVEFORM SELECT screen allows the clinician to select two waveforms at a time. Positive values (above zero on the vertical axis) relate to the inspiratory phase of ventilation, and negative values relate to the expiratory phase. Pressure/volume and flow/volume loops are also available, along with reference loop storage. The pressure/volume graphic loop displays V_T on the vertical axis and airway pressure on the horizontal axis. The flow/volume graphic loop displays flow on the vertical axis and V_T on the horizontal axis. The FREEZE screen provides mobile target and reference cursors, allowing the clinician to pause and evaluate significant events. New software allows C_{20} and dynamic compliance values as well as ventilator settings to be measured. The TREND feature is provided with ten selectable parameters and can be set for 15-minute or 1-, 2-, 4-, 8-, or 24-hour windows.[14]

Special Features

Leak Compensation

Leak compensation is used to stabilize baseline pressure, prevent autocycling, and optimize assist sensitivity in the presence of leaks. Although, it should only be used with leaks around artificial airways. It is not recommended for patients with minimal respiratory effort and no leak because some patients cannot trigger appropriately with the leak compensation active. Leak compensation is only functional in the volume-cycled modes. When pressure decreases 0.25 cm H_2O below baseline, the leak compensation feature introduces small amounts of flow into the circuit, attempting to reestablish baseline pressure. The amount of leak compensation necessary is sensed by the exhalation valve pressure transducer, so the flow-control valve returns to the determined value after each ventilation. The amount of flow is reevaluated every 8 milliseconds. With the assist sensitivity set at -1 cm H_2O, the maximum amount of flow available is 5 L/min; with the assist sensitivity set at -2 to -5 cm H_2O, the maximum amount of flow available is 10 L/min. After any power-up, leak compensation is on; this is the default setting. The leak compensation is turned on and off by pressing the SELECT button until the desired feature is displayed in the digital window (top left digital display).

Partner IIi Monitor

The Bird Partner IIi Monitor is a microprocessor-controlled volume monitor with a variable-orifice, differential-pressure, flow-measuring device that is placed in the patient circuit near the upper airway (for the infant sensor only). It measures effective inspiratory and expiratory volumes, digitally displays measured values (V_T, rate, $\dot{V}_E$, and the real-time flow signal [only with the infant sensor]) and alarm parameters (high rate, low minute ventilation), and provides an adjustable APNEA alarm (10 to 60 seconds in 5-second increments) (see Figure 11-21). The APNEA button is located on the rear panel of the monitor. The clinician can view the current apnea setting by pressing this red button and seeing the displayed value in the TIDAL VOLUME window. If the APNEA button is repeatedly pressed, the clinician can adjust the apnea setting.

The monitor can be used with the infant or the pediatric sensor. The infant sensor is placed at the proximal airway and circuit wye and can only be used with artificial airways with an internal diameter $\leq$4.5 mm (Figure 11-23). The sensor (*B*) is placed with the arrow pointing toward the patient (*A*) and the monitoring tubes (*C*) facing upward to prevent accumulation of condensation or secretions within the lines. (See Box 11-12 for an important clinical note about cleaning the infant sensor.) The gas inlet on the back of the monitor connects to a 50-psi source and is used to inject gas (at 12 mL/min) through the pressure line

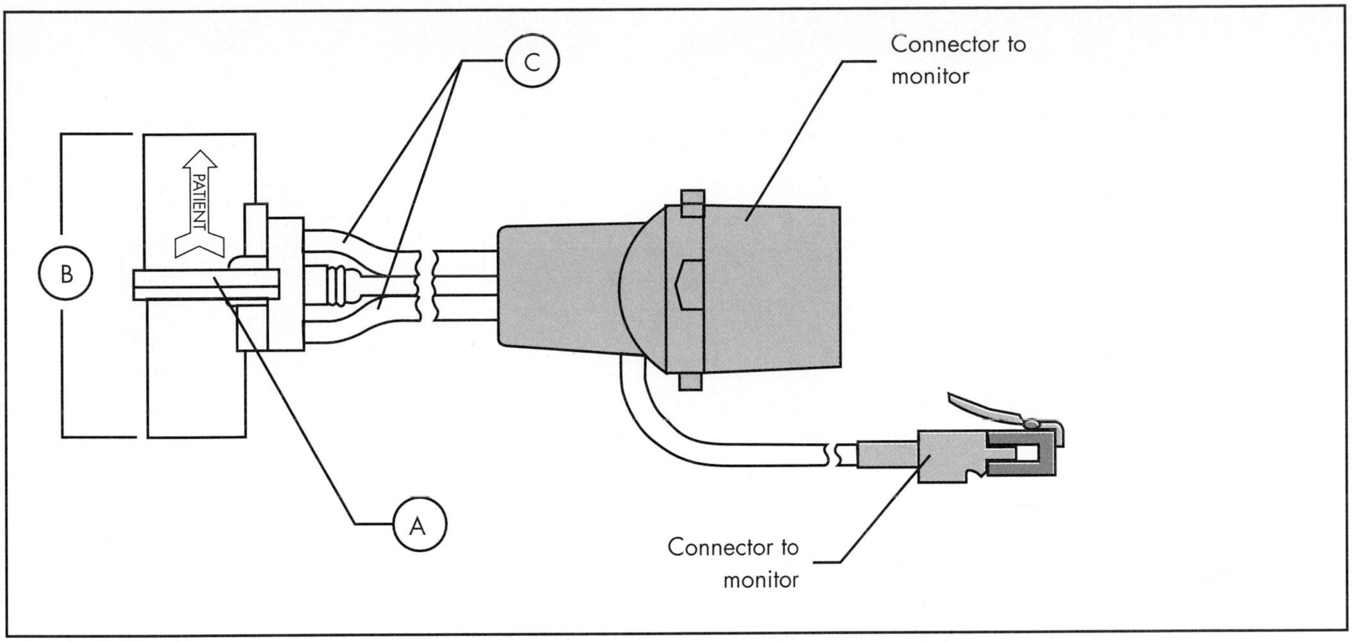

Figure 11-23 Infant sensor used with the Partner IIi monitor and the VIP Bird. (Courtesy Bird Products Corp., Palm Springs, Calif.)

BOX 11-12

Important Clinical Note

The infant flow sensor should be cleaned every 24 hours to maintain accurate V_T measurements and flow-triggering capabilities. The sensor can be sterilized in a cold solution or a gas. Steam autoclaving or pasteurization cannot be used because the high temperatures will damage the flow element.

BOX 11-13

Use of a Capnograph with an In-Line Sensor

When using capnographic monitoring, place the end-tidal CO_2 sensor between the infant sensor and the patient circuit wye to provide optimal flow-triggering capabilities. Special connectors are available to facilitate the additional monitoring. The infant sensor has less than 1 mm of dead space.

to prevent obstructions within the line and water from entering the differential-pressure transducer. The gas flow is synchronized with the expiratory phase so that no additional volume is delivered to the patient during inspiration. The V_T readout is the effective V_T because the sensor is placed at the patient airway. Box 11-13 explains the use of a capnograph with an infant flow sensor.

The pediatric sensor (Figure 11-24, *B*) is placed just in front of the expiratory valve with the sensor pointing in the direction of gas flow. The V_T readout includes compressible volume and effective V_T. V_T measurements are derived from the flow measurement. As flow passes through the sensor and past the variable-orifice flow element, which resides between two chambers, the flow element bends in the direction of flow, creating a small pressure difference between the two chambers. The differential-pressure transducer measures the pressure difference between the two chambers and sends an analog signal to the microprocessor, which compares the signal to a calibration curve and translates the value to a volume.[13] (This happens in all Bird sensors.)

DRAGER BABYLOG 8000 INFANT VENTILATOR

The Dräger Babylog 8000 Infant Ventilator (Dräger Corporation, Telford, Penn.) is used to mechanically ventilate premature babies and infants (Figure 11-25). The weight limit for use of this ventilator is 20 kg. The Babylog is electrically and pneumatically powered and pneumatically and microprocessor-controlled. The incorporation of a hot-wire anemometer at the patient wye allows the Babylog to monitor flow at the endotracheal tube level, thereby improving patient/ventilator synchrony.[15]

Noteworthy Internal Functions

The compressed air and oxygen sources pass through a filter and a non-return valve before entering the pressure regulators (Figure 11-26). The two gas sources then enter

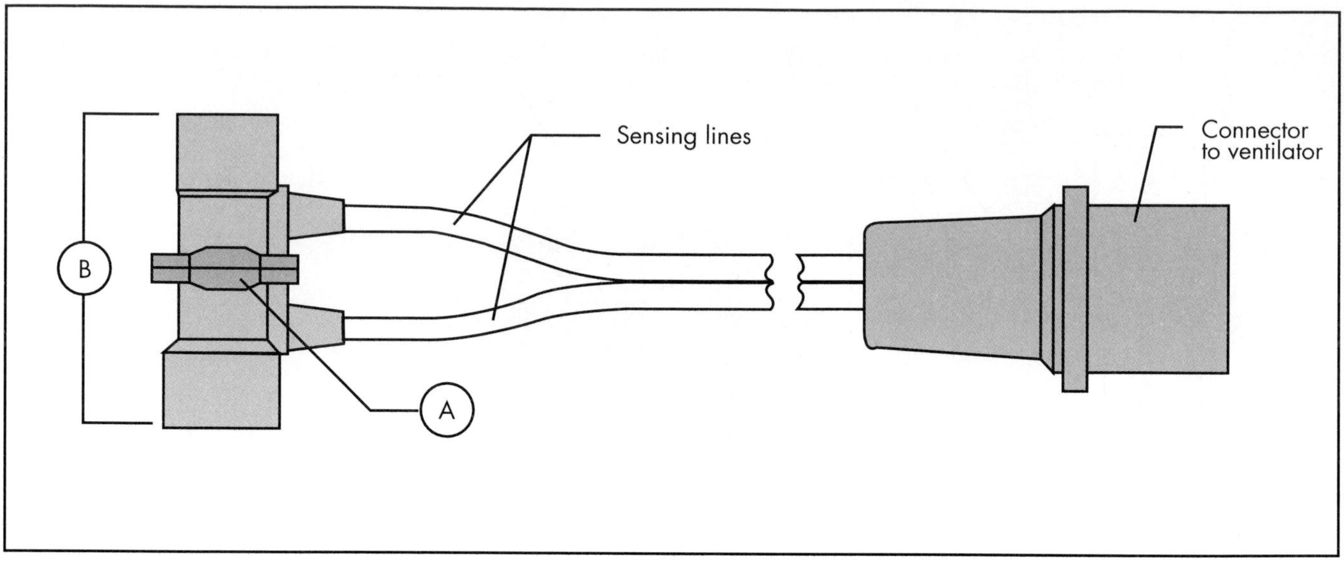

Figure 11-24 Pediatric sensor used with Partner IIi monitor and VIP Bird. (Courtesy Bird Products Corp., Palm Springs, Calif.)

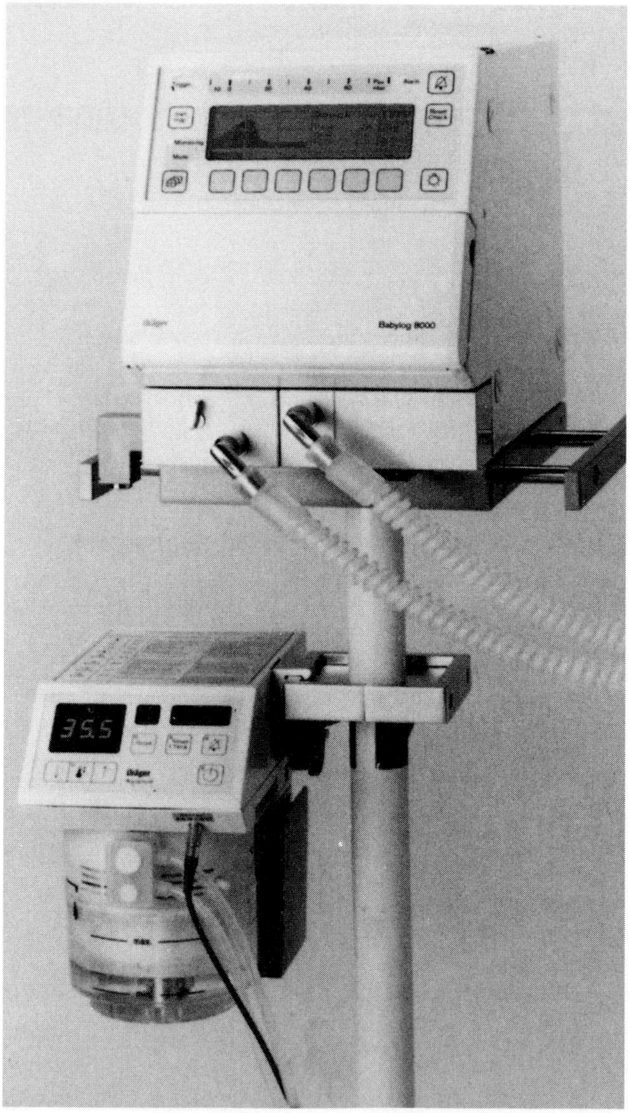

Figure 11-25 The Dräger Babylog 8000 Infant Ventilator. (Courtesy Dräger Corp., Telford, Pa.)

the solenoid valves and flow adjusters, which blend and control the gas flowing through the inspiratory limb of the patient circuit. If there is a gas supply or electrical failure, the patient can spontaneously breathe room air through the filter and the non-return valve. Expiratory gas flow from the patient circuit is regulated by a pneumatic exhalation valve. The pneumatic safety valve directs excessive pressure build-up in the ventilator system through the exhalation valve.

Overview of Control and Alarm Panel

Figure 11-27 is a diagram of the control and alarm panel, which contains a rotary dial panel and a display/**soft key** panel. The dial panel has buttons for the operating modes (CPAP and CMV) and rotary dials for the ventilator parameters. An activated mode is indicated by an illuminated LED on its button. The button must be pressed until the green LED is continuously illuminated in order for the mode to be activated. This is a safety feature in place to prevent accidental mode changes. Illuminated, green LEDs indicate mandatory parameters to be set for a certain mode of ventilation. If a parameter has been internally limited or needs attention, its green LED flashes.

The rotary dial panel contains six dials: OXYGEN CONCENTRATION % (21% to 100%); INSPIRATORY TIME (0.1 to 2.0 seconds); EXPIRATORY TIME (0.2 to 30 seconds); INSPIRATORY FLOW (1 to 30 L/min); INSPIRATORY PRESSURE LIMIT (10 to 80 cm H_2O); and PEEP (0 to 15 cm H_2O). Table 11-17 provides parameter specifications for the Dräger Babylog 8000.

The screen and soft key panel on the top of the ventilator serves various functions. The WAVEFORM display window displays scalar waveforms of either pressure or flow over time. The MEASURED VALUES window digitally displays minute ventilation, oxygen concentration, peak in-

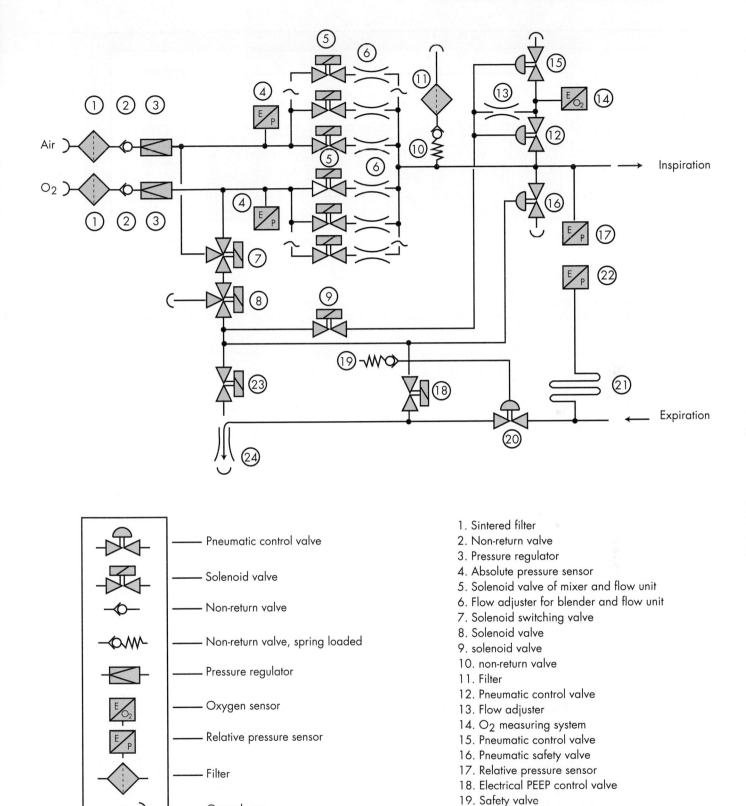

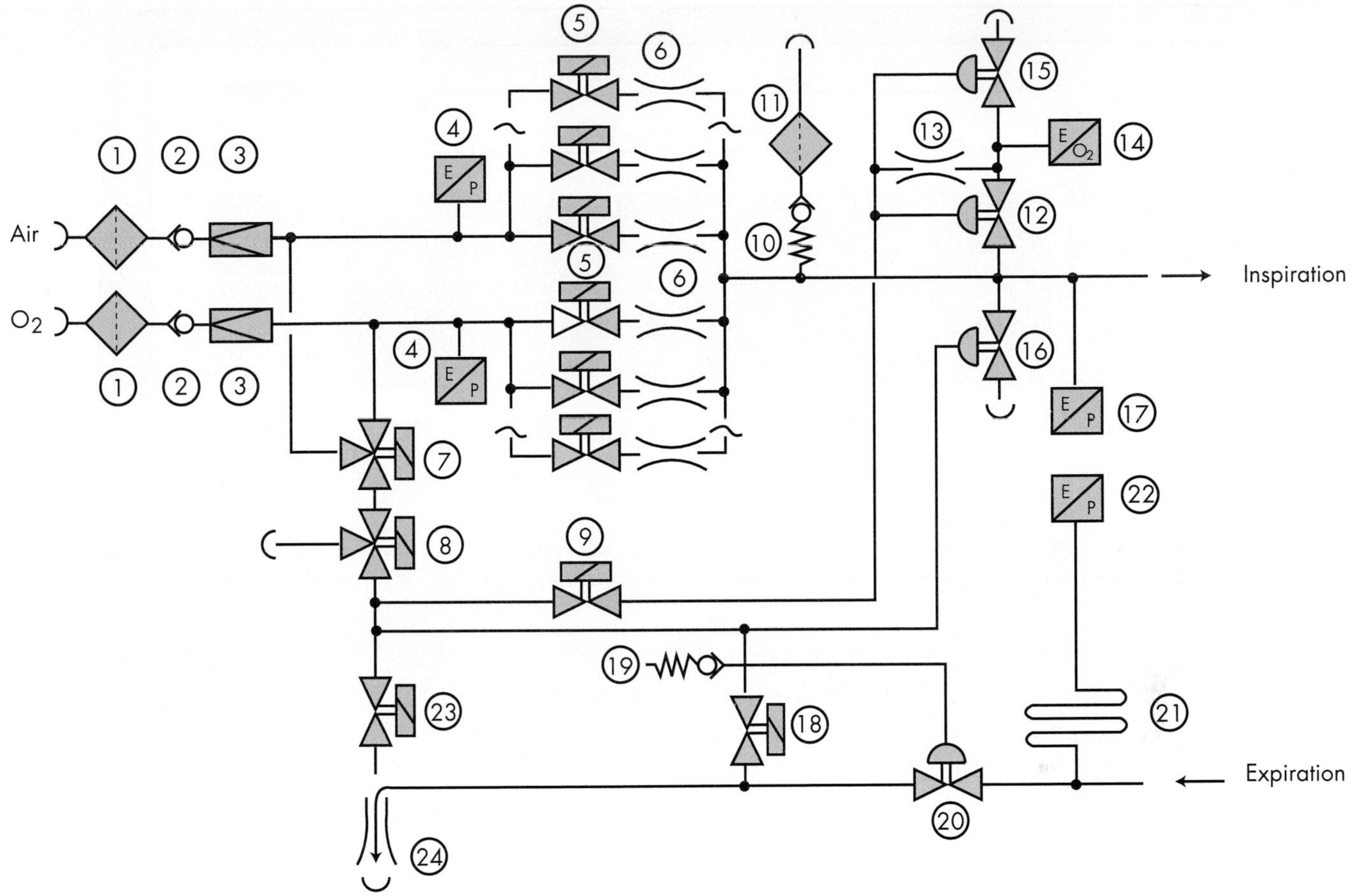

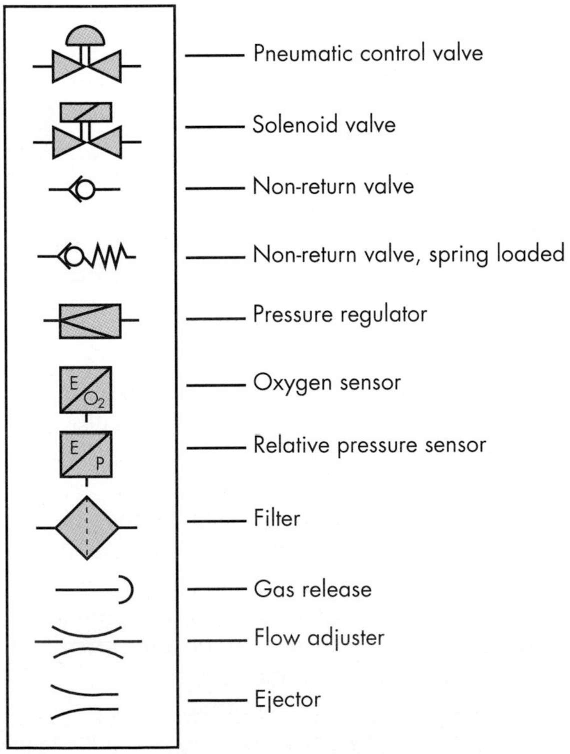

1. Sintered filter
2. Non-return valve
3. Pressure regulator
4. Absolute pressure sensor
5. Solenoid valve of mixer and flow unit
6. Flow adjuster for blender and flow unit
7. Solenoid switching valve
8. Solenoid valve
9. solenoid valve
10. non-return valve
11. Filter
12. Pneumatic control valve
13. Flow adjuster
14. O_2 measuring system
15. Pneumatic control valve
16. Pneumatic safety valve
17. Relative pressure sensor
18. Electrical PEEP control valve
19. Safety valve
20. Expiration valve
21. Bactericidal labyrinth
22. Relative pressure sensor
23. Solenoid valve
24. Ejector

Figure 11-26 The internal pneumatic circuit of the Dräger Babylog 8000 Infant Ventilator. (Courtesy Dräger Corp., Telford, Pa.)

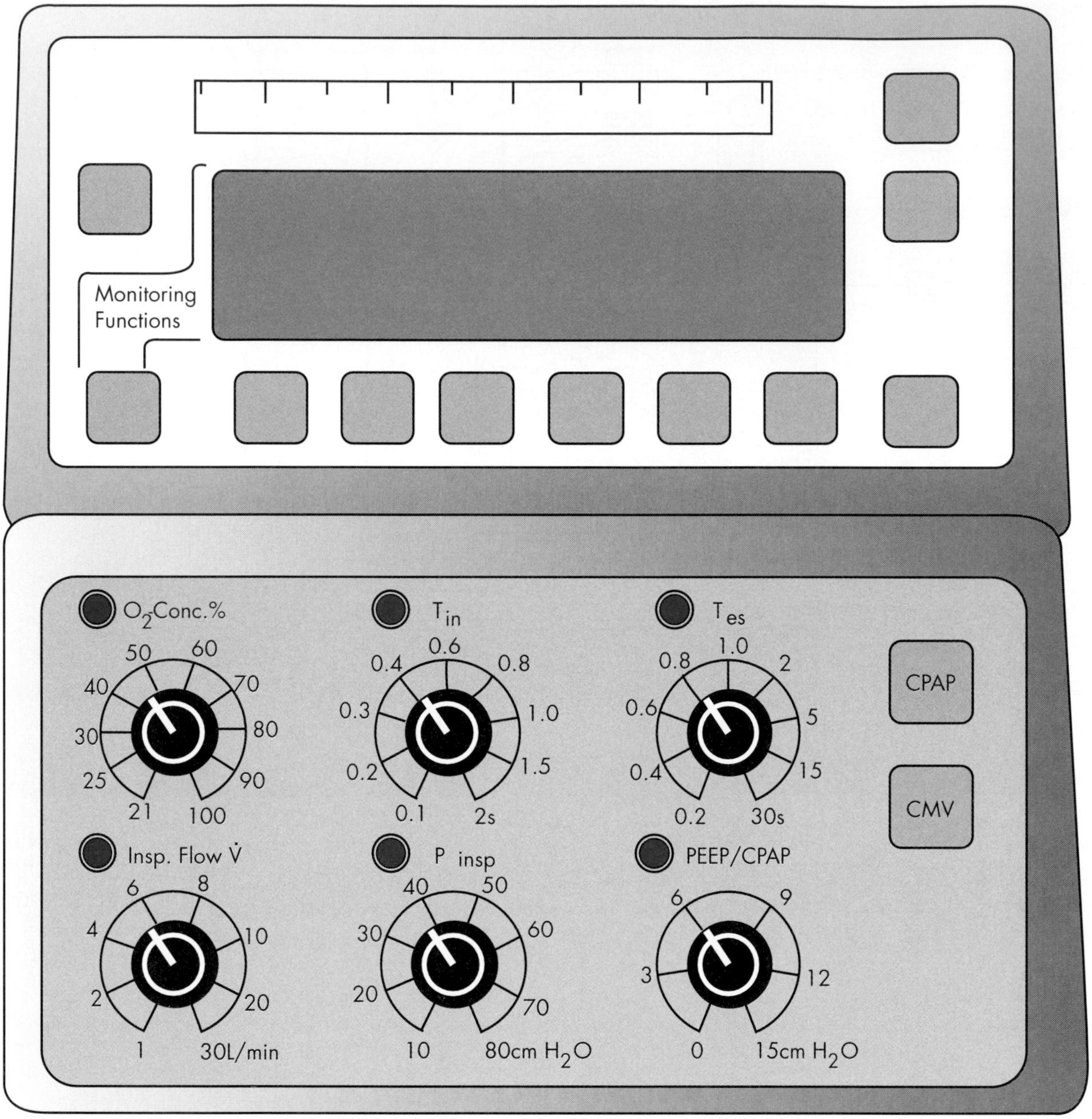

Figure 11-27 The control and alarm panel of the Babylog 8000 Infant Ventilator. (Courtesy Dräger Corp., Telford, Pa.)

spiratory pressure, mean airway pressure, and PEEP. The current mode of ventilation and other pertinent information are displayed on the far right in the STATUS window. The soft keys are used to select ventilator modes and functions, as well as access other windows. The MENU keys are at the bottom of the screen. The screen functions are selected from their respective submenus on the MONITORING AND FUNCTIONS menu. Green LEDs indicate whether MONITORING or FUNCTIONS has been selected. The MANUAL soft key is above the monitoring LED and activates a manual breath or extends an existing breath in progress. The maximum inspiratory time available is 5 seconds. Text messages are displayed as pop-up windows at the top of any screen.

The ALARM SILENCE and RESET/CHECK soft keys are on the top right panel. The ALARM SILENCE control silences the alarm for 2 minutes, and the RESET/CHECK control allows the clinician to view messages and clear them from the screen. A red alarm light flashes when a warning or caution message is displayed on the screen.

Inspiratory and expiratory pressure sensors calculate the airway pressure, which is then displayed as a real-time airway pressure measurement on an **illuminated bar graph** at the top of the monitor. The yellow LED illuminates when inspiration is triggered.

The OXYGEN CONCENTRATION alarm limits are set internally at ±4%. The alarm limits for PEEP and inspiratory pressure are also set internally by the microprocessor. The

TABLE 11-17

Specifications for the Babylog 8000 Infant Ventilator

Inspiratory time	0.1 to 2.0 seconds
Expiratory time	0.2 to 30 seconds
Inspiratory flow	1 to 30 L/min
Expiratory flow	1 to 30 L/min
Peak inspiratory pressure	10 to 80 cm H_2O
PEEP/CPAP	0 to 15 cm H_2O
Oxygen concentration	21% to 100%
Rate	2 to 150 breaths/min
Trigger mechanism	Flow/volume trigger
Alarms	Loss of PEEP/CPAP; high pressure; high minute ventilation; low minute ventilation; minute-ventilation delay; and apnea

LOSS OF PEEP/CPAP limit is −4 cm H_2O (minimum of −2 cm H_2O). The HIGH-PRESSURE alarm limit is automatically set to the inspiratory pressure + 10 cm H_2O, or the PEEP/CPAP + 4 cm H_2O. If excessive pressure builds up in the circuit, the exhalation valve opens to allow exhalation. Adjustable alarm limits include HIGH MINUTE VENTILATION, LOW MINUTE VENTILATION, MINUTE VENTILATION DELAY (0 to 30 seconds), and APNEA (5 to 20 seconds).

The ventilator alarms are arranged in order of importance and grouped into ADVISORY, WARNING, and ALARM messages that are digitally displayed on the ventilator screen, eliminating the guesswork of troubleshooting alarm conditions. Incidents such as OBSTRUCTED ENDOTRACHEAL TUBE, KINKED CIRCUIT, and APNEA are clearly identified on the ventilator screen. Each level has a distinctive tone that indicates its level of importance. Every message is recorded in the **message log,** which can store the last 100 entries. The log records the time of occurrence, the displayed text, and the response.

Modes of Ventilation

The mandatory breaths in A/C and SIMV are time- or patient-triggered, pressure-targeted, and time-cycled. The operator sets the following parameters: T_I, T_E, inspiratory flow, inspiratory pressure, PEEP, and trigger sensitivity. Mandatory breaths are volume-triggered when a patient's spontaneous inspiratory volume is greater than or equal to the set trigger volume (set at ≥2), or else the mandatory breath is time-triggered.

Continuous flow supports spontaneous respiratory efforts between the mandatory breaths in the CPAP mode. The amount of continuous flow available is determined by either the INSPIRATORY FLOW control or the **VARIABLE INSPIRATORY VARIABLE EXPIRATORY (VIVE)** FLOW option.

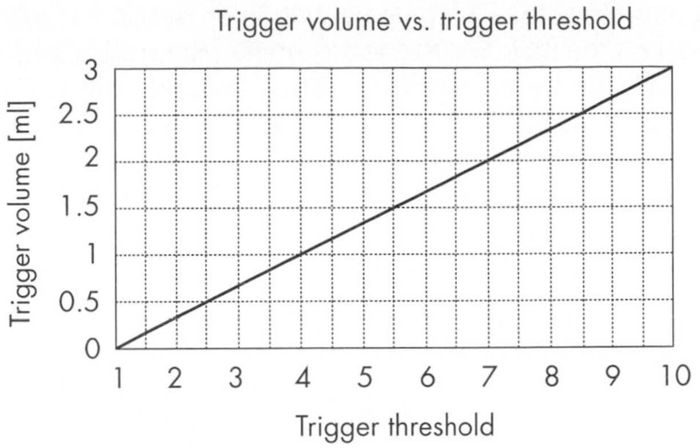

Figure 11-28 The trigger sensitivity setting on the Babylog 8000 Infant Ventilator.

With VIVE, you may independently set a higher flow than necessary for mandatory breaths during the expiratory phase, so that a patient with increased spontaneous demands can get extra flow during the expiratory phase; and then during the inspiratory phase, the flow will go back to the preset flow for the mandatory breath (e.g., 5 L/min on inspiration and 8 L/min on expiration). There is a Venturi in the expiratory channel to prevent autoPEEP with high expiratory flows.

Trigger sensitivity is set up by accessing the main MENU function and selecting the TRIGGER button. The trigger sensitivity ranges from 1 to 10, with 1 as the most sensitive trigger and 10 as the least sensitive. The 1 to 10 trigger scale corresponds to a volume of 0 to 3 mL. The lowest setting (1) is recommended, and a yellow TRIGGER LED illuminates with each triggered breath. If the trigger sensitivity is at 1 when the Babylog measures a 0.25 L/minute (straight flow trigger) flow change, then the mechanical breath is synchronized. Settings above 1 indicate that the Babylog is evaluating the system for flow changes but waits until a particular volume moves across the flow sensor before synchronizing the breath with the patient's inspiratory effort (see Figure 11-28).

The IMV breath is pressure-targeted, time-triggered, pressure- or flow-limited, and time- or pressure-cycled. The operator sets the following parameters: oxygen concentration, T_I, T_E, inspiratory flow, inspiratory pressure, and PEEP. The mandatory rate is calculated by adding the set T_I and T_E and dividing the sum into 60 seconds. The mandatory breath is time-triggered based on the rate calculation.

Nasal CPAP can be applied, but the flow measurement must be disabled by disconnecting the connector from the flow sensor and pressing the RESET/CHECK button. The operator sets the following parameters: oxygen concentration, inspiratory flow, and PEEP.

Graphics Displays

Real-time pressure and flow scalar waveforms are displayed on the monitoring screen. The waveforms are accessed by pressing either the $\overline{\text{P}}$AW or FLOW button on the GRAPH submenu on the main MONITORING menu. The scale is automatically set by the ventilator. The displayed flow scalar waveform indicates the inspiratory flow pattern above the baseline and the expiratory flow pattern below. FREEZE and TREND options are also available. The TREND feature stores a 24-hour window.

Special Features

A built-in **NiCd battery** is automatically recharged during ventilator operation. The ventilator must run for at least 30 minutes for the battery's full charge to be available.

The oxygen analyzer runs an automatic calibration every 24 hours, but this can also be done manually under the CAL submenu on the FUNCTION menu. The calibration takes about 5 minutes to complete. The flow-sensor calibration is accessed through the CAL submenu on the FUNCTION menu. To calibrate the flow sensor, just follow the instructions on the screen. Minute ventilation and apnea monitoring are only possible with a calibrated flow sensor. Flow-sensor calibration should be performed each time the ventilator is turned on and after sensor assembly and replacement.

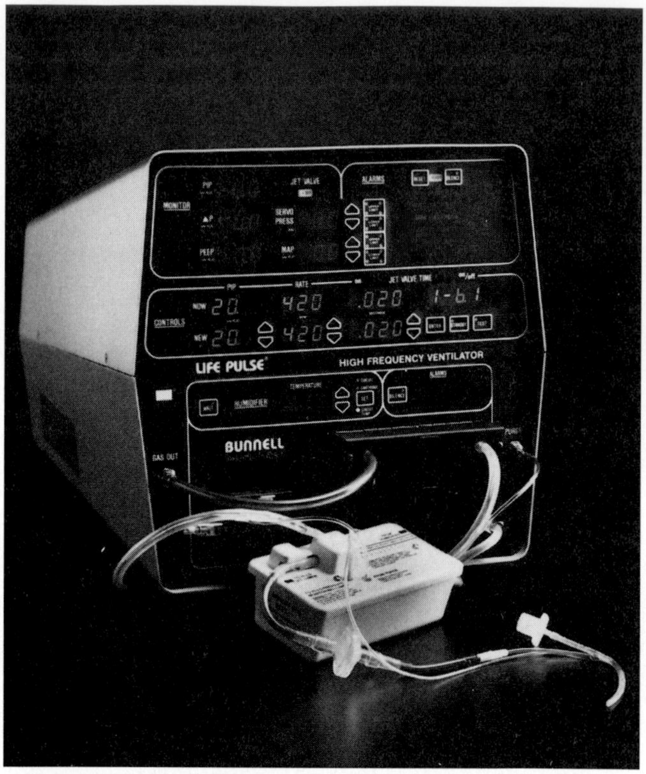

Figure 11-29 The Bunnell Life Pulse High-Frequency Jet Ventilator. (Courtesy Bunnell, Inc., Salt Lake City.)

Bunnell Life Pulse High-Frequency Jet Ventilator

The Bunnell Life Pulse High-Frequency Jet Ventilator (HFJV; Bunnell, Inc., Salt Lake City) (Figure 11-29) is indicated for patients with severe respiratory distress syndrome complicated by pulmonary air leak who are not aided with conventional mechanical ventilation strategies and for patients with pulmonary interstitial emphysema. The Bunnell HFJV is a microprocessor-controlled, pressure-limited, time-cycled, constant flow **high-frequency jet ventilator** that works parallel with a conventional ventilator. The conventional ventilator provides background conventional ventilation (if desired), supplies gas for spontaneous breathing, and regulates the PEEP level.[16]

Overview of Control and Alarm Panel

The ON/OFF button is on the middle left of the front panel. When pressed, it turns the ventilator on (green light displayed) and off (no light). Figure 11-30 is a diagram of the seven components of the ventilator, including the following sections: monitoring; alarms; controls; patient box; rear panel; disposable cartridge/circuit; and humidifier monitor, alarms, and controls.

The ventilator monitoring displays provide pertinent patient and ventilator performance information. They are on the top left front panel of the control panel and are as follows: PIP, ΔP (PIP − PEEP), PEEP, SERVO PRESSURE, and $\overline{\text{P}}$AW. These four patient pressures are sensed at the distal end of the Hi-Lo Jet tube (Mallinckrodt Inc., St. Louis) or LifePort endotracheal tube adaptor (Bunnell, Inc.) (if used) and measured by an electronic transducer in the patient box. The displays are averages calculated over a short time and do not reflect alveolar pressure. Mean airway pressure can be increased by increasing PIP, respiratory rate, PEEP, and the rate and V_T of the sigh breaths. The PEEP level is controlled by the conventional ventilator.

The SERVO PRESSURE measurement (0 to 20 psig) is the amount of internal pressure required to generate the PIP displayed in the NOW display and is a clinical indicator of changes in lung characteristics or acute changes (e.g., tension pneumothorax, endotracheal tube leak, and atelectasis). For example, decreased lung compliance results in decreased servo pressure because less gas is required to meet the set PIP. Increases in lung compliance or the development of a pneumothorax may result in elevated servo pressures.

The jet valve ON/OFF lights on the top left front panel (monitor panel) indicate the communication between the ventilator and the pinch valve (in the patient box). The ON light shows that the valve is signaled to open for inspiration. The OFF light indicates that the valve is signaled to close for expiration. The ON and OFF lights alternate idly.

The ventilator alarm limits displays are on the top right front panel and include the following: SERVO PRESSURE

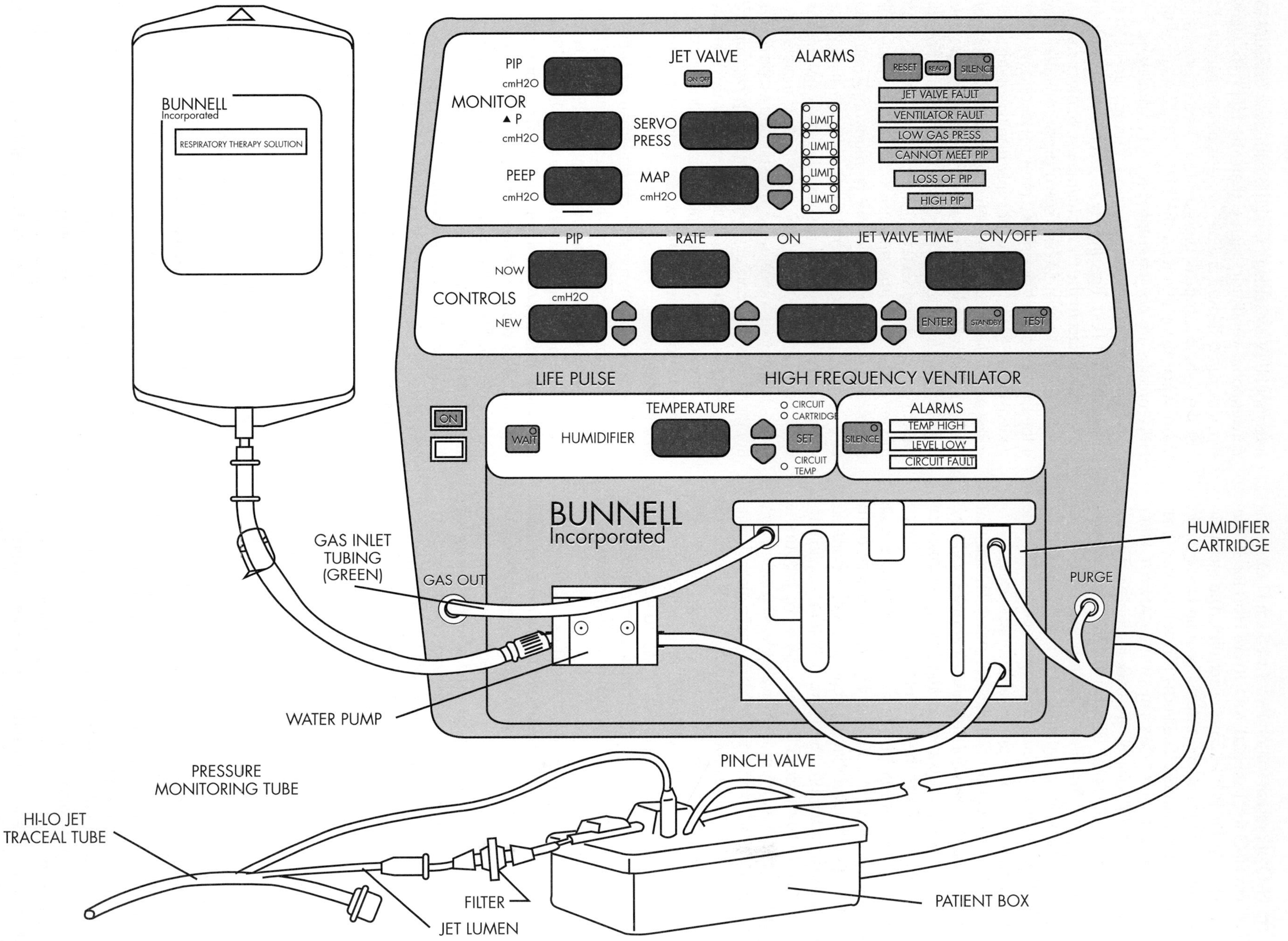

Figure 11-30 Seven components of Bunnell Life Pulse High-Frequency Jet Ventilator. (Courtesy Bunnell, Inc., Salt Lake City.)

(±1 cm H_2O of present value); $\bar{P}$AW (±1.5 cm H_2O); HIGH PIP (>5 cm H_2O for 1 second, or >10 cm H_2O for 30 seconds); and LOSS OF PIP (<25% of set PIP). The mean airway pressure and the servo pressure upper and lower limits can be manually adjusted. The HIGH PIP, JET VALVE FAULT, VENTILATOR FAULT, LOW GAS PRESSURE, CANNOT MEET PIP, and LOSS OF PIP alarms are back-lit displays. The JET VALVE FAULT alarm alerts the clinician that the pinch valve in the patient box is not functioning appropriately. The microprocessor is continuously monitoring the pinch valve and activates the alarm when malfunctions are detected. The Life Pulse stops operating if the pinch valve is not cycling.

The VENTILATOR FAULT alarm alerts the clinician that there is a problem with the Life Pulse electronics or valves. A numerical code is displayed in the JET VALVE ON/OFF time window to indicate the type of failure.

The LOW GAS PRESSURE alarm alerts the clinician that the gas supply is less than 30 psig. The CANNOT MEET PIP alarm alerts the clinician that the ventilator is either unable to consistently deliver breaths at the set PIP or is unable to deliver pressure to the set PIP while the servo pressure is increased to the maximum level available. This alarm can result from a leak in the humidifier cartridge/patient circuit, an incomplete circuit/jet tube connection, a defective or damaged jet endotracheal tube (e.g., kinked tube, improper position, occlusion, or leak), an inability to reach present settings on a larger patient (12 to 20 kg), a patient breathing asynchronously, or an ineffective pinch valve opening action that results in higher servo pressures to meet current settings.

The RESET and ALARM SILENCE (60 seconds) buttons, as well as the READY light are above the ventilator alarm displays. The RESET button has the machine recalculate automatic upper and lower limits for the servo pressure and $\bar{P}$AW parameters and should be used when changes are made on the conventional ventilator and Life Pulse adjustments are not made. When the RESET button is pressed, the READY light turns off and SERVO PRESSURE and $\bar{P}$aw alarm indicators are inactive. The Life Pulse calculates new alarm limits; then the READY light goes on, and all alarms are reactivated. The READY light indicates when the machine has stabilized after start-up or reset and calculated alarm limits, and is ready for full operation. The SILENCE button stops audible alarms for 60 seconds, but the alarm will resume after this time if the condition has not been resolved. A red light goes on in the corner of the SILENCE button when the silence function is in effect.

The ventilator control parameters and displays are on the middle front panel and include: PIP (8 to 50 cm H_2O); RATE (240 to 660 breaths/minute); JET ON TIME (inspiratory time; .02 to 0.034 seconds); and ON/OFF RATIO (1:1.6 to 1:12). The NOW displays indicate current operating settings. The NEW display in the control area allows the operator to adjust set parameters and see the changes before actually entering new parameters. Some operators may interrupt HFJV by setting the sigh breath peak pressure (on conventional ventilator) higher than the HFJV to aggressively recruit collapsed alveoli, whereas other operators adjust the sigh breath peak pressure (on conventional ventilator) equal to or less than the HFJV PIP setting so that HFJV breaths are not interrupted for other situations.

The operating mode selection buttons are ENTER, STANDBY, and TEST. Pressing the ENTER button changes the NOW parameters to the NEW parameters. In older software versions, inappropriately high servo pressure would occur if the ENTER button was pressed prior to connection of the patient circuit to the patient, possibly resulting in high pressures and delivery of excessively high tidal volumes. Software upgrades made this no longer possible. A LOSS OF PIP alarm occurs if the ENTER button is pressed before the patient circuit is connected to the patient. The STANDBY mode is used when the operator wants to interrupt HFJV temporarily (e.g., for suctioning or monitoring the effectiveness of conventional ventilation), although airway pressures are monitored and displayed alarms are inactive while in the standby mode. Red lights and an audible alarm every 30 seconds indicate that the standby mode is functioning, as it is automatically with ventilator power-up. The TEST mode is an automatic test that checks the ventilator systems and circuitry for proper function during standby and should not be performed while a patient is connected to the jet ventilator.

The disposable humidifier cartridge/patient breathing circuit is a closed system that provides humidity to, heats, and monitors the gas exiting the ventilator (Figure 11-31, *A* and *B*). The humidifier cartridge heats and humidifies the gas before it is delivered to the patient. The cartridge receptacle holds the humidifier cartridge in place when the latch is closed. The water in the cartridge is warmed by an aluminum heater plate.

The gas out and purge pneumatic connectors on the front panel are different sizes to prevent improper connections. The short, green, gas-inlet tubing connects gas flow from the ventilator to the cartridge. When the water-level sensors detect a decrease in the water level, the clear, water-inlet tubing transfers water via the built-in pump, thus filling the humidifier cartridge. Water is transferred from a non-pressurized source (e.g., a solution bag or bottle) to the pressurized humidifier cartridge by the water pump. The water level is automatically regulated by the water-level sensor pins in the cartridge. The purge port supplies gas to the **purge valve,** which is located in the patient box. The purge gas is used to remove moisture or mucus from the monitoring line of the Hi-Lo Jet tube or Life Port adaptor. The small, clear, second lumen of the patient circuit connects to this port.

The HUMIDIFIER WAIT button turns off the heater and water pump, allowing easy removal and replacement of the cartridge/circuit. A red light in the corner of this button flashes to indicate activation of the wait feature. To resume normal function, simply press the button again.

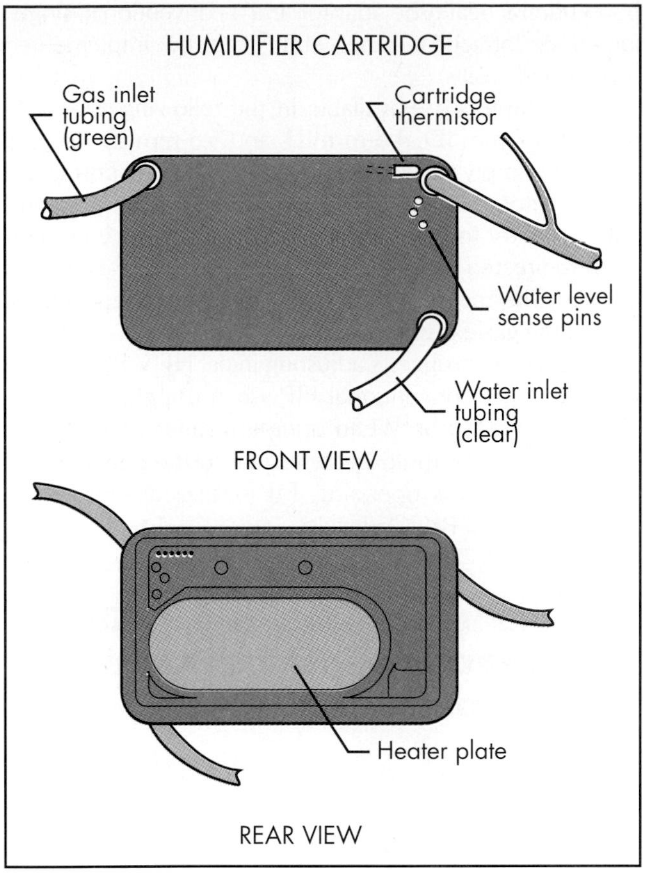

Figure 11-31 The humidifier cartridge/patient breathing circuit of the Bunnell Life Pulse High-Frequency Jet Ventilator.

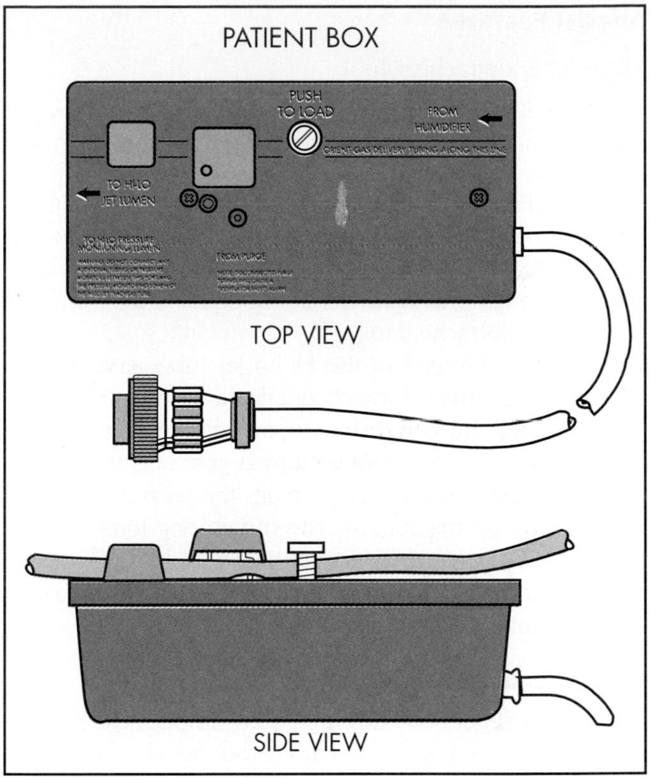

Figure 11-32 The patient box on the Bunnell Life Pulse High-Frequency Jet Ventilator.

Thermistors are located in the patient breathing circuit and cartridge connection to ensure adequate gas-temperature delivery to the patient. The available temperature range is from 32° to 42° C.

The temperature is displayed in three separate windows, which are labeled as CIRCUIT (desired), CARTRIDGE (desired), and CIRCUIT TEMPERATURE (actual temperature). The SET button selects the temperature setting/measurement to be displayed. The window display automatically returns to the CIRCUIT TEMPERATURE display reading as the default. The humidifier system has a separate SILENCE button (i.e., separate from the ventilator ALARM SILENCE button) and various back-lit alarm messages that alert the clinician of any temperature/water level changes and electrical problems within the cartridge/circuit.

The patient box is a satellite component that contains the pinch valve, purge valve, and pressure transducer (Figure 11-32). It is designed to be placed near the patient's head for accurate pressure monitoring and jet pulse delivery. The patient box electrical cable connects to the rear panel of the ventilator. An **electromagnetic** solenoid activates the pinch valve. The pinch valve breaks the flow of pressurized gas into small bursts with a pinch-and-release action on the silicone tubing of the patient breathing circuit. The PUSH TO LOAD button opens the valve to allow correct placement of the silicone tube within the patient box, as well as repositioning of the silicone tubing. The silicone tubing should be moved 2 mm every 8 hours to prevent areas of wear and tear. A bacteria filter is present downstream from the pinch valve to provide particle filtration. Note that Santoprene (Monsanto) has replaced the silicone tubing in newer units, eliminating the need for repositioning and filtering. A millimeter measuring guide is printed on the patient box as a visual aid. The purge valve maintains a moisture-free pressure monitoring line by allowing pressurized gas from the ventilator to pass through the line. A 10-millisecond burst of gas is put through the monitoring line every 10 seconds. The pressure transducer measures tracheal pressure and sends the information to the microprocessor.

The rear panel contains the mixed gas input connection, oxygen sensor connection, hour meter, circuit breaker, ALARM VOLUME control, patient box connector, analog output, and **dump valve** outlet. The gas input fitting connects the ventilator to an oxygen blender in order to provide varied oxygen concentrations. A 30- to 100-psig supply source is required. The oxygen sensor connection allows continuous monitoring of FiO_2. The dump valve is a safety valve that releases internal pressure.

Special Features

Hi-Lo Jet Endotracheal Tube

The triple-lumen **Hi-Lo Jet tracheal tubes** (Mallinckrodt Critical Care, Argyle, NY) are uncuffed and range in size (in 0.5-mm increments) from 2.5- to 6.0-mm inner diameter (ID) (Figure 11-33). The external diameter is about equal to the external diameter of a half-size larger standard endotracheal tube. For example, a 3.0-mm ID Hi-Lo Jet tube has an external diameter about equal to a 3.5-mm ID standard endotracheal tube.[16]

The triple lumena of the Hi-Lo Jet tube serve various functions. The main lumen contains a 15-mm connector that provides the connection point for the conventional ventilator circuit wye. The jet lumen connects the patient box to the patient breathing circuit; the jet pulses are delivered through this lumen. The monitoring lumen monitors pressures at the distal end of the Hi-Lo Jet tube; this lumen is connected to the TO Hi-Lo Pressure Monitoring Lumen connection on the patient box.

Life Port Endotracheal Tube Adaptor

The development of the Life Port Endotracheal Tube Adaptor (Figure 11-34) has eliminated the requirement of intubating/reintubating patients with the specialized jet tube before HFJV initiation. With the use of this double-port endotracheal tube adaptor and a conventional, single-lumen endotracheal tube, HFJV can be implemented quickly and easily.

The adaptors are available in the following sizes: 2.5-mm ID, 3.5-mm ID, 4.5-mm ID, and 5.5-mm ID. To initiate HFJV, simply replace the 15-mm standard endotracheal tube adaptor with the Life Port adaptor. The jet port provides an entry for gas from the jet ventilator. The inspired gas is redirected through a nozzle, which increases the gas velocity. The momentum of the gas is converted to pressure as the gas exits the nozzle.

Bunnell, Inc. suggests adjusting initial HFJV PIP to 10% more than the conventional PIP when using the 2.5-mm ID Life Port adaptor. When using the larger adaptors, the initial HFJV PIP should be set equal to the conventional PIP. Once HFJV is operating, PIP settings are titrated to produce desired $PaCO_2$ levels.

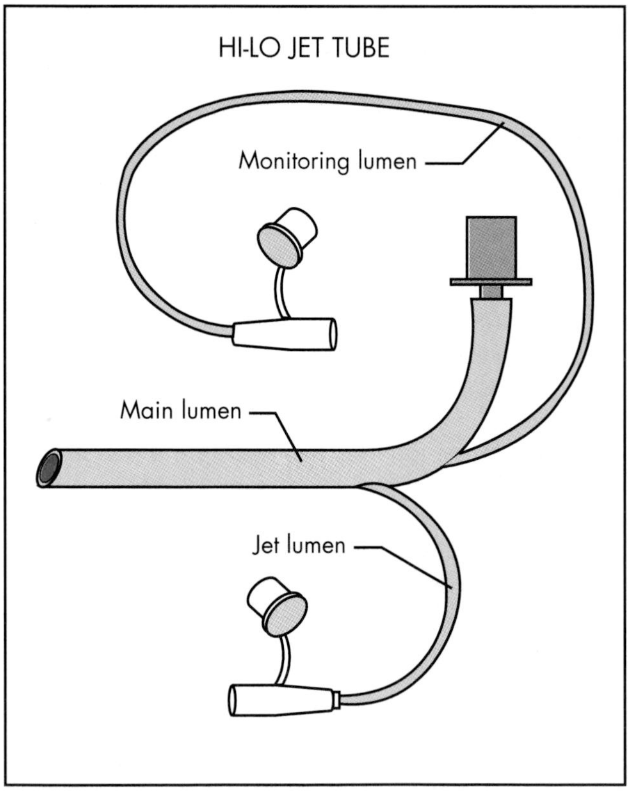

Figure 11-33 Triple-lumen Hi-lo Jet tracheal tubes for use in high-frequency jet ventilation. (Courtesy Mallinckrodt Critical Care, Argyle, NY.)

SensorMedics 3100 and 3100A High-Frequency Oscillatory Ventilators

The 3100 model was the first of the two high-frequency oscillators introduced by the SensorMedics Corporation of Yorba Linda, Calif. for use with neonates. An improved model, the 3100A, soon followed, replacing the 3100 (Figure 11-35, *A*). Both of these models have been used extensively to treat acute respiratory failure in infants. The 3100A is also used for older pediatric patients and adults.

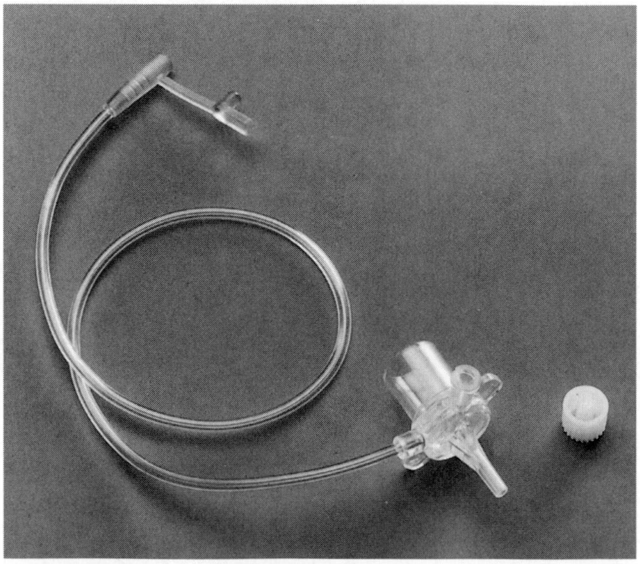

Figure 11-34 Bunnell Life Port Endotracheal Tube Adaptor for use in high-frequency jet ventilation. (Courtesy Bunnell, Inc., Salt Lake City)

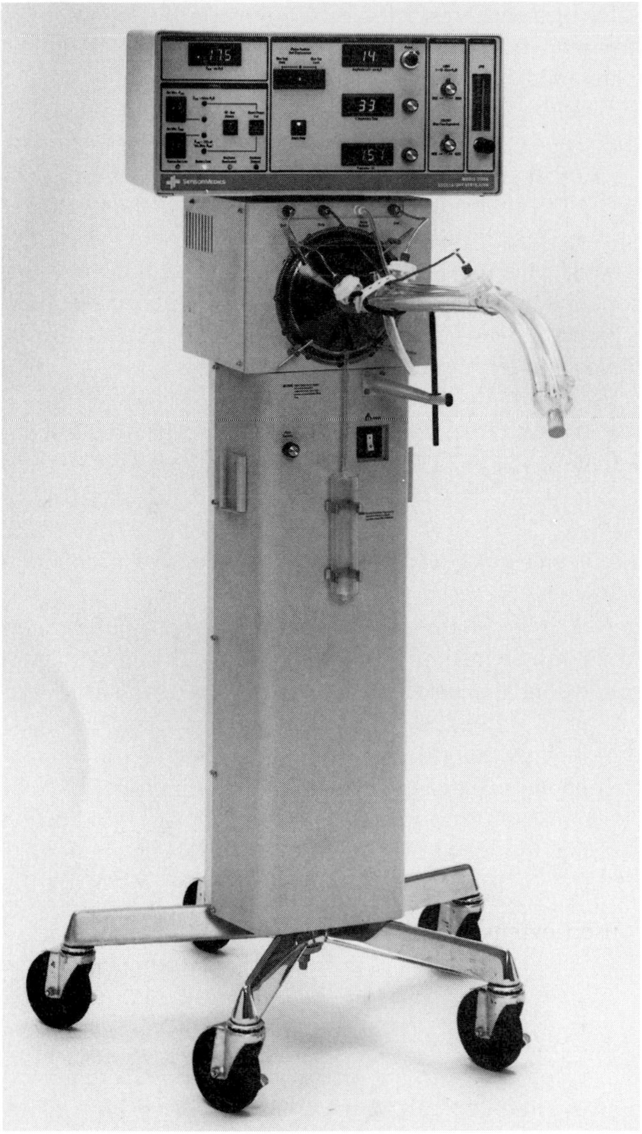

A

Noteworthy Internal Functions

The core of the SensorMedics models is the **oscillator subsystem,** or the **piston assembly** (Figure 11-36). The system incorporates an electronic **control circuit,** or **square-wave driver,** which powers a linear drive motor. This motor consists of an electrical coil within a magnet, similar to a permanent magnet speaker. When a positive polarity is applied to the square-wave driver, the coil is driven forward. The coil is attached to a rubber bellows, or diaphragm, to create a piston. When the coil moves forward, the piston moves toward the patient airway, creating the inspiratory phase. When the polarity becomes negative, the electrical coil and the attached piston are driven away from the patient, creating an active expiration.[17]

The amount of **polarity voltage** applied to the electrical coil determines the distance that the piston is driven toward/away from the patient airway. Therefore increasing the polarity voltage increases the piston movement, or amplitude. Piston excursion is limited, however, by resistance from the pressure within the patient circuit and the oscillator subsystem, which limits the piston stroke to 365 mL. The total time for a piston stroke is a few milliseconds. When oscillations are at low frequencies, the piston has enough time to travel the available excursion length during either the inspiratory or expiratory phase and remain at its maximum position until it begins to move in the opposite direction. Conversely, as oscillating frequency is increased, the excursion time of the piston becomes a greater percentage of the breath phase. The percentage of time the piston remains completely forward or backward decreases. At very high frequencies, the polarity to the coil changes so rapidly that the piston does not have time for a complete excursion and arrival at its maximum position. In fact, it may only travel a fraction of its potential distance before changing direction. Therefore volume delivered by the piston is decreased as oscillatory frequency is increased.

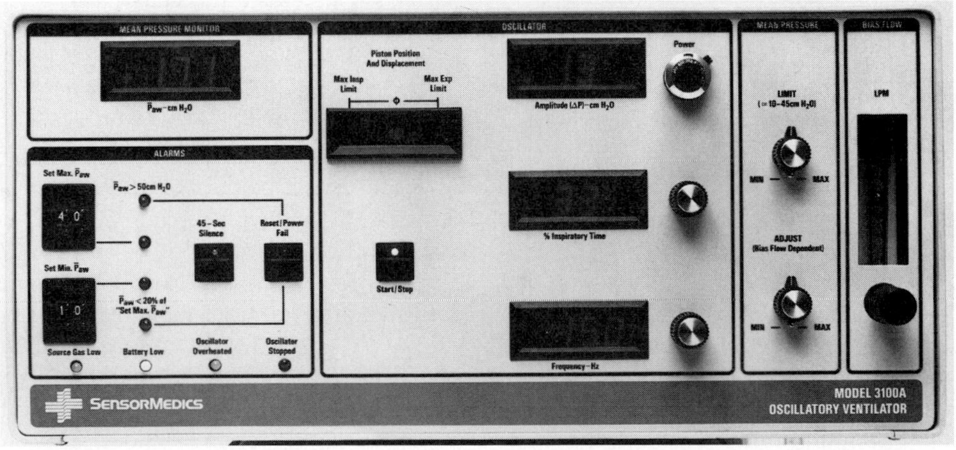

B

Figure 11-35 **A,** SensorMedics Model 3100A High-Frequency Oscillator. **B,** Control panel of the 3100A. (SensorMedics Corp., Yorba Linda, Calif.)

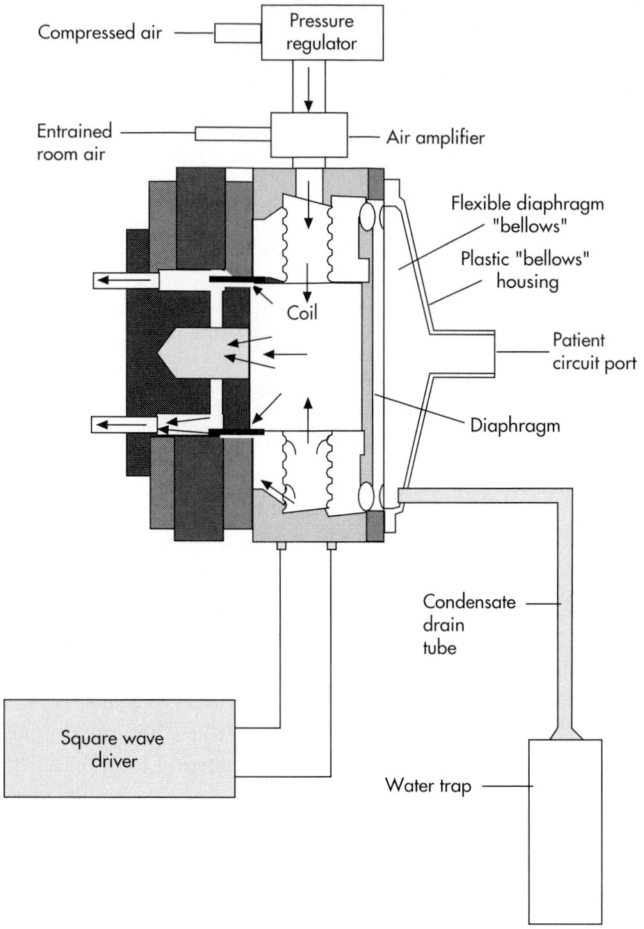

Figure 11-36 The piston assembly of the SensorMedics Model 3100A High-Frequency Oscillator. (Courtesy SensorMedics Corp., Yorba Linda, Calif.)

Although the engineering of the piston subsystem is designed to produce as little friction as possible, the rapid movement of the piston generates some heat. Therefore a Venturi type of air amplifier is used to introduce cooling air around the electrical coil on the 3100A. A separate compressed air source of at least 30 psig serves this system, which consists of a regulator and a Venturi. The regulator reduces air flow to 15 L/min, and the Venturi entrains 45 L/min of room air. This provides 60 L/min of cooling air for the subsystem.

Circuit Design

Figure 11-37 shows the basic circuit of the 3100A. After exiting the back panel of the ventilator and passing through a humidifier, blended gas enters the patient circuit at the **bias flow** inlet. Flow is set using the BIAS FLOW control on the front panel (see Figure 11-35, *B*). The gas mixture fills the space in front of the piston and flows past both the limit valve and the endotracheal tube connection. Gas then passes the dump valve and exits through either the control valve or a small restricted orifice next to the control valve housing. The oscillating piston moves the circuit gas in forward and backward directions toward the airway. The rate of bias flow, the pressure maintained at the airway, and the speed and excursion of the piston are all set by the clinician.

Any standard humidifier can be used with the 3100 and 3100A. Circuits are designed to accommodate heater sensors to provide servo-controlled temperature at the airway. Heated-wire circuits are available to reduce water condensation. All circuits incorporate a water outlet, tubing, and a water trap that permits water condensate to drain away from the piston.

Controls (see Figure 35, *B*)

On/Off

The ventilator's ON/OFF switch is on the front of the unit, below and to the right of the piston (Figure 11-35, *A*). If power to the unit is OFF, or electrical power is interrupted while the ventilator is in operation, an audible alarm sounds, and the red POWER FAILURE LED on the front control panel illuminates. This alarm can only be silenced by pressing the RESET button on the front panel. With any interruption in ventilator operation, pressurization of the circuit's three mushroom valves stops immediately, allowing the circuit to vent to the atmosphere. This venting permits the patient to breathe room air. The proximity of the vented dump valve to the airway enables the patient to breathe room air with minimal resistance from the ventilator circuit.

Piston Centering

The piston's forward and backward excursions are limited by two **mechanical stops.** If time and amplitude allow the piston to encounter one of the stops, it remains stationary for the duration of the inspiratory or expiratory time, and then changes direction. An infrared sensor is used to track piston movement between the mechanical stops. Piston movement is displayed on a bar graph on the control panel. The left end of the bar graph is marked MIN INSP LIMIT and the right is MAX INSP LIMIT. The dot represents the piston's center position.

The **PISTON CENTERING** control (Figure 11-35, *A*, below and left of the diaphragm) adjusts an electrical counterforce to the piston. This counter-force acts in opposition to the $\bar{P}$AW on the front side of the piston. This opposing counter-force has a centering effect on the piston. At a constant $\bar{P}$aw, as the PISTON CENTERING control is turned clockwise, the piston moves toward the maximum inspiratory limit, which is one of the mechanical stops. The oscillator should not be operated so that the piston is driven against a mechanical stop for an extended time. The piston should be kept in the center of the bar graph to maintain piston efficiency and maximize the life of the oscillator mechanism.

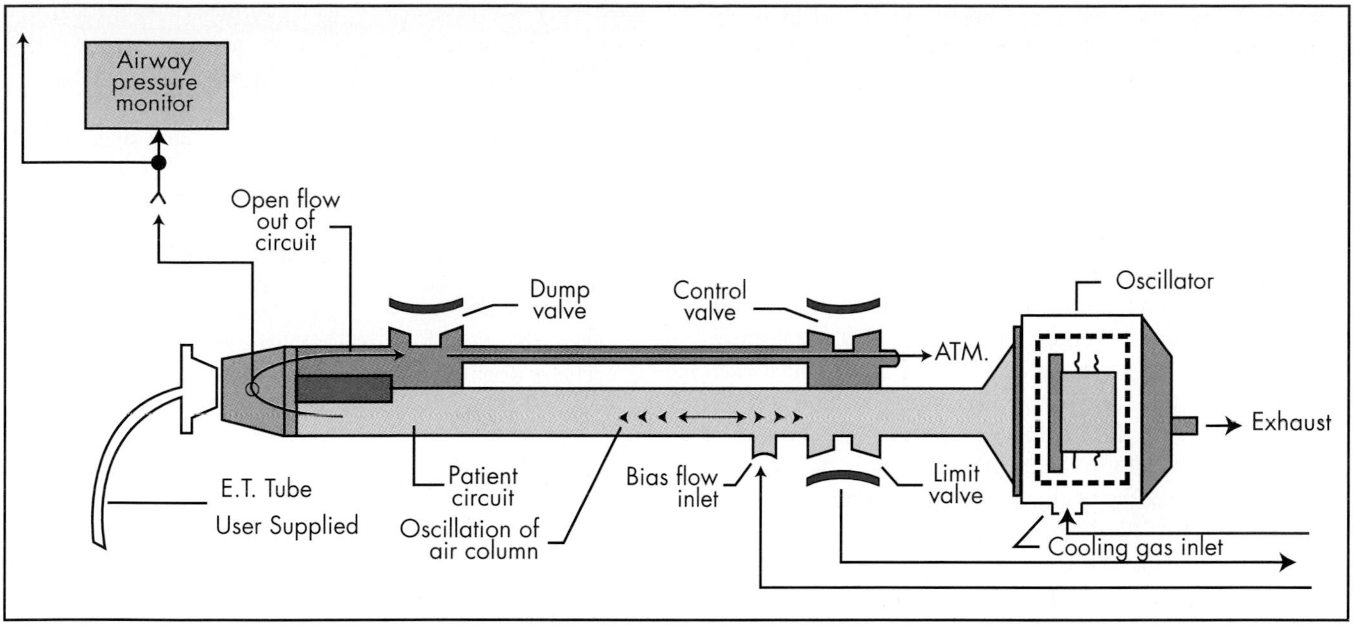

Figure 11-37 The basic breathing circuit of the SensorMedics Model 3100A High-Frequency Oscillator. (SensorMedics Corp., Yorba Linda, Calif.)

Adjusting other controls, such as the MEAN PRESSURE ADJUST or POWER control, changes the piston position. The clinician should check and adjust piston centering after changing other settings.

Bias Flow

The BIAS FLOW control sets the rate of continuous flow through the patient circuit. Adjusting this control counterclockwise increases flow to an internal limit of 40 L/min. Flow is indicated by a ball float within a glass tube graduated in 5-L/min increments.

FiO_2

A standard air/oxygen blender is used to provide blended gas to the ventilator. A minimum pressure of 30 psig is required. The gas mixture is adjusted to the desired FiO_2 before it enters the ventilator.

Mean Pressure Adjust

The MEAN PRESSURE ADJUST control adjusts the mean airway pressure ($\overline{P}aw$). This control varies the resistance placed on the control valve, which is the mushroom valve on the patient circuit at the terminus of the expiratory limb. $\overline{P}aw$ is digitally displayed in the MEAN PRESSURE MONITORING window. Although the MEAN PRESSURE ADJUST control is the primary determinant of $\overline{P}aw$, other controls also affect it. For example, increasing bias flow increases $\overline{P}aw$. Changes to the POWER, FREQUENCY, T_I, and PISTON CENTERING controls also change the $\overline{P}aw$. Therefore if a change in $\overline{P}aw$ occurs because another control has been adjusted, the MEAN PRESSURE ADJUST control should be used to return the $\overline{P}aw$ to the desired level.

Mean Pressure Limit

The MEAN PRESSURE LIMIT control is normally used to set a limit that the $\overline{P}aw$ cannot exceed. Adjustable to a maximum of 45 cm H_2O, this control can be used to protect the patient from an inadvertent rise in mean airway pressure. This control sets a pressure in the limit valve, which is a mushroom valve close to the bias flow inlet of the patient circuit. If the pressure within the circuit exceeds this pressure, the limit valve opens to vent excess pressure to the atmosphere.

An alternative use of the MEAN PRESSURE LIMIT control is to set it above the mean airway pressure that would otherwise exist using only the MEAN PRESSURE ADJUST control. Using the control this way assures the clinician that $\overline{P}aw$ will not exceed that prescribed, regardless of changes made in bias flow, T_I %, or frequency. However, the clinician should be aware that control changes resulting in an uncentered piston can change $\overline{P}aw$, regardless of where the MEAN PRESSURE LIMIT control is set. Increasing the power or amplitude can also increase $\overline{P}aw$.

Power/ΔP

The POWER control determines the amount of polarity voltage applied to the oscillator's subsystem electrical coil. Turning this control clockwise increases the forward and backward displacement of the piston, therefore increasing oscillatory pressure (ΔP), or amplitude, and delivered volume. Pressure is adjustable from approximately 7 to 90 cm H_2O.

The extent to which the ΔP increases depends on the resistance the piston encounters to forward movement. For example, when the oscillator is used with a patient with extremely low pulmonary or chest wall compliance, the piston meets a high resistance in the inspiratory phase. Increasing the POWER setting increases ΔP, but not proportionally according to the amount of resistance the piston encounters from the $\bar{P}aw$. Therefore if a low level of $\bar{P}aw$ is used, ΔP adjustments for the same change in power are greater than if a high level of $\bar{P}aw$ is used.

% Inspiratory Time

The fraction of time that the piston is in the inspiratory position is determined by the % INSPIRATORY TIME control. For example, if the control is set at 33%, the piston spends 33% of the breath cycle in the inspiratory position and the remaining 67% in the expiratory position. The control is adjustable from 30% to 50%. The setting is digitally displayed in the window to the left of the control.

Changing the T_I affects the symmetry of the oscillator waveform. For example, if the clinician decreases the % INSPIRATORY TIME control from 50% to 33%, the amount of time for the piston to travel during the inspiratory phase may be limited. This is especially true at high frequencies. Therefore the ΔP and $\bar{P}aw$ could be affected by changes in the T_I %.

Frequency

The FREQUENCY control sets the oscillatory frequency, or breaths per minute, in Hertz. One Hertz is equal to 60 cycles, or 60 breaths per minute. The control is adjustable from 3 to 15 Hertz, and the setting is digitally displayed in the window to the left of the control.

As frequency is increased, the excursion of the piston is limited by the time allotted for each breath cycle. Therefore changes in the frequency affect mean airway pressure and ΔP (Boxes 11-14 and 11-15).

Start/Stop

The START/STOP control either enables or disables oscillator operation. Pressing this button lights the green OSCILLATOR STOPPED LED if the ventilator's microprocessor determines that the unit is safe to operate. This control only allows the oscillator to begin operating if the start-up procedure was properly performed.

Reset

The RESET button sets or resets the unit's SAFETY and POWER FAILURE alarms. Alarm-triggering conditions must be corrected before reset can occur. This button does not function unless the ventilator has been enabled with the START/STOP button.

Certain alarm conditions, such as the $\bar{P}aw$ $<$20% SET MAX $\bar{P}aw$ alarm, cause the circuit dump valve to immediately deflate. When the clinician presses the RESET button, the dump valve reinflates. It is necessary to hold down the RESET button until the airway pressure is $>$20% of that on the SET MAX $\bar{P}aw$ thumb wheel, or reset may not occur.

BOX 11-14

Altering Oscillator Frequency

A patient is on the SensorMedics 3100A at a frequency of 15 Hz. The clinician decides to lower the frequency to 10 Hertz. Doing this allows the piston more travel time, resulting in greater piston displacement, or more volume delivered to the patient. (The exact amount of the volume increase is unknown.) In some patients, an inadvertent (and unknown) increase in V_T may contribute to volutrauma. Therefore the clinician should always use caution when altering the oscillatory frequency.

BOX 11-15

Adjusting Controls

Many of the controls on the 3100 affect more than one parameter. For example, when adjusting the amplitude with the POWER control, the change in piston thrust changes the level of mean airway pressure. When the frequency is adjusted, changes in amplitude, piston position, and mean airway pressure occur. Therefore the clinician should use caution when making a setting change and carefully readjust the other settings that might also change.

The RESET button also is used to silence the ventilator's battery-powered audible POWER FAILURE alarm when the unit is turned off or the electrical power is interrupted.

Alarms

45-Second Silence

For most alarm conditions, the audible portion can be silenced for 45 seconds by pressing the 45-SEC SILENCE button. When activated, the button's yellow LED illuminates, and stays lit until the silent period elapses.

When the oscillator is turned off at the POWER switch or stops because of a power interruption, the audible alarm can only be silenced with the RESET button.

Set Maximum and Minimum $\bar{P}aw$

The SET MAX $\bar{P}aw$ and SET MIN $\bar{P}aw$ thumb wheel switches enable the clinician to set maximum and minimum limits for $\bar{P}aw$. Because endotracheal tube leaks or spontaneous breathing may cause $\bar{P}aw$ to drift, a safety range should be set. When either limit is reached, a red LED next to the corresponding thumb wheel lights, and an audible alarm sounds. The ventilator continues to operate, but the alarm condition persists until the MEAN

PRESSURE ADJUST control is readjusted or new alarm limits are set.

$\bar{P}$aw <20% Set Max $\bar{P}$aw

Conditions causing a sharp drop in $\bar{P}$aw (to a level less than 20% of the value set on the SET MAX $\bar{P}$aw thumb wheel) trigger a $\bar{P}$aw <20% SET MAX $\bar{P}$aw alarm. When this alarm is triggered, the oscillator stops, the red LED lights to indicate this alarm condition, and the audible alarm sounds. Bias flow continues to be delivered to permit spontaneous ventilation.

$\bar{P}$aw > 50 cm H_2O

The $\bar{P}$AW > 50 CM H_2O alarm is activated if mean airway pressure rises above 50 cm H_2O for any reason. When this alarm activates, the dump valve opens, causing the oscillator to stop. The red LED lights to indicate this alarm condition, and an audible alarm sounds. Although the audible alarm can be silenced with the 45-sec silence button, the oscillator will not resume operation until the RESET button is pressed and held until mean airway pressure exceeds 20% of that on the SET MAX $\bar{P}$aw thumb wheel.

Power Failure

The battery-powered POWER FAILURE alarm is activated if the POWER switch to the ventilator is turned off or electrical power is interrupted. If the unit's main circuit breaker is tripped or the main power supply fails, this alarm condition would also occur. The POWER FAILURE LED lights and the alarm sounds. Both can be stopped by pressing the RESET button.

When power is restored to the ventilator, the circuit must be occluded (Box 11-16) and the RESET button pressed and held until mean airway pressure exceeds 20% of that on the SET MAX $\bar{P}$aw thumb wheel. Only then will oscillations resume.

Battery Low

The yellow BATTERY LOW LED lights when the battery serving the POWER FAILURE alarm is low. No audible alarm is activated.

Source Gas Low

The yellow SOURCE GAS LOW LED lights whenever gas pressure from the blender falls below 30 psig. This LED also lights if the pressure drops below 30 psig in the separate compressed air source for cooling the piston subsystem. The most common cause of this alarm condition is obstruction of the inlet filter cartridge with dirt. If this problem is not corrected, the piston subsystem is likely to overheat, resulting in piston failure.

Oscillator Overheated

The yellow OSCILLATOR OVERHEATED LED lights when the oscillator coil temperature reaches 175° C. No audible alarm sounds. Failure to correct this problem can result in piston failure.

BOX 11-16

Returning the Oscillator to Operation after Disconnect

When alarm conditions occur, especially those that shut down the oscillator, the clinician should immediately remove the patient from the circuit and provide manual ventilation. Once the cause of the alarm condition is corrected, the airway connector should be plugged, and oscillations restarted using the RESET button. Plugging the circuit and restarting oscillations is necessary to confirm safe operation. Once this is done, the plug is removed, and the connection is immediately hand-occluded. Then the circuit is quickly reconnected to the patient's airway.

Troubleshooting

The array of audio/visual alarms help the clinician to troubleshoot specific problems with the SensorMedics ventilators. The instruction manual also provides a troubleshooting guide.

Circuit leaks are most likely to occur at the many connection points. For example, the pressure line running from the airway wye to the front of the unit could be loose. Lines running from the front to each of the mushroom valves can be the source of leaks. All of these lines have Luer connections that should be tight. Although rare, any of the mushroom valves can rupture, causing the unit to stop oscillating and alarm.

When a circuit not equipped with heater wires is used, water pooling can occur at any low point in the circuit. If the patient is positioned below the circuit, excessive condensate can run into the patient airway. Care should be taken to keep water drained from the circuit.

The clinician should note any unusual knocking coming from the piston. If the SensorMedics is operated for long periods of time at very low frequencies, the piston can start to fail. If the piston housing is not connected to a compressed air source, or if the unit is operated without sufficient piston centering, the piston wears more rapidly than normal. Usually piston failure can be detected by a knocking sound and by drifting in the mean airway pressure and amplitude levels.

Every clinician who uses SensorMedics oscillators should be able to perform a system calibration and check. An outline of this procedure is printed on the top left side of the unit. If problems are noted in maintaining desired settings, the patient should be removed from the ventilator and the procedure performed. Doing so often reveals the source of the problem.

Summary

The ventilators discussed in this chapter are widely and exclusively used in pediatric settings. Some models covered elsewhere in this text are equipped to effectively monitor and ventilate the largest adults as well as the smallest infants, and this capability is a trend in newer ventilator designs.

Many ventilators that were originally designed to be used for adults are easily adapted to pediatric and, in some cases, neonatal situations. In many clinical settings, a staff that works with patients of all ages (and sizes) is accustomed to providing mechanical ventilation to this wide variety of patients. In such settings, a ventilator that is easily adapted to need is a cost and time savings in staff technical training.

Infant and pediatric ventilators will continue to develop, particularly to provide better monitoring capabilities. Additional developments in specialized applications unique to the neonatal/pediatric population are certain, including ventilatory support to spontaneously breathing patients and high-frequency technology. Recently, some clinicians have shown interest in ventilators capable of delivering subambient oxygen concentrations, and others have envisioned systems capable of providing specialty gases (e.g., nitric oxide and heliox). Someday units providing liquid ventilation may be on the market. Prototype closed-loop systems that monitor arterial blood and expired gases and adjust their own ventilator settings are being tested and have been in the planning stages for years.

Like all technology, necessity drives the scope and the direction of advancement. As clinical problems present themselves, technical innovations render ever more sophisticated solutions. Other factors, such as other medical advances, economics, demographics, and even ideology, continue to affect the infant/pediatric ventilator market.

References

1. Chatburn RL: Principles and practices of neonatal and pediatric ventilation, Respir Care 36:573, 1991.
2. Betit P, Thompson JE, and Benjamin PK: Mechanical ventilation. In Koff PB, Eitzman D, and Neu J, editors: Neonatal and pediatric respiratory care, ed 2, St Louis, 1993, Mosby.
3. Aladdin Infant Flow System instruction manual, Reno, Nev., 1994, Hamilton Medical, Inc.
4. Sechrist Model IV-100B Infant Ventilator operator's manual, Anaheim, Calif., 1984, Sechrist Industries, Inc.
5. Bourns Infant Pressure Ventilator Model BP200 instruction manual, form P/N 50000-10200, Riverside Calif., 1974, Allied Healthcare Products, Inc.
6. Bear Cub Infant Ventilator Model BP2001 instruction manual, form P/N 50000-10220, Riverside, Calif., 1982, Allied Healthcare Products, Inc.
7. Bear Cub 750vs Infant Ventilator instruction manual, form P/N 51-10641-00, Riverside, Calif., 1996, Allied Healthcare Products, Inc.
8. Infant Star Neonatal Ventilator operating instructions, form P/N 9910005, San Diego, 1986, Infrasonics, Inc.
9. Infant Star 500 Ventilator operating instructions, San Diego, 1996, Infrasonics, Inc.
10. Infant Star 950 Ventilator operating instructions, San Diego, 1996, Infrasonics, Inc.
11. Infant Star 100 Neonatal Ventilator operating instructions, San Diego, 1995, Infrasonics, Inc.
12. Infant Star 200 Neonatal-Pediatric Ventilator operating instructions, San Diego, 1995, Infrasonics, Inc.
13. VIP Bird Infant-Pediatric Ventilator instruction manual, Palm Springs, Calif., 1991, Bird Products, Inc.
14. VIP Graphics instruction manual, Palm Springs, Calif., 1991, Bird Products. Inc.
15. Dräger Babylog 8000 operator's manual, ed 1 (United States), Chantilly, Va., 1993, Dräger, Inc.
16. Life Pulse High Frequency Jet Ventilator operator's manual, Salt Lake City, 1991, Bunnell, Inc.
17. 3100A High Frequency Oscillatory Ventilator operator's manual, form P/N 767124, Yorba Linda, Calif., 1991, SensorMedics Corp.

Internet Resources

1. Thermo Respiratory Group Home Page: www.sensormedics.com
2. Nellcor Puritan Bennett Infant and Pediatric Ventilators: www.nellcorpb.com/product/ventilators/infant_pediatric.html
3. Hamilton Medical: www.hamilton-medical.ch
4. Dräger Neonatal Care Systems: www.draeger.com/english/mt/mt-p/index.htm
5. Sechrist Respiratory Products—Introduction: www.sechristind.com/intro_rp.html

Review Questions

See Appendix A for answers.

1. Which of the following best describes the TPTV mode?
   a. TPTV is a pressure-triggered, flow-cycled mode
   b. TPTV is a time-triggered, time-cycled mode
   c. TPTV is a time-triggered, patient-triggered, and flow-cycled mode
   d. TPTV is a flow-triggered, pressure-cycled mode
2. The Aladdin Infant Flow System incorporates an alarm system for which of the following conditions?
   a. spontaneous respiratory rate falling outside of set parameters
   b. FiO_2 reading different from set FiO_2
   c. apnea
   d. spontaneous minute volume falling outside of set parameters
3. If a patient's endotracheal tube becomes completely plugged while being ventilated on the Healthdyne 105 ventilator, which of the following will occur?
   a. the ventilator's high-pressure alarm will be activated
   b. the ventilator's low minute volume will be activated
   c. the ventilator's insufficient expiratory time alarm will be activated
   d. no ventilator alarm will be activated
4. On the Sechrist IV-100B, a timed mandatory breath is initiated when the back-pressure switch sensing line is occluded by which of the following?

a. OR/NOR fluidic valve
b. solenoid valve
c. pneumatic needle valve
d. scissors valve

5. On the Bourns BP200 infant ventilator, the MAX INSP TIME control:
   a. overrides both the I:E RATIO and RATE control settings
   b. overrides the I:E RATIO control setting regardless of the ventilator rate setting
   c. provides a back-up inspiratory time in case the I:E RATIO control setting is inadvertently changed
   d. overrides the I:E RATIO control setting and determines the actual inspiratory time of mandatory breath (only at ventilator rate settings less than 10 breaths/min)
6. When added to the Bear Cub 2001 Infant Ventilator, the Bear Cub Enhancement Module (CEM) adds which of the following capabilities to the ventilator?
   a. SIMV
   b. assist/control
   c. tidal volume monitoring
   d. all of the above
7. Which of the following best describes the volume limit feature of the Bear Cub 750vs ventilator?
   a. activates an alarm if tidal volume decreases to a preset level
   b. phases out mandatory breaths from the ventilator when spontaneous breaths fall within certain parameters
   c. allows the PIP to adjust itself upward or downward to maintain the patient's tidal volume within set parameters
   d. sets a ceiling for volume delivered by mechanical breaths
8. The purpose of the background flow feature on the Infant Star 500 and 950 ventilators is to:
   a. maintain a minimum gas flow past humidifier temperature probes to prevent inspiratory gas from overheating
   b. compensate for leaks around the endotracheal tube
   c. maintain a gas flow sufficient for spontaneous inspiratory demands but low enough to minimize circuit PEEP
   d. provide a back-up flow of blended gas to the patient in case the demand valve fails
9. The Infant Star 950 ventilator differs from the Sensormedics 3100A in which of the following ways?
   a. the Infant Star creates gas pulses rather than piston-generated mechanical oscillations
   b. the Infant Star can provide both conventional and high-frequency ventilation
   c. when operating in one of its high-frequency modes, the Infant Star can provide greater flows, mean airway pressures, and oscillatory frequencies
   d. both A and B
10. The tracking relief pressure valve on the Infant Star 100 and 200 ventilators serves which of the following functions?
    a. automatically sets a high-pressure safety limit
    b. prevents the operator from setting the safety pressure-relief valve too high
    c. automatically sets an appropriate PIP level
    d. prevents the operator from setting the minimum inspiratory pressure alarm too low
11. Termination sensitivity is an added feature on the VIP Bird ventilator that:
    a. allows the clinician to adjust the flow termination point of the breath
    b. operates in all modes
    c. can be adjusted from 0 to 25% in increments of 5%
    d. A and C
12. On the VIP Bird, the termination sensitivity setting flashes when the:
    a. breath is terminated at the set value
    b. breath is time-cycled
    c. breath is both flow-triggered and flow-cycled
    d. expiratory time is deemed too short by the ventilator's microprocessor
13. On the VIP Bird, leak compensation is:
    a. available in all modes
    b. only available in volume-cycled modes
    c. used to stabilize baseline pressure in the presence of leaks
    d. B and C
14. The Bunnell Jet Ventilator:
    a. operates in tandem with a conventional ventilator
    b. requires the use of the Hi-Lo Jet tube
    c. delivers rates of 240 to 660 insufflations/minute
    d. A and C
15. The triple lumen Hi-Lo Jet tube:
    a. is the type of only endotracheal tube that can be used with the Bunnell Jet ventilator
    b. ranges in size from 2.5 to 6.0 mm ID
    c. must be replaced with a standard endotracheal tube when the patient is switched to conventional ventilation
    d. all of the above
16. The Dräger Babylog 8000 Infant Ventilator:
    a. is used to ventilate premature and term infants
    b. has a weight limit of 10 kilograms
    c. has a built-in battery
    d. all of the above
17. The POWER control on the Sensormedics 3100A is primarily used to change the:
    a. mean airway pressure
    b. frequency
    c. bias flow
    d. amplitude
18. If the frequency on the Sensormedics 3100A is increased from 10 to 15 Hertz and no other settings are changed, which of the following will occur?
    a. inspiratory time will increase
    b. volume delivered by the piston will decrease
    c. amplitude will increase
    d. none of the above

CHAPTER 12

CHAPTER OUTLINE

Home-Care and Transport Devices

Kevin Lord

CHAPTER LEARNING OBJECTIVES

Upon completion of this chapter, the reader should be able to:

1. Compare the transport ventilators described and provide a list of their common characteristics.
2. Explain the factors that determine tidal volume (V_T), rate, and flow for each ventilator described.
3. Discuss the desirable characteristics of a transport ventilator.
4. Explain how PEEP is applied and used for each ventilator.
5. Describe the oxygen system for each ventilator and how it regulates and monitors the fraction of inspired oxygen (FiO_2).
6. List alarm capabilities for all ventilators.
7. Explain the flow of the gas source through the internal mechanisms of each ventilator.
8. Describe what type of individuals would be best-suited for home-care ventilation.
9. Compare and contrast the differences between positive- and negative-pressure ventilators.
10. Describe the benefits of NIPPV over traditional ventilation.

KEY TERMS

Antisuffication Valve
Caudal
Cephalad
Chest Cuirass
External PEEP Valve
Internal Regulator
Iron Lung
Microprocessor
Pneumatic System
Pneumobelt
Poppet Valve
Potentiometer
Pressure-Relief Valve
Rocking Bed
Solenoid Valve

Because of the special requirements of ventilating patients during transport and in home- or extended care environments, a variety of ventilators have been developed for these settings. The first part of this chapter reviews some ventilators specifically intended for transporting patients who require ventilatory support. The second section focuses on ventilators and ventilatory aids used in home- and extended care facilities.

Transport Ventilators

Although transporting mechanically ventilated patients for diagnostic or therapeutic procedures is common, it is also associated with a degree of risk. Every attempt should be made to ensure that monitoring, ventilation, oxygenation, and patient care are constant during movement, but this is difficult to maintain for individual being manually ventilated for an extended time. Alterations in any of these constants can lead to hyper- or hypoventilation, hypoxemia, acid/base imbalances, and dysrhythmias, ultimately affecting the patient's safety and well-being.

Today, ventilators are developed to meet the specific needs of patient transport. They are designed as compact, lightweight units (compared with the traditional ICU ventilators) that maintain a reliable power source. The complexity of the machine has been reduced without compromising patient support.

This chapter presents the design of specific transport ventilators instead of their applications to patient use. The American Association for Respiratory Care (AARC), however, has developed a clinical practice guideline specifically addressing the purpose, indications, methods of providing, and complications associated with transporting mechanically ventilated patients (Box 12-1).

Bird Avian

The Avian transport ventilator (Figure 12-1; Bird Products, Inc.) is a microprocessor-controlled ventilator primarily used for transporting pediatric and adult patients. It can function in four modes: control, assist/control (A/C), synchronized intermittent mandatory ventilation (SIMV), and continuous positive airway pressure (CPAP) ventilation. It is lightweight (11 lbs) and portable (10″ × 12″ × 5″).

Power Source

The Avian is electrically and pneumatically powered and requires both sources to properly perform all of its operations. The electronic system can use three possible power sources:

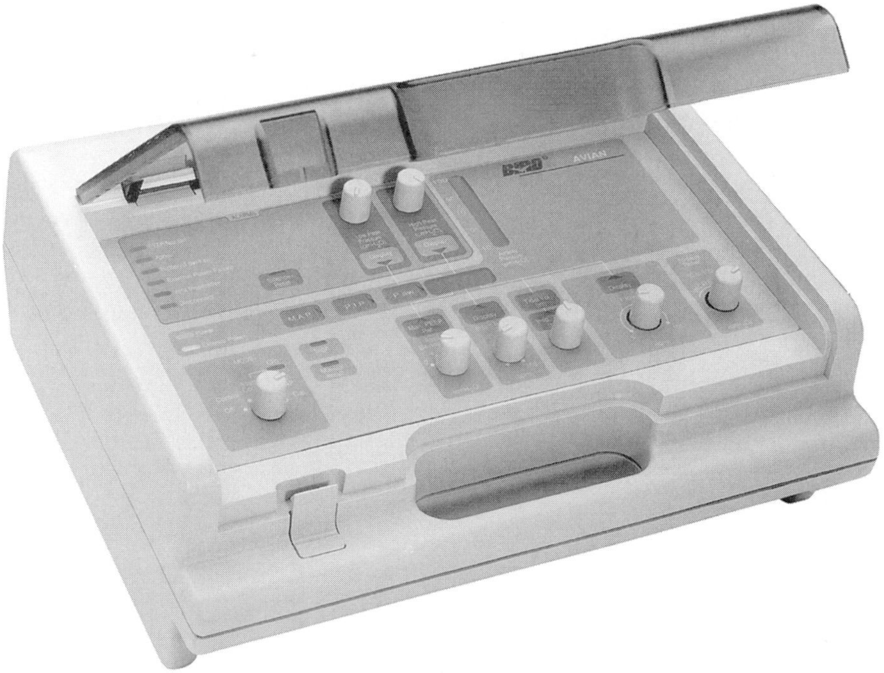

Figure 12-1 The Bird Avian Ventilator. (Courtesy Bird Products Corp., Palm Springs, Calif.)

BOX 12-1

Clinical Practice Guidelines

Transport of the Mechanically Ventilated Patient

Definition/Description

Patient transport is the preparation, the movement to and from, and the time spent at an allocated destination.

Indications

Transportation of mechanically ventilated patients should only be undertaken after a careful evaluation of the risk:benefit ratio.

Transportation should be undertaken on the attending physician's order.

Contraindications

Contraindications include the inability to provide adequate oxygenation, sustain acceptable cardiopulmonary status, and maintain an adequate airway.

Precautions and/or Complications

Hazards and complications of transport include the following:

- Hyperventilation during manual ventilation, resulting in respiratory alkalosis, cardiac dysrhythmias, and hypotension.
- Loss of PEEP/CPAP, resulting in hypoxemia.
- Position changes that result in hypotension, hypercarbia, and hypoxemia.
- Equipment failure, resulting in inaccurate data or loss of monitoring capabilities.
- Inadvertent disconnection of intravenous pharmacologic agents, resulting in hemodynamic instability.
- Accidental extubation.
- Accidental removal of vascular access.
- Loss of oxygen supply, resulting in hypoxemia.

Limitations

The literature suggests that nearly two thirds of all transports for diagnostic studies fail to yield results that affect patient care.

Monitoring

Monitoring provided during transport should be maintained at the level of stationary care.

For complete guidelines see AARC clinical practice guidelines: transport of the mechanically ventilated patient, Resp Care 38:1169, 1993.

- An internal 6-volt DC battery
- An external 12-volt DC battery
- A standard AC outlet

The internal battery can sustain ventilator operation for about 11 hours and requires about 18 hours to fully recharge. The external DC battery must be able to maintain an output of 11 to 30 volts to sustain ventilator operation, and the AC power option requires an adaptor to properly function.

The pneumatic system requires a medical-grade high-pressure source gas that can deliver 40 to 60 psi and has minimum flow-rate capabilities of 100 L/min. The source may be a cylinder, wall outlet, or oxygen/air blender with a DISS connector.

Internal Mechanisms

Source gas enters through the gas inlet port at the top of the ventilator. The pressure is reduced to a constant working pressure of 30 psi to ensure optimal machine function. When a mandatory breath is delivered, the gas flow moves from the regulator to the main solenoid valve, which controls inspiratory flow. Gas flows from the main solenoid valve to the flow-control poppet valve, which has two functions. It regulates and maintains gas flow to the patient based on the desired control settings; and it involves a potentiometer valve, which is attached to the flow-control poppet valve, measures changes in valve position, and relays this information to the microprocessor. This allows V_T to be calculated during mandatory breath delivery.

Before it leaves the internal circuit for the patient circuit, the source gas passes a one-way check valve, the pressure-relief valve, and the proximal airway pressure line. The pressure-relief valve is a safety feature that prevents airway pressure from exceeding a set value. If this occurs, the excess pressure and volume are vented to room air. The proximal airway line allows for communication with the airway pressure transducer and monitors the airway pressure and pressure alarms.

The demand valve provides flow for spontaneous breaths that are initiated in the SIMV or CPAP modes. The effort required to trigger the demand valve is determined by the sensitivity setting. (Mandatory breath triggering is determined by the sensitivity setting as well. Once triggered, gas flows through the demand orifice and through a fixed resistor that regulates flow to 60 L/min. Because the check valve is bypassed, the exhalation valve stays open, allowing any excess flow to be vented to the atmosphere.

A removable PEEP valve can be attached to the outlet port of the exhalation valve. The Avian automatically compensates the sensitivity or the trigger mechanism for the addition of PEEP so that work of breathing does not increase.

Controls and Alarms

The front panel of the Avian contains several controls for setting parameters, as well as for monitoring patient data and alarms.

Mode Control Knob

The MODE selector has five possible settings: OFF, CONTROL, ASSIST/CONTROL, SIMV/CPAP and CAL. The OFF setting turns the ventilator off and triggers the VENT INOP alarm, which can be silenced by the ALARM SILENCE/RESET button. The visual alarm, however, continues to flash for 30 minutes. The CAL setting lets the operator calibrate the airway pressure transducer to properly read "O" at ambient pressure. The other modes are presented in the discussion of modes of ventilation later in this chapter.

Control Parameters

The CONTROL parameters include the following functions:

- Tidal volume
- Inspiratory time
- Rate
- Flow
- PEEP

The TIDAL VOLUME function is active when the machine is operating in volume-targeted ventilation. It allows the operator to set a range of 50 to 2000 mL for a mandatory breath. When the machine is initially turned on, the unit defaults to volume-targeted ventilation with volume-cycling, which requires a V_T setting in all modes except CPAP.

Mandatory breaths can be changed from volume to time-cycling by using the T_V/T_I control. To activate time-cycled ventilation, the TIDAL VOLUME/INSPIRATORY TIME button must by pressed and the T_I set. The new selection is displayed in the monitor window. To activate the new setting, press the TIDAL VOLUME/INSPIRATORY TIME button a second time. If you want to change the inspiratory time setting, enter the new setting, and then press the DISPLAY button. Remember that when the Avian is initially turned on, the default setting is for volume-cycled–not time-cycled ventilation. When time-cycled ventilation is desired, this change must be made every time the power is turned on.

The RESPIRATORY RATE control in the center of the control panel allows for time-triggering of a mechanical breath (0 to 150 breaths/min). The FLOW control on the bottom right regulates the maximum flow delivered to the patient on all mandatory breaths (5 to 100 L/min).

The PEEP valve is a separate attachment to the exhalation valve. To access this function, press the MANUAL PEEP REFERENCE button on the front panel and hold it for 3 seconds until the "A" in the display window disappears. This allows the operator to manually set the PEEP range from 0 to 20 cm H_2O. If the PEEP value deviates by more than 5 cm H_2O from the desired setting, an audible alarm is activated, and the display window reads "PEEP Not Set," alerting the operator to the problem.

> **BOX 12-2**
>
> **Decision Making & Problem Solving**
>
> A patient is being ventilated with the Bird Avian in the A/C mode. V_T is 0.6 L; rate is 10 breaths/min; PIP is 25 cm H_2O; and the HIGH PEAK PRESSURE alarm is set at 35 cm H_2O. A decision is made to switch to pressure-limited ventilation. Where should the respiratory therapist set the HIGH PEAK PRESSURE alarm and the PRESSURE-RELIEF control to still achieve approximately the same V_T?
>
> See Appendix A for the answer.

The ASSIST SENSITIVITY control allows the operator to set a threshold trigger sensitivity for all breath types (-2 to -8 cm H_2O). The sensitivity is automatically PEEP-compensated. For example, if PEEP is 5 cm H_2O and the sensitivity is -2 cm H_2O, the breath triggers when an inspiratory effort drops the baseline pressure to 3 cm H_2O.

The PRESSURE-RELIEF control is in the middle, right part of the control panel. It is designed to allow the operator to set the maximum acceptable pressure in the circuit during a mandatory breath and can serve one of two purposes. It is a safety feature, and should be set 5 to 15 cm H_2O above the HIGH PEAK PRESSURE alarm in case it fails. It also functions as a pressure-limiting control when set to the desired limit, and the high peak pressure alarm is set at 5 to 15 cm H_2O above the pressure-relief setting. Its adjustable range is 10 to 100 cm H_2O. This control is a spring-loaded valve with no electronic input, so it is a secondary safety feature for high circuit pressures if there is an electronic failure (Box 12-2).

The SIGH function is on the front left part of the control panel. When activated, it delivers a breath 1.5 times the V_T or T_I setting, depending on which is active. The maximum limits are 3 seconds for T_I and 2000 mL for V_T. Sigh frequency is once every 100 breaths or once every 7 minutes, whichever comes first.

The MANUAL BREATH control allows the operator to deliver a mandatory breath at the current ventilator settings. When activated, the breath rate timer is reset so that a time-triggered breath will not occur until the next full cycle.

Airway Pressure Alarms

The Avian lets the operator set and monitor high and low airway pressures. The HIGH PEAK PRESSURE alarm establishes the maximum pressure allowed in the patient circuit during all breaths. This alarm is at the top central part of the control panel, has an allowable range of 1 to 100 cm H_2O,

BOX 12-3

Recoverable Alarms on the Avian

- Loss of electrical power
- Mode switch momentarily turned off
- Power voltage out of range

and cannot be set below the PEEP setting. When the set pressure level is exceeded, inspiration stops and the machine cycles into exhalation, venting the remaining volume and pressure to room air.

The LOW PEAK PRESSURE alarm is only active during mandatory breaths in the control, A/C and SIMV modes. It is in the middle of the top of the control panel and has an allowable range of 2 to 50 cm H_2O. It is activated when a patient does not exceed the alarm settings during the inspiratory phase of each breath.

Additional Alarms

Additional alarms that are monitored include the following:

- DISCONNECT
- VENTILATOR INOPERATIVE
- EXTERNAL POWER LOW/FAIL
- BATTERY LOW/FAIL
- ALARM/SILENCE RESET
- I:E RATIO
- APNEA

The DISCONNECT alarm is at the bottom of the alarm section on the control panel. It monitors the airway pressure in the patient circuit and is activated if the pressure does not exceed 2 cm H_2O above the baseline pressure during a mandatory breath.

The VENTILATOR INOPERATIVE alarm is in the alarms section of the control panel and has two conditions: recoverable and nonrecoverable. The nonrecoverable alarm is usually due to a software problem or CPU malfunction. The machine must be turned off, and the ALARM/SILENCE button pressed to silence the alarm. The patient must be disconnected and manually ventilated until the problem is resolved. For a list of the recoverable problems, see Box 12-3. When any one of the recoverable problems occurs, the machine returns to normal working function once the condition has been rectified.

The EXTERNAL LOW/FAIL alarm is activated when the external power supply connected to the ventilator is operating outside of the acceptable range (11 to 30 DC for an external battery). The machine automatically switches to the internal battery. When the internal battery voltage falls below 5.6 ± 0.2 volts and no external supply is connected, the BATTERY LOW/FAIL alarm is activated. The battery life remaining depends on the machine settings.

The ALARM/SILENCE RESET button is in the alarm section on the control panel. When it is activated, this control silences the alarm for a certain time (depending on the problem) and resets the visual alarm in the display window.

The Avian does not allow I:E ratios greater than 1:1 to occur. If any combination of T_I or V_T, flow, and breath rate creates a $T_I > 50\%$ of the TCT, the ventilator generates an audio/visual alarm. This alarm cannot be reset until the problem is alleviated. In the meantime, the ventilator continues to function with a T_I of 50% of the TCT.

The APNEA alarm is also in the alarm section of the control panel and is activated when 20 seconds elapse with no breath detection (spontaneous or mandatory). The audio/visual alarms are activated, and the ventilator resorts to a back-up rate of 12 breaths/min in the A/C mode, using the set parameter. The back-up ventilation can be terminated by pressing the ALARM/RESET button.

Modes of Ventilation

The Bird Avian offers the following four modes of ventilation: control, A/C, SIMV, and CPAP. As already mentioned, the machine may be set to volume- or time-cycled ventilation, but the default setting is volume-cycled. Therefore when operating in any modes but CPAP, the operator must be aware of how the machine is cycling. In the control mode, T_I or V_T, flow, and breath rate are all active, offering a time- or volume-cycled, volume-targeted breath. The assist sensitivity setting is not functional in this mode.

The A/C mode allows the patient to initiate mechanical breaths, and thereby control the total breath rate of the ventilator. All other functions set in the control mode are still active in this mode except for ASSIST/SENSITIVITY. When operating in A/C, the patient must generate an inspiratory effort greater than the set sensitivity to initiate a breath.

The SIMV mode allows for spontaneous breathing between the volume-targeted mandatory breaths. All previous functions are still active, and PEEP and sigh operations are added.

When operating in the CPAP mode, the control function is turned to SIMV, the rate is set to "0," and the PEEP valve is adjusted to the desired setting. All breaths are spontaneous and completely controlled by the patient. If the patient fails to trigger the ventilator within 20 seconds (not an adjustable time period), the APNEA alarm is activated, and the ventilator reverts to back-up ventilation. Back-up ventilation consists of 12 breaths/min with all set controls operational in the A/C mode. To terminate this function, the ALARM SILENCE/RESET button must be pressed.

Oxygen Source

The Avian operates from a 100% gas source, therefore the oxygen percentage depends upon the gas powering the

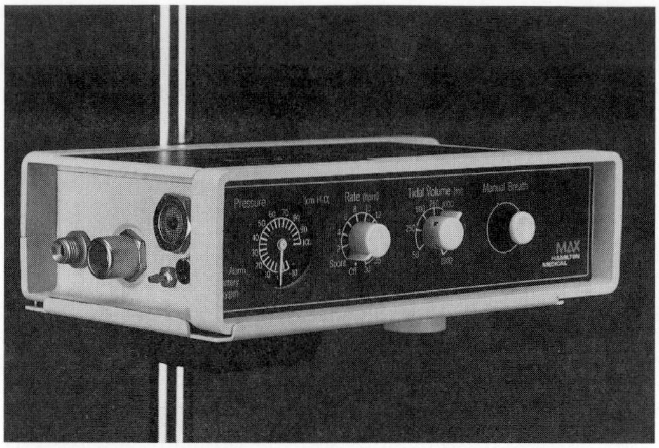

Figure 12-2 The Hamilton MAX Ventilator. (Courtesy Hamilton Medical, Reno, Nev.)

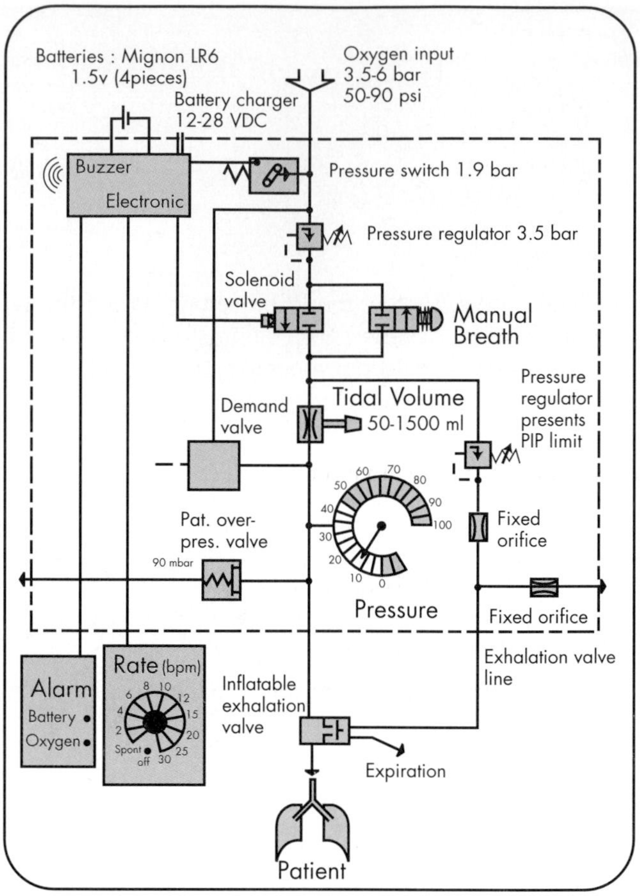

Figure 12-3 A MAX flow diagram. (Courtesy Hamilton Medical, Reno, Nev.)

BOX 12-4

Decision Making & Problem Solving

A respiratory therapist is asked to transport a ventilated patient from the ICU to x-ray using the MAX ventilator. The respiratory rate is 15 breaths/min with no additional spontaneous breaths, and the V_T is 500 mL. The oxygen E cylinder has 1200 psi available, and the estimated time of the trip (one-way) is 30 minutes. Does the therapist have to change to a full cylinder to make the round trip?

See Appendix A for the answer.

ventilator. To vary FiO_2, the unit should use an air/oxygen blender for its gas power.

HAMILTON MEDICAL MAX

The Hamilton Medical, Inc. MAX (Figure 12-2) is used to ventilate pediatric or adult patients during transport. It uses IMV ventilation to provide time- or patient-triggered, volume-targeted, and time-cycled mandatory breaths that are delivered with a constant flow. Spontaneous breaths are pressure-triggered and pressure-limited. The device is lightweight (~5 lbs) and compact (11.5″ × 6″ × 3″).

Power Source

The MAX is electrically controlled and pneumatically powered, and requires energy supplies for both systems to properly operate. The electronic system normally uses four 1.5-volt, AA batteries to power the control panel and solenoid valve. As an alternate electrical power source, an external DC battery source with an input range of 12 to 28 volts and a minimum of 150 mA can be used. The MAX can also be connected to a standard 120-volt AC outlet with a 12-volt converter.

The pneumatic system is designed to use 100% medical-grade oxygen as its primary source gas. For proper operation, it requires a pressure of 50 to 90 psi from a cylinder, wall outlet, or oxygen/air mixer. If compressed gas is used instead of oxygen, there can be an increase in V_T by as much as 10% due to the difference in densities between the two gases. The internal components of the ventilator do not consume any gas during operation, providing the operator more accuracy in predicting the length of time a cylinder may last in transport (Box 12-4).

Internal Mechanisms

The source gas enters through a connection on the side panel (Figure 12-3) and is routed through an internal regulator that precisely adjusts the pressures to 50 psi. After passing through the regulator, the flow is guided to an electronically controlled solenoid valve. During mandatory breaths, this valve opens for a set period of 1 second, thus fixing the T_I. Next, the source gas branches, directing flow to a second flow-control valve and pressure regulator. The

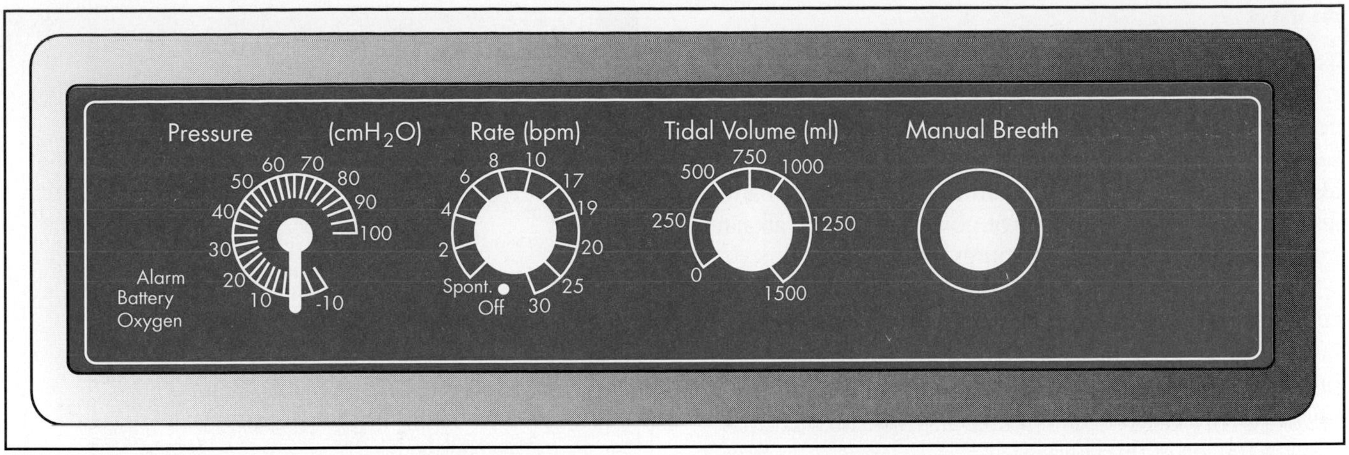

Figure 12-4 The MAX front control panel.

flow-control valve regulates the flow/V_T that is to be delivered to the patient. The pressure regulator functions as a pressure-relief valve, limiting the maximum allowable pressure in the patient circuit. The pressure relief is factory-set at 45 cm H_2O, but can be manually changed from 10 to 100 cm H_2O inside the machine.

When spontaneous breaths are initiated, the patient must open the pneumatically controlled demand valve. This differs from mechanical breaths in the following two ways:

- It requires the patient to provide an inspiratory effort sufficient to drop circuit pressure -1 to -2 cm H_2O below ambient pressure to generate inspiratory flow. When PEEP is required, it becomes increasingly difficult for the patient to trigger a spontaneous breath because the ventilator does not compensate for PEEP.
- The demand valve is powered by the source gas and can provide flows up to 145 L/min.

When a manual breath is delivered, the electronically powered solenoid valve is bypassed and gas enters directly into the circuit (see description of manual breath in the following section on controls).

Controls

Figure 12-4 provides a view of the controls located on the front panel. The three primary controls are the rate, tidal volume and manual breath control.

Rate

The rate control allows mandatory breaths to be set from 2 to 30 breaths/min. It also has a spontaneous setting in which mandatory breaths stop and all breaths are spontaneously triggered breaths (preset sensitivity of -1 to -2 cm H_2O). Under these conditions, the patient determines the rate and V_T of each breath. Note that this setting provides no back-up mandatory rate. The OFF position of this control stops mandatory and patient-triggered breaths and inactivates the alarm system (see the discussion of alarms at the end of this section).

> **BOX 12-5**
>
> **Manual Inhalation Button**
>
> There is no maximum length of time that the MANUAL INHALATION button can be pressed, but the patient is protected from overinflation by the internal safety pop-off valve (set at 45 cm H_2O).
>
> If there is an electrical power failure, the transport team can ventilate a patient with manual breaths because pneumatic power can still provide flow delivery. The MANUAL BREATH control does not require electricity to work. It diverts the gas around the electronically controlled solenoid valve (see Figure 12-3).

Tidal Volume

The MAX is a flow-controller, so V_T delivery is a function of flow and T_I. Thus when the V_T is adjusted, it is the flow rate (variable from 0 to 90 L/min) that is actually being adjusted. The face panel, however, displays incremental changes in adjustable volumes of 50 to 1500 mL for mandatory breaths.

Manual Breath

By depressing the MANUAL BREATH button, a positive-pressure breath can be delivered at any time. Volume delivery depends on how long the button is pressed. Once the manual button is released, inspiration is terminated. For example, if it is pressed for 1 second, the set V_T will be delivered because the normal T_I is fixed at 1 second (Box 12-5).

Pressure Gauge

The pressure gauge on the left side of the front panel is calibrated in cm H_2O (-10 to 100 cm H_2O) and allows the operator to view the active pressure in the circuit, PEEP, and the maximum pressure change from baseline.

Alarms

The MAX has two alarms (LOW BATTERY and LOW OXYGEN) and a pressure-limit feature. If there is a low battery condition, a constant visual indicator illuminates and a pulsating tone sounds simultaneously. The LOW BATTERY alarm indicator is activated when the rechargeable batteries have less then 10 minutes of power left or the alkaline batteries have less than 30 minutes left.

The LOW OXYGEN indicator also has audio/visual indicators that are activated when the input pressure source falls below 27 psi and alert the operator to the insufficient pressure from the source gas. Note that there is no built-in O_2 analyzer. The LOW OXYGEN light indicates the pressure level at the gas source inlet.

There is no low-pressure alarm for circuit leaks, but there is an audible alarm for excessive high pressures. Excessive pressures are limited by the internal pressure alarm system that is part of the exhalation valve circuit assembly. This internal pressure system acts as a pressure relief, venting excessive flow through the exhalation valve to room air when circuit pressure exceeds the set value (and sounding a noise concurrently). It limits pressure delivery but does not end inspiration. As previously mentioned, the pressure-relief limit is preset by the manufacturer at 45 cm H_2O and can be internally adjusted from 10 to 100 cm H_2O.

Modes of Ventilation

The design of the Hamilton MAX provides only one mode of ventilation: IMV; but the unit is set up to allow for control, and spontaneous (CPAP) as well. When the patient does not trigger any additional breaths above the set rate, the ventilator operates in a control mode fashion with the V_T and breath rate controlled by the ventilator.

When the RATE is set to SPONTANEOUS, there is no set mandatory breath rate. All spontaneous breaths are pressure-triggered, pressure-limited, and pressure-cycled. The ventilator provides inspiratory flow when the patient generates sufficient pressure to open the demand valve (-1 to -2 cm H_2O). Inspiration ends when the circuit pressure rises above the required pressure to maintain an open demand valve. This setting in spontaneous ventilation can act as CPAP, or rather as EPAP (expiratory airway pressure), when an external PEEP valve is added to the expiratory valve outlet. The MAX does not have an internal mechanism for PEEP compensation. Any additional rise in baseline pressure will require the patient to generate a negative pressure of -1 to -2 plus the additional baseline pressure. If high PEEP levels are used, this could increase the patient's work of breathing (Box 12-6).

During ventilation, mandatory breaths are delivered minimally at the rate set on the rate control.

When the MAX is used in the IMV mode, mandatory breaths are patient- or time-triggered, volume-targeted, and time-cycled. Adequate spontaneous inspiratory efforts that occur between the mandatory breaths are delivered as spontaneous breaths. (Note that if the patient is in the middle of a spontaneous inspiration and the ventilator determines it is time for another mandatory breath, the mandatory breath is delivered on top of the spontaneous breath.) The mandatory breaths are not synchronized with the patient's spontaneous efforts. If breaths are not synchronous and breath stacking ensues, the operator can increase the mandatory breath rate to override the spontaneous rate and reduce the chance of any additional breath stacking.

BOX 12-6

Decision Making & Problem Solving

A patient is being transported with the MAX ventilator. The rate is set at 10 breaths/min, and the V_T is at 500 mL. An expiratory CPAP valve has been added to the exhalation valve outlet; the CPAP is set at 7 cm H_2O. The respiratory therapist observes the pressure manometer and notices that the pressure drops to -1 to -2 cm H_2O at the beginning of inspiration, peaks at 25 cm H_2O, and then goes to 7 cm H_2O during exhalation. What accounts for the observed pressure changes, and what can be done to correct them?

See Appendix A for the answers.

Oxygen Source

Because the MAX operates from a high-pressure gas source, oxygen delivery depends on the gas powering the ventilator. When oxygen is the source gas, FiO_2 is 1.0. When air is used, it is 0.21. To provide variable oxygen concentrations, connect the unit to an air/oxygen blender.

DRÄGER MICROVENT

The Dräger Microvent (Figure 12-5) is a time- or patient-triggered, volume-targeted ventilator primarily used for transporting adult patients. It may also be used on pediatric patients weighing over 33 lb. The Microvent can function in four modes: control, A/C, SIMV, PSV, and CPAP. It is lightweight (9.5 lb) and portable (8.5″ × 4.7″ × 8.1″).

Power Source

The Dräger Microvent requires an electrical and a pneumatic power source to properly operate. The electronic system can use the following three separate power sources:

- An AC outlet
- An external, 12-volt battery
- An internal, rechargeable or non-rechargeable battery

The internal battery has a lifespan of about 2 hours when fully charged and requires about 5 hours for recharging. When approximately 10 minutes of operating time is left, the message "charge NiCd" is illuminated in the display window. When the ventilator is connected to one of the two external power sources, the green POWER CONNECTED status light goes on and the internal battery pack begins charging. This occurs regardless of whether the ventilator is on or off. The internal battery is essential to the operation of the machine; without it the ventilator cannot function.

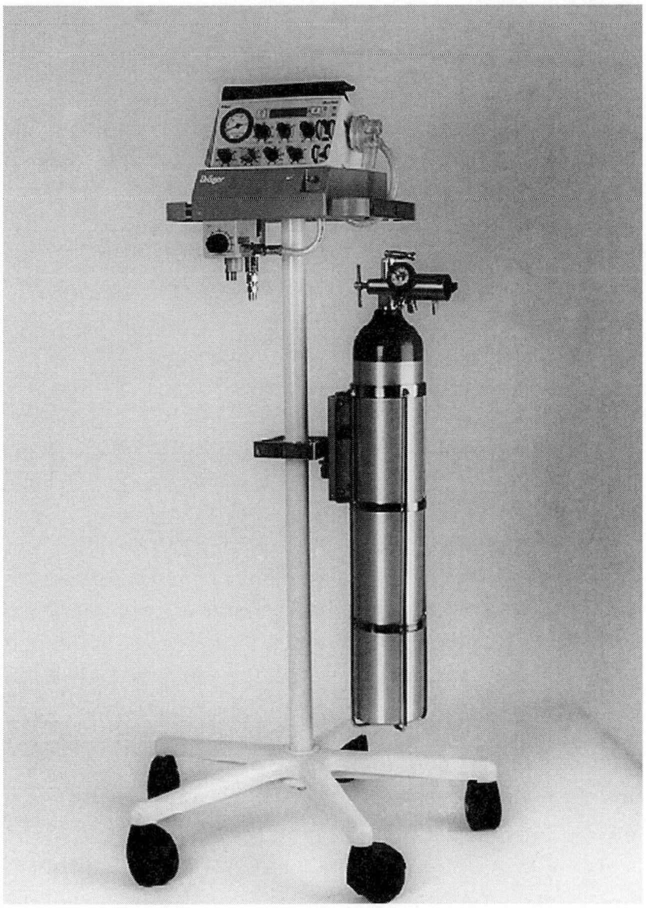

Figure 12-5 The Dräger Microvent Ventilator. (Courtesy Dräger, Inc., Telford, Pa.)

The pneumatic component requires medical-grade gas at 38 to 84 psi. The source may be a cylinder, wall outlet, or oxygen/air mixer, as long as it contains a DISS connector. The ventilator consumes 1 L/min of gas for its pneumatic functions. When estimating the longevity of an oxygen cylinder during transport, do not forget to add this factor to your calculations (Box 12-7).

Internal Mechanisms

The source gas enters through the inlet filter at the rear of the machine (Figure 12-6) and is immediately reduced to a constant working pressure. From the regulator, flow is diverted to the PEEP and exhalation valves to be primed and also to the inspiratory/expiratory (I/E) valve. The source gas is then routed to the electronically controlled pressure regulator, which governs the rate and pattern of gas flow to the patient. From the pressure regulator, gas passes a one-way check valve and is then sent to the patient circuit. A flow sensor at the wye connector of the patient circuit monitors inspiratory and expiratory minute ventilation and patient airway pressures.

The Microvent provides a continuous, 10-L/min flow of gas through the patient circuit (bias flow). This flow is provided by the demand valve and is intended to help reduce the patient's work of breathing for spontaneously triggered breaths. If the patient requires a flow above 10 L/min, the demand valve can provide flows up to 120 L/min. If the gas supplies fail, ambient air can be drawn in through an antisuffocation valve.

BOX 12-7

Calculation of Cylinder Duration for the Microvent

For the estimated cylinder duration for the Microvent in the control mode, use the following formula:

$$\text{Expected time of operation} = \frac{\text{pressure of gas supply (liters)}}{\text{minute ventilation} + 1 \text{ (liters/min)}}$$

Pressure of gas supply = tank pressure × conversion factor

For example:

2200 psi = tank pressure
0.28 = conversion factor for an E cylinder
pressure of gas supply = (2200 psi) (0.28) = 622 L

The reason that 1 is added to the minute ventilation is to account for the consumption of 1 L of gas/min. Suppose an E cylinder has a pressure reading of 1800 psi. The patient is breathing 10 times per minute at a set V_T of 0.5 L. How long will is take for the tank to be completely empty?

volume of gas supply = (1800 psi)(0.28) = 504 L
minute ventilation = rate × VT
= (10 breaths/min)(0.5 L) = 5 L

$$\text{expected time of operation} = \frac{504 \text{ L}}{(5 + 1) \text{ liters/minute}}$$
= 84 min

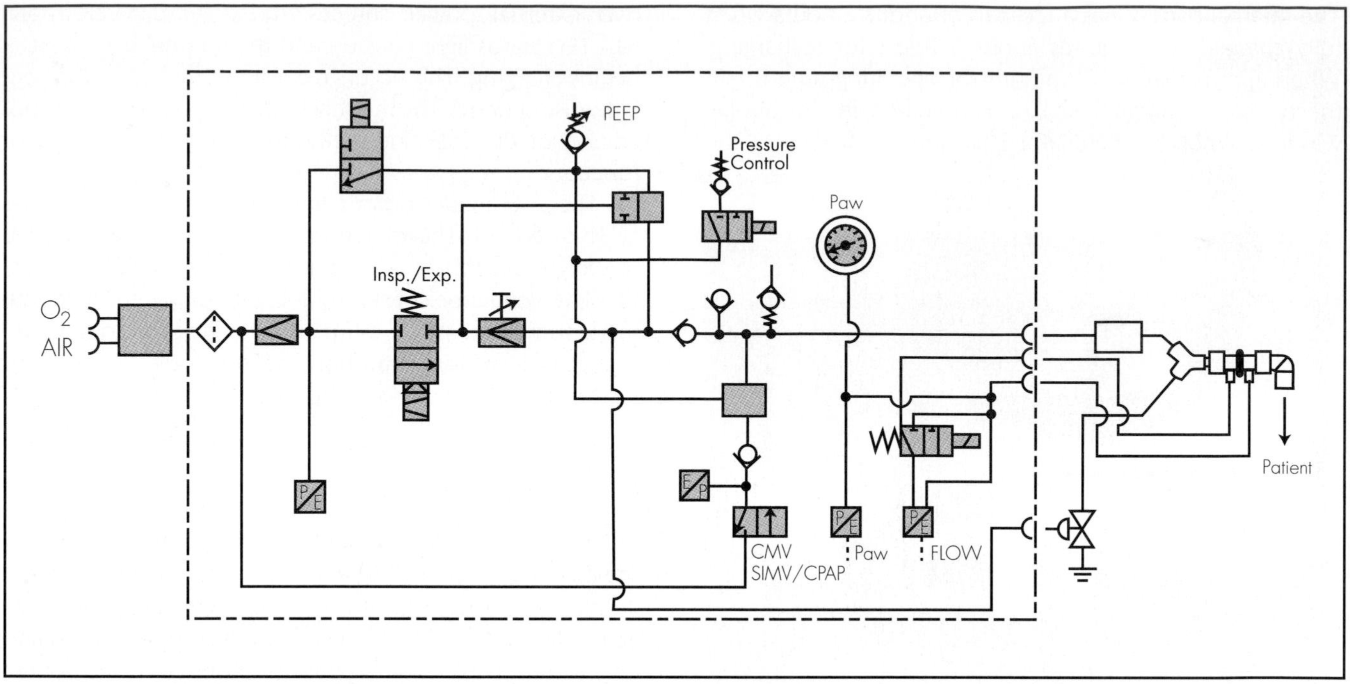

Figure 12-6 A Microvent flow diagram. (Courtesy Dräger, Inc., Telford, Pa.)

Controls

The front panel of the Microvent is easy to operate and contains a pressure monitor, liquid crystal display (LCD), alarm controls and indicators, and the basic unit controls (Figure 12-7).

Pressure Gauge

The pressure manometer is on the top left part of the control panel and continuously monitors airway pressure (10 to 80 cm H_2O).

Liquid Crystal Display

An LCD at the top center part of the front panel shows the measured parameters, alarms, and advisory messages that are monitored and detected by the unit.

The pressure gauge, which is on the top left part of the front control panel provides continuous measurements of airway pressure in centimeters of water.

The three controls in the middle-front of the panel are the VENTILATOR RATE, V_T, and T_I. The respiratory rate is active in control, A/C, and SIMV modes. The knob setting is to the left of the three controls. It maintains the set number of mandatory breaths in the control mode, the minimum number of mandatory breaths in the A/C mode, and the maximum number in SIMV. The adjustable range is 0 to 60 breaths/min.

The V_T control is in the middle of the three controls and regulates the volume delivered to the patient during each mandatory breath. It has an adjustable range of 100 to 1500 mL.

The T_I control is on the far right of the three controls and regulates the length of time spent in inspiration. It has an adjustable range of 0.2 to 3 seconds. The V_T combined with the T_I are responsible for the delivered flow on mandatory breaths.

Pressure Support and PEEP

The PRESSURE SUPPORT and PEEP parameters are just below the previously discussed controls. The PRESSURE SUPPORT control is on the left of the two function knobs and has an operational range of 0 to 35 cm H_2O. It only functions during spontaneous breaths and must be set higher than the CPAP/PEEP level or it will not function. The level of pressure support provided to the patient during each breath is determined by the difference between the pressure support and the PEEP settings (Box 12-8).

The PEEP/CPAP control, which is on the lower-right part of the control panel has an operational range of 0 to 18 cm H_2O and functions in all modes of ventilation. To use the CPAP mode, the operator must place the mode selector in SIMV and turn the rate to setting to "0" breaths/min.

Alarms

The Microvent can monitor several parameters and alert the operator to fluctuations that exceed set values (Box 12-9).

High Peak Pressure Alarm and Pmax

The PMAX control is on the bottom left of the front panel and limits upper airway pressure (20 to 80 cm H_2O).

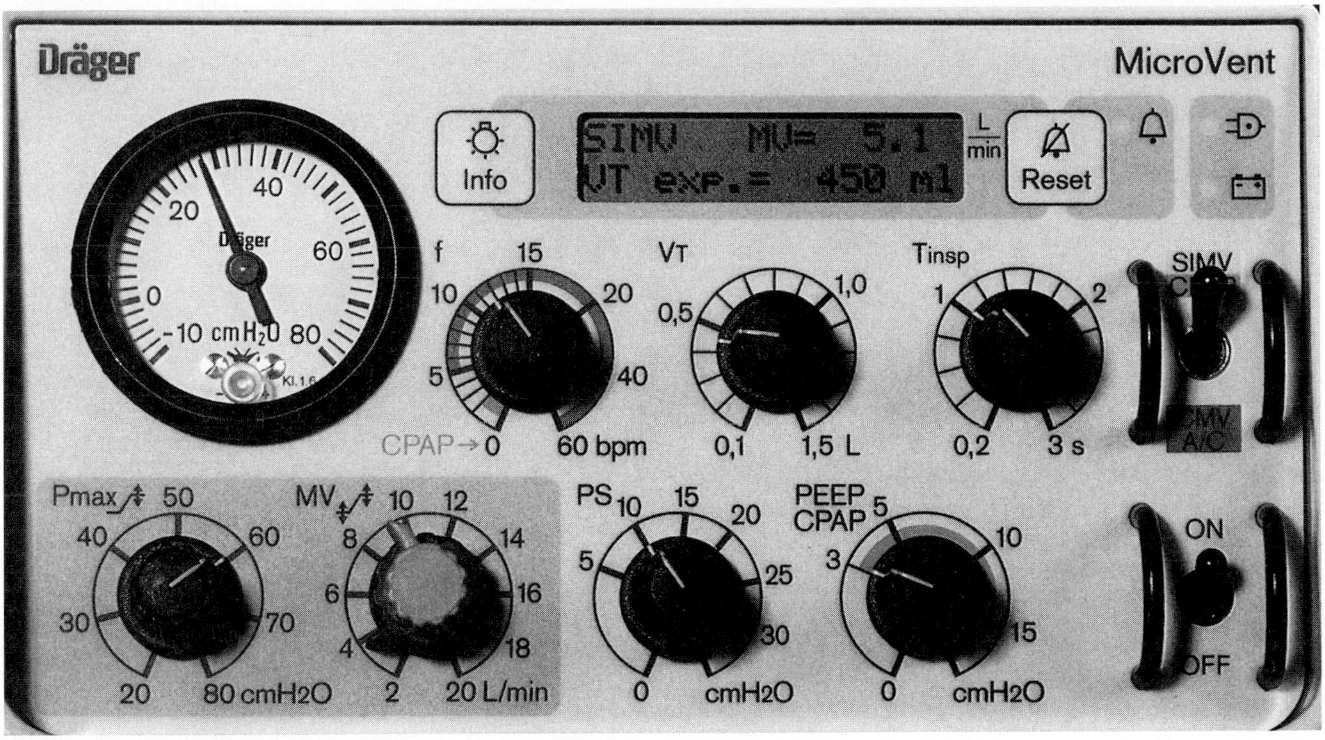

Figure 12-7 The Microvent control panel. (Courtesy Dräger, Inc., Telford, Pa.)

BOX 12-8

Decision Making & Problem Solving

In the CPAP mode, the PEEP is set at 5 cm H_2O, and the pressure support is at 15 cm H_2O. What is the actual amount of pressure support that the patient receives with each spontaneous breath?

See Appendix A for the answer.

BOX 12-9

Microvent Alarms

- High peak pressure (Pmax)
- Low airway pressure
- High PEEP
- Apnea
- High and low minute ventilation
- Power system alarms (O_2 pressure low, power failure, charge NiCd)

When circuit pressure exceeds the set Pmax level, the HIGH PEAK PRESSURE alarm (audio/visual) is activated. The I/E solenoid valve closes, which stops inspiration and allows the remainder of the breath to be vented to room air.

Low Airway Pressure and High PEEP Alarms

The LOW AIRWAY PRESSURE and HIGH PEEP alarms (audio/visual) are set by the manufacturer and alert the operator when violated. The LOW AIRWAY PRESSURE alarm is activated when the pressure in the patient circuit fails to reach 5 cm H_2O within 15 seconds of the previous mandatory breath. The HIGH PEEP alarm is activated when airway pressure fails to drop below 22 cm H_2O during exhalation.

Apnea Alarm

The apnea alarm is only functional during CPAP (SIMV rate = 0 breaths/min). When the patient fails to make a sufficient effort to trigger the ventilator within 15 seconds, the alarm is activated. It does not have an adjustable range.

High and Low Minute Ventilation Alarms

HIGH and LOW MINUTE VENTILATION settings are adjustable from 2 to 20 L/min and alert the operator when the patient exceeds the set parameters.

Power System Alarms

The power system alarms include O_2 PRESSURE LOW, POWER FAILURE, and CHARGE NICD. The O_2 PRESSURE LOW alarm activates when the gas inlet pressure falls below 22 psi, indicating that the gas source is not providing enough pressure to the ventilator for proper function. The POWER FAILURE and CHARGE NICD alarms are activated when the external power supply fails or the internal battery has less than 10 minutes of operational power left.

Reset Button

The RESET button at the top right part of the front panel can be used to silence alarms for 2 minutes when pressed.

Modes of Operation

The Microvent offers the following modes of ventilation:

- CMV
- A/C
- SIMV
- CPAP
- PSV

In CMV, rate, V_T, and T_I are all active, offering time-triggered, volume-targeted, and time-cycled breaths. All breaths are ventilator-controlled.

When in the A/C mode, the mode selector switch remains in CMV. To access the A/C function, the operator must press the INFO key until the display message reads "CMV–A/C." In this mode, rate, V_T, and T_I are all functioning. The A/C mode allows mandatory breaths to be patient-triggered (flow), and there is no adjustable sensitivity control to set. The ventilator responds to a 4 L/min decrease in baseline flow to trigger a mandatory breath.

When the Microvent is in the SIMV mode, mandatory breath delivery is the same as that in A/C with one exception. In A/C, every patient effort that exceeds the trigger sensitivity level (4 L/min) results in a mandatory breath. In SIMV, the mandatory breath rate is limited to the RATE control setting. An asterisk appears in the display window with the delivery of every triggered mandatory breath. The patient may breathe spontaneously between these breaths.

To use CPAP on the Microvent, the mode indicator remains in the SIMV setting, but the rate is adjusted to "0." When in CPAP, all breaths are spontaneous, requiring the patient to generate a -1 cm H_2O pressure to trigger the ventilator. (Note that mandatory breaths are flow-triggered, and spontaneous breaths are pressure-triggered.) PEEP and PRESSURE SUPPORT are active controls in CPAP. The pressure support setting must always be greater than PEEP to operate. If there is an apneic period ($>$15 seconds), the ventilator initiates a backup rate of 8 breaths/min at the set V_T and T_I. It is important to set these controls even when the rate is set to 0 because of their use in an apneic event.

Oxygen Source

The Microvent operates from two gas sources, therefore the oxygen percentage depends upon the FiO_2 setting on the external blender. (To ensure accurate FiO_2s, monitor the circuit with an oxygen analyzer.) There is no entrainment feature.

DRÄGER OXYLOG 2000

The Oxylog 2000 (Figure 12-8) is a time- or patient-triggered, volume-targeted ventilator used primarily for emergencies and transporting adult or pediatric patients weighing at least 33 lb. The Oxylog can function in three modes: control, SIMV, and CPAP. It is lightweight (9.5 lb) and portable (8.5″ × 4.7″ × 8.1″).

Power Source

The Dräger Oxylog requires an electrical and a pneumatic source to properly function. The electronic system can use the following three separate power sources:

- An AC outlet
- An external 12-volt battery
- An internal rechargeable or non-rechargeable battery

When the ventilator is connected to one of the two external power sources, the green POWER CONNECTED status light goes on and the internal battery pack starts charging—regardless of whether the ventilator is on or off. The internal battery is essential to the operations of the machine. It has a functional lifespan of about 6 hours when fully charged and requires about 8 hours to recharge to maximum capacity. When approximately 10 minutes of operation are left, a message in the display window reads: "Charge NiCd."

The pneumatic component requires a high-pressure medical-grade gas (oxygen or air) supplied in a range of 38 to 84 psi. The source may be a cylinder, wall outlet, or oxygen/air blender with a DISS connector. The internal

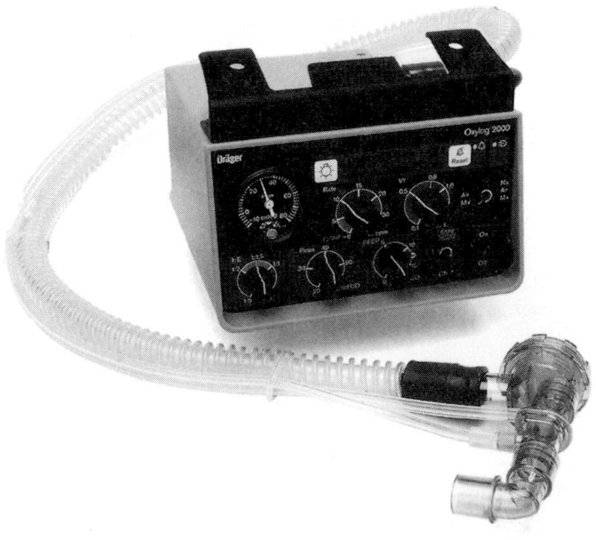

Figure 12-8 The Dräger Oxylog 2000 Ventilator. (Courtesy Dräger, Inc., Telford, Pa.)

> **BOX 12-10**
>
> ### The Oxylog 2000 Air/Mix Injector
>
> When the AIR/MIX switch is on, the gas source passes through the internal injector, which draws ambient air from the room to dilute the mixture to 60%. This conserves gas use by 50% and allows for prolonged transport when a limited source gas is used.

pneumatic components of the ventilator consume 1 L/min of gas to support their functions. It is necessary to include this factor in the calculation for cylinder duration. The Oxylog is also equipped with an oxygen-conserving device, an air/mix injector (Box 12-10).

Internal Mechanisms

The gas source enters through the inlet port at the rear of the machine (Figure 12-9) and is immediately filtered and reduced to a constant working pressure by a regulator. From the regulator, the flow is diverted to the PEEP and exhalation valves to be primed and then to the inspiratory/expiratory (I/E) valve. The I/E valve regulates the release of inspiratory flow in a time-cycled fashion. Next, the gas source passes an electronically controlled pressure regulator, which governs the rate and pattern of flow before it passes through one of the following two valves:

- A pneumatic control valve that supplies the patient with a 100% gas source.
- An injector that supplies the patient with a 60% gas source.

The route is determined by the position of the AIR/MIX switch (see Box 12-10). After its route through the pneumatic valve or the injector, the gas flows to the patient circuit.

To initiate a spontaneous breath, the patient must open the demand valve by generating a minimum pressure change of -1 cm H_2O. During a spontaneous breath, gas from the demand valve bypasses the injector that is regulated by the AIR/MIX switch. As a result, all spontaneous breaths are provided at 100% source gas. The maximum flow for a spontaneous breath is 120 L/min.

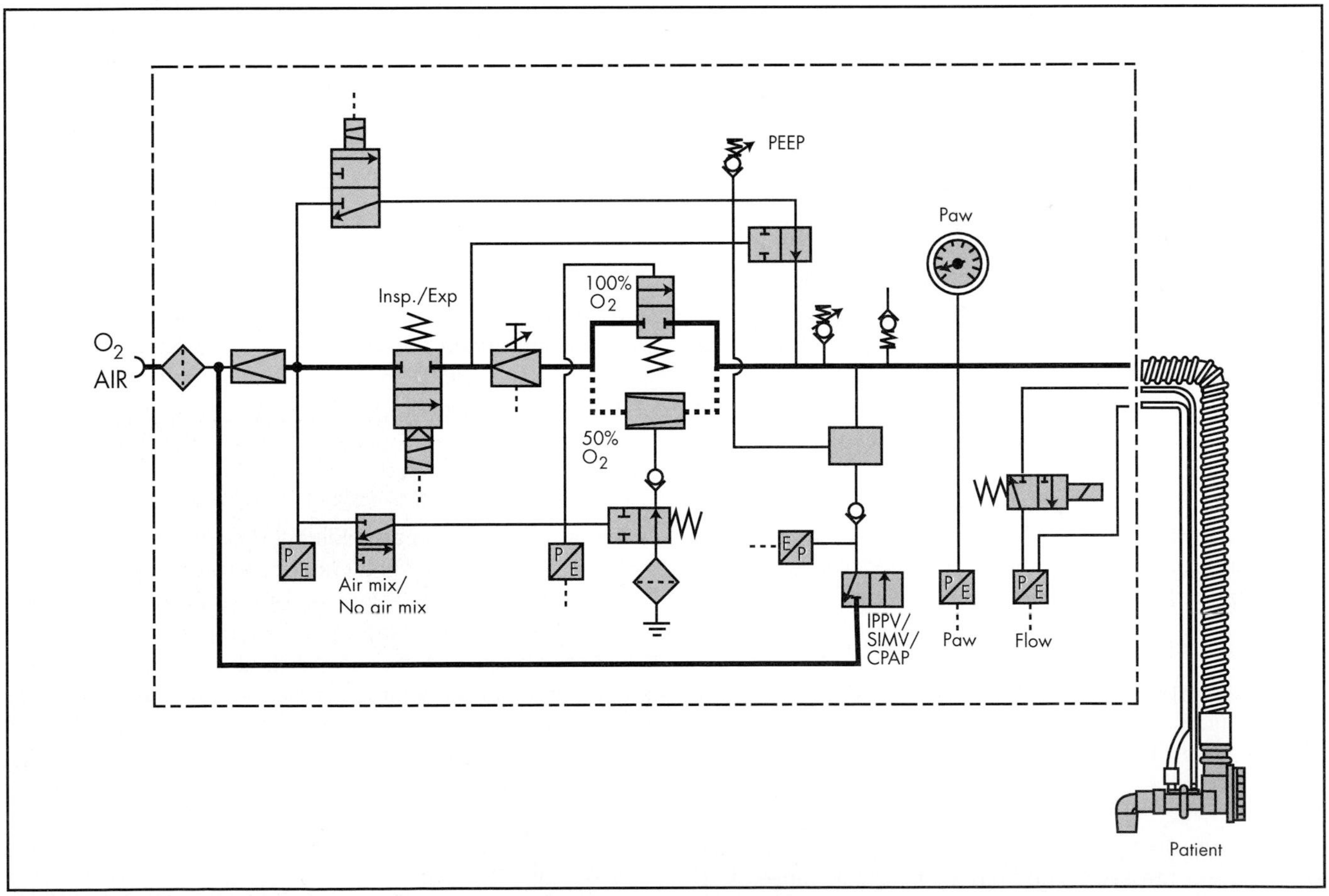

Figure 12-9 An Oxylog 2000 flow diagram. (Courtesy Dräger, Inc., Telford, Pa.)

TABLE 12-1

The Oxylog 2000 color-coded settings

	Range (kg)	Minute ventilation	Ventilator rate
Green (infants)	10 to 20 kg	0.1 to 0.3 L	30 to 40 breaths/min
Blue (children)	20 to 40 kg	0.3 to 0.8 L	20 to 30 breaths/min
Brown (adults)	above 40 kg	0.8 to 1.5 L	5 to 20 breaths/min

Courtesy Dräger, Inc., Telford, Pa.

Controls and Alarms

The controls and alarms on the Oxylog 2000 are simple and easy to operate.

Pressure Monitoring Gauge

The pressure gauge is on the top left part of the control panel and provides continuous measurements of airway pressure in centimeters of water.

Control Parameters

The control parameters include the following: V_T, rate, I:E ratio, and PEEP. The V_T knob, which is in the middle of the control panel, regulates the volume delivered to the patient during each mandatory breath (100 to 1500 mL). The V_T is also color-coded for quick setting (see the discussion of additional features in this section or Table 12-1 for a complete explanation).

The RATE control knob is to the left of the volume setting and functions to regulate the set number of mandatory breaths in the control mode and the minimum number of mandatory breaths in SIMV. The ventilator has an adjustable range of 5 to 60 breaths/min in the control and SIMV modes. When the MODE selector is placed in SIMV and the rate is less than 5 breaths/min, the ventilator switches to CPAP.

The I:E control knob is at the bottom-left of the control panel and has an operational range of 1:3 to 2:1 ± 5%. The Oxylog allows for IRV in the control mode, which is not a common feature for transport ventilators. In the SIMV mode, the I:E ratio is determined by the rate setting (see Table 12-2 for complete details).

The PEEP control is located on the lower middle part of the control panel and has an operational range of 0 to 15 cm H_2O. The PEEP control is functional in all modes.

Alarms and Alarm Reset

The Oxylog provides HIGH and LOW AIRWAY PRESSURE alarms, HIGH and LOW MINUTE VENTILATION alarms, and POWER SOURCE alarms.

High-Pressure Alarm

The high-pressure alarm labeled PMAX is on the lower left part of the control panel and has an adjustable range of 20 to 60 cm H_2O. When airway pressures exceed the PMAX setting, a red ALARM status light starts blinking and an intermittent audible alarm is triggered. Simultaneously, the inspiratory flow stops, and the exhalation valve opens. When the problem is corrected, the audible alarm is silenced, but the visual display must be manually reset with the ALARM RESET button at the top right of the control panel. The ALARM RESET can also be used to silence audible alarms for 2 minutes. If the problem is corrected, the RESET button clears the display screen.

TABLE 12-2

I:E Ratio in the SIMV Mode for the Oxylog 2000

Frequency setting	Effect
0	No ventilator breaths (CPAP)
5 to 12 breaths/min	Fixed T_I (2 seconds)
12 to 40 breaths/min	Fixed T_I (1:1.5)
	I:E = 1:1.5 seconds

Courtesy Dräger, Inc., Telford, Pa.

Low-Pressure Alarms

The LOW-PRESSURE alarm does not have a control knob. It is activated when the pressure in the patient circuit does not reach at least 10 cm H_2O pressure in 20 seconds after the previous mandatory breath. An audio/visual alarm is activated that is not functional in the CPAP mode.

High and Low Minute Ventilation Alarms

Minute ventilation is an additional parameter that is monitored by the Oxylog. The Oxylog monitors expired minute ventilation through the flow sensor near the expiratory valve and ensures that the patient is being properly ventilated. The current reading is shown in the display window. A fluctuation outside of set parameters may activate the audio/visual alarm. If the expiratory minute volume falls below 40% of the inspiratory minute volume, the alarm activates. Hosing and connections should be checked for any possible problems because a leak is suggested.

Apnea Alarm

The APNEA alarm is only functional in the CPAP mode. When the patient does not make sufficient effort to open the demand valve within 15 seconds, an audio/visual alarm is activated.

Power System

The pneumatic system has an O_2 PRESSURE LOW alarm that is activated when the gas inlet pressure falls below 28 psi. This indicates that the gas source is not providing sufficient pressure for proper ventilator function. The electronic system has a POWER FAILURE and a CHARGE NICD alarm that are activated when the external power supply fails or the internal battery has less than 10 minutes of power left.

Modes of Ventilation

The Dräger Oxylog offers control, SIMV, and CPAP modes. In the control mode, the ventilator requires that the V_T, rate, and I:E ratio be set. The unit is then time-triggered. To trigger a mandatory breath, the machine requires the patient to initiate a 4-L/min change in flow. To trigger gas flow for spontaneous breaths in the SIMV mode, the patient must generate a pressure change of -2 cm H_2O below baseline to open the demand valve. As in the control mode, V_T and rate are set and active in SIMV, but the I:E ratio is not; it is determined by the rate setting (see Table 12-2).

The third option of ventilation is CPAP. In CPAP, only the PEEP control is set. To trigger flow delivery in this mode, the patient must be able to generate a pressure change of -2 cm H_2O below baseline. The air/mix switch is nonfunctional because all breaths come from the demand valve, which bypasses the air/mix injector.

Oxygen Source

The Oxylog operates from a 100% gas source. The FIO_2 is not only dependent on the gas source being used, but also on the AIR/MIX switch and the mode selected for use. The AIR/MIX switch allows the operator to choose from 1.0 to 0.60 FIO_2 when oxygen is the gas source. The air/mix function is only operational for mandatory breaths. All spontaneous breaths receive 100% of the source gas. Attaching a gas blender to regulate FIO_2 gives the operator more control over oxygen delivery.

NEWPORT MEDICAL INSTRUMENTS E100I

The Newport E100I (Figure 12-10) is a pressure- or time-triggered, volume- or pressure-targeted, and time-cycled ventilator that is gas powered and electronically controlled. It is used for infant, pediatric, and adult patients and can operate in A/C, SIMV, and spontaneous modes. The E100i is lightweight (13 lb) and portable (10.5″ × 9.5″ × 6.5″).

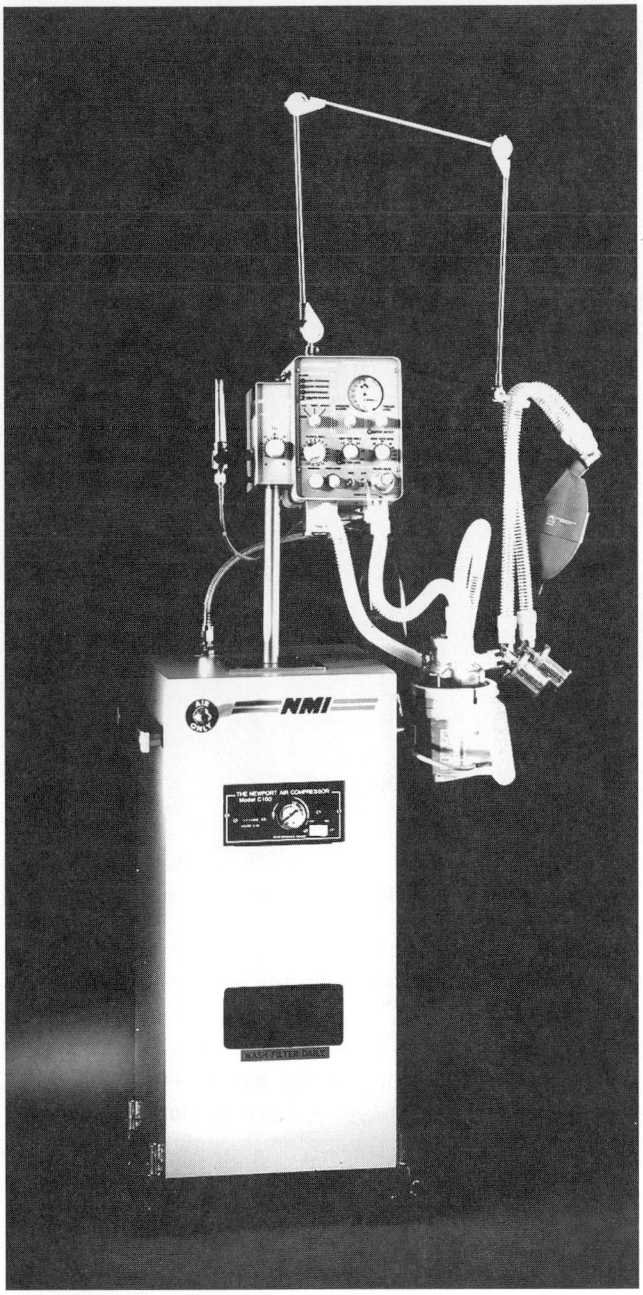

Figure 12-10 **A,** the Newport E100i (Courtesy Newport Medical Instruments, Inc., Newport Beach, Calif.)

Power Source

The E100i requires both an electrical and a pneumatic power source to properly function. The electronic system requires AC power (110 or 220 volts) or power supplied by the external back-up battery. The back-up battery can operate for about 4 hours and can be used in times of transport or power failure. The battery pack is recharged when the ventilator is powered by AC—regardless of whether the power is on or off.

The pneumatic system requires two medical-grade gases supplied to an air/oxygen mixer at 35 to 90 psi (50

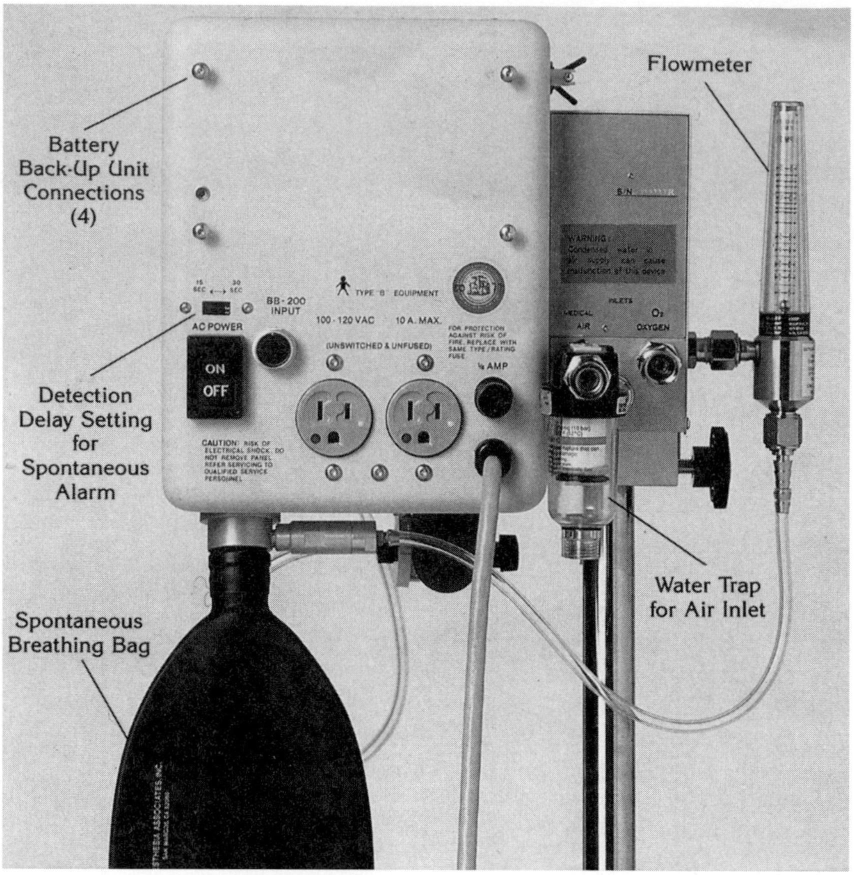

Figure 12-10 (continued) **B,** rear ventilator panel. (Courtesy Newport Medical Instruments, Inc., Newport Beach, Calif.)

psi is nominal). The air and oxygen sources may be a cylinder or wall outlet. If one source gas runs out before the other, an automatic crossover valve in the air/oxygen mixer allows the ventilator to continue operating on the remaining source gas. If this occurs, the FiO_2 may be altered.

Internal Mechanisms

The source gases entering the air/oxygen mixer (Figure 12-11) are immediately reduced to a working pressure of 28 psi. The route of the mixed gas for mandatory breaths starts at the opening of an electronically controlled solenoid valve. This valve opens based on the set respiratory rate and closes after the set T_I on the front panel. The pressure in the line during inspiration when the solenoid valve is open then opens the pneumatic "Humphrey interface" valve, which supplies gas to the main flow control. The main flow controller regulates the flow delivered to the patient circuit.

The amount of flow delivered through the patient circuit for spontaneous breathing is determined by the position of the CONSTANT FLOW switch and the auxiliary flowmeter setting. When switched on, the CONSTANT FLOW switch delivers 9 to 12 L/min to the reservoir bag and into the patient breathing circuit between mandatory or manual breaths. The auxiliary flowmeter attached to the air/oxygen mixer can be used in place of the continuous flow control or as a supplement to provide flows above 12 L/min to the patient. The reservoir bag should be used to ensure proper adjustment of flow from the flowmeter and continuous flow switch. This bag should not completely deflate at any time during periods of spontaneous breathing. (Note that using excessive flows during spontaneous breathing may contribute to an increase in expiratory resistance, and thereby increase the potential for auto-PEEP.)

If all electrical and pneumatic systems fail, the patient may draw ambient air into the breathing circuit through an emergency intake valve when no other flow is available. The patient effort required to open this valve is approximately -2.0 cm H_2O.

Controls

Exception for the APNEA ALARM DELAY switch, all of the Newport E100i ventilation alarm settings and visual alarm indicators are on the front panel (Figure 12-12).

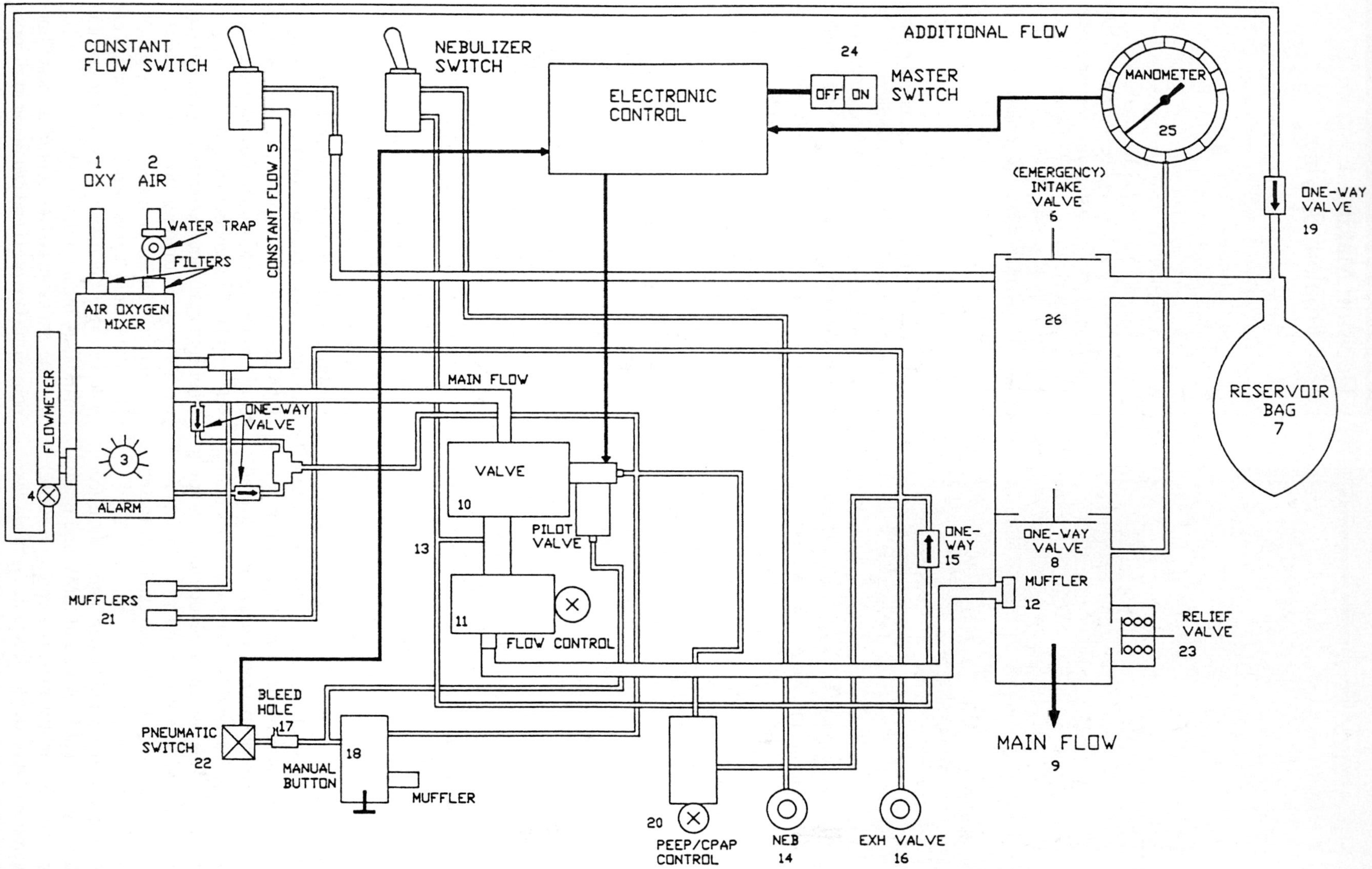

Figure 12-11 A pneumatic schematic of the Newport E100i. (Courtesy Newport Medical Instruments, Inc., Newport Beach, Calif.)

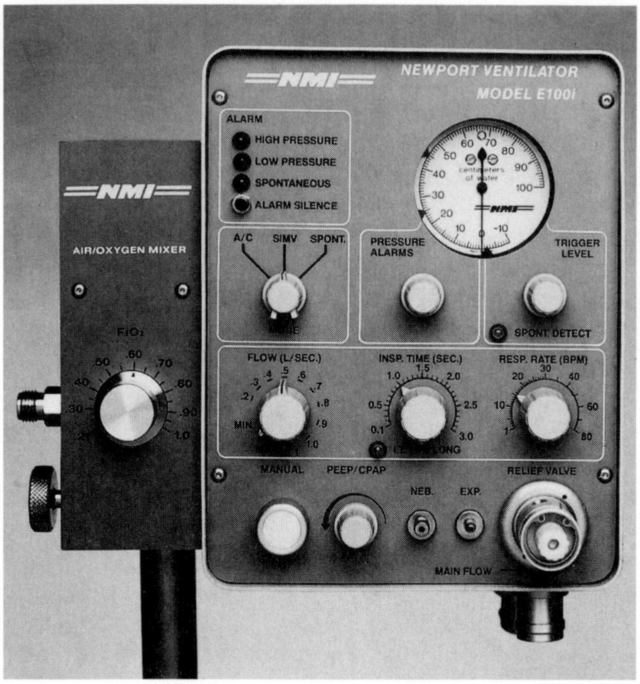

Figure 12-12 Newport E100i front control panel. (Courtesy Newport Medical Instruments, Inc., Newport Beach, Calif.)

BOX 12-11

Decision Making & Problem Solving

The respiratory therapist is ventilating a patient with a Newport E100i. The settings are: PEEP = 10 cm H_2O; mode = CPAP (spontaneous); FiO_2 = 0.40; sensitivity = +1 cm H_2O. The spontaneous alarm is sounding continuously. The respiratory therapist recognizes the alarm and assesses the patient for spontaneous breaths. The therapist counts 12 chest rises within 1 minute, but the alarm is still sounding, and notices that the pressure manometer drops to +6 cm H_2O with each inspiratory breath. What may be a possible solution?

See Appendix A for the answer.

Control Parameters

The primary controls are MANDATORY FLOW, T_I, RESPIRATORY RATE, PEEP/CPAP, and TRIGGER SENSITIVITY. When the E100i is set up to deliver volume-targeted mandatory breaths, V_T is determined by the mandatory flow and the T_I setting (V_T = flow [L/sec] × T_I [sec]). Mandatory flow is adjustable from 0.1 to 1.6 L/second (3 to 100 L/min) with the control knob on the left side of the face panel. The MANDATORY FLOW control is a needle valve that lets the operator meter mixed-gas delivery during mandatory breaths.

The T_I control for mandatory breaths is adjustable from 0.1 to 3.0 seconds and located in the middle of the E100i face panel. The T_I setting determines the length of time the mandatory flow is delivered during every time- or pressure-triggered mandatory breath in A/C or SIMV. The Newport E100i does not allow for inverse I:E ratios. If the T_I and rate settings result in an inverse I:E ratio, a visual alarm ("IT too long") notifies the operator of the problem. T_I is then limited to 1:1, and the mandatory flow and rate are delivered as set. The mandatory delivered V_T, however, is less than the mandatory set V_T. This discrepancy is due to the T_I limitation set by the I:E parameters of the machine. To reestablish the desired V_T, the mandatory flow can be increased or the T_I can be reduced.

The RATE control is on the middle right part of the E100i face panel. It is operational in A/C and SIMV and is adjustable from 1 to 120 breaths/min. This control regulates the time-triggered activation of the electronic solenoid valve (see the discussion of internal mechanisms in this section).

The PEEP/CPAP control regulates the internal PEEP valve on the Newport E100i and allows for an adjustable range of 0 to 25 cm H_2O in all modes. When PEEP is used during transport, a small amount of additional flow is required to maintain airway pressure, and this is considered when the operational time of the cylinder is assessed. In addition to the changes in cylinder duration, the trigger sensitivity should also be adjusted relative to the new baseline pressure so that the patient incurs no additional work of breathing.

The TRIGGER SENSITIVITY control in the top right corner of the face panel determines the pressure change required to trigger a mandatory breath. It must always be set lower than baseline pressure to prevent autotriggering and must also be set for breath detection in CPAP (Box 12-11).

Additional Controls

The additional E100i controls include the MANUAL INFLATION button, the pressure-relief valve, and the CONSTANT FLOW switch. The MANUAL BREATH control is pneumatically controlled and can therefore be used if there is an electric power failure. This control bypasses the electronic solenoid valve (see the discussion of internal mechanisms) and delivers the set flow and FiO_2 for as long as the button is pressed. The set limit of the pressure-relief valve prevents overinflation and limits the flow delivered to the patient. The ventilator continues to deliver flow when the pressure-relief setting is met, however, delivered flow that would cause the pressure to rise above the pressure-relief setting is vented to ambient air instead of to the patient. The HIGH-PRESSURE alarm sounds when its setting is exceeded, but will *not* cause the breath to cycle into expiration when a mandatory breath is delivered.

The PRESSURE-RELIEF control is located at the bottom right of the face panel and can be set in all modes of ventilation to limit the maximum pressure in the patient circuit from

0 to 100 cm H_2O. Exceeding this value does not end inspiration, but vents excess flow from the patient circuit to room air (see the modes of ventilation section).

The CONSTANT FLOW switch on the left side of the ventilator delivers 9 to 12 L/min of mixed gas flow to the patient circuit between mandatory breaths.

Alarms

The front panel of the Newport E100i has a visual alarms section that alerts the operator to HIGH- and LOW-PRESSURE alarm violations and periods of patient apnea (SPONTANEOUS alarm). All of the visual alarms are accompanied by audible alarms. The HIGH-PRESSURE alarm is active in all modes. When the pressure setting (0 to 100 cm H_2O) is reached, the inspiratory phase of a time- or pressure-triggered mandatory breath ends. This does *not* apply to manual inflation, however, because during a manual breath, the alarm is activated but the ventilator does not cycle into expiration. The LOW-PRESSURE alarm is only active in the A/C and SIMV modes. It is activated if the airway pressure does not exceed the LOW-PRESSURE alarm setting during a time- or pressure-triggered mandatory breath. The one knob used to set both the HIGH- and LOW-PRESSURE alarm settings is in the upper middle part of the face panel. The HIGH- and LOW-PRESSURE alarm settings are coupled together when the knob is rotated. To independently adjust the HIGH-PRESSURE alarm setting, the operator must pull out the control knob before rotating it.

The SPONTANEOUS alarm is only functional in the spontaneous mode. It is activated when patient inspiratory efforts fail to lower airway pressure to the trigger sensitivity setting within 15 or 30 seconds. The operator controls the specific time period with a switch on the back panel. This alarm is designed to alert the operator of apneic episodes during spontaneous ventilation.

Additional Alarms

The E100i offers additional audible-only alarms, including AC and DC POWER FAILURE, AIR/O_2 LOW SOURCE GAS PRESSURE, and LOW BATTERY. The POWER FAILURE alarm is a continuous pulsating alarm that is activated when there is a loss of electric power. The AIR/O_2 LOW SOURCE GAS PRESSURE alarm is also a continuous alarm that is activated when the air or oxygen source gas pressure falls below 35 psi. The LOW BATTERY alarm is activated when about 20 minutes of normal battery back-up power are left. It is also a continuous alarm and is only terminated when the problem is resolved.

Modes of Ventilation

The Newport E100i offers A/C, SIMV, and spontaneous modes. In both A/C and SIMV, mandatory breaths may be volume- or pressure-targeted. When using volume-targeted A/C, the operator must set the trigger level, flow, T_I, and rate. Mandatory breaths are either time- or pressure-triggered, and the set V_T is determined by the flow and T_I settings.

When the E100i is in the volume-targeted SIMV mode, mandatory breath delivery is the same as that in A/C with one exception. In A/C, every patient effort that exceeds the trigger sensitivity level results in a mandatory breath. In SIMV, the mandatory breath rate is limited to the RATE control setting. The patient can breathe any additional breaths beyond the set rate from the mixed gas of the constant flow switch or auxiliary flowmeter. The spontaneous V_T completely depends on patient effort.

In the spontaneous mode (CPAP), no mandatory breaths are delivered. All spontaneous breaths depend on patient effort, and flow is provided by the CONSTANT FLOW switch and the auxiliary flowmeter. Although the patient is not required to trigger a spontaneous breath, it is important that the trigger level is set so that all spontaneous breaths are detected by the ventilator. If the E100i does not detect a patient inspiratory effort within the set apnea time, the SPONTANEOUS alarm is activated (see the discussion of alarms in this section for further detail). The delivered FiO_2 is determined by that set on the air/oxygen blender.

The E100i lets the operator pressure-target mandatory breaths in both A/C and SIMV, operating (in principle) similar to pressure control ventilation (see Chapter 9). When the parameters for pressure-limited ventilation are set, the PRESSURE-RELIEF control is set at the desired pressure limit, and the HIGH-PRESSURE alarm is fixed *above* that setting. This is important so that the HIGH-PRESSURE alarm setting does not end inspiration. After the pressure in the patient circuit reaches the PRESSURE-RELIEF control setting, the excess flow is vented to room air in order to maintain the set pressure limit (a plateau) until the T_I has expired. Changes in patient compliance or resistance can affect the V_T delivered.

Oxygen Source

The Newport E100i is equipped with an integral air/oxygen mixer that requires medical-grade oxygen and compressed air. It precisely regulates the delivered FiO_2 into the patient circuit for all mandatory breaths and inflations as well as for spontaneous breaths.

IMPACT UNI-VENT 750

The Uni-Vent 750 (Figure 12-13) is a pressure- or time-triggered, volume-targeted, pressure- or time-cycled microprocessor-controlled ventilator used primarily for transport. It is 9″ × 11.5″ × 4.5″ and weighs about 12.5 lb. This ventilator allows control, AIC, and SIMV modes to be used.

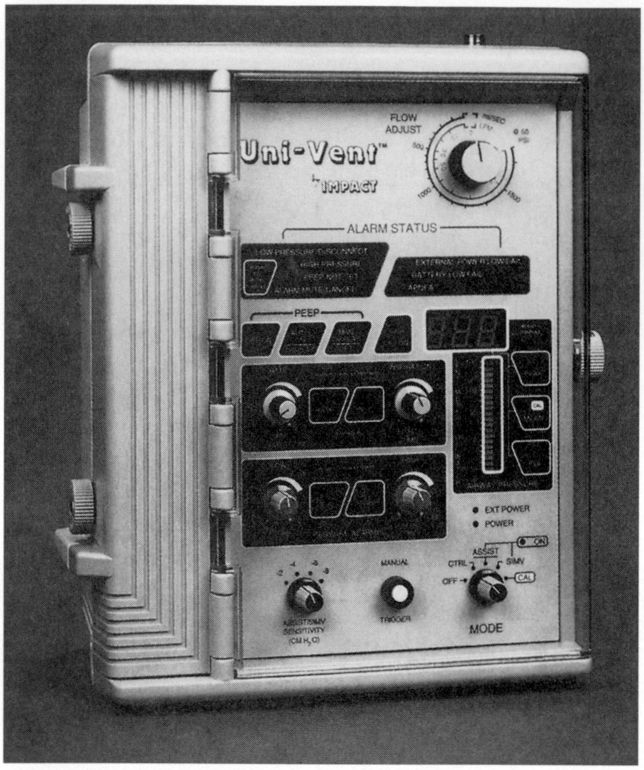

Figure 12-13 The Impact Uni-Vent 750 Ventilator. (Courtesy Impact Instrumentation, Inc., West Caldwell, NJ.)

Power Source

The Uni-Vent 750 requires dual energy supplies to properly perform. The electronic system requires one of the following three sources to power the microprocessor and its electrical components:

- An internal DC battery
- An external DC battery
- A 120-volt AC outlet (with a converter)

The internal battery has an estimated life of 9 hours. The pneumatic system requires a high-pressure source gas at 50 to 100 psi to properly perform. The source may be a cylinder, wall outlet, or oxygen/air blender.

Internal Mechanisms

The internal elements (Figure 12-14) of the pneumatic system receive the source gas from the oxygen inlet on the rear panel and route the gas through an internal regulator that precisely adjusts the pressure to 50 psi. After passing the regulator, the gas flow is guided through two parallel circuits. The first circuit, which contains two main inspiratory flow valves, is used during control and A/C modes. If one valve does not close when the machine cycles into expiration, the second valve stops gas flow to the patient and prevents overinflation. This is a safety feature of the system. During a patient- or time-triggered breath, the inspiratory flow solenoid opens and gas flow passes the flow-control valve and is directed to the patient. The Uni-Vent has no V_T setting. The volume delivered to the patient depends on the set T_I and flow.

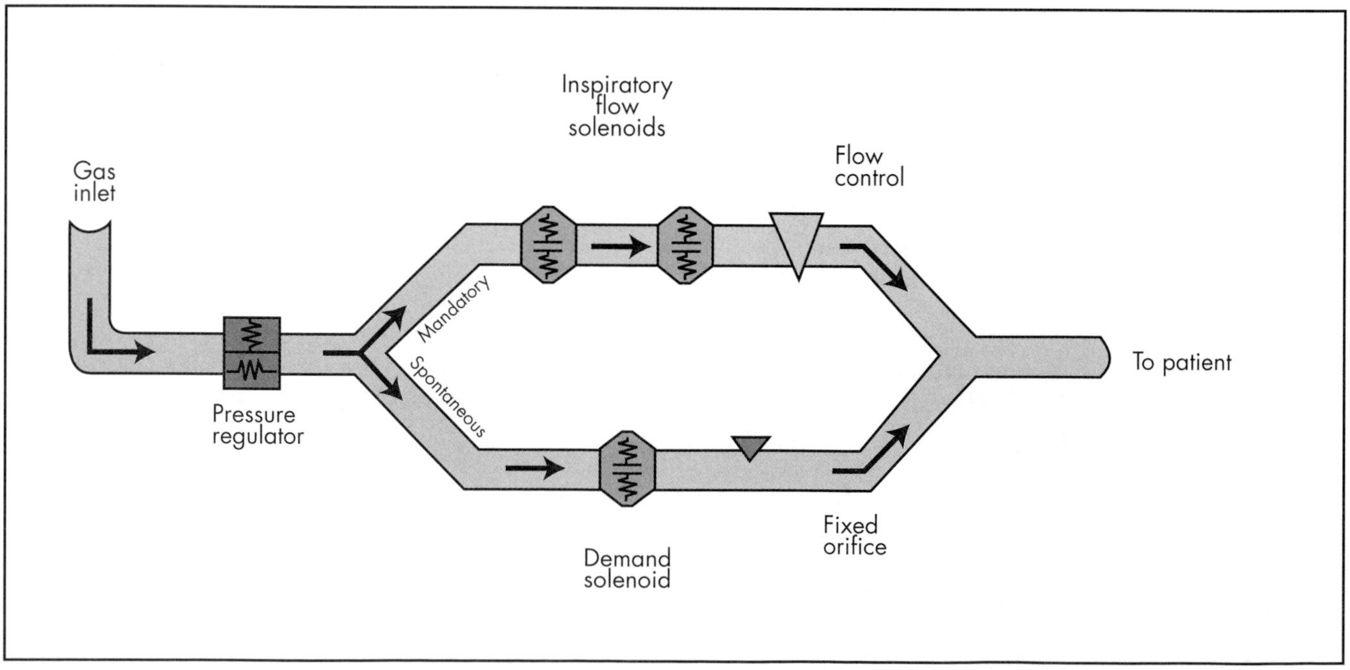

Figure 12-14 A Uni-Vent 750 flow diagram.

When spontaneous breaths are initiated, the flow through the system is directed to the pneumatically controlled demand valve. The demand valve has an opening pressure of -1 cm H_2O below baseline. Once the demand valve is opened, the gas source passes through a fixed orifice, which limits the peak flow to the patient to 60 L/min for spontaneous breaths.

When using disposable patient circuits, a separate anti-asphyxia valve must be attached at the patient connection to allow for spontaneous breaths in case of valve failure. The nondisposable circuits have a patient valve instead of an exhalation valve (Figure 12-15). The patient valves in the nondisposable units serve the purpose of the exhalation valve and also contain the anti-asphyxia valve.

The Uni-Vent 750 requires that an external PEEP valve is attached to the exhalation valve. The ventilator compensates for added PEEP with one of two mechanisms: automatic or manual. In the automatic mode, the microprocessor analyzes the patient circuit's pressure waveforms over three consecutive breaths to determine the level of PEEP. This process of updating the PEEP in the patient circuit is a continuous one. The manual process requires the operator to enter the PEEP value directly into the microprocessor using the keypad. When the operator chooses to use the manual method, the PEEP NOT SET ALARM is inactivated.

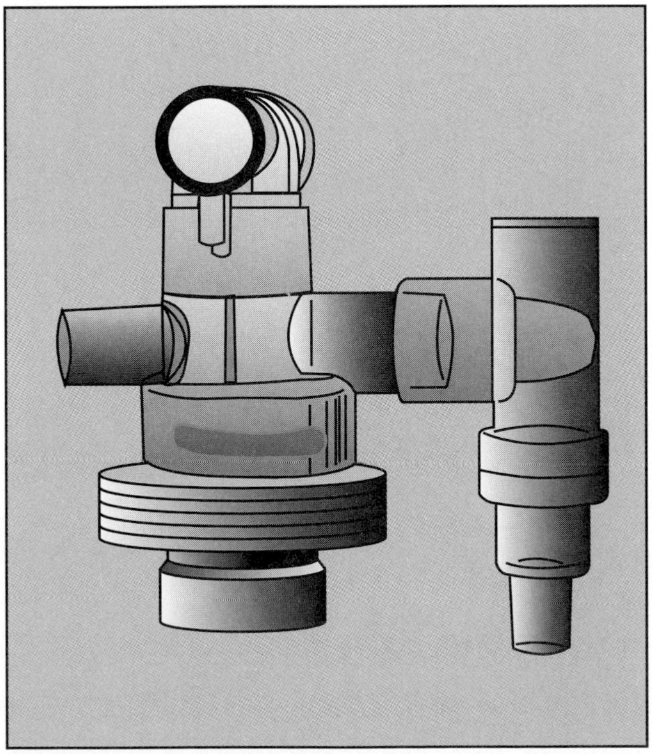

Figure 12-15 The Uni-Vent 750 patient valve. (Courtesy Impact Instrumentation, Inc., West Caldwell, NJ.)

Controls and Alarms

The Uni-Vent contains several controls for setting and monitoring parameters and alarms.

Rate

The respiratory RATE control is active in control, A/C, and SIMV modes of ventilation and time-triggers a mandatory breath in each of these modes. It has an adjustable range of 1 to 150 breaths/min. This function, in combination with T_I, controls the I:E ratio of the ventilator.

Flow Adjust

The FLOW ADJUST control allows for adjustable flow rates from 50 to 1500 mL/sec (3 to 90 L/min). If the flow setting is insufficient for the inspiratory demands of the patient, then the anti-asphyxiation valve allows for room air to be entrained for additional flow. When this occurs, the valve creates a whistling sound, alerting the operator to the problem. (Note that opening of the anti-asphyxiation valve and entrainment of room air can alter the FiO_2 delivered to the patient.)

Manual Breath

The MANUAL BREATH button can be used to deliver a positive-pressure breath whenever the operator deems fit and is operational in all modes. When activated, the ventilator delivers a breath at the set flow rate for as long as the operator holds the button. This control is designed to be operational if there is a CPU or electronics failure. The breath timer is reset after a full exhalation period elapses, therefore preventing the stacking of a time-delivered breath.

Airway Pressure Alarms

There are two airway pressure alarms on the 750 that can be adjusted and monitored. They are the HIGH-PRESSURE and the LOW-PRESSURE/DISCONNECT alarms. The HIGH-PRESSURE alarm is activated when the airway pressure exceeds the set HIGH-PRESSURE alarm for 2 seconds during a single breath. It also acts as a pressure relief for the ventilator. If the high-pressure setting is surpassed, the ventilator vents the excess flow to the atmosphere and allows for the set T_I to complete its cycle. The adjustable range of this function is 15 to 100 cm H_2O.

The LOW-PRESSURE/DISCONNECT alarm detects leaks and disconnections in the patient circuit and has an adjustable range of 0 to 50 cm H_2O. If the patient fails to meet the low-pressure setting, or if the airway pressure fails to reach $+1$ cm H_2O at the time of the next mandatory breath, the alarm is activated.

Additional Alarms

Three additional alarms on the Uni-Vent are the APNEA, the PEEP NOT SET, and the INVERSE I:E alarms. The APNEA alarm is activated when the patient fails to trigger a spontaneous or mandatory breath in 19 seconds (nonadjustable). The ventilator defaults to a back-up rate of 12 breaths/min and uses the current set V_T. The APNEA alarm is only operational in the assist and SIMV modes.

The PEEP NOT SET alarm is activated when the end-expiratory pressure fails to return to the set value by +2 to −1 cm H_2O for three consecutive breaths. This alarm is inactivated when the manual instead of the automatic mode is used to set PEEP.

The Uni-Vent 750 does not allow for IRV. Any combination of rate and T_I that creates a longer inspiratory than expiratory period activates the INVERSE I:E alarm. The ventilator defaults to exhalation and elicits an audio/visual alarm that cannot be deactivated until the problem is corrected.

Power Alarms

The Uni-Vent 750 has two power alarms: EXTERNAL POWER LOW/FAIL and BATTERY LOW/FAIL. The EXTERNAL POWER LOW/FAIL alerts the operator when the external power source is disconnected or fails. The BATTERY LOW/FAIL alarm is set off when the internal battery voltage falls below 11 volts or is defective and will not recharge.

Modes of Ventilation

The Uni-Vent 750 offers three modes of ventilation: control, assist (A/C), and SIMV. In the control mode, the machine delivers time-triggered, volume-targeted breaths based on the set rate, T_I, and flow. Although if necessary, the patient is able to take spontaneous breaths between the mandatory breaths through the anti-asphyxia valve (see Figure 12-16). In a sense, this is like an IMV mode.

The A/C mode lets the patient initiate mechanical breaths and ultimately control the total breath rate of the ventilator (time-triggered + patient-triggered). All other functions that were set in control mode are still active in this mode with the addition of assist sensitivity. Breaths are patient- or time-triggered, volume-targeted, and time-cycled.

When the SIMV mode is used, the patient can breathe spontaneously through the internal demand valve and receive mandatory breaths through the main inspiratory valve. All controls set in the A/C mode are set and functional in SIMV. Spontaneous breaths must generate a pressure change of 1 cm H_2O to open the internal demand valve and provide flow to the patient (Box 12-12).

Oxygen

The Uni-Vent operates from a 100% gas source, therefore the oxygen percentage depends on the gas powering the ventilator. An alternative to regulating the FiO_2 is to use a gas blender. There is no entrainment feature on this ventilator.

BOX 12-12

Control and IMV Modes on the Uni-Vent 750

In the control mode, the patient receives time-triggered mandatory breaths from the machine. Between these breaths, the patient can breathe spontaneously from the anti-asphyxia valve in the patient circuit.

In the SIMV mode, the mandatory breaths are patient- or time-triggered. Between mandatory breaths, the patient breathes spontaneously from the internal demand valve.

In the control mode, spontaneous breaths are at room air (FiO_2 0.21). In the SIMV mode, spontaneous breaths receive the FiO_2 provided by the gas source.

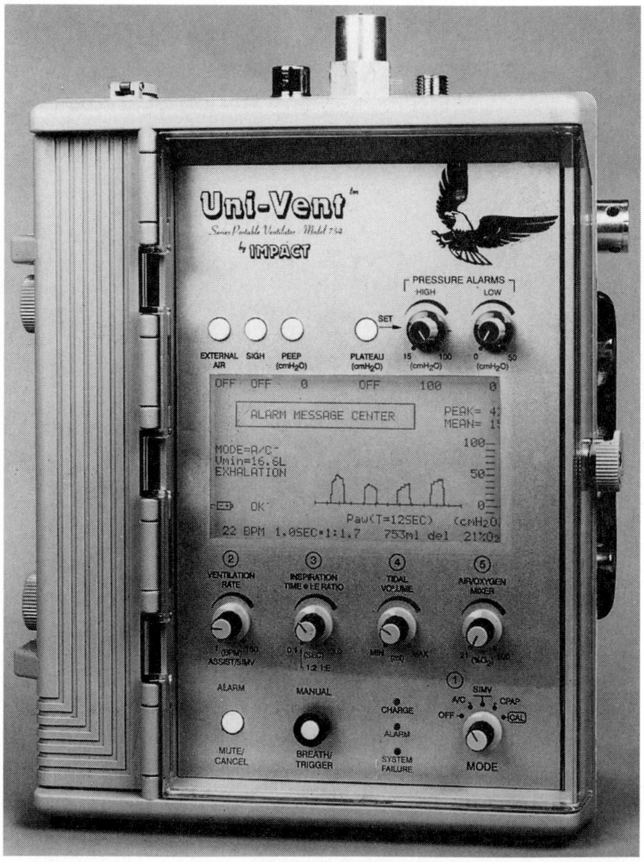

Figure 12-16 The Uni-Vent 755 Eagle, the latest transport ventilator from Impact. (Courtesy Impact Instrumentation, Inc., West Caldwell, NJ.)

IMPACT UNI-VENT EAGLE 755

The Eagle 755 (Figure 12-16) is a recent addition to Impact's Uni-Vent line. It is an updated version of the 750 model, retaining the same basic size and weight of its predecessor (9″ × 11.5″ × 4.5″ and about 13 lb). Improvements include a direct V_T setting and an updated alarm package, which features scroll knobs that allow HIGH- and LOW-PRESSURE alarms to be set directly on the digital bar graph and back-up ventilation that is activated during apneic periods. In addition to the back-up ventilation, the 755 also gives the operator the option of pressure plateau ventilation. When operating in this mode, the ventilator limits the pressure allowed in the airways, but does not end inspiration until the desired V_T is delivered. If the pressure in the airways reaches the set pressure limit before the entire V_T is delivered, a pressure plateau occurs, venting the excess flow until the ventilator delivered the entire V_T. The 755 also has an LCD display that lets the operator view all settings continuously along with real-time pressure waveforms, a built-in compressor with a blender and an FiO_2 display, an interactive operator demonstration mode, and an internally calibrated and adjustable PEEP control.

SUMMARY OF TRANSPORT VENTILATORS

When transporting patients, take particular care to ensure optimal monitoring of patient status, ventilation, oxygenation and patient care. Choosing and using the right equipment are part of the therapist's responsibilities. The ideal transport ventilator is small, lightweight, and able to withstand the rigors of transport while providing adequate ventilation the whole time.

Home-Care Ventilators

Home care began in the United States over 100 years ago.[1] Individuals discharged from the hospital that still required routine care were the primary candidates for this emerging sector of medicine. Today it is one of the fastest growing areas of health care. With the continued rise in the cost of caring for patients in the acute or extended care environment, home care is a realistic alternative for individuals battling primarily chronic diseases.

The following section focuses on the technical aspects of the equipment available for home-care ventilation. The supportive measures include primarily positive-pressure ventilators, which are the most commonly used, and noninvasive positive-pressure ventilators.

NELLCOR PURITAN BENNETT COMPANION 2801

The Nellcor Puritan Bennett Companion 2801 (Figure 12-17) is an updated model of the 2800 with a new front panel and several upgrades. The airway pressure and exhalation valve connections are of different sizes, and the high and low airway pressures are calibrated for an increase in accuracy and ease in use. Additional upgrades include increases in the range settings for peak flow, peak inspiratory pressure, low inspiratory pressure, APNEA alarm, and sensitivity.

The Companion 2801 is an electronically powered, rotary-piston–driven, microprocessor-controlled ventilator that is primarily used for home-care support (for a review of rotary-driven pistons see Chapter 9). Its dimensions are 12 3/4″ × 10 5/8″ × 13 1/4″ and it weighs about 31 lb. The 2801 produces a sinusoidal flow waveform for any mandatory breath in any of its working modes: control, A/C, and SIMV.

Power Source

The Companion 2801 can prioritize and then choose from the following three power sources:

- A standard AC outlet
- An external DC battery
- An internal DC battery

A standard electrical AC outlet is the primary energy source for routine daily operations. An external DC source is what the machine automatically switches to if there is a power failure. If neither AC nor external DC

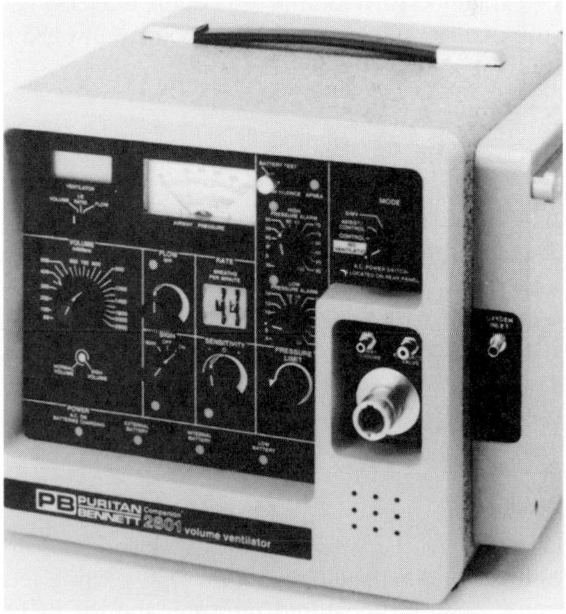

Figure 12-17 The Bennett Companion 2801. (Courtesy Bennett Group, Boulder, Co.)

power is available, then the ventilator uses the internal battery. It is of the lowest priority because it has a maximum working capacity of only about 30 to 60 minutes, depending on ventilator settings. As soon as an AC outlet is available or an external battery is attached, the ventilator automatically switches to the available source with the highest priority rating.

During use, the 2801 is continuously recharging the internal battery. When the ventilator is not in use, it must be connected to an external power source and the mode switched to NO VENTILATION for the internal battery to charge. It takes about 4 hours to recharge a totally depleted battery.

Internal Mechanisms

The Companion 2801 delivers a breath by drawing in room air through the intake filter and check valve at the rear of the machine. The gas source then enters into the piston chamber during the exhalation phase of the respiratory cycle. When the piston begins the forward stroke (inspiration), the gas source moves from the piston chamber past a second check valve, an adjustable relief valve, and the exhalation manifold before entering the patient circuit. The adjustable relief valve monitors the internal pressure and does not allow it to increase above the set value. When pressures exceed this setting, the excess pressure is vented to room air (see the discussion of pressure limit ventilation in the section on modes of ventilation).

The exhalation valve is at the external PEEP valve and regulates the direction of flow during inspiration and expiration. It is primed for operation by a branch of the main internal circuit before passing the second check valve. It closes the expiration valve during inspiration, directing gas flow to the patient, and opens during expiration to allow the exhaled breath to be released.

Control Panel and Alarms

The front panel of the Companion 2801 (Figure 12-18) is divided into several sections and includes the MODE switch, a monitor section, parameter controls, and an alarm section.

Mode Control

The MODE selector is at the top right corner of the control panel. The 2801 lets the operator select control, A/C, or SIMV. These settings are described further in the discussion of modes of ventilation.

Display Features

The Companion 2801 has two display capabilities: the airway pressure manometer (10 to 80 cm H_2O), which lets the operator view the measured pressure, and the LCD, which displays one of three possible parameters. A switch just beneath the LCD allows the operator to choose between VOLUME, I:E RATIO, and FLOW.

Control Parameters

The main control parameters include V_T, rate, flow, and sensitivity. The V_T control is on the middle left part of the control panel and sets the delivered V_T to the patient during a mandatory breath (50 to 2500 mL).

The respiratory RATE function on the middle of the control panel uses a two-digit rotary thumb wheel (see Figure 12-18) that lets the operator select a range from 1 to 69 breaths/min.

The FLOW function is in the middle of the control panel and regulates peak flow to the patient (20 to 120 L/min).

The SENSITIVITY setting is on the bottom right of the control panel and is active in the A/C and SIMV modes. This control allows the patient to pressure-trigger a mandatory or spontaneous breath (−10 to 10 cm H_2O).

Additional Controls

Additional functions include PRESSURE LIMIT and SIGH.

The PRESSURE LIMIT control is at the bottom right of the control panel and limits the maximum amount of pressure in the airway. The machine allows for an adjustable range of 10 to 100 cm H_2O.

The SIGH VOLUME setting is an additional knob on the V_T control. When the sigh function is switched to ON, the ventilator delivers three consecutive sigh breaths every 10 minutes. The sigh volume cannot be set below the V_T or two times more than the V_T.

PEEP

There is no PEEP control on the Companion 2801. If the operator wants to provide PEEP to the patient, an external PEEP valve must be attached to the exhalation manifold. When using PEEP, the sensitivity must be adjusted to account for the increase in baseline pressure. The ventilator does not compensate for PEEP (Box 12-13).

Airway Pressure Alarms

The Companion 2801 lets the operator control settings that regulate and monitor airway pressure, including the HIGH-PRESSURE alarm and the LOW-PRESSURE alarm. The HIGH-PRESSURE alarm is a separate control setting that allows for an adjustable range of 25 to 100 cm H_2O. When the setting is exceeded, an audio/visual alarm is activated, and inspiration stops. Any remaining volume is vented through the exhalation valve to room air. A continuous pulsating alarm sounds until the problem is resolved.

The LOW-PRESSURE alarm is in the middle right part of the control panel and has an adjustable range of 2 to 32 cm H_2O. This alarm is activated if the pressure in the circuit does not achieve the desired setting for two consecutive breaths or 15 seconds—whichever comes first. A continuous pulsating alarm sounds until the problem is resolved.

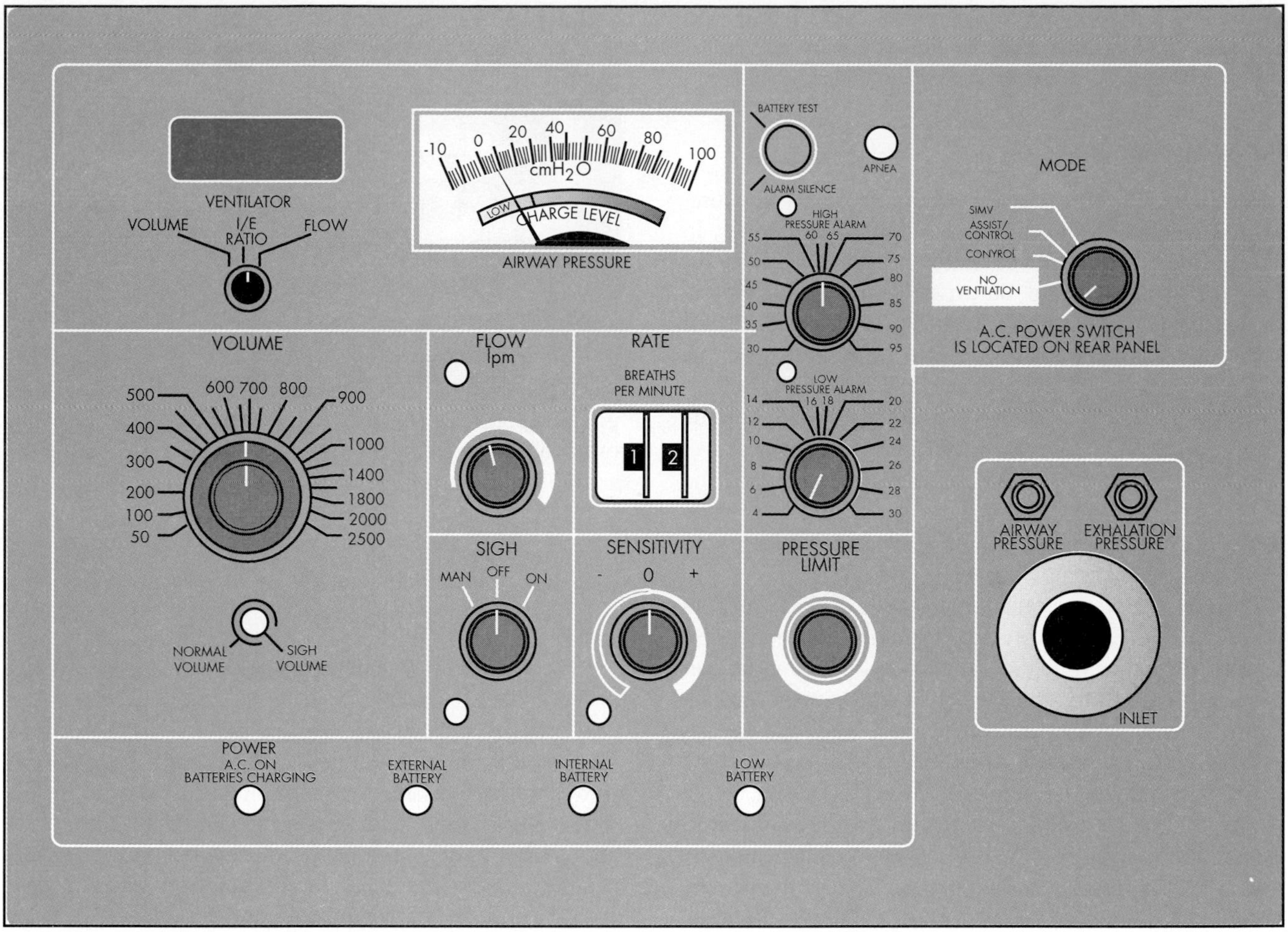

Figure 12-18 The Companion front panel.

BOX 12-13

Decision Making & Problem Solving

A respiratory therapist is called by the wife of a patient who is using the Companion 2801. The patient has recently resumed spontaneous breathing (A/C mode, V_T = 0.5, rate = 9 breaths/min, PEEP = 5 cm H_2O).

The wife states, "My husband seems to have trouble getting a breath started from the machine. When he breathes in, the pressure gauge goes to −1 cm H_2O, then it goes up to 20 cm H_2O, and then back down to 5 cm H_2O when he breathes out." What do you think is the problem?

See Appendix A for the answers.

Additional Alarms

Additional alarms include APNEA, LOW BATTERY, POWER SWITCHOVER, and FLOW.

The APNEA alarm LED illuminates if the patient does not trigger a breath within 15 seconds (nonadjustable) while the SIMV mode is used. If the rate is set below 8 breaths/min and an apneic period is detected (15 seconds), then an alarm sounds. A back-up rate of 12 breaths/min is initiated if the apnea persists for longer than 30 seconds. For the ventilator to return to the original settings, the patient must trigger two breaths within 10 seconds. The visual alarm stays lit until the ALARM SILENCE/BATTERY TEST button is pressed.

The low battery alarm is activated when the power source in use falls below 11.9 volts of DC current. A pulsating alarm continues until the problem is resolved or the ALARM SILENCE/BATTERY TEST button is pressed. This alarm is also triggered when the internal battery falls below the set voltage of 11.9 volts. Every 15 minutes the ventilator tests the internal battery. If it does not meet the minimum standard of 11.9 volts, an alarm sounds for 5 seconds. The visual alarm is also activated and remains lit until the ALARM SILENCE/BATTERY TEST button is pushed.

The POWER SWITCHOVER alarm activates when the ventilator automatically switches from a higher priority power source to a lower one. The pulsating alarm continues to sound until the ALARM SILENCE/BATTERY TEST button is pressed. There is no alarm activated when the ventilator switches from a lower to a higher priority power source.

The FLOW alarm is an audio/visual alarm that is activated when the I:E ratio is more than 1:0.8 or the ventilator fails to deliver the set number of breaths.

Modes of Ventilation

The Companion 2801 can provide volume- or pressure-targeted ventilation in control, A/C, or SIMV modes. In volume-targeted control ventilation, the operator sets V_T, flow, and respiratory rate. Because this mode does not allow any patient interaction, the SENSITIVITY control is not functional, and the ventilator operates with time-triggering.

The A/C mode lets the patient to initiate volume-targeted mandatory breaths as well as set a minimum back-up rate. The V_T, FLOW, RATE, and SENSITIVITY controls are all active.

When operating in SIMV, all controls used with the A/C mode are active. The patient is allowed to breathe spontaneously and independently of the ventilator between mandatory volume-targeted breaths.

Pressure-targeted ventilation operates during a mandatory breath in any of the previously mentioned modes. It is activated by setting the PRESSURE LIMIT control at the current plateau pressure and the V_T higher than normal requirements. When a breath is delivered, the set pressure is reached and an inspiratory pressure plateau occurs until the set V_T is delivered. Once the plateau is reached, all additional volume is vented to room air. This mode functions similarly to, but not exactly as PCV. The factor that differentiates this mode from traditional PCV is that the ventilator is volume-, not time-cycled. The machine remains in inspiration until the full V_T is delivered, regardless of whether it is to the patient or to room air. Fluctuations in V_T delivery to the patient are expected.

Oxygen Source

An oxygen accumulator must be attached to increase the FiO_2 above room air. The accumulator is a mixing chamber that provides a reservoir of mixed gas and lets the operator increase the delivered FiO_2. The accumulator is not a calibrated device, an O_2 analyzer should be used.

INTERMED BEAR 33

The Bear 33 (Figure 12-19) is a microprocessor-controlled, volume ventilator used primarily for home-care support. It is 7.5″ × 14″ × 12.8,″ weighs 32 lb, and offers control, A/C, and SIMV modes.

Power Source

The Bear 33 is an electrically powered ventilator. When the POWER switch on the front panel is turned on, the machine automatically selects from the following three power sources:

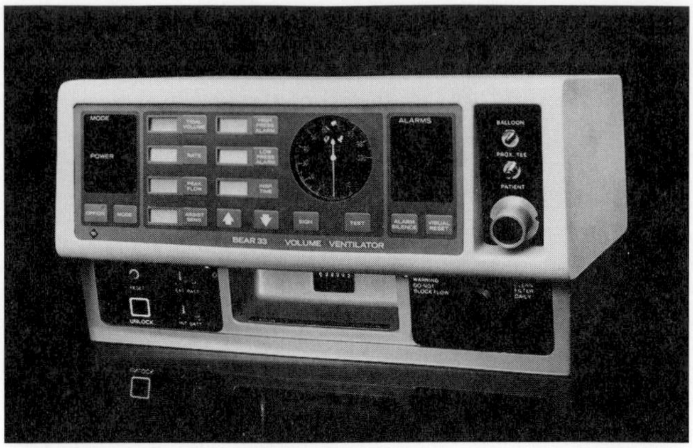

Figure 12-19 The Bear 33 Ventilator. (Courtesy Bear Medical Systems, Riverside, Calif.)

- An AC outlet
- An external DC battery
- An internal DC battery

The AC outlet, which has top priority, is a standard 110- or 220-volt AC outlet. The external DC battery gets second priority, and the internal DC battery is ranked third. The ventilator is programmed to select the highest priority power source available for use at all times. Note that when the internal battery is in use, it has an expiration time of about 1 hour, so it should only be used as a back-up power source in case of emergencies. As soon as an AC outlet becomes available or an external battery is attached, the ventilator automatically switches to the available source with the highest priority.

Internal Mechanisms

Room air is drawn into the ventilator through the gas inlet filter (Figure 12-20). It then passes through the one-way check valve and enters into the cylinder assembly during the backstroke (expiration phase) of the piston. Once the piston begins the upstroke (inspiration), the air passes through the output check valve en route to the patient circuit. This check valve is a one-way valve that prevents air from reentering the cylinder assembly. Before the gas source enters the patient circuit, it passes the set pressure-relief valve and the bypass check valve. The set pressure-relief valve limits the maximum pressure the ventilator can generate. When the pressure in the patient circuit exceeds the high-pressure setting, a solenoid valve is activated, and the exhalation valve vents the remaining breath to room air. All mandatory breaths are delivered in a characteristic sine-wave pattern.

For spontaneous breaths, the bypass check valve lets the patient draw in room air through the inlet port while the piston is positioning for the next mandatory breath. The

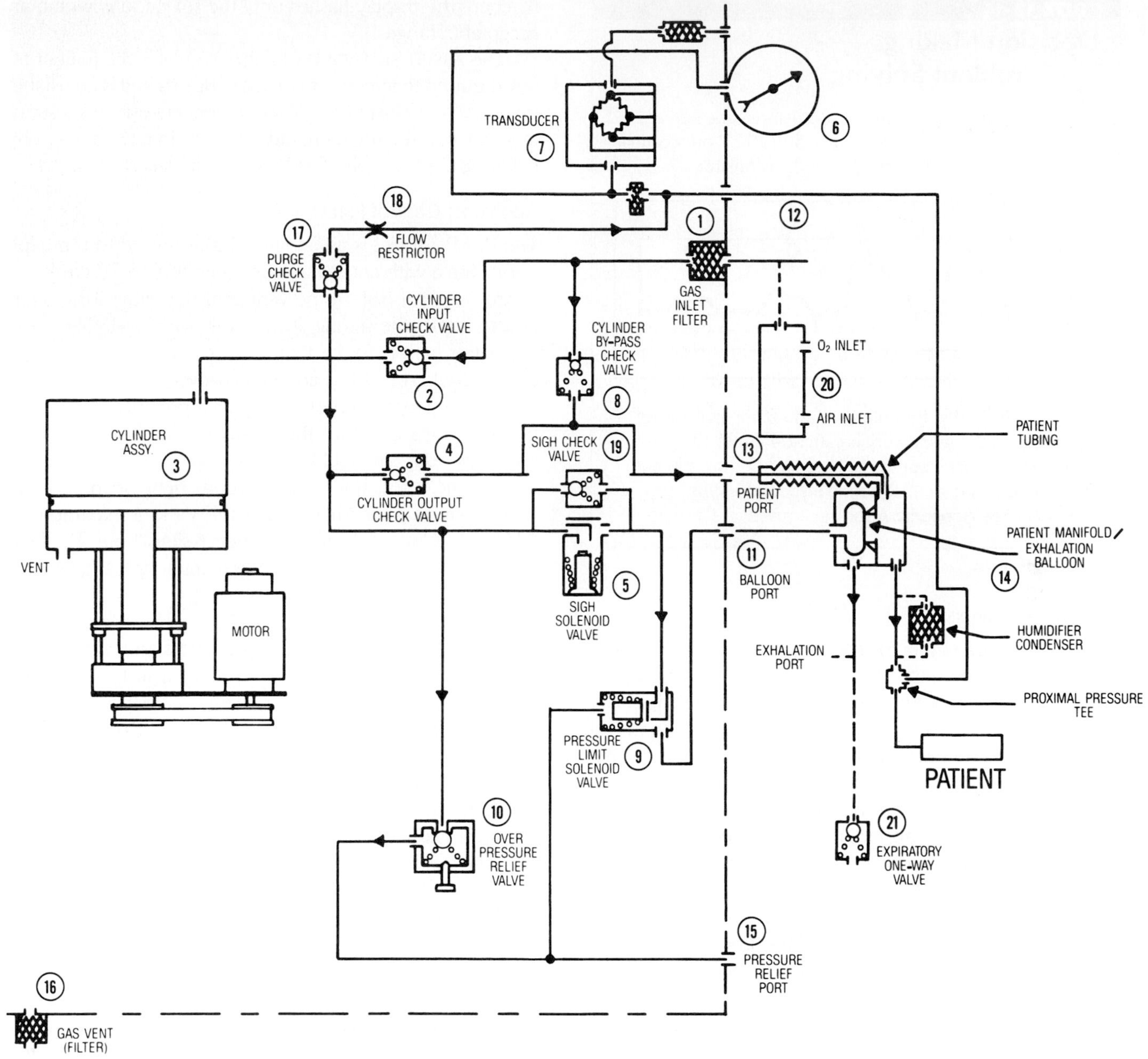

Figure 12-20 A pneumatic schematic of the Bear 33. (Courtesy Bear Medical Systems, Riverside, Calif.)

patient must overcome the resistance of the circuit, including PEEP, and generate pressures more negative than −0.2 cm H_2O in order to open this valve. An additional gas source for spontaneous breaths is room air drawn past the deflated exhalation balloon in the exhalation valve assembly. This additional source becomes void when an external PEEP valve is added to the port.

The PEEP valve on the Bear 33 is not part of the ventilator's internal mechanisms. An external valve must be attached to the patient manifold if PEEP is to be applied, which can cause an increase in the patient's work of breathing. The Bear 33 does not offer any compensatory mechanism for spontaneous breaths when PEEP is applied. The higher the PEEP level, the more difficult it is for the patient to trigger a spontaneous breath. (Note that this is not the case for mandatory breaths because the assist sensitivity can be adjusted to compensate for the additional PEEP when the patient triggers a mandatory breath [Box 12-14].)

Control Panel and Alarms

The Bear 33 has a conservative control panel (Figure 12-21) that allows the operator access to parameter functions and alarm settings.

BOX 12-14

Decision Making & Problem Solving

The figure below shows a pressure/time curve during SIMV ventilation with +5 of PEEP on a patient being ventilated with a Bear 33 ventilator.

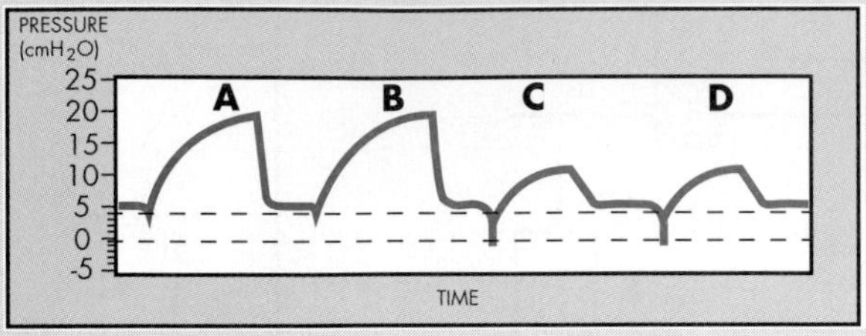

Note that for breaths *A* and *B*, the patient triggered the mandatory breath at 4 cm H_2O. However, spontaneous breaths *C* and *D* show pressure decreasing to −0.2 during inspiration. Why?

See Appendix A for the answer.

Control Parameters

The control parameters for the Bear 33 include V_T, RATE, PEAK FLOW, and ASSIST SENSITIVITY. The V_T control is at the top left part of the control panel and has an adjustable range of 100 to 2200 mL. To change the setting, use the up and down arrow keys. If an inappropriate V_T is set, the display blinks until an acceptable setting is chosen.

The RATE control is on the middle left part of the control panel and has an adjustable range of 2 to 40 breaths/minute. It is functional in all modes of ventilation.

The PEAK FLOW control is in the middle left part of the control panel and regulates the maximum flow delivered to the patient (20 to 120 L/min). This function is only active during mandatory breaths. If the set peak flow limit is reached, the display flashes until the selection is within an acceptable range.

The ASSIST SENSITIVITY control regulates the patient effort required to initiate a mandatory breath and is adjustable from −9 to 19 cm H_2O. When the patient initiates a spontaneous breath, the demand valve is bypassed, thereby negating the function of assist sensitivity (see Box 12-14).

Additional Control Parameters

The PEEP control is an additional attachment to the expiratory valve with an operational range of 0 to 20 cm H_2O. There is no control on the ventilator that allows the operator to adjust the setting; it must be done manually at the exhalation valve. (Note that the assist sensitivity must be adjusted when PEEP is added; however, the patient must be able to generate enough negative pressure on spontaneous breaths to return the airway pressure back to baseline plus −0.2 cm H_2O.)

The SIGH function at the bottom right of the control panel delivers a breath 1.5 times the V_T to a maximum of 3300 mL. When activated, it delivers 6 sighs/hour. The Bear 33 also lets the operator deliver a manual sigh at any time.

Airway Pressures

The Bear 33 has two separate pressure alarms and an APNEA alarm. The HIGH-PRESSURE alarm is in the center of the top of the control panel and adjustable from 10 to 80 cm H_2O. If the patient exceeds this setting on any given breath, a visual indicator is activated. An audio alarm is only triggered if the setting is exceeded for two consecutive breaths. When the high-pressure setting is reached, inspiration ends. If at any time the airway pressure exceeds 80 cm H_2O, the audible and visual alarms are activated immediately. This is a nonadjustable alarm limit.

The LOW-PRESSURE alarm is at the center of the top of the control panel and has an operable range of 3 to 70 cm H_2O. The visual alarm is activated when the inspiratory

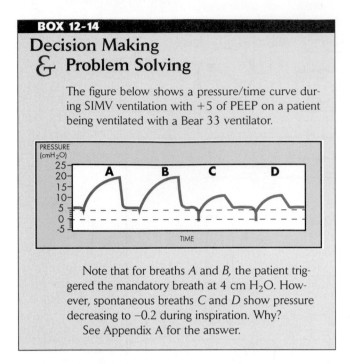

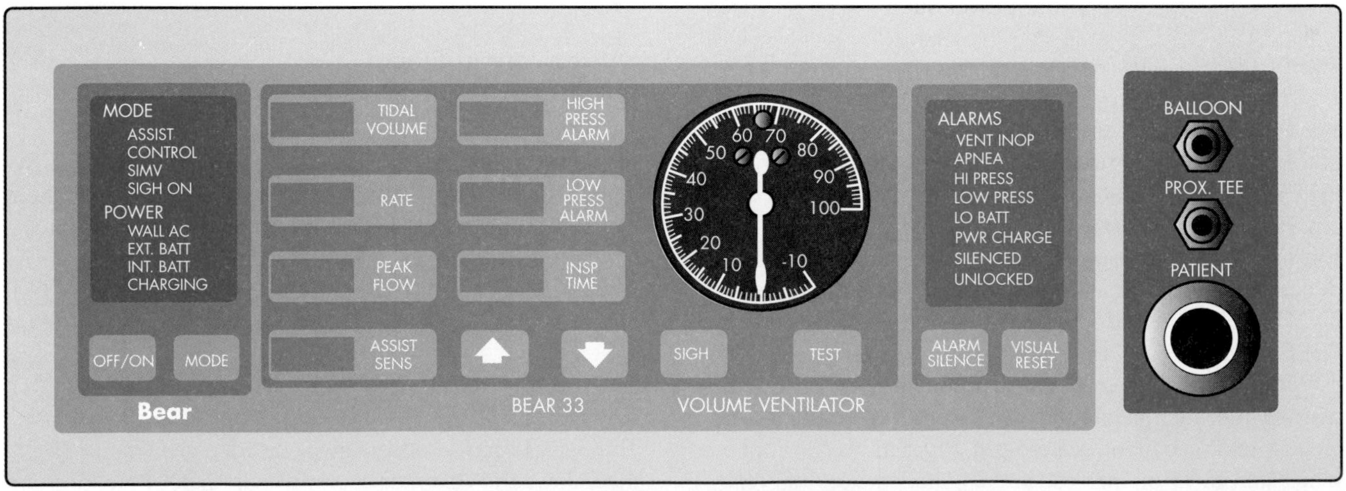

Figure 12-21 The Bear 33 front control panel. (Courtesy Bear Medical Systems, Riverside, Calif.)

BOX 12-15

Causes of the Ventilator Inoperative Alarm

1. Failure to cycle.
2. High or low T_I. The ventilator does not allow for inverse I:E ratios. This alarm is activated when the T_I is less than 0.25 seconds or greater than 4.99 seconds. The I:E ratio is calculated based on the V_T, flow, and rate settings.
3. Timing circuit failure.
4. Internal power supply failure.
5. Internal battery supply insufficient to drive ventilator.

pressure fails to reach the desired setting. If the patient does not attain the low-pressure setting on two consecutive breaths, the visual indicator stays lit and the audible alarm sounds. The visual alarm remains illuminated until manually reset, even if the patient generates a sufficient pressure on following breaths.

Operational Alarms

The following alarms monitor the ventilator's function and electronic power supply and include the VENT INOPERATIVE, LO INTERNAL BATTERY, POWER CHANGE, and APNEA alarms. The VENT INOPERATIVE alarm is audio/visual and is activated when one of the conditions presented in Box 12-15 occurs.

The LO INTERNAL BATTERY alarm is activated when the internal battery has about 25% or less of operating power. It can be silenced for 60 seconds with the ALARM SILENCE button or deactivated by changing to another power source.

The POWER CHANGE alarm activates when the power supply has been switched to a lower priority source, for example from AC to internal battery. The audible alarm automatically resets when the power supply is reinstated. If this is not done, the operator must manually reset the alarm with the ALARM RESET button.

The APNEA alarm is not an adjustable control and is not on the front panel. It has a fixed setting of 20 seconds. If no spontaneous or mechanical breaths are detected within this time, the audio/visual alarm activates. Detection of spontaneous breaths is irrelevant of the sensitivity setting.

Modes of Ventilation

The Bear 33 offers the control, A/C, and SIMV modes.

When in the control mode, the V_T, rate, and peak flow controls are set. The ventilator is time-triggered and does not use the assist sensitivity feature. Unlike traditional ventilators, however, the Bear 33 allows for spontaneous breathing that is not synchronized to occur between mandatory breaths (i.e., IMV). This is made possible by the bypass check valve (see Figure 12-20 or refer to the discussion of internal mechanisms in this section).

The A/C mode lets the patient initiate mandatory breaths. V_T and flow are both active in this mode, in addition to trigger sensitivity. When the ventilator "assists" the patient's breath, an "A" appears on the sensitivity display. The ventilator does not cycle into inspiration if triggered in the first 750 milliseconds from the beginning of expiration of the previous mandatory breath.

When operating in the SIMV mode, the patient is able to breathe spontaneously between mandatory breaths. The mode operates by generating an "assist window" that remains open until a patient-initiated, mandatory breath occurs. While the window is open, any effort sufficient to overcome the sensitivity setting triggers a mandatory breath. After a mandatory breath has been given, the window closes for a time to allow for spontaneous breaths by the patient. The rate setting is the factor that influences the time period available for mandatory and spontaneous breaths.

Oxygen Source

In order to increase the FiO_2 above 0.21, an oxygen accumulator must be attached.[7] The accumulator is a mixing chamber that provides a reservoir of mixed gas and lets the operator increase the delivered FiO_2. The accumulator is not a calibrated device, so periodic checks with an O_2 analyzer are important.

LIFECARE PLV-100 AND PLV-102

The Lifecare PLV-100 (Figure 12-22) and PLV-102 (Figure 12-23) volume ventilators are lightweight microprocessor-based units ideally suited for long-term home use. Their compact size and variable power sources make them highly portable, thus giving the advantage of mobility to the patient and caregiver.

Power Source

Both the PLV-100 and PLV-102 are designed to operate on the most practical power source available. The preferred power source is a 120-volt AC electrical current, but if there is a power failure, both ventilators automatically select a 12-volt DC external battery if connected. This external battery can power the ventilator up to 24 hours depending on the ventilator's rate, volume, and pressure settings. The higher these settings, the shorter the time provided by the battery. If the external power source is not connected, these units use a 12-volt DC internal battery. This internal battery is intended for emergency use only because it can only provide about 1 hour of power,

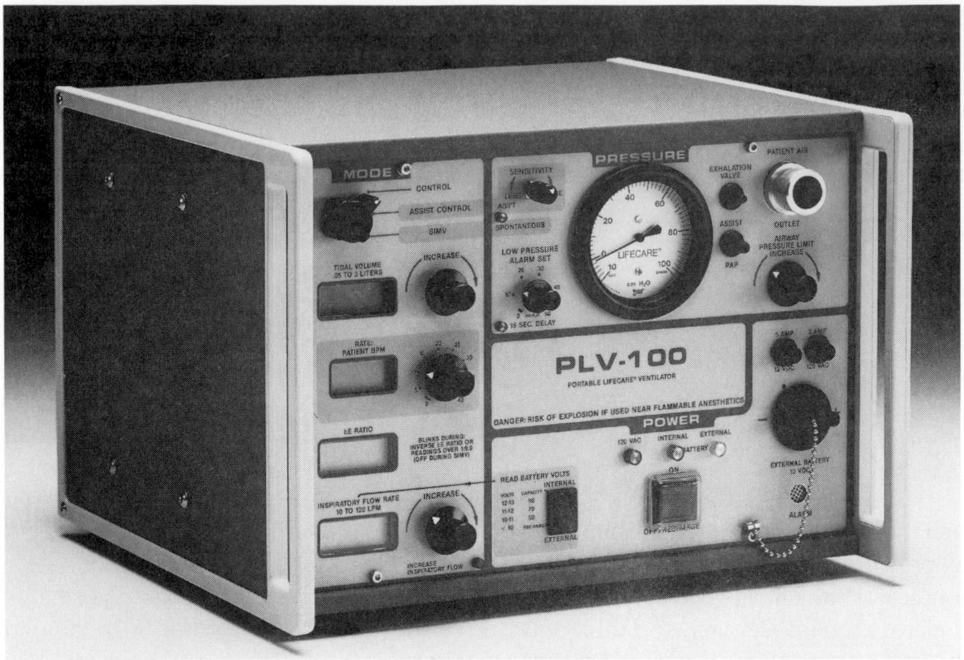

Figure 12-22 The Lifecare PLV-100. (Courtesy Respironics, Pittsburgh.)

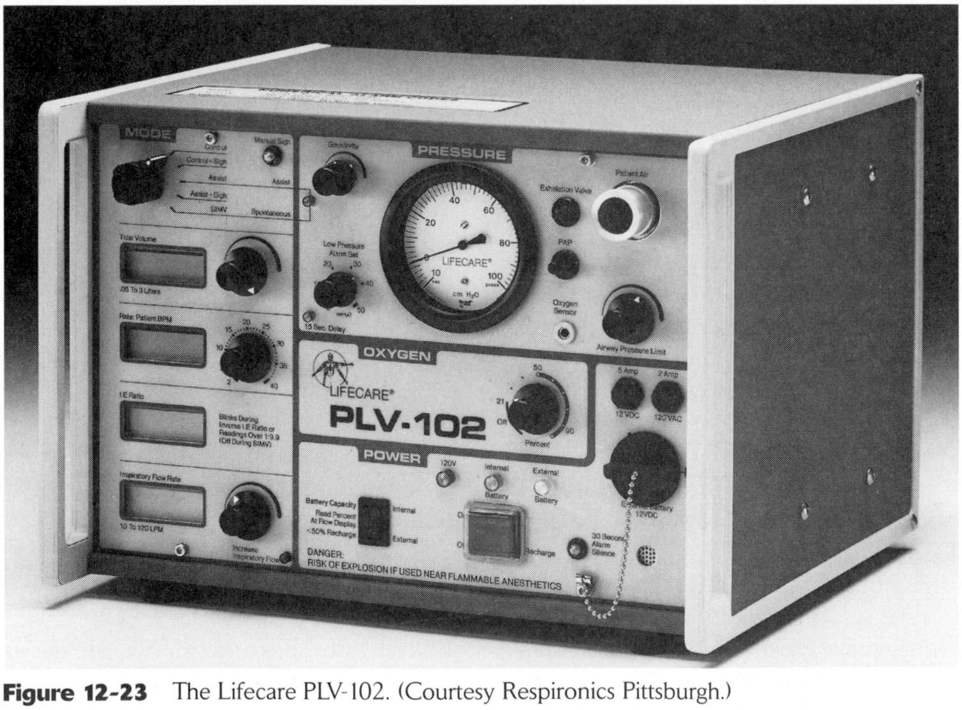

Figure 12-23 The Lifecare PLV-102. (Courtesy Respironics Pittsburgh.)

depending on the ventilator's rate, volume, and pressure settings. The internal battery is automatically recharged whenever the ventilator is operating on a 120-volt AC power source. Each time the external or internal DC power source is selected, the ventilator sounds a 3-second alarm to alert the operator to verify the DC battery voltage level to ensure that safe operating time remains. This voltage level can be easily obtained by the READ BATTERY VOLTS indicator on the front panel of both machines.

Both ventilators are programmed to provide a complete check of the microprocessor system, front panel digital displays, LEDs, audible alarms, and pressure transducer operation. This is a 5-second diagnostic sequence of checks that takes place each time the ventilators are turned on.

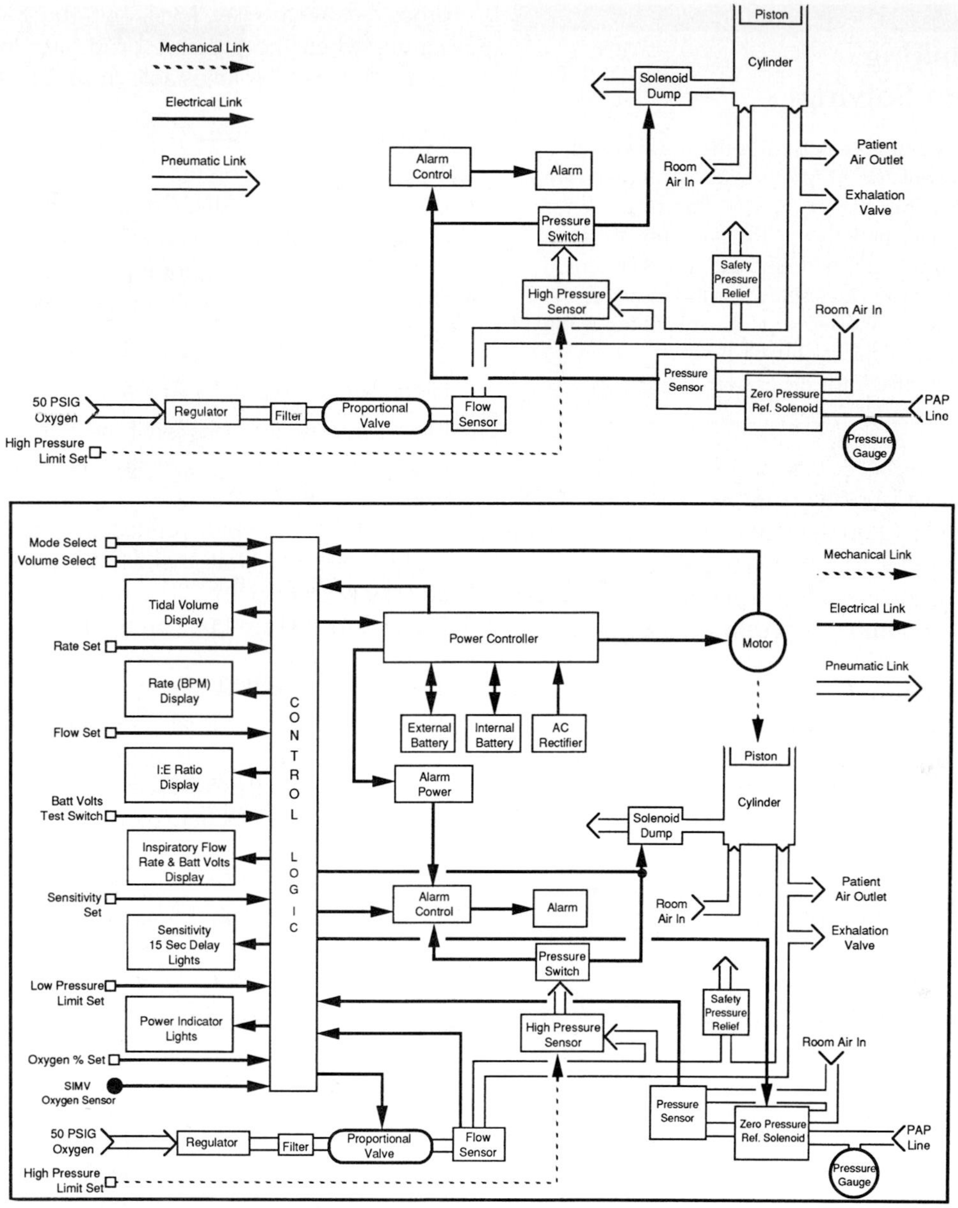

Figure 12-24 A pneumatic schematic of the Lifecare PLV-102. (Courtesy Respironics, Pittsburgh.)

Internal Mechanisms

The delivery of gas flow to the patient is provided by a rotary piston driven by a brushed motor and controlled by a microprocessor (Figure 12-24). The piston draws gas into the housing on the downstroke through a check valve and an air intake filter on the back of the machine. On the upstroke, the piston compresses the gas and pushes it out to the patient circuit and exhalation valve. The gas also passes a safety pressure-relief valve and a pressure transducer. Pressure is monitored by the proximal airway pressure line, which provides feedback to the microprocessor system. Because the drive mechanism is a rotary piston, gas is delivered in a characteristic sine-wave flow pattern with a sigmoidal pressure curve.

Controls

Both the PLV-100 and PVL-102 are volume-targeted ventilators. Actual volume delivery to the patient is determined by the backward and forward stroke of the rotary piston. By adjusting the TIDAL VOLUME control on the front panel of the machine, the operator is actually setting the length of the piston's backward stroke. As the piston's forward stroke occurs, the set V_T is delivered to the patient. The set V_T is shown on a LCD display adjacent to the V_T control. The V_T is adjustable from 0.05 to 3.0 liters.

The inspiratory phase of both ventilators is either pressure- or time-triggered, volume-targeted, and time-cycled. A SENSITIVITY control determines the amount of patient inspiratory effort relative to patient airway pressure required

BOX 12-16

Decision Making & Problem Solving

A patient is being ventilated in the hospital with a PLV-102 ventilator in preparation for home-care ventilation. The patient has a threshold-resistor PEEP valve attached distal to the exhalation valve on a disposable circuit. The PEEP setting is 7 cm H_2O.

The respiratory therapist measures exhaled V_Ts at 0.5 mL when the set V_T is 0.7 mL. What is the possible cause of this problem?

See Appendix A for the answer.

to trigger an "assisted" breath. This control is adjustable from +3 to −6 cm H_2O on the PLV-100 and from +18 to −5 cm H_2O on the PLV-102. If the patient has no spontaneous effort, inspiration begins as a result of the elapsed time between the set number of breaths. The rate range for both ventilators is 2 to 40 breaths per minute.

The AIRWAY PRESSURE LIMIT control establishes the maximal airway pressure allowed during the inspiratory phase. When the set pressure limit is reached, excess pressure is vented to the atmosphere through the piston safety valve as the motion of the piston continues. Thus the set pressure limit is not exceeded and T_I remains constant. The airway pressure limit is adjustable from 5 to 100 cm H_2O on the PLV-100 and from 10 to 100 cm H_2O on the PLV-102.

PEEP/CPAP

If the operator wants PEEP/CPAP on either the PLV-100 or PLV-102, an external threshold resistor valve can be added to the patient circuit. This valve should be placed proximal to the exhalation valve if a disposable circuit with an exhalation valve diaphragm is in use.[2] Placing the PEEP valve distal to this type of exhalation valve can cause incomplete sealing of the exhalation diaphragm, which results in a significant loss of delivered V_T. The application of PEEP/CPAP may also require readjustment of the machine sensitivity so that the patients can assist without significantly increasing their work of breathing (Box 12-16).

Alarms

Both the PLV-100 and PLV-102 have audio and/or visual alarms for low pressure, apnea, high pressure, inverse I:E ratios, increased inspiratory flow, switch to battery, low external battery, low internal battery, power failure, microprocessor failure, and ventilator malfunction.

Low-Pressure Alarm

This alarm is activated when a patient's proximal airway pressure falls below the set low airway pressure level. An LED on the front panel lights immediately after pressure drops below this set level, but the audible alarm only sounds when the pressure drop lasts more than 15 seconds. This alarm is adjustable from 2 to 40 cm H_2O.

Apnea Alarm

This alarm is incorporated in the LOW-PRESSURE alarm and occurs only in the SIMV mode. It is activated if the machine does not sense a spontaneous breath from the patient within 15 seconds, or if proximal airway pressure falls below the set low airway pressure level for more than 15 seconds.

High-Pressure Alarm

This alarm is activated anytime ventilating pressure exceeds the set high-pressure limit. As mentioned previously, excess pressure is vented to the atmosphere through the piston chamber. When ventilating pressure falls below the set high-pressure limit, the alarm resets itself. This alarm is adjustable from 5 to 100 cm H_2O on the PLV-100 and from 10 to 100 cm H_2O on the PLV-102.

Inverse I:E Ratio Alert

This alarm is only a visual alarm and is activated whenever T_I exceeds T_E, or whenever the I:E ratio is $<$ 1:9.9. It is inactivated during the SIMV mode because of the patient's spontaneous breaths between mandatory breaths.

Increase Inspiratory Flow Alert

This alarm is also only a visual alarm and is activated if the set inspiratory flow rate is not sufficient to meet the other set parameters of V_T and respiratory rate. Under these conditions, the inspiratory flow automatically increases.

Switch to Battery Alert

This is a 3-second audible alarm that sounds whenever the ventilator switches to internal or external DC power from an AC power source. This way, the operator is alerted that limited operation time remains.

Low External Battery Alarm

This alarm is an audio/visual alarm that is activated when the external battery voltage falls below 9.5 volts when in use.

Low Internal Battery Alarm

This is an audio/visual alarm that is activated when the internal battery voltage falls below 9.5 volts when in use.

Power Failure Alert

This is an audible alarm that is activated whenever the ventilator is turned on and all power sources are exhausted or disconnected.

Microprocessor Failure Alarm

This is a continuous audible alarm that is activated when the ventilator fails to pass its diagnostic self-test on start-up.

When this alarm is activated, the piston motor is locked out to prevent uncontrolled piston motion.

Ventilator Malfunction

This is an audible "fast beep" alarm that is activated whenever the ventilator's pressure transducer or piston system fails.

In addition to these standard alarms, the PLV-102 has an OXYGEN SYSTEM alarm. This visual alarm is activated whenever the oxygen flow is inadequate or the source pressure falls below 35 psi. This alarm is also activated if oxygen flow is detected during the exhalation phase of a breath because this indicates either a defective flow sensor or oxygen flow at an inappropriate time.

Modes of Ventilation

Control, A/C, and SIMV modes are available on both the PLV-100 and PLV-102. In the control mode, all patient breaths are delivered by the ventilator at a preset V_T, rate, and inspiratory flow. Based on these settings, the T_I is determined and the I:E ratio is displayed on the front panel of the machine. In the A/C mode, the patient's spontaneous effort may pressure-trigger the ventilator to deliver assisted breaths above the minimal rate setting, but the V_T and inspiratory flow rate remain constant at preset values. The I:E RATIO display varies depending on the rate the patient is assisting. In the SIMV mode, the ventilators deliver breaths according to a set minimum respiratory rate, V_T, and inspiratory flow rate, however the patient may breathe spontaneously between these mandatory machine breaths. The patient's spontaneous breaths may come through the air intake valve (on the back panel of the machines), or through a continuous flow H-valve assembly added to the ventilator circuit. The ventilator synchronizes the delivery of mandatory machine breaths with the patient's trigger effort by allowing a 6-second window of time before mandatory breath delivery. If the patient makes an assist effort during this time window, the ventilator's microprocessor responds to this effort and delivers a mandatory SIMV breath.

In addition to the control, A/C, and SIMV modes, two additional modes have been added to the PLV-102 ventilator: control + sigh and A/C + sigh. In either of these modes, a sigh breath at 150% of the set V_T is delivered every 100 breaths.

Oxygen Source

Administering oxygen with the PLV-100 ventilator may be accomplished by bleeding in oxygen through an inlet adapter attached to the patient circuit, or through an accumulator placed at the gas intake port. The addition of oxygen through an inlet adapter increases delivered V_T, and FiO_2 varies depending on the delivered minute volume. In addition, extra flow into the circuit from the oxygen flowmeter may necessitate adjustment of the machine's sensitivity in order for the patient to trigger assisted breaths.

Oxygen-enriched gas can be obtained on the PLV-102 by attaching a high-pressure oxygen hose to the DISS inlet on the back panel of the machine. As oxygen enters, it passes through a proportional valve and flow sensor before going to the internal inspiratory circuit. Based on the set V_T and set oxygen percentage, the microprocessor system controls the proportional valve to deliver the desired FiO_2. When using low V_Ts (<300 mL) and high oxygen percentages (>50%), the accuracy of oxygen delivery cannot be guaranteed.

In the SIMV mode, the use of an oxygen sensor is recommended for more precise control of oxygen levels during spontaneous breathing. The sensor provides feedback to the ventilator's microprocessor system, allowing oxygen to be titrated into the circuit during inspiration of a spontaneous breath. This sensor should be placed in-line with the ventilator circuit, between the humidifier and at least 18 inches from the H-valve or patient outlet. Regardless of mode, oxygen is only delivered during inspiration. The oxygen percent can be set by turning the oxygen % knob on the front of the PLV-102.

AEQUITRON LP6 AND LP10

The LP6 Plus (Figure 12-25) is an identical machine to the LP10 except for the PRESSURE LIMIT control, which gives the operator the option of PCV.

The Aequitron LP6 Plus and LP10 are microprocessor-controlled, volume-targeted ventilators primarily used for

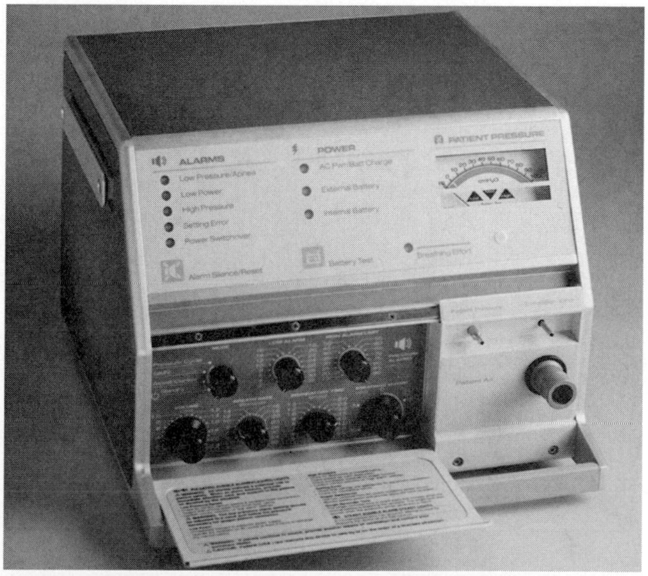

Figure 12-25 The LP6 Plus. (Courtesy Nellcor Puritan Bennett, Pleasanton, Calif.)

home-care ventilation. They are compact (9.25″ × 13.5″ × 12.5″) and lightweight (33 lb) and their versatility in ventilation provides for volume- or pressure-targeted A/C and SIMV modes for pediatric and adult patients (Figure 12-26).

Power Source

Both machines operate on a standard 110- or 220-volt electrical outlet. If there is a power failure or an inability to use an AC outlet, the following alternative power sources are available:

- An external 12-volt battery
- An internal 12-volt battery

The internal 12-volt battery is intended as an emergency back-up only and is able to supply power for 30 to 60 minutes when fully charged. A POWER light display on the front panel enables the operator to see which power source is currently in use. When the AC light is green, the ventilator is using a wall outlet while charging the internal battery. A constant amber light indicates that an external power source in use, and a flashing amber light signifies that the internal battery is in use. When the internal battery is in use, and audible alarm sounds every 5 minutes to remind the operator that the battery is in use. When approximately 5 minutes of energy are left, the LOW POWER alarm rings continuously, signaling the need to change power sources. After using the internal battery, it is imperative to recharge it for at least 3 hours.

Internal Mechanisms

The LP10 uses a rotary drive piston, which delivers a sinusoidal flow waveform to the patient (Figure 12-26). The piston draws gas into the housing through the inlet filter port by means of a downward stroke of the piston. The gas

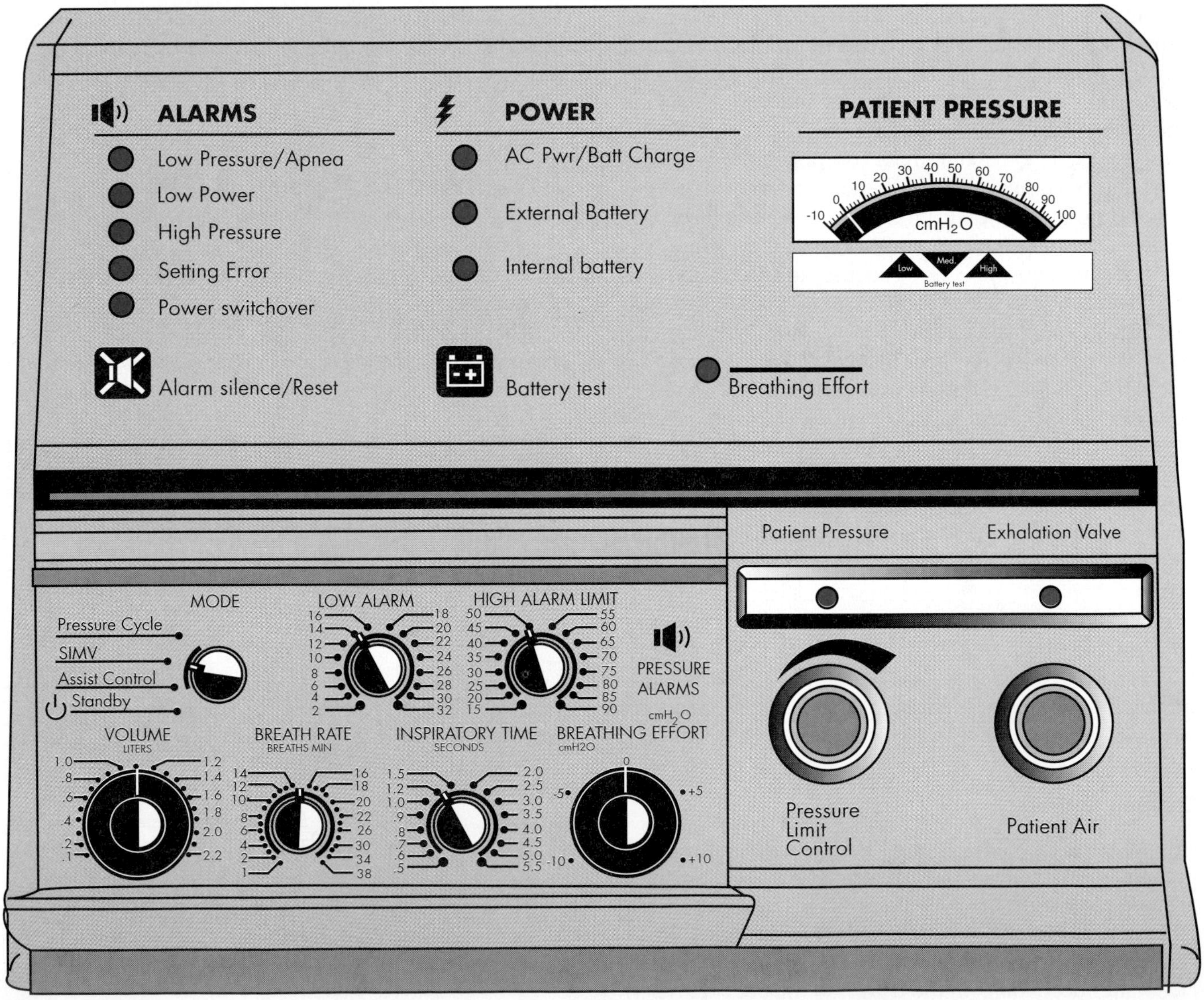

Figure 12-26 The LP10 front control panel. (Courtesy Nellcor Puritan Bennett, Pleasanton, Calif.)

passes a one-way check valve before entering the piston chamber. On the upstroke, the compressed gas moves through another one-way valve and out to the patient circuit and exhalation valve, passing the pressure transducer. The pressure transducer monitors airway pressures and relays the information to the microprocessor (Figure 12-27).

Control Panel and Alarms

The front panel of the LP10 (Figure 12-26) contains several controls for setting parameters and monitoring patient data and alarms.

Tidal Volume

The TIDAL VOLUME control is on the bottom left of the control panel. It has an operational range of 100 to 2200 mL that is adjustable in 100-mL increments.

Rate

The RATE control is on the bottom left part of the control panel (1 to 38 breaths/min) and sets the minimum number of mandatory breaths in A/C and the maximum number of mandatory breaths in SIMV.

Inspiratory Time

The INSPIRATORY TIME control is at the bottom middle of the control panel (0.5 to 5.5 seconds).[3] The T_I and rate are responsible for the T_E and the I:E ratio. The machine does not allow an inverse I:E ratio to be set. If the operator uses inappropriate settings that create an inverse I:E ratio, an alarm sounds and the ventilator delivers the set number of breaths at an I:E ratio of 1:1 (Box 12-17).

BOX 12-17

Decision Making & Problem Solving

The respiratory therapist is using an LP10 to ventilate a home-care patient. The set rate is 15 breaths/min; the T_I is 2.5 seconds; and the V_T is 700 mL. Will the patient receive the full 2.5 seconds of inspiration?

See Appendix A for the answer.

Breathing Effort (Trigger Sensitivity)

The function of this control is to set the threshold required by the patient to trigger a mandatory breath. It has an operational range of −10 to +10 cm H_2O. The BREATHING EFFORT should be adjusted for increased levels of PEEP to prevent any unnecessary increases in the patient's work of breathing.

PEEP

The LP10 does not have an internal PEEP control, but an external valve can be attached to the exhalation manifold. The ventilator allows for PEEP compensation for mandatory breaths by adjusting the trigger sensitivity up to +10 cm H_2O. If the trigger sensitivity is set above the PEEP setting, autocycling may occur. For example, if PEEP is 6 cm H_2O, and sensitivity is +7 cm H_2O, the unit can autocycle.

Alarms

The LP10 monitors several parameters. When the parameters fall outside their acceptable ranges, the ventilator

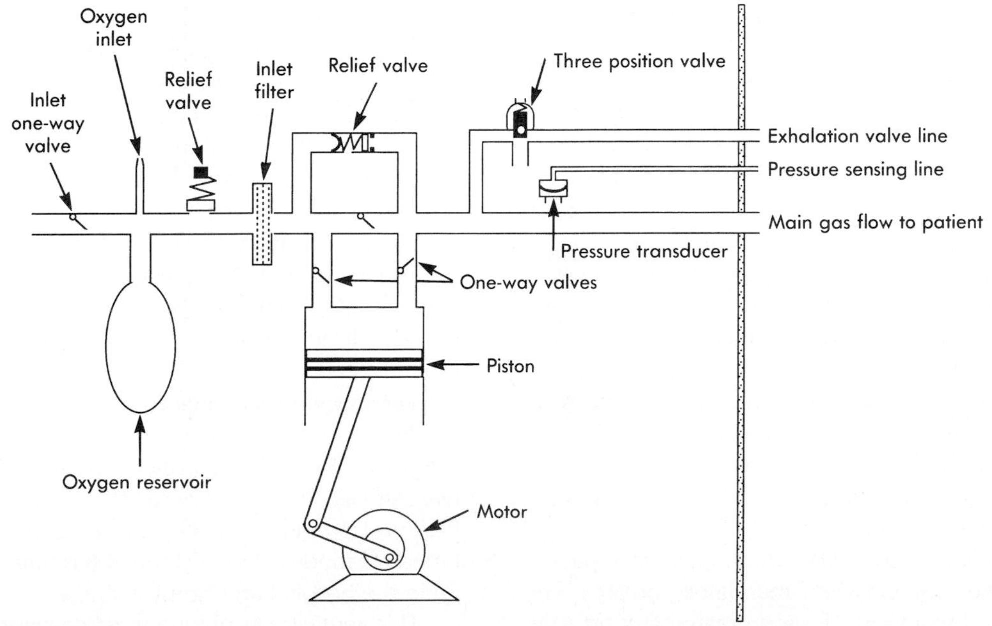

Figure 12-27 A functional diagram of the Aequitron LP6 Plus. (Courtesy Nellcor Puritan Bennett, Pleasanton, Calif.)

alarms to alert the operator to the specific problem. The first of these alarms is the HIGH ALARM/LIMIT, which is only active when the ventilator is working in a volume-targeted mode *without* the PRESSURE-LIMIT control function. When the ventilator is using the PRESSURE-LIMIT control, the alarm only sounds if the pressure-limit valve fails to open. During pressure-cycle ventilation, the HIGH ALARM/LIMIT is used to determine the desired pressure level. It only alarms if the set pressure level is exceeded by 10 cm H_2O or more in this mode.

The LOW-PRESSURE control is at the top middle of the control panel and has an adjustable range of 2 to 32 cm H_2O. When this alarm is activated, the LOW PRESSURE/APNEA light goes on. The problems most commonly associated with this alarm are leaks in the circuit and lack of patient spontaneous breathing efforts. If the set rate is less than 6 breaths/min and the patient fails to trigger a breath within 10 seconds, the LOW PRESSURE/APNEA alarm sounds, and a back-up rate of 10 breaths/min starts. The delivered V_T is the same as that set on the control panel.

There are two basic alarms that monitor the LP10 power sources: the LOW POWER alarm and the POWER SWITCHOVER alarm. The LOW POWER alarm, which is a continuous audible alarm, is activated when approximately 5 minutes of power are left in the internal battery. The POWER SWITCHOVER alarm is activated when the ventilator switches from an AC outlet or an external DC source to the internal battery. Both features are in the ALARMS section of the control panel.

Modes of Ventilation

When using the A/C mode, the operator sets V_T, breath rate, T_I, and trigger sensitivity. In this mode, the patient can initiate mandatory breaths at or above the set rate, but every breath is at the set V_T.

The A/C mode also offers the ability of time-cycled, pressure-limited breaths (PCV). When the PRESSURE LIMIT control function is active, it alters the pressure waveform of the ventilator, allowing for a plateau to occur during inspiration when the set pressure level is achieved. The ventilator vents the excess pressure for the duration of the inspiratory cycle. The PRESSURE LIMIT control is not calibrated; it operates off of a spring-loaded valve. Before the parameters are set, the patient should be disconnected. The operator then occludes the patient wye connector, and rotates the dial until the desired pressure is achieved. After the patient has been reconnected, it is important to closely monitor the pressure because there may be a fall in the set pressure. Further adjustment of the PRESSURE LIMIT control may be necessary if this occurs.

The volume-targeted SIMV mode lets the patient breathe spontaneously between mandatory breaths. The operator sets V_T, breath rate, T_I, and breathing effort (trigger sensitivity). When operating in the SIMV mode, the operator can also use the PRESSURE LIMIT control, which operates the same in SIMV as in A/C.

The pressure-cycle mode operates by limiting the maximum pressure allowed in the patient circuit during inspiration. The ventilator assists or controls the patient- or time-triggered breaths. When the set pressure determined by the high alarm limit is achieved, *inspiration stops*. There is *no* plateau phase. A HIGH-PRESSURE alarm only sounds if the pressure in the airway exceeds the pressure setting by more than 10 cm H_2O.

Oxygen Source

The LP10 can deliver oxygen concentrations greater than 21% by two methods. It bleeds oxygen directly into the patient circuit and can deliver FiO_2s up to 0.4 with this method, but it is important to remember that additional volume is being added to the circuit as well. Be sure to consider this when setting the volume control. The second method of increasing FiO_2 is by delivering oxygen directly into the rear panel air inlet port. This method can provide an FiO_2 of 1.0. When delivering additional oxygen to the LP10, the FiO_2 must be measured as close to the patient as possible with an oxygen analyzer. The machine does not provide a means of measuring FiO_2.

RESPIRONICS BIPAP S/T

The BiPAP unit was the first to provide bi-level positive airway pressure (hence the acronym *BiPAP*). The unit currently has four models: S, S/T, S/T-D, and S/T-D30. The S model was the original BiPAP model, offering bi-level support only in the spontaneous mode. The next ventilator, the S/T, offered spontaneous and timed ventilation, providing the clinician with the ability to use time-triggered and time-cycled breaths. All other basic functions stayed the same as on the S model. The S/T-D and S/TD-30 improved upon the machine's diagnostic abilities and allowed the unit to interface with a recorder to log parameters. The underlying distinction between the S/T-D30 and S/T-D model is the maximum airway pressure the device is able to deliver. The S/T-D30 allows for a maximum pressure of 30 cm H_2O, compared with 20 cm H_2O for the S/T-D model. All discussion of the BiPAP unit here is limited to the S/T version.

The machine is a low-pressure, electrically driven, electrically controlled device. It is 7 3/4 × 9 × 12 3/16 in., weighs 9.5 lb, and can work in the IPAP (Inspiratory Positive Airway Pressure), EPAP (Expiratory Positive Airway Pressure), spontaneous (S), spontaneous/timed (S/T), and timed (T) modes of ventilation. It has traits that make it useful in the hospital and home settings.

This ventilator is unique in its delivery of V_T and flow, and in its internal mechanics. The machine is either flow- or time-triggered, pressure-limited, and flow- or time-cycled and can deliver a square or a decelerating waveform. Because it is used with a mask for its working operations, it uses a flow transducer in series with the patient air outlet to continuously adjust the instantaneous flows to account for leaks (see the discussion of controls in this section).

Power Source

The BiPAP has two potential power sources: AC current or an external DC battery. It neither contains an internal battery nor requires a pneumatic source.

Internal Mechanisms

The unique internal workings of the BiPAP are driven by a blower that is controlled by the microprocessor. Room air is drawn into the unit through the filter on the front panel of the machine and is then directed to the pressure-controlling valve. This electronically controlled valve has two regulating factors: an electric current and a magnetic field. They both function in combination with the microprocessor and flow transducer to react to and compensate for changes in flow and pressure to maintain the desired settings. Once the source gas leaves the pressure-controlling valve, it passes through the flow transducer and then to the patient.

The BiPAP uses a single-circuit patient circuit with an exhaust port and a pressure line to monitor patient flows and pressure changes. The exhaust port may be one of several different types: the Whisper Swivel (most common), Castle Port, or NRV valve. The purpose of these ports is to exhaust CO_2 to room air, and under no circumstance should they be occluded. The occlusion may cause rebreathing of dead space air and improper ventilation of the patient. The proximal pressure line relays information to the microprocessor on the status of flow and volume changes within the patient circuit.

Leak Compensation

Because the BiPAP is flow-triggered for spontaneous breaths, there is a mechanism in place to compensate for the variations in the amount of air leak around the airway interface. There are three mechanisms that continuously monitor and adjust the baseline flow: total flow rate adjustment, expiratory flow rate adjustment, and tidal volume adjustment. Total flow rate adjustment is used when the operator first turns the machine on, or when gross leaks may occur. It establishes a baseline flow as quickly and as accurately as possible so that the flow transducer recognizes spontaneous efforts (i.e., a decrease in baseline flow by 40 mL/sec for 30 msec). The expiratory flow rate and tidal volume adjustments monitor additional parameters, such as no flow conditions and inspiratory and expiratory tidal volumes, in order to fine-tune flow on a breath-to-breath basis.

Control Panel

The BiPAP front panel (Figure 12-28) consists of an ON/OFF switch and a tubing connector for the patient circuit and the proximal pressure line. The remaining functions can be found on the back panel unless the unit is a S/T-D or S/T-D 30 model with the detachable control panel (see the discussion of additional features in this section).

The rear control panel contains the IPAP and EPAP settings, the FUNCTION selector knob, the RATE control knob, and the % IPAP control knob (see Figure 12-28).

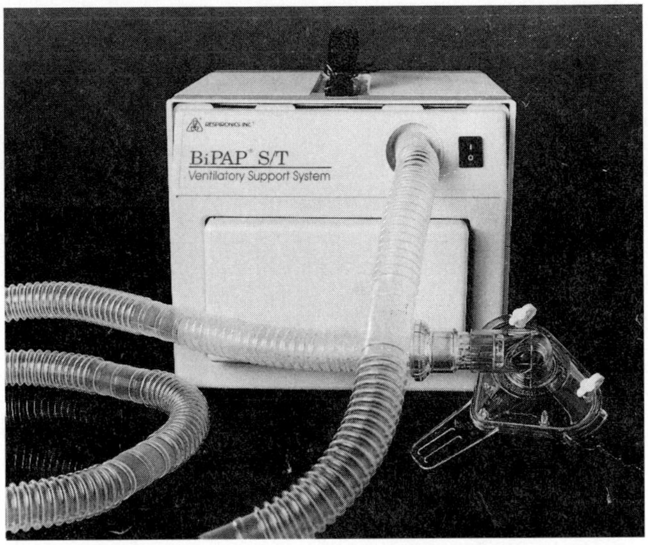

A

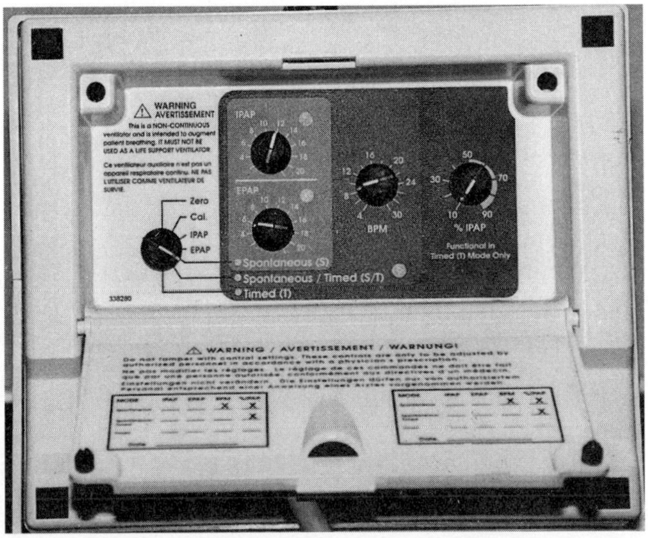

B

Figure 12-28 **A,** front panel of the BiPAP S/T-D; **B,** rear panel. (Courtesy Respironics, Pittsburgh.)

BOX 12-18

Decision Making & Problem Solving

The respiratory therapist notices that the ventilator is not cycling from IPAP to EPAP. The current settings are IPAP = 8 cm H_2O; EPAP = 8 cm H_2O; rate = 10 breaths/min; % T_I = 25%; mode = S/T. What is the problem?

See Appendix A for the answer.

BOX 12-19

Decision Making & Problem Solving

A patient is being supported by the BiPAP in the S/T mode with a rate setting of 6 breaths/min. The spontaneous respiratory rate of the patient is 20 breaths/min. How many time-triggered breaths are delivered to the patient?

See Appendix A for the answer.

IPAP

The IPAP control knob lets the operator set the inspiratory positive airway pressure and is operational in all modes. It is can deliver pressures of 4 to 20 cm H_2O.

EPAP

The EPAP control knob lets the operator set the expiratory positive airway pressure. The machine does allow the EPAP pressures to be set higher than the IPAP pressures. If this happens, IPAP levels are delivered throughout inspiration and expiration until proper adjustments are made (CPAP). This function is operational in all modes and has an adjustable range of 4 to 20 cm H_2O (Box 12-18).

BPM Control (Breaths per Minute)

The BPM control knob lets the operator set the minimal respiratory rate (4 to 30 breaths/min) and is functional in the S/T and T modes. When a timed breath is delivered, the LED under the BPM control is illuminated.

% IPAP Control

This control lets the operator control the fraction of time spent in inspiration during the respiratory cycle. It is only active in the T mode, can be set from 10% to 90%, and is capable of inverse I:E ratios.

Modes of Ventilation

This knob sets the mode the ventilator's mode: timed, spontaneous/timed, spontaneous, or CPAP (IPAP or EPAP).

When the MODE knob is set to the TIMED position, IPAP, EPAP, rate, and % IPAP are activated. The mandatory breaths are time-cycled from inspiration to expiration. The patient may take additional spontaneous breaths over the set rate, but the ventilator does not cycle to the IPAP pressure level but maintains flow to maintain the EPAP setting.

In the spontaneous/timed (S/T) mode, IPAP, EPAP, and rate are set. The machine is flow-triggered by the patient or time-triggered based on the rate setting and the rate of the patient's spontaneous efforts. If the patient's spontaneous rate is equal to or greater than the set rate, all breaths are spontaneously triggered. If the patient fails to trigger a breath within the determined time interval, a time-triggered breath is delivered. In S/T, the RATE control does not guarantee a set number of mandatory breaths, but a set number of breath periods—regardless of whether they are patient- or machine-triggered (Box 12-19).

The spontaneous mode requires IPAP and EPAP pressures to be set; all breaths are flow-triggered and flow-limited by the patient. In this mode, the unit functions like PEEP with pressure support. Every breath depends on patient effort, and pressure is maintained in both the inspiratory and expiratory phases of the respiratory cycle.

Although there is no CPAP position on the MODE selector knob, the machine functions as such when in either the IPAP or EPAP position. When the MODE selector is set to IPAP, the ventilator maintains the pressure set at the IPAP control throughout inspiration and expiration. When the selector is in the EPAP position, the ventilator performs similarly, using the EPAP control setting vs. the IPAP setting. Because pressure is maintained at one pressure level throughout the respiratory cycle, the unit functions as if in a CPAP mode, regardless of the control setting used.

Additional Features

Additional features (Figure 12-29) include the detachable control panel (DCP) and the airway pressure monitor, which are both available on the S/T-D and S/T-D 30 models.[3] The DCP lets the operator control all functions on the rear panel and also includes a selectable display feature. This display feature is an LCD that can provide IPAP or EPAP pressure readings, estimates of exhaled V_T, and estimated circuit leak information to the clinician.

The airway pressure monitor (APM) can continuously monitor circuit pressure. It contains an alarm package that alerts the operator when high and low pressure limits are exceeded, the battery power is low, and the machine is inadvertently turned off. The APM and the DCP enhance BiPAP's patient monitoring.

Oxygen Source

The Respironics BiPAP machine uses room air under normal conditions, but can be modified to increase FiO_2 delivery.

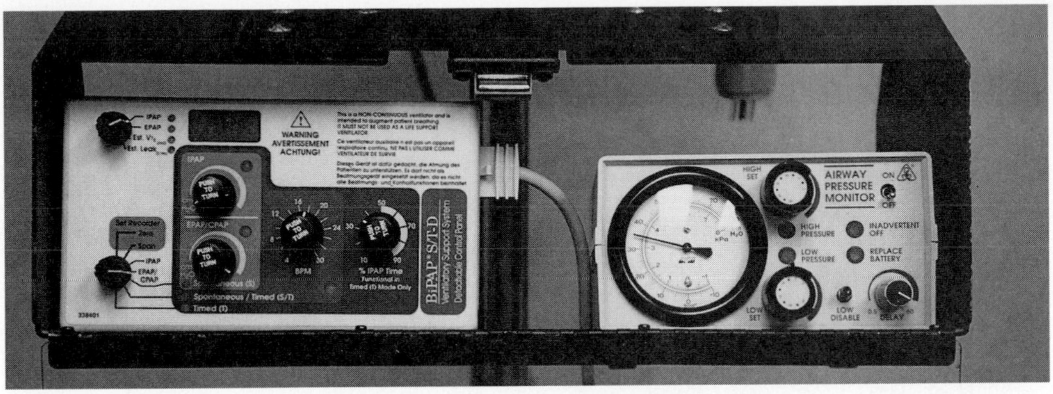

A B

Figure 12-29 BiPAP. **A,** airway pressure monitor (APM); **B,** detachable control panel (DCP). (Courtesy Respironics, Pittsburgh.)

Oxygen may be bled directly into the patient's mask or into an oxygen-enrichment attachment that can be purchased from Respironics. The oxygen-enrichment device is attached to the tubing connector, allowing increased FiO_2 delivery.

HEALTHDYNE QUANTUM PSV

The Quantum PSV (Figure 12-30) is a blower-driven ventilator capable of working in the CPAP, spontaneous, and spontaneous/timed modes. Because of its size (8 × 2.75 × 3 in.) and weight (6.7 lb), it is commonly used in both the hospital and home settings.

Power Source

Unlike many home ventilators, the Quantum PSV only uses one power source, a standard 120-volt AC electrical outlet.

Internal Mechanisms

The Quantum PSV uses a blower-driven, valve-controlled system (Figure 12-31) that can provide various pressure levels to the patient to facilitate airway patency. The machine is either flow- or time-triggered, pressure-limited, and flow- or time-cycled. It uses a flow transducer to continuously adjust the flow output to account for leaks around the patient's mask.

Air is entrained through the inlet filter and passes by the flow sensor, which relays information to the microprocessor that indicates the current status of flow moving to the patient circuit. Next it goes through the controlling valve, which regulates flows and pressures. The controlling valve is electronically governed based on the IPAP, EPAP, rise time, rate, and % I time settings (see the discussion of the control panel in this section for information on specific settings). To flow-trigger a breath, the patient only needs to generate a flow change of 0.25 L/sec. Once in inspiration, the unit measures the peak inspiratory flow and determines 75% of that value. Then it uses this measurement (75%) to determine the flow rate at which to cycle into exhalation. The flow sensor's continuous feedback of information to the microprocessor allows the Quantum PSV to adapt to small or large patient demand changes.

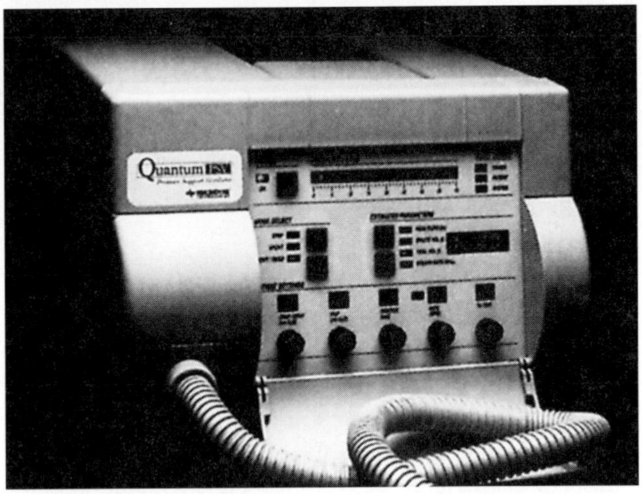

Figure 12-30 The Healthdyne Quantum PSV Ventilator. (Courtesy Respironics, Pittsburgh.)

Control Panel

The Quantum PSV allows for a variety of functions, all of which can be managed with the control panel (see Figure 12-31). The controls that maybe adjusted to accommodate the patient needs are:

1. CPAP/EPAP
2. IPAP
3. % I TIME
4. Rise TIME
5. RATE

The CPAP/EPAP setting is at the lower left of the control panel (2 to 25 cm H_2O). The machine does not let the

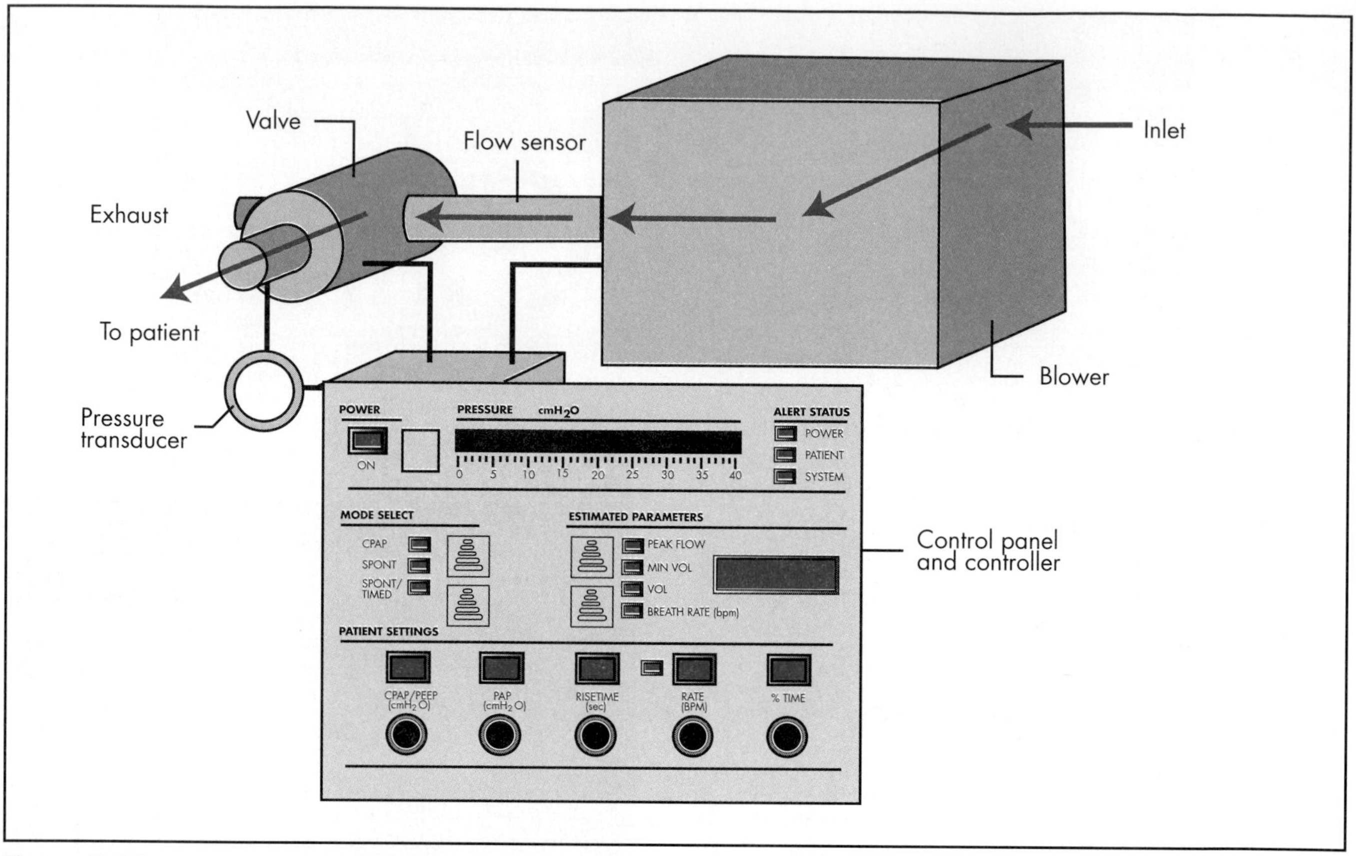

Figure 12-31 A Quantum PSV flow diagram. (Courtesy Respironics, Pittsburgh.)

operator set the EPAP pressures higher than the IPAP pressures. For example, if the IPAP level is 5 cm H_2O and the EPAP level is 7 cm H_2O, then the EPAP level is automatically reduced to 5 cm H_2O and a state of CPAP exists. If this happens, the CPAP mode indicator light flashes.

The IPAP control sets the IPAP (2 to 30 cm H_2O) and should always be set above the EPAP setting, unless in the CPAP mode.

The % I TIME control is only functional in the spontaneous/timed mode. It allows the operator to determine the amount of time spent in inspiration relative to the TCT (10% to 90%). The Quantum allows for inverse I:E ratio ventilation. When the ventilator is initially changed from CPAP or spontaneous to spontaneous/timed, the % I TIME defaults to a setting of 33% until the operator enters the desired setting.

The RISE TIME lets the operator control the rate at which pressure change occurs between IPAP and EPAP, which ultimately affects the pressure curve. It has an operational range of 0.1 to 0.9 seconds and maximizes patient comfort by easing from one phase of the breath cycle into the other. The % I TIME must be set higher than the rise time, or the RISE TIME control flashes, limiting the rise time to maintain the desired T_I. The RISE TIME setting is lowered by using the lowest possible setting, but always remains below the inspiratory time percent (Box 12-20).

BOX 12-20

Decision Making & Problem Solving

The respiratory rate on the Quantum PSV is set at 30 breaths/min; the % T_I is at 0.8 seconds; and the rise time is 0.9 seconds. The therapist notices that the RISE TIME control light is flashing. What is wrong with the current settings?

See Appendix A for the answer.

The RATE control (4 to 40 breaths/min) is at the bottom right of the control panel and is only operational in the spontaneous/timed mode. When the operator changes the ventilator to the spontaneous/timed mode, there is a default setting of 10 breaths/min that automatically appears. Other desired rates have to be entered.

Estimated Parameters

The Quantum estimates the following parameters and presents them in the display window: PEAK FLOW, TIDAL VOLUME, MINUTE VOLUME, and BREATH RATE (all measured on inspiration). The peak flow parameter has a measurable range of 0 to 4.99 L/sec and is determined after the baseline flow and leaks have been measured. Any value above 4.99 L/sec causes the PEAK FLOW display to flash.

The TIDAL VOLUME (0 to 4.99 L) is calculated based on inspiratory flow and T_I. Any value above 4.99 L causes the TIDAL VOLUME display to flash.

The BREATH RATE parameter is an estimate of the spontaneous breath rate plus the timed breath rate (0 to 99 breaths/min) that takes the average of the last four breaths. Any measurement greater than 99 breaths/min causes the display to flash.

The minute volume (0 to 99.99 L/min) is calculated by multiplying the total respiratory rate by the V_T (both estimated parameters).

If the patient does not trigger a breath for more than 20 seconds, all of the estimated parameter windows show "---."

Modes of Ventilation

The Quantum PSV offers three options of ventilatory modes: CPAP, spontaneous, and spontaneous/timed. CPAP is established by setting the EPAP level to the desired pressure setting. The blower and controlling valve work to sustain the flow and pressure selected by the operator to maintain patient comfort.

The spontaneous mode requires an IPAP setting greater than the EPAP setting. The patient flow-triggers the ventilator by reducing the baseline flow by 0.25 L/sec to cycle the machine from EPAP to IPAP. The BREATH RATE and % I TIME settings determine the time spent in IPAP and EPAP. The V_T depends on patient effort.

When operating in the spontaneous/timed mode, the following controls must be set: EPAP, IPAP, RATE, RISE TIME, and % I TIME. The ventilator guarantees that a minimum number of breaths is delivered to the patient, and the rise time and percentage of inspiratory time can be adjusted to improve patient comfort. This mode lets patients initiate and take spontaneous breaths. If the patient does not meet the number of set breaths, the ventilator initiates and delivers a breath.

Oxygen Source

The Quantum delivers room air under normal conditions, but can be modified to increase the F_{IO_2}. A T-adaptor can be placed between the mask and the hose to bleed oxygen into the mask. There is no F_{IO_2} adjuster, so periodic checks with an O_2 analyzer are required to monitor the delivered oxygen.

NONINVASIVE SUPPORT AIDS

Noninvasive support aids are designed to assist the patient with inspiration and/or expiration without applying pressure to the airways.

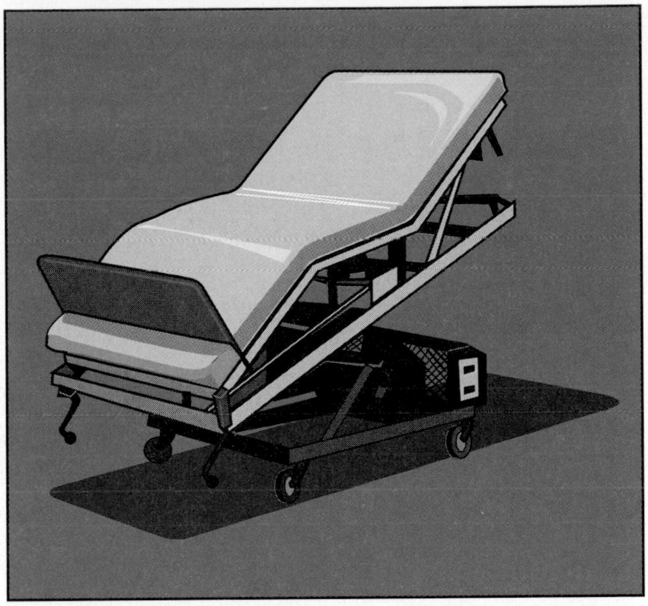

Figure 12-32 A rocking bed.

Rocking Bed

The rocking bed (Figure 12-32) uses gravity to aid and assist in the ventilation of patients with diaphragmatic weakness or paralysis. It functions based on the diaphragm and the abdominal contents, moving with gravity in a see-saw motion. When the bed tilts the head down, the abdominal contents move cephalad (toward the head), aiding in expiration. When the head returns to an upward position, the contents move caudal (toward the feet), aiding in inspiration. The rocking bed can move in a 60-degree arc at 8 to 34 cycles/min.[5] Rates of 12 to 16 cycles/min with a rocking position of near horizontal to 40-degrees feet down are optimal for most people. Although not everyone is able to tolerate the noise and motion, the rocking bed is still a viable means of aiding ventilation.

Pneumobelt

The pneumobelt is a device that consists of three separate parts: a bladder, an adjustable corset, and a positive-pressure generator. It applies a positive pressure over the abdomen during expiration, thereby forcing the diaphragm cephalad. This forced expiratory maneuver decreases functional residual capacity (FRC) and returns the diaphragm to a better length-tension relationship. This allows for an increase in V_T on ensuing inspiratory efforts. (Note that all inspiratory maneuvers are unaided and depend fully on patient effort.)

Before the pneumobelt is attached, the patient should find a comfortable, upright, sitting position. Because effectiveness of the device depends on gravity, the patient must sit at a trunk angle >30 degrees from horizontal.[6] The fit

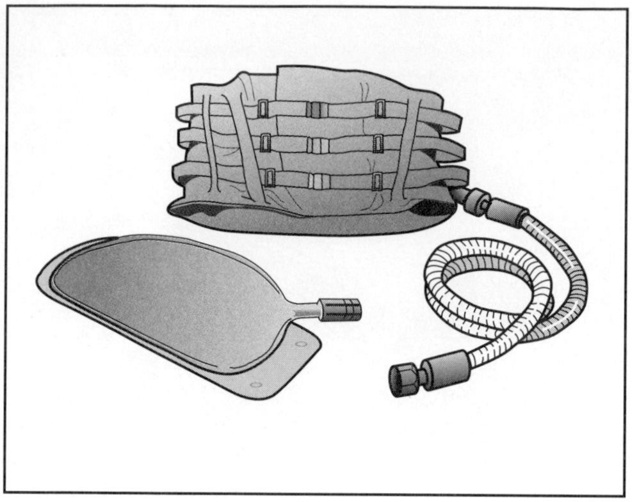

Figure 12-33 A pneumobelt. **A,** corset; **B,** bladder.

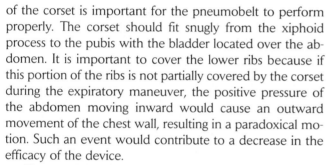

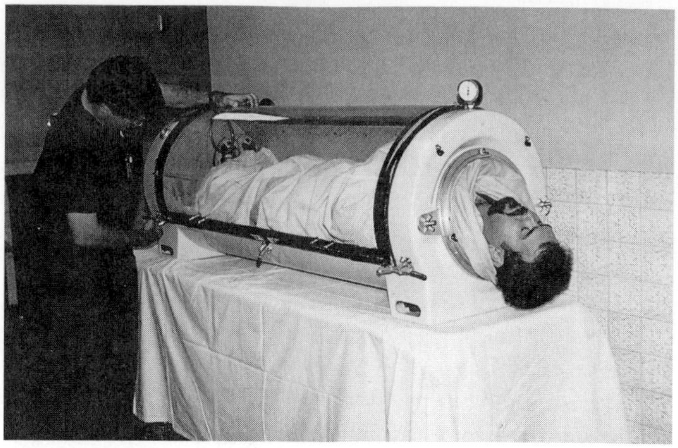

Figure 12-34 A body respirator (iron lung).

of the corset is important for the pneumobelt to perform properly. The corset should fit snugly from the xiphoid process to the pubis with the bladder located over the abdomen. It is important to cover the lower ribs because if this portion of the ribs is not partially covered by the corset during the expiratory maneuver, the positive pressure of the abdomen moving inward would cause an outward movement of the chest wall, resulting in a paradoxical motion. Such an event would contribute to a decrease in the efficacy of the device.

The next step of pneumobelt operation is to determine what inflation pressures to start with. It is not uncommon to start peak inflation pressures at 20 cm H_2O and steadily increase them until an adequate V_T is achieved. Normally, pressures of 30 to 50 cm H_2O are sufficient for acceptable support.[17] The pneumobelt augments V_Ts from 300 to 1200 mL when operated properly. The positive-pressure generator required to run the pneumobelt is of no specific brand or type; any one will do.

Negative-Pressure Ventilators

The following discussion focuses on two main types of negative-pressure ventilators: the iron lung and the chest cuirass, which attempt to mimic normal respiratory mechanics. During inspiration, negative pressure is applied outside the chest cavity, creating a pressure gradient that allows for air flow into the lungs. The greater the pressure gradient, the greater the V_T. Although negative pressure ventilation (NPV) reduces the side effects of positive-pressure ventilation, it is not without its own problems. NPV has been found to increase the risk of influx, induce obstructive sleep apnea, and generate rib fractures and hypotension. In addition, it is noisy; it is hard to ensure a proper seal with it; patient care is hampered; and it creates a feelings of uneasiness in the patient.

NPV has the following three basic modes, depending on the generator's capabilities:

1. Inspiratory negative pressure only
2. Inspiratory negative pressure/positive expiratory pressure
3. Continuous negative pressure

The mode using inspiratory negative pressure only is the most common. Negative pressure only is generated on inspiration to assist or deliver a breath, and exhalation is allowed to occur passively via elastic recoil of the lung. The next mode, negative inspiratory pressure/ positive expiratory pressure, uses positive expiratory pressure similarly to PEEP on traditional positive-pressure ventilators. This mode is not commonly used and has been found to contribute to patient discomfort. The third available option is continuous negative pressure. Negative pressure applied during end-expiration is referred to as NEEP. In addition to aiding in inspiration, NEEP facilitates expiration while allowing for increased respiratory rates and venous return. Its side effects additionally include the risk of airway collapse and ensuing increases in FRC. For these reasons, this later mode of ventilation is not often used. The following devices are machines that use negative pressure to ventilate the patient.

Body Respirator

The body respirator, or the iron lung (Figure 12-34), is a long cylinder that encases the patient from neck to toe, only exposing the head to ambient pressure. The airtight seal created at the neck allows the device to generate subatmospheric pressure around the thorax. The pressure gradient that develops is what lets the body respirator aid or deliver a negative-pressure breath to the patient.

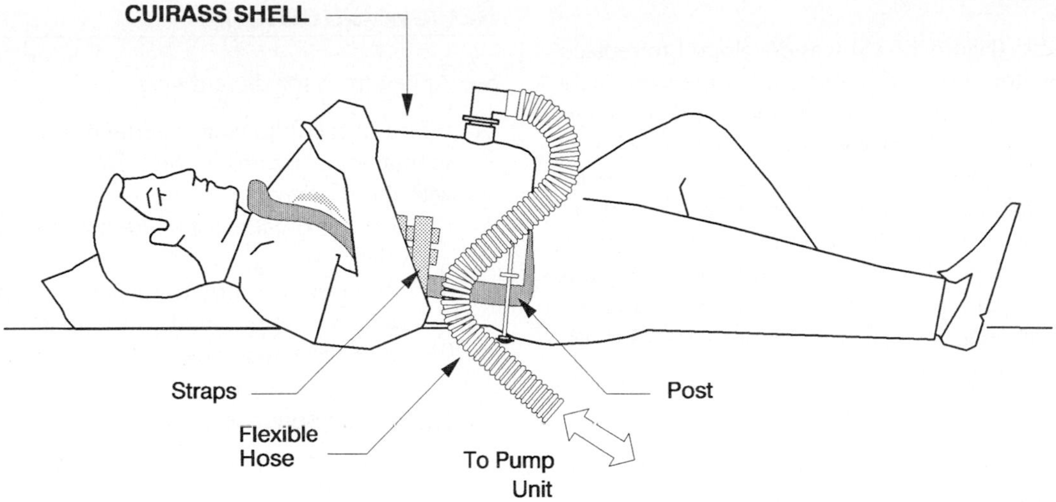

Figure 12-35 A cuirass shell used for negative-pressure ventilation. The patient is placed in the supine position, and the cuirass is stabilized with straps and posts. The method of ventilation is identical to that of the chest shell unit. (Redrawn from Dupuis Y: Ventilators: theory and clinical application, ed 2, St Louis, 1992, Mosby.)

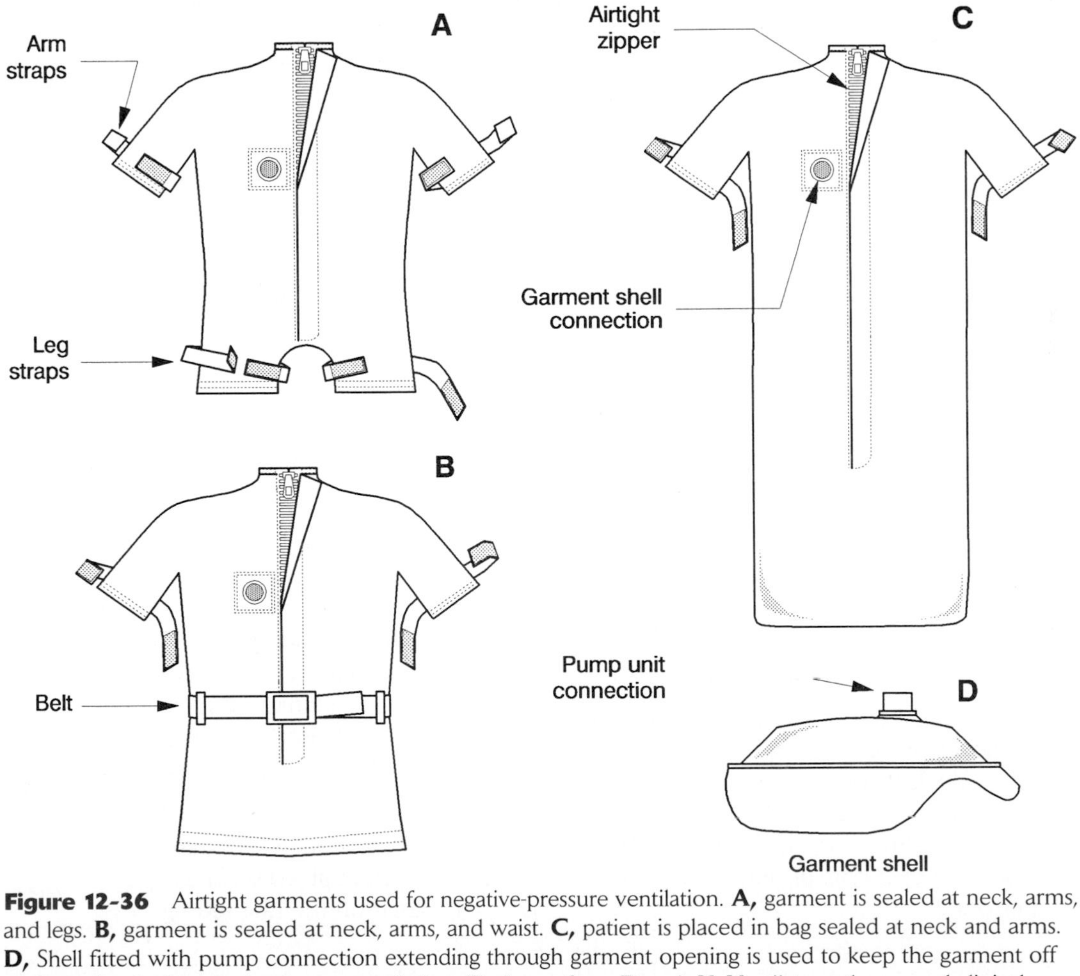

Figure 12-36 Airtight garments used for negative-pressure ventilation. **A,** garment is sealed at neck, arms, and legs. **B,** garment is sealed at neck, arms, and waist. **C,** patient is placed in bag sealed at neck and arms. **D,** Shell fitted with pump connection extending through garment opening is used to keep the garment off of the patient's chest and enhance ventilation. (Redrawn from Dupuis Y: Ventilators: theory and clinical application, ed 2, St Louis, 1992, Mosby.)

Chest Cuirass

The chest cuirass (Figure 12-35) was developed to replace the body respirator; it is smaller and less cumbersome. The cuirass is a rigid shell that covers the thorax and abdomen and is secured to the patient with abdominal straps. A 2- to 3-inch barrier is used between the chest wall and the actual cuirass so that there is no restriction during inspiration. A tight seal is essential for the device to function properly. Therefore, for optimal performance, a custom shell should be made for the patient. A shell that conforms to the patient will have fewer leak problems. This device works with any negative-pressure pump.

Additional NPVs

Additional NPVs are the poncho, the raincoat, and the pneumosuit (Figure 12-36), which use NPV while aiding in patient comfort. The pneumosuit uses a negative-pressure generator and an iron-mesh cage that encapsulates the chest cavity in addition to the suit. The cage allows for a 2- to 3-inch barrier between the chest wall and the suit to prevent negative pressure from being directly applied to the thorax. A seal is made at the neck and extremities (which extremities is determined by the type of suit used), and maintaining these seals is the most common problem associated with this device.

Summary of Home-Care Equipment

With increasing life expectancy and our ability to support diseases once thought to be untreatable, home care is a viable alternative to hospital care. Indihar[7] did a cost-based study comparing five different sites of chronic ventilator care. When comparing the step-down unit in a hospital with home care supported by the family, the costs were reduced by approximately one third. Cost is not the only reason for home-care ventilation, but it is a major reason why it is being so vigorously researched.

When choosing positive-pressure ventilators, invasive or noninvasive techniques, negative-pressure ventilators, or supportive aids, it is important that the patient and family are well-informed of the operations of the machine. They should be aware of the possible problems that might arise and of all the additional power sources available. When looking at supportive devices for the home, choose one that is simple and operator-friendly with clear alarms to alert the operator of any malfunctions. It is important to remember that the primary operators of home-care devices are nonmedical personnel.

Review Questions

See Appendix A for the answers.

1. Which of the following statements is(are) true about spontaneous breaths in the SIMV and CPAP modes with the Bird Avian?
   I. Flow for breaths is provided by the demand valve.
   II. The effort required to trigger spontaneous breaths is determined by the sensitivity setting.
   III. An H-valve assembly with reservoir bag is added to the patient circuit for spontaneous breaths.
   IV. Spontaneous breaths can receive a flow of up to 60 L/min.
   a. III only
   b. I and II only
   c. II, III, and IV
   d. I, II, and IV only
2. The PEEP NOT SET indicator illuminates on the Bird Avian, indicating which of the following?
   a. PEEP is not in use on this patient
   b. The PEEP value deviates from the actual PEEP by more than 5 cm H_2O
   c. PEEP is not available on this ventilator
   d. The sensitivity needs readjusting because the PEEP has been changed
3. Which of the following statements is(are) true about the Hamilton MAX?
   I. The sensitivity is PEEP-compensated.
   II. There is a LOW INSPIRATORY PRESSURE alarm available.
   III. The sensitivity is not adjustable.
   IV. The FiO_2 is adjustable.
   a. III only
   b. I and IV only
   c. I, II and III only
   d. I, II, III, and IV
4. When using the Dräger Microvent, the HIGH PEEP alarm might be activated with which of the following circumstances?
   a. PEEP > Pmax.
   b. There is a leak in the circuit, and PEEP is in use.
   c. There is a kink in the expiratory line.
   d. There is water in the expiratory line.
5. The APNEA alarm on the Oxylog 2000 is:
   a. Adjustable from 10 to 30 seconds
   b. Constant at 15 seconds
   c. Constant at 20 seconds
   d. Based on the rate setting

6. The APNEA alarm on the Uni-Vent 750 is activated; which of the following is(are) true?
   I. An apnea period of 15 seconds has been detected.
   II. The ventilator is either in the A/C or SIMV mode.
   III. A back-up rate of 12 breaths/min at the current settings for V_T delivery starts.
   IV. The anti-asphyxia valve opens, letting the patient breathe spontaneously from room air.
   a. IV only
   b. I and IV only
   c. II and III only
   d. I, II, and IV
7. The POWER SWITCHOVER alarm on the Companion 2801 activates when the:
   a. Ventilator switches to a lower priority source
   b. Unit goes from battery to AC power
   c. Internal battery has <11 volts left
   d. Operator turns the ventilator off
8. During ventilation with the Bear 33, a patient's peak inspiratory pressure exceeds the HIGH-PRESSURE alarm setting. Which of the following will occur?
   a. The excess pressure vents into the room
   b. An alarm sounds
   c. Inspiration ends
   d. A plateau pressure is sustained until the percentage of T_I is reached
9. The INCREASE INSPIR FLOW light on the Lifecare PLV 102 is on. Which of the following statements is(are) true?
   a. The patient's inspiratory flow demand exceeds the set flow
   b. The operator tried set a flow lower than the available flow range
   c. The machine detects airtrapping (auto-PEEP)
   d. Flow is not sufficient to meet the set parameters of V_T, f, and I:E limitations
10. A constant amber light is illuminated on the front panel of the LP10, indicating:
    a. An external power source is in use
    b. PEEP is active
    c. The sensitivity is turned off
    d. The internal battery voltage is adequate
11. The CPAP light on the Quantum PSV is flashing, indicating:
    a. The unit is in the CPAP mode
    b. A HIGH CPAP alarm is active
    c. EPAP is set higher than IPAP
    d. The CPAP level must be set
12. All spontaneous breaths on the Respironics BiPAP S/T are flow-triggered—true or false?
13. The range for the PEEP control on the Companion 2801 is 0 to 30cm H_2O—true or false?
14. The Bird Avian can be time- or volume-cycled—true or false?
15. The Newport E100i can provide either volume- or pressure-targeted mandatory breaths—true or false?
16. When an APNEA alarm activates on the Bear 33, back-up ventilation begins at 12 breaths/min at the set V_T—true or false?
17. You can check the battery voltage on the Lifecare PLV 102 by using the READ BATTERY VOLTS indicator—true or false?

References

1. Dunne PJ and McInturff SL: Respirator home care: the essentials, Philadelphia, 1998, F.A. Davis Co.
2. Gietzen JW, Lund JA, and Swegarden JL: Effect of PEEP placement on function of home-care ventilators, Respir Care 36:1093, 1991.
3. LP10 Volume Ventilator with Pressure Limit clinician's manual, Minneapolis, 1991, Aequitron Medical.
4. BiPAP clinical manual, S/T and S/T-D, Murrysville, Pa., 1990, Respironics, Inc.
5. Quantum PSV operator's manual, Marrieta, Ga., 1997, Healthdyne Technologies.
6. Tobin MJ: Principles and practice of mechanical ventilation, New York, 1994, McGraw-Hill.
7. Indihar SF: Cost of comparison care for chronic ventilator patients, Chest 99:260, 1991.

Bibliography

American Association for Respiratory Care: Clinical practice guideline: transport of the mechanically ventilated patient, Resp Care 38:1169, 1993.

Avian operators manual 4 248C, Palm Springs, Calif., 1995, Bird Products Corp.

Bach JR: The prevention of ventilatory failure due to inadequate pump function, Resp Care 42:403, 1997.

Branson RD, Hess DR, and Chatburn RL: Respiratory care equipment, Philadelphia, 1995, J.B. Lipponcott.

Companion 2801 operator's instructing manual, Marietta, Ga., 1997, Healthdyne Technologies.

Dupuis YG: Ventilators: theory and clinical application, St Louis, 1986, Mosby.

Emerson Negative-Pressure Ventilator, Cambridge, Mass., 1961, J.H. Emerson Co.

Intermed Bear 33 clinical instruction manual 50000-10133, Riverside, Calif., 1987, Bear Medical Corp.
Kacmarek RM, et al: Imposed work of breathing during synchronized intermittent mandatory ventilation provided by five home care ventilators, Respir Care 36:1093, 1991.
Kacmareck RM and Spearman CB: Equipment used for ventilatory support in the home, Respir Care 31:311, 1986.
MAX operator's manual 610253, Reno, Nev, 1991, Hamilton Medical.
Micovent operator's manual, Chantilly, Va., 1995, Dräger Inc.
Newport E100 operator's manual OPR100, Rev B, Newport Beach, Calif., Newport Medical Instruments.
Oxylog operator's instruction manual, Chantilly, Va., 1995, Dräger Inc.
Pilbeam SP: Mechanical ventilation: physiological and clinical applications, ed 2, St Louis, 1986, Mosby.
PLV-100 operating manual, Westminster, Co., 1990, Lifecare Inc.
PLV-102 operating manual, Westminster, Co., 1990, Lifecare Inc.
Uni-Vent 750/750M operator's manual, Rev B, West Caldwell, NJ, 1991, Impact Instrumentation Inc.

Internet Resources

1. Dräger Inc.:
   http://www.draeger.com
2. Hamilton Medical Inc.:
   http://www.hammed1.com
3. Nellcor Puritan Bennett:
   http://www.nellcorpb.com
4. Sensormedics, Inc.:
   http://www.sensormedics.com
5. Siemens Medical Systems, Inc.:
   http://www.siemens.vents

CHAPTER 13

CHAPTER OUTLINE

KEY TERMS

Acid-Fast Bacteria
Aerobes
Airborne
Airborne Precautions
Anaerobes
Autoclave
Bacilli
Bactericide
Chemical Sterilant
Cleaning
Cocci
Contact Precautions
Decontamination
Diplobacilli
Diplococci
Direct Contact
Disinfection
Droplet Precautions
Eukaryotic
Facultative
Fomites
Fungicide
Germicide
Gram-Negative
Gram-Positive
Gram Stain
High-Level Disinfection
Indirect Contact
Infection Surveillance
Intermediate-Level Disinfection
Isolation Techniques
Low-Level Disinfection
Normal Flora
Nosocomial
Pasteurization
Pathogenic
Prokaryotic
Spirochetes
Standard Precautions
Staphylococci
Sterilization
Streptobacilli
Streptococci
Transmission-Based Precautions
Universal Precautions
Vehicles
Vectors
Vibrio
Virucide

Principles of Infection Control

J. M. Cairo

CHAPTER LEARNING OBJECTIVES

Upon completion of this chapter, the reader should be able to:

1. Identify the major groups of microorganisms associated with nosocomial pneumonia.
2. List four factors that can influence the effectiveness of a germicide.
3. Define *high-level disinfection, intermediate-level disinfection,* and *low-level disinfection.*
4. Describe the process of pasteurization and its application to the disinfection of respiratory care equipment.
5. Explain how quaternary ammonium compounds, alcohols, acetic acid, phenols, glutaraldehyde, hydrogen peroxide, and iodophores and other halogenated compounds are used as disinfectants.
6. Name the four physical methods commonly used to sterilize medical devices.
7. Discuss the principle of ethylene oxide sterilization.
8. Identify infection-risk devices used in respiratory care.
9. Compare standard precautions with transmission-based precautions.
10. Describe three components of an effective infection surveillance program.

Preventing **nosocomial** infections is a formidable task for respiratory therapists. It is particularly challenging because devices used for respiratory care are potential reservoirs and **vehicles** for the transmission of infectious microorganisms. Additionally, many patients receiving respiratory care, especially those of extreme age or who are recovering from thoracoabdominal surgery, have an increased risk of developing nosocomial pneumonia. Underlying diseases, depressed sensorium, and immunosuppression can also add to the risk of developing a nosocomial infection.[1]

This chapter is a review of the aspects of microbiology and infection control that respiratory care practitioners must understand to prevent nosocomial pneumonia. Specifically, the following are described here: 1) the microorganisms that are most often associated with nosocomial pneumonia; 2) the accepted methods for **cleaning,** disinfecting, and sterilizing reusable respiratory care equipment; 3) the proper use of **isolation techniques** to prevent person-to-person transmission of microorganisms; and 4) effective methods of **infection surveillance.**

PRINCIPLES OF CLINICAL MICROBIOLOGY

Microbiology is the study of microorganisms such as bacteria, viruses, protozoa, fungi, and algae. All of these organisms, with the possible exception of algae, are **pathogenic** and therefore can produce infectious diseases in susceptible hosts.[4] Clinical microbiology is primarily concerned with the isolation, identification, and control of these pathogenic, or disease-producing, organisms.

Clinical microbiology is put into effect when a patient shows symptoms and signs of an infection. Diagnosis of an infectious disease requires isolating the suspected pathogen from the site of infection. The specimen is then inoculated onto agar or into a broth containing vital nutrients. In many cases, the organism is allowed to grow at body temperature in a specially designed incubator. Note that the collection process must be performed with care and use of aseptic techniques to avoid microbial contamination from adjacent tissue and **normal flora.** Normal flora, which are microorganisms normally found in or on a particular body site, do not normally cause infectious disease, but it is important to recognize that these organisms can present problems because they can overgrow the pathogen and produce erroneous results.

Identification of microorganisms is most often accomplished by directly examining the specimen through microscopy with the aid of biological staining and culturing techniques. Metabolic and immunologic tests may also help clinical microbiologists to discern the nature of the invading microbe, especially as relates to its susceptibility to antibiotics.

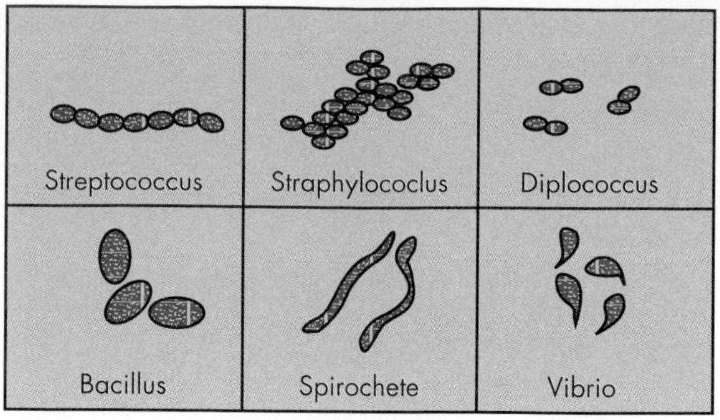

Figure 13-1 The morphology of bacteria: *a,* streptococcus; *b,* staphylococcus; *c,* diplococcus; *d,* bacillus; *e,* spirochete; *f,* vibrio comma.

Control of pathogenic microorganisms relates to eliminating infections and preventing the spread of infectious diseases. Infections are usually eradicated by enhancing the host's innate immunity with antibiotics and immunizations. **Decontamination** of diagnostic and therapeutic medical equipment, furniture, and commonly used items and surfaces, as well as the use of barrier precautions (i.e., isolation precautions) are examples of infection control techniques.

A variety of microorganisms can be isolated from the hospital environment. A brief description of the major groups of pathogenic organisms associated with nosocomial pneumonia follows. More detailed information about the science of microbiology can be found in the references listed at the end of the chapter.[1,2,3]

Survey of Microorganisms

Bacteria

Bacteria are **prokaryotic,** unicellular organisms that range in size from 0.5 to 50 μm. Bacteria are generally classified according to their morphology (shape) and their staining and metabolic characteristics. Certain bacteria are also capable of producing endospores, which are intermediate bacterial forms that develop in response to adverse condition. As is discussed later in this chapter, bacterial endospores can regenerate to vegetative cells when conditions improve.

As Figure 13-1 shows, the primary bacterial shapes are **cocci** (spherical), **bacilli** (rodlike), and **spirochetes** (spiral). Cocci that occur in irregular clusters are called **staphylococci.** Cocci and bacilli that occur in pairs are called **diplococci** and **diplobacilli,** respectively; chains of cocci and bacilli are called **streptococci** and **streptobacilli,** respectively.

Classifying bacteria according to their staining characteristics is usually accomplished with simple staining techniques, such as the **Gram stain** and the **acid-fast stain.**

BOX 13-1

Decision Making & Problem Solving

Laboratory examination of a sputum sample from a febrile patient with a productive cough (purulent, blood-streaked sputum) reveals the presence of Gram-positive diplococci and many segmented neutrophils. Suggest a possible diagnosis based on these findings.

See Appendix A for the answer.

A Gram stain separates bacteria into two general classes: those that retain an initial gentian violet stain after an alcohol wash (**Gram-positive**), and those that do not retain the initial violet stain (**Gram-negative**). Gram-positive organisms appear blue or violet; Gram-negative organisms have a red appearance that results from a counterstain of the red dye safranin. Notable Gram-positive pathogens are *Bacillus anthracis, Streptococcus pneumoniae, Staphylococcus aureus, Corynebacterium diphtheriae,* and *Clostridium* sp. (e.g., *C. botulinum, C. perfringes, C. tetani*). Gram-negative pathogens include *Pseudomonas aeruginosa, Eschericia coli, Klebsiella pneumoniae, Haemophilus influenzae, Serratia marcescens, Bordatella pertussis, Neisseria meningitidis,* and *Legionella pneumophila.*[3] Box 13-1 provides a clinical scenario that shows how Gram stains can be used in the differential diagnosis of lower respiratory tract infections.

Acid-fast stains (also called Ziehl-Neelsen stains) are used to identify bacteria that belong to the genus *Mycobacteria.* These microbes retain a red (carbol-fuchsin) dye after an acid wash, thus ***acid-fast bacteria*** is used synonymously with *Mycobacteria. Mycobacteria tuberculosis* organisms are responsible for pulmonary, spinal, and miliary tuberculosis (TB). The incidence of tuberculosis has increased dramatically during the past decade, especially in patients infected with the human immunodeficiency virus (HIV; see the following discussion of viruses).

Metabolic characterization of bacteria usually involves identifying the substrate requirements for growth or the production of specific enzymes by the microbe. For example, bacteria that require oxygen for growth are called **aerobes,** and those that can grow without oxygen are called **anaerobes. Facultative** bacteria can survive with or without oxygen. Enzyme markers that are commonly quantified include catalase and coagulase.

As mentioned, certain bacteria form endospores under adverse conditions. Endospores are metabolically active life forms that can maintain their viability in the presence of dryness, heat, and poor nutrition. Their robust nature makes them especially resistant to disinfectants and a constant source of concern for infection control personnel. The most notable sources of bacterial endospores are from the aerobic *Bacillus* sp. and the anaerobic *Clostridium* sp.

Table 13-1 lists some commonly encountered bacterial genera along with a summary of their morphologic, staining, and metabolic characteristics.

Viruses

Viruses are submicroscopic parasites that consist of a nucleic acid core surrounded by a protein sheath and range in size from 20 to 200 nm. Viruses are typically described as nonliving because they must invade a living organism in order to replicate. Viruses are generally classified according to their structure (i.e., icosahedral, helical, or complex) and nucleic acid content (i.e., DNA or RNA). They can also be differentiated by the type of host that they invade (i.e., animal, plant, or bacteria).

The most commonly encountered pathogenic viruses are listed in Table 13-2 and include the influenza viruses, paramyxoviruses, adenoviruses, rhinoviruses, enteroviruses, herpes viruses, rubella viruses, hepatitis virus, and human immunodeficiency viruses. Viruses are responsible for a number of respiratory illnesses including the common cold, croup, tracheobronchitis, bronchiolitis, and pneumonia. The hepatitis and HIV viruses are particularly important pathogens because they are spread by **direct contact** (i.e., through sexual contact or blood and serum). Universal isolation precautions were designed to prevent the transmission of these types of infections. Isolation precautions for blood-borne pathogens are discussed in detail later in this chapter.

Rickettsiae and *Chlamydiae* spp.

These unusual microorganisms are intracellular parasites. *Rickettsiae* and *Chlamydiae* spp. are both less than a µm in diameter. Their complex structure makes them resemble bacteria, but they act like viruses because they require a living host to replicate.[4] *Rickettsiae* sp. are transmitted by insects (e.g., lice, fleas, ticks), and *Chlamydiae* sp. are transmitted by contact or the **airborne** route. Common Rickettsial diseases include typhus, Rocky Mountain spotted fever, and Q fever. (Note that Q fever is spread by the aerosol route rather than by insect vectors.) Chlamydial infections are also associated with pneumonia, sinusitis, pharyngitis, and bronchiolitis.[4]

Protozoa

Protozoa are unicellular eukaryotes that occur singly or in colonies. Protozoan infections are common in tropical climates, especially where sanitation is poor or lacking. Common examples of protozoan infections include amebiasis, malaria, and trypanosomiasis.[4] The most important protozoan that can invade the lung and cause pneumonia is *Pneumocystis carinii. Pneumocystis* pneumonia is common in immunocompromised patients—particularly those infected with HIV. Note that although *Pneumocystis* sp. are classified as protozoans, they are more closely related to fungi.[5]

TABLE 13-1

Commonly encountered bacteria along with morphologic, staining, and metabolic characteristics

Genera	Gram stain	Shape/configuration	Aerobic/anaerobic	Species
Bacillus	Positive	Rod, chain	Aerobic	*B. anthracis*
Bordetella	Negative	Rod	Aerobic	*B. pertussis*
Clostridium	Positive	Rod, separate, chain, pairs, palisade	Anaerobic	*C. tetani, C. botulinum, C. perfringens*
Corynebacterium	Positive	Rod, palisade	Aerobic	*C. diphtheriae*
Diplococcus	Positive	Coccus, encapsulated pairs	Aerobic	*D. pneumoniae*
Staphylococcus	Positive	Coccus, clusters	Aerobic	*S. aureus*
Streptococcus	Positive	Coccus, chain	Aerobic	Groups A, B, C, & D
Mycobacterium	Positive	Rod, separate or "cords"	Aerobic	*M. tuberculosis, M. leprae*
Neisseria	Positive	Coccus, pairs	Aerobic	*N. meningitidis*
Proteus	Negative	Rod, separate	Aerobic	*N. mirabilis, N. vulgaris*
Pseudomonas	Negative	Rod, separate	Aerobic	*P. aeruginosa*
Serratia	Negative	Rod, separate	Aerobic	*S. marcescens*
Escherichia	Negative	Rod, separate	Aerobic, facultatively anaerobic	*E. coli*
Klebsiella	Negative	Rod, separate	Aerobic	*K. pneumoniae*
Haemophilus	Negative	Rod, separate	Aerobic	*H. influenzae, H.* haemolyticus, H. *parainfluenzae*
Salmonella	Negative	Rod, separate	Aerobic, facultatively anaerobic	*S. typhi, S. enteritidis*

From Kacmarek RM, Mack CW, and Dimas S: The essentials of respiratory care, ed 3, St Louis, 1990, Mosby.

TABLE 13-2

Commonly encountered viruses

Virus	Transmission route	Diseases
INFLUENZA	Respiratory tract	Tracheobronchitis Pneumonia Susceptibility to bacterial pneumonia
PARAMYXOVIRUSES		
Mumps	Respiratory tract	Parotitis Orchitis Pancreatitis Encephalitis
Measles (rubeola)	Respiratory tract	Rash, systemic illness Pneumonia Encephalomyelitis
Parainfluenza	Respiratory tract	Upper respiratory disease Croup, pneumonia
Respiratory syncytial	Respiratory tract	Bronchitis Bronchiolitis Pneumonia
ADENOVIRUSES	Respiratory tract Conjunctivae	Tracheobronchitis Pharyngitis Conjunctivitis
RHINOVIRUSES	Respiratory tract	Rhinitis Pharyngitis
ENTEROVIRUSES		
Coxsackie	Respiratory tract Gut	Systemic infections Meningitis Tracheobronchitis Myocarditis
Polio	Gut	CNS damage (including anterior horn cells; paralysis)
HERPESVIRUSES		
Herpes simplex	Oral Genital Eye	Blisters—latent infection Keratoconjunctivitis
Varicella Herpes zoster	Respiratory tract	Vesicles—all ectodermal tissues (skin, mouth, respiratory tract)
Cytomegalo-virus	Not known	Usually disseminated disease in newborn and immune deficient
RUBELLA	Respiratory tract	Systemic mild illness, rash, congenitalanomalies in embryo
HEPATITIS	Blood, body fluids	Hepatitis Systemic disease
RABIES	Bites, or saliva on cut	Fatal CNS damage
HIV	Blood, body fluids	AIDS

From Scanlan CL, Spearman CB, and Sheldon RL: Egan's fundamentals of respiratory care, ed 6, St Louis, 1995, Mosby.

Fungi

Fungi are **eukaryotic** organisms that include molds and yeast. Molds consist of chains of cells or filaments called hyphae and reproduce asexually by forming spores. Yeasts are unicellular fungi that reproduce sexually or asexually by budding. Fungal infections or mycoses can occur in normal healthy individuals, but they are more prevalent in patients with compromised immune function (i.e., opportunistic infections). Fungal infections in otherwise healthy individuals are usually caused by *Histoplasma capsulatum, Coccidioides immitis,* and *Blastomyces dermatitidis.* Opportunistic fungal infections are typically caused by *Candida albicans* and *Aspergillus fumigatus.*[3,4]

Transmission of Infectious Diseases

Three elements must be present for infectious material to spread: a source of pathogen, a mode of transmission for

TABLE 13-3

Routes of infectious disease transmission

Mode	Type	Examples
Contact	Direct	Hepatitis A Venereal disease HIV Staphylococcus Enteric bacteria
	Indirect	Pseudomonas Enteric bacteria Hepatitis B and C HIV
	Droplet	Measles Streptococcus
Vehicle	Waterborne	Shigellosis Cholera
	Foodborne	Salmonellosis Hepatitis A
Airborne	Aerosols	Legionellosis
	Droplet nuclei	Tuberculosis Diphtheria
	Dust	Histoplasmosis
Vectorborne	Ticks and mites	Rickettsia, Lyme's disease
	Mosquitos	Malaria
	Fleas	Bubonic plague

From Scanlan CL, Spearman CB, and Sheldon RL: Egan's fundamentals of respiratory care, ed 6, St Louis, 1995, Mosby.

the infectious agent, and a susceptible host. Nosocomial pneumonia is most often caused by bacteria; viruses and fungi contribute to a lesser extent. The most common source of pathogenic microorganisms is infected patients, but contaminated water, food, and medications are also sources of infectious material.

Infectious particles can be transmitted by four routes: contact, vehicles, airborne, and vectors (Table 13-3). Direct contact occurs when the infectious organism is physically transferred from a contaminated person to a susceptible host through touching or sexual contact. **Indirect contact** involves transfer of the infectious agent to a susceptible host via a fomite (e.g., clothing, surgical bandages, instruments, or equipment).[2] Transfer of infectious materials by vehicles most often occurs through contaminated water and food, although intravenous fluids, blood and blood products, and medications can also occasionally harbor infectious particles.[6] Airborne or respiratory transmission involves the transfer of infectious particles through aerosol droplets and dust particles. Infectious agents are transferred by the vector route when an insect transfers the infectious particle from a host to susceptible individual.[4] Transmission of infections by vectors is rarely associated with nosocomial infections. See Box 13-2 to test your understanding of infection transmission.

BOX 13-2

Decision Making & Problem Solving

As was already discussed, infectious agents can be transmitted by a variety of means, including contact, vehicles, airborne, and vector routes. Identify the most probable means of transmission for the following infectious particles.

- *Pseudomonas aeruginosa* organisms
- HIV
- *Mycobacteria tuberculosis* organisms
- *Rickettsiae* sp.

See Appendix A for the answers.

A variety of mechanical and immunological factors usually protect the host from becoming infected with pathogenic organisms.[6] Alterations of mechanical barriers occurring when skin and mucous membranes are breached during surgery, endotracheal intubation, or placement of indwelling catheters can significantly increase an individual's risk of developing a nosocomial infection. Defects in immune function that occur because of an underlying disease or as a result of therapeutic interventions (e.g., radiation therapy or pharmacological therapies) can also increase the risk for infection. Table 13-4 lists several conditions, possible precipitating causes, and common pathogens associated with hospitalized patients at risk for developing nosocomial infections.

Infection Control Methods

The purpose of any hospital infection control program is to prevent the spread of nosocomial infections. The two most important concepts to understand about infection control are decontamination of patient care items and isolation precautions.

Decontamination, or the removal of pathogenic microorganisms from medical equipment, is accomplished by cleaning, **disinfection,** and **sterilization** with an appropriate **germicide** (i.e., an agent that destroys pathogenic microorganisms). Cleaning is the removal of all foreign material, particularly organic matter (e.g., blood, serum, pus, and fecal matter) from objects with hot water, soap, detergent, and enzymatic products. Disinfection is the removal of all pathogenic microorganisms except bacterial endospores. Liquid chemicals and **pasteurization** are the most common disinfection methods used. Sterilization is the elimination of all forms of microbial life. It can be accomplished by either physical or chemical processes.

TABLE 13-4

Medical conditions and common pathogens in hospitalized patients with increased susceptibility to nosocomial infections

Condition	Possible cause	Common pathogens
Skin and mucosal barrier disruption	Burns	*Staphylococcus aureus*
	Foley catheter	*Pseudomonas aeruginosa*
	IV catheter	*Enterobacteriaceae* species
	Surgical wound	Candida
	Endotracheal tube	
Neutropenia	Oncochemotherapy	*P aeruginosa*
	Drug reactions	*Enterobacteriaceae species*
	Autoimmune process	*Staphylcoccus epidermidis*
	Leukemia	*Staphylcoccus aureus,* Aspergillus
Disruption of normal flora	Antibiotic therapy	*Clostridium difficle*
	Oncochemotherapy	Candida
Altered T-cells	Cushing's syndrome	Mycoplasma tuberculosis
	Corticosteroid therapy	Fungal infections
	Hodgkins' disease	Herpes viruses
	AIDS	*Pneumocystis carinii*
	Organ transplantation	Toxoplasmosis
Hypogammaglobulinemia	Nephrotic syndrome	*Streptococcus pneumoniae*
	Multiple myeloma	*Hemophilus influenzae*
		Enterobacteriaceae species
Hypocomplementemia	Systemic lupus erythematosus	*Neisseria menigitidis*
	Liver failure	*Streptococcus pneumoniae*
	Vasculitis	*Enterobacteriaceae* species

From Chatburn RL: Decontamination of respiratory care equipment: what can be done, what should be done, Respir Care 34(2):98, 1989.

Factors Influencing the Effectiveness of Germicides

As was just stated, germicides are agents used to destroy pathogenic microorganisms. They destroy these microorganisms by damaging their cell membranes, denaturing their protein, or disrupting their cellular processes.[2] **Bactericides** destroy all pathogenic bacteria; **virucides** destroy viruses; and **fungicides** kill fungi. Note that *germicide* is a general term used to describe agents that destroy pathogenic microorganisms on living tissue and inanimate objects; *disinfectant* is used to describe agents that destroy pathogenic microorganisms on inanimate objects only.[7]

A number of factors can affect disinfection and sterilization, including the number, location, and innate resistance of the microorganisms; the concentration and potency of the germicide; the duration of exposure to the germicide; and the physical and chemical environment in which the germicide is used.[8] A brief discussion of several key points to remember when using germicides follows.

Number and Location of Microorganisms

The amount of time required to kill microorganisms is roughly proportional to the number of microorganisms present. Cleaning helps to reduce the number of microbes to a manageable number. The location of the microorganisms can also influence the effectiveness of a germicide because physical barriers can prevent contact of the germicide and the microbe. Thus it is imperative that the germicidal agent has direct contact with any part of the device that is exposed to potential pathogens. Therefore proper disassembly (and assembly) of equipment during the decontamination process can be a limiting factor when assessing the effectiveness of a physical or chemical agent.

Microbial Resistance

The presence of microbial capsules can increase a microorganism's resistance to disinfection and sterilization. This resistance is generally overcome by increasing the exposure time of the germicide to the microbe. Bacterial spores are the most resistant microbes, followed by my cobacterium, nonlipid or small viruses, fungi, lipid or medium viruses, and vegetative bacteria (e.g. *Staphylococcus* and *Pseudomonas* spp.). The resistance of Gram-positive and Gram-negative microorganisms to disinfection and sterilization is similar, except for *Pseudomonas aeruginosa,* which shows greater resistance to some disinfectants.[9,10]

Concentration and Potency of the Germicide

In general, a disinfectant's potency increases as its concentration increases. (Iodophors are an exception to this statement.) It is important to remember, however, that

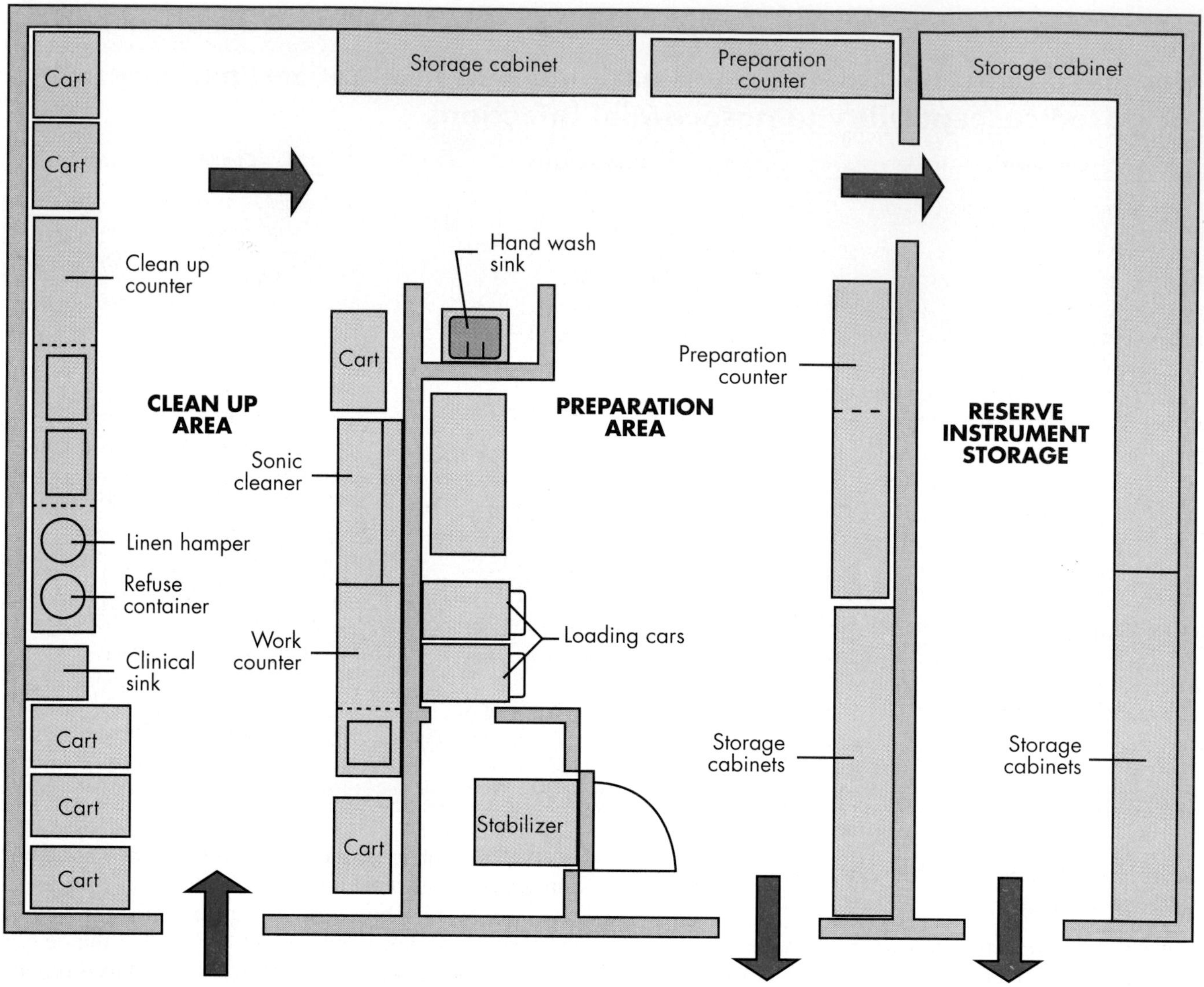

Figure 13-2 Schematic illustrating a typical cleaning area for respiratory care equipment. (Redrawn from Perkins JJ: Principles and methods of sterilization in health sciences, Springfield, Ill., 1978, Charles Thomas.)

germicides are affected differently by concentration adjustments. That is, diluting a germicide influences the amount of time required for disinfection or sterilization.

Physical and Chemical Factors

The effectiveness of a germicide depends on the temperature, pH, and relative humidity of the environment in which it is used. Generally, the activity of most germicides increases as the temperature increases. Increasing the pH improves the antimicrobial activity of some disinfectants (e.g., glutaraldehyde and quaternary ammonium compounds); increasing alkalinity of other agents decreases their effectiveness (e.g., phenols, hypochlorites, iodine). Relative humidity is an important determinant of the activity of gaseous disinfectants (e.g., ethylene oxide and formaldehyde).

Cleaning

Cleaning is the first step in the decontamination process. Figure 13-2 is a schematic of a typical cleaning area for respiratory care equipment. Note that the space is divided into dirty and clean areas with separate entries and exits. This design helps to ensure that clean equipment is not mixed or contaminated with soiled items.

The cleaning process usually begins with disassembly of the equipment to help ensure that dirt and organic matter are removed from surfaces that are not necessarily visible when the device is assembled. Ultrasonic systems are sometimes used for cleaning equipment with crevices that are difficult to clean. These ultrasonic devices create small bubbles that can penetrate and dislodge dirt and organic material, particularly in hard-to-reach crevices.

As stated, cleaning is usually done with soaps, detergents, and enzymatic products. Soaps and detergents contain amphipathic molecules that help dissolve fat and grease by reducing surface tension so that water can penetrate the organic matter. The amphipathic nature of these agents relates to their ability to dissolve both polar and nonpolar molecules. That is, they can dissolve polar or water-soluble (hydrophilic) substances, as well as nonpolar or water-insoluble (hydrophobic) substances. Soaps are not bactericidal but may be combined with a disinfectant. Detergents are weakly bacteriocidal against Gram-positive organisms but they are not effective against tubercle bacilli and viruses.[4]

Cleaning can be done by hand with a scrub brush or with an automatic system. These automatic systems are similar to dishwashers found in the home. Dirty equipment goes through a series of wash and rinse cycles before automatically undergoing pasteurization or cold disinfection.

Once the equipment is cleaned, it should be dried to remove residual water because moisture can alter the effectiveness of disinfectants and sterilizing agents. For example, water can dilute the disinfectant or change its pH.[7] Residual moisture can also combine with ethylene oxide to form ethylene glycol, a toxic chemical that is difficult to remove.[4] To avoid recontamination, equipment should be reassembled in a clean area separate from the area for processing soiled equipment. Clean equipment should never be allowed to sit on open counters for a prolonged time.

Disinfection

By definition, disinfection differs from sterilization because it lacks sporicidal properties.[8] Disinfection can be accomplished by physical and chemical methods. Pasteurization is the most common physical method of disinfection. Quaternary ammonium compounds, alcohols, acetic acid, phenols, iodophores, sodium hypochlorite, glutaraldehyde, and hydrogen peroxide are examples of chemical disinfectants. Table 13-5 lists some commonly used disinfectants and their germicidal properties.

It is important to note that certain disinfectants (e.g., hydrogen peroxide, peracetic acid, and glutaraldehyde) can eliminate spores with sufficient exposure time (i.e., 6 to 10 hours). Disinfectants that can eliminate spores are called **chemical sterilants. High-level disinfection** occurs when chemical sterilants are used at reduced exposure times (<45 min). High-level disinfectants kill bacteria, fungi, and viruses, but do not kill high-level bacterial spores. **Intermediate-level** disinfectants remove vegetative bacteria, tubercle bacteria, viruses, and fungi, but do not necessarily kill spores. **Low-level** disinfectants kill most vegetative bacteria, some fungi, and some bacteria. Box 13-3 summarizes the properties of an ideal disinfectant.

Pasteurization

Pasteurization uses moist heat to coagulate cell proteins. The exposure time required to kill vegetative bacteria depends on the temperature. Two techniques are commonly used: the flash process and the batch process. In the flash process, the material to be disinfected is exposed to moist heat at 72° C for 15 seconds. With the batch process, equipment is immersed in a water bath heated to 63° C for 30 minutes. The batch process can kill all vegetative bacteria and some viruses, including HIV. The flash process is used to pasteurize milk and other heat-labile liquids. Most respiratory care equipment can withstand the conditions of the batch process.

Quaternary Ammonium Compounds

Quaternary ammonium compounds (Quats) are organically substituted ammonium compounds that are cationic detergents containing four alkyl or heterocyclic radicals and a halide ion. The halide may be substituted by a sulfate radical. They are thought to interfere with the bacteria's energy-producing enzymes, denature its essential cell proteins, and disrupt the bacterial cell membrane.[8,11,12] Quats are bactericidal, fungicidal, and virucidal against lipophilic viruses. They are not sporicidal or tuberculocidal or virucidal against hydrophilic viruses. They are inactivated by organic material and their effectiveness is reduced by cotton and gauze pads, which may absorb some of their active ingredients.[8] Quats are routinely used to sanitize noncritical surfaces (e.g., floors, walls, and furniture) and can generally retain their activity for as long as 2 weeks if they are kept free of organic material.[7]

Alcohols

Ethyl and isopropyl alcohol are the two most common alcohols used for disinfection. Both are bactericidal, fungicidal, and virucidal and do not kill bacterial spores. The optimum concentrations of both alcohols range from 60% to 90%. Their ability to disinfect decreases significantly at concentrations below 50%.[8]

It is thought that alcohols kill microorganisms by denaturing proteins. This is a reasonable hypothesis considering that absolute ethyl alcohol, a dehydrating agent, is less bactericidal than an ethyl alcohol and water mixture because proteins are denatured more quickly in the presence of water.[13] Although alcohols have been shown to be effective in fairly short periods (<5 min), the Centers for Disease Control (CDC) recommend that exposure times of 15 minutes be required for 70% ethanol.[7]

Alcohols are used to disinfect rubber stoppers of multiple-use medication vials, oral and rectal thermometers, stethoscopes, and fiberoptic endoscopes. They can also be used to clean the surfaces of mechanical ventilators and areas used for medication preparation.[8] Alcohols are good solvents, and therefore can remove shellac from

TABLE 13-5

Germicidal properties of disinfectants and sterilization agents

			Inactivates*					
Germicide	**Use-dilution**	**Level of disinfection**	**Bacteria**	**Lipophilic viruses**	**Hydrophilic viruses**	**M. *tuberculosis***	**Mycotic agents**	**Bacterial spores**
Isopropyl alcohol	60% to 95%	Int	+	+	−	+	+	
Hydrogen peroxide	3% to 25%	CS/High	+	+	+	+	+	±
Formaldehyde	3% to 8%	High/Int	+	+	+	+	+	±
Quaternary ammonium compounds	0.4% to 1.6% aqueous	Low	+	+	−	−	±	
Phenolic	0.4% to 5% aqueous	Int/Low	+	+	±	+	±	
Chlorine	100 to 1000 ppm free chlorine	High/Low	+	+	+	+	+	±
Iodophors	30 to 50 ppm free iodine	Int	+	+	+	±	±	
Glutaraldehyde	2%	CS/High	+	+	+	+	+	±

TABLE 13-5 (Cont'd)

Germicidal properties of disinfectants and sterilization agents

Important characteristics									Approximate cost (in dollars)	
Shelf life >1 week	Corrosive/ deleterious effects	Residue	Inactivated by organic matter	Skin irritant	Eye irritant	Respiratory irritant	Toxic	Easily obtainable	Purchase ($)/gal	Cost ($)/gal at use-dilution
+	±	−	+	±	+	−	+	+	3.70 (70%)	3.70 (70%)
+	−	−	±	+	+	−	+	+	24.50 (6%)	24.50 (6%)
+	−	+	−	+	+	+	+	+	38.42 (37% wt)	3.84 (3.7% wt)
+	−	−	+	+	+	−	+	+	10.77	.04 (0.4%)
+	−	+	±	+	+	−	+	+	9.70–15.70	.06 (0.4%) .08 (0.8%)
+	+	+	+	+	+	+	+	+	1.00 (5.25%)	.10 (0.5%)
+	±	+	+	±	+	−	+	+	10.10 10%	.05 (0.05%)
+	−	+	−	+	+	+	+	+	6.50–14.00	6.50–14.00

*Inactivates all indicated microorganisms with a contact time of 30 min or less, except bacterial spores, which require 6–10 hr contact time.

Abbreviations: *Int,* intermediate; *CS,* chemical sterilant; +, yes; −, no; ±, variable results.

From Rutala WA: Disinfection, sterilization, and waste disposal. In Wenzel RP, editor: Prevention and control of nosocomial infections, Baltimore, 1997, Williams and Wilkins.

BOX 13-3

Properties of an Ideal Disinfectant

Broad Spectrum
Should have a wide antimicrobial spectrum

Fast Acting
Should produce a rapid kill

Not Affected by Environmental Factors
Should be active in the presence of organic matter (e.g., blood, sputum, feces) and compatible with soaps, detergents, and other chemicals encountered in use

Nontoxic
Should not be irritating to the user

Surface Compatibility
Should not corrode instruments and metallic surfaces and should not cause the deterioration of cloth, rubber, plastics, and other materials

Residual Effect on Treated Surface
Should leave an antimicrobial film on the treated surface

Easy to Use

Odorless
Should have a pleasant odor or no odor to facilitate its routine use

Economical
Cost should not be prohibitively high

Solubility
Should be soluble in water

Stability
Should be stable in concentrate and use dilution

Cleaner
Should have good cleaning properties

From Rutala WA: Disinfection, sterilization, and waste disposal. In Wenzel RP, editor: Prevention and control of nosocomial infections, Baltimore, 1997, Williams and Wilkins.

equipment surfaces. They can cause swelling and hardening of rubber and plastic tubes after prolonged and repeated use.

Acetic Acid

Acetic acid (white household vinegar) is used extensively as a method for decontaminating home-care respiratory care equipment. It is also used in hospitals, but on a limited basis. Because of its acidic nature (pH ~2), its presumed mechanism of bactericidal action is lowering a microbe's intracellular pH thus inactivating its energy-producing enzymes.

The optimum concentration of acetic acid is 1.25%, which is the equivalent of one part 5% white household vinegar and three parts water. It has been shown to be an effective bactericidal agent (particularly against *Pseudomonas aeruginosis*), but its sporicidal and virucidal activity has not been documented.[14]

Peracetic acid, or peroxyacetic acid, is acetic acid to which an oxygen atom has been added. It has been shown to be an excellent disinfectant with sterilization capabilities.[4] Peracetic acid is a strong oxidizing agent that kills microbes by denaturing proteins, disrupting cell wall permeability, and oxidizing cellular metabolites.[15] Its strong oxidizing action is also a shortcoming because it can corrode brass, iron, copper, and steel.[8]

Phenols

Carbolic acid, the prototype of these six-carbon aromatic compounds, was first used as a germicide by Lister in his pioneering work on antiseptic surgery.[8] Although carbolic acid is no longer used as a disinfectant, chemical manufacturers have synthesized numerous phenol derivatives that have been shown to be effective bactericidal, fungicidal, virucidal, and tuberculocidal agents. (Note that these derivatives are not sporicidal.) Phenol derivatives contain an alkyl, phenyl, benzyl, or halogen substituted for one of the hydrogen atoms attached to the aromatic ring. Commonly used phenols include orthophenylphenol and orthobenzylparachlorophenol.

Phenols kill microbes by denaturing proteins and injuring the cell wall. They are primarily used as surface disinfectants for floors, walls, and countertops. Phenols are readily absorbed by porous material, and residual disinfectant can cause skin irritation. They have been associated with hyperbilirubinemia in neonates when used as disinfectants in nurseries.[16]

Iodophors and Other Halogenated Compounds

An iodophor is a solution that contains iodine and a solubilizing agent or carrier. This combination results in a chemical that provides a sustained release of free iodine in an aqueous solution.[8] The best known iodophor is povidone-iodine, which is used as an antiseptic and disinfectant.

Iodophors penetrate the cell wall of microorganisms, and their mode of action is thought to be disruption of protein and nucleic metabolisms. They are bactericidal, tuberculocidal, fungicidal, and virucidal, but are not effective against bacterial spores. Note that solutions formulated for antiseptic use are not suitable for disinfectant use because antiseptic solutions contain significantly less free iodine than those formulated as disinfectants.

Sodium hypochlorite contains free available chlorine in an aqueous solution. Three forms of chlorine are present in the sodium hypochlorite mixture: free chlorine (Cl_2), hypochlorite anion (OCl^-), and hypochlorous acid (HOCl). It has been suggested that these forms of chlorine kill microbes by interfering with cellular metabolism, denaturing proteins, and inactivating nucleic acids.[8,17,18] Sodium hypochlorite (household bleach) demonstrates a range of -cidal activities. A 1:100 dilution is bactericidal, tuberculocidal, and virucidal in 10 minutes, and fungicidal in 1 hour. The CDC recommends that a 1:10 dilution is used to clean blood spills.[4,19] It is not, however, sporicidal. Although sodium hypochlorite is inexpensive and relatively fast-acting, it is corrosive to metals. It forms bischloromethyl ether (a carcinogen) when it comes in contact with formaldehyde and trihalomethane when hot water is hyperchlorinated. It has a limited shelf life and is inactivated by organic matter.

Glutaraldehyde

Glutaraldehyde solutions are some of the most common disinfectants used in respiratory care departments. As stated, these solutions can be used as chemical sterilants if exposure time is extended. They kill microbes by alkylating hydroxyl, sulfhydryl, carboxy, and amino groups of microorganisms, which ultimately interferes with protein synthesis.[8] Alkaline and acid glutaraldehyde solutions are commercially available.

Alkaline glutaraldehyde is packaged as a mildly acidic solution (2% glutaraldehyde) that is activated with a bicarbonate solution, yielding a solution with a pH of 7.5 to 8.5. It is bactericidal, fungicidal, tuberculocidal, and virucidal with an exposure time of 10 minutes. It is sporicidal with an exposure time of 6 to 10 hours. The average shelf life of alkaline glutaraldehyde is 14 days to 1 month. It is irritating to skin and mucous membranes (particularly the eyes). The Occupational Safety and Health Administration (OSHA) therefore limits exposure of workers to 0.2 ppm airborne alkaline glutaraldehyde. Gloves should be worn to avoid dermatitis.[20,21]

Acid glutaraldehyde, which has a pH of 2.7 to 3.7, is available as a 2% solution that does not require activation and comes ready-to-use. Acid glutaraldehyde is similar to alkaline glutaraldehyde in its -cidal activity; it is bactericidal, tuberculocidal, and fungicidal. Note that exposure time must be extended to 20 minutes for acid glutaraldehyde to be tuberculocidal. The activity of an acid glutaraldehyde solution can be enhanced by warming it to 60° C. At this temperature, acid glutaraldehyde is bactericidal, fungicidal, and virucidal in 5 minutes; tuberculocidal in 20 minutes; and sporicidal in 60 minutes.[4] Acid glutaraldehyde is not irritating to skin and mucous membranes like alkaline glutaraldehyde. Its shelf life is approximately 30 days.

Hydrogen Peroxide

Commercially available 3% solutions of hydrogen peroxide are effective disinfectants of bacteria (including Mycobacteria), fungi, and viruses, and are active within 10 minutes at room temperature. Higher concentrations (6% to 25%) and prolonged exposure are required for sterilization. Hydrogen peroxide is sporicidal in 6 hours at 20° C; it is effective against spores in 20 minutes at 50° C.[8]

Hydrogen peroxide kills microorganisms by forming hydroxyl radicals that can attack membrane lipids, nucleic acids, and other essential compounds. Note that catalase-positive aerobes and facultative anaerobic bacteria can inactivate metabolically produced hydrogen peroxide by degrading it into water and oxygen.

Sterilization

Like disinfection, sterilization techniques are generally divided into physical and chemical methods. Physical methods most often rely on heat, specifically dry heat, boiling water, steam under pressure (**autoclave**), and incineration. Ionizing radiation (i.e., gamma and x-rays) has also been shown to be an effective method of sterilization; however, this method is used on a limited basis in the hospitals. The most commonly used chemical for sterilization is ethylene oxide. See Table 13-5 for a comparison of the advantages and disadvantages of various sterilization methods.

Heat

Probably the simplest and surest means of destroying microorganisms is burning or incineration. This method is reserved for items that are disposable or are so contaminated that their reuse is prohibited.[4] Besides destroying the material that is being sterilized, it should be recognized that incineration creates air pollution.

Dry heat is another effective method of heat sterilization. Its use is limited to items that are not heat-sensitive. Temperatures must be maintained between 160° to 180° C for 1 to 2 hours for sterilization. Dry heat is routinely used to sterilize laboratory glassware and surgical instruments, but cannot be used for heat-sensitive items made of rubber or plastic.

Boiling water kills vegetative bacteria and most viruses in 30 minutes; but its effectiveness against spores, especially those of thermophilic organisms, is somewhat questionable. Boiling water is commonly used to sterilize metal surgical instruments. Like dry heat, its use is prohibited with heat-sensitive equipment. Because water boils at a lower temperature at high altitudes, exposure time must be prolonged when using this form of sterilization at high elevations.[4,6] Steam under pressure, or autoclaving, is a highly effective and inexpensive method of sterilization. Of the aforementioned techniques, autoclaving is probably the most versatile. It is routinely used on laboratory glassware,

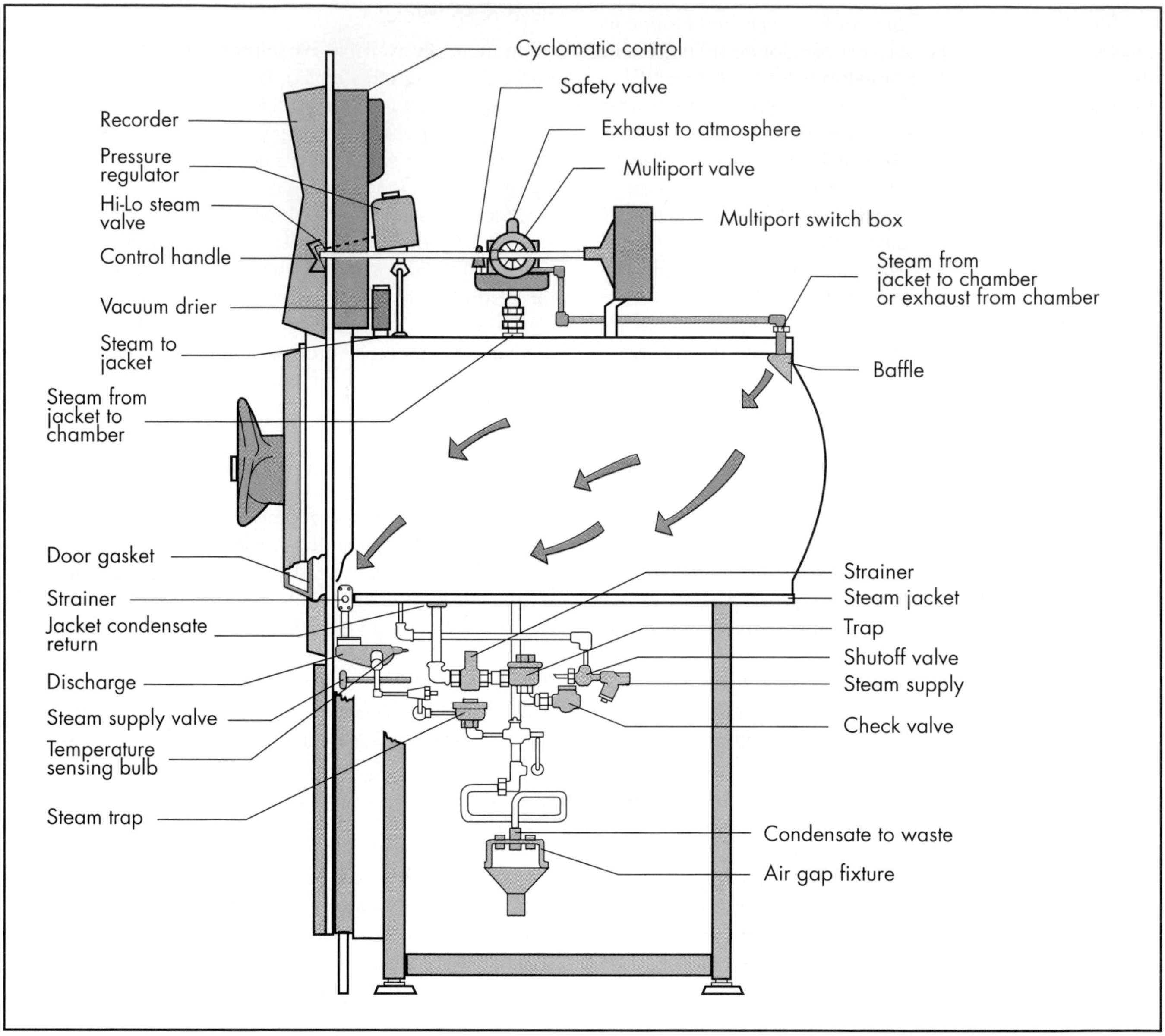

Figure 13-3 Components of an autoclave. From Perkins JJ: Principles and methods of sterilization in health sciences, Springfield, Ill., 1978, Charles Thomas.

surgical instruments, liquids, linens, and other heat- and moisture-resistant materials.

The technique of autoclaving is fairly simple. Items to be autoclaved are cleaned and wrapped in linen, gauze, or paper. They are then placed in a chamber like the one shown in Figure 13-3, which is closed and secured. It is evacuated of air, moisture is added (100% humidity), and the pressure inside is raised to 15 to 20 psig. Air is evacuated from the chamber because residual air prolongs the penetration time of steam, thus increasing the total autoclave cycle time. Pressure is used to raise the temperature of the steam, which is critical because the amount of time required to achieve sterilization depends on the temperature inside of the autoclave. For example, at atmospheric pressure, steam has a temperature of 100° C. At 15 psig it has a temperature of 121° C, and at 20 psig it has a temperature of 132° C. At 121° C, all microbes and spores are killed within 15 minutes; at 132° C, killing occurs in 10 minutes.

Because the process of autoclaving depends on several factors, heat-sensitive and biological indicators are routinely used to ensure quality control during the process. Heat-sensitive tape that is used for packaging materials for autoclaving changes color when it is exposed to a given temperature for a prescribed amount of time. The most common biological indicators for autoclaving are strips of paper that are impregnated with *Bacillus stearothermophilus* spores. These strips should be used weekly (at a minimum) to ensure that the autoclave is working properly.

Ethylene Oxide

Ethylene oxide (ETO) is a sterilant that has been used since the 1950s. It is a colorless gas that is flammable and explosive. It kills microorganisms by alkylating proteins, DNA, and RNA, thus interfering with cellular metabolism.[11] ETO was originally combined with chlorofluorocarbons (CFCs), which acted as a stabilizing agent. Under provisions of the Clean Air Act of 1993, CFCs were phased out in 1995 because of their detrimental effect on the ozone layer. Currently, ETO is used alone or in combination with different stabilizing agents, such as carbon dioxide or hydrochlorofluorocarbons.

ETO kills all microorganisms and spores, with bacterial spores being more resistant than vegetative microbes. The effectiveness of ETO depends on the gas concentration (450 to 1200 mg/L), the temperature (29° C to 65° C), the humidity (45% to 85% relative humidity), and the exposure time (2 to 5 hours).[8] Generally, increases in ETO concentration and temperature shorten sterilization time.

All equipment to be sterilized with ETO must be free of water because water interferes with the sterilization process. Additionally, equipment must be packaged in ETO-permeable materials, such as paper, muslin, or plastic bags made of polyethylene or polypropylene. The actual process of automated ETO sterilization consists of several stages: a preconditioning phase and a gas-injection phase, exposure of the item to the ETO, evacuation of gas from the chamber, and an air-washing period.[8] After sterilization, all equipment exposed to ETO must be aerated before use. Note that the aeration time is usually not considered part of the sterilization time and is usually accomplished by mechanical aeration for 8 to 12 hours at 50° to 60° C. Aeration at room temperature is considered dangerous because of ETO's toxicity.

Biological indicators, similar to those used for autoclaving, must be used to monitor the effectiveness of the ETO. *Bacillus subtilis* spores are generally used for this purpose. Figure 13-4 shows a typical device for monitoring sterilization. *Bacillus subtilis* organisms imbedded in a paper strip are housed within a plastic capsule inside of a glass ampule containing a growth medium (e.g., tryptic soy broth).[8] The ampule is placed among the materials to be sterilized. After the sterilization cycle, the ampule is crushed and the paper strip is immersed in the liquid. The strip is then incubated according to manufacturer directions. Microbe growth is indicated by changes in the turbidity of the growth medium after incubation.[2]

Inhalation of ETO has been associated with nose and eye irritation, dyspnea, headache, nausea, vomiting, dizziness, and convulsions.[22] Direct contact with ETO causes skin irritation and burns. The OSHA and the Joint Commission for Accreditation of Hospital Organizations (JCAHO) provide general guidelines for the safe use of ETO. The current OSHA standard for ETO exposure is 1 ppm in 8 hours with a maximum short-term exposure of 5 to 10 ppm for 15 minutes.[23,24]

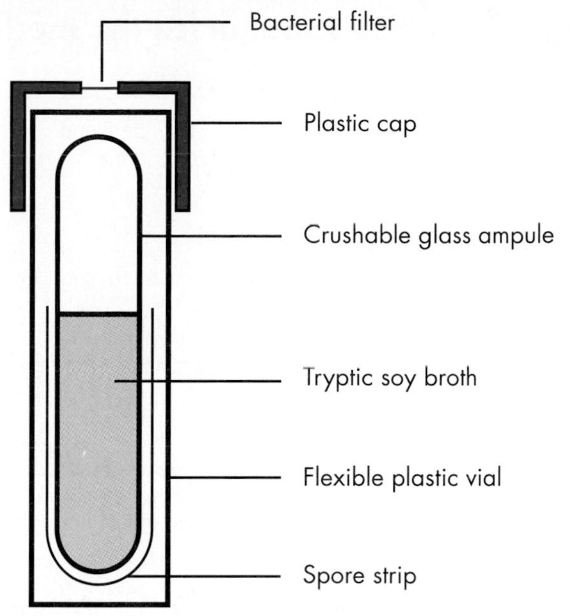

Figure 13-4 Biological sterilization indicators: the capsule contains a strip impregnated with bacterial spores, a pH indicator, and a culture medium (e.g., tryptic soy broth). After sterilization, the ampule is crushed, releasing culture medium onto the strip containing the spores. Incomplete sterilization is indicated if the capsule turns yellow. (Redrawn from Boyd and Hoeri: Basic medical microbiology, ed 3 Boston, 1986, Little, Brown.)

Identifying Infection-Risk Devices

It is unnecessary to sterilize all patient-care items. Whether a medical device should be cleaned and disinfected or sterilized depends on its intended use. In 1968, E. H. Spaulding[25] devised a classification scheme that could be used by infection-control professionals in the planning of disinfection and sterilization methods for patient-care items and equipment. Spaulding's classification system placed devices into three categories based on the degree of risk of infection involved in their use. The categories are critical, semicritical, and noncritical. Critical items must be sterilized because they are introduced into sterile tissue or the vascular system (e.g., surgical instruments, implants, cardiac and urinary catheters, heart-lung and hemodialysis equipment, and needles). Because semicritical items (e.g., ventilator tubing) come in contact with intact mucous membranes, a minimum of high-level disinfection is recommended. Respiratory care and anesthesia equipment, endoscopes, and thermometers are semicritical items. High-level disinfection is

TABLE 13-6

Infection-risk categories for medical equipment

Category	Description	Examples	Processing
Critical	Devices introduced into the bloodstream or other parts of the body	Surgical devices Cardiac catheters Implants Heart-lung and hemodialysis components	Sterilization
Semicritical	Devices that contact intact mucous membranes	Endoscopes Tracheal tubes Ventilator tubing	High-level disinfection
Noncritical	Devices that touch only intact skin or do not contact patient	Face masks Blood-pressure cuffs Ventilators	Detergent washing Low-intermeiate level disinfection

Adapted from Chatburn RL: Decontamination of respiratory care equipment: what can be done, what should be done, Respir Care 34(2):98, 1989. In Scanlan CL, Spearman CB, Sheldon RL: Egan's fundamentals of respiratory care, ed 6, St Louis, 1995, Mosby.

effective against blood-borne pathogens (i.e., HIV, Hepatitis B virus) and *Mycobacteria tuberculosis.* Noncritical items come in contact with intact skin, but not mucous membranes. Intact skin acts as an effective barrier to most microorganisms, so sterility is not critical. Common examples of noncritical items are face masks, ventilators, stethoscopes, and blood pressure cuffs. Table 13-6 lists examples of medical devices and how they are classified by Spaulding's system. Box 13-4 contains a summary of the guidelines for processing reusable respiratory care equipment. Box 13-5 describes several strategies for preventing the spread of pathogenic organisms by in-use respiratory care equipment (e.g., nebulizers, ventilator circuits, manual resuscitators, and oxygen therapy apparatuses). Box 13-6 provides a test of your understanding of the principles of infection control techniques.

Isolation Precautions

In 1996, the CDC, in cooperation with the Hospital Infection Control Practices Advisory Committee (HIPAC), revised its guideline for isolation precautions in hospitals.[26] The revised guideline contains information on the history of isolation practices, along with recommendations for isolation precautions in hospitals. The recommendations for isolation techniques are intended for acute-care hospitals, although some of the precautions are applicable to subacute or extended-care facilities.

The revised recommendations contain two levels of precautions: **standard precautions** and **transmission-based precautions.** Standard precautions are to be used with all hospitalized patients, regardless of their diagnosis or presumed infection status.[26] Standard precautions represent a combination of **universal precautions** and body substance isolation (BSI) precautions, and apply to blood, all body fluids (secretions and excretions [except sweat]), nonintact skin, and mucous membranes. Standard precautions are designed to reduce the risk of transmission of microorganisms from both recognized and unrecognized sources of infection in hospitals.[26]

Transmission-based precautions are designed to interrupt transmission of known or suspected pathogens that can be transmitted by airborne or droplet routes, or by direct contact with skin and contaminated surfaces. Transmission-based precautions are for the care of patients with highly transmissible or epidemiologically important pathogens that necessitate additional precautions to stop their transmission. Box 13-7 gives a synopsis of the various types of isolation precautions and a list of conditions requiring each type of precaution. Table 13-7 lists clinical syndromes or conditions warranting additional precautions to prevent the transmission of epidemiologically important pathogens upon confirmation of diagnosis.

Fundamentals of Isolation Protection

Hand washing is the most important prevention strategy to protect health-care workers from being infected by contacting infected patients. It also reduces the risk of health-care workers transmitting infectious microorganisms from one patient to another or from a contaminated to a clean site on the same patient.[27,28,29] Routine hand washing should comprise a soap and water wash with a rubbing action to create a lather over both hands for longer than 10 seconds. Hands should be rinsed thoroughly and dried with disposable or single-use towels or an air drier.[30] Hand washing should be performed with an antimicrobial agent after contacting patients colonized with virulent microorganisms.[31] Hands should be washed before caring for any

BOX 13-4

Guidelines for Processing Reusable Respiratory Care Equipment

All reusable respiratory care equipment should undergo low- or intermediate-level disinfection as part of the initial cleaning.

All reusable breathing circuit components (including tubing and exhalation valves, medication nebulizers and their reservoirs, large volume jet nebulizers and their reservoirs) should be considered semicritical items.

Semicritical items should be sterilized between patient use; heat-stable items should be autoclaved, and heat-labile items should undergo ETO sterilization.

If sterilization is not feasible, semicritical items should undergo high-level disinfection or pasteurization.

The internal machinery of ventilators and breathing machines need not be routinely sterilized or disinfected between patients.

Respirometers and other equipment used to monitor multiple patients should not directly touch any part of a ventilator circuit or a patient's mucous membranes. Rather, disposable extension pieces and low-resistance HEPA filters should be used to isolate the device. If the device cannot be isolated from the patient or circuit, it must be sterilized or receive high-level disinfection before use on other patients.

Once they have been used on one patient, nondisposable resuscitation bags (BVMs) should be sterilized or receive high-level disinfection before use on other patients.

From Scanlan CL, Spearman CB, and Sheldon RL: Egan's fundamentals of respiratory care, ed 6, St Louis, 1995, Mosby. Derived from Chatburn RL: Decontamination of respiratory care equipment: what can be done, what should be done, Respir Care 34(2)98, 1989; and AARC Technical Standards and Safety Committee: Recommendations for respiratory therapy equipment: processing, handling, and surveillance, Respir Care 22:928, 1977.

BOX 13-5

Strategies for Preventing the Spread of Pathogenic Organisms by In-Use Respiratory Care Equipment[2,6,34,36-38]

- Nebulizers should always be filled with sterile distilled water. Large-volume nebulizers should be filled completely before initial use. When replenishing fluid, any fluid remaining in the nebulizer should be emptied, and the reservoir filled completely.
- Large-volume jet nebulizers and medication nebulizers, as well as their reservoirs and tubing should be changed or replaced every 24 hours with equipment that has undergone high-level disinfection.
- Avoid using humidifiers and nebulizers that create droplets for purposes of room humidification.
- In-use ventilator circuits, including their humidifiers and nebulizers, should be changed every second or third day (48 to 72 hours). If a heat-moisture exchanger bacterial filter (i.e., artificial nose) is used instead of a water humidifier, changing the circuit between patients may be satisfactory.
- Water condensation in ventilator and nebulizer tubing should be discarded and not drained back into the reservoir.

BOX 13-6

Decision Making & Problem Solving

The hospital infection control committee notifies your department that the incidence of nosocomial pneumonia in the recovery room increased significantly during the month of December. It has been suggested that the source of the pneumonia could be reusable large-volume jet nebulizers. How would you determine if in-use large volume jet nebulizers are responsible for this outbreak of pneumonia? How could you monitor the effectiveness of the sterilization of these devices?

See Appendix A for the answers.

patient, but it is particularly important that hands are washed before and after performing invasive procedures or touching wounds or patients at a high risk of infection.

Gloves are worn for several reasons: 1) to protect the health-care worker from contact with blood and body fluids (i.e., blood-borne pathogens); 2) to be a barrier so that resident and transient microorganisms on the hands of health-care workers are not transferred to patients during patient care or medical or surgical procedures; and 3) to prevent health care workers to indirectly transmit pathogens from an infected patient to another patient.[27,32] It is important to remember that hand washing is essential after removing gloves following each patient contact because hands can be contaminated during glove removal. Defects or tears in gloves can also contaminate the hands.[33,34]

Gowns and other protective apparel (e.g., shoe covers) are worn to prevent contamination of clothing and protect the skin of personnel from blood and body fluid exposure.[26] This protective apparel should be impermeable to liquids and worn only once, then discarded. Wearing gowns and protective apparel is mandated by OSHA's final rule on blood-borne pathogens.[31]

Face shields or masks with protective eyewear should be worn whenever there is a possibility of blood or body fluid being splashed or sprayed. They may also be mandated in special circumstances stated in the OSHA Bloodborne

BOX 13-7

Infection-Control Precautions and Patients Requiring Them

Standard Precautions

Use standard precautions for the care of all patients

Airborne Precautions

In addition to standard precautions, use airborne precautions for patients known or suspected to have serious illnesses transmitted by airborne droplet nuclei. Examples of such illnesses include:

- Measles
- Varicella (including disseminated zoster)*
- Tuberculosis†

Droplet Precautions

In addition to standard precautions, use droplet precautions for patients known or suspected to have serious illnesses transmitted by large particle droplets. Examples of such illnesses include:

Invasive *Haemophilus influenza* type b disease (meningitis, pneumonia, epiglottitis, and sepsis)

Invasive *Neisseria meningitidis* disease (meningitis, pneumonia, and sepsis)

Other serious bacterial respiratory infections spread by droplet transmission, including:

- Diphtheria (pharyngeal)
- Mycoplasma pneumonia
- Pertussis
- Pneumonic plague
- Streptococcal pharyngitis, pneumonia, or scarlet fever in infants and young children

Serious viral infections spread by droplet transmission, including:

- Adenovirus*
- Influenza
- Mumps
- Parvovirus B19
- Rubella

Contact Precautions

In addition to standard precautions, use contact precautions for patients known or suspected to have serious illnesses easily transmitted by direct patient contact or by contact with items in the patient's environment. Examples of such illnesses include: gastrointestinal, respiratory, skin, or wound infections or colonization with multidrug-resistant bacteria (judged by the infection control program based on current state, regional, or national recommendations to be of special clinical and epidemiologic significance).

Enteric infections with a low infectious dose or prolonged environmental survival, including: *Clostridium difficile* organisms.

For diapered or incontinent patients: enterohemorrhagic *Eschericha coli, Shigella,* hepatitis A, or rotavirus.

Respiratory syncytial virus, parainfluenza virus, or interoviral infections in infants and young children.

Skin infections that are highly contagious or that may occur on dry skin, including;

- Diphtheria (cutaneous)
- Herpes simplex-virus (neonatal or mucocutaneous)
- Impetigo
- Noncontained abscesses, cellulitis, or decubiti
- Pediculosis
- Scabies
- Staphylococcal furunculosis in infants and young children
- Zoster (disseminated or in the immunocompromised host)*

Viral/hemorrhagic conjunctivitis

Viral hemorrhagic infections (Ebola, Lassa, or Marburg)

From Garner JS: Guideline for isolation precautions in hospitals, Infect Control Hosp Epidemiol 17:53, 1996.

*Certain infections require more than one type of precaution.

†See CDC Guidelines for Preventing the Transmission of Tuberculosis in Health-Care Facilities.[20]

Pathogen Final Rule.[31] Face masks are used to prevent the spread of large particle droplets that are transmitted by close contact (e.g., when working with patients who are coughing or sneezing), although the efficacy of wearing a mask to prevent transmitting *Mycobacterium tuberculosis* organisms has been questioned.[35] Respiratory protective devices are now required to prevent the inhalation of airborne droplet nuclei. A wide range of respirators that meet NIOSH standards are available to prevent the inhalation of droplet nuclei. Face shields or protective eyewear should be worn during all invasive procedures (i.e., when obtaining arterial blood gas samples and inserting intravascular catheters).

Patient care equipment and articles that can potentially be **fomites** for transmitting infectious particles (e.g., needles, scalpels, and other sharp objects) should be disposed in specially designated containers. Disposable medical gas therapy devices, such as nebulizers and tubing, should be disposed by being placed in a sturdy bag or container. Reusable items should be sterilized or disinfected by standard procedures to avoid transmitting infectious microorganisms from patient-to-patient. Disposable items should be disposed of according to hospital and applicable government regulations. Take care not to contaminate the outside of the bag when being handled or transported.

Fluids and medications that are used to treat patients should be sterile. Thus only sterile water should be used to fill nebulizers and humidifiers. Unused portions of large bottles of sterile water should be discarded within 24

TABLE 13-7

Clinical syndromes and conditions warranting additional empiric precautions to prevent the transmission of infectious diseases.*

Clinical syndrome or condition†	Potential pathogens‡	Empiric precautions
Diarrhea		
Acute diarrhea with a likely infectious cause in an incontinent or diapered patient	Enteric pathogens§	Contact
Diarrhea in an adult with a history of recent antibiotic use	*Clostridium difficile*	Contact
Meningitis	*Neisseria meningitidis*	Droplet
Rash or exanthems, generalized, etiology unknown		
Petechial/ecchymotic with fever	*Neisseria meningitidis*	Droplet
Vesicular	Varicella	Airborne & Contact
Maculopapular with coryza & fever	Rubeola (measles)	Airborne
Respiratory infections		
Cough/fever/upper lobe pulmonary infiltrate in an HIV-negative patient or a patient at low risk for HIV infection	*Mycobacterium tuberculosis*	Airborne
Cough/fever/pulmonary infiltrate in any lung location in an HIV-infected patient or a patient at high risk for HIV infection	*Mycobacterium tuberculosis*	Airborne
Paroxysmal or severe persistent cough during periods of pertussis activity	*Bordetella pertussis*	Droplet
Respiratory infections, particularly bronchiolitis & croup, in infants and young children	Respiratory syncytial or parainfluenza virus	Contact
Risk of multi-drug–resistant microorganisms		
History of infection or colonization with multi-drug–resistant organisms	Resistant bacteria‖	Contact
Skin, wound, urinary tract infection in a patient with a recent hospital or nursing home stay in a facility where multi-drug–resistant organisms are prevalent	Resistant bacteria‖	Contact
Skin or wound infection		
Abscess or draining wound that cannot be covered	*Staphylococcus aureus* Group A streptococcus	Contact

*Infection control professionals are encouraged to modify or adapt this table according to local conditions. To ensure that appropriate empiric precautions are always implemented, hospitals must have systems in place to evaluate patients routinely according to these criteria as part of their preadmission & admission care.

†Patients with the syndromes or conditions listed below may present with atypical signs or symptoms (e.g. pertussis in neonates and adults may not have paroxysmal or severe cough). The clinician's index of suspicion should be guided by the prevalence of specific conditions in the community, as well as clinical judgment.

‡The organisms listed under this column are not intended to represent the complete, or even most likely, diagnosis, but rather are possible etiologic agents that require additional precautions until they can be ruled out.

§These pathogens include enterohemorrhagic *Escherichia coli, Shigella,* hepatitis A, & rotavirus.

‖Resistant bacteria judged by the infection control program, based on current state, regional, or national recommendations, to be of special clinical or epidemiological significance.

From Garner JS: Guideline for isolation precautions in hospitals, Infect Control Hosp Epidemiol 17:52, 1996.

hours. Single-dose ampules of sterile water and normal saline are ideal for small-volume nebulizers. Multidose vials should be stored according to manufacturer's specifications (e.g., refrigerated after opening). Single- and multi-dose vials should not be used beyond the date on the label.[2]

Standard Precautions

As was stated, standard precautions are a synthesis of previous CDC guidelines for universal precautions and body substance isolation techniques. Hands should be washed between tasks and procedures on the same patient to prevent cross-contamination of different body sites.[26] A plain, non-antimicrobial soap may be used for routine hand washing; and antimicrobial agents or waterless antiseptic agents are used for specific circumstances, as defined by the infection control committee of the hospital.[26] Gloves, masks, protective eyewear, and gowns should be worn when there is a chance of contacting blood, body fluids, secretions, excretions, and contaminated items. Needles and other sharp objects should be handled with care to prevent injuries. Needles should not be recapped; when it is necessary to recap a syringe, both hands should never be used, instead use the one-hand "scoop" technique or a mechanical device to recap syringe needles safely.[27]

Airborne Precautions

Airborne precautions have two major components: 1) placement of the infected patient in an area with appropriate air handling and ventilation; 2) use of respiratory protective devices by health-care workers and visitors entering the patient's room.[26,27] Measles, chickenpox (primary *Varicella zoster*), and tuberculosis are illnesses that require airborne precautions. Because *Varicella zoster* organisms can also be transmitted by direct contact, infected patients may also require contact isolation.

Droplet Precautions

Droplet precautions are designed to prevent the transmission of microorganisms contained in droplets that are generated by sneezing, coughing, or talking, or during procedures such as bronchoscopy and suctioning.[26] Precautions include gloves, masks, and protective eyewear. Special air handling and ventilation are not required. *Haemophilus influenzae* type b organisms and *Neisseria meningitidis* organisms are transmitted by this route. Other serious infections are adenovirus, influenza, parvovirus B19, pertussis, streptococcal pharyngitis, pneumonia, and scarlet fever.[27]

Contact Precautions

Contact precautions are recommended for patients infected with pathogenic organisms that can be spread by direct patient contact or contact with items in the patient's environment.[26] Contact precautions require the patient to be isolated in a private room with a bath. Masks, gloves, and gowns should be used when caring for these patients. Illnesses requiring contact isolation include gastrointestinal, respiratory, and skin infections. Some of the organisms responsible for these illnesses are *Clostridium difficile, Shigella* sp., Hepatitis A, respiratory syncytial virus, and the parainfluenza virus. Patients colonized with multi-drug–resistant organisms of special clinical and epidemiological significance also require contact isolation. Box 13-8 provides a problem-solving exercise on isolation precautions typically required in the clinical setting.

BOX 13-8

Decision Making & Problem Solving

You are on call in the emergency room when one adult and two children are admitted after a house fire. The children incurred only minor cuts and bruises, but the adult sustained third-degree burns over 60% of his body. What precautions should you take when treating burn patients?

See Appendix A for the answer.

Surveillance

Ongoing surveillance is required to ensure that an infection control program is providing adequate protection for patients and health-care providers. Surveillance typically consists of three components: monitoring equipment-processing procedures, sampling in-use equipment routinely, and microbiologically identifying suspected pathogens.[4] Equipment processing is monitored using the aforementioned chemical and biological indicators. In-use equipment can be routinely sampled with sterile cotton swabs, liquid broth, and aerosol impaction. Swabs can be used to obtain samples from easily accessible surfaces of respiratory care equipment. Liquid broth can be used to obtain samples when cotton swabs cannot reach many parts of the equipment (e.g., inside tubing). Aerosol impaction is used to sample the particulate output of nebulizers.

Microbiological identification requires the hospital's clinical laboratory staff to work with clinicians to identify infectious organisms. Clinical microbiologists can provide information about nosocomial infections from direct smears and stains, cultures, serological tests, and antibiotic susceptibility testing. Identifying the cause of a nosocomial infection is essential to prevent and minimize hospital epidemics.[4]

Summary

Three elements must be present for an infectious disease to spread: a source of pathogens, a mode of transmission of the infectious agent, and a susceptible host. Nosocomial pneumonia is most often due to bacteria, but viruses, protozoa, and fungi contribute to a lesser extent. Most nosocomial bacterial pneumonias are described as polymicrobial, with Gram-negative bacilli being the predominant microbes identified.

There are four routes of transmission of infectious materials: contact, vehicles, airborne, and vectors. Nosocomial pneumonia can be spread by any of these routes. Contact, vehicle, and airborne transmission are the most common routes in hospital settings. Infection-control methods involve cleaning, disinfecting, and sterilizing respiratory care equipment, along with isolation precautions, which are the primary means of stopping the spread of nosocomial pneumonia.

The effectiveness of an infection control program should be monitored routinely with mechanical, chemical, and biological indicators. These indicators are readily available, easy to use, and ultimate proof that patients are not being exposed to microorganisms that can cause hospital-acquired infections.

Review Questions

See Appendix A for the answers.

1. Which of the following organisms is a Gram-negative bacteria often associated with nosocomial pneumonia?
   a. *Pseudomonas aeruginosa*
   b. *Diplococcus pneumoniae*
   c. *Clostridium botulinum*
   d. *Staphylococcus aureus*
2. *Mycobacterium tuberculosis* organisms are:
   a. Gram-negative bacilli
   b. Anaerobic infection
   c. Acid-fast bacteria
   d. Spore-producing bacteria
3. All of the following are transmitted through the respiratory route except:
   a. Rubella
   b. Rhinoviruses
   c. Varicella
   d. HIV
4. Name three elements that must be present for infectious materials to spread.
5. Which of the following disinfectants can be used as a chemical sterilant?
   a. Povidone-iodine
   b. Acetic acid
   c. Glutaraldehyde
   d. Isopropyl alcohol
6. Indicate whether each of the following is a critical (C), semicritical (S), or noncritical (N) risk of infection.

   _____ Ventilator tubing

   _____ Swan-Ganz catheter

   _____ Blood pressure cuff

   _____ Endoscope (bronchoscope)

   _____ Endotracheal tubes
7. Which of these clinical conditions warrants additional precautions to prevent the spread of epidemiologically significant pathogens?
   a. Meningitis
   b. Pertussis
   c. Measles
   d. Diarrhea in an adult with a history of recent antibiotic use
8. The best method to sterilize a bronchoscope is:
   a. With ethylene oxide
   b. A 10-hour soak in 2% glutaraldehyde
   c. A 20-minute soak in 70% isopropyl alcohol
   d. With steam autoclave
9. Which of the following methods should not be used to sterilize plastic oxygen masks?
   a. Ethylene oxide
   b. Steam autoclave
   c. 70% isopropyl alcohol
   d. 2% alkaline glutaraldehyde
10. Which of the following conditions requires the application of contact precautions?
    a. Legionellosis
    b. Diphtheria
    c. Hepatitis
    d. Rubella
11. Which of the following are potential causes of skin and mucosal barrier disruption?
    I. Foley catheters
    II. IV catheters
    III. Endotracheal tubes
    IV. Burns
       a. I and II only
       b. II and III only
       c. I, II, and IV only
       d. I, II, III, and IV
12. Which of the following organisms are associated with nosocomial pneumonia?
    I. *Klebsiella* sp.
    II. *Pseudomonas* sp.
    III. *Chlamydia* sp.
    IV. Influenza virus
       a. I and II only
       b. I and III only
       c. II and III only
       d. I, II, and IV only

References

1. Delost MD: Introduction to diagnostic microbiology, St Louis, 1997, Mosby.
2. Scanlan CL, Spearman CB, and Sheldon RL: Egan's fundamentals of respiratory care, ed 6, St Louis, 1995, Mosby.
3. Niederman MS, Sarosi GA, and Glassroth J: Respiratory infections: a scientific basis for management, Philadelphia, 1994, Saunders.
4. Pilbeam SM: Microbiology. In Kacmarek RM, Mack CW, and Dimas S, editors:The essentials of respiratory care, St Louis, 1990, Mosby.
5. Zimmerman PE and Martin WJ: Pneumocystis carinii. In Niederman MS, Sarosi GA, and Glassroth J, editors: Respiratory infections: a scientific basis for management. Philadelphia, 1994, Saunders.
6. Schaberg DR: How infections spread in the hospital, Respir Care 34(2):81, 1989.
7. Chatburn RL: Decontamination of respiratory care equipment: what can be done, what should be done, Respir Care 34(2):8, 1989.
8. Rutala WA: Disinfection, sterilization, and waste disposal. In Wenzel RP, editor: Prevention and control of nosocomial infections, Baltimore, 1997, Williams & Wilkins.
9. Favero MS, et al: Gram-negative water bacteria in hemodialysis systems, Health Lab Sci 12:321, 1987.
10. Rutala WA and Cole EC: Ineffectiveness of hospital disinfectants against bacteria: acollaborative study, Infect Control 8:501, 1987.
11. Sykes G: Disinfection and sterilization, 2 ed, London, 1965, E and FN Spon, Ltd.
12. Petrocci AN: Surface active agents: quaternary ammonium compounds. In Block SS, editor: Disinfection, sterilization, and preservation, ed 3, Philadelphia, 1983, Lea and Febiger.
13. Morton HE: Alcohols. In Block SS, editor: Disinfection, sterilization, and preservation, ed 3, Philadelphia, 1983, Lea and Febiger.
14. Chatburn RE, Kallstrom TJ, and Bajaksouzian MS: A comparison of acetic acid with a quaternary ammonium compound for the disinfection of hand-held nebulizers, Respir Care 33:179, 1988.
15. Block SS: Peroxygen compounds. In Block SS, editor: Disinfection, sterilization, and preservation, ed 3, Philadelphia, 1983, Lea and Febiger.
16. Rutala WA: APIC guideline for selection and use of disinfectants, Am J Infect Control 18(2):99, 1990.
17. Bloomfield SF and Uso EE: The antibacterial properties of sodium hypochlorite and sodium dichloroisocyanurate as hospital disinfectants, J Hosp Infect 6:20, 1985.
18. Favero MS and Bond WW: Chemical disinfection of medical and surgical materials. In Block SS, editor: Disinfection, sterilization, and preservation, ed 3, Philadelphia, 1983, Lea and Febiger.
19. United States Department of Labor: Bloodborne pathogens and acute care facilities, *OSHA* 3128, 1992.
20. Gorman SP, Scott EM, and Russell AD: A review: antimicrobial activity, uses, and mechanisms of action of glutaraldehyde, J Appl Bacteriol 48:161, 1980.
21. Fisher AA: Reactions to glutaraldehyde with particular reference to radiologist and x-ray technicians, Cutis 28:113, 1981.
22. Gross JA, Haas MI, and Swift TR: Ethylene oxide neurotoxicity: report of four cases and review of the literature, Neurology 29:978, 1979.
23. Occupation Safety and Health Administration: Occupational exposure to ethylene oxide—OSHA, Final standard, Fed Register 49(122):25734, 1984.
24. Kruger DA: What is 5 ppm? Understanding and complying with the new ETO STEL (short term exposure limit) regulation, J Health Material Manage 7(2):34, 1989.
25. Garner JS: Guideline for isolation precautions in hospitals, Infect Control Hosp Epidemiol 17:53, 1996.
26. Beekman SE and Henderson DK: Controversies in isolation policies and practices. In Wenzel RP, editor: Prevention and control of nosocomial infections, Baltimore, 1997, Williams & Wilkins.
27. Larson E: APIC guideline for handwashing and hand antisepsis in health care settings, Am J Infect Control 23:251, 1995.
28. Garner J and Favero M: Guideline for handwashing and hospital environmental control, United States Department of Health and Human Services Public Health Service, Centers for Disease Control, 7:59, 1986.
29. Donowitz LG: Infection control for the health care worker, Baltimore, 1994, Williams & Wilkins.
30. Garner JS and Favero MS: Guideline for handwashing and hospital environmental control, Infect Control 7:231, 1986.
31. Department of Labor, Occupational Safety and Health Administration: Occupational exposure to bloodborne pathogens: final rule, Federal Register 56:64175, 1991.
32. Olsen R, et al: Examination gloves as barriers to hand contamination and clinical practice, JAMA 350, 1993.
33. Doebbeling B, et al: Removal of nosocomial pathogens from the contaminated glove: implications for glove reuse and handwashing, Ann Inter Med 109:394, 1988.
34. Cadwallader HL, Bradley CR, and Ayliffe GA: Bacterial contamination and frequency of changing ventilator circuits, J Hosp Infect 5(1):65, 1990.
35. Centers for Disease Control: Guidelines for preventing the transmission of tuberculosis in health-care settings, with special focus on HIV-related issues, MMWR 39(RR-17):1, 1990.
36. Gallagher J, Stangeways JE, and Allt-Graham J: Contamination control in long term ventilation: a clinical study using a heat and moisture exchanging filter, Anesthesia 42(5):476, 1987.

Bibliography

1. Bartlett JG, et al: Bacteriology of hospital-acquired pneumonia, Arch Intern Med 146:868, 1986.
2. Boucher RM: Cidex and sonacide compared, Respir Care 22:790, 1977.
3. Centers for Disease Control: Guides lines for preventing the transmission of tuberculosis in health-care settings, with special focus on HIV-related issues, MMWR 39(RR-17):1, 1990.
4. Fargon JY, et al: Nosocomial pneumonia in patients receiving continuous mechanical ventilation: perspective analysis of 52

episodes with use of a protected specimen brush and quantitative culture techniques, Am Rev Respir Dis 139:871, 1989.
5. Hierholzer WJ: Guideline for prevention of nosocomial pneumonia, Respir Care 39(12):1191, 1994.
6. Spaulding EH: Chemical disinfection of medical and surgical materials. In Lawrence CA and Block SS, editors: Disinfections, sterilization, and preservation, ed 3, Philadelphia, 1968, Lea and Febiger.

Internet Resources

1. Guideline for Prevention of Nosocomial Pneumonia: http://aepo-xdv-www.epo.cdc.gov/wonder/prevguid/p0000451/p0000451.htm
2. The University of Michigan hospitals–Infection control manual: http://www.med.umich.edu/ics/icm/index.htm
3. Joint Commission on Accreditation of Health Care Organizations: http://www.jcaho.org
4. Handwashing Compliance Control Center: http://users.aol.com/comcontrol/comply.htm
5. Centers for Disease Control and Prevention: http://www.cdc.gov
6. National Center for Infectious Diseases: http://www.cdc.gov/ncidod/ncid.htm
7. The United Kingdom Communicable Disease Surveillance Centre: http://www.open.gov.uk/cdsc/cdschome.htm
8. Federation of American Scientist: http://www.fas.org/promed

CHAPTER 14

CHAPTER OUTLINE

KEY TERMS

Alpha Waves
Apnea/Hypopnea Index
Apnea Index
Arousal Response
Beta Waves
Central Sleep Apnea
Cheyne-Stokes Respiration
Circadian Cycle
Collodion
Delta Waves
Holter Monitoring
International 10-20 EEG System
K-Complexes
Mixed Sleep Apnea
Non-REM Sleep
Obstructive Sleep Apnea (OSA)
Polysomnography
Relatively Low-Voltage, Mixed-Frequency (RLVMF) Waves
REM Sleep
Sleep Spindles
Theta Waves

Sleep Diagnostics

J.M. Cairo

CHAPTER LEARNING OBJECTIVES

Upon completion of this chapter, the reader should be able to:

1. Describe the various stages of sleep in adults and children.
2. Discuss the physiologic effects of sleep on cardiopulmonary function in healthy individuals.
3. List the most common measurements recorded during polysomnography.
4. Summarize the clinical and laboratory criteria used to diagnose obstructive, central, and mixed apnea.
5. Describe various strategies that can be used to monitor arterial oxygen saturation, nasal-oral airflow, and respiratory effort of patients with obstructive sleep apnea syndrome.
6. Explain the physiologic consequences of obstructive sleep apnea.
7. Name several common diseases associated with central sleep apnea.

The effect of sleep on breathing has received considerable attention in the past 30 years. Much of this attention relates to an increased awareness of sleep-related disorders and improved technology for assessing neurologic and cardiopulmonary functions during sleep. The physiologic effect of sleep on breathing is normally of little consequence in healthy individuals. Its effect on patients with altered respiratory function (i.e., those afflicted with chronic pulmonary diseases) can be profound, however, and lead to significant consequences.

Physiology of Sleep

Sleep is part of a cyclical phenomenon (i.e., **circadian cycle**) controlled by an endogenous pacemaker that remains active even in an isolated environment free of time cues.[1] Sleep in itself is a nonhomogenous phenomenon comprising two distinct states: non-rapid eye movement (non-REM) sleep and rapid eye movement (REM) sleep. As seen in Table 14-1, these states can be defined by electrographic and behavioral criteria, such as brain-wave activity, oculomotor activity, responsiveness to external stimuli, and muscle tone.[2,3]

Non-REM sleep, or quiet sleep, consists of four stages, which are thought to represent progressively deeper levels of sleep. At sleep onset (non-REM Stage 1), normal sleepers can be easily aroused because they alternate between wakefulness and sleep. The electroencephalogram (EEG) shows **alpha** and **beta waves,** which are present during wakefulness, diminishing as the sleeper's EEG converts to **relatively low-voltage, mixed-frequency (RLVMF) waves** (Figure 14-1, *A*). (Note that alpha waves are rhythmical waves that occur at a frequency of 8 to 13 per second, whereas beta waves occur at frequencies of 14 to 80 cycles per second.[4]) Skeletal muscle tone changes only slightly from waking levels; eye movements throughout non-REM sleep are slow, rolling, pendulous, and disconjugate.[5]

Stage 1 sleep lasts for only a brief time and is followed by a transition to Stage 2 non-REM sleep, which is identified by the appearance of **sleep spindles** and **K-complexes** on the sleeper's EEG (Figure 14-1, *B*). Sleep spindles are waveforms with waxing and waning amplitude that occur at a frequency of 9 to 13 cycles per second. K-complexes are large, vertical, slow waves that have an amplitude of at least 75 microvolts with an initial negative deflection.[5] Arousal thresholds (i.e., the level of stimuli required to change to a "lighter" stage of sleep or wakefulness) are higher in Stage 2 than those in Stage 1.

The deepest stages of non-REM sleep (Stages 3 and 4) are referred to as slow-wave sleep because of the presence of large **delta waves** that appear when the sleeper enters these stages (Figure 14-1, *C*). Delta waves include all EEG waves with a frequency less than 3.5 cycles per second.[5] It is important to recognize that the distinction between Stage 3 and Stage 4 is somewhat arbitrary because both appear almost identical on EEGs. For example, most clinicians define the beginning of Stage 3 as that period when slow waves constitute from 20% to 50% of the EEG recording. Stage 4, on the other hand, is identified by the presence of slow waves for at least 50% of the EEG recording.[2,5] The arousal threshold during Stages 3 and 4 is considerably higher than during Stages 1 and 2 of non-REM sleep.

After about 70 to 100 minutes of non-REM sleep, the normal sleeper enters **REM sleep.** During this phase of sleep, there is an increase in cerebral activity, as evidenced by the presence of a RLVMF pattern on EEG with a burst of **theta waves** (see Figure 14-1, *D*). Theta waves have a sawtooth appearance and occur at a frequency of 4 to 7 cycles per second.[4,5] It is generally accepted that dreaming occurs during REM sleep because sleepers who awaken after dreaming during REM sleep can recall their dreams. Although dreaming does occur during non-REM sleep, those dreams are usually not remembered. Eye movements during REM sleep are rapid, and conjugate eye movements are present. The arousal threshold (i.e., skeletal muscle tone) during REM sleep varies and may actually be absent.

TABLE 14-1

Behavioral and electrographic characteristics of sleep-wake states

Characteristic	Wake	Sleep: Non-REM	Sleep: REM
Eye lids	Open or closed	Closed	Closed
Eye movements	Slow or rapid	Slow or absent	Rapid
Responsiveness to external stimuli	Simple or complex	Simple	Often absent
Electroencephalogram	Low voltage, high frequency	High-voltage, low-frequency	Low-voltage, high-frequency
Electromyogram	High-level tonic activity	Lower-level tonic activity	Absence of tonic activity
Electroculogram	Slow or rapid movements	Slow or rapid movements	Rapid movements

From Phillipson EA: Sleep disorders. In Murray JF and Nadel JE: Textbook of respiratory medicine, Philadelphia, 1997, Saunders.

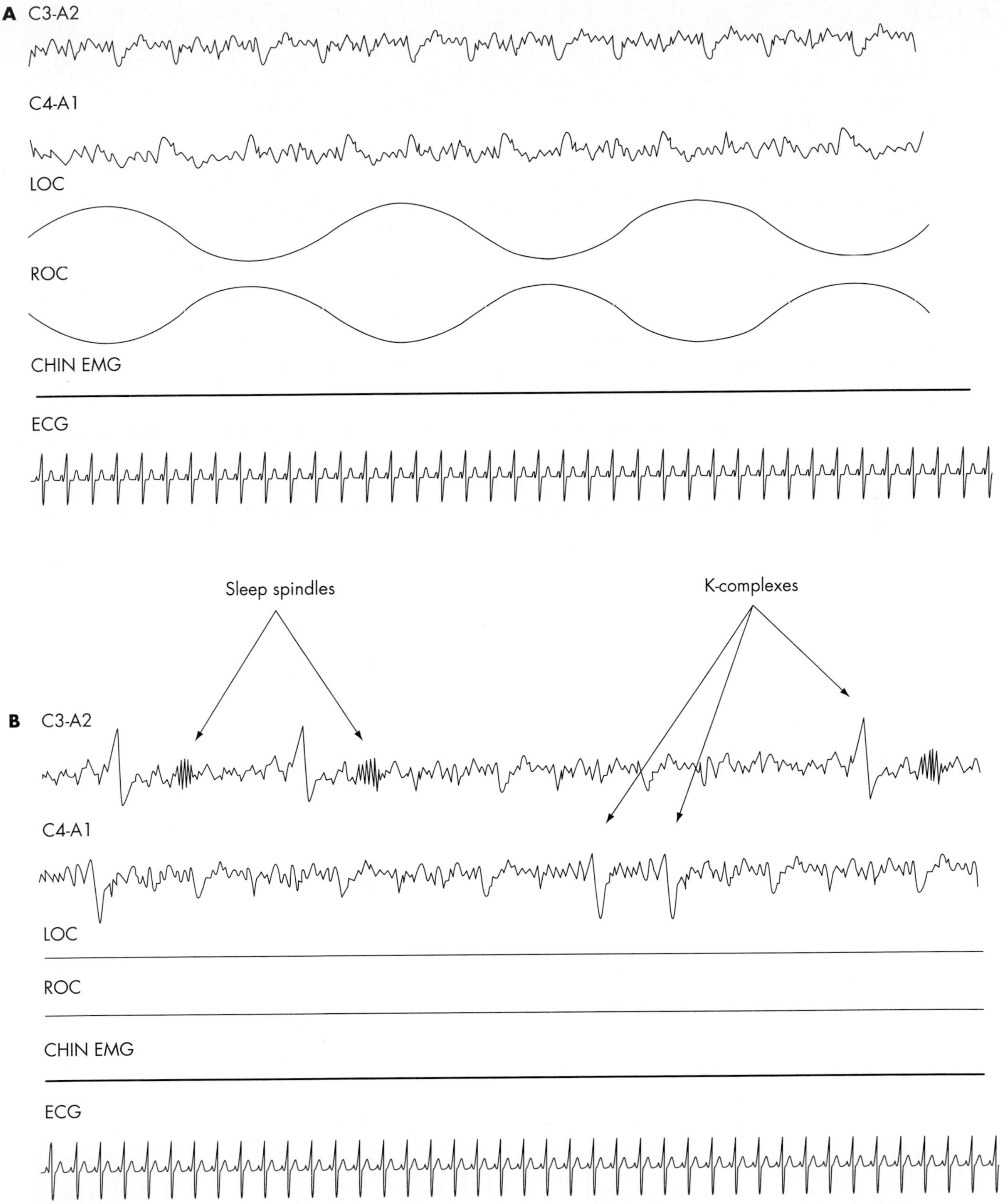

Figure 14-1 **A,** Stage 1 sleep. Stage 1 is characterized by a relatively low-voltage, mixed-frequency EEG; slow, rolling eye movements (*LOC* and *ROC* relate to eye movements that are left of center and right of center, respectively.); and tonic EMG activity. **B,** Stage 2 sleep. Stage 2 is characterized by relatively low-voltage background EEG activity; sleep spindles and K-complexes; absence of eye movements; and tonic EMG activity.

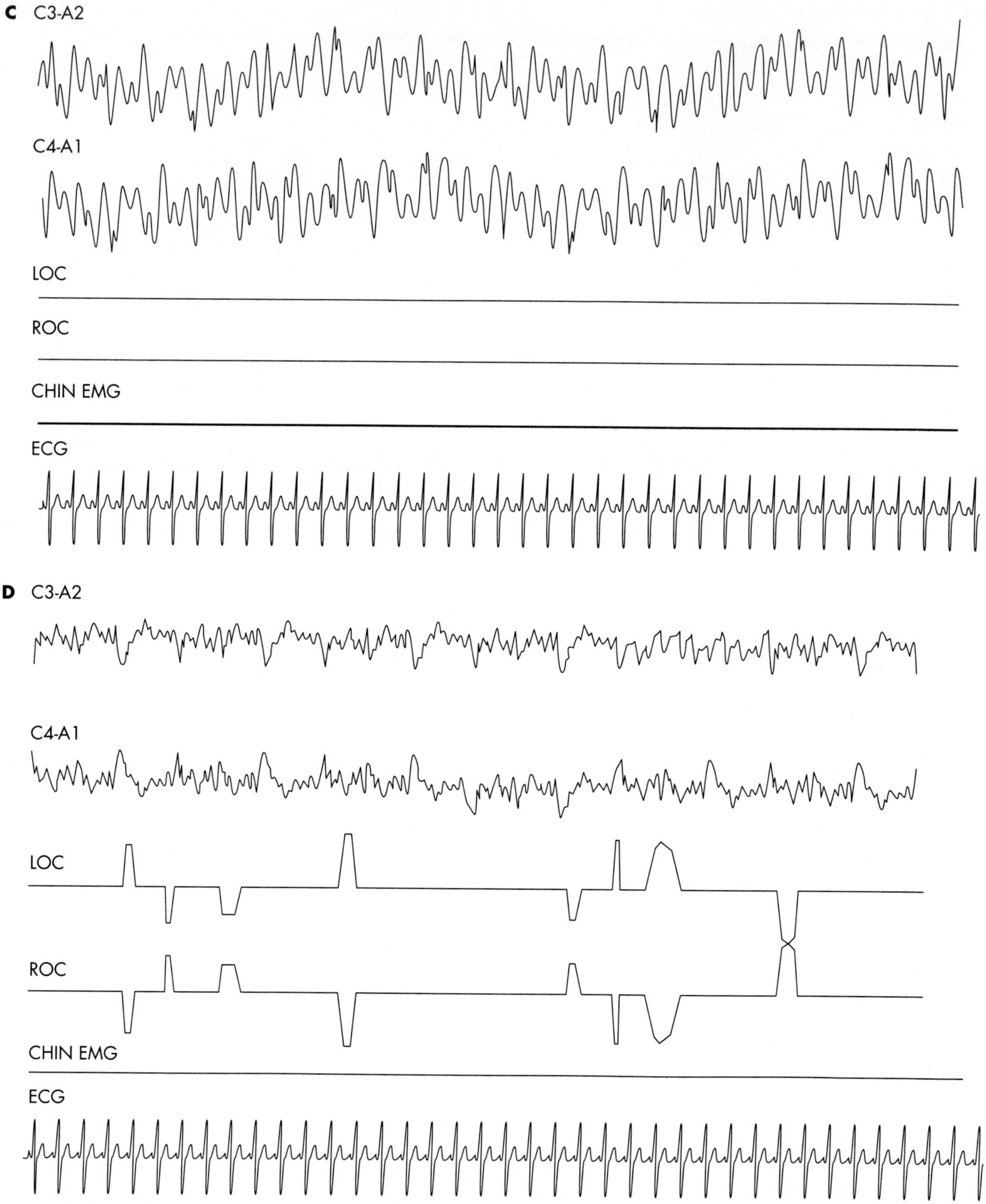

Figure 14-1 (continued) **C,** Stage 4 sleep. Stage 4 is characterized by high-voltage, slow-wave EEG activity; absence of eye movements; and tonic EMG activity. **D,** REM sleep. REM sleep is characterized by relatively low-voltage, mixed-frequency background EEG activity, with a burst of notched theta waves; rapid, saccadic, conjugate eye movements; and chin muscle tone significantly decreased from waking and NREM sleep levels. (Redrawn from Sheldon SH, Spire JP, and Levy HB: Pediatric sleep medicine, Philadelphia, 1992, Saunders.)

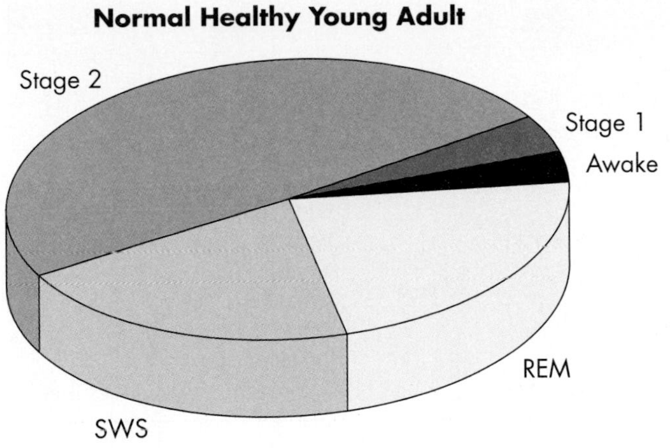

Stage	Percent of Total Recording Time
Wake after sleep onset	Less than 5%
Stage-1	2% to 5%
Stage-2	45% to 55%
Slow-wave sleep	13% to 23%
REM	20% to 25%

Figure 14-2 Sleep stage distribution in normal healthy adults. (Redrawn from Sheldon SH, Spire JP, and Levy HB: Pediatric sleep medicine, Philadelphia, 1992, Saunders.)

BOX 14-1

How Much Sleep Do We Need?

It is generally accepted that the amount of sleep that an individual requires is influenced by their age. Infants typically require about 16 hours a day, and teenagers need 8 or 9 hours per night on average. For most adults, 7 to 8 hours a night seems to be sufficient, although some people only require about 5 hours per day, and others require as many as 10 hours of sleep each day. As they get older (>60 years of age), people tend to sleep more lightly and for shorter time periods. What may not be obvious is that we continue to need about the same amount of sleep that we required in early adulthood.

Certain conditions can also influence the amount of sleep that we require. That is, we have an increased need for sleep while recovering from an acute illness, such as a cold or the flu. Women in their first trimester of pregnancy often need several more hours of sleep than usual. The amount of sleep a person needs also increases when there has been a deprival of sleep in previous days. Getting too little sleep creates a "sleep debt," which ultimately must be repaid. Although we may think that we can adapt to getting less sleep than we need, sleep deprivation can severely alter our judgment, reaction time, and other neurologic functions.

See the National Institute of Neurological Disorders and Stroke website: *http://www.ninds.nih.gov* for more details.

(It is interesting that if the arousal stimulus is incorporated into the dream content, arousal is less likely.[5])

During a typical night of sleep, a normal adult sleeper cycles between non-REM sleep and REM sleep about every 90 to 120 minutes.[1] Slow-wave sleep (non-REM Stages 3 and 4) is most prominent during the first half of the night and decreases as the night progresses. REM sleep, on the other hand, becomes longer and more intense throughout the sleep period, with the longest and most intense REM sleep occurring in the early morning hours.

Figure 14-2 illustrates the average amount of time that a healthy adult spends in each sleep state. Normally 4 to 6 cycles of sleep stages occur per night. Although there are variations between sleepers, these averages are a good approximation of the time distribution of non-REM sleep, REM sleep, and wakefulness during a typical night of sleep (Box 14-1).

The classic states of non-REM and REM sleep are not easily identified at birth with standard electroencephalographic (EEG), electromyographic (EMG), and electroculographic (EOG) analysis. Although similarities exist between the sleep states that occur in newborns and adults, sleep stages during the neonatal period are generally categorized as active sleep, quiet sleep, and intermediate sleep. Active sleep is comparable to REM sleep; quiet and intermediate sleep states have many of the same characteristics of non-REM. It is worth noting that infants enter active sleep first instead of entering into quiet sleep like adults do. Between 6 to 8 weeks of age, infant sleep becomes more predictable; and by 12 weeks of age, the various stages of non-REM sleep and REM sleep are recognizable. By 12 months of age, infants exhibit the classic sleep stages seen in adults. As mentioned, sleep-state distribution for healthy adult sleepers during a typical 8-hour period of sleep usually involves non-REM and REM sleep states alternating cyclically every 90 to 120 minutes, with periods of REM sleep lasting from 10 to 30 minutes. In contrast, infants spend considerably more time in REM sleep than adult sleepers (i.e., during various stages in development, infants may spend as much as 75% of their sleep in REM).[1,5]

Effect of Sleep on Breathing

The effects of sleep on breathing are summarized in Table 14-2. As the sleeper passes through the various stages of non-REM sleep, there is a progressive reduction in chemosensitivity and respiratory drive. The reduction in respiratory drive that occurs during the early stages of non-REM sleep (Stages

TABLE 14-2

Physiologic effect of sleep on respiration

Feature	Sleep Stages 1 and 2	Sleep Stages 3 and 4	REM sleep
Pattern of breathing	Periodic	Stable	Irregular
Apneas	Short, central	Rare	Short, central
$PaCO_2$	Variable	↑ 2–8 mm Hg above wakefulness	Variable, similar to Stages 3, 4
Ribcage muscles	Active	Active	Inhibited
Diaphragm	Active	Active	Active
Upper airway muscles	Active	Active	Inhibited
Chemoresponsiveness	↓ compared with wakefulness	↓ compared with Stages 1, 2	↓ compared with Stages 3, 4
Arousability to respiratory stimuli	Low thresholds	Low thresholds	High thresholds

From Phillipson EA: Sleep disorders. In Murray JF and Nadel JE: Textbook of respiratory medicine, Philadelphia, 1997, Saunders.

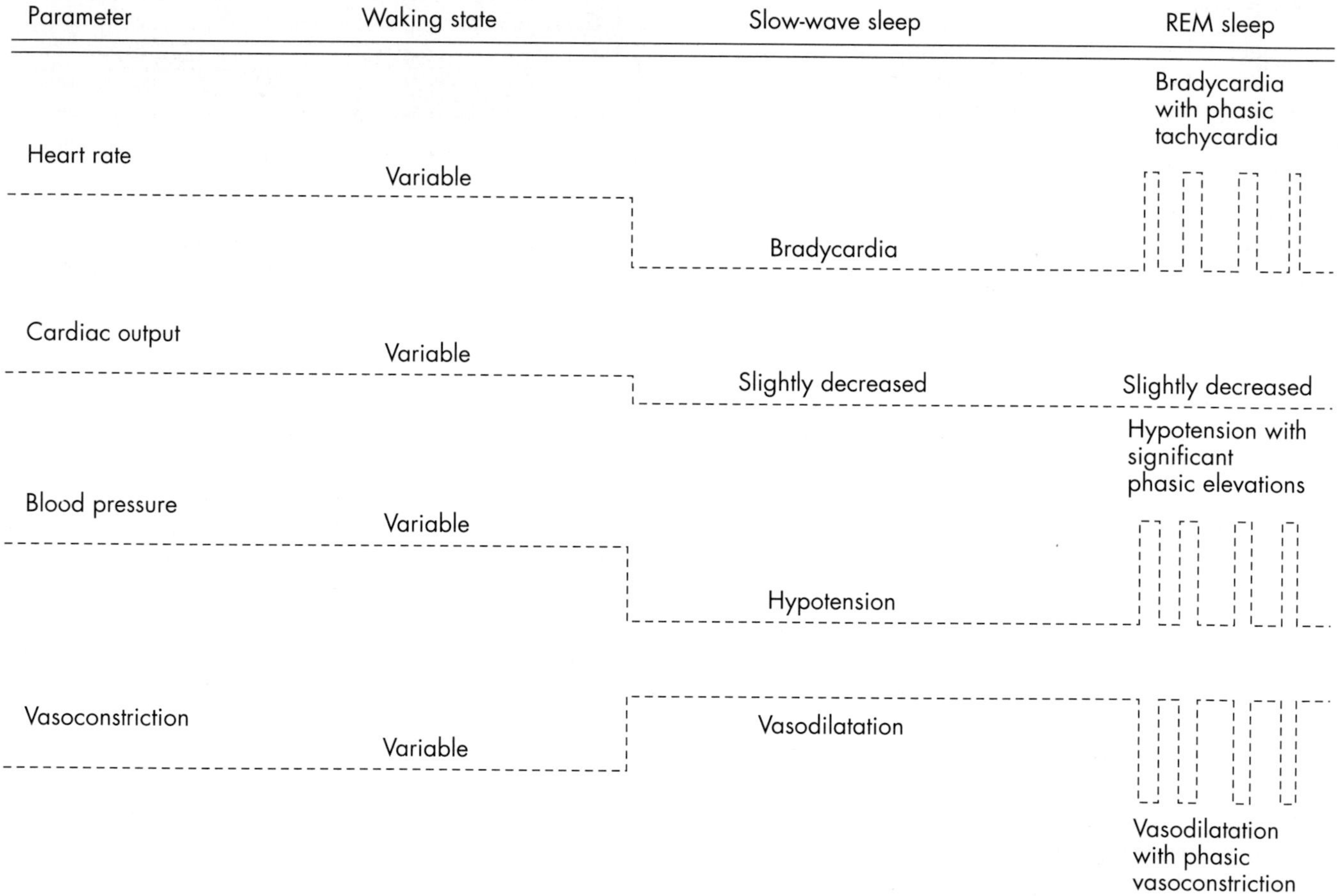

Parameter
Waking state
Slow-wave sleep
REM sleep
Bradycardia with phasic tachycardia
Heart rate
Variable
Bradycardia
Cardiac output
Variable
Slightly decreased
Slightly decreased
Hypotension with significant phasic elevations
Blood pressure
Variable
Hypotension
Vasoconstriction
Variable
Vasodilatation
Vasodilatation with phasic vasoconstriction

Figure 14-3 The effect of sleep on cardiovascular function in awake and sleep states. (Redrawn from Sheldon SH, Spire JP, and Levy HB: Pediatric sleep medicine, Philadelphia, 1992, Saunders.)

1 and 2) predisposes the person to apneic periods (i.e., **Cheyne-Stokes respiration**) when fluctuating between being awake and asleep. With the establishment of non-REM slow-wave sleep (Stages 3 and 4), nonrespiratory inputs are minimized, and minute ventilation is regulated by metabolic control. Minute ventilation decreases by 1 to 2 L/min when compared with wakefulness. As a consequence, the partial pressure of arterial carbon dioxide ($PaCO_2$) rises by 2 to 8 mm Hg, and the partial pressure of oxygen in the arteries (PaO_2) decreases by 5 to 10 mm Hg.

As the sleeper enters into REM sleep, breathing becomes irregular as the ventilatory response to chemical and mechanical respiratory stimuli is further reduced and even transiently abolished. Skeletal muscle activity, along with the intercostal and accessory muscles of respiration, is decreased, and the upper airway muscles are inhibited. This inhibition leads to an increase in upper airway resistance, but inhibition of the intercostal and accessory muscles is associated with diminished thoracoabdominal coupling and short periods of central apnea for durations of 10 to 20 seconds. $PaCO_2$ and PaO_2 levels are variable, but are generally similar to those in the latter stages of non-REM sleep.

Effect of Sleep on Cardiovascular Function

The effects of sleep on cardiovascular function are shown in Figure 14-3. In most individuals, both heart rate and blood pressure are generally reduced during sleep. Reductions in heart rate average about 5 to 10 beats/minute during non-REM sleep and up to 15 beats/minute during REM sleep. Blood pressure shows a moderate decrease of 10 to 15 mm Hg during non-REM sleep and up to 25 mm Hg during REM sleep. Alterations in heart rate seen during sleep seem to parallel sleep-related alterations in blood pressure. These variations are especially evident during REM sleep, when arterial blood pressure varies to a greater extent than during non-REM sleep.[5] Changes in blood pressure during REM sleep are characterized as sharp increases in mean arterial pressure, which are superimposed on a relatively hypotensive state.

Cardiac output is usually only slightly reduced during non-REM sleep when compared with the waking state. The reduction in cardiac output, however, is more pronounced during REM sleep (e.g., approximately a 10% reduction).[5] Changes in cardiac output that are seen during sleep are not accompanied by changes in stroke volume, which tend to remain similar to values measured while the person is in a quiet, awake state.[5]

DIAGNOSIS OF SLEEP APNEA

The ability to wake from sleep or to rouse to a lighter stage of sleep requires activation of higher neurological centers (i.e., the reticular activating system and cortex).[2] Such activation results in an immediate increase in respiratory drive, activation of the upper airway muscles, stimulation of the cough reflex, and initiation of behavioral responses, specifically increases in skeletal muscle tone.[2,4] If these **arousal responses** do not occur, sleep apnea or alveolar hypoventilation can result.

Diagnosis of sleep apnea is based on information derived from patient history and physical examination and from laboratory studies that focus on sleep structure and cardiorespiratory function. The medical history and physical examination provide information that can be used to determine whether patients are at risk for sleep apnea and if they demonstrate the common symptoms and signs associated with various sleep-related disorders. Laboratory studies range from simple overnight monitoring of arterial blood gases with pulse oximetry and transcutaneous monitoring to analyzing cardiopulmonary and neuromuscular function with **polysomnography.**

TABLE 14-3

Laboratory investigation of respiratory disturbances during sleep

Type of test	Variable measured*	Technique
Screening	SaO_2	Ear oximeter
	PCO_2	Transcutaneous sensor
	Heart rate, rhythm	Holter monitoring
Standard polysomnography	EEG	Surface electrodes
	EOG	Surface electrodes
	Submental EMG	Surface electrodes
	Tibialis EMG	Surface electrodes
	Breathing pattern	Surface transducers
	SaO_2, PCO_2	Ear oximeter, transcutaneous sensor
	Electrocardiogram	Standard electrodes
Special procedures	Intrapleural pressure	Esophageal catheter
	Diaphragm EMG	Esophageal or surface electrodes
	Esophageal pH	Esophageal electrodes
	Arterial blood gases	Arterial catheter
	Pulmonary arterial pressure	Swan-Ganz catheter
	Systemic blood pressure	Arterial catheter

From Phillipson EA: Sleep disorders. In Murray JF and Nadel JE: Textbook of respiratory medicine, Philadelphia, 1997, Saunders.

Polysomnography

Although patient history and physical examination can provide evidence that a patient may be afflicted with sleep apnea, the data may be equivocal and thus lead the clinician to under- or overestimate the severity of the patient's sleep-disordered breathing. For this reason, laboratory assessment of patients suspected to have sleep apnea should be performed to ensure a definitive diagnosis.

Table 14-3 summarizes the various laboratory procedures that can be used to investigate physiologic function during sleep. Although screening tests can provide valuable information about cardiopulmonary function during sleep, they do not allow for sleep staging and quantification of patient arousal or awakening during the course of the study. It is gen-

BOX 14-2

Clinical Practice Guidelines

Polysomnography

Indications

Polysomnography may be indicated for patients demonstrating any of the following conditions:

- COPD with an awake PaO_2 >55 mm Hg whose illness is complicated by pulmonary hypertension, right heart failure, polycythemia, or excessive daytime sleepiness
- Restrictive ventilatory impairment secondary to chest-wall and neuromuscular disturbances whose illness is complicated by chronic hypoventilation, polycythemia, pulmonary hypertension, disturbed sleep, morning headaches, or daytime somnolence and fatigue
- Disturbances of respiratory control with an awake $PaCO_2$ >45 torr, or patients whose illness is complicated by pulmonary hypertension, polycythemia, disturbed sleep, morning headaches, or daytime somnolence and fatigue
- Nocturnal cyclic brady- or tachyarrhythmias, nocturnal abnormalities of atrioventricular conduction, or ventricular ectopy that appears to increase in frequency during sleep
- Excessive daytime sleepiness or insomnia
- Snoring, which is associated with observed apneas and/or excessive daytime sleepiness

Contraindications

There are no absolute contraindications to polysomnography when indications are clearly established. Risk:benefit ratios should be assessed, however, if medically unstable inpatients are to be transferred from the clinical setting to a sleep laboratory for overnight polysomnography.

Precautions/Complications

- Skin irritation may occur as a result of the adhesive used to attach electrodes to the patient.
- At the conclusion of the study, adhesive remover is used to dissolve adhesive on the patient's skin. Adhesive removers (e.g., acetone) should only be used in well-ventilated areas.
- Engineering (or qualified biomedical personnel) must certify the integrity of the polysomnographic equipment's electrical isolation.
- The adhesive used to attach EEG electrodes, (e.g., collodion) should not be used to attach electrodes near the patient's eyes and should always be used in well-ventilated areas.
- Due to the high flammability of collodion and acetone, they should be used with caution, especially with patients requiring supplemental oxygen.
- Collodion should be used with caution in small infants and patients with reactive airway disease.
- Patients with parasomnias or seizures may be at risk for injury related to movements during sleep. Institution-specific policies and guidelines describing personnel responsibilities and appropriate responses should be developed.

Assessment of Need

Polysomnography should be used to assess oxygenation, cardiac status, and sleep continuity in those patients who are suspected of having sleep-related respiratory disturbances, periodic limb-movement disorders, or any of the sleep disorders described in the International Classification of Sleep Disorders Diagnostic and Coding Manual.

Assessment of Test Quality

- Polysomnography should either confirm or eliminate a diagnosis of a sleep-related respiratory disturbance.
- Documentation of findings, suggested therapeutic intervention, and/or other clinical decisions resulting from polysomnography should be noted on the patient's chart.
- Each laboratory should devise and implement indicators of quality assurance for equipment calibration and maintenance, patient preparation and monitoring, scoring methodology, and scoring variances between technicians.

For a complete copy of this guideline, see American Association for Respiratory Care: Clinical practice guideline: polysomnography, Respir Care 40(12):1236, 1995.

erally accepted that polysomnography is the gold standard for identifying the type and severity of sleep apnea. Polysomnography usually includes all-night audio/video monitoring of the patient, as well as recordings of ECGs, respiratory activity, EEGs, EOGs, and electromyograms (EMG).[6] (Box 14-2 summarizes the AARC Clinical Practice Guideline for Polysomnography.) Besides being used to determine whether a patient demonstrates sleep apnea or hypopnea, polysomnography can also provide valuable information about the most effective means of treating these patients.

Electrocardiography

Cardiac activity, including heart rate and rhythm, is usually monitored with at least two ECG leads (e.g., Lead II and a modified chest lead). It is important to recognize that monitoring two ECG leads can only provide limited information about the electrical activity of the heart. If more information about the patient's ECG is required, a 12-lead ECG or **Holter monitoring** may be indicated.

Electroencephalography

An EEG is a recording of fluctuations in the electric potentials of cortical neurons. These electric potentials are transmitted from the cortex through the coverings of the brain to the scalp, where electrodes placed at various points on the scalp are used to sense the sum of the potentials in the underlying cortex. EEGs provide valuable information on the integrity of the central nervous system

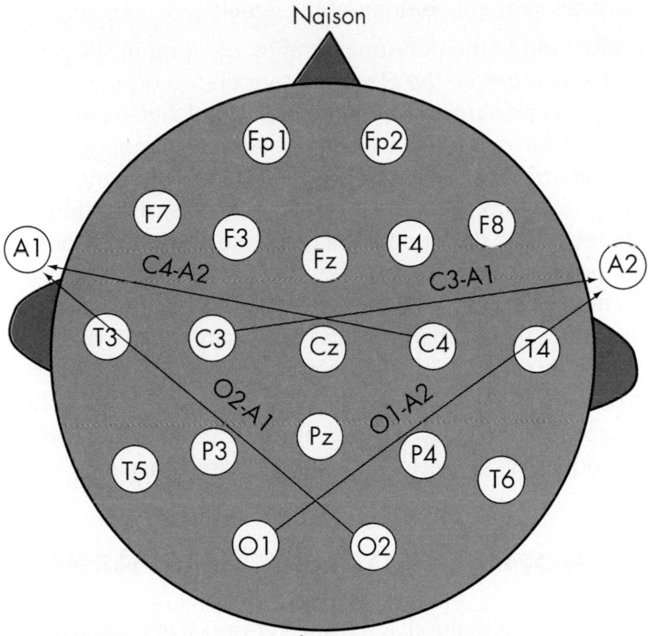

Figure 14-4 A standard polysomnographic EEG montage. (Redrawn from Sheldon SH, Spire JP, and Levy HB: Pediatric sleep medicine, Philadelphia, 1992, Saunders.)

and form the basis for identifying the various sleep stages that the patient enters during the sleep study.

To ensure that the information is meaningful and can be compared with that of different laboratories, a standardized system for electrode placement is used to record EEGs during sleep studies. The standard EEG montage used for polysomnography is based on the **International 10-20 EEG system** (Figure 14-4).[5,7] Note that modified EEG recordings that are typically used to stage sleep may not identify seizure disorders; so in cases where seizures are suspected, more elaborate EEG recordings, as well as a neurological consultation, may be necessary.

To place electrodes properly, one should first mark where they will be placed on the scalp. It is important to recognize that improper placement of these electrodes can severely affect the validity of the sleep study and lead to erroneous data. The scalp should be cleaned with alcohol to minimize electrical impedance. The cup-shaped electrodes are filled with conductive paste or jelly and affixed to the scalp with cotton or gauze. The electrodes can be affixed to the scalp with tape or glue, or they can be anchored to the scalp by placing a piece of gauze soaked in **collodion** over the electrode (notice that the gauze can be dried with compressed air after it has been positioned over the electrode). Once the electrodes are affixed to the patient, the electrode wires are then plugged into a junction box, which is coupled to the polygraph recorder.

Respiratory Activity

Assessment of respiratory activity during sleep usually involves measuring oxygen saturation, nasal-oral airflow, and respiratory effort. Oxygen saturation can be easily assessed using pulse oximetry or transcutaneous monitoring. (See Chapter 8 for a detailed discussion of noninvasive blood gas monitoring.) The pulse oximeter probe is placed on an earlobe, finger, or toe. Although transcutaneous monitoring can be used to assess oxygenation during sleep, the transcutaneous probe must be repositioned intermittently (every 2 to 4 hours), and may therefore interfere with the patient's sleep and lead to inadvertent arousal during the study. Indwelling arterial catheters can also be used to assess arterial blood gases, but the risks outweigh the benefits of using this approach and may lead to unnecessary complications.

Nasal-oral airflow is typically measured by a thermistor or thermocouple device at the airway opening. The most common problems with these devices relate to probe position (i.e., the technician may have to reposition the probe frequently and adjust the amplifier sensitivity, thus disturbing the patient's sleep and reducing the validity of the study).

Respiratory effort can be measured by recording rib cage and abdominal movements, measuring intrapleural pressure changes, or measuring airflow at the airway opening with a pneumotachograph. A variety of devices are available for measuring rib cage and abdominal movements, including strain gauge or piezoelectric belts placed around the chest or abdomen, respiratory inductance plethysmography, and impedance pneumography. Intrapleural pressure changes can be measured with an esophageal balloon catheter positioned in the upper third of the esophagus that is connected to a standard strain-gauge pressure transducer.

Remember that although all of these techniques can provide measurements of respiratory effort, techniques that restrict patient movement can compromise test results. Techniques that make the patient uncomfortable can ultimately decrease patient compliance during the study.

Electromyography

Electromyographic recording of various skeletal muscles can be accomplished during sleep using surface electrodes similar to those used for electrocardiograms. Monitoring EMG signals can provide information about the patient's sleep-wake behavior and also allows arousal responses and sleep movements to be quantified. EMG signals recorded from the intercostal muscles can also be used to assess respiratory movements, which is a rather cumbersome technique considering the alternative methods of measuring respiratory activity that were discussed in the previous section.

Three electrodes are typically affixed to the chin with tape. Two of these electrodes are placed between the tip of the chin and the hyoid bone, lateral to each other and 2 cm apart; a third electrode is placed in the center of the chin. The submental EMG signal recorded from these electrodes is used to detect activation of the muscles that expand the upper airways (e.g., the genioglossus and the geniohyoid).[8] When leg movements are to be assessed, two surface electrodes are taped about 3 to 5 cm apart on each leg over the tibialis anterior muscle.

Electrooculography

Recording eye movements during sleep allows the non-REM and REM sleep states to be identified. Electrodes are placed on the skin surface in the periorbital region, specifically about 1 cm lateral to the outer canthi of the eyes and offset from the horizontal plane (i.e., 1 cm above the horizontal plane on one side and 1 cm below the horizontal plane on the other side). With this configuration, horizontal, vertical, and oblique eye movements can be detected. Figure 14-5 shows how these movements are recorded. Note that the height or depth of the deflection depends on the movement of the eyes relative to the fixed electrodes and is described as being either right-of-center (ROC) or left-of-center (LOC).[5]

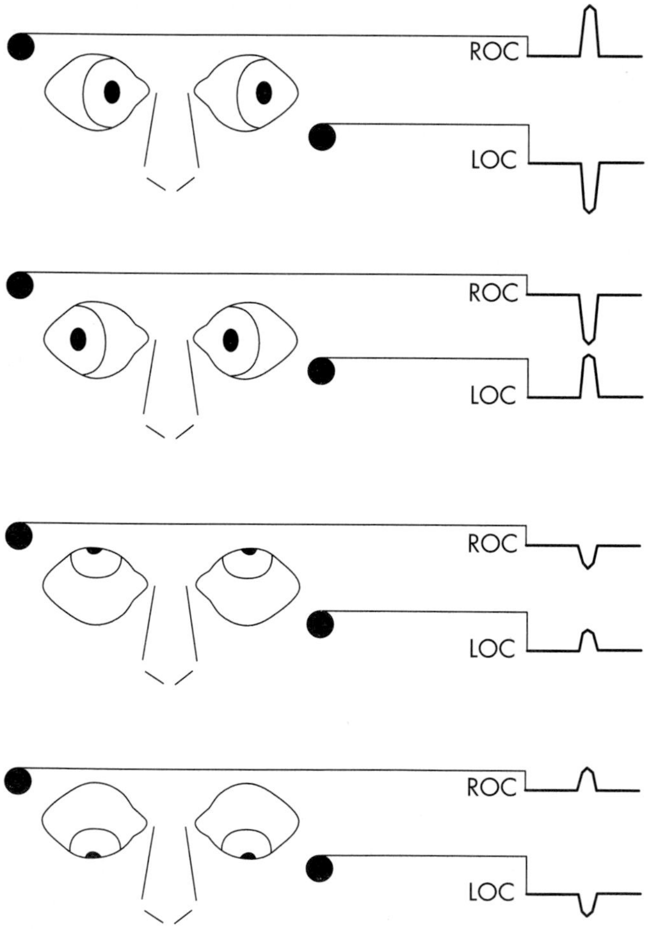

Figure 14-5 Electrooculogram electrode placement. ***ROC*** indicates eye movement to the right of center; ***LOC*** indicates eye movement to the left of center. (Redrawn from Sheldon SH, Spire JP, and Levy HB: Pediatric sleep medicine, Philadelphia, 1992, Saunders.)

Calibration of Polysomnography Signals

Calibration of the polysomnography equipment should be performed before the electrodes are placed on the patient using manufacturer's recommendations (check the user's manual for details on calibrating various channels). Once the electrodes and sensors are affixed to the patient, a presleep calibration should be performed. This calibration lets the technician determine if all of the electrodes and sensors are positioned properly, if the amplifier settings are appropriate for retrieving meaningful data, and if there are any recording device malfunctions (i.e., chart recorder is functioning improperly). It also provides a series of baseline references for awake measurements. Documenting all calibrations is essential because if calibration is performed inadequately, the test results are ultimately invalid.

PATHOPHYSIOLOGY OF SLEEP APNEA

Sleep apnea is defined as repeated episodes of complete airflow cessation for longer than 10 seconds.[9] Hypopnea, in contrast, is usually defined as a reduction in airflow by 50% or more for 10 seconds, with some residual airflow and a physiologic consequence (i.e., arterial oxygen desaturation).[10,11] To compare the frequency of apnea with that of

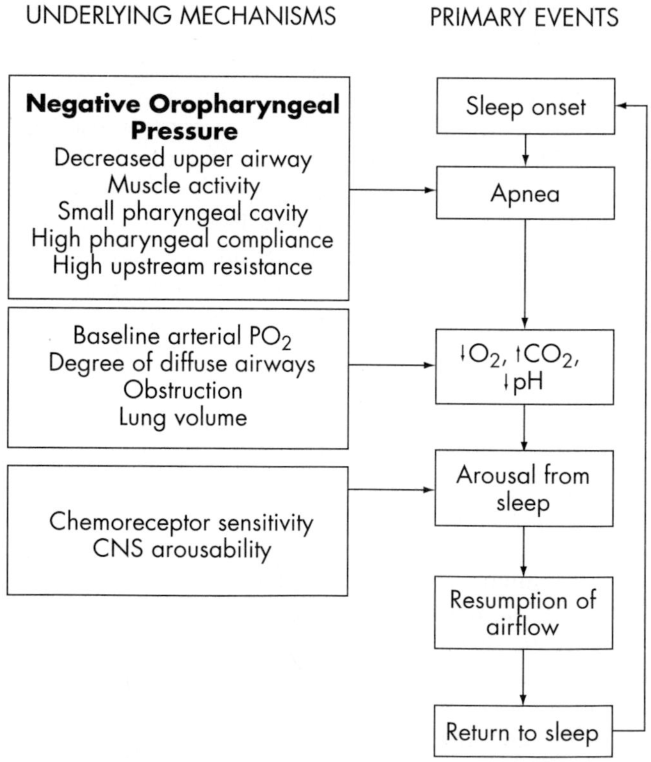

Figure 14-6 The primary sequence of events in OSA, along with the pathogenic mechanisms that contribute to these events. (Redrawn from Bradley TD and Phillipson EA: Pathogenesis and pathophysiology of the obstructive sleep apnea syndrome, Med Clin North Am 69:1169, 1985.)

hypopnea during a sleep study, an **apnea index** (AI) or an **apnea/hypopnea index** (AHI) is usually calculated. The AI is the number of apneic periods observed divided by the total number of hours of sleep; the AHI includes both apneic and hypopneic episodes for the total number of hours of sleep. Normative data of asymptomatic individuals from Guilleminault and Dement[12] suggest that males average about seven apneic episodes per 8 hours of sleep, and females only average about two episodes per 8 hours of sleep.

Sleep apnea syndrome is considered to be present if apnea occurs in excess of five times per hour of sleep.[10,11] As such, three types of sleep apnea are generally described: **obstructive sleep apnea (OSA), central sleep apnea,** and **mixed sleep apnea.** OSA is characterized by the lack of airflow due to occlusion of the upper airways despite continued respiratory efforts. Central sleep apnea is characterized by the absence of airflow and respiratory efforts. Mixed sleep apnea has characteristics of both central and obstructive sleep apnea, with the central event usually preceding the obstructive event.

Obstructive Sleep Apnea

In OSA, airflow at the airway opening ceases due to complete occlusion of the upper airway. Occlusion of the upper airway may occur with posterior movements of the tongue and palate. As these structures move posteriorly, they come into apposition with the posterior pharyngeal wall, resulting in occlusion of the nasopharynx and the oropharynx.[2] Figure 14-6 shows the sequence of events that typically occur in OSA. Notice that obstruction of the upper airways initiates the primary sequence of events. Then apnea and progressive asphyxia develop until there is arousal from sleep, restoration of upper airway patency, and resumption of airflow. With relief of asphyxia, the person quickly returns to sleep—only to have the sequence of events repeat itself over and over. In fact, the sequence can repeat itself several hundred times per night.[13]

As seen in Figure 14-7, OSA is associated with several physiologic consequences and clinical features.[14] The physiologic consequences of OSA include the development of cardiac arrhythmias, pulmonary and systemic hypertension,

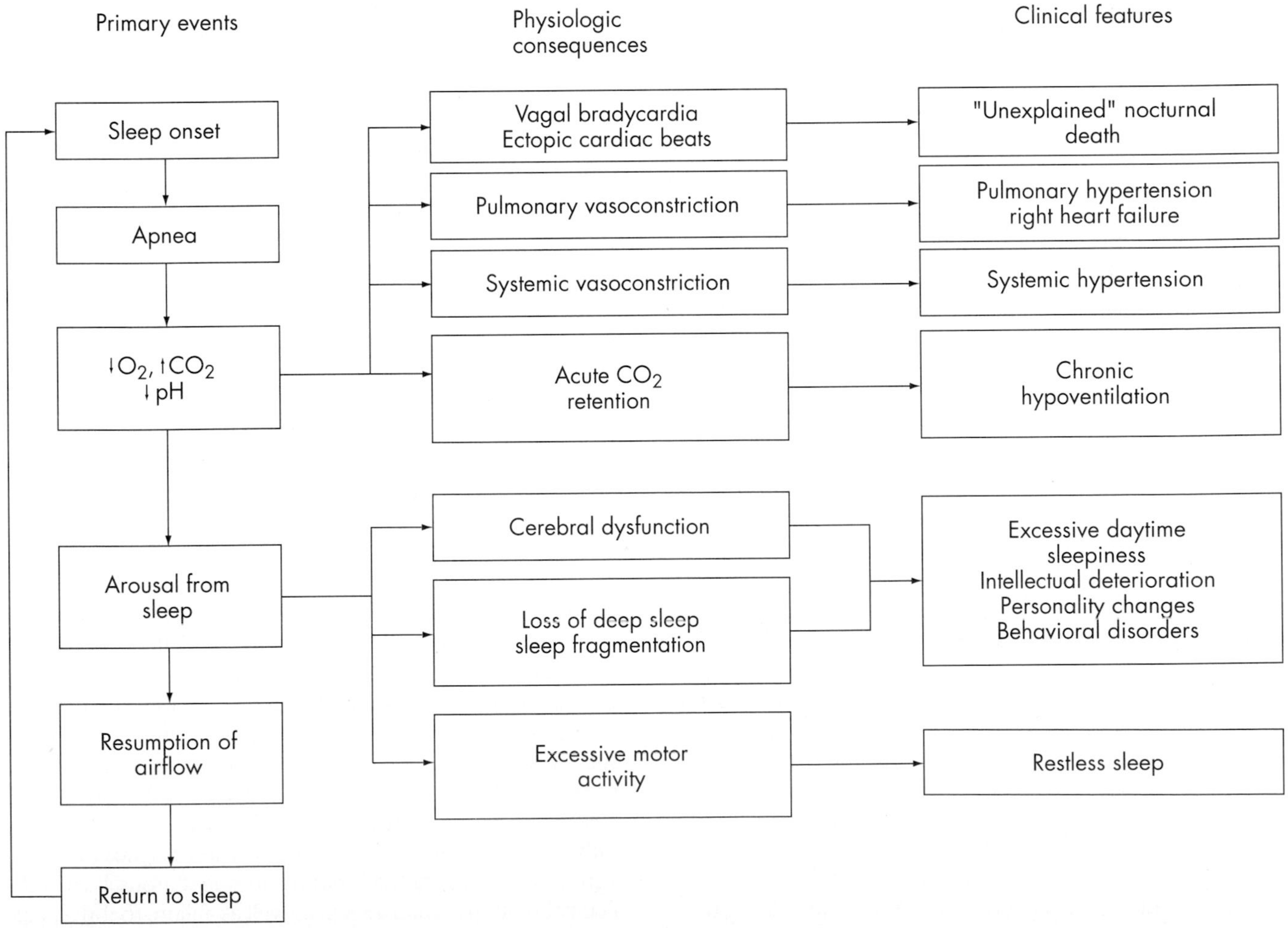

Figure 14-7 The physiologic response and clinical features that result from sleep apnea. (Redrawn from Phillipson EA: Sleep disorders. In Murray JF and Nadel JA, editors: Respiratory medicine, ed 2, Philadelphia, 1994, Saunders.)

BOX 14-3

Standard Definition of Obstructive Sleep Apnea

1 Patient complains of excessive sleepiness or insomnia. Occasionally, patients are unaware of the clinical features observed by others.
2. Patient experiences frequent episodes of obstructed breathing during sleep.
3. Associated features include loud snoring, morning headaches, a dry mouth upon awakening, and chest retraction during sleep in young children.
4. Polysomnographic monitoring demonstrates more than five obstructive apneas >10 seconds each in duration per hour of sleep, and one or more of the following:
   - Frequent arousal from sleep associated with apneas
   - Bradytachycardia
   - Arterial oxygen desaturation in association with the apneic episode—with or without a multi-sleep latency of less than 10 minutes
5. OSA can be associated with other medical disorders (e.g., tonsillar enlargement).
6. Other sleep disorders can be present (e.g., periodic limb movement disorder or narcolepsy).

From Diagnostic Steering Committee: The international classification of sleep disorders: diagnostic and coding manual, ed 2, Lawrence, Kan., 1997, Allen Press.

BOX 14-4

Decision Making & Problem Solving

Mr. H is a 62-year old automobile mechanic with a 60-pack per year history of smoking cigarettes. He was referred to the sleep laboratory after he was involved in an automobile accident when he reportedly fell asleep while driving home from work. He is unaware of any chronic abnormalities with his sleep pattern, but he does acknowledge that he has experienced excessive daytime sleepiness. His wife reports that she has noticed that he snores throughout the night and his sleep has become increasingly restless during the past 6 months. In fact, his wife reports that his snoring has become loud enough to disturb her sleep, and jokes that if his snoring gets any louder the neighbor may begin to complain. She also reports that his snoring episodes are more frequent and considerably louder if he has a night cap (i.e., consumes an alcoholic drink) before going to sleep. Does this patient demonstrate any history and physical findings that suggest the presence of OSA? Briefly describe a diagnostic strategy to properly diagnose his condition.

See Appendix A for the answer.

acute hypercapnia, cerebral dysfunction, loss of deep sleep and sleep fragmentation, and excessive motor activity. These physiologic alterations can result in turn in restless sleep, excessive daytime sleepiness, personality and behavioral changes, intellectual deterioration, right-heart failure, and unexplained nocturnal death.[2]

The most common symptoms associated with OSA in adult patients include chronic loud snoring, gasping or choking episodes during sleep, excessive daytime sleepiness, morning headaches, and personality and cognitive deterioration related to fatigue from lack of sleep. Box 14-3 contains the standard definition of OSA, which was published by the American Sleep Disorders Association.[15] Patients at the greatest risk of developing OSA are those who are obese (particularly those demonstrating nuchal obesity [i.e., neck size >17 inches for men and >16 inches for women] and nasopharyngeal narrowing). Systemic hypertension also adds to the risk of OSA. The symptoms of OSA may be worse when patients ingest central nervous system depressants (i.e., sedatives, hypnotics, etc.) or consume alcohol, especially when it is ingested close to bedtime. Partial sleep deprivation, such as occurs with shift work, may also affect patients with moderate OSA symptoms. Respiratory allergies and environmental factors, such as smoking and ascent to altitude, can augment the symptoms of patients with mild OSA.

Figure 14-8 shows the key polysomnographic events that occur during the apneic episode of a patient with OSA. Although there is a cessation of airflow, respiratory efforts continue, as evidenced by movement of the rib cage and the abdomen. During the apneic episode, there is a fall in oxygen saturation. Box 14-4 presents the case of a patient with OSA.

The criteria for defining OSA in children are not as well established as those for adults.[10] In children, OSA is best identified by combining phasic oxygen desaturation, hypercarbia, and intermittent paradoxical respiratory efforts. (Note that oxygen desaturation of less than 92% is generally considered abnormal in children, depending on their baseline oxygen saturation. Brief oxygen desaturations of >4% occur infrequently in children, and thus should be considered abnormal. Measurements of end-tidal partial pressure of carbon dioxide [$PetCO_2$] can also provide evidence of sleep-disordered breathing in children. It has been suggested that $PetCO_2$ values of >45 torr for at least 60% of the total sleep time or $PetCO_2$ values >13 torr above baseline values indicate sleep-disordered breathing.)[10] Other criteria that should be noted when diagnosing sleep apnea in children include snoring, frequent arousal, and difficulty breathing while asleep, as well as, failure to thrive, cor pulmonale, or neurobehavioral disturbances.[16]

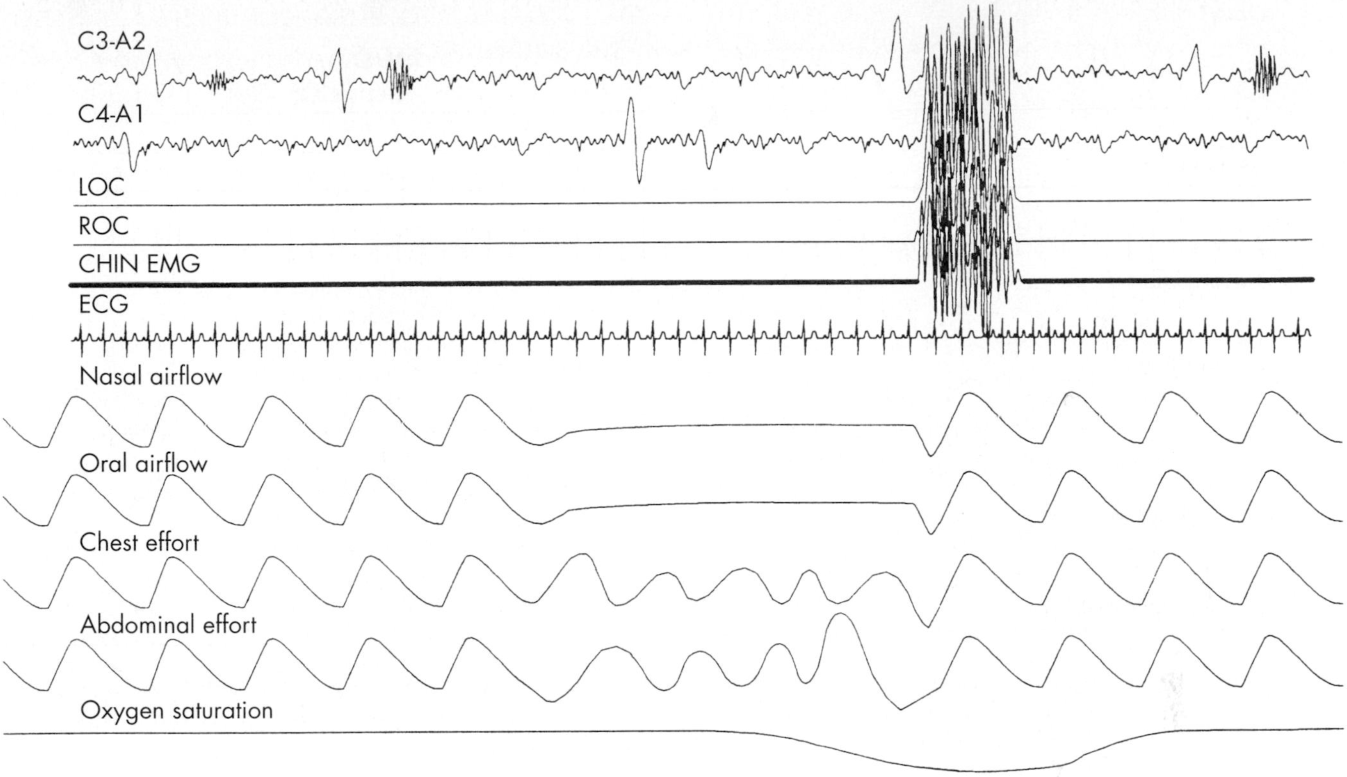

Figure 14-8 Polysomnographic tracings of a patient demonstrating OSA during REM sleep. The patient exhibited constant loud snoring, paradoxical movement of the chest and abdomen, and recurrent complete airway obstructions, leading to oxygen desaturation. (Redrawn from Sheldon SH, Spire JP, and Levy HB: Pediatric sleep medicine, Philadelphia, 1992, Saunders.)

Central Sleep Apnea

Central sleep apnea includes several disorders associated with cessation of respiratory drive and a complete loss of EMG activity of the respiratory muscles. Several mechanisms that have been proposed to account for these alterations involve defects in respiratory control or muscle function, transient fluctuation in respiratory drive, and reflex inhibition of central respiratory drive.[2] Central sleep apnea is associated with central alveolar hypoventilation, neuromuscular diseases involving the respiratory muscles, and central nervous system diseases, but it can occur secondary to hyperventilation, such as occurs when a person ascends to high altitudes. Central sleep apnea is also a common finding in patients who experience esophageal reflux or upper airway collapse. It is important to mention only about 10% of apneic patients seen in most sleep laboratories have central sleep apnea, thus our knowledge of this disorder is somewhat limited when compared with the information available about OSA.[17]

Patients with central sleep apnea typically report gasping for air and shortness of breath upon awakening from a central sleep apneic episode. Depression, as assessed both subjectively and by formal testing, is a common finding among patients with central sleep apnea. It is interesting to note that patients with central sleep apnea do not normally report insomnia and hypersomnolence like those with OSA. Patients with central sleep apnea typically have a normal body habitus, although obese patients may also demonstrate this form of sleep apnea.

Figure 14-9 shows an example of a polysomnographic tracing for a patient with central sleep apnea. As with OSA, there is a complete cessation of airflow that lasts for 10 seconds or longer. In contrast to OSA, airflow cessation is associated with a cessation in respiratory effort, and thus no movement of the rib cage or abdomen.

Mixed Sleep Apnea

Most patients who experience central sleep apnea also demonstrate evidence of OSA. In fact, because these two types of apnea typically coexist, most authors define central sleep apnea as occurring in individuals in whom more than 55% of the apneic episodes are central in origin. The exact cause of mixed apnea is unclear at this time; but it has been suggested that the mechanisms responsible for central and obstructive sleep apnea may be related because several studies have shown that the upper airway muscles behave like respiratory muscles. That is, the upper airway muscles contract and dilate the pharynx when the diaphragm is stimulated.[18]

Polysomnography provides clear evidence of the presence of mixed apnea. As Figure 14-10 shows, airflow

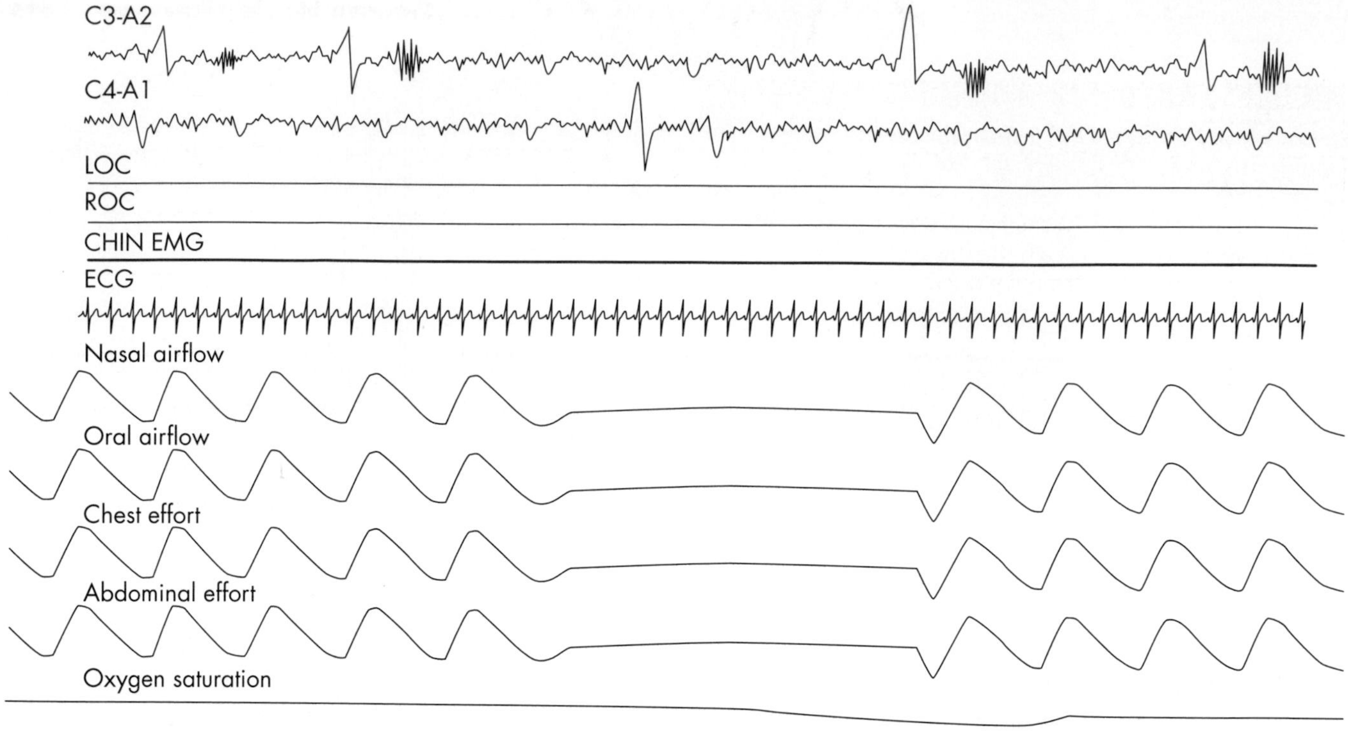

Figure 14-9 Polysomnographic tracings of a patient with central sleep apnea. Note that during the apneic episode there is complete cessation of nasal and oral airflow with concomitant absence of respiratory effort (i.e., no movements of chest or abdomen). (Redrawn from Sheldon SH, Spire JP, and Levy HB: Pediatric sleep medicine, Philadelphia, 1992, Saunders.)

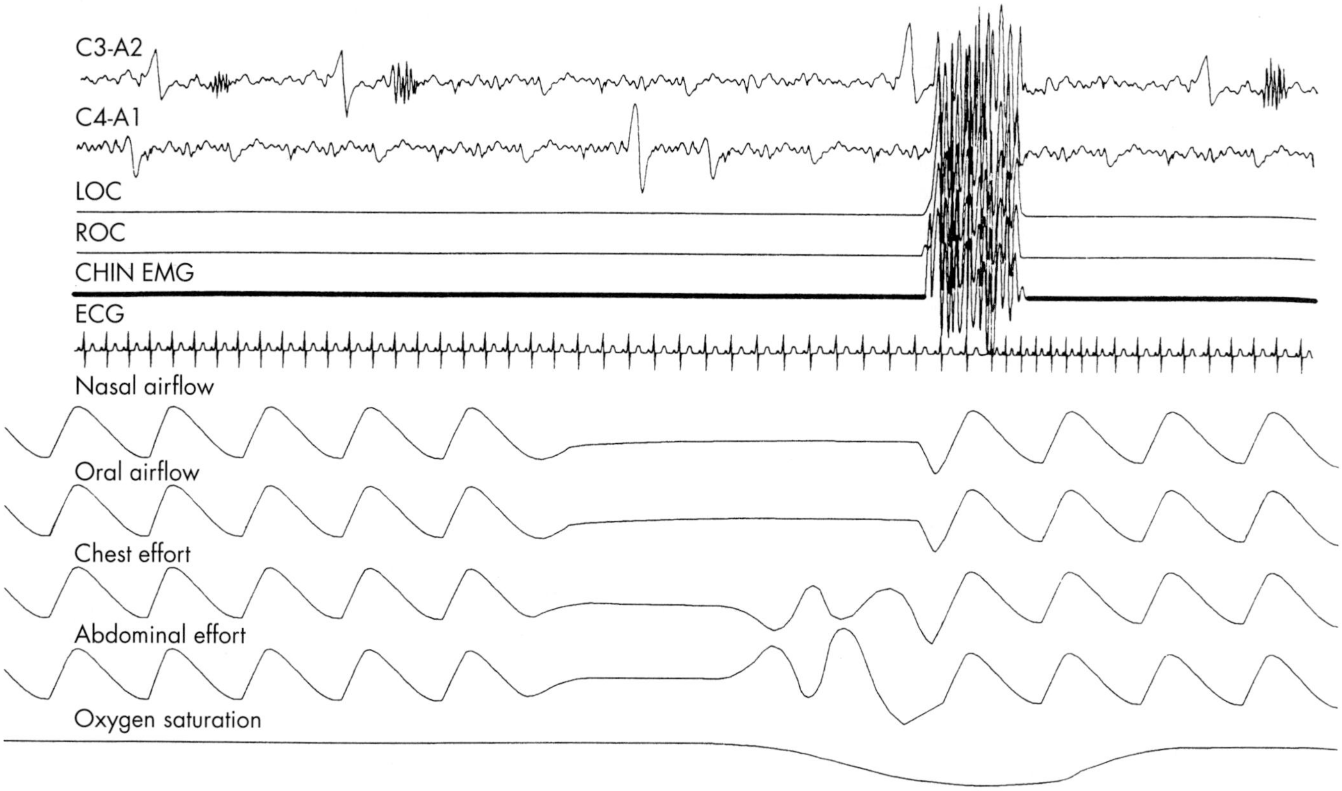

Figure 14-10 Polysomnographic tracings from a patient with mixed apnea. There is cessation of airflow at the nose and mouth. Initially, there is an absence of respiratory effort (central component), followed by at least two cycles of respiratory effort with continued absence of airflow (obstructive component). Significant oxygen desaturation is also present. Note that the EEG, EOG, and EMG signals are obscured by motion artifacts. (Redrawn from Sheldon SH, Spire JP, and Levy HB: Pediatric sleep medicine, Philadelphia, 1992, Saunders.

BOX 14-5

Decision Making & Problem Solving

The following polysomnogram was obtained from a 45-year old post-polio patient who was referred to the sleep laboratory for diagnosis of sleep apnea. She complains of restless sleep, morning headaches, chronic fatigue, and daytime sleepiness. Interpret these findings.

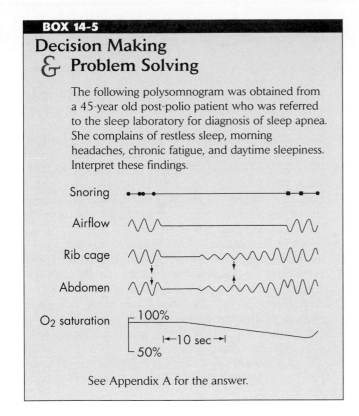

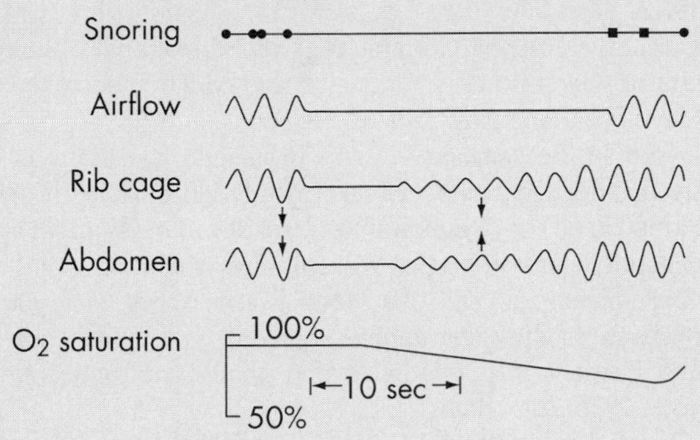

See Appendix A for the answer.

cessation is preceded by a central apneic event (i.e., no movement of the rib cage or abdomen). The obstructive component can be ascertained by observing that there is a resumption of respiratory effort, although there is still a cessation of airflow. With arousal from sleep, the apneic event ends and airflow resumes as the airway opens (Box 14-5).

Summary

The physiologic effects of sleep on breathing are normally of little consequence in healthy individuals. In patients with altered respiratory function, however, sleep can have profound effects on physiologic function, which—if left untreated—can lead to dire consequences. Recent advances in our understanding of sleep structure and ability to assess cardiopulmonary and neuromuscular function during sleep have greatly improved our ability to recognize and treat sleep-related disorders.

Three types of sleep apnea are described: obstructive, central, and mixed. OSA is characterized by airflow cessation at the airway opening, even though the patient continues to make respiratory efforts. Central sleep apnea involves a complete cessation of respiratory efforts and airflow, and mixed apnea includes characteristics of both obstructive and central apnea. In patients with mixed apnea, the central apneic component typically precedes the obstructive event.

Diagnosis of sleep apnea is based on clinical findings, including patient history and physical examination, along with laboratory studies. Obtaining a complete history and physical examination is the first step of identifying if an individual is at risk for sleep apnea. Overnight monitoring of arterial blood gases with pulse oximetry or transcutaneous electrodes or polysomnography is then performed to make a definitive diagnosis of sleep apnea.

Although there is some controversy about the best strategy to use when attempting to diagnose sleep apnea, it is generally agreed that polysomnography is the gold standard for evaluating the presence and severity of sleep apnea. Polysomnography, which involves recording various electrogenic potentials (e.g., ECGs, EEGs, respiratory activity, and EOGs) can also be used to select the most effective management strategy once sleep apnea is identified in a patient.

Review Questions

See Appendix A for the answers.

1. Which of the following are characteristic findings of Stage 2 of non-REM sleep?
   I. Sleep spindles and K-complexes on EEG
   II. Slow pendulous and disconjugate movements of the eyes
   III. A relatively low threshold for arousal from sleep
   IV. Adult patients typically enter this stage of sleep after about 90 minutes of non-REM sleep
   a. I and II only
   b. II and IV only
   c. I, II, and III only
   d. II, III, and IV only
2. The classic states of non-REM and REM sleep are not easily identified at birth using standard polysomnography—true or false?
3. Describe the impact of sleep on breathing in a healthy adult.
4. Which of the following changes in cardiovascular function occurs during sleep?
   a. Heart rate increases by about 5 to 10 beats/minute during non-REM sleep
   b. Blood pressure decreases by as much as 25 mm Hg during REM sleep
   c. Cardiac output increases only slightly during non-REM sleep
   d. Stroke volume remains constant during non-REM and REM sleep
5. When performing polysomnography, it is suggested that the technician monitor a minimum of at least two modified ECG leads—true or false?
6. List three variables that should be monitored to assess respiratory activity during polysomnography.

7. Which of the following are typical history and physical findings in patients with OSA?
   I. Chronic loud snoring
   II. Excessive daytime sleepiness
   III. Personality changes
   IV. Obesity
   a. I and III only
   b. II and IV only
   c. I, II, and III only
   d. I, II, III, and IV

8. Describe the physiologic consequences of OSA.

9. Which of the following are associated with central sleep apnea?
   I. Alveolar hypoventilation
   II. Myasthenia gravis
   III. Stroke
   IV. Angina pectoris
   a. I and II only
   b. II and III only
   c. I, II, and III only
   d. I, III, and IV only

10. Which of the following findings will a patient demonstrate during periods of mixed apnea with hypoxemia?
    a. Systemic hypotension
    b. Increased cardiac output
    c. Decreased heart rate
    d. Pulmonary hypertension

References

1. Guilleminault C and Dement WC: General physiology of sleep. In Crystal RG and West JB, editors: The lung: scientific foundations, New York, 1991, Raven Press, Ltd.
2. Phillipson EA: Sleep disorders. In Murray JF and Nadel JA, editors: Respiratory medicine, ed 2, Philadelphia, 1994, Saunders.
3. Aserinsky E and Kleitman N: Regularly occurring periods of eye motility and concomitant phenomena during sleep, Science 118:273, 1953.
4. Guyton AC and Hall JE: Human physiology and mechanisms of disease, ed 6, Philadelphia, 1996, Saunders.
5. Sheldon SH, Spire JP, and Levy HB: Pediatric sleep medicine, Philadelphia, 1992, Saunders.
6. American Association for Respiratory Care: Clinical practice guideline: polysomnography, Respir Care 40(12):1236, 1995.
7. Jasper HH: The ten-twenty system of the International Federation, Electroencephalogr Clin Neurophysiol 10:371, 1958.
8. Funsten AW and Suratt PM: Evaluation of respiratory disorders during sleep, Clinics in Chest Medicine 10(2): 1989.
9. Strollo PJ and Fernandez KS: Disorders of sleep. In Scanlan CL, Wilkins RL, and Stoller JK, editors: Egan's fundamentals of respiratory care, ed 7, St Louis, 1998, Mosby.
10. Phillips BA, Anstead MI, and Gottlieb DL: Monitoring sleep and breathing: methodology, Clin Chest Med 19(1):203, 1998.
11. Arand DL and Bonnet MH: Sleep-disordered breathing. In Burton GC, Hodgkin JE, and Ward JJ: Respiratory care: a guide to clinical practice, ed 4, Philadelphia, 1997.
12. Guilleminault C and Dement WC: Sleep apnea syndromes and related sleep disorders. In Williams RL and Karacan I, editors: Sleep disorders: diagnosis and treatment, New York, 1978, Wiley and Sons.
13. Bradley TD and Phillipson EA: Pathogenesis and pathophysiology of the obstructive sleep apnea syndrome, Med Clin North Am 69:1169, 1985.
14. Phillipson EA: Sleep apnea, Med Clin North Am 23:2314, 1982.
15. Diagnostic Steering Committee: The international classification of sleep disorders: diagnostic and coding manual, ed 2, Lawrence, Kan., 1997, Allen Press.
16. Dyson M, Beckerman RC, and Brouillette RT: Obstructive sleep apnea syndrome. In Beckerman RC, Brouillette RT, and Hunt CE, editors: Respiratory control disorders in infants and children, Baltimore, 1992, Williams and Wilkins.
17. Guilleminault C, Van den Hoed J, and Mitler M: Clinical overview of the sleep apnea syndrome. In Guilleminault C and Dement WC, editors): Sleep apnea syndromes, New York, 1978, Alan R. Liss, Inc.
18. Onal E, Lopata M, and O'Connor T: Pathogenesis of apnea in hypersomnia-sleep apnea syndrome, Am Rev Respir Dis 125:167, 1982.

Internet Resources

1. American Association for Respiratory Care: http://www.aarc.org
2. American Sleep Disorders Organization: http://www.asda.org
3. The Sleep Medicine Homepage: http://www.users.cloud9.net/~thorpy
4. Sleep Net: http://www.sleepnet.com
5. National Jewish Medical and Research Center: http://www.njc.org
6. The Association of Polysomnographic Technologists: http://www.aptweb.org/index.htm
7. University of Pennsylvania Obstructive Sleep Apnea Page: http://www.med.upenn.edu/health/pf_files/penntoday/v6n1/sleep.html
8. National Heart Lung and Blood Institute—Facts about sleep apnea: http://www.nhlbi.nih.gov/nhlbi/sleep/gp/sleepapn.htm
9. National Institute of Neurological Disorders and Stroke—Understanding sleep: http://www.ninds.nih.gov/HEAINFO/DISORDERS/SLEEP/brain-basics-sleep.HTM

APPENDIX A

Answers to Decision Making & Problem Solving Boxes and Review Questions

Author's Note

Decisions made in the clinical setting vary considerably between individuals and hospitals. There is usually more than one acceptable solution to a problem in patient care. The answers provided here represent only one or two possible choices of treatment. Readers are encouraged to talk these cases over with instructors, mentors, and other colleagues.

CHAPTER 1

Decision Making & Problem Solving Boxes

Box 1-6

You can calculate the volume of gas in his lungs as he descends the pond by applying Boyle's law. We know that at sea level, where pressure surrounding the diver equals 1 atm (atmospheric pressure), the volume in his lungs equals 3000 mL. As the diver descends, the pressure surrounding him increases by 1 atm for every 33 feet. Thus, at 33 feet, the pressure exerted on the diver equals 2 atm. We can calculate the volume of gas in his lungs using the following variation of Boyle's law,

$$V_2 = V_1P_1/P_2$$
$$V_2 = (3000\text{ mL})\ (1\text{ atm})/(2\text{ atm})$$
$$V_2 = 1500\text{ mL}$$

At a depth of 66 feet, the pressure exerted on the diver equals 3 atm and his volume is calculated as,

$$V_2 = V_1P_1/P_2$$
$$V_2 = (3000\text{ mL})\ (1\text{ atm})/(3\text{ atm})$$
$$V_2 = 1000\text{ mL}$$

Thus at 33 feet below the surface of the pond, the pressure to which the diver is exposed equals 2 atm, causing the diver's lung volume to decrease to one half (1500 mL) of the original volume at 33 feet and one third (1000 mL) of the original volume at 66 feet.

Box 1-7

According to Gay-Lussac's law, the pressure of a gas within a cylinder is directly related to the temperature at which the cylinder is exposed. Increasing this temperature therefore causes a proportional increase in the pressure of the gas within the cylinder. Thus, in this example, if the fire is not controlled and the temperature in the basement rises, the pressure within the cylinders can increase, creating an explosive hazard. Moving the cylinders therefore removes the hazardous condition.

Box 1-8

In this problem, P_1 = 760 mm Hg; V_1 = 6L; T_1 = 273K; T_2 = 37° C (310 K); P_2 = 3 atm or 2280 mm Hg; V_2 = unknown. Thus,

$$P_1V_1/T_1 = P_2V_2/T_2$$
$$V_2 = P_1V_1T_2/P_2T_1$$
$$V_2 = [(760\text{ mm Hg})(6\text{ L})(310\text{ K})] / [(2280\text{ mm Hg})(273\text{ K})]$$
$$V_2 = 2.27\text{ L}$$

Box 1-9

Various conditions can cause a reduction in the rate of oxygen diffusion across the alveolar-capillary membrane. Decreasing the surface area of the membrane (e.g., resection of a lobe of the lung), increasing the thickness of the alveolar-capillary membrane (e.g., pulmonary fibrosis or the presence of pulmonary edema), and reducing the partial pressure gradient for oxygen between the alveoli and the blood flowing through the pulmonary capillary (e.g., reducing the partial pressure of inspired oxygen, such as when one ascends the high altitude) will reduce the rate at which oxygen crosses the alveolar-capillary membrane.

Review Questions

1. (a) 98.6° F; (b) 12° C; (c) 310 K; (d) 298 K
2. (a) 2.94 kPa; (b) 1034 cm H_2O; (c) 33 cm H_2O; (d) 3 atm
3. PO_2 = 158 mm Hg; PN_2 = 585 mm Hg; PCO_2 = 0.22 mm Hg
4. c

5. 793.15 mm Hg
6. 2.4 L
7. The density of oxygen = 32/22.4 = 1.43 g/L. The density of carbon dioxide = 44/22.4 = 1.973 g/L.
8. b
9. a, c, or d
10. d
11. 2 A
12. (1) Ensuring that all devices attached to patients are electrically grounded; (2) ensuring equipment circuit interrupters are functioning; (3) ensuring that all electrical devices used with a microshock-sensitive patient are well-insulated and connected to outlets with a common, low-resistance ground.

CHAPTER 2

Decision Making & Problem Solving Boxes

Box 2-2

(1) Frozen carbon dioxide (dry ice); (2) Heliox; (3) Oxygen; (4) Nitric oxide.

Box 2-5

There is an apparent leak at the connection. The valve stem should first be closed, then the connection between the cylinder outlet and the regulator tightened.

Box 2-9

Turn off the zone valve that controls oxygen flow from the main oxygen supply to the affected area (in this case, the fifth floor of the north wing). Call for assistance to provide E cylinders of oxygen for patients requiring oxygen therapy.

Review Questions

1. b or c
2. d
3. c
4. d
5. d
6. c
7. a
8. b
9. b
10. d
11. a
12. b
13. c
14. a
15. False; see Box 2-8.

CHAPTER 3

Decision Making & Problem Solving Boxes

Box 3-4

The flow rate of oxygen is 6 L/min or 100 mL/sec (6000mL/60 sec). If the expired gas is exhaled in the first 1.5 sec of expiration, then 0.5 sec are available for filling the anatomic reservoir, which is approximately 50 mL for this patient. The anatomical reservoir includes the nose, nasopharynx, and oropharynx, which is about one third of the patient's deadspace, or 150 mL (1 mL for every pound is a good estimate of the amount of deadspace in a normal subject). The patient's inspiration lasts 1 sec, so he will inspire 100 mL of 100% oxygen. Therefore the anatomical reservoir and the inspiratory flow deliver 150 mL of 100% oxygen to the patient. The remaining 350 mL of tidal volume will be entrained room air, which has an FiO_2 of about 0.20. This 350 mL of room air contains 70 mL of 100% oxygen (350 mL × 0.20 = 70 mL).

The delivered FiO_2 can now be estimated:

50 mL of 100% oxygen from the anatomical reservoir.
100 mL of 100% oxygen (O_2 flow = 100 mL/sec).
350 mL of 21% oxygen (350 mL × 0.20 = 70 mL).
220 mL of 100% oxygen/500 mL tidal volume.
Estimated delivered FiO_2 = 0.44.

Box 3-5

These are common complaints of patients who use nasal cannulas for long-term oxygen therapy. You could suggest that he consider using a transtracheal oxygen (TTO) device. These devices are more comfortable for patients requiring long-term oxygen therapy and are generally well-tolerated by patients. Just as important, they are cosmetically more pleasing to most patients than nasal cannulas. If the patient agrees to try the TTO device, you must teach him how to properly care for it. Adequate education is an essential part of ensuring patient compliance with any type of long-term oxygen therapy device.

Box 3-8

You should remove the helium-oxygen mixture, switch the patient to 100% oxygen (i.e., non-rebreathing mask), and immediately notify the physician of the patient's condition. You should recheck the concentration of oxygen delivered from the cylinder. It is possible that the contents of the cylinder were "unmixed," and thus the FiO_2 delivered to the patient was actually much less than expected.

Review Questions

1. The easiest way to determine the number of stages in a regulator is to count the number of pressure-relief valves. Each chamber should have its own pressure-relief valve.
2. c
3. False
4. c
5. d
6. c
7. b
8. (1) Pneumothorax, (2) sinusitis, (3) seizures, (4) optic neuritis, (5) hypercapnia.

9. d
10. c
11. The actual flow delivered to the patient is 18 L/min because you must multiply the indicated flow by the correction factor of 1.8. Thus 1.8 × 10 L/min = 18 L/min.
12. d
13. (1) Flushed skin; (2) full and bounding pulse; (3) the presence of premature ventricular contractions (PVCs); (4) hypertension; (5) muscle twitching.

Chapter 4

Decision Making & Problem Solving Boxes

Box 4-10

The most appropriate device for a 4-year old child is a small-volume nebulizer. If possible, the aerosol should be administered through a mouthpiece to provide improved deposition of the medication. Although an MDI treatment could be suggested, this type of device may not be the most effective means of delivering aerosols to younger pediatric patients.

Box 4-11

Sample devices might include the Circulaire, RespirGard II, or Pari IS2. MMAD should be in the 1 to 3 micron range.

Box 4-15

A heated bland aerosol device with a MMAD of 1 to 5 microns, or a heated-wick device.

Box 4-16

The problem is that the device is unable to meet the inspiratory flow needs of the patient. As a consequence, he must entrain room air, which reduces the FIO_2 that is being delivered. You can correct this situation by choosing a high-flow aerosol generator, such as a Misty-Ox device. Alternatively, you could connect two low-flow aerosol nebulizers together with a Brigg's adapter to increase flow. The key point is to choose an aerosol delivery device that can provide an inspiratory flow that will exceed the patient's inspiratory flow needs.

Box 4-17

A fitted respirator mask, gloves, and goggles will probably be adequate. A gown is also useful protection, but may not be practical in the home-care setting.

Review Questions

1. a
2. a
3. c
4. a
5. b
6. c
7. a
8. d
9. (1) Simple HMEs, (2) heat and moisture exchanging filters, (3) hygroscopic condenser humidfiers, and (4) hygroscopic condenser humidifiers with filters.
10. b
11. b
12. b
13. b
14. b
15. c

Chapter 5

Decision Making & Problem Solving Boxes

Box 5-1

Two devices that can be used in this emergency situation are laryngeal mask airways (LMA) and the Combitube.

Box 5-2

There are several possibilities. The tube could be in the esophagus, the patient's cardiac output could be low, or there could be no perfusion of blood through the lungs, as might occur as a result of a massive pulmonary embolus.

Box 5-3

First, the airway should be clear of any excessive secretions. The cuff is then deflated, which may necessitate suctioning the patient if secretions that were above the cuff become dislodged. The inner cannula is then removed, and the tracheostomy tube opening is occluded. The patient is evaluated to determine upper airway function.

Review Questions

1. a
2. c
3. c
4. b
5. b
6. a
7. d
8. a
9. d
10. a
11. (1) Detection of CO_2 with a capnograph; (2) auscultation of bilateral breath sounds and no audible sounds over the gastric region when the patient is artificially ventilated; (3) lateral chest radiograph.
12. b
13. d
14. d
15. b
16. c

Chapter 6

Decision Making & Problem Solving Boxes

Box 6-3

This is a fairly common problem encountered by respiratory therapists. Most patients who have undergone abdominal surgical procedures avoid taking deep breaths because of the intense pain that occurs when the diaphragm pushes on the abdominal contents. This patient should be started on an aggressive plan that includes bronchial hygiene and lung expansion therapy to prevent postoperative atelectasis and pneumonia. The plan could include incentive spirometry, cough training (with instructions on splinting), aerosol therapy, and possibly chest physiotherapy and postural drainage.

Box 6-6

Although the patient is a candidate for antibiotic therapy as a medical treatment, respiratory care is needed to help clear secretions and reexpand lung bases that seem to be either secretion filled and/or atelectatic. Because the patient is unable to cooperate to perform therapies such as incentive spirometry and/or coughing and deep breathing, IPPB is an appropriate form of therapy in this case. This therapy might be accompanied by an beta adrenergic agent and a mucolytic to help mobilize secretions so that they can be cleared with suctioning. Postural draining and percussion might also be beneficial, particularly because this patient is not mobile.

Box 6-7

This is a primary indication for using IPV. Although it is a relatively new lung expansion technique, early studies indicate that IPV can be a useful bronchial hygiene technique for treating cystic fibrosis patients. Because of the acute nature of the patient's present illness, it is reasonable to give an initial IPV treatment and then reassess the patient in 1 to 2 hours. If the treatment improved gas exchange, as evidenced by physical assessment and pulse oximetry, further treatments would be indicated, thus preventing impending respiratory failure, which would require endotracheal intubation and mechanical ventilation. Other therapeutic modalities that might be considered would include aerosol therapy, chest physiotherapy and postural drainage, and PEP therapy.

Review Questions

1. a
2. c
3. b
4. (1) Upper abdominal surgery; (2) thoracic surgery; (3) presence of a restrictive lung defect associated with quadraplegia or a dysfunctional diaphragm; and (4) to prevent atelectasis in patients with COPD who are scheduled for surgery.
5. The patient should raise the three balls within the plastic housing of the device by taking slow deep breaths through the mouthpiece connected to the Triflo device. The patient should hold each breath for 3 to 5 seconds while raising the three balls. The patient should perform this maneuver for 5 to 10 breaths per session and repeat each session hourly while awake.
6. b
7. This patient is a good candidate for incentive spirometry; he is alert and cooperative. Although he does experience some pain when he takes deep breaths, he should be able to take deep breaths (vital capacity > 10 mL/kg).
8. d
9. d
10. c
11. 100%
12. b
13. (1) Underwater seals; (2) weighted ball resistors; (3) spring-loaded valve resistors; and (4) magnetic valve resistors.
14. d

CHAPTER 7

Decision Making & Problem Solving Boxes

Box 7-1

There are several things that could interfere with the operation of the device: (1) The mouthpiece is connected to wrong side of the device, and thus the exhaled gas cannot be measured in this configuration. (2) The patient did not perform the test properly because either the technique was not clearly explained to him or he did not give a good effort. (3) The device was not plugged in to the electrical outlet. (4) The patient's exhaled gas is leaking around the mouthpiece.

Box 7-2

Lung volume measurements by body plethysmography are an application of Boyle's law (i.e., when temperature is constant, volume and pressure are inversely related: $P_1V_1 = P_2V_2$).

Box 7-4

The FVC, $FEV_{1.0}$, and $FEF_{25\text{-}75}$ are considerably reduced. The $FEV_{1.0}/VC$ is also reduced. The RV and FRC are elevated indicating the presence of airtrapping. These findings are consistent with an individual with moderate to severe COPD.

Box 7-7

One possible explanation for this type of problem is that there is a leak in the sampling line. This problem can also occur when moisture builds up in the sampling line.

Review Questions

1. a
2. c
3. c
4. b
5. b
6. b

7. c
8. a
9. c
10. d
11. Inert gas techniques measure communicating lung volumes; body plethysmographs measure thoracic gas volumes (including gas trapped behind closed airways). For patients with airtrapping, the N_2 washout techniques underestimate the true FRC by the amount of trapped air present.
12. d
13. c
14. d
15. b

CHAPTER 8

Decision Making & Problem Solving Boxes

Box 8-2

The presence of an air bubble will cause the PCO_2 to be lower than normal and the PO_2 to be higher than normal. The reason for this discrepancy is that room air has a PCO_2 of about 0.3 mm Hg and a PO_2 of approximately 150 mm Hg (see Chapter 3 for a full discussion of partial pressures of gases in room air).

Box 8-3

The interpretation of respiratory alkalosis is probably correct. The PO_2 results, however, need to be evaluated by another method because capillary PO_2 does not always correlate well with PaO_2

Box 8-4

Neither the SpO_2 nor the calculated SaO_2 accurately reflect the true oxygen saturation when CO poisoning is suspected. SpO_2 can be falsely high. SaO_2 is calculated by the ABG analyzer's microprocessor; PaO_2 is a measure of dissolved (not bound) O_2. The patient's blood sample should be run on a CO-Oximeter, which directly measures the oxyhemoglobin saturation and carboxyhemoglobin levels. For example, suppose that the CO-Oximeter measured the following: O_2 Hb = 83%; COHb = 15%; and thus HHb = 2%. Assume that the total hemoglobin equals 15 gm%. Then 83% of 15 gm% of Hb = 12.45 gm%; 15% of 15 gm% = 2.25 gm%; 2% of 15 gm% = 0.3 gm%. Notice that the pulse oximeter only detects the levels of O_2Hb and HHb. That is, the pulse oximeter reading suggests that only 2% of the hemoglobin is unsaturated and that 98% is saturated with oxygen. So 98% of the 15 gm% of Hb represents 14.7 gm% O_2Hb. Therefore the pulse oximeter overestimates the true level of oxyhemoglobin by about 2.25 gm%.

Review Questions

1. a
2. b
3. c
4. c
5. a
6. a
7. d
8. a
9. b
10. b
11. d
12. a
13. Quality control may be defined as a system that includes analyzing control samples (with known values of pH, PCO_2, PO_2), assessing the results of these measurements against defined limits, identifying problems, and specifying corrective actions.

    Quality assurance involves proficiency testing, which provides a dynamic process of identification, evaluation, and resolution of problems that affect blood gas measurements.
14. a
15. a
16. c

CHAPTER 9

Decision Making & Problem Solving Boxes

Box 9-10

In an OR/NOR device, the splitter configuration directs the main gas flow straight down to outlet O2. In the proportional amplifier, the splitter configuration appears to split the gas flow, directing part of it to O2 and part to O1.

Box 9-14

The pressure must drop to +10 cm H_2O minus the sensitivity setting (i.e., 10 − 1 = +9 cm H_2O). Inspiration starts when the pressure drops to +9 cm H_2O or 1 cm H_2O below baseline pressure.

Box 9-15

Base flow = 6 L/min − trigger flow. Measured flow must drop to 4 L/min.

Box 9-21

Technically, it is incorrect to call them volume cycled if volume cycling is defined as the measurement of volume and the ending of inspiratory flow when the volumc was achieved. A classic example of this is the MA-1 because the rising of the bellows and the contact of a switch near the top of the bellows ends inspiration (i.e., until the volume leaves the bellows [a volume device] inspiration does not end). This is an example of true volume cycling.

One could argue, however, that the measurement of flow over time is a volume measurement because volume = time/flow. Modern flow-controlling valves are very accurate in their flow delivery. Should we split hairs over this issue? What is most important in the clinical setting? We're interested in volume ventilation or delivery of a tidal volume. We would want to know that the volume left the ventilator at the end of inspiratory flow. This is the case.

Both are correct. One is technically correct by very strict standards and definition. The other is correct based on common clinical usage and an acceptance that flow/T_I = volume.

Box 9-28

We know that PSV is patient-triggered, and that patients determine their own tidal volume based on their lung characteristics and their inspiratory effort, as well as by the set pressure. The ventilator algorithm that ends the breath does so when a predetermined flow that is a percentage of peak flow is reached. It can be argued that the programmer designed the algorithm so that the ventilator knows the patient's inspiration is ending (i.e., flow is declining). Therefore the programming is based on what the patient's breath is doing. So you could argue that it really is the patient's breathing pattern that determines all phases of a pressure-supported breath.

Box 9-31

No, the ventilator will measure a minute ventilation of 7.5 L/min (25 breaths/min × V_T of 0.3 = 7.5 L/min), which is well above the set minimum of 4.0 L/min. The patient has an increased work of breathing. Unless the high rate alarm is set, the operator will be unaware of the patient's problem.

Box 9-39

Problem 1: It seems that inspiratory flow is inadequate because pressures are dropping so low during inspiration. The patient may be opening the safety pop-in valve. Check the gas source to be sure it is on and connected and that the flow is adequate.

Problem 2: There is probably a leak in the system.

Review Questions

1. Pneumatic and electric
2. This is a closed-loop or intelligent system.
3. b
4. Pressure-limited ventilation, pressure-controlled ventilation, and pressure-targeted ventilation
5. c
6. False
7. Controlled volume ventilation is time-triggered, volume-targeted (limited), and time- or volume-cycled. The flow curve is constant (rectangular), and the volume and pressure curves are ascending ramps.
8. Patient-triggering; pressure or flow are the most common variables in patient triggering.
9. There is a leak in the circuit.
10. There seems to be an increase in Raw.
11. CPAP is only for spontaneously breathing patients. The term PEEP implies that mechanical ventilation is also in use.
12. d
13. b
14. High-frequency oscillatory ventilation
15. c
16. b
17. b

Chapter 10

Decision Making & Problem Solving Boxes

Box 10-2

The patient would be able to open the demand valve as long as the −1 cm H_2O pressure is detected, but spontaneous breaths may be unrecognized by the assist transducer. The rate displayed would only show mandatory—not spontaneous—breaths. Also, the exhaled volume display would only update with each mechanical breath, although all volumes since the last mechanical breath would be added together, thus giving a high volume reading.

Box 10-3

The ventilator bases mandatory breath delivery on a time period equal to 60 breaths/sec (4 breaths/min), or 15 seconds. The next mandatory breath will be delivered at the beginning of the next 15-second interval or about 15 seconds after the last mandatory breath. The apnea alarm will sound if the apnea time has been set at less than 15 seconds.

Box 10-6

With a constant flow of 1 L/sec and a V_T of 0.5 L, the inspiratory time is 0.5 seconds (T_I = flow/V_T).

T_I will increase if the curve is changed to a descending ramp. With a descending ramp, the peak flow of 60 L/min is only delivered at the beginning of the breath and gradually slows to 50% of its value. The easiest way to determine the new T_I is to check the digital readout on the monitoring screen for T_I.

Box 10-11

The Insp/Exp Hold pad is pressed twice until "E HLD" is displayed in the monitor window. Next the select key is pressed and held. The expiratory pressure (auto-PEEP) will be displayed in the window.

Box 10-15

The ventilator will switch to the A/C mode if apnea ventilation is activated. The rate will become whatever rate is set on the apnea back-up rate control. The tidal volume will become whatever is set on the tidal volume control. Normal operation can be resumed if the patient begins to spontaneously breathe again (two consecutive breaths with V_T > 50% of set) or the operator presses the alarm reset button and activates the control setting for breath rate.

Box 10-23

First, these settings are pretty absurd for any patient and are only given here to demonstrate a point.

The "limited" alert tells the therapist that an incompatible settings condition exists. Check the T_I, V_T, and flow to see if the V_T can be delivered in the T_I determined by the set variables. TCT = 60/20 = 3 sec. Flow = 20 L/min, or 0.33 L/sec. T_I = V_T/flow plus inspiratory pause = 0.7 L/(0.33 L/sec) plus 1.2 sec = 3.32 sec. This means that the T_I would exceed TCT, which is an impossible condition.

The inspiratory flow definitely needs to be increased, and the use of a 1.2-second inspiratory pause should be questioned.

Box 10-24

The breath was flow-cycled. The breath ended when flow dropped to the set peak flow value of 60 L/min. Tidal volume delivery was about 0.8 L, which was higher than the set value of 0.65 L.

Box 10-31

(1) PCV is active in the CMV mode. The operator only has to set the pressure limit using the press.control knob to establish the desired ventilating pressure. To check this setting, press the Paw touch pad below the measured values window and read the P_{peak} value.

(2) The manufacturer recommends using the plateau pressure from a volume-targeted breath and adding 3 cm H_2O. In this case, $P_{plateau}$ was 16 cm H_2O. A starting pressure would be about 19 cm H_2O.

(3) The $\dot{V}_E$ in volume ventilation was 6.5 L/min (0.65 L × 10 breaths/min = 6.5 L). You could start at a liter above and below the previous target, using 5.5 L/min (low alarm) and 7.5 L/min (high alarm). Then see how much the patient's $\dot{V}_E$ fluctuates once PCV is initiated. The exact amount for setting high and low $\dot{V}_E$ alarms is strictly up to clinicians and the institutions in which they practice.

(4) Tidal volume delivery can be checked by pressing the touch pad marked with a "T,V_T,f,R,C" below the measured values window. The measured expired V_T ("VTe") will appear in the window.

Box 10-34

(1) The flow waveform is constant because the ventilator is in volume-targeted ventilation.

(2) The inspiratory time of a mandatory breath is calculated as follows:

CMV rate = 15 breaths/min
60 sec ÷ 15 breaths/min = 4 sec is the mandatory breath cycle time. TCT/(sum of I:E) = inspiratory time
I:E is 1:3. I + E = 4
4 seconds/4 = 1 second; inspiratory time is 1 second

(3) Flow is 60 L/min, or 60 L/(60 sec) = 1 L/sec. V_T = 0.5 L. Time for delivery of volume = V_T/flow = 0.5 ÷ (1 L/sec).

Time for delivery of volume = 0.5 sec.
T_I = 1 second.
Pause time will be T_I − time for volume delivery, or 1.0 sec − 0.5 sec = 0.5 sec pause time.

(4) The time interval between mandatory breaths will be 60 sec ÷ 4 breaths/min, or 15 seconds.

Box 10-41

(1)

$$T_I = 2 \text{ sec}$$
$$TCT = 6 \text{ sec (60 sec/10 breaths per min)}$$
$$T_E = TCT - T_I = 6 \text{ sec} - 2 \text{ sec} = 4 \text{ sec}$$
$$I{:}E = 2{:}4 \text{ or } 1{:}2$$

(2) At a flow of 60 L/min (1 L/sec), the ventilator can deliver 0.5 L in 0.5 sec. (T_I = V_T/flow in seconds.)

(3) Set T_I is 2 sec. V_T is delivered in 0.5 sec. The Dräger will time cycle the breath. An inspiratory pause will occur after a V_T delivery equal to 1.5 sec.

Box 10-43

Within only 4 hours, the ventilator is unable to deliver the set V_T using the previously set pressure. This suggests a change in patient lung characteristics. The respiratory therapist should evaluate the patient to determine the cause. Does the patient have a pneumothorax? Is the endotracheal tube becoming occluded? It is more appropriate here to further assess the patient and find out what is wrong than to make an immediate ventilator change.

Box 10-46

Disconnecting the patient may increase the risk of infection, which is one reason why closed suction catheters are used.

Box 10-51

To complete the setting of an alarm value, you must press the dial knob to activate the new setting.

Box 10-54

In APRV, both pressure and time levels are treated as straight CPAP. In PCV+ you have the option of adding PS to the expiratory phase of the breaths. Conceptually, you should not need PS during the release phase of APRV because you are not in that phase long enough to use it. T_{low} is a very short time period.

Box 10-55

Inspiratory pause is 15% of TCT (45% − 30% = 15%).
Expiratory time is 55% (30% + 15% + 55% = 100%).

Box 10-56

The % cycle time is based on 100%. By adding inspiration and expiration from the desired I:E ratio, you get a value of 5. This is divided into 100%: 100% ÷ 5 = 20%. The I portion is 1 unit, or 20%. The E portion is 4 units, or 4 × 20% = 80%. With the T_I control (dark blue) set at 20%, and the T_E control (light blue) set right next to it, the result is 20% T_I and 80% T_E: 20%:80% = 1:4.

Box 10-58

The therapist might not have held the PCV touch pad down for the 2 seconds required.

Box 10-59

The therapist should check the option or DIP switches at the back of the ventilator. The number 3 switch should be in the on position.

Box 10-64

The ventilator will increase the pressure support level in 1 cm H_2O increments until the exhaled $\dot{V}_E$ equals or exceeds the MMV setting.

In this example, both $\dot{V}_E$ and $\dot{V}_A$ decreased. The patient's respiratory rate increased, perhaps in the patient's effort to maintain $\dot{V}_E$. This increased the work of breathing (WOB) for the patient. To alert the clinician that rate is increasing, it is important to set the high rate alarm. It should be placed at a value that the clinician deems appropriate for the patient and the situation.

Box 10-70

(1) TCT = 60 sec ÷ (10 breaths/min) = 6 sec.
T_I = 25% of 6 sec, or 1.5 sec.
Flow = V_T/T_I = 0.5 L/1.5 sec
= 0.33 L/sec, or about 20 L/min.

(2) If the rate is turned to 12 breaths/min, the new TCT will be 5 sec. 25% of 5 sec = 1.25 sec. With the same tidal volume, the new flow will be 0.4 L/sec, or 24 L/min. It makes sense that the flow would need to be faster to get the same V_T delivered in a shorter time.

(3a) $T_I = V_T$/flow. (Convert flow to liters/second.) T_I = 0.8 ÷ (1 L/sec) = 0.8 sec for inspiration.

(b) When P-SIMV is selected, the ventilator is in a pressure-targeted mode. When configured for peak flow, this function only works in volume ventilation. T_I depends at what level the respiratory therapist sets that control.

(4a) Because these configurations do not apply in PCV, we will assume volume ventilation. TCT = 4 sec. I:E is 1:3 and consists of 4 parts (1 + 3); inspiration is 1 part. Each part is 1 second long (4 sec/4 parts). So, T_I = 1 sec.

(b) Peak flow cannot be calculated from this information when PCV is in use. Flow depends on the pressure setting, the patient's lung conditions, and any patient effort.

(c) If the unit is configured for I:E, then the ratio is constant—even if an inspiratory pause is added. With an I:E of 1:3, T_I stays at 1.0 sec (T_E = 3 sec). An added pause of 0.5 sec shortens delivery time to 0.5 sec. The breath must be delivered in a shorter time so that peak flow has to increase.

Box 10-76

When APV is used during pressure-targeted ventilation (A/C or SIMV), its upper pressure limitation is Pmax − 10 cm H_2O. In this example, Pmax was set at 35 cm H_2O. The ventilator had to deliver 25 cm H_2O to achieve the target volume: 35 cm H_2O − 10 cm H_2O = 25 cm H_2O. The alarm will activate. The therapist might want to increase Pmax to as much as 45 cm H_2O. This would limit pressure to 35 cm H_2O, which is probably the highest pressure advisable to avoid lung injury. (Remember that the ventilator has taken into account changes in patient lung compliance to determine the pressure needed to deliver the target V_T.)

Box 10-78

Problem 1: $\dot{V}_E$ will be 100 mL/min/kg, or 6 L/min (60 kg × 100 mL/kg)

Problem 2: $\dot{V}_E$ will be 200 mL/min/kg IBW × 50%, 5 kg × 200 mL/kg = 1.0 L; 50% of 1 L/min = 0.5 L/min.

10-83

This is an exercise in observation. There are several things that don't match.

V_T: the graph shows a V_T of about 720 mL, but the digital exhaled V_T is 800. Two possible causes for this difference are presence of a leak and difference due to tubing compliance correction. It is probably not a leak because the volume curve returns to zero at end-exhalation (see Chapter 9). If it is because of tubing compliance, you would expect the graph to be higher because the ventilator must increase volume delivery above the set value to compensate for tubing compliance loss.

Flow waveform: The waveform on the ventilator setting is constant, but the one in the graph looks like a sine wave. The flow setting is 60 L/min, and the graphics flow is about this same amount.

Inspiratory plateau is at 0 sec on the digital screen, but the graph shows a plateau. Notice that the flow drops to zero at the end of exhalation, and the volume curve also plateaus. What is unusual about the peak pressure and the plateau pressure is that they are equal, which means that there is no airway resistance present. Perhaps the ventilator is attached to a test lung with zero airway resistance.

The I:E ratio is 1:5, but the graphics ratio looks like IRV with I > E.

The rate is set and measured as 12 breaths/min, but in the graph three breaths occur in a 6-second period, which translates to 30 breaths/min. None of these breaths are patient-triggered because there is no negative deflection before a breath that shows on the pressure/time curve.

Can you find any other discrepancies? So much for our original assumption that the data corresponded to the graphs. It certainly doesn't.

Box 10-84

Water in the proximal pressure line can interfere with accurate pressure readings and is one of the possible causes of a high PEEP/CPAP alarm. Others include the following: a kinked or blocked expiratory line; an exhalation valve that is not properly assembled; and an increase in machine rate that results in air trapping (auto-PEEP).

Box 10-88

It is important to set a low-pressure alarm appropriately in PCV to alert you to such a situation. Although low-pressure alarms sometimes indicate a leak, the graphs in Figure 10-67 do not (see Chapter 9 for troubleshooting with graphics). To improve volume delivery, the therapist can either increase the pressure to increase the volume delivery, possibly helping to achieve the desired V_T in the set T_I; or the therapist can lengthen T_I to provide enough time for the desired pressure to be delivered, thus improving volume delivery. However, increasing T_I will affect the I:E ratio.

Box 10-94

Linear drive pistons produce constant (rectangular) waveforms (see Chapter 9). Unless the microprocessor is programmed to change the forward speed and action of the piston, this unit will only produce a constant flow waveform during volume ventilation.

Box 10-96

Because you are in the process of setting up a mode, the flashing indicator suggests that you forgot to press the key. You must press the tidal volume key, adjust the value using the control knob (if you want to change V_T, and press Accept; or you must press the key and accept the previous setting. All flashing keys must be pressed before you can initiate a new mode.

Box 10-102

For the "DECR RESP RATE FIRST" message to appear, T_I must be > 75% of TCT.

TCT is 60 sec/rate = 60 sec/20 breaths/min = 3 sec
$T_I = V_T/\text{flow} = 1.0$ L/(30 L/min)
A flow of 30 L/min is 0.5 L/sec
$T_I = 2$ sec
75% of 3 sec = 2.25 sec. Because $T_I = 2$ sec is < 2.25 sec., the error message will not appear.

Box 10-108

Volume added will be 2 mL/cm $H_2O \times 30$ cm $H_2O = 60$ mL

V_T delivered to the circuit will be
600 mL + 60 mL = 660 mL.

The exhaled V_T will read 600 mL because the computer will subtract the 60 mL of volume that was added.

Box 10-110

The alarm is set incorrectly. The patient was originally in CMV, and the alarm setting was appropriate, but it was not changed when the patient was switched to SIMV. The alarm is being activated because the spontaneous V_T is lower than the alarm setting. The alarm should be set slightly below the average spontaneous V_T.

Box 10-112

If the patient ceases to trigger a breath at a rate of 2 breaths/min, a maximum of 60 seconds could elapse before a machine-triggered mandatory breath would occur. The longest interval that can be set for an apnea period is 60 seconds. Fortunately, a prudent respiratory therapist would have set an apnea interval of no more than 20 seconds so that apnea ventilation would begin long before the 60-second interval had elapsed (see the section on special functions in Chapter 10 for a description of apnea ventilation).

Box 10-114

Problem 1— 10 breaths/min = TCT of 6 sec (60 sec ÷ 10 breaths/min). With an I:E ratio of 1:1, total units in a breath are 1 + 1 = 2. Each unit is 6 sec ÷ 2 units = 3 sec. $T_I = 3$ sec.; $T_E = 3$ sec. If the rate is changed to 15 breaths/min and T_I is constant, then TCT = 60 sec ÷ 15 breaths/min = 4 sec. With T_I contstant at 3 sec, the $T_E = TCT - T_I$, or 4 sec − 3 sec = 1 sec. The ratio is 3:1.

Problem 2— Old T_I was 3 sec. When rate is increased from 10 to 15 breaths/min and I:E is constant at 1:1, then TCT is 4 sec. With an I:E of 1:1, total units in a breath are 1 + 1 = 2. Each unit is 4 sec ÷ 2 units = 2 sec. $T_I = 2$ sec.; $T_E = 2$ sec.

Box 10-119

Problem 1: The therapist should increase the flow on the front panel flowmeter until the gauge no longer displays significant negative pressure during inspiration.

Problem 2: The therapist should check the patient's ventilatory pattern to be sure the patient is not coughing. If the patient is not, the inspiratory flow of gas set on the front panel flow meter should be reduced.

Box 10-122

The flow is only 30 L/min. With a T_I of only 0.5 seconds and a low flow, there is not enough time for the ventilator to reach the PIP setting for this patient. Of course, this is influenced by patient lung characteristic and patient effort. A flow of 30 L/min may be adequate to achieve the target pressure in a patient with low compliance, but in this case, you should first increase the flow and then reevaluate breath delivery.

Box 10-125

The pressure drop is probably the result of a very small leak in the circuit. The low-pressure alarm activates because the pressure has dropped below the trigger sensitivity level during exhalation and exceeded the time alloted.

Box 10-128

During pressure-targeted ventilation, increasing T_I increases mean airway pressure. During volume-targeted ventilation, however, you might increase PEEP to increase mean airway pressure. If you increase T_I during volume-targeted ventilation, you will also increase V_T delivery unless you make correspondingly decrease flow. Remember that with the Wave during volume ventilation, $V_T = \text{flow} \times T_I$.

Box 10-133

Check the toggle switch for adult/infant $\dot{V}_E$ ranges because sometimes this is incorrectly positioned. If it is in the infant setting, a $\dot{V}_E$ of 6 L/min will give a high-ventilation alarm.

Box 10-134

Turn the oxygen up to 100%, but remember to turn the oxygen control back to its original setting afterward. You could press the gas change button briefly to flush the system with 100% oxygen, but this must be done with caution.

When the gas change button is pressed, the patient is not being ventilated. Circuit pressure is maintained at 20 cm H_2O, which subjects the patient to high flows and effectively creates 20 cm H_2O of PEEP.

Box 10-135

The ventilator will not permit the T_I to exceed 80% of the TCT. In this case, TCT was 5 seconds; 0.8 × 5 sec = 4.0 sec. T_I would be 4 sec, and T_E would be 1 sec. This is an extreme example of an inverse ratio (4:1). It would be rare to see this used in an actual patient case.

Box 10-137

Question 1: The tidal volume is determined by the inspiratory pressure level, the characteristics of the patient's lungs, and how much of an inspiratory effort the patient makes. Tidal volume is variable in pressure support.

Question 2: 19 cm H_2O, or the PEEP level plus the inspiratory pressure level.

Question 3: Pressure support is designed to stop inspiratory flow if pressure rises above the inspiratory pressure + PEEP + 3 cm H_2O. The upper pressure limit also acts as a safety back-up to release pressure level.

Question 4: The inspiratory gas flow will stop when the ventilator measures a T_I equal to 80% of the total cycle time. With a set rate of 15 breaths/min, TCT is 4 seconds. Inspiration will end at 3.2 seconds.

Box 10-138

The flashing yellow light next to the pause time% control indicates that an attempt has been made to exceed the 80% T_I limit. The ventilator will shorten the pause time so that the T_I is 80%. In this case, because the T_I = 80%, there will be no pause.

Box 10-145

As the patient's rate drops below 12 breaths/min, the ventilator determines that it is not maintaining the set $\dot{V}_E$ even though it is maintaining V_T. To compensate, it will increase the pressure to increase the delivered V_T, thus increasing $\dot{V}_E$.

In this example, the patient's rate dropped to 8 breaths/min. The volume was 500 mL. The machine measures a $\dot{V}_E$ of 4.0 L/min, and the set value is 6.0 L/min. The machine will increase volume delivery (by increasing pressure) to a maximum of 150% of the set value. In this case, the ventilator would go as high as 750 mL of V_T to keep the $\dot{V}_E$ at 6.0 L/min, the set value. Don't forget that in VS the ventilator cannot alter the rate. $\dot{V}_E$ can be higher than the set value, but not lower.

Box 10-146

SIMV cycle time = 60 sec/SIMV frequency
= 60/3 = 20 sec.
SIMV period = 60 sec/CMV frequency = 60/15 = 4 sec.
Spontaneous period = 20 sec − 4 sec = 16 sec.

Bear 3 Review Questions

1. b
2. a
3. a
4. c
5. b
6. b; the trigger sensitivity must be set appropriately and the patient's inspiratory effort must be sufficient to activate it.
7. c
8. False; it must detect a volume lower than the set low expired volume for the number of consecutive breaths set on the detection delay control.
9. False; it does not determine volume delivery in spontaneous modes (CPAP and PSV).
10. True
11. Water may have accumulated on the flow sensor because it is not mounted vertically. This may have caused the abnormal readings to occur.

Bear 1000 Review Questions

1. d
2. c
3. d
4. b; if only one gas is available, the delivered FIO_2 may be altered. The alarm will activate if either of the gas sources drops below 27.5 psi, so technically, choice a is also correct, although it is not the best answer.
5. This is both true and false. It is true that the Bear 1000 normally operates with air/O_2 high pressure sources and electrical power. If an air compressor has been added to it, however, it can use the air compressor as a high-pressure gas source. If the compressor is the only high-pressure gas source, it cannot deliver a high oxygen percentage.
6. True
7. The lock control may be active. If the LED near the lock control is illuminated, the control needs to be pressed to unlock the panel and allow the tidal volume to be adjusted.
8. Unless the LED next to the V_T control is illuminated, it cannot be adjusted. One likely problem is that the ventilator is in a ventilatory mode in which the V_T control is not active, such as PSV or PCV.
9. No. The sharp rise in pressure that then falls to a plateau indicates that the flow is too rapid at the beginning of inspiration and the pressure sloping feature should be used to adjust it.
10. Volume output = volume added + set volume
Volume output = (25 × 3 mL/cm H_2O) + 0.7 = 0.775 L
11. Because the breath flow cycles and volume delivery is higher than set, the patient must be actively breathing.

Bird 8400STi Review Questions

1. c
2. c
3. a; reaching the set high-pressure limit ends inspiration and causes an audio/visual alarm.
4. b
5. a
6. d
7. d
8. True
9. False; only units that have had the PCV option added will provide this mode.
10. The patient triggers the breath, as suggested by the dip in pressure before inspiration begins. The ventilator reaches the set pressure and sustains it. The patient must have received at least the set $\dot{V}_I$ because there was no rise in pressure at the end of inspiration, which would have occurred if flow had been sustained (see Figure 10-15). Expiration occurs normally.

T-Bird Review Questions

1. a
2. a
3. a; the ventilator automatically indicates when DC power voltage drops. When the external battery is depleted, the ventilator will automatically switch to the internal battery.
4. a; if the inspiratory hold is not held long enough or the unit cannot get a stable reading, it cannot measure plateau pressure and calculate static compliance.
5. a
6. d
7. False; the T-Bird does not require a high-pressure gas source to function.
8. True
9. True
10. Both ventilators flow cycle out of inspiration when V_T delivery is achieved. The Bear 1000 flow cycles at 30% of the measured peak flow delivered during inspiration. The T-Bird AVS III flow cycles when the actual flow value equals the set peak flow.

Evita Review Questions

1. a; pressure support and rise time are not functional in CMV or in SIMV.
2. b; there is not a touch pad for PCV. It is active in either the CMV or SIMV modes.
3. c; if flow is zero at the end of inspiration, pressure has equilibrated. When there is no pressure gradient, there is no flow.
4. c; PSV normally flow cycles out of inspiration. In this instance it is time cycling. The unit was unable to detect flow dropping off. A leak in the system is a common cause of continued flow delivery.
5. c; the special feature called occlusion pressure can be used to assess a patient's neuromuscular drive.
6. d
7. d
8. True
9. True
10. APRV provides two levels of CPAP (P_{high} and P_{low}; see Figure 10-30) and is intended for use with spontaneously breathing patients. The operator can adjust both pressure levels and the time each level of pressure is applied (see the section on APRV in this chapter).

Dräger E-4 Review Questions

1. d
2. a
3. a; with PPS, the more the patient demands of support, the more the ventilator supplies, and vice-versa.
4. d
5. True
6. False; Pmax is a function that limits the amount of pressure that can be provided, particularly with mandatory breath delivery during volume ventilation.
7. False; Neoflow is a feature available for the upgraded version (2.n) of the Evita 4 that allows the unit to be used in neonatal ventilation.
8. The unit's front panel contains touch pads, a dial (rotary) knob and a computer screen. On the computer screen are images or icons. Some are shaped like knobs and called soft or cyber knobs, and some are shaped like touch pads and called soft or cyber pads. All these dials and knobs are used to control the unit.
9. Touch the soft pad for V_T on the computer screen to select it (changes from green to yellow). Use the rotary knob to choose the desired value for V_T. Press the rotary knob when the desired value is visible to activate that value, and the color changes back.
10. This is a top priority warning, indicating that the set high-frequency respiratory rate limit has been exceeded.

Evita 2 Dura Review Questions

1. d
2. c
3. b; the low airway pressure alarm is automatically set at 5 cm H_2O above the baseline pressure (PEEP).
4. c
5. b; only low or medium priority alarms will reset if the problem is corrected.
6. True; the purpose of this special function is to measure end-expiratory pressure (auto-PEEP level).
7. False; the Evita 2 Dura is not equipped for neonatal ventilation. Otherwise, both ventilators require you to select the type of patient you are going to ventilate during the initial set-up.
8. True; after a parameter touch pad is pressed, it flashes to indicate that it is activated and can be changed.
9. When an alarm event occurs, either exclamation points or a red or yellow light flashes at the upper right corner of the unit. The number of exclamation points (one, two, or three) or the color that appears designates the level of alarm priority. In addition, an alarm message is displayed at the upper right corner of the computer screen to provide information on the type of alarm limit that has been exceeded. If a low or medium priority alarm occurs and the problem is corrected, the alarm (lights, message, and audible) switches off. Warning messages, however, must be acknowledged by pressing the alarm reset touch pad.
10. Although the setting of the parameter is slightly different because of the difference in the control panels, the function of Pmax in the Evita 2 Dura is the same as in the E-4. Pmax operates in CMV, SIMV, and MMV modes. When Pmax is operational, the unit will guarantee the set V_T, but limits the pressure delivered during the breath.

The pressure in the circuit rapidly reaches the maximum pressure setting (Pmax,), inspiration continues for the set inspiratory time (time-cycled), but the amount of pressure in the circuit does not go above this setting. Flow rises rapidly during inspiration, plateaus, and then becomes a descending flow waveform. The V_T will remain constant at the set value as long as flow drops to zero before the end of inspiration. If flow does not drop to zero for the pressure being provided by the unit, then the volume cannot be guaranteed and a volume not constant alarm is activated.

Hamilton AMADEUS Review Questions

1. c; this flow doubles the rate of the source gases.
2. b; the PEEP is 8 cm H_2O (dark blue), and the P_{peak} is 25 cm H_2O (light blue). PS is the difference between the two.
3. d; the trigger and cycle functions are the same for both. PCV is pressure-targeted, and A/C is volume-targeted in this example. All breaths in any mode are limited by the upper pressure limit setting. Pressure support is not available in A/C.
4. b
5. False; it is the descending ramp.
6. True
7. 6 L/min
8. Total cycle time = 60 sec ÷ (10 breaths/min) = 6 seconds T_I = 1.5 sec; pause time = 0.6 seconds; so, the total T_I = 2.1 seconds. (Note that when pause is selected it lengthens inspiratory time.) T_E = TCT − T_I; T_E = 6 seconds − 2.1 seconds = 3.9 seconds. I:E = 2.1:3.9 sec = 1:1.9, or about 1:2.
9. Either the flow sensor has been reversed in its position or it needs calibration.
10. The control for this is the option, or DIP, switch 9 on the back of the ventilator. In the off position, the flow waveform is constant; to get the descending ramp, the switch must be on. The ventilator will have to be turned off and then on again before the microprocessor will detect this change.

Hamilton VEOLAR^{FT} Review Questions

1. b; 80 L/min (precisely 79.8 L/min). The flow for the 50% descending ramp is 1.33 times the peak flow during a constant waveform.
2. b
3. a; CMV = 15 breaths/min, and % cycle time = 33 %. The CMV is not usually set <15 breaths/min during SIMV because of its effect on inspiratory flow.
4. d; if the patient becomes disconnected in PSV, this alarm may occur because the internal reservoir tank pressure drops while the ventilator tries to compensate for the large leak due to the disconnection.
5. c; there is no PCV inspiratory pressure knob on the VEOLAR^{FT}.
6. True
7. False; the flush control flushes the circuit at 60 L/min with the oxygen percentage set on the O_2 % control.
8. True; the nebulizer may increase V_T slightly.
9. E% = 75% (100% − 25%); TCT = 60 sec ÷ (15 breaths/min) = 4 sec; T_I = 1 sec; T_E = 3 sec; I:E = 1:3. These are set values; however, if a breath is patient-triggered, it can actually shorten T_E.
10. When hold is pressed during exhalation, it stops the delivery of the next breath (valve closes when inspiratory flow is detected) and keeps the exhalation valve closed to measure end-expiratory pressure or auto-PEEP. To read this value, select the PEEP touch pad in the monitoring section.

Hamilton GALILEO Review Questions

1. d
2. c; for volume ventilation, one of these three can be selected when the unit is first started by pressing the M knob when the ventilator is turned on. If peak flow is chosen, T_I will still be the cycling mechanism in PCV and PSV breaths.
3. a; because the patient is apneic, breaths must be time-triggered. They are pressure-targeted, but will adjust to guarantee the desired volume delivery.
4. c
5. False; the highest pressure would be the high pressure alarm, which is normally set above the pressure level for breath delivery.
6. True
7. The commonly adjusted parameters for any mode appear on the screen. The operator selects the desired parameter, such as tidal volume, by scrolling through the choices using knob C. When the desired parameter is highlighted, the operator pushes knob C to select the parameter. The icon for the parameter then changes from yellow to red. By rotating knob C, the operator changes the numeric value of the parameter. For example, if V_T is highlighted (yellow) and selected (red), the value for V_T can be increased or decreased by rotating knob C. The operator confirms the changes when knob C is pressed, or it will not become active.
8. The actual values for any of the alarm parameters are represented by a green horizontal line on the bargraph for the parameter.
9. $\dot{V}_E$ delivery in the adult is 0.1 L/min/kg IBW when the $\dot{V}_E$ support is set at 100%. For a 50 kg adult, the $\dot{V}_E$ will equal 5 L/min.
10. They are very similar except for the way in which the pressures are set. On the VEOLAR^{FT}, the PS level plus CPAP equals the peak pressure. For example, if P_{peak} is 20 cm H_2O and CPAP is set at 5 cm H_2O, the PS

level is 15 cm H_2O (P_{peak} − CPAP). In the GALILEO if you want 15 cm H_2O of PS and the patient is receiving 5 of CPAP, set PS at 15 cm H_2O. P_{peak} will be 20 cm H_2O (PS + CPAP).

Adult Star Review Questions

1. b; the graphic waveform reads the actual volume of gas passing through the expiratory flow sensor and is not corrected for tubing compliance, so this is a good answer. A patient circuit leak would give an exhaled V_T that is lower than the set value. If the expiratory flow sensor was out of calibration, the exhaled V_T on the screen could be more or less that the set value depending on the calibration procedure, so choice c is also a possible cause here. Water in the proximal pressure line would interfere with pressure readings, not volume readings.
2. a; the ventilator will function from the air source. If the set O_2% is > 21%, delivered oxygen will be lower than set.
3. b; II is true. The Adult Star 2000 does not require an external flowmeter because it comes with a nebulizer. As long as this option is provided to the Star 1500, it will also use the internal nebulizer function. The nebulizer does not alter V_T or O_2%. It automatically shuts off after 30 minutes.
4. c
5. d
6. c
7. a; PCV with a constant I:E ratio requires the use of the A/C mode and is called PCV I:E ratio cycling.
8. False; sighs are not available with PCV or with CPAP.
9. False; loops are only accessible through the respiratory mechanics option but are not a part of the standard graphics package.
10. Screen 1, the ventilator setting screen, and Screen 3, the graphic monitoring screen.

Nellcor Puritan Bennett 740 Review Questions

1. d; this is a high priority alarm indicating that the O_2% has fallen at least 10% below the set O_2% for 30 seconds or more and that the pressure in the source O_2 high-pressure line is too low.
2. b; a maintenance check is due in 24 hours.
3. c
4. d; 100% O_2 provides 100% oxygen for 2 minutes. Using the alarm silence key silences audible alarms for 2 minutes during bedside procedures, as long as the ventilator is in a normal state (no alarms).
5. c; constant illumination of the alarm indicator means that an alarm condition has autoreset. The message window is telling you that this was a high-pressure alarm in which circuit pressure exceeded the set high-pressure limit. Actually, the patient might need suctioning, but needs to be assessed before this can be concluded.
6. c
7. False; when not in use, the ventilator should be in the standby mode to allow the battery to charge. This requires that it be plugged into an AC power source, turned on, and placed into standby using the menu function.
8. False; it only works in the spontaneous mode.
9. True
10. Apnea ventilation will not begin because it is only available in the spontaneous mode. Because the minimum respiratory rate of 3 breaths/min is the lowest possible setting for both A/C and SIMV, a mandatory breath will occur before the apnea time would have elapsed (it actually elapses at 20.2 seconds). However, you would expect a low $\dot{V}_E$ alarm to occur as long as you had set the low $\dot{V}_E$ alarm correctly.

Nellcor Puritan Bennett 7200 Review Questions

1. b
2. a
3. d; the manufacturer advises you to review apnea parameters when modes are changed. When switching from CMV to SIMV, give a mandatory breath to avoid delay in breath delivery particularly with low SIMV rates and when apnea time is set high.
4. d
5. It increases. For example, if flow is set at 60 L/min (1 L/sec), V_T is 1.0 L, and flow is constant, then T_I is 1 second ($T_I = V_T$/flow). However, when you change to a descending ramp, the peak flow is 60 L/min at the beginning of inspiration and descends to 5 L/min at the end of inspiration. Because flow decreases, T_I must increase for the same flow and V_T setting.
6. b; the low V_T alarm will activate because it is set above the spontaneous V_T. The apnea alarm will not activate because the patient's spontaneous rate is adequate.
7. b; I, II, and IV are not in Option 30/40.
8. c
9. c; the T_I is constant at 1.0. The new TCT (6 breaths/min) is 10 seconds. T_E = TCT − T_I, or T_E = 10 sec − 1 sec = 9 sec. The new I:E ratio will be 1:9.
10. Set trigger flow at 2 L/min for this size patient. The base flow must be about twice this value (4 L/min), but the lowest available setting is 5 L/min (maximum is 20 L/min).

Newport Breeze E150 Review Questions

1. The best answer is c because the most likely cause of this problem is the trigger sensitivity setting. Because the ventilator was just turned on, the therapist might not be sure of the trigger setting.

   The answer is not a because spontaneous flow helps maintain baseline pressure in A/C, and indirectly affects triggering. In fact, if the spontaneous flow is set too low, it could potentially cause auto-triggering if baseline pressure is not being maintained.

Choice b is wrong because this ventilator does not have a control mode.

The answer is not d because a low inspiratory flow would affect breath delivery after inspiration had started but not prior to inspiration.

2. a; use of the built-in nebulizer function increases the gas flow to the patient by about 6 L/min. The amount is included in the reported digital V_T display.
3. The best answer is c because the pressure-relief valve will allow circuit pressure to reach the set value but will not end inspiration. Pressure will plateau for the remainder of inspiration.

   The answer is not a because if the high-pressure limit were reached, inspiration would end abruptly, even if the alarm silence was pressed.

   It is not c because for a pressure-targeted mode, you could still get a plateau pressure like this, but you would not see the set V_T in the display window. Instead, you would see the expiratory time.

   It is not d because if there were a leak, it would not allow pressure to build and plateau.
4. d; the low CPAP alarm has replaced the apnea alarm. When the low CPAP alarm is set, the apnea alarm is automatically deactivated. The ventilator has detected that circuit pressure has fallen below the set value for a minimum of 4 seconds. A small leak is the most likely cause because some pressure is still present in the circuit.
5. c
6. b; technically, you could set the pressure-relief valve close to peak pressures measured during volume ventilation and use it to achieve a plateau. When pressure in the circuit reaches the pressure-relief valve setting, however, gas will vent from the circuit, thereby reducing volume delivery.
7. b; one of the high-pressure gas sources has lost pressure.

   The answer is not a because if you switch from A/C power and the internal battery is charged and now in use, it will sound every 5 minutes, not continuously.

   It is not c because when the ventilator has been turned on, an alarm sounds briefly and then turns off.

   If the pressure relief valve is activated the only sound you might hear is gas escaping from the valve, but there is no alarm, so choice d is not correct.
8. True
9. False; the E150 does not have a tidal volume control.
10. First, the therapist should check the sensitivity setting to be sure it is adjusted to the baseline and fine-tuned to be as sensitive as possible to patient effort. Then the set spontaneous flow setting should be checked because it may be too high for patient need and may be interfering with the ventilator sensing patient effort. In addition, there might be a leak in the circuit.

Wave E200 Review Questions

1. a
2. a; the high-pressure–relief valve is normally set above the high-pressure alarm. It limits pressure but does not end inspiration. Because pressure is released to the air, volume delivery will decrease. It does not have an alarm.
3. Either a or b are correct, although it is probably better to add an external gas source for nebulization than to change the mode of ventilation to the patient. You would have to monitor the effects of the extra flow on pressures, flows, and volumes. The E200 nebulizer does not work during pressure-control ventilation.
4. d
5. d; either of these could cause this situation.
6. b; setting the switch to 3:1 will allow IRV to reach that limit. Changing other settings is irrelevant.
7. True
8. True
9. A 10% discrepancy from delivered V_T is not alarming. It may be the result of a knob setting being slightly off. Another possibility is that the pressure-relief valve setting is reached during the volume-targeted breath.
10. T_I is constant on the Wave and is based on what is set on the front panel. When you use an inspiratory pause, this actually shortens the time during which inspiratory flow can occur. To achieve the target V_T (based on set flow and T_I), the actual flow increases over the set value. The increase in flow results in a small increase in pressure.

Servo 900C Review Questions

1. c
2. c
3. b
4. d; the working pressure must be adequate to deliver the tidal volume at the desired flow for the patient and be above the peak pressure for the patient.
5. c; the breaths/min control must be set higher than the SIMV rate setting. When it is set lower than the SIMV rate, the ventilator uses the rate set on the breaths/min control.
6. b; the total cycle time is 6 seconds. Inspiratory time will be 38% (33% + 5%) of 6 seconds, or 2.28 seconds.
7. True
8. True; the set apnea time is 15 seconds.

9. V_T = (12 L/min) ÷ 12 breaths/min = 1.0 L; TCT = 60 sec ÷ (12 breaths/min) = 5 sec. T_I = 0.2 × 5 sec = 1 sec. Flow = (12 L/min) × (100%/20%) = 60 L/min.
10. During PC, the inspiratory pressure control determines the target pressure, and this value is added to the set baseline (PEEP) level.

Siemens Servo 300 Review Questions

1. c
2. d
3. a; the CMV rate must be set higher than the SIMV rate, or the CMV set rate becomes the actual rate and the indicator flashes.
4. a
5. d; when a patient becomes apneic and the unit switches to PRVC with volume support, all the listed events occur. The machine uses the set parameters, including the set rate, to deliver PRVC.
6. a; if the leak is large enough to prevent the flow from dropping to 5% of the measured peak flow, then the breath will time-cycle at 80% of TCT. Reaching the pressure limit would also end a PS breath, but this would probably not occur in this situation.
7. True
8. False
9. The Servo 300 gives four test breaths when PRVC is initiated. It measures pressures and volumes in order to calculate the system compliance and uses this information to determine the pressure required to deliver the desired volume.
10. The ventilator will sound an alarm, and the message "LIMITED PRESSURE" appears in the window. The ventilator will not let the pressure rise higher than the upper pressure limit setting minus 5 cm H_2O.

    For this patient, this indicates that more pressure is required to deliver the same volume. The patient's lung characteristics may have changed. For example, the airway resistance may have increased because of secretions in the airway, or the lung compliance may have decreased from a lung problem such as a pneumothorax or developing pulmonary edema. The patient should be carefully evaluated to determine the cause and then treated appropriately.

CHAPTER 11

Decision Making & Problem Solving Boxes

Box 11-7
The flow is inadequate for the ventilator to deliver the set PIP within the selected inspiratory time. Therefore the low inspiratory pressure alarm will be activated. Increasing the flow should resolve this problem.

Box 11-8
The ventilator rate of 78 bpm permits a TCT of 0.77 seconds. If T_I is set at 0.5 seconds, a T_E of only 0.27 seconds is possible (0.77 seconds − 0.5 seconds = 0.27 seconds). Therefore the insufficient expiratory time alarm will be activated. For rates below 100 bpm, a T_E less than 0.3 seconds will trigger this alarm.

Review Questions

1. b
2. b
3. d
4. b
5. b
6. d
7. d
8. c
9. d
10. a
11. d
12. b
13. d
14. d
15. b
16. a and d
17. d
18. b

CHAPTER 12

Decision Making & Problem Solving Boxes

Box 12-2
The high peak pressure alarm is about 35 cm H_2O, and the pressure-relief control is at 25 cm H_2O to allow the therapist to start at approximately the same V_T as was set in the volume control mode.

Box 12-4
Yes. The E cylinder can provide approximately 45 minutes of ventilation.

Rate = 15 breaths/min. V_T = 500 mL. Cylinder pressure = 1500 psi. Tank factor (E cylinder) = .28.

$$\text{Estimated duration} = \frac{\text{(cylinder pressure) (tank factor)}}{\text{minute ventilation}}$$

$$\text{(Cylinder pressure) (tank factor)} = (1500\ \text{psi})\ (.28) = 336\ \text{L}$$

$$\text{Minute ventilation} = (\text{rate})\ (V_T) = (15\ \text{breaths/min})\ (0.5\ \text{L}) = 7.5\ \text{L/min} = \frac{336\ \text{L}}{7.5\ \text{L/min}} = 44.8\ \text{min}$$

Box 12-6
The sensitivity is set by the manufacturer at −2 cm H_2O. The patient must create a drop in the circuit pressure to

−2 cm H_2O to trigger a volume-targeted breath. The peak pressure is the sum of the pressures associated with delivery of the set volume plus the baseline pressure. During exhalation, the pressure drops to the value set on the PEEP valve. To overcome this problem, the operator can increase the breath rate to reduce the work of breathing required by the spontaneously triggered breaths.

Box 12-8

10 cm H_2O of the pressure support. The pressure support delivered to the patient is the difference between pressure support and PEEP: 15 − 5 = 10 cm H_2O.

Box 12-11

Adjust the sensitivity >6 cm H_2O but <10 cm H_2O so that the ventilator recognizes the spontaneous efforts. Although the patient is not required to trigger the ventilator for spontaneous breaths, it is important that the trigger sensitivity is set at the appropriate level to recognize every patient effort to prevent unnecessary activation of the spontaneous alarm.

Box 12-13

The sensitivity has to be adjusted. Before the patient took spontaneous breaths, the sensitivity did not need to be set.

Box 12-14

The Bear 33 does not compensate for PEEP on spontaneous breaths. The trigger sensitivity allows for adjustments to mandatory, not spontaneous, breaths. When the patient triggers a spontaneous breath, the demand valve must be opened at −0.2 cm H_2O below atmospheric pressure, regardless of what the baseline pressure is.

Box 12-16

There are several possible answers. There could be a small leak in the circuit, or the measuring device (respirometer) is inaccurate. The V_T setting on the ventilator may be out of calibration, but most likely, the PEEP attachment is in the wrong position. It should be placed proximal to the exhalation valve when a disposable circuit is used.

Box 12-17

No. The total cycle time is 4 seconds with an inspiratory time of 2.5 seconds. The inverse I:E ratio alarm will sound and limit the I:E ratio to 1:1, thereby limiting the inspiratory time.

Box 12-18

The machine will not cycle from inspiration to expiration when the EPAP setting is equal to or greater than the IPAP setting. Until the IPAP setting is increased or the EPAP setting is decreased, the pressure will remain constant in the circuit (CPAP = 8 cm H_2O) at the IPAP setting.

Box 12-19

None. If the rate setting is 6, the total respiratory cycle is 10 seconds. Because the patient is breathing 20 times a minute, or once every 3 seconds, the time interval for a time triggered breath is never exceeded, and no time-triggered mandatory breath is delivered.

Box 12-22

The rise time setting is greater than the % I time. Because this has occurred, the % I time will remain the same, but the rise time setting will be decreased to the maximum setting below the % I time.

Review Questions

1. d
2. b
3. a
4. c; the high PEEP alarm activates if the pressure fails to drop to <22 cm H_2O in 15 seconds after mandatory breath delivery. A kink in the main expiratory line may cause this to occur.
5. b
6. c; the apnea period is preset at 19 seconds and is not adjustable. The ventilator does engage in back-up ventilation.
7. a
8. c; inspiration ends (pressure cycling), and a visual indicator lights, but an audible alarm will not sound unless two consecutive breaths exceed the pressure-limit setting.
9. d
10. a
11. c
12. True
13. False; it does not have a PEEP control.
14. True
15. True
16. False; it has no back-up ventilation.
17. True

CHAPTER 13

Decision Making & Problem Solving Boxes

Box 13-1

The clinical manifestations described point to a diagnosis of pneumonia. The laboratory findings suggest a bacterial pneumonia; *Streptococcus pneumoniae* sp. are most commonly associated with bacterial pneumonia.

Box 13-2

(1) Pseudomonas aeruginosa is a highly motile, gram-negative bacillus found in the human gastrointestinal tract. It is a contaminant in many aqueous solutions (vehicle route).

(2) Human immunodeficiency virus is primarily transmitted through the exchange of body fluids (e.g., sexual contact) with an HIV-infected individual.

(3) Tuberculosis is a chronic bacterial infection that is almost exclusively transmitted within aerosol droplets produced by the coughing or sneezing of an individual with active tuberculosis.

(4) *Rickettsiae* spp. are small pleomorphic coccobacilli. *Rickettsia spp.* are responsible for diseases that are transmitted by lice, fleas, ticks, and mites.

Box 13-6
First, determine if the device is contaminated. Microbiological identification requires that the hospital's clinical laboratory staff work with the staff of the respiratory care department to determine if infectious organisms are in the devices in question. The clinical microbiologist can provide information about nosocomial infections from direct smears and stains, cultures, serological tests, and antibiotic susceptibility testing.

Ongoing surveillance is required to ensure that an infection control program is adequately protecting patients and health care providers. Surveillance typically consists of the following: equipment processing quality control, routine sampling of in-use equipment, and microbiological identification. Equipment processing is monitored with chemical and biological indicators. Routine sampling of in-use equipment can be done with sterile cotton swabs, liquid broth, and aerosol impaction. Aerosol impaction is an effective method for sampling the particulate output of nebulizers.

Box 13-8
Most major burn wounds become infected during the first 48 to 72 hours after the incident. Care should therefore be directed to minimizing situations where wound colonization can occur. For this reason, the most effective strategy is to use strict contact isolation procedures.

Review Questions

1. a
2. c
3. d
4. (1) A source of pathogens, (2) a mode of transmission of the infectious agent, and (3) a susceptible host.
5. c
6. Semicritical—ventilator tubing; critical—Swan-Ganz catheter; noncritical—blood pressure cuff; semicritical—endoscope (bronchoscope); semicritical—endotracheal tubes.
7. b
8. b
9. b
10. c
11. d
12. a

CHAPTER 14

Decision Making & Problem Solving Boxes

Box 14-4
Several important facts suggest that Mr. H may have a sleep-related disorder: he has been referred to the laboratory after an automobile accident when he "fell asleep at the wheel." He also reports excessive daytime sleepiness, and his wife says that he snores and that his sleeping pattern has become increasingly restless during the last 6 months. It is also mentioned that he has a long history of smoking cigarettes (possibly indicating the presence of some chronic respiratory problem, such as small airway disease) and that alcohol seems to exacerbate his snoring episodes. All of these findings suggest that Mr. H might have obstructive sleep apnea.

An effective strategy here would be to schedule this patient for an overnight sleep study involving polysomnography. This information, coupled with a complete history and physical examination, should allow for a diagnosis of sleep apnea if that is the case. Furthermore, the results of these studies will provide valuable information on the severity of the disorder, thus helping you to devise an appropriate treatment plan.

Box 14-5
This is a typical polysomnographic recording of a patient with mixed sleep apnea. Notice that an initial central apnea is followed by an obstructive apnea that usually produces significant oxygen desaturation.

Review Questions

1. c
2. True
3. As the sleeper passes through the various stages of non-REM sleep, there is a progressive reduction in chemosensitivity and respiratory drive. The reduction in respiratory drive that occurs during the early stages of non-REM sleep (Stages 1 and 2) predisposes the person to periods of apnea (i.e., Cheyne-Stokes respiration) as he or she fluctuates between being awake and asleep. With the establishment of non-REM slow-wave sleep (Stages 3 and 4), nonrespiratory inputs become minimized, and minute ventilation is regulated by metabolic control. Minute ventilation decreases by 1 to 2 L/min when compared with wakefulness. As a consequence, $PaCO_2$ rises by 2 to 8 mm Hg, and PaO_2 decreases by 5 to 10 mm Hg.

   As the sleeper enters REM sleep, breathing becomes irregular as the ventilatory response to chemical and mechanical respiratory stimuli are further reduced and even transiently abolished. There is decreased skeletal muscle activity, including inhibition of the upper airway muscles and the intercostal and accessory muscles of respiration. Inhibition of the upper airway muscles leads to an increase in upper airway resistance, and inhibition of the intercostal and accessory muscles is associated with diminished thoracoabdominal coupling and short periods of central apnea (10 to 20 seconds in duration). $PaCO_2$ and PaO_2 levels are variable but are generally similar to those during the latter stages of non-REM sleep.

4. b
5. True
6. (1) Oxygen saturation; (2) nasal-oral airflow; (3) respiratory effort.
7. d
8. See Figure 14-8 for the answer to this question.
9. c
10. d

GLOSSARY

100% O_2 suction A control on the Nellcor Puritan Bennett 7200 ventilator that causes the ventilator to deliver 100% O_2 for 2 minutes. Intended for use prior to patient suctioning.

absolute humidity The actual mass or content of water in a measured volume of air. It is usually expressed in grams per cubic meter, or pounds.

absolute zero The temperature at which no molecular motion occurs: -273° C, or 0 K.

absorbance sensor An apparatus designed to react to physical stimuli from light or other radiant energy.

accelerating waveform A pressure- or flow-time tracing that indicates upward or increasing movement (acceleration) of the pressure or flow value over time.

accumulator A device that allows a volume of gas to be held for a period and then releases the gas at a preset rate. Used as a timing or limiting mechanism.

accuracy The state or quality of being precise or exact.

acid-fast bacteria Of, or pertaining to, certain bacteria (especially *Mycobacteria* spp.) that retain red dyes after an acid wash.

acoustics The science of sounds.

actual bicarbonate The concentration of HCO_3^- that is present in the plasma of anaerobically drawn blood. It is derived from measurements of pH and $PaCO_2$ using the Henderson-Hasselbalch equation.

adaptive pressure ventilation (APV) A closed-loop (servo-controlled) mode of ventilation available on the Hamilton GALILEO ventilator that provides pressure-targeted ventilation with a volume guarantee.

adaptive support ventilation (ASV) A closed loop mode of ventilation available on the Hamilton GALILEO that uses pressure-targeted ventilation to ensure a certain minute volume. The ventilator predicts tidal volume and respiratory rate based on the patient information entered by the operator, constantly monitors patient and ventilator parameters, and adjusts breath delivery to establish the least amount of work possible for the patient.

adhesion The physical property by which unlike substances are attracted and hold together; also refers to the abnormal formation of fibrous tissues (resulting from inflammation or injury) that bind together body structures that are normally separate.

adjustable reducing valve See *adjustable regulator.*

adjustable regulator A valve that allows the user to determine (adjust) pressure limits.

adjustable restrictor A mechanism that governs flow or pressure with a series of variable-sized orifices.

aerobe A microorganism that lives and grows in the presence of free oxygen.

aerosol A suspension of solid or liquid particles in a gas.

aerosol mask A device covering both the nose and mouth that is used to deliver aerosols in respiratory care.

airborne Carried in the air via aerosol droplets, droplet nuclei, or dust particles.

airborne precautions Safeguards designed to reduce the risk of airborne transmission of infectious agents.

air-dilution Adding air to a primary gas to reduce the oxygen concentration of the primary gas.

air-dilution control A mechanism that allows the user to set the amount of air dilution in a device.

air-entrainment mask An oxygen mask that uses a Venturi or Pitot type of device to provide precise concentrations of high-flow oxygen to a patient.

air foil A device that acts like an airplane wing to generate pressure differences by creating areas of high and low resistance in an airstream.

air inlet regulator A regulator that determines the inlet pressure on a gas system or ventilator.

air-mix control Another name for an air-dilution control. Used in the Bird Mark and Bennett TV and PR series respirators.

airway pressure Pressure achieved in the patient airway.

airway pressure release ventilation (APRV) A mode of ventilation during which the patient breathes spontaneously at an elevated baseline that is periodically "released" to allow expiration.

airway resistance (Raw) A measure of the impedance to ventilation caused by gas movement through the airways. It is computed as the change in pressure along a tube divided by the gas flow through the tube.

alarm A signal that is a warning of danger, such as a high-pressure or apnea alarm.
alarm silence A control button that silences audible alarms for approximately 60 seconds or until it is pressed a second time.
Allen test A test for the patency of the radial artery. The patient's hand is formed into a fist while the therapist compresses the ulnar and radial arteries. Compression continues while the fist is opened. If blood perfusion through the ulnar artery is adequate, the hand should flush and resume normal (pink) coloration when the ulnar artery compression is released.
alpha wave One of the four types of brain waves, characterized by a relatively high voltage or amplitude and a frequency of 8 to 13 cycles per second. Alpha waves are the "relaxed waves" of the brain and are the majority of the waves recorded by electroencephalograms. Compare *beta wave, delta wave,* and *theta wave.*
alternating current (AC) An electric current that reverses direction, according to a consistent sinusoidal pattern. Compare *direct current.*
alternating supply system A gas supply system that has two supplies of compressed gas (primary and secondary). The secondary system is used when the primary system fails.
alveolar ventilation (V_A) The volume of air that ventilates all the perfused alveoli, measured as minute volume in liters per minute. This figure is also the difference between total ventilation and dead space ventilation. The normal average is from 4 to 5 liters/min.
ambient compartment In the Bird Mark ventilator series, the portion of the ventilator casing that is open to the environment, and hence to ambient pressures.
ambient inlet filter A portion of an air entrainment device that removes dust particles and other debris from the entrained air before it enters the gas circuit.
AMBU (air-mask-bag-unit) A type of manual resuscitator consisting of a pliable bag, a one-way valve system, and either a mask or an artificial airway connector.
American Standard Indexing A type of safety system for high-pressure gas connections. American Standard connections are noninterchangeable to prevent the interchange of regulator equipment between gases. American Standard Indexing includes separate systems for large and small cylinders.
ammeter An instrument for measuring the strength of an electric current in terms of amperes.
amorphous solids A solid, such as glass or margarine, in which the constituent atoms and molecules are arranged in a fashion that is not rigid. In contrast, the constituent particles of crystalline solids are more rigidly arranged.
amperometric Refers to measuring an electric current at a single applied potential.
amplitude The height of a waveform; usually indicative of intensity.
anaerobe A microorganism that grows and lives in the absence of oxygen.
analog pressure manometer A back-up method of verifying digitally displayed pressure values (peak, mean, and plateau pressure).
analyte Any substance that is measured; usually applied to a component of blood or other body fluid.
AND/NAND gate A monostable fluidic element with two control ports and two outlet ports.
anemometer A gauge for determining the force or speed and sometimes the direction of the wind or air.
aneroid barometer See *aneroid manometer.*
aneroid manometer A pressure-measuring device that compares a reference pressure to an observed pressure (using one of several methods).
aneroid manometer assist indicator (cycle indicator) A light that signals a pressure change in an aneroid manometer indicating that the patient has generated a negative pressure (assist effort).
anti-suffocation valve An internal, subambient relief valve on a ventilator that opens if the ventilator cannot provide a breath to the patient. The patient can then inhale, open the valve, and receive room air.
AP series A Bennett ventilator series used for IPPB administration. AP stands for air-compressor powered.
apnea alarm A system that warns that the patient is not breathing or being ventilated.
apneic period A reference to a setting that is adjustable from 2 to 60 seconds to warn that a patient is not breathing.
apneic ventilation Emergency back-up ventilation triggered when no patient breath is detected for a certain period of time.
apneustic flow time A reference to a control on the old Bird Mark series ventilators that limited the length of apnea or no flow allowed by the ventilator.
Archimedes's principle States that when an object is submerged in a fluid, it will be buoyed up by a force equal to the weight of the fluid that is displaced by the object.
arousal response A response to sensory stimulation to induce active wakefulness.
artificial nose See *heat and moisture exchanger.*
assist A mode of ventilation in which every breath is patient-triggered.
assist and sensitivity mechanism A device that sets the maximum effort a patient must make (sensitivity) before the ventilator triggers (assists).
assisted breaths Breaths in which the patient begins inspiration, but the ventilator controls the inspiratory phase and ends inspiration.
assist/control (A/C or ACV) mode Continuous mandatory ventilation (CMV) in which the minimum breathing rate is predetermined, but the patient can initiate ventilation at an increased rate with a set tidal volume or pressure.

assist/control pressure-targeted A mode of ventilation in which the operator selects a pressure for inspiration. Breaths can be patient- or time-triggered.
assistor A ventilator that lets the patient initiate inspiration.
assistor/controller A ventilator that can function as an assistor or as a controller.
atmospheric barometric pressure The force exerted by the air column extending from the measuring site to the edge of space (i.e., 760 mm Hg at sea level). Sometimes called ambient pressure.
atmospheric-to-subatmospheric pressure gradient The difference in the force exerted by the ambient pressure and that exerted in a negative-pressure system. May be called driving pressure.
atom The smallest division of an element that exhibits all the properties and characteristics of that element, including neutrons, electrons, and protons. The number of protons in the nucleus of every atom of a given element is the same and is called its atomic number.
atomic theory The concept that all matter is composed of submicroscopic atoms that are in turn composed of protons, electrons, and neutrons. A chemical element is identified by the number of protons in its atoms.
autoclave An apparatus that uses steam under pressure to sterilize articles and equipment.
Autoflow A dual mode of ventilation that provides pressure-targeted breaths with volume guarantee whenever volume ventilation (CMV, SIMV, MMV) is simultaneously selected in the Dräger E-4 ventilator. It also alters the function of the inspiratory and expiratory valves, allowing patients to receive whatever inspiratory flow they demand—up to 180 L/min in any volume mode—regardless of the volume settings.
Automode A ventilator feature (available on the Servo 300A) designed to switch from a control to a support mode of ventilation if the patient triggers two consecutive breaths. The ventilator remains in the support mode as long as the patient keeps triggering breaths.
auto-PEEP Abnormal and usually undetected residual pressure above atmospheric remaining in the alveoli at end-exhalation due to dynamic air trapping. Also called intrinsic PEEP.

Babington/hydrosphere nebulizer A type of nebulizer in which a thin film of water flowed over a hollow glass sphere with a slit in it, through which a high-flow gas stream was passed, creating a high-density aerosol.
bacilli Aerobic or facultatively aerobic, spore-bearing, rod-shaped microorganisms of *Bacillaceae* spp.
back pressure A reduction in the pressure gradient secondary to downflow resistance.
back-pressure compensation Any method that allows accurate pressures and flows to be read.
back-pressure switch A fluidic element with one control port that has a loop with a built-in restriction and two outlet ports.
back-up rate A control rate set on a ventilator to take over if a patient's assisted ventilation falls below the desired rate.
back-up ventilation (BUV) A mode of volume ventilation (available on the Nellcor-Puritan Bennett 7200 ventilators) with a minimum breath rate that goes into effect if the patient becomes apneic.
bacteria filter A device designed to remove particles and bacteria from the system. Usually rated in pore size or in microns.
bactericide Any drug or other agent that kills bacteria.
baffle Any obstruction in an aerosol's path that breaks the aerosol into smaller particles.
base excess/deficit The number of millimoles of strong acid or base required to titrate a blood sample to a pH of 7.4, a PCO_2 of 40 mm Hg, and a temperature of 37° C.
base flow The flow added to the circuit during exhalation in order to provide flow triggering; see also *bias flow.*
baseline pressure The pressure level at which inspiration begins and ends.
beam deflection The change in the direction of a beam or jet of gas when it is hit with another jet of gas moving through a fluid device.
bell factor In a water-sealed spirometer, the number of milliliters of gas that must be displaced to cause a kymograph pen to move 1 millimeter.
bellows accumulator A device used to store a volume of gas that will be pressurized for delivery to the patient. Usually a bag or bellows.
bellows chamber The inside of a bellows containing a volume of gas.
bellows potentiometer A mechanism that senses the volume displacement of a bellows and releases the contents at a preset value, usually through an electrical signal.
Bennett Cascade A specialized, heated passover humidifier employing a water-air froth as a humidifying technique.
Bennett circuit The patient gas delivery tubing that includes all of the tubing and ancillary devices from the machine to the patient and back.
Bennett MA-1 ventilator A mechanical volume ventilator (*M*echanical *A*ssistor-*1*) previously manufactured by the Puritan-Bennett Corporation.
Bennett PR ventilators Bennett *P*ressure *R*espirator series (1 and 2) pneumatically powered assistor/controllers. No longer produced.
Bennett valve A drumlike device with pressure/flow sensitive vanes that controlled gas pressure and flow in the Bennett PR and AP series respirators.
Berman airway An upper airway device (oropharyngeal airway) used to provide air passage distal to the tongue by keeping the base of it away from the back of the throat.
beta wave One of the four types of brain waves, characterized by relatively low voltage and a frequency of more than 13 cycles per second. Beta waves are the "busy waves" of the brain. Compare *alpha wave; delta wave;* and *theta wave.*

bias alert A message provided on the T-Bird AVS ventilator that informs the operator of the bias flow setting after self-testing at start-up.
bias flow Flow in the circuit during the expiratory phase of mechanical ventilation that makes fresh gas immediately available when the patient inhales. Bias flow also reduces the ventilator's response time for triggering a breath.
bilevel continuous positive airway pressure (BiPAP) A variant of continuous positive airway pressure in which both inspiratory and expiratory pressures are set by the operator.
bilevel positive airway pressure (BiPAP) A spontaneous breath mode of ventilatory support that allows separate regulation of the inspiratory and expiratory pressures. Also called bilevel pressure assist or bilevel pressure support.
BiPAP Abbreviation for bilevel continuous positive airway pressure.
bistable A special type of fluidic control unit that acts as a switch mechanism.
bleed hole A small hole in the center body of the Bird Mark series respirators that allowed pressure equalization across the center body, or a small hole in an accumulator device that allowed the measured escape of gas to "dump" the accumulator contents.
bleed regulator An adjustable bleed hole.
blowers A mechanical device sometimes used to control volume delivery in a mechanical ventilator (e.g., a rotating vane that produces a flow of gas).
body humidity The absolute humidity in a volume of gas saturated at a body temperature of 37° C; equivalent to 43.8 mg/L.
body plethysmography A method of studying alveolar pressures, lung volumes, and airway resistance. The patient sits or reclines in an airtight compartment and breathes normally. The pressure changes in the alveoli are reciprocated in the compartment and recorded automatically by the body plethysmograph.
body tank respirator Iron lung; a type of negative-pressure ventilator.
boiling point The temperature at which a liquid begins to turn to a gas. For water at 1 atm: 100° C, 212° F, or 373° Absolute.
Boothby-Lovelace-Bulbulian (BLB) mask An apparatus for administering oxygen; consists of a mask fitted with an inspiratory-expiratory valve and a rebreathing bag.
Bourdon flowmeter A flowmeter that incorporates a Bourdon gauge.
Bourdon gauge A device that indicates pressure measurements from the use of a hollow, coiled tube that attempts to straighten in response to increased pressure.
Bourdon regulator A regulator that incorporates a Bourdon gauge.
BPM (breaths per minute) Respiratory rate. Usually a digital or analog indicator on the ventilator control panel.
Brownian movement The random movement of molecules/particles caused by being struck by other molecules/particles.
BTPS Abbreviation for body temperature, ambient pressure, saturated (with water vapor).
bubble humidifier A device that increases the water content of a gas by passing it through a volume of water.
buffer base The total blood buffer capable of binding hydrogen ions. Normal buffer base (NBB) ranges from 48 to 52 mEq/L.

calorimetry A method of determining energy expenditure by using the measurements of the amount of heat radiated and absorbed by an organism.
capillary blood gases (CBGs) Gases dissolved in the blood that are obtained from a capillary sample. Results include pH, PCO_2, and PO_2 values, which may differ from arterial blood gas values.
capillary mesh A netlike web with small openings that are used to measure flow and resistance in monitoring devices.
capillary system Microscopic tubes that connect arteries and veins and provide perfusion to tissues and cells.
capnogram A tracing that shows the proportion of carbon dioxide in exhaled air.
capnograph A device that measures and provides a graphic representation of the amount of carbon dioxide in a gas sample. A mainstream capnograph analyzes gas at the airway. With a sidestream capnograph, however, the gas to be analyzed is aspirated from the airway through a narrow-bore polyethylene tube and transferred to a sample chamber.
cardiopulmonary resuscitation (CPR) A basic emergency procedure for life support involving artificial respiration and manual external cardiac massage.
cascade humidifier A bubble humidifier in which gases travel down a tower and pass through a grid into a chamber of heated water. The displaced water rises above the grid, forming a liquid film that is converted to froth as the gas also rises from the chamber through the grid. The process results in an airflow that can have a relative humidity of up to 100% (see *Bennett Cascade*).
caudad Toward the tail or end of the body; away from the head.
Celsius (C) Temperature scale in which 0° is the freezing point of water and 100° is the boiling point of water at sea level.
center body The metallic divider in the mid portion of the Bird Mark series that was a site for gas channels and control devices.
central sleep apnea Absence of breathing as the result of medullary depression, which inhibits respiratory movement; becomes more pronounced during sleep. Compare *mixed sleep apnea* and *obstructive sleep apnea*.
central processing unit (CPU) The component of a computer that controls the encoding and execution of instructions. Mainly consists of an arithmetic unit, which performs arithmetic functions, and an internal memory, which controls the sequencing of operations. Also called processor.

centrifugal nebulizers A humidification device in which a spinning disk with vanes on it breaks water into particles.
cephalad Toward the head.
ceramic switch Part of the Bird Mark series ventilators that controls flow through the gas channels. Consists of a ceramic tube with offset grooves and holes that selectively match up with gas channel inlets in the center body.
chamber An accessory to enhance aerosol deposition from a metered dose inhaler.
check valve A device usually consisting of a one-way valve that prevents back or retrograde gas flow.
chemical analyzer A device that measures the amount of a specific gas in a system by measuring the results of chemical reactions.
chemical potential energy Potential energy stored in a chemical bond, such as petroleum reserves of coal, gas, or oil.
chemical sterilant Any chemical agent that destroys all living organisms, including viruses, in a material.
chemiluminescence monitoring A type of nitrogen oxide monitoring system routinely used during nitric oxide administration. It involves the quantification of gas-specific photoemission. See also *electrochemical monitoring.*
chest cuirass The shell-like part of a negative-pressure ventilator.
chest shell piece The rigid portion of a cuirass type of negative-pressure ventilator that covers the thorax.
Cheyne-Stokes respiration An abnormal, repeating pattern of breathing characterized by progressive hypopnea alternating with hyperpnea and ending in a brief apnea.
child adult mist (CAM) tent An environmental enclosure that controls oxygen concentration, humidity, and temperature.
circadian rhythm A pattern based on a 24-hour cycle, especially the repetition of certain physiologic phenomena, such as sleeping and eating.
CIRC alarm Circuit integrity warning. Denotes a leak or disconnection in the patient circuit.
Clark electrode The electrode most commonly used to measure the partial pressure of oxygen.
cleaning The removal of all foreign material, especially organic matter (e.g., blood, serum, pus, and fecal matter) from objects with hot water, soaps, detergents, and enzymatic products.
closed-circuit calorimeter See *indirect calorimeter.*
closed-loop system A hardware/software combination that controls a mechanical or electronic process without user input.
clutch plates In the Bird Mark series, the steel plates that are connected by a wire shaft and suspended between two magnets. The clutch plates act as on/off switches for gas flow.
Coanda effect A term in fluidics that refers to the side-wall attachment phenomenon of gas streams.
cocci Bacteria that are round, spherical, or oval, such as gonococci, pneumococci, staphylococci, and streptococci.
cohesion The attractive force between like molecules.
collodion A clear or slightly opaque, highly inflammable liquid composed of pyroxylin, ether, and alcohol. It dries to a strong, transparent film that is used as a surgical dressing.
combined power ventilator A ventilator that requires both pneumatic and electric sources for operation. The electric source often powers a microprocessor.
combined pressure device A ventilator that employs both positive and negative pressure during breath delivery. For example, a high-frequency oscillator delivers positive pressure on inspiration and negative pressure on expiration.
combined pressure gradient The additive pressure difference in a multipart system, such as the combined air-to-arterial-to-cell pressure difference.
Combitube A double-lumen device designed to provide a patent upper airway when inserted blindly after failed intubation or in a comatose patient with airway difficulties.
compensated leak alarm A warning that activates when the leak compensation mechanism is engaged.
compensator valve A system designed to provide additional flow or volume to overcome the effects of leaks in a pressurized system.
compound A substance composed of two or more different elements, chemically combined in definite proportions, that cannot be separated by physical means.
compressibility factor A mathematical expression of the reduction of volume delivery in a ventilator setting in response to increased pressure in the system.
compressor A machine that uses electrical power to move a piston, fan, or bellows, which in turn reduces the volume of air and increases its pressure.
compressor-driven unit A mechanical ventilator that is powered by an air compressor.
concentration gradient In open or communicating systems, the difference between the amount of a substance in part of the system and the amount of the same substance in another part of the system.
condensation Change of state from gas to liquid, such as with water vapor condensation.
constant positive airway pressure See *continuous positive airway pressure (CPAP).*
constant positive-pressure breathing (CPPB) A mode of ventilation in which the ventilating pressures are always elevated above zero.
contact precautions Safeguards designed to reduce the risk of transmission of epidemiologically important microorganisms by direct or indirect contact.
continuous flow CPAP system A continuous positive airway pressure (CPAP) system incorporating a constant flow of gas.
continuous flow IMV system A volume ventilator with the addition of an intermittent mandatory ventilation circuit that incorporates a constant flow of gas. The one-way valve going toward the patient circuit is kept open by

the continuous flow and does not have to be opened by the patient. Also called a closed-circuit IMV system.
continuous-flow ventilation (CFV) A mode of ventilation in which a gas stream constantly passes through the airway and is hence available.
continuous mandatory ventilation (CMV) A mode of ventilation that provides control or assist/control ventilation. Breaths are time- or patient-triggered, volume- or pressure-targeted, and volume- or time-cycled.
continuous nebulizer A nebulizer that runs during the entire ventilatory cycle.
continuous positive airway pressure (CPAP) A method of providing positive pressure for spontaneously breathing patients without mechanical assistance (i.e., mandatory breath delivery). A technique for increasing functional residual capacity and arterial oxygenation.
continuous supply system A mechanism that delivers a gas or an aerosol throughout the ventilatory cycle.
control mode Continuous mandatory ventilation (CMV) in which the breathing frequency is determined by the ventilator without patient initiation according to a preset cycling pattern (time-triggered ventilatory support).
control panel The user interface, with the controls for the operator to set desired parameters.
control pressure manometer A gauge that indicates the maximum or control pressure in a ventilator system.
control pneumatic logic circuit A fluidic circuit that controls the operation of other circuits.
control variables Four elements of breath delivery including flow, volume, pressure, and time. The elements are controlled and/or limited by the ventilator. Numerical values for each element are set on the front panel of the ventilator by the operator.
controlled expiratory time A system that controls rate or end-expiration by limiting expiratory time.
controller A type of ventilator that will not allow spontaneous breathing.
convoluted tube A tube that has many bends and turns.
counterweight A weight used to offset the effects of pressure on a system.
coupling chamber In an ultrasonic nebulizer, the water-filled space between the ultrasonic source and the solution to be nebulized. It transmits the ultrasonic waves from the transducer to the medication chamber.
CPAP Abbreviation for continuous positive airway pressure. A method of pressurized gas delivery whereby the patient breathes spontaneously without mechanical assistance at pressures above ambient.
critical pressure The pressure above which a material cannot exist as a gas.
critical temperature The temperature below which a material cannot exist as a gas.
cryogenic Producing extremely low temperatures.
cuirass The shell-like part of a negative-pressure ventilator.
cupped-disk valve A type of valve that looks like a shallow bowl. The convex side of the disk fits into an orifice, sealing it to end inspiration and inspiratory flow delivery, and begin the expiratory phase during mechanical ventilation.
cyber knob The term given by Dräger for the icons on the monitor screen of the Dräger E-4 ventilator that are shaped like knobs and used to control the unit.
cyber pad The term given by Dräger for the icons on the monitor screen of the Dräger E-4 ventilator that are shaped like touch pads and used to control the unit.
cycle rate control The part of the ventilator that determines the length of the ventilatory cycle.
cycle variable The phase variable that is measured and used to end inspiration; the element of breath delivery that determines the end of inspiration; see *control variables.*

dead space ventilation Ventilation characterized by respirated gas volume that does not participate in gas exchange. Alveolar dead space is characterized by alveoli that are ventilated but are not perfused.
dead space volume (V_D) The amount of volume during ventilation which is not involved in gas exchange because of lack of pulmonary perfusion to the area.
decelerating taper (ramp) A flow curve in which the flow gradually decreases over time.
decelerating waveform See *decelerating taper.*
decompression port A gas channel that relieves pressure in part of the gas circuit.
decontamination The process whereby contaminants are removed from objects, usually by simple physical means (e.g., washing).
default Failure to do something when required or expected.
delay time control A device that controls the back-up rate on a ventilator by setting a maximum time between cycles.
delta wave The slowest of the four types of brain waves, characterized by a frequency of less than 3.5 cycles per second and a relatively high voltage. Delta waves are "deep-sleep waves" associated with a dreamless state from which an individual is not easily aroused. Compare *alpha wave*; *beta wave*; and *theta wave.*
demand-flow accelerator servo An automatic device that increases patient gas flow in response to patient effort.
demand-flow CPAP system A continuous positive airway pressure (CPAP) system in which the patient must open a one-way valve to receive gas flow from a warmed and humidified blended gas source.
demand-flow IMV system An intermittent mandatory ventilation system in which the patient is required to perform the work of opening a one-way valve. Also called a parallel flow IMV or open-circuit IMV.
demand sensitivity system A subsystem that sets the level of inspiratory effort needed to trigger a ventilator into the inspiratory phase.

demand valve A mechanism that provides pressurized gas when the patient makes an inspiratory effort.
density An expression of the amount of mass per unit of volume a substance possesses.
Diameter Index Safety System (DISS) A safety system for compressed gas fittings. The DISS is used in respiratory care when equipment is connected to a low-pressure gas source (less than or equal to 200 psi).
diameter restrictor A device that controls or reduces flow by reducing the diameter of the flow path.
diaphragm compressor A gas delivery system that operates to reduce gas volume by increasing pressure via movement of a flexible diaphragm.
diaphragm/leaf valves Comparatively thin, flat valves that have many applications in respiratory care. They may separate high- and low-pressure areas, as one-way valves or as back flow prevention devices.
diaphragm valve See *diaphragm/leaf valves.*
diplobacilli Bacilli that occur in pairs.
differential area gas blending valve A gas-mixing device that changes the proportions of a gas mixture by varying the size of each gas inlet port.
differential output The difference between the output of O_1 and O_2 in a fluidic element.
diffuser A device used to mix or dissipate gases. Also a device to muffle the sound of a loud turbine or compressor.
diffuser humidifier A device that forces gas flow through a porous material submerged in water, causing the gas to form many bubbles that rise to the surface of the gas.
diffusion The physical process whereby atoms or molecules tend to move from an area of higher concentration or pressure to an area of lower concentration or pressure.
Digital Communications Interface (DCI) A function on the Nellcor Puritan Bennett 7200 ventilator that provides data reports including data logs, chart summary reports, ventilator status reports, and host reports.
digital flowmeter A flowmeter on the panel of the Newport Breeze E150 that displays and controls the flow during spontaneous breaths and is used to stabilize baseline pressure between mandatory breaths in assist/control.
diluter regulator A mechanism that controls the entrained air in an oxygen diluter system.
diplococcus A member of the *Coccaceae* family that occur in pairs because of incomplete cell division. Diplococci are often found as parasites of saprophytes. Also used to describe bacteria of the *Coccaceae* family that occur as pairs of cocci.
dipole-dipole interaction The interaction of equal and opposite electrical charges.
direct-acting valve A device that provides volume or flow by direct action from a control knob or device, such as the valve connected to a water faucet. As the faucet is turned, the valve opens or closes.
direct contact Mutual touching of two individuals or organisms. Many communicable diseases may be spread by direct contact between infected and healthy persons.
direct drive piston A piston whose movement is governed by linear (straight line) movement of a shaft that is connected to the piston head. Also called a linear drive piston. Compare with *rotary drive piston.*
diode A high-vacuum type of electron tube with a cold anode and a heated cathode that is used as a rectifier of alternating current.
direct current (DC) Current flowing in one direction. Compare *alternating current.*
direct-drive piston ventilator A ventilator that incorporates a linear drive piston.
disconnect ventilation An emergency mode of ventilation available on the Nellcor Puritan Bennett 7200 ventilator that activates when the microprocessor detects inconsistencies in airway pressures, PEEP, and the gas delivery pressure in the pneumatic system, which can occur in conditions such as tubing disconnects or plugged tubing.
disinfection The process of destroying at least the vegetative phase of pathogenic microorganisms by physical or chemical means.
display window A monitoring screen on the front panel of a ventilator that displays ventilator parameters.
DISS See *Diameter Indexed Safety System.*
Doppler effect The apparent change in frequency of sound or light waves emitted by a source as it moves away from or toward an observer. The frequency increases as the source moves toward the observer and decreases as it moves away (e.g., the rising pitch of a approaching train and the falling pitch of a departing train). The Doppler effect is also observed in electromagnetic radiation (e.g., light and radio waves).
double circuit A type of ventilator with two distinct gas flows, one of which provides power to deliver a breath, and the other is the actual flow delivered to the patient's airway.
double-lumen endotracheal tube (DLET) A specialized endotracheal tube that allows the right and left lungs to be ventilated separately (i.e., independent lung ventilation).
double-stage reducing valve A pressure-control device that lowers line pressure to working pressure in two steps. Generally from 2200 psig to 750 psig to 50 psig.
drag turbine The name of the flow control device in the T-Bird AVS ventilator.
drive mechanism Refers to the method by which gas flow to the patient is achieved with a mechanical ventilator.
droplet precautions Safeguards designed to reduce the risk of transmitting infectious agents by droplet.
drum vane The air foils on the Bennett valve in the PR, TV, and AP series respirators, which act as sensitivity and flow-cycling mechanisms.
dry powder inhaler A type of metered dose inhaler that delivers a drug as a powder rather than as a liquid aerosol.
dry-rolling seal spirometer A type of device measuring volume changes in the airway opening. Consists of a

canister containing a piston sealed to it with a rolling diaphragmlike seal.
dual modes of ventilation a phrase used to describe pressure-targeted ventilation that also guarantees delivery of a set volume.
dual OR/NOR gate See *OR/NOR fluidic switch.*
duckbill/diaphragm/fishmouth valves Valves made of elastic materials that have a slit in the middle, which opens when pressurized to allow gas flow.
dump port A mechanism that allows expired gas to exit the ventilator. May be part of the expiration valve.

EGTA See *esophageal gastric tube airway.*
elastic potential energy The potential energy stored in a compressed spring that will be converted into kinetic energy when the spring is allowed to uncoil.
electrical analyzer A type of gas analyzer that detects changes in electrical current in response to varying gas concentrations.
electrically powered Energy supplied by the activity of electrons or other subatomic particles in motion. Also a mechanical device or ventilator requiring electricity to operate.
electricity A form of energy expressed by the activity of electrons and other subatomic particles in motion, as in dynamic electricity, or at rest, as in static electricity. Electricity can be produced by heat; generated by a voltaic cell; or produced by induction, rubbing on nonconductors with dry materials, or chemical activity.
electrochemical Pertains to the electrical effects that accompany chemical action and the chemical activity produced by electrical influence.
electrochemical monitoring A type of monitoring system routinely used when oxgen or nitric oxide is administered. Gases diffusing across a semipermeable membrane react with an electrolyte solution, generating a current flow between two polarized electrodes as electrons are liberated or consumed. See also *chemiluminescence monitoring.*
electrochemical sensor An apparatus designed to react to physical stimuli that accompany chemical activity produced by electrical influence.
electrode A contact for the induction or detection of electrical activity. Also a medium for conducting an electrical current from the body to physiologic monitoring equipment.
electromagnetic frequency interference (EFI) The disruption of the operation of a device due to electromagnetic waves in the vicinity.
electromechanical transducer A mechanical device that is activated by electricity and capable of converting one form of energy into another. Commonly used to measure physical events.
electromechanical valve A mechanical valve system that responds to an electrical signal; also called an electrically powered mechanical valve.
electromotive force (EMF) The electrical potential, or the ability of electric energy to perform work. Usually measured in joules per coulomb, or volts. Any device, such as a storage battery, that converts some form of energy into electricity is a source of EMF.
electronic capacitance transducer An electronic component that changes one form of energy to another based on the strength of the electrical charge stored in the unit.
electronic logic In the Bear 3 ventilator, the term applied to the control mechanism that governs ventilator operation.
electronically controlled PEEP valve A PEEP valve whose pressure limits are maintained by electrically operated valves.
element One of more than 100 primary, simple substances that cannot be broken down into any other substance by chemical means. Each atom of any element contains a specific number of protons in the nucleus and an equal number of electrons outside the nucleus. The nucleus contains a variable number of neutrons. An element with a disproportionate number of neutrons may be unstable, in which case the nucleus undergoes radioactive decay into a more stable elemental form.
endotracheal tube A type of artificial airway inserted through the mouth or nose and the larynx into the trachea.
energy expenditure The metabolic cost (in calories or kilojoules) of various forms of physical activity.
entrainment device A device designed to add ambient gas into a primary gas stream. Usually a jet/Venturi device.
entrainment nebulizer A nebulizer designed to entrain gas or liquids into the primary gas stream. See *entrainment device.*
entrainment reservoir The part of an entrainment nebulizer that contains the substance to be entrained and nebulized.
EOA See *esophageal obturator airway.*
esophageal gastric tube airway (EGTA) A type of artificial airway that consists of a double lumen tube that passes through a tight-fitting face mask and extends through the mouth into the esophagus (this portion has an inflatable cuff above the distal opening). The oral portion of the airway has a ventilation tube with holes through which gas from a resuscitation device ventilates the lungs.
esophageal obturator airway (EOA) A type of artificial airway used in emergency situations. Consists of a blind tube that passes through a tight-fitting face mask and extends through the mouth into the esophagus (this portion has an inflatable cuff). The oral portion of the airway has holes through which gas from a resuscitation device is forced into the lungs.
EST See *extended self-test.*
eukaryotic Of or pertaining to cells with true nuclei bounded by a nuclear membrane and capable of mitosis.
evaporation The process by which liquids change into the vapor state. This occurs because of changes in temperature, pressure, and vapor pressure gradients.
exhalation timer A control that determines the length of the expiratory portion of the respiratory cycle.

exhalation valve A one-way valve system through which exhaled gases exit the ventilator and its circuit.
exhalation valve leak alarm A device that warns that the integrity of the exhalation valve has failed.
exhausted fuel cell alarm A warning that the sensing mechanism in a fuel cell gas analyzer is not functional.
expiratory flow cartridge In the Bird Mark series, an accumulator cartridge that used an adjustable and controlled leak to vary expiratory time.
expiratory flow gradient control A device that allows for adjustment of expiration by manipulation of back pressure and expiratory pressure gradients.
expiratory hold A mechanical ventilator control that delays mandatory breath delivery when it is pressed during the end of exhalation, used for measuring auto-PEEP.
expiratory hold (end-expiratory pause) The time at the end of exhalation after a mandatory breath during which the ventilator delays delivery of another mandatory breath for the purpose of measuring end-expiratory pressure. Usually performed to check for auto-PEEP.
expiratory pause See *expiratory hold.*
expiratory positive airway pressure (EPAP) The pressure measured in a patient circuit during exhalation. A parameter that can be set during bilevel positive airway pressure (BiPAP) ventilation that governs pressure delivery during exhalation.
expiratory resistance control An adjustable device that allows back pressure to increase forces opposing expiratory flow.
expiratory retard A device or control designed to increase the resistance to exhaled gas flow, which increases the pressure maintained in the circuit during exhalation and can increase expiratory time.
expiratory servo valve The device that controls the expiratory scissors valve in the Siemens 900 series ventilators.
expiratory tidal volume The volume from a normal inspiration to a normal expiration measured from a patient's exhaled air.
expiratory time The length of time of the expiratory portion of a breath. From the end of inspiration to the beginning of the next inspiration.
expiratory time accumulator See *expiratory flow cartridge.*
expiratory time control See *expiratory flow cartridge.*
expiratory timer See *expiratory flow cartridge.*
expiratory trigger sensitivity (ETS) The adjustable control available on the Hamilton GALILEO ventilator used to establish the percent of peak flow at which pressure support or spontaneous breaths will cycle out of inspiration.
extended self-test (EST) A series of tests that are part of the normal maintenance procedure for the Nellcor Puritan Bennett 7200 ventilator and that trained personnel perform between patient uses.
external battery A direct current power source sometimes used by ventilators as an alternative power supply when the normal electrical power source is not available.
external circuit The portion of the pneumatic circuit consisting of tubing from a ventilator to a patient. Also called patient circuit or ventilator circuit.
external IMV reservoir A reservoir bag or tubing that provides a volume of gas at a predetermined FiO_2 in a sufficient amount to accommodate the patient's volume.
external IMV system A reservoir, tubing, gas source, and valve system attached to the outside of a ventilator. Sometimes referred to as an H-valve assembly because of its design.
external PEEP valve A threshold or flow resistor added to the exhalation valve assembly of a ventilator or breathing device (e.g., resuscitation valve) to provide positive pressure during exhalation.
extreme extension See *sniffer's position.*

facultative Not obligatory; having the ability to adapt to more than one condition (e.g., a facultative anaerobe that can live with or without oxygen).
Fahrenheit (F) A temperature scale in which the boiling point of water is 212° and the freezing point of water is 32° at sea level.
fail-safe valve A safety measure designed to provide a way for the patient to breathe if the gas delivery devices fail.
fail-safe baseline metering orifice A variable metering device whose orifice opens during failure of power or pressure.
feedback channel In pneumatic or fluid devices, a mechanism that provides a signal or flow to a control device.
feedback line See *feedback channel.*
fenestrated tracheotomy tube A tracheotomy tube with a hole or "window" (*fenestra* in Latin) on the posterior wall of the outer cannula above the cuff. This allows the patient to speak when the inner cannula is removed, the cuff is deflated, and the tracheostomy tube is occluded at the connector. Fenestrated tubes aid in weaning patients from the artifical airway.
fetal hemoglobin (HbF) A hemoglobin variant that has a greater affinity for oxygen than adult hemoglobin. HbF is gradually replaced over the first year of life by HbA (adult hemoglobin).
FiO_2 (fraction of inspired oxygen) The ratio (amount) of oxygen to the total volume of a gas mixture; expressed as a decimal.
fishmouth valve See *duckbill/diaphragm/fishmouth valves.*
fixed orifice A hole in a device that has a specific, unchanging size.
fixed-performance oxygen-delivery system Oxygen therapy equipment that supplies inspired gases at a consistent preset oxygen concentration. Also called a high flow system.
fixed restrictor A device that is designed to produce a set back pressure (resistance) that inhibits forward flow.
flapper A type of valve system that employs a lightweight diaphragm to occlude an orifice.

flap vane In the Nellcor Puritan Bennett PR, AP, and TV series ventilators, the winglike protrusions extending from the Bennett valve's internal cylinder that react to the force of airflow to cycle the device.

Fleisch pneumotachometer A device that operates on the principle that the flow of gas through the device is proportional to the pressure drop that occurs as the gas flows across a known resistance (a bundle of brass capillary tubes arranged in parallel.)

flip-flop device See *flip-flop unit.*

flip-flop unit A fluidic element that contains two outlets and two control ports. The main flow switches flow from one outlet to the other when a signal gas pulse acts on the main flow.

floating-island nebulizer A type of aerosol production device in which the jet assembly floats underneath a pontoon assembly in a reservoir of water. Also called a Win-Liz nebulizer after the wives of the inventors.

flow acceleration cartridge In the Bird Mark series, a pneumatic device designed to increase inspiratory flow.

flow-and-volume augmented breaths in the Bear 1000 A function that provides additional flow or volume when the patient's inspiratory effort drops pressure below the set baseline pressure.

flow-by option A feature available on the Nellcor Puritan Bennett 7200 ventilator that provides continuous flow during the expiratory phase to provide fresh gas at the beginning of inspiration and reduce the ventilator response time to patient inspiratory effort (also see bias flow and base flow).

flow control See *flow control valve.*

flow control valve A device that controls and adjusts inspiratory flow on a ventilator, thus affecting respiratory rate and/or volume.

flow-dependent incentive spirometer A device that encourages a patient to take slow, deep breaths. The patient is encouraged to achieve a specific air flow during inspiration by using a visual cue that indicates air flow.

flow-dependent valve A device that responds to low flow by halting inspiration. The operating principle of the Bennett valve in the AP, PR, and TV series Nellcor Puritan Bennett respirators. A flow-dependent valve measures and displays the inspiratory flow that the patient achieves during a maximum sustained inspiratory effort.

flowmeter A device that controls and measures a flow of gas or liquid. Usually stated in volume per unit of time.

flow rate control See *flow control.*

flow resistor See *flow restrictor.*

flow restrictor A device that reduces the flow of a fluid/gas out of a system by providing an in-stream obstruction, usually in the form of a orifice of reduced size, thus causes back pressure in the system. Increases or decrease in gas flow result in increases or decreases in the back pressure created by the restrictor.

flow restrictor/regulator See *flow restrictor.*

flow sensor A mechanism that detects the movement of a volume of gas.

flow transducer An electronic device that changes one type of signal to another type proportionate to the flow that passes through it.

flow trigger The amount the flow must drop from the base flow value to trigger a breath during mechanical ventilation.

flow triggering When the ventilator detects a drop in gas flow then inspiration is set to occur.

flow waveforms The graphic pattern produced when flow is plotted against time.

fluid logic A method for delivering gas flow that uses fluidic elements that do not require moving parts (see fluidics).

fluidic Referring to hydrodynamic principles used to direct gas flow through circuits, resulting in switching of flow directions and signal amplification. Also used in pressure and flow sensing.

fluidic-breathing assistor A device that uses the principles of fluidics to augment the patient's ventilatory efforts.

fluidic drive A type of pneumatically powered ventilator or device that uses fluidic principles (elements). A mechanism to provide the primary power source for gas delivery using fluidics.

fluorescent sensor An optical blood gas sensor that uses dyes that fluoresce when struck by light in the ultraviolet or near-ultraviolet visible range. The pH, PCO_2, or PO_2 of arterial blood can be determined by using these devices.

fomite Nonliving material, such as bed linens or equipment, that may transmit pathogenic organisms.

fractional distillation of liquid air A method of reducing air to its component gases using pressure and temperature changes. See *Joule-Kelvin-Thompson method.*

fractional hemoglobin saturation The amount of oxyhemoglobin measured divided by the amount of all four types of hemoglobin present, written as follows: Fractional $O_2Hb = O_2Hb \div (HHb + O_2Hb + COHb + MetHb)$.

FRC See *functional residual capacity.*

freezing point The temperature at which a liquid becomes a solid.

French scale A measurement scale commonly used to delineate the external diameter of catheters; 1 French unit equals approximately 0.33 mm.

French sizes See *French scale.*

froth A mixture of liquid and gas that forms a dense layer of bubbles, increasing the gas/liquid surface area.

functional hemoglobin saturation The oxyhemoglobin concentration divided by the concentration of hemoglobin capable of carrying oxygen, written as follows: Functional $O_2Hb = O_2Hb \div (HHb + O_2Hb)$.

functional residual capacity (FRC) The total amount of gas left in the lungs after a normal, quiet exhalation.

fungicide An agent destructive to fungi.

fusible plug A type of pressure-relief mechanism made of a metal alloy that melts when the temperature of the gas in the tank exceeds a predetermined temperature. Fusible plugs operate on the principle that as the pressure in a tank increases, the temperature of the gas increases, which causes the plug to melt. The melting of the plug releases excess pressure.

galvanic analyzer An electric analyzer that measures gas concentrations by measuring the change in resistance of electric current in both reference and sampling circuits.
gas A fluid state of matter with the least organization and definition.
gas-collector exhalation valve A device that allows expired gases to be collected through a one-directional port.
gas streaming Asymmetric velocity profiles that occur when gas flows in both directions through a conductive airway (tube) at the same time as exhaled gas travels on the outside of the tube and inspired gas moves down the center.
geometric standard deviation (GSD) A measure of the variability of particle diameters within an aerosol. The higher the GSD, the more (larger *and* smaller) particles are present.
Geudel airway An upper airway device (oropharyngeal airway) used to provide air passage distal to an obstructing tongue.
germicide A drug that kills pathogenic microorganisms.
glucose oxidase An enzyme used to coat electrodes when measuring glucose.
gmw See *gram molecular weight.*
gram molecular weight (gmw) A chemical measurement for the mass of a chemical equal to the atomic weight of its chemical components (expressed in grams); sometimes called the combining weight.
Gram negative Having the pink color of the counterstain used in Gram's method of staining microorganisms. This property is a primary method of characterizing organisms in microbiology.
Gram positive Retaining the violet color of the stain used in Gram's method of staining microorganisms. This property is a primary method of characterizing organisms in microbiology.
Gram stain The method of staining microorganisms using a violet stain and an iodine solution; decolorizing with an alcohol or acetone solution; and counterstaining with safranin. The retention of either the violet color of the stain or the pink color of the counterstain is a primary means of identifying and classifying bacteria. Also called Gram's method.
graphics A visual representation of monitored parameters, such as pressure, volume, and flow per unit time. See *scalars.*
gravitational potential energy The potential energy an object can gain by falling, as a result of gravity.

Haldane effect The influence of hemoglobin saturation and oxygen on carbon dioxide dissociation.
hardware The mechanical, magnetic, and electronic design, structure, and devices of a computer. Compare *software.*
heat and moisture exchanger (HME) A passive, disposable device that humidifies and warms incoming gases in patients receiving mechanical ventilation using the principles of condensation and evaporation. Also called an artificial nose.
heated blow-by humidifier A type of pass-over humidifier that exposes gas flow to a heated water reservoir, where heat and moisture are transferred into the gas stream.
heated wire See *heated wire circuit.*
heated wire circuit A type of ventilator circuit in which the inspiratory tubing is heated to reduce water vapor "rain-out" (condensation).
heliox A low-density therapeutic mixture of helium with at least 20% oxygen; used in some institutions as part of large airway obstruction treatment.
Henderson-Hasselbalch equation The chemical formula relating pH, pKa, and the ratio of the conjugate base (bicarbonate) to the weak acid (carbonic acid).
HFFI See *high-frequency flow interrupter.*
HFJV See *high-frequency jet ventilation.*
HFO See *high-frequency oscillation.*
HFV See *high-frequency ventilation.*
high breathing rate alarm A ventilator warning system that indicates rapid respirations exceeding the desired rate.
high-frequency flow interrupter (HFFI or HIFI) A type of high-frequency ventilator that provides rapid gas pulses to the airway (up to 30 Hz) by periodically interrupting a high-flow gas stream.
high-frequency flow interruption See *high-frequency flow interrupter.*
high-frequency jet ventilation (HFJV) A type of high-frequency ventilator that provides a jet gas pulse to the airway via a small-lumen catheter within the endotracheal tube at rates of about 100 to 200 pulses/min.
high-frequency oscillation (HFO) A type of high-frequency ventilator that cycles at rates of 60 to 3000 times per minute.
high-frequency oscillatory ventilation (HFOV) See *high-frequency oscillation.*
high-frequency percussive ventilation (HFPV) Ventilation that incorporates the beneficial characteristics of a conventional positive-pressure ventilator and a jet ventilator. Can be compared with time-cycled, pressure-limited ventilation in which high-frequency pulsations (up to 100 to 225 cycles/min, or 1.7 to 4 Hz) are injected into the airway through a Venturi during the inspiratory phase.
high-frequency positive pressure ventilation (HFPPV) A mode of ventilatory support with rates from 60 to 100/minute and small tidal volumes (often approaching anatomic dead space) using a low-compliance patient circuit.
high-frequency ventilation (HFV) A method of ventilation at rates >80 times per minute. See also *high-frequency jet ventilation* and *high-frequency oscillation.*

high-level disinfection Using chemical sterilants at reduced exposure times (less than 45 minutes) to kill bacteria, fungi, and viruses. High-level disinfection does not kill a high level of bacterial spores. Compare *intermediate-level disinfection* and *low-level disinfection.*

Holter monitoring Making prolonged (usually 24 hours) electrocardiograph recordings on a portable tape recorder while the patient, wearing appropriate monitoring leads, conducts normal daily activities.

hood An environmental control device that covers the head and regulates the humidity, gas concentration, and temperature of inspired gases.

hot film anemometer A flow-sensing device used in some ventilators that works by measuring the temperature of the gas flow. Similar to hot-wire flow transducers.

humidity The amount of water vapor in a system expressed as weight/volume (e.g., grams/liter). Also water in the molecular form.

humidity deficit A condition in which the available humidity is less than the potential humidity; that is, the percentage relative humidity is less than 100 (e.g., the humidity deficit at a body temperature of 37° C is compared with its capacity of 44 mg/L).

hydrogen bonding The attractive force of compounds in which a hydrogen atom covalently linked to an electronegative element (e.g., oxygen, nitrogen, or fluorine) has a large degree of positive character relative to the electronegative atom, thereby causing the compound to have a large dipole.

hydrometer A device that determines the specific gravity or density of a liquid by comparing its weight with that of an equal volume of water. A calibrated hollow glass device is placed in the liquid being examined, and the depth to which the device settles in the liquid is noted.

hydrophobic The property of repelling water molecules.

hygroscopic The property of attracting and binding water molecules.

hyperbilirubinemia Above-average amounts of the bile pigment bilirubin in the blood; often characterized by jaundice, anorexia, and malaise.

hypertonic A solution of water and chemicals whose solute to solvent ratio exceeds that of normal body fluids. For salt water, this is greater than 0.9% NaCl.

ideal gas A gas acting as if it exactly follows all of the gas laws.

I:E ratio control A ventilator control that regulates the proportions of inspiratory and expiratory time during a respiratory cycle.

I:E ratio limit control A mechanism that prevents high inspiratory to expiratory (I:E) ratios; usually above 1:1.

IMV (pressurized breaths) See *intermittent mandatory ventilation.*

indirect calorimeter A device used for energy expenditure. (With a closed-circuit calorimeter, the patient breathes into and out of a container prefilled with oxygen. Oxygen consumption is determined by measuring the volume of oxygen the patient uses. With an open-circuit calorimeter, the volume of oxygen is determined by measuring the volumes of inspired and expired gases along with the fractional concentrations of oxygen in the inspired and expired gases. The volume of oxygen is then determined by calculating the difference between the amount of oxygen in the inspired gas and the amount in the expired gas.)

indirect contact Contacting a susceptible host with a contaminated intermediate object (usually inanimate) in the patient's environment.

indirect-drive piston A ventilator power mechanism in which the power gas is driven by a piston but does not go to the patient. For example, the power gas may compress a bellows that contains the patient gas volume.

inertia The tendency of objects to resist changes in position unless acted upon by an outside force (from Newton's laws).

inertial impaction The deposition of particles by collision with a surface; the primary mechanism for pulmonary deposition of larger particles (usually over 5 μm in diameter). Large particles tend to travel in a straight line and collide with surfaces in their pathway (e.g., airway branches, baffles).

infection surveillance The procedures of a hospital or other health facility to minimize the risk of spreading of nosocomial or community-acquired infections to patients or staff members.

inflating port An orifice through which ventilating gas flows.

injector A device that adds a quantity of liquid or gas to a main flow source. See *jet.*

inspiratory controls Mechanisms that determine the length and timing of inspiratory gas flow.

inspiratory flow rate control A ventilatory mechanism that sets the gas volume delivered per unit of time during inspiration.

inspiratory hold (plateau) A ventilatory maneuver in which delivered volume is held in the lungs before exhalation. Inspiratory gas flow stops, and the expiratory valve is maintained briefly in the closed position, thus keeping the delivered volume (and pressure) in the lungs. Commonly used to measure plateau pressure for the calculation of static compliance.

inspiratory interrupter switch A control device that terminates inspiration.

inspiratory pause See *inspiratory hold.*

inspiratory positive airway pressure (IPAP) The pressure measured in a patient circuit during inspiration. A parameter that can be set during bilevel positive airway pressure (BiPAP) ventilation and governs pressure delivery during inspiration.

inspiratory pressure calibration control Allows the inspiratory pressure limit to be set.

inspiratory pressure level The maximum amount of pressure allowed during mechanical ventilation.

inspiratory pressure-time product (PTP) The integration of the area within the curve during inspiration on a pressure/time graph.

inspiratory pressure-relief control A device that sets the "pop-off" pressure on a mechanical ventilator.

inspiratory time (T_I) See *inspiratory time control.*

inspiratory time control Sets the length of inspiration either directly or as a fraction of the I:E ratio.

inspiratory time percent The proportion of the respiratory cycle time devoted to inspiration.

inspiratory timer A control that determines the time allowed for inspiration.

insulator A nonconducting substance that is a barrier to heat or electricity passage.

intensive care unit (ICU) A hospital unit in which patients requiring close monitoring and care are housed for as long as necessary.

intermediate level disinfection Removing vegetative bacteria, tubercle bacteria, viruses, and fungi, but not necessarily killing spores. Compare *high-level disinfection* and *low-level disinfection.*

intermittent mandatory ventilation (IMV) (pressurized breaths) A time-triggered ventilatory mode that permits spontaneous ventilation and intersperses required pressurized breaths at predetermined intervals. See also *synchronized intermittent mandatory ventilation.*

intermittent (inspiratory) positive-pressure breathing (IPPB) A treatment modality in which the inspiratory pressure is elevated above atmospheric but is allowed to return to atmospheric during exhalation. Another term applied to mechanical ventilation.

intermittent positive-pressure ventilation (IPPV) Intermittent positive-pressure breathing done continuously as a form of mechanical ventilation.

internal battery A direct current power source sometimes used by ventilators as an alternative power supply when an alternating current source is not available.

internal demand valve A device that is triggered to provide gas flow when patient effort decreases pressure or flow below a certain baseline.

internal mechanism A device inside a ventilator or piece of equipment that functions in the operation of the equipment.

internal regulator A device inside a ventilator for adjusting pressure delivery.

International 10-20 EEG system The standard pattern for electrode placement on the scalp to record EEGs during sleep studies.

intrinsic positive end expiratory pressure (PEEPi) The level of pressure in the airway as a result of pressure trapped in the lung at the end of exhalation. Also called auto-PEEP.

invasive Characterized by a tendency to spread or infiltrate. Also refers to the use of diagnostic or therapeutic methods that require access to the inside of the body.

inverse ratio ventilation (IRV) Ventilation in which inspiratory time exceeds expiratory time. See *pressure-controlled inverse ratio ventilation* and *volume controlled-inverse ratio ventilation.*

in vitro Occurring in a laboratory apparatus (of a biological reaction).

in vivo Occurring in a living organism (of a biological reaction).

IPPB flow Gas flow during IPPB breaths.

iron lung A negative-pressure ventilator. Also called a tank ventilator, artificial lung, or Drinker respirator.

isolation procedures Infection control measures that combine barrier-type precautions (e.g., hand washing and the use of gloves, masks, and/or gowns) with the physical separation of infected patients in specific disease categories in order to disrupt transmission of pathogenic microorganisms.

isolation techniques See *isolation procedures.*

isotonic A solution of water and chemicals whose solute concentration equals that of plasma.

jet A device using a gas-entrainment mechanism to mix gases or add aerosols to a mainstream gas flow.

jet humidifier A humidifier that uses the jet principle to add water vapor to the main gas flow.

jet nebulizer A nebulizer that uses the jet principle to add water droplets to the main gas flow; contains a baffle.

jet Venturi A jet used to produce a pressure drop for entraining gas or fluid.

joule A unit of energy or work in the meter-kilogram-second system. It is equivalent to 10^7 ergs, or 1 watt second.

Joule-Kelvin effect A physical phenomenon in which the rapid expansion of a gas without the application of external work causes a cooling of the gas. Used in the liquefication of air to produce oxygen and nitrogen. Also called the Joule-Thompson effect.

Joule-Kelvin-Thompson method See *fractional distillation of gases.*

Joule-Thompson effect See *Joule-Kelvin effect.*

K complexes Large vertical slow waves with amplitudes of at least 75 microvolts with an initial negative deflection.

Kelvin (K) An absolute temperature scale calculated in centigrade units from the point at which molecular activity apparently ceases (-273.15° C). To convert Celsius degrees to Kelvin, add 273.15.

kilowatt Unit of measure of electrical power (1000 watts).

kinetic activity Molecular motion uses energy and produces heat as a by-product.

kinetic energy The energy a body possesses by virtue of its motion.

kinetic flowmeter A flow-regulation device that incorporates a spindle or plunger in place of a floating ball as a flow indicator.
kymograph A device for graphically recording lung volume changes during spirometry. See *water-sealed spirometers.*

laryngeal mask airway (LMA) A custom-formed, soft mask with a hollow tube fitting into the pyriform sinuses directly above the larynx. Used to establish and maintain a patent upper airway.
laryngoscope An endoscope for examining the larynx.
latent heat The amount of heat needed for a substance to change its state of matter.
leaf-type valve See *leaf valve.*
leaf valve A thin membrane that overlays an orifice and that when closed prevents fluid (gas or liquid) transmission through the opening.
Levy-Jennings charts The most common method of recording quality control data. These charts allow the operator to detect trends and shifts in performance and thus can help avoid problems associated with reporting inaccurate data due to analyzer malfunction.
light-emitting diode (LED) An electronic component that emits light when exposed to current flow. Used in instruments to display digital data.
limiting variable An element of breath delivery including flow, volume, pressure, or time given a set maximum value by the operator that cannot be exceeded during the breath.
linear-drive piston A piston whose movement is governed by linear (straight line) movement of a shaft that is connected to the piston head. See *direct drive piston.*
liquefaction The conversion of a substance into its liquid form.
liquid crystal A type of data display surface that indicates data by turning parts of the display on (dark) or off (light).
liquid crystal display See *liquid crystal.*
lock-out cartridge A control that inhibits (locks out) the functions of other controls or systems.
loop A graphic display of two variables plotted on the x (horizontal) and y (vertical) axis that is circlelike. Pressure/volume and flow/volume loops are most commonly used.
low battery alarm A warning that the power (charge) remaining in a battery is below acceptable limits.
low inlet gas alarm A warning that system pressure is below optimal pressure standards.
low-level disinfection Killing most vegetative bacteria, some fungi, and some bacteria. Compare *high-level disinfection* and *intermediate-level disinfection.*
low-pressure reducing valve A pressure-regulating system designed to operate below 50 psig.
low-pressure regulator A low-pressure–reducing valve combined with a flowmeter.
low-residual-volume, high-pressure cuff A type of endotracheal or tracheostomy tube seal that uses low volumes at high pressures to achieve an airtight seal.
low-resistance/high-compliance system A system in which the forces resisting flow are low and the volume change per unit of pressure exerted is high.
Luer-Loc A glass or plastic syringe with a simple screw-lock mechanism that securely holds the needle in place. Also called Luer syringe.

Macintosh blade A curved laryngoscope blade, as opposed to a straight Miller type of blade.
macroshock A shock from an electric current of 1 mA or greater that is applied externally to the skin.
magnetic valve resistors A type of threshold resistor containing a bar magnet that attracts a ferromagnetic disc seated on the expiratory port of a pressurized circuit.
magnetic PEEP valve A valve that maintains a positive end-expiratory pressure by means of a magnetically activated component.
magnetism The branch of physics dealing with magnets and magnetic phenomena; also called magnetics.
main solenoid The master control device governing flow in a gas-delivery system.
mainstream capnograph See *capnograph.*
mainstream nebulizer A nebulizer that introduces the jet stream into the main gas flow.
mandatory breath A breath initiated and ended by the mechanical ventilator . Mandatory breath delivery is completely determined by the ventilator.
mandatory minute ventilation (MMV) A closed-loop (servo-controlled) mode of ventilation that guarantees delivery of a set minute volume by monitoring patient spontaneous minute volume and supplementing breaths as necessary to achieve the set minute volume.
mandatory minute volume See *mandatory minute ventilation.*
manifold A system of interconnected devices (e.g., a gas manifold). Two or more cylinders connected to regulators and a metering device or a breathing manifold. The externally mounted exhalation valve, tubing, and nebulizer, which make up a portion of the ventilator circuit.
manometer ports Orifices from which pressure readings are obtained by connecting pressure manometers.
manual trigger A device whose function is activated by hand.
mass median aerodynamic diameter (MMAD) Regarding aerosol particles, the diameter at which the mass is equally divided. That is, 50% of the particles are lighter than the MMAD and 50% are heavier.
mass spectrometry A sophisticated analysis technique used to analyze the composition of substances by examining a stream of charged particles to separate elements on the basis of atomic mass.
maximum expiratory flow A pulmonary function measurement of the patient's ability to exhale quickly and forcefully (in liters/second).
maximum inspiratory time control The mechanism that determines the length of inspiration allowed.

maximum motor current The highest electrical current the motor will tolerate.
maximum pressure control Sets the highest allowable ventilator pressure. Also called pressure-limit control.
maximum pressure limit (Pmax) The upper pressure value that can be delivered during inspiration. In the Hamilton GALILEO, the Pmax setting also establishes a reference point for pressure delivered during servo-controlled modes of ventilation.
mean airway pressure (MAP) The average pressure occurring in the airway during a complete respiratory cycle. Mathematically, the area below the pressure/time curve for one breathing cycle divided by the breath cycle time.
measured variables One or more of the four elements of a breath (pressure, flow, volume, and time) monitored during ventilation.
mechanics The branch of physics dealing with the motion of material bodies and the phenomena of the action of forces on them.
melting point The temperature at which solids begin to turn into liquids.
membrane concentrator An oxygen concentrator that separates oxygen from air by means of a selectively permeable membrane.
mercury barometer A device for measuring atmospheric pressure by the change in the height of a mercury column.
message window A monitoring screen on the front panel of a ventilator used to display messages.
metered dose inhaler (MDI) A small pressurized cartridge that contains a propellant and a medication. When the cartridge is activated, a precise amount of aerosolized medication is delivered.
microcuvette A small transparent tube or container with specific optical properties. The chemical composition of the container determines the vessel's use (e.g., Pyrex glass for examining materials in the visible spectrum, or silica for those in the ultraviolet range).
microprocessor A small, compact computer designed to monitor and control specific functions.
microprocessor-controlled Regulated by a small, compact computer.
microshock A shock from a usually imperceptible electrical current (<1 milliampere) that is allowed to bypass the skin and follow a direct, low-resistance pathway into the body.
microswitches Small, control devices that institute or halt processes.
Miller blade A straight laryngoscope blade, as opposed to a curved Macintosh blade.
mini-fluid amp A device that increases the strength of a fluidic signal.
minimum minute volume See *mandatory minute volume.*
minimal occluding volume (MOV) The least amount of air needed to achieve a seal in a cuffed endotracheal or tracheostomy tube.
minute ventilation The total ventilation per minute. The product of tidal volume and respiratory rate, as measured by expired gas collection for 1 to 3 minutes. The normal value is 5 to 10 liters per minute. Also called minute volume.
minute volume control The mechanism that sets the minute volume delivered by a ventilator.
mixed sleep apnea Repeated episodes of complete airflow cessation for more than 10 seconds during sleep, with characteristics of both obstructive sleep apnea and central sleep apnea. In mixed sleep apnea, the central event usually precedes the obstructive event.
mixer A device that blends or mixes two gases to provide a precise mixture (concentration) of the gases.
mixture A substance composed of ingredients that are not chemically combined and do not necessarily occur in a fixed proportion.
molecular sieve A term used to describe components of a type of oxygen concentrator that filters air and chemically removes nitrogen and some trace gases from the air.
molecule The smallest unit that exhibits the properties of an element or compound. A molecule is composed of two or more covalently bonded atoms.
monitor To observe and evaluate a body function closely and constantly. Also, a mechanical device that provides a visual or audio signal or a graphic record of a particular function (e.g., a cardiac or fetal monitor).
monoplace hyperbaric chamber A hyperbaric unit rated for single occupancy.
monostable A fluidic device or element that can direct gas flow to only one outlet unless the gas flow is acted upon by a separate gas pulse.
multiplace hyperbaric chamber A walk-in hyperbaric unit that provides enough space to treat two or more patients simultaneously.
multistage reducing valve See *multistage regulator.*
multistage regulator A pressure-reducing valve that has more than one level of pressure reduction between system pressure and working pressure.
mustache cannula A type of reservoir nasal cannula that can reduce oxygen supply use when compared with a continuous-flow nasal cannula.

nasal cannula An oxygen-delivery device characterized by small, hollow prongs that are inserted into the external nares.
nasal catheter An oxygen delivery device consisting of a narrow, hollow tubing that is inserted through the nose into the nasopharynx.
nasal trumpet A type of artificial airway. Also called a nasal, or nasopharyngeal, airway.
nasopharyngeal airway A type of artificial airway inserted through the nose with the distal tip in the posterior part of the oropharynx. Also called nasal trumpet or nasal airway.

nasotracheal intubation Using the nose as the entry point for placement of tubes or catheters in the trachea.
nebulizer A type of aerosol production device that consists of an "atomizer," or JET, and a baffle or baffles.
nebulization controls Devices on ventilators that regulate the time and/or intensity of the flow output from a connector used to power a nebulizer.
nebulizer controls See *nebulization controls.*
nebulizer solenoid A switch mechanism that turns the nebulizer on or off.
nebulizer system The parts of a device that produce, control, and deliver aerosols to the patient.
negative end-expiratory pressure (NEEP) See *negative expiratory pressure.*
negative expiratory pressure A mode of ventilation in which a small suction is exerted during expiration to assist expiratory flow, reduce mean airway pressure, and decrease expiratory time.
negative extrathoracic pressure A subatmospheric pressure applied to the external chest wall. Used in negative-pressure ventilators.
negative-pressure capability The ability of a device to generate subambient pressures.
negative-pressure control The mechanism that regulates the application of negative pressures in a device.
negative-pressure jet A Venturi or Pitot device that reduces pressure by air entrainment.
negative-pressure Venturi See *negative-pressure jet.*
negative-pressure ventilator A machine that provides ventilation by generating less pressure than ambient (atmospheric) around the thorax while maintaining the upper airway at ambient. The iron lung and chest cuirass are examples.
Nernst equation An expression of the relationship between the electrical potential across a membrane and the concentration ratio between permeable ions on either side of the membrane.
newton An SI unit of force that would impart an acceleration to 1 kg of mass of 1 meter per second.
nonconstant flow generator A ventilator that reacts to back pressure and resistance by varying the inspiratory flow pattern.
nonforced vital capacity The maximum amount of air that can be slowly exhaled after a maximum inspiration. Also called slow vital capacity.
noninvasive Pertains to a diagnostic or therapeutic technique that does not require the skin to be broken or a cavity or organ of the body to be entered (e.g., obtaining a blood pressure reading by auscultation with a stethoscope and sphygmomanometer).
nonlinear drive piston See *rotary drive piston.*
non-rapid eye movement sleep See *non-REM sleep.*
nonrebreathing valve A valve that opens, allowing gas to flow to the patient, then closes, allowing exhaled air to exit by another route. Examples are spring-loaded and diaphragm valves. Diaphragm valves are further subdivided into duckbill (or fishmouth) valves and leaf type of valves.
non-REM sleep Non-rapid eye movement sleep. Four observable, progressive stages of sleep that represent three fourths of a typical sleep period and are collectively called non-REM sleep. The remaining sleep time is usually occupied with REM sleep, during which dreaming occurs.
normal body humidity At BTSP, 47 mm Hg vapor pressure or 43.8 gm H_2O/L of air.
normal flora Microorganisms that live on or within a body to compete with disease-producing microorganisms and provide a natural immunity against certain infections.
normal rate control The system that sets the normal breathing frequency on a ventilator.
nosocomial Pertaining to or originating in a hospital (e.g., a nosocomial infection).

obstructive sleep apnea (OSA) A condition in which five or more apneic periods (≥10 seconds each) occur per hour of sleep and that is characterized by occlusion of the oropharyngeal airway with continued efforts to breathe. Compare *central sleep apnea* and *mixed sleep apnea.*
occlusion pressure ($P_{0.1}$) or **airway occlusion pressure** See $P_{0.1}$.
ohm A unit of measurement of electrical resistance. One ohm is the resistance of a conductor in which an electrical potential of 1 volt produces a current of 1 ampere.
one-point calibration Adjusting the electronic output of an instrument to a single known standard to help ensure quality assurance. It should be performed before analyzing an unknown sample, unless the analyzer is programmed to automatically perform a one-point calibration at regular intervals (e.g., every 20 to 30 minutes).
open-circuit calorimeter See *calorimeter.*
open-loop system A microprocessor-controlled system that provides clinical data or advice but defers to the user to take the appropriate action.
open-top tent An environmental control enclosure used for small children; features an open top to facilitate CO_2 washout.
optical encoder The name of the device on the T-Bird ventilator that sends information about the turbine speed to the microprocessor in order to control the precise flow delivered to the patient.
optical plethysmography A technique for measuring blood volume changes in a specific body part (e.g., a digit or earlobe). These blood volume changes are then used to define systolic and diastolic time periods during the cardiac cycle.
optics A field of study that deals with the electromagnetic radiation of wavelengths that are shorter than radio waves but longer than x-rays.
O_2 relay An electronic or mechanical device that controls oxygen flow into a delivery system.

OR/NOR gate A monostable, fluidic element with one control port and two outlet ports.
oropharangeal airway An artificial airway that is inserted into the mouth until the distal tip is behind the base of the tongue, providing an open channel to the laryngopharynx.
outflow valve A control device that regulates the gas exiting a system.
outlet manifold Part of the exhalation valve on a ventilator.
outlet valve A safety valve on a piped-gas system that prevents the high-pressure gas from free-flowing.
over-pressure alarm A warning that the pressures in a system have exceeded predetermined levels.
over-pressure relief A device that allows pressure to be released from a system that has exceeded desired pressure limits.
over-pressure–relief valve See *over-pressure relief.*
oximeter A device that monitors the amount of oxygen in a (physiologic) system. See *pulse oximeter* and *CO-oximeters.*
oxygen analyzer A device used to determine the concentration of oxygen in a gas mixture.
oxygen blender A device that mixes oxygen with air or other gases to provide precise oxygen concentrations.
oxygen concentrator A device that increases the oxygen content of inspired gas by enriching or concentrating the oxygen in air.
oxygen control A device in a ventilator that regulates the oxygen concentration delivered to the patient.
oxygen controller/blender See *oxygen blender.*
oxygen exhaust port An opening through which oxygen-enriched gas is expelled to the atmosphere.
oxygen inlet regulator A pressure-control device that governs the pressure of the oxygen entering a system.
oxygen percentage control See *oxygen control.*
oxygen percentage valve A metering device that regulates the proportion of oxygen in the delivered gas.
oxygen sensor The monitoring probe of an oxygen analyzer.
oxygen system The equipment and devices that distribute, control, and monitor oxygen from the bulk storage unit to the site of patient use.

$P_{0.1}$ The mouth pressure 100 msec after the start of a patient's inspiratory effort that is measured in a closed (occluded) system; a measure of the output of the respiratory center.
$PaCO_2$ Partial pressure of arterial carbon dioxide.
P_ACO_2 Partial pressure of alveolar carbon dioxide.
PaO_2 Partial pressure of arterial oxygen.
P_AO_2 Partial pressure of alveolar oxygen.
paramagnetic Of or pertaining to a characteristic that causes a substance to be attracted to magnetic fields.
parameter A value or constant used to describe or measure a set of data representing a physiologic function or system (e.g., the use of blood acid-base relationships as parameters for evaluating the function of a patient's respiratory system).
partial pressure The absolute pressure exerted by one gas in a mixture of gases.
partial-rebreathing mask A kind of oxygen mask that allows patients to reinhale the first third of their exhaled breath.
particle filter A device that removes particulate matter from an area or gas stream.
particle inertia The tendency of a particle to maintain a direction and speed of motion unless acted on by another force.
pass-over humidifier A humidification system in which the patient gas supply flows over a water supply. See *blow-by humidifier.*
pasteurization The process of applying moist heat, usually to a liquid such as milk for a specific time to kill or retard the development of pathogenic bacteria.
pathogenic Capable of producing disease.
patient circuit The portion of the pneumatic circuit consisting of tubing from a ventilator to a patient. Also called external, or ventilator, circuit.
patient disconnect alarm A system warning that the patient is not connected to the ventilator; a low-pressure alarm.
patient triggering When pressure, flow, or volume begin the breath; that is, the patient controls the beginning of inspiration.
peak flow A measurement of the maximum amount of gas that can be forcefully exhaled after a maximum inspiration; expressed in liters per minute.
peak flow control A control on the front panel of a ventilator used to set the maximum flow delivered during a mandatory inspiration.
peak flow meter A device that regulates the maximum flow a ventilator delivers.
peak flow setting See *peak flow control.*
peak inspiratory pressure (PIP) A measurement of the maximum pressure in the patient circuit that occurs during delivery of a mandatory breath from a ventilator. Also called peak pressure (Ppeak).
peak pressure See *peak inspiratory pressure.*
pedestal ventilator A term used in reference to a Bennett PR series respirator.
PEEP See *positive end-expiratory pressure.*
PEEP/CPAP pressure-control valve A mechanism that regulates the pressure limits of the PEEP/CPAP devices in a ventilator system.
PEEP exhalation valve An exhalation valve fitted with a PEEP device.
pendant cannula A type of reservoir nasal cannula that can reduce oxygen supply use when compared with a continuous-flow nasal cannula. The reservoir is attached as connecting tubing that is a conduit to a pendant, which hangs below the chin.

pendelluft Movement of gas from "fast" to "slow" filling spaces during breathing. Alternatively, the ineffective movement of gas back and forth (accompanied by mediastinal shifting) from a healthy lung to one with a flail segment; caused by a crushing chest injury.

percent pause time A ventilator control that uses a percentage of the inspiratory time to provide a pause at the end of inspiration, usually lengthening inspiratory time and allowing for an inspiratory hold.

pH Abbreviation for potential hydrogen, a scale representing the relative acidity (or alkalinity) of a solution, in which a value of 7.0 is neutral, below 7.0 is acid, and above 7.0 is alkaline.

pH electrode See *Sanz electrode.*

P_{H_2O} Partial pressure of water vapor; 47 mm Hg at BTSP.

phase variables During breath delivery, the variables controlled by the ventilator that are responsible for each of the four parts of a breath, including triggering (begins inspiratory flow), cycling (ends inspiratory flow), and limiting (places a maximum on a control variable: pressure, volume, flow, and/or time).

photoplethysmography The use of light waves to detect changes in the volume of an organ or tissue. Pulse oximeters use this principle to measure the arterial pulse.

physical analyzer A gas analyzer that uses the principles of physics (heat, electrical flow, etc.) to measure gas concentration.

piezoelectric quality The ability of a substance to change shape in response to and at the frequency of an electrical current, thus changing electrical energy into mechanical energy.

Pin Index Safety System (PISS) A standardized scheme to prevent accidental mismatching of reducing valves and pressurized gases in small capacity cylinders (E or smaller).

PISS See *Pin Index Safety System.*

piston bag A baglike reservoir that contains a volume of gas to be delivered to the patient when compressed by a piston.

piston compressor A gas source in which a volume of gas is reduced in volume and pressurized by a piston.

plateau pressure ($P_{plateau}$) The pressure measured in the patient circuit of a ventilator during an inspiratory hold maneuver. Also the pressure needed to overcome the elastic component of the lungs (static compliance) during breath delivery.

pneumatic Pertaining to air or gas.

pneumatically powered Supplied energy by high-pressure gas or air.

pneumatic circuit A series of tubing that directs the gas flow in a ventilator and from a ventilator to a patient.

pneumatic drive mechanism A method of operating a ventilator using pressurized gas as a power source.

pneumatic expiratory timing device A gas-powered device that controls expiratory time (e.g., using a controlled leak to deflate a diaphragm and open an inspiratory valve).

pneumatic nebulizer A device that produces an aerosol cloud using a pressurized gas source as the propellant.

pneumatic system An air or gas system.

pneumatic timing mechanisms See *pneumatic expiratory timing device.*

pneumobelt A corset with an inflatable bladder that fits over the abdominal area. The bladder is connected by a hose to a ventilator that delivers positive pressure at an adjustable rate and pressure. Used to assist in the respiratory rehabilitation of patients with high cervical injuries to alleviate strain.

pneumotachometer A device that measures the flow of respiratory gases. The pressure gradient is directly related to flow, thus allowing a computer to derive a flow curve measured in liters per minute.

pneumotachygraph An instrument that incorporates a pneumotachometer to record variations in respiratory gas flow.

polarographic electrode A device that employs the flow of electric current between the negative (cathode) and positive (anode) electrodes to measure a physical phenomenon such as the partial pressure of oxygen in the blood. See *arterial blood gas analysis.*

polysomnography The measurement and recording of variations in airflow, EEG, EOG, and arterial blood gases during sleep. Used in the diagnosis of sleep apnea.

poppet assembly A spool-shaped device used to open or close an orifice in response to pressure differences.

poppet valve See *poppet assembly.*

positive end-expiratory pressure (PEEP) A form of therapy applied during mechanical ventilation that elevates the baseline pressure at which inspiration is delivered. PEEP increases functional residual volume and mean airway pressure to improve oxygenation.

positive intrapulmonary pressure A condition where the pressure in the lungs is maintained at levels above physiologic.

positive-pressure ventilator A device that applies positive pressure to the lungs to improve gas exchange.

POST See *power-on self-test.*

potential energy The energy a body possesses by virtue of its position.

potentiometer An electronic device in which the output signal varies in strength with the strength of the input signal.

potentiometric Refers to measuring voltage.

power A source of physical or mechanical force or energy. Force or energy that can be put to work (e.g., electric power).

power failure alarm A warning device that indicates that the main power source of a piece of equipment has failed. Also known as a power disconnect alarm.

power indicators Monitoring lights or diodes that illuminate to give information about a device's power source.

power-on self-test (POST) An essential test started by the microprocessor as soon as the ventilator is turned on that lasts about 5 seconds. The unit must complete this test before it is functional.

power source The origin of physical or mechanical force or energy. Force or energy that can be put to work (e.g., electric power).

power transmission system Gas or electrically powered mechanical devices that generate a pressure gradient to provide all or part of the work of breathing for a patient. Also called a drive mechanism.

precision/imprecision In measurement, precision is freedom from random errors; imprecision is inaccuracy due to random error.

precision metering device See *proportional metering device.*

preset minute volume The set amount of gas to be delivered in a minute through a ventilator.

preset reducing valve See *preset regulator.*

preset regulator A device that decreases the pressure from a gas supply system to a predetermined lower pressure.

preset working pressure A predetermined pressure at which pneumatically powered devices function efficiently and safely. Usually below 60 psig.

pressure The amount of force exerted per unit of area.

pressure augmentation (PAug) A servo-control (closed-loop) mode of pressure-targeted ventilation that guarantees volume delivery on a breath-by-breath basis.

pressure and sensitivity adjustments Mechanisms that let the operator select the pressure and sensitivity values on a mechanical ventilator.

pressure capacitance chamber A device that increases or decreases pressure against a pressure-relief valve in the Bio-Med MVP-10 ventilator.

pressure compartment In the Bird Mark series, the right side of the respirator in which superambient pressures could develop and be transmitted to the patient.

pressure control The mechanism that determines the pressure level generated by the ventilator.

pressure-control ventilation (PCV) A mode of ventilation in which the maximum preset pressure is delivered, regardless of the volume achieved.

pressure-controlled inverse ratio ventilation (PCIRV) Pressure-targeted, time-cycled ventilation in which the inspiratory time exceeds the expiratory time.

pressure differential devices Mechanisms that operate by attempting to balance pressures within the device.

pressure differential transducer A device whose output signal strength depends on the difference between two or more input pressures.

pressure-equalization passage In the Bird Mark series, a hole in the center body that allows for equalization of pressure between the pressure and ambient sides of the respirator.

pressure limit control A dial or button that allows the operator to determine the preset maximum pressure a ventilator will deliver.

pressure-limited A descriptive term indicating that a maximum pressure has been set that cannot be exceeded. Also see *pressure-targeted ventilation* and *pressure ventilation.*

pressure-limited resuscitators Emergency ventilation devices that have a preset maximum inspiratory pressure.

pressure-limited ventilation A mode of ventilation in which inspiration is stopped when a selected pressure value is reached.

pressure ramp (Pramp) A ventilator control that determines how rapidly the set pressure is achieved during inspiration. Also called pressure sloping.

pressure-regulated volume control (PRVC) The name given to a mode of ventilation on the Siemens Servo 300 ventilator that provides pressure-targeted, time-cycled ventilation that is volume guaranteed.

pressure release Baseline ventilation in which elevated baseline pressures are periodically allowed to fall to baseline or a pressure-relief safety valve is activated.

pressure-relief valve A safety device that vents pressure in excess of a preset value to atmosphere.

pressure sensor A device that detects pressure or pressure changes.

pressure slope A ventilator control that adjusts the rate at which the set pressure is reached during inspiration. Also called pressure sloping. See *pressure ramp.*

pressure support See *pressure-support ventilation.*

pressure-support ventilation (PSV) A mode of ventilatory support designed to augment spontaneous breathing. Patient-triggered, pressure-targeted, flow-cycled ventilation.

pressure switch A device that responds to changes in or the presence of a pressure signal by instituting an action within the ventilator system.

pressure-targeted ventilation A form of ventilation in which the operator selects a specific pressure for delivery of inspiration.

pressure transducer A mechanism that converts a pressure signal to another form of energy, usually electric.

pressure triggering Inspiration begins when the ventilator senses a drop in circuit pressure.

pressure ventilation Setting a desired pressure. Also called pressure-limited ventilation, pressure-controlled ventilation, and pressure-targeted ventilation.

prokaryotic Of or pertaining to an organism that does not contain a true nucleus surrounded by a nuclear membrane. Characteristic of lower life forms, such as bacteria, viruses, and blue-green algae. Division of the organism occurs through simple fission.

proportional amplifier A fluidic control device that boosts or reduces output signal strength in proportion to the strength of the input signal.

proportional assist ventilation (PAV) A method of assisting spontaneous ventilation in which the practitioner adjusts the amount of work the ventilator will perform.

proportional manifold A mechanism that directs blended gas through a series of solenoids to control flow in the Infrasonics Infant Star ventilator.

proportional metering device A mechanism used to provide precise mixtures of gases. As the amount of one gas increases at a given total flow, the amount of the second gas decreases proportionately.
proportional solenoid A valve designed to modify gas flow. Typically, an electrical current flows through an electromagnet, creating a magnetic field that controls a plunger. The plunger governs the valve opening and gas delivery.
proportioning valve A system in which two or more valves vary the amounts of the gases they control entering the gas delivery system. This determines the final composition of the gas mixture.
proximal airway pressure gauge A gauge that indicates the proximal airway pressure.
proximal pressure line A line in the patient circuit to monitor airway pressures at the wye connector.
PSV See *pressure-support ventilation.*
PSVmax The amount of pressure-support ventilation delivered to achieve a desired volume.
pulse demand oxygen delivery system A system that only delivers oxygen to the patient during inspiration (on demand).

quality assurance Any evaluation of services provided and the results achieved as compared with accepted standards.
quality control A planned, systematic approach to designing, measuring, assessing, and improving performance.
quenching A process of removing or reducing an energy source, such as heat or light. Also, stopping or diminishing a chemical or enzymatic reaction.
quick-connect adapter A device that allows rapid connection and disconnection of compressed gas appliances to high-pressure gas delivery systems.
quick-connect outlet See *quick-connect adapter.*

radio frequency interference (RFI) The disruption of the operation of a device due to specific types of radio waves in the vicinity.
rapid eye movement sleep See *REM sleep.*
rapid shallow breathing (RSB) index A weaning parameter mathematically defined as the spontaneous respiratory rate divided by the spontaneous tidal volume.
rate The frequency of occurrence stated in incidents per unit of time (e.g., 16 per minute).
rate control A device that allows the number of breaths per minute to be selected.
ratio light A visual warning indicating that the I:E ratio is not within predetermined limits.
real gas A gas that does not fit all of the kinetic theories, as compared with an ideal gas.
rebreathing mask A gas-delivery system in which expired gases are oxygen-enriched and inhaled again by the patient. Characterized by a reservoir bag and a series of one-way valves.
reducing valve A mechanism that decreases the delivery pressure of a gas to a lower the "working" pressure.
reference electric potential A constant electrical voltage against which electrical flow in a sampling chamber is compared during gas analysis.
reference potentiometer A device that compares a predetermined, preset signal to other signals within an electrical or fluidic system.
reference pressure A preset pressure level to which other pressures are compared within a control system.
reference pressure-support bias pressure A condition in the Bear-3 ventilator in which spring tension in the adjustable pressure-support regulator equals the PEEP pilot pressure plus the pressure-support setting. This increases the machine-side pressure in the regulator, maintaining pressure support.
relative humidity The ratio of actual to potential water vapor in a volume of gas (i.e., how much *is present* as opposed to how much *could be* present).
REM sleep Rapid eye movement sleep. Sleep periods, lasting from a few minutes to half an hour, during which dreaming occurs. REM sleep periods alternate with non-REM sleep periods.
reservoir bag A pliable container that holds a volume of premixed gas for use in succeeding ventilations or as a back-up.
reservoir system A collection of bags or tubes that form a device to contain a supply of gas or liquid for later use.
residual volume (RV) The volume of gas remaining in the lungs after a complete exhalation.
respiration rate control The mechanism that controls the number of respirations per minute in a ventilator.
respiratory mechanics Measurable values used to evaluate the capacity for spontaneous breathing, which includes parameters such as maximum inspiratory pressure (MIP, also called negative inspiratory force [NIF]), vital capacity (VC), tidal volume (V_T), respiratory rate (f), compliance (C), and airway resistance (Raw).
respiratory system compliance The distensibility of the lungs and chest wall, which is determined by dividing the tidal volume by the pressure. Normal compliance averages 0.1 L/cm H_2O.
rheostat An electronic device that allows for variable control of the amount of electrical current flowing from the device.
rocker arm assembly The mechanism that determines piston stroke length to control tidal volume in the Bennett M25A and M25B portable ventilators.
rocking bed A device that rocks a patient from 15 to 30 degrees. Rocking moves the abdominal contents, and the resulting diaphragmatic movement assists lung ventilation.
rotary blower A kind of fan or compressor in which a fanlike device spins at high speeds to produce a pressurized gas flow.
rotary compressor See *rotary blower.*
rotary drive piston A piston that is connected to a wheellike device, the movement and speed of which gov-

erns it. Also called nonlinear drive piston. Compare *direct- or linear- drive piston.*
rotary vane respirometer A volume recording device that measures the movement of a drumlike cylinder with blade- or wing-shaped extensions (air foils).

safety valve A device that protects a patient-breathing system from complete closure, leading to suffocation, by allowing access to air. Also, a device that prevents excessive pressure in a patient-breathing system.
sample chamber In gas analyzers, the reservoir in which the observed gas (that to be analyzed) is held and compared with the reference gas.
Sanz electrode The standard electrode that measures pH. Composed of two half-cells that are connected by a potassium chloride bridge.
scalars Graphic displays of pressure, volume, and flow over time.
secondary equipment Oxygen-delivery equipment extending from the wall outlet or reducing valve to the patient apparatus.
sedimentation The deposition of insoluble materials at the bottom of a liquid or out of suspension in an aerosol.
semipermeable membrane A biologic or synthetic membrane that only permits the passage of certain molecules (e.g., based on size or electrical charge).
sensing port A connection or opening through which gas pressure, flow, or concentrations are sampled or measured.
sensing/servoing Venturi A Venturi device with known pressure gradients, allowing comparisons with unknown pressures.
sensitivity See *sensitivity setting.*
sensitivity control See *sensitivity setting.*
sensitivity setting A setting on a ventilator that determines the amount of patient inspiratory effort necessary to start inspiration. Also called trigger sensitivity and sensitivity control.
separation bubble A low-pressure vortex.
sequencing switch Used in the Bird Mark 7A and 8A respirators to regulate flow through control ports. See *ceramic switch.*
service verification test (SVT) A test procedure used on the T-Bird ventilator to evaluate unit function.
servo-controlled A closed-loop system in which a microprocessor compares a set parameter with a measured parameter and alerts the operator and/or makes specific changes to the set value based on its findings.
servo-controlled flow valve A servo valve that varies and controls gas flow in response to feedback from a flow transducer.
servo valve A scissorlike device that controls flow through the patient circuit in the Siemens Servo 900 ventilators.
set tidal volume The preset or desired volume of a ventilator, usually calculated based on the patient's physical characteristics.
Schmitt trigger An integrated circuit made up of several proportional devices (three proportional amplifiers and two flip-flop valves) connected in a series. Often used in pressure-cycled fluidic ventilators.
sidestream A gas analyzer that extracts a small sample of gas from the main gas flow for analysis. A nebulizer in which the aerosol cloud is formed outside of the main gas flow.
sidestream capnograph See *capnograph.*
sidestream nebulizer See *sidestream.*
Siggaard-Anderson nomogram A graph for calculating actual and standard bicarbonate, buffer base, and base excess concentrations.
sigh rate The frequency, in sigh breaths per hour, that will be delivered by a ventilator.
sigh system The portion of a ventilator dedicated to the production and timing of sigh breaths.
silica gel A crystalline chemical compound that is reversibly hydrophilic. It absorbs water and water vapor; a drying agent.
simple humidifier A device that uses unsophisticated methods of adding water vapor to inhaled gases (e.g., bubble or pass-over type of humidifiers).
simple mask A device consisting of a gas supply line and a conelike appliance that fits over the mouth and nose of the patient.
SIMV See *synchronized intermittent mandatory ventilation.*
SIMV breaths/min The number of synchronized mandatory respirations delivered per minute.
SIMV cycle time The length of time between mandatory synchronized inspirations.
SIMV system The part of a ventilator mechanism devoted to producing and monitoring SIMV breaths.
SIMV volume ventilator A ventilator that can deliver volume-targeted breaths in the SIMV mode.
sine waveform A graphic representation of the relationship between amplitute and time in which amplitute demonstrates repetitive peaks and valleys.
sine-wavelike curve See *sine waveform.*
single circuit A ventilator whose source gas powers the machine and is also the gas delivered to the patient's airway.
single-circuit ventilator See *single circuit.*
single-stage reducing valve See *single-stage regulator.*
single-stage regulator A pressure-reducing system that lowers primary equipment pressure to working pressure (approximately 50 psig) in one step.
sinusoidal Of or pertaining to the shape of a sine wave.
sleep spindles Waveforms with waxing and waning amplitude that occur at a frequency of 9 to 13 cycles per second.
slip/stream nebulizer See *sidestream nebulizer.*
slope Any inclined line, surface, position; a slant.
sloping To have an upward or downward inclination. To take an oblique direction, incline, or slant. Also see *pressure slope* and *pressure ramp.*

slow vital capacity See *nonforced vital capacity.*
small-volume nebulizer (SVN) A pneumatic aerosol generator. It may be used with a gas-flow circuit used for IPPB therapy or mechanical ventilation, or as a hand-held nebulizer powered by low-flow oxygen or compressed air.
SmartTrigger The name given to the trigger function on the Bear 1000 ventilator in which the ventilator selects the signal that is most sensitive to the patient's effort with the quickest response.
smart window The name given to part of the display screen on the Dräger E-4 ventilator that gives information about ventilating parameters.
sniffer's position Extension of the occiput with flexion of the lower cervical spine; the optimal position to establish and maintain a patent upper airway, as well as for oral intubation. Also called extreme extension.
software The programs, data, routines, etc. for a digital computer. Compare *hardware.*
solenoid A magnetically operated, electrically powered, switching device in which an electrically charged coil moves in a cylinder.
solenoid valve A valve whose position is controlled by a solenoid.
solubility coefficient An expression of the ability of a liquid to hold dissolved solids or gases.
spacer An accessory to enhance aerosol from a metered dose inhaler.
specific gravity The ratio of the weight of one volume of a substance to the weight of the same volume of water. Usually expressed in grams per liter or grams per cubic meter.
spinning disk A kind of nebulizer in which a volume of water is broken into particles by the action of a rapidly revolving, toothed disk. Also called a centrifugal humidifier.
spirochete Any bacterium of the genus *Spirochaeta* that is motile and spiral-shaped with flexible filaments. Spirochete organisms include those responsible for leptospirosis, relapsing fever, and syphilis.
spirograph A graphic representation of lung volumes and ventilatory flow rates.
spirometer A device that measures lung volumes and flow rates.
spirometer alarm A low volume or patient disconnect warning device.
splitter configuration Part of a fluidic element consisting of an intersection point, toward which the main gas flow is directed. The gas flow hits the splitter, causing the gas stream to split and follow two separate pathways.
spontaneous bag A reservoir device that holds gas to be inhaled during patient-initiated, unassisted respirations.
spontaneous breaths Breaths initiated and ended by the patient with no ventilatory support provided. The ventilatory muscles must assume all responsibility for breathing.
spontaneous indicator (demand indicator) A visual or audio signal denoting patient-initiated breathing.
spring and disk release valve A valve whose opening is governed by the ability of a pressure greater than that caused by a spring's pressure on a movable, disk-shaped valve cover.
spring disk A spring of a predetermined tension attached to a flat disk. Used to occlude orifices until the spring tension is exceeded by another pressure source.
spring-loaded bellows A power transmission system for a ventilator that uses a spring to apply force and increase the pressure delivered to the patient.
spring-loaded device A device that functions based on its ability to overcome the tension imposed by a spring.
spring-loaded disk PEEP valve A positive end-expiratory pressure valve that allows for pressure relief when the expiratory pressure exceeds the spring disk's spring tension.
spring-loaded resistors A type of threshold resistor that relies on a spring to hold a disc or diaphragm down over the expiratory port of a pressurized circuit.
spring-loaded valve A valve that functions based on its ability to overcome the tension imposed by a spring.
square waveform A graphic representation of two variables that form a boxlike shape. Also called a constant, or rectangular, waveform.
square-wave flow curve A flow-time diagram that takes the form of a box, indicating a constant flow delivered during inspiration.
standard bicarbonate The plasma concentration of HCO_3 in mEq/liter that would exist if the PCO_2 were normal (40 torr).
standard precautions Guidelines recommended by the Centers for Disease Control and Prevention to reduce the risk of transmission of blood-borne and other pathogens in hospitals. Standard precautions apply to blood and all body fluids, secretions, and excretions (excluding sweat) regardless of whether they contain blood; nonintact skin; and mucous membranes.
***Staphylococcus* spp.** A genus of nonmotile, spherical Gram-positive bacteria. Some species are normally found on the skin. Certain species cause severe purulent infections or produce an enterotoxin, which may cause nausea, vomiting, and diarrhea. Life-threatening staphylococcal infections may arise in hospitals.
static compliance A lung characteristic associated with the elastic properties of the lungs such that a delivered volume is associated with a specific delivered pressure under conditions of no gas flow. Mathematically expressed as the change in volume divided by the change in pressure.
Stead-Wells spirometer A type of water-sealed device that uses a plastic instead of a metal bell to measure volume changes in the airway opening.
stepper motor A microprocessor-controlled motor with multiple possible positions. Used to open valves or gas flow channels for quick response to microprocessor signals.
sterilization The complete destruction of all microorganisms, usually by heat or chemical means.
Stoke's law The physical law governing the rainout of aerosol particles in the lung through sedimentation.

streptobacilli Chains of bacilli.
***Streptococcus* spp.** A genus of nonmotile, Gram-positive cocci classified by serologic type (Lancefield groups A through T), hemolytic action (alpha, beta, gamma), reaction to bacterial viruses (phage types 1 to 86), and when grown on blood agar. The various species occur in pairs, short chains, and chains. Some are facultative aerobes; some are anaerobic. Some species are also hemolytic, but others are nonhemolytic. Many species cause disease in humans.
subambient pressure-relief valve In the Bear 5 and Bear 1000 ventilators, a safety bypass system that lets the patient breathe ambient air if ventilator power fails or inspiratory circuit pressure exceeds 120 cm H_2O.
subambient-pressure valve See *subambient pressure-relief valve.*
subambient overpressure pressure-relief valve (SOPR) See *subambient pressure-relief valve.*
subambient relief valve An internal anti-suffocation valve. If the ventilator cannot provide a breath, the patient can inhale, open the valve, and receive room air.
sublimation The direct transition of a substance from solid to the gas or vapor state.
sulfhemoglobin A form of hemoglobin containing an irreversibly bound sulfur molecule that prevents normal oxygen binding.
supercooled liquid An amorphous solid (e.g., margarine).
supply pressure The driving or operating pressure of a gas-powered device.
sustained maximum inspiration (SMI) A therapeutic breathing maneuver in which patients are coached to inspire from the resting expiratory level up to their inspiratory capacity (IC), with an end-inspiratory pause.
synchronized intermittent mandatory ventilation (SIMV) A mode of ventilation in which the patient breathes spontaneously with mandatory breaths periodically imposed after an inspiratory effort.
synchronous period The period during which a mandatory breath may be imposed.
system failure alarm A warning device that signals that the mechanism being monitored has ceased functioning.
Système International (SI) An internationally accepted scientific system of expressing length, mass, and time in base units (IU) of meters, kilograms, and second, replacing the old centimeter-gram-second system (CGS). The SI system includes the ampere, kelvin, candela, and mole as standard measurements.

tank ventilator Another name for the iron lung.
Taylor dispersion The enhanced mixing of gases associated with the turbulent flow of high velocity gases moving through small airways and their bifurcations.
temperature A measure of molecular activity or motion. Also a reference to the reactive hotness or coldness of a material.
temperature correction Attaining body temperature within a normal range.
terminal flow control A control on the Bennett PR-2 that lets the operator provide a minimum flow to compensate for leaks during inspiration.
thermal conductivity The physical ability of a substance to conduct heat. This principle is used in oxygen analyzers and flow sensors.
thermal flowmeter A device that measures gas flow using a temperature-sensitive, temperature-resistive element.
thermodynamics The science of the interconversion of heat and work.
thermometer An instrument for measuring temperature. Usually consists of a sealed glass tube that is marked in degrees of Celsius or Fahrenheit and contains liquid such as mercury or alcohol. The liquid rises or falls as it expands or contracts according to changes in temperature.
theta wave One of the four types of brain waves, characterized by a relatively low frequency of 4 to 7 cycles per second and a low amplitude of 10 μU. Theta waves are the "drowsy waves" that appear in electroencephalograms when the individual is awake but relaxed and sleepy. Compare *alpha wave, beta wave,* and *delta wave.*
Thorpe tube See *Thorpe-tube flowmeter.*
Thorpe-tube flowmeter A type of flowmeter in which the gas stream suspends a steel ball in a tapered tube. As the ball obstructs a greater proportion of the cross-section of the tapered tube, flow is reduced.
Thorpe-tube/reducing-valve regulator A combination of a pressure-reducing valve and a Thorpe-tube type of flowmeter that can regulate both pressure and flow.
three-point calibration Adjusting the electronic output of an instrument to two known standards, as in a two-point calibration, and then adding a third standard intermediate to the other two to ensure linearity of the response. It should be performed every 6 months or whenever an electrode is replaced.
three-way exhalation valve solenoid An electronic device that determines the direction of flow in an expiratory valve.
threshold resistance Usually the amount of pressure needed to overcome resistance to flow.
threshold resistor In positive airway therapy, a device against which a patient exhales. The pressure generated by a threshold resistor can be set to provide specific expiratory pressures independent of flow.
timing flip-flop A fluidic control device that is an on/off switch.
tonicity An expression of the amount of solute in a solution.
total cycle time (TCT) The time required for both inspiration (T_I) and expiration (T_E). Also called total respiratory cycle and ventilatory cycle time.
total lung capacity (TLC) The total amount of gas in the lungs after a maximum inspiration.

total volume output In ventilators, the sum of nebulizer gas volume and ventilatory gas volume.
tracheal button A device used to provide a temporary seal in a tracheostomy; used to keep the stoma patent.
tracheostomy tube An artificial airway surgically inserted into the trachea through the neck.
transcutaneous electrode A monitoring electrode that measures or indicates changes in physiologic conditions across the skin.
transmission-based precautions In hospitals, safeguards designed for patients documented or suspected to be infected with highly transmissible or epidemiologically important pathogens for which additional precautions (beyond standard precautions) are needed to interrupt transmission. There are three types of transmission-based precautions: airborne precautions, droplet precautions, and contact precautions, which may be combined for diseases with multiple transmission routes. Whether these types are used singularly or in combination, they are to be used in addition to standard precautions.
trigger The manner in which a ventilator determines when to begin inspiration (e.g., time-triggering or patient-triggering).
trigger sensitivity The amount of patient effort needed to begin inspiratory gas flow from a ventilator. Usually determined by measured pressure or flow changes.
trigger variable That which begins inspiration. A ventilator may be time-, pressure-, flow-, or volume-triggered.
triple-stage reducing valve A pressure-reducing system that reduces pressure from 2200 to 750 psig, then to 50 psig.
turbine An engine or motor driven by the pressure of steam, water, air, etc. against the curved vanes of a wheel or set of wheels fastened to a driving shaft.
two-point calibration Adjusting the electronic output of an instrument to two known standards to ensure quality assurance. Usually performed at least three times daily, usually every 8 hours.

ultrasonic nebulizer (USN) A device that uses high-intensity sound waves to break water into very fine particles.
ultrasonic transducer A mechanism that converts electrical energy into sound waves by means of a piezoelectric crystal.
underwater jet humidifier A device that adds water vapor to a carrier gas by injecting a high-velocity gas stream below the surface of a water reservoir, causing a large amount of small bubbles to form and rise to the water surface.
underwater seal resistor A type of threshold resistor in which tubing attached to the expiratory port of a pressurized circuit is submerged beneath a column of water.
universal precautions An approach to infection control designed to prevent transmission of bloodborne diseases, such as human immunodeficiency virus and hepatitis B, in health-care settings. Universal precautions were initially developed in 1987 by the Centers for Disease Control and Prevention in the United States and in 1989 by the Bureau of Communicable Disease Epidemiology in Canada. The guidelines for universal precautions include specific recommendations for use of gloves, masks, and protective eyewear when contact with blood or body secretions containing blood is anticipated.
upper pressure limit The maximum amount of pressure allowed to be delivered by a ventilator. See also *maximum pressure limit* and *pressure limit.*
user interface The control panel; where the operator sets the controls. Also called the front panel.
user verification test (UVT) A ventilator test on the T-Bird AVS that allows the operator to review several ventilator functions, such as a lamp test, a filter test, and a leak test.

van der Waals forces Physical intermolecular forces that cause molecules to be attracted to each other.
vapor A transition state between a liquid and a gas during which, through application of pressure/temperature changes, the transition may be reversed.
vaporization The process whereby matter in its liquid form is changed into its vapor or gaseous form.
vapor pressure The force exerted by vapors on a gas or a mixture of gases.
variable performance oxygen-delivery system Oxygen therapy equipment that delivers oxygen at a flow that only provides part of the patient's inspired gas needs. Also called a low-flow system.
variable pressure control A closed-loop mode of ventilation available on the Cardiopulmonary Corp. Venturi ventilator that is pressure-targeted, time-cycled, and volume guaranteed.
variable pressure support A closed-loop mode of ventilation available on the Cardiopulmonary Corp. Venturi ventilator that is patient-triggered, pressure-targeted, flow-cycled, and volume-guaranteed.
variable restrictor A device that reduces flow by incorporating an adjustable orifice.
vector An animal carrier, especially an insect, of infectious organisms.
vehicle Any substance, such as food or water, that can be a mode of transmission for infectious agents.
ventilator A mechanical device that moves gases into and out of the lungs.
ventilator circuit The portion of the pneumatic circuit consisting of tubing from a ventilator to a patient. Also called external circuit or patient circuit.
ventilator inoperative alarm See *ventilator inoperative system.*
ventilator inoperative system A system that warns of the nonfunctional status of a ventilator.
ventilatory cycle time The time it takes from the beginning of one inspiration to the beginning of the next in-

spiration. Also called the total cycle time and the total respiratory cycle.

ventilatory pattern The rate, volume, flow, and pressure characteristics of breathing over a period.

Venturi A device that incorporates a jet device to create pressure flow and admixture changes in a gas stream. Also called an air-entrainment device.

Venturi gate Part of a mechanism in the Bird Mark series ventilators that balanced spring tension on a valve cover with driving pressure to adjust flow through a Venturi device.

Venturi PEEP valve A Venturi whose output pressure opposes gas flow through a one-way valve to increase end-expiratory pressure.

vernier A control that can initiate small changes in a system. Usually a dial that can be adjusted in small increments.

vibrio A bacterium that is curved and mobile. Cholera and several other epidemic forms of gastroenteritis are caused by members of this genus.

virucide Any agent that destroys or inactivates viruses.

viscosity The thickness of a fluid; its ability to flow.

vital capacity (VC) The total amount of air that can be exhaled after a maximum inspiration. The sum of the inspiratory reserve volume, the tidal volume, and the expiratory reserve volume.

volt (V) The unit of electrical potential. In an electric circuit, a volt is the force required to send 1 ampere of current through 1 ohm of resistance, or the difference in potential between two points on a conductor carrying a charge of 1 ampere when there is a dissipation of 1 watt between them.

voltmeter An instrument, such as a galvanometer, that measures (in volts) the differences in potential between different points of an electric circuit.

volume-assured pressure support (VAPS) A pressure-targeted mode of ventilation that guarantees volume delivery with each breath. It is a servo-control (closed-loop) mode that is similar in function to pressure augmentation.

volume control A dial or setting that determines the volume to be delivered by a mechanical ventilator.

volume-controlled inverse ratio ventilation (VCIRV) A volume-targeted, volume- or time-cycled mode of ventilation in which inspiratory time exceeds expiratory time.

volume-displacement incentive spirometer A device that encourages a patient to take slow, deep breaths (as in sighing or yawning) to inspire a preset volume of air. The device measures and visually displays the volume of air that the patient inspires during a sustained maximum inspiration.

volume-displacement device The mechanism by which some ventilators deliver a positive-pressure breath. The device may be a piston, bellow, concertina bag, or similar "bag-in-chamber" mechanism.

volume hold A ventilator control or a maneuver where a volume of gas is held in the patient's lungs for a period of time so static pressure can be read or gas distribution improved.

volume limit A setting that sets the maximum deliverable volume on a ventilator.

volume support A closed-loop mode of ventilation available on the Siemens Servo 300 ventilator that is patient-triggered, pressure-targeted, flow-cycled, and volume guaranteed.

volume ventilation Setting a desired tidal volume in breath delivery. Also called volume-limited ventilation, volume-controlled ventilation, and volume-targeted ventilation.

volume targeted ventilation A form of ventilation in which the operator selects a specific volume for delivery of inspiration.

vortex shedding A characteristic of flow systems in which changes in flows that contact air foils are proportionate to the velocity of the gas, thus allowing for pressure, flow, and volume to be determined.

water-weighted diaphragm A PEEP device in which a water column placed in contact with the diaphragm of an expiration valve creates a PEEP pressure equal to the height of the water column.

watt A unit of power, equivalent to work done at the rate of 1 joule per second.

weighted ball resistors A type of resistor in which a steel ball is placed over a calibrated orifice that is attached directly above the expiratory port of a pressurized circuit.

Wheatstone bridge A particular arrangement of multiple resistors in an electrical circuit.

wick humidifier A type of humidification system in which the flow is exposed to a water-saturated cloth, paper, or polyethylene membrane.

Wood's metal A metal alloy commonly used in fusible plugs.

work of breathing The amount of force needed to move a given volume into the lung with a relaxed chest wall. It can be reduced when applied properly with mechanical ventilation.

Wye connector An adapter shaped like the letter Y that connects the endotracheal tube adapter to the main inspiratory and expiratory lines of a patient circuit used for mechanical ventilation.

zone valve A valve that controls gas flow to specific areas served by a bulk gas system.

Frequently Used Formulas and Values

Gas Laws

Definitions of standard conditions

	Temperature (°C)	Pressure (mm Hg)	Water Vapor
STPD	Zero	760	Zero
ATPD	Ambient	Atmospheric	Zero
ATPS	Ambient	Atmospheric	Saturated
BTPS	37	Atmospheric	47 mm Hg

Gas Cylinders

Oxygen cylinder factors for common cylinder sizes

D Cylinder	0.16
E Cylinder	0.28
G Cylinder	2.41
H Cylinder	3.14
K Cylinder	3.14

Flow Rates, and Mixing Air and Oxygen

Air to oxygen ratios and total flows of several common venturi devices*

%	Oxygen flow rate (L/min)	Air/Oxygen Ratio	Total Flow (L/min)
24%	4	25.3:1	105
28%	4	10.3:1	45
31%	6	6.9:1	47
35%	8	4.3:1	42
40%	8	3:1	32
50%	12	1:7:1	32
60%	24	1:1	48
70%	24	0.6:1	38

Formulas Used with Gas Laws

Boyle's law (solving for pressure): $P_2 = \frac{P_1 \times V_1}{V_2}$

Boyle's law (solving for volume): $V_2 = \frac{P_1 \times V_1}{P_2}$

Charles's law (solving for volume): $V_2 = \frac{V_1 \times T_2}{T_1}$

Gay–Lussac's law (solving for pressure): $P_2 = \frac{P_1 \times T_2}{T_1}$

Combined gas law:

$$V_2 = \frac{V_1 \times P_1 \times T_2}{P_2 \times T_1} \text{ (solving for volume)}$$

Combined gas law:

$$P_2 = \frac{V_1 \times P_1 \times T_2}{V_2 \times T_1} \text{ (solving for pressure)}$$

Combined gas law:

$$T_2 = \frac{P_2 \times V_2 \times T_1}{P_1 \times V_1} \text{ (solving for temperature)}$$

Combined gas law:

$$V_2 = \frac{V_1 \times [P_1 - (P_{H_2O} @ T_1)] \times T_2}{[P_2 - P_{H_2O} @ T_2)] \times T_1}$$

$$\text{Density} = \frac{\text{GMW}}{22.4 \text{ L}}$$

$$\text{Density} = \frac{[(\text{GMW of gas \#1} \times \%) + (\text{GMW of gas \#2} \times \%)]}{22.4 \text{ L}}$$

Formulas Used with Cylinders and Liquid Oxygen

$$\text{Cylinder factor} = \frac{\text{cubic feet in full cylinder} \times 28.3}{\text{pressure of full cylinder}}$$

$$\text{Duration (minutes)} = \frac{\text{gauge pressure (psig)} \times \text{cylinder factor}}{\text{oxygen flow rate (liters/minute)}}$$

$$\text{Duration of liquid oxygen cylinder (min)} = \frac{\text{liquid } O_2 \text{ capacity (L)} \times 860 \times \text{gauge reading (\%)}}{\text{oxygen flow rate (L/min)}}$$

$$\text{Duration (min)} = \frac{\text{weight of liquid } O_2 \text{ remaining (pounds)} \times 344}{\text{oxygen flow rate (liters/minute)}}$$

Formula Used When Mixing Air and Oxygen

$$O_2\ (\%) = \frac{(\text{air flow} \times 21\%) + (O_2 \text{ flow} \times 100\%)}{\text{total gas flow}} \times 100$$

Formulas Used When Calculating Humidity

$$\text{RH (\%)} = \frac{\text{content}}{\text{capacity}} \times 100$$

$$\text{BH (\%)} = \frac{\text{content}}{\text{capacity @ 37° C}}$$

$$\frac{\text{capacity @ 37° C} - \text{absolute humidity}}{\text{humidity deficit}}$$

$$\text{AH} = \frac{\text{water output (milliliters/minute)} \times 1000 \text{ mg/ml}}{\text{gas flow in liters/minute}}$$

$$PiO_2 \text{ (in mm Hg)} = [(Pb - P_{H_2O}) \times FiO_2]$$

Formulas Used with Mechanical Ventilation

Ideal body weight in pounds (men) = 106 + 6(Ht − 60)

Ideal body weight in pounds (women) = 105 + 5(Ht − 60)

Normal spontaneous tidal volume = 7–9 mL/kg of ideal body weight

Mechanical ventilation tidal volume = 10–15 mL/kg of ideal body weight

V_T (lost due to compressed gas) = (peak − PEEP) × TCF

V_T (delivered) = V_T (set) − V_T (lost)

$\dot{V}_E$ (liters/minute) = V_T (liters/breath) × f (breaths/minute)

$$V_T \text{ (liters/breath)} = \frac{\dot{V}_E \text{ (liters/minute)}}{\text{f (breaths/minute)}}$$

$$\dot{V}_I \text{ (liters/minute)} = \frac{V_T \text{ (liters)}}{T_I \text{ (seconds)}} \times 60$$

$$T_I \text{ (seconds)} = \frac{V_T \text{ (liters)}}{\dot{V}_I \text{ (liters/minute)} \div 60}$$

$$\text{TCT (seconds)} = \frac{60 \text{ sec/min}}{\text{frequency (breaths/minute)}}$$

I:E ratio = 1:($T_E \div T_I$)

total parts = I + E

T_I = TCT ÷ total parts

T_E = TCT − T_I

Formulas Used with Compliance and Resistance

$$C_{dyn} = \frac{V_T}{\text{peak} - \text{PEEP}}$$

$$C_{stat} = \frac{V_T}{\text{plateau} - \text{PEEP}}$$

$$R_{AW} = \frac{\text{peak} - \text{plateau}}{\dot{V}_I} \times 60$$

Formulas Used When Calculating Dead Space

$$V_D/V_T = \frac{PaCO_2 - P\bar{e}CO_2}{PaCO_2}$$

$$V_D \text{ (physiologic)} = \frac{PaCO_2 - P\bar{e}CO_2}{PaCO_2} \times V_T$$

V_D (physiologic) = V_D (anatomic) + V_D (alveolar)

V_D (anatomic) = 1 mL/lb of ideal body weight.

V_T = V_D (physiologic) + V_A [per breath]

$\dot{V}_E$ = $\dot{V}_D$ (physiologic) + $\dot{V}_A$ [per minute]

$\dot{V}_E$ = Vt × f

$\dot{V}_D$ (physiologic) = V_D (physiologic) × f

$\dot{V}_A$ = V_A × f

INDEX

A

B

C

D

E

F

G

H

I

P

Q

R

S

T

U

V

W

X

Z

INFANT VENTILATORS

Table includes optional software functions but not optional hardware such as graphic screens, analyzers or monitors.
OPT = optional
HFO = high frequency oscillation
HFJ = high frequency jet
• = can be adjusted to provide

		INFANT VENTILATORS	Bear Cub 200	Bear Cub BP 2001	Bear Cub 750vs	Bird VIP	Dräger Babylog 8000	Healthdyne 105 Infant	Nellcor Puritan Bennett Infant Star	Nellcor Puritan Bennett Infant Star 100	Nellcor Puritan Bennett Infant Star 200	Nellcor Puritan Bennett Infant Star 500	Nellcor Puritan Bennett Infant Star 950	Sechrist 100B	Sechrist IV 200	HIGH-FREQUENCY VENTILATORS	Bunnell Life Pulse (HFJ)	Sensormedics 3100A (HFO)
MODES	MODES (others)												HFO				HFJ	HFO
	Volume Targeted A/C (includes C)		•	•	•	√	√	•						•	•			
	Volume Targeted SIMV (includes IMV)		•	•	•	√	√	•	•	•	•	•	•	•	•			
	Pressure Targeted A/C (includes C)		√	√	√	√	•	√	√	√	√	√	√	•	•			
	Pressure Targeted SIMV (includes IMV)		√	√	√	√	√	√	√	√	√	√	√	•	•			
	Pressure Support (PSV)					√	√											
	Time-triggered, Pressure-limited Time-cycled Ventilation (TPTV)		√	√	√	√	√	√	√	√	√	√	√	√	√			
	Pressure Targeted Ventilation with Volume Guarantee (Dual Control)																	
	Dual Control (per breath)																	
	Dual Control (over several Breaths)																	
	Mandatory Minute Volume																	
	Proportional Assist Ventilation*																	
	Airway Pressure Release Ventilation																	
TRIGGER MECH.	TRIGGER MECHANISM																	
	Time		√	√	√	√	√	√	√	√	√	√	√	√	√		√	√
	Manual		√	√	√	√	√	√	√	√	√	√	√	√	√			
	Pressure					√												
	Flow			√	√	√	√											
	Volume						√											
	Abdominal movement						OPT		OPT			OPT	OPT					
FLOW WAVEFORM	FLOW WAVEFORM (in volume vent.)																	
	Constant (rectangular or square)		√	√	√	√	√	√	√	√	√	√	√	√	√		√	
	Descending Ramp					√												
	Sine																	√
	Ascending Ramp																	
SPECIAL FEATURES	SPECIAL FEATURES																	
	Adjustable Slope (ramp)						√		•	•	•	•	•					
	Graphics (optional [opt])				OPT	OPT	√											
LUNG MECH.	LUNG MECHANICS TESTING																	
	Compliance					OPT												